Textbook of
Pediatric Infectious Diseases

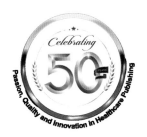

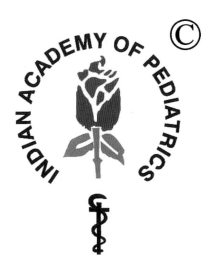

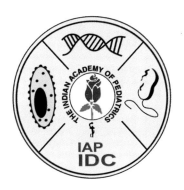

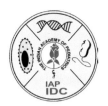
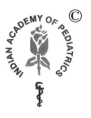

Textbook of
Pediatric Infectious Diseases

Second Edition

Emeritus Editor

A Parthasarathy

Distinguished Professor
The Tamil Nadu Dr MGR Medical University, Chennai
Retd Senior Clinical Professor
Department of Pediatrics
Madras Medical College, Chennai
Deputy Superintendent
Institute of Child Health and Hospital for Children
Chennai, Tamil Nadu, India

Editor-in-Chief

Ritabrata Kundu

Professor
Department of Pediatrics
Institute of Child Health
Kolkata, West Bengal, India

Vijay N Yewale

Director and Consultant Pediatrician
Dr Yewale's Multispecialty Hospital for Children
Navi Mumbai
Honorary Pediatric Consultant
Mathadi Hospital Trust, Navi Mumbai
Head, Department of Pediatrics
Apollo Hospitals, Navi Mumbai, Maharashtra, India

Executive Editors

Ashok Rai

Consultant Pediatrician
Surya Superspecialty Hospital, Varanasi
Kilkari Institute of Child Health, Varanasi
Director, Indian Institute of Cerebral Palsy and Handicapped Children, Varanasi
Honorary IMA Professor of Pediatrics and Faculty
Heritage Institute of Medical Sciences, Varanasi, Uttar Pradesh, India

Digant D Shastri

CEO and Senior Pediatrician
Killol Children Hospital and NICU
Surat, Gujarat, India

Chief Academic Editor

Jaydeep Choudhury

Associate Professor
Institute of Child Health
Kolkata, West Bengal, India

Academic Editors

Abhay K Shah

Senior Consultant Pediatrician
Children Hospital, Ahmedabad, Gujarat, India

Dhanya Dharmapalan

Consultant Pediatrician
Dr Yewale's Multispecialty
Hospital for Children
Navi Mumbai, Maharashtra, India

Kheya Ghosh Uttam

Assistant Professor
Institute of Child Health
Kolkata, West Bengal, India

Sanjay Krishna Ghorpade

Director and Professor
Department of Pediatrics
Postgraduate Institute of Pediatrics and
Niramay Hospital and Research Center
Satara, Maharashtra, India

Shyam Kukreja

Director and Head
Department of Pediatrics
Max Superspecialty Hospital
Patparganj, New Delhi, India

Vasant Khalatkar

Consultant Pediatrician and Neonatologist
Khalatkar Hospital
Nagpur, Maharashtra, India

Forewords

Digant D Shastri, Santosh T Soans

JAYPEE BROTHERS MEDICAL PUBLISHERS
The Health Sciences Publisher
New Delhi | London | Panama

Jaypee Brothers Medical Publishers (P) Ltd

Headquarters

Jaypee Brothers Medical Publishers (P) Ltd
4838/24, Ansari Road, Daryaganj
New Delhi 110 002, India
Phone: +91-11-43574357
Fax: +91-11-43574314
Email: jaypee@jaypeebrothers.com

Overseas Offices

J.P. Medical Ltd
83 Victoria Street, London
SW1H 0HW (UK)
Phone: +44 20 3170 8910
Fax: +44 (0)20 3008 6180
Email: info@jpmedpub.com

Jaypee-Highlights Medical Publishers Inc
City of Knowledge, Bld. 235, 2nd Floor
Clayton, Panama City, Panama
Phone: +1 507-301-0496
Fax: +1 507-301-0499
Email: cservice@jphmedical.com

Jaypee Brothers Medical Publishers (P) Ltd
Bhotahity, Kathmandu
Nepal
Phone: +977-9741283608
Email: kathmandu@jaypeebrothers.com

Website: www.jaypeebrothers.com
Website: www.jaypeedigital.com

© 2019, Jaypee Brothers Medical Publishers

Inquiries for bulk sales may be solicited at: jaypee@jaypeebrothers.com

Textbook of Pediatric Infectious Diseases

First Edition: 2013

Second Edition: 2019

ISBN 978-93-5270-250-3

Printed at Replika Press Pvt. Ltd.

Contributors

A Balachandran
Senior Pediatrician and Pulmonologist
Mehta's Children Hospital
Chennai, Tamil Nadu, India
dr_abalachandran@hotmail.com/
drabc52@gmail.com

A Parthasarathy
Distinguished Professor
The Tamil Nadu Dr MGR Medical
University, Chennai
Retd Senior Clinical Professor of Pediatrics
Madras Medical College, Chennai
Deputy Superintendent
Institute of Child Health and Hospital for
Children
Chennai, Tamil Nadu, India
apartha2020@gmail.com

Abhay K Shah
Senior Consultant Pediatrician
Children Hospital
Ahmedabad, Gujarat, India
drabhaykshah@yahoo.com

Agni Sekhar Saha
Consultant Neonatologist and Pediatrics
Fortis Hospital
Kolkata, West Bengal, India

Ajay Kalra
Erstwhile Professor of Pediatrics
Sarojini Naidu Medical College
Former Head, Department of Pediatrics
Institute of Medical Sciences
Agra, Uttar Pradesh, India
drajaykalra@yahoo.com

AK Dutta
Director Professor
Department of Pediatrics
Lady Hardinge Medical College
New Delhi, India
drdutta@gmail.com

Alok Kumar Deb
Scientist-D/Epidemiology Division
National Institute of Cholera
and Enteric Diseases
Kolkata, West Bengal, India

Anil K Prasad
Head
Department of Respiratory Virology
V Patel Chest Institute (1972-2002.)
University Professor and Head (1987-2002)
of Respiratory Virology, V Patel Chest
Institute, Delhi,
University Professor Medical Microbiology,
Delhi University (1993-96)
New Delhi, India

Anju Aggarwal
Associate Professor
Department of Pediatrics
University College of Medical Sciences
and Guru Tegh Bahadur Hospital
New Delhi, India
aanju67@gmail.com

Anuradha De
Professor
Department of Microbiology
Lokmanya Tilak Municipal
Medical College and Hospital
Mumbai, Maharashtra, India
dr_anuradhade@yahoo.com

Apurba Ghosh
Director and Professor
Department of Pediatrics
Institute of Child Health
Kolkata, West Bengal, India
apurbaghosh@yahoo.com

Ashish Pathak
Professor
Department of Pediatrics
RD Gardi Medical College
Ujjain, Madhya Pradesh, India
Post-doctoral fellow
Department of International Maternal and
Child (IMCH), Uppsala University
Uppsala, Sweden

Ashok Kapse
Pediatrician
Kapse Children Hospital
Surat, Gujarat, India
ashok.kapse@mail.com

Ashok Rai
Consultant Pediatrician
Surya Superspecialty Hospital, Varanasi
Kilkari Institute of Child Health, Varanasi
Director
Indian Institute of Cerebral Palsy and
Handicapped Children, Varanasi
Hon. IMA Professor of Pediatrics and
Faculty, Heritage Institute of Medical
Sciences, Varanasi, Uttar Pradesh, India
drashokrai@gmail.com

Ashutosh Marwah
Senior Consultant
Department of Pediatric and
Congenital Heart Diseases
Escorts Heart Institute and Research
Center, New Delhi, India

Atul Kulkarni
Consultant Pediatrician
Department of Pediatrics
Ashwini Sahakari Rugnalaya
Solapur, Maharashtra, India
dratulkulkarni@rediffmail.com

Baldev S Prajapati
Professor
GCS Medical College
Hospital and Research Center
Ahmedabad, Gujarat, India
baldevprajapati55@gmail.com

Dhanya Dharmapalan
Consultant Pediatrician
Dr Yewale's Multispecialty
Hospital for Children
Navi Mumbai, Maharashtra, India
drdhanyaroshan@gmail.com

Digant D Shastri
CEO and Senior Pediatrician
Killol Children Hospital and NICU
Surat, Gujarat, India
drdigant@hotmail.com

Geoff Kahn
Research Associate
International Vaccine Access Center (IVAC)
Johns Hopkins Bloomberg
School of Public Health
Baltimore, Maryland, USA

Hitt Sharma
Additional Director (Medical Affairs)
Serum Institute of India Ltd.
Pune, Maharashtra, India
drhis@seruminstitute.com

Ira Shah
Professor (Addl) Pediatrics and Head
Pediatric Infectious Diseases and
Pediatric GI, Hepatology
Incharge, Pediatric HIV, TB, Liver Clinics
BJ Wadia Hospital for Children, Mumbai
Consultant Pediatric Infectious Diseases
(PID) and Hepatology, Nanavati Hospital
Mumbai, Maharashtra, India
irashah@pediatriconcall.com

Janani Sankar
Senior Consultant
KanchiKamakoti Childs Trust Hospital
Chennai, Tamil Nadu, India
janani.sankar@yahoo.com

Jaydeep Choudhury
Associate Professor
Department of Pediatrics
Institute of Child Health
Kolkata, West Bengal, India
drjaydeep_choudhury@yahoo.co.in

Jesson Unni
Editor-in-Chief
IAP Drug Formulary
Consultant Pediatrician
Dr Kunhalu's Nursing Home
Kochi, Kerala, India
jeson@asianetmedia.com

K Pandian
Pediatric Neurologist Consultant
KanchiKamakoti Childs Trust Hospital
Chennai, Tamil Nadu, India
pandian7@yahoo.com

Ketan Bharadva
Masoom Children's Hospital and Child
Development and Rehab Unit
Neo Plus Neonatal and Pediatric
Intensive Care Unit
Surat, Gujarat, India
doctorketan@gmail.com

Kheya Ghosh Uttam
Assistant Professor
Institute of Child Health
Kolkata, West Bengal, India
kheyauttam@yahoo.co.in

Lalitha Kailas
Professor and Head
Department of Pediatrics
SAT Hospital
Government Medical College
Thiruvananthapuram, Kerala, India
lalithakailas@hotmail.com

Lois Privor-Dumm
Director
Alliances and Information
International Vaccine Access Center (IVAC)
Johns Hopkins Bloomberg School of
Public Health, Baltimore, Maryland, USA

M Govindaraj
Professor in Pediatrics, Indira Gandhi
Institute of Child Health
South Hospital Complex
Bengaluru, Karnataka, India
drgovindraj@yahoo.co.in

M Indra Shekhar Rao
Director
Division of Pediatrics and Neonatology
Professor of Pediatrics, NMC
Navodaya Hospital for Women and
Children, Secunderabad
Former Head
Pediatrics, Osmania Medical College
Med Superintendent, Institute of Child
Health Niloufer Hospital
Hyderabad, Telangana, India

M Vijayakumar
Consultant
Pediatric Nephrologist
Mehta's Children Hospital
Chennai, Tamil Nadu, India
doctormvk@gmail.com

MK Sudarshan
Dean
Principal and Professor
Community Medicine
Kempegowda Institute of Medical
Sciences
Bengaluru, Karnataka, India
mksudarshan@gmail.com

Malathi Sathiyasekaran
Consultant Pediatric Gastroenterologist
KanchiKamakoti Childs Trust Hospital
Sundaram Medical Foundation and
Apollo Hospitals
Chennai, Tamil Nadu, India
mal.bwcs@gmail.com

Monjori Mitra
Associate Professor
Department of Pediatrics
Institute of Child Health
Kolkata, West Bengal, India
monjorimr@gmail.com

Narendra Rathi
Consultant Pediatrician
Rathi Children Hospital
and Maternity Home
Akola, Maharashtra, India
drnbrathi@hotmail.com

Naveen Jain
Coordinator
Department of Neonatology
Associate Professor
Kerala Institute of Medical Sciences
Thiruvananthapuram, Kerala, India
naveen_19572@hotmail.com

Naveen Thacker
Director
Deep Children Hospital and
Research Center
Kutch, Gujarat, India
drnaveenthacker@gmail.com

Nigam Prakash Narain
Professor
Department of Pediatrics
Patna Medical College and Hospital
Patna, Bihar, India
nigampn@gmail.com

Niranjan Mohanty
Professor and Head
Department of Pediatrics
Srirama Chandra Bhanja Medical
College and Hospital
Cuttack, Odisha, India
drnmohanty@yahoo.co.in/
mohantyniranjan84@gmail.com

Nupur Ganguly
Associate Professor
Department of Pediatric Medicine
Institute of Child Health
Kolkata, West Bengal, India
nupur_diya@yahoo.com

P Ramachandran
Professor
Department of Pediatrics
Sri Ramachandra University
Chennai, Tamil Nadu, India
ramachandran_dr@rediffmail.com

Parang Mehta
Consultant Pediatrician
Mehta Hospital
Surat, Gujarat, India
drparang@gmail.com

Prabhas Prasun Giri
Assistant Professor
Department of Pediatrics
Institute of Child Health
Kolkata, West Bengal, India

Priyankar Pal
Associate Professor
Department of Pediatrics
Institute of Child Health
Kolkata, West Bengal, India
priyankar70@dataone.in

Rajal B Prajapati
Associate Professor
Department of Pediatrics
Smt NHL Municipal Medical College
Ahmedabad, Gujarat, India

Rajesh G Patel
Consultant Pediatrician
City Hospital
Mumbai, Maharashtra, India

Rajesh Kumar
Senior Resident
Department of Pediatrics
Patna Medical College and Hospital
Patna, Bihar, India

Rajeshwar Dayal
Professor and Head
Department of Pediatrics
Sarojini Naidu Medical College
Agra, Uttar Pradesh, India
r_dayal123@rediffmail.com

Rajniti Prasad
Professor and Head
Department of Pediatrics
Institute of Medical Sciences
Banaras Hindu University
Varanasi, Uttar Pradesh, India
rajnitip@gmail.com

Raju C Shah
Professor and Head
Gujarat Cancer Society
Medical College
Ahmedabad, Gujarat, India
rajucshah@gmail.com

Rakesh Kumar
Assistant Professor
Department of Pediatrics
Advanced Pediatric Center
Postgraduate Institute of Medical
Education and Research
Chandigarh, India
drrakesh.pgi@gmail.com

Ranjana Kumar
Senior Specialist
Program Manager South East Asia
Program Delivery Team, GAVI Alliance
Secretariat
Chemin Des Mines
Geneva, Switzerland

Ritabrata Kundu
Professor
Department of Pediatrics
Institute of Child Health
Kolkata, West Bengal, India
rkundu22@gmail.com

Rohit Agrawal
Director and Consultant Pediatrician
Chandrajyoti Children Hospital
Mumbai
Visiting Consultant
Kohinoor Hospital
Mumbai, Maharashtra, India

S Balasubramanian
Senior Consultant Pediatrician
KanchiKamakoti Childs Trust Hospital
Chennai, Tamil Nadu, India
sbsped@gmail.com; sbsped53@sify.com

S Venkat Reddy
Consultant Pediatrician
Division of Pediatrics and Neonatology
Navodaya Hospital for Women and
Children
Secunderabad, Telangana, India

S Yamuna
Pediatrician and Adolescent Physician
Child and Adolescent Clinic
Director
Center for Excellence in Parenting
Chennai, Tamil Nadu, India
dryamunapaed@yahoo.com

Sailesh Gupta
Consultant Pediatrician
Arushree Children Hospital
Mumbai, Maharashtra, India
guptasailu@gmail.com

Sandipan Dhar
Associate Professor
Department of Pediatric Dermatology
Institute of Child Health
Kolkata, West Bengal, India
drsandipan@gmail.com

Sangeeta Sharma
Head
Department of Pediatrics
Lala Ram Sarup Institute of
Tuberculosis and Respiratory Diseases
New Delhi, India
sangeetasharma2000@gmail.com

Sanjay Krishna Ghorpade
Director and Associate Professor
Department of Pediatrics
Postgraduate Institute of Pediatrics and
Niramay Hospital and Research Center
Satara, Maharashtra, India
drghorpadesanjay@gmail.com

Sankaranarayanan VS
Head and Senior Consultant
Department of Pediatrics
Gastroenterology
KanchiKamakoti Childs Trust Hospital
Chennai, Tamil Nadu, India
drvssankaranarayanan@gmail.com

Sankar Sengupta
Professor and Head
Department of Microbiology
Institute of Child Health, Kolkata
Executive Director
Desun Hospital and Heart Institute
Kolkata, West Bengal, India
*dr_shankars@yahoo.com/
dr.sankars@gmail.com*

Santanu Bhakta
Assistant Professor
Institute of Child Health
Kolkata
Fellow in Pediatric Pulmonology
Kolkata, West Bengal, India
santanu.bhakta@rediffmail.com

Savitri Shrivastava
Consultant
Department of Pediatrics and
Congenital Heart Diseases
Escorts Heart Institute and Research
Center
New Delhi, India

Shivananda
Ex Director
Indira Gandhi Institute of Child
Health, Bengaluru, Karnataka, India

Shyam Kukreja
Director and Head
Department of Pediatrics
Max Superspecialty hospital
Patparganj, New Delhi, India

Somu Sivabalan
Consultant
Pediatrician and Pulmonologist
Velammal Hospital
Chennai, Tamil Nadu, India
sivabalan.somu@gmail.com

Srinivas G Kasi
Consultant Pediatrician
Kasi Clinic
Bengaluru, Karnataka, India
sgkasi@gmail.com

SS Kamath
Consultant Pediatrician
Welcare Hospital
Kochi, Kerala, India
sskamath@vsnl.net/sachikamath@gmail.com

Suhas V Prabhu
Visiting Pediatric Consultant
PD Hinduja National Hospital
Mumbai, Maharashtra, India
suhaspra@hotmail.com

Sumanth Amperayani
Registrar of Pediatrics
Department of Respiratory Medicine and
Asthma Clinic
KanchiKamakoti Childs Trust Hospital
Chennai, Tamil Nadu, India

Sushil Kumar Kabra
Professor
Pediatric Pulmonology Division
Department of Pediatrics
All India Institute of Medical Sciences
New Delhi, India
skkabra@hotmail.com

Sutapa Ganguly
Professor and Head
Department of Pediatric Medicine
Malda Medical College and Hospital
Malda, West Bengal, India
sutapaganguly@hotmail.com

Swati Y Bhave
Executive Director
Association of Adolescent and
Child Care in India (AACCI), Mumbai
Senior Visiting Consultant
Indraprastha Apollo Hospital
New Delhi, India
sybhave@gmail.com

T Jacob John
Professor Emeritus
Department of Pediatrics
Christian Medical College
Vellore, Tamil Nadu, India
tjacobjohn@yahoo.co.in

Tanu Singhal
Consultant in Pediatrics and
Infectious Disease
Kokilaben Dhirubhai Ambani Hospital
and Medical Research Institute
Mumbai, Maharashtra, India
tanusinghal@yahoo.com

TU Sukumaran
Professor
Department of Pediatrics
Pushpagiri Institute of Medical
Sciences
Thiruvalla, Kerala, India
tusukumaran@gmail.com

Upendra Kinjawadekar
Consultant Pediatrician and
Neonatologist
Kamalesh Mother and Child Hospital
Navi Mumbai, Maharashtra, India
upen228@yahoo.co.in

V Poovazhagi
Assistant Professor
Department of Pediatrics
Institute of Child Health and
Hospital for Children
Chennai, Tamil Nadu, India
poomuthu@yahoo.com

Vasant Khalatkar
Senior Consultant Pediatrician
Children Hospital
Ahmedabad, Gujarat, India

Vijay N Yewale
Director and Consultant Pediatrician
Dr Yewale's Multispecialty Hospital for
Children, Navi Mumbai
Honorary Pediatric Consultant
Mathadi Hospital Trust, Navi Mumbai
Head, Department of Pediatrics
Apollo Hospitals
Navi Mumbai, Maharashtra, India
vnyewale@gmail.com

Vipin M Vashishtha
Director and Consultant Pediatrician
Mangla Hospital and Research Center
Bijnor, Uttar Pradesh, India

Yashwant Patil
Consulting Pediatrician
Associate Professor in Pediatrics
Datta Meghe Institute of Medical
Sciences
Nagpur, Maharashtra, India
dryashwantpatil@gmail.com

YK Amdekar
Medical Director
BJ Wadia Hospital for Children
Mumbai, Maharashtra, India
ykasya@gmail.com

Foreword

It is a proud privilege for me to write the foreword for the second edition of *Textbook of Pediatric Infectious Diseases.* I consider it as a great honor not only as I served the Indian Academy of Pediatrics (IAP) Infectious Diseases Chapter as Chairperson in 2013, but also being on the editorial board of the first edition of this textbook too.

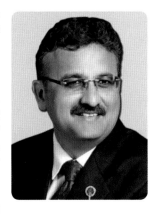

In the Indian subcontinent, infectious diseases account for a major chunk of child health problems and hence there is a dire need for a textbook on this subject in Indian context. Looking to the need, in 2013 during the golden jubilee year, the first edition of IAP—*Textbook of Pediatirc Infectious Diseases* was published and within short span, it has become popular amongst readers. Hence, the need for the revised edition arise. Considering this, IAP Infectious Diseases Chapter, 2017 team under the leadership of Dr Ashok Rai and Dr Vasant Khalatkar took initiative to come out with the second edition of the textbook.

In the current publication, all-important aspects of pediatric infectious diseases are being addressed very diligently through 10 core chapters with each chapter having in detailed description on individual conditions. A chapter on IAP protocols on management of common infectious diseases will surely contribute in facilitating protocol-based approach and annexures on intravenous fluid therapy and drug dosage will help the clinician in minimizing the errors.

My sincere compliments and congratulations to all the authors who as a part of their sense efforts to disseminate the knowledge, have contributed chapters for this prestigious publication. I congratulate the entire editorial board, lead by the emeritus editor Dr A Parthasarathy for his untiring efforts to bring out the second edition and my special compliments to other editorial board members—Drs Ashok Rai, Ritabrata Kundu, Vijay N Yewale, Jaydeep Choudhury, Shyam Kukreja, Vasant Khalatkar, Abhay K Shah, Dhanya Dharmapalan and Kheya Ghosh Uttam.

I am sure that this new edition of the book will be as popular as the previous edition amongst the postgraduate students, teaching faculties as well as practicing pediatricians. I wish this landmark publication great success and wish it will contribute in the minimizing menace of infectious diseases to child health.

Digant D Shastri
President
Indian Academy of Pediatrics, 2019

Foreword

Infectious diseases form the bulk of the healthcare issues affecting children. Hence, it is incumbent on every pediatrician to be very thorough with the correct diagnosis and effective treatment of the wide variety of infections that kids are prone to.

The second edition of *Textbook of Pediatric Infectious Diseases* provides an exhaustive listing of all types of infectious diseases one might come across. Going through the contents, I was highly impressed by the completeness of the endeavor, which is evident in the detailed coverage, it has given to every type of malady without missing anything. Even more amazing is the fact that this book brings together all the best talents in the field, with the editors and authors list being a virtual Who's Who of pediatrics. This alone should speak volumes for the authenticity of the material. The contents are also well organized for easy reading, reference and comprehension.

The recent spate of comeback of many diseases, which were considered to be long gone, is a grim reminder that infectious diseases cannot be wished away. The war on microbes is a never ending one and the sooner we accept it, the better equipped we will be for fighting it. A combination of science and strategy should form the core of our battle plan. Continuous and persistent effort is required if we are to make a discernible difference in the emerging scenario. The IAP Infectious Diseases Chapter has been rendering yeoman's service in this regard and the good work should go on.

I wish to congratulate all those who strived for compiling and bringing out this book, which is poised to be an excellent weapon in our fight against infectious diseases. I hope this book will readily gain the widespread exposure, it deserves among clinicians and academics alike.

Santosh T Soans
President
Indian Academy of Pediatrics, 2018

Prologue

It is a matter of pride and pleasure for us to write the prologue for *Textbook of Pediatric Infectious Diseases*, an official publication of Indian Academy of Pediatrics—Infectious Diseases Chapter.

Academics and advocacy are two important wings of Indian Academy of Pediatrics (IAP). It has always been an endeavor of IAP to update the skill and knowledge of its members by various scientific programs and publications related to child health. Infectious Diseases Chapter of IAP is also committed and focused to this noble mission. Infectious Diseases Chapter is one of the most vibrant chapters of IAP, known for its various scientific publications and other scientific activities. This publication will definitely make a positive and fruitful impact on pediatricians as far as rational management and prevention of infectious diseases are concerned.

Infectious diseases contribute a major chunk of cases in our day-to-day practice. It also contributes tremendously to child mortality and morbidity. In spite of the availability of modern therapeutic and preventive modalities, thousands of children die in our resource-poor country because of various infections. In view of all these aspects, Infectious Diseases Chapter of IAP has decided to come out with an important publication *Textbook of Pediatric Infectious Diseases*. A large number of luminaries and experts of National and International repute have contributed to this noble cause initiated by Infectious Diseases Chapter of IAP.

It gives us immense pleasure to present the 2nd edition of our prestigious *"Textbook of Pediatric Infectious Diseases"*. In this edition, the authors have done their best to modify and upgrade the contents. We express our gratitude to all the contributors, editors and office bearers of IAP for their cooperation and contribution for this project. We also take this opportunity to thank Dr A Parthasarathy, Emeritus Editor for his constant guidance and encouragement, Dr Ritabrata Kundu and Dr Vijay N Yewale, Editors-in-Chief for shaping this book in present format.

This book has been designed in an excellent manner to solve the queries of pediatricians regarding most of the infectious disease problems. We are sure that this book will be very useful for clinicians in their day-to-day practice and will be an effective tool in solving their problems.

Vijay N Yewale	**Ashok Rai**	**Vasant Khalatkar**
Chairman 2016	Chairman 2017	Honorary Secretary 2016-17
Infectious Diseases Chapter	Infectious Diseases Chapter	Infectious Diseases Chapter

Preface

We are proud to bring out the 2nd edition of *Textbook of Pediatric Infectious Diseases,* a dream project of Infectious Diseases Chapter of Indian Academy of Pediatrics. Infectious diseases are assuming more and more importance in our daily practice with the emergence and reemergence of diseases.

The entire text of the 2nd edition has been revised extensively. The book gives latest information about the magnitude of infectious diseases burden along with the contribution of vaccine preventable diseases. Antimicrobial resistance and new infectious agents are the two main challenges in our country. Both these topics have been covered in the revised edition.

Infection in immune compromised with prophylaxis has been aptly covered. Besides infections of the organs and systems, also, specific common infections, which are part of day-to-day practice have been included. Short but comprehensive approach to common protozoal, parasitic and fungal infection, emerging infections like *Rickettsia*, *Leptospira* and *Brucella* have been included so that they can be diagnosed in time to save lives.

One of the important contents is the inclusion of guidelines and protocols of Infectious Diseases Chapter, which have been published in the preceding years. It enables the reader to understand the most comprehensive way to diagnose and treat the diseases which are common problems of our country.

Finally, we have also covered principles of immunization which is one of the important pillars to control infectious diseases. Immunization both in immune compromised and competent and the important information about the common drug dosage have been included. In short, we have tried to cover all the aspects of infectious diseases. The editorial board would be happy if this book is useful not only to the practicing pediatricians; but also to the students.

A Parthasarathy
Ritabrata Kundu
Vijay N Yewale
Ashok Rai
Digant D Shastri

Acknowledgments

We are grateful to the Chairperson and the members of the Executive Board of the Indian Academy of Pediatrics (IAP) Infectious Diseases Chapter for the initiation of the project of bringing out the second edition of *Textbook of Pediatric Infectious Diseases* for the medical students and practitioners. The first edition was released in the Golden Jubilee Pedicon, Kolkata, 2013.

The editors are grateful to the executive board of the IAP Infectious Diseases Chapter for giving them the opportunity to bring out the second edition of this prestigious book. Sincere appreciation and thanks go to the various contributors and chapter editors who have contributed to the second edition under the guidance of Dr A Parthasarathy.

The meticulous guidance and cooperation provided by Dr Santosh T Soans, President 2018; Dr Digant D Shastri, President Elect 2019; Dr Bakulesh Jayant Parekh, Honorary Secretary-General 2016–17 of IAP are gratefully acknowledged.

Our grateful thanks to Mrs Nirmala, Mr R Janardhanan, Dr Pratibha, Ms Shruthi Pavana, Ms Swathi Pavana, Mr P Balaji, Ms Kavitha, Ms Kavya and Ms Mahiya, for secretarial assistance and to Mr D Prakash, Mr Ajay Kumar, Mr Shukla, Mr Sathiyathasan and Mrs Umadevi Sathish, for help rendered in scrutiny and formatting of manuscripts, typesetting the editorial corrections, correspondence assistance, etc. to the Editor-in-Chief at Chennai during the preparation of the first edition of the book.

Our sincere and grateful thanks go to M/s Jaypee Brothers Medical Publishers (P) Ltd., New Delhi, India, especially Shri Jitendar P Vij (Group Chairman), Mr Ankit Vij (Managing Director), Ms Chetna Malhotra Vohra (Associate Director–Content Strategy), Mrs Samina Khan (PA to Director-Publishing), and other members of Jaypee Brothers Medical Publishers (P) Ltd., New Delhi, India, for their untiring coordination efforts in the production of the book. Special thanks to Ms Payal Bharti for all the coordination throughout the production process.

All attempts have been made to acknowledge the sources of information and illustrations. Inadvertent omission, if any, is regretted.

Editorial Board

Contents

General Topics

A Parthasarathy

1.1	MAGNITUDE OF INFECTIOUS AND VACCINE-PREVENTABLE DISEASES IN CHILDREN AND ADOLESCENTS IN INDIA

A Parthasarathy, Hitt Sharma

INTRODUCTION

The WHO 2016 country specific report for India on prevalence of six vaccine-preventable diseases (VPDs), which were targeted for elimination in 1985 through the Universal Immunization Program, is alarming. Although majority of the states have achieved good control of these diseases through sustained and high immunization coverage, there are still many states in the North-Eastern region of the country which could achieve only 30–40% routine immunization coverage. These states with low immunization coverage levels contribute to the maximum number of reported VPDs cases, thus responsible for their heavy burden in the Indian country profile. Thanks to creativity, professionalism and perseverance in the National Polio Surveillance Program today, WHO has removed India from the list of polio-endemic countries in the world with the last case of polio reported from India as of January 13, 2010. However, regarding other pediatric infectious diseases, only little data is available due to lack of countrywide effective surveillance system.

DEMOGRAPHY

Table 1.1.1 depicts the demography and vital statistics figures pertaining to the years 1980–2016 with comparative figures for the years 1980, 1990, 2000 and 2012–2016.

REPORTED CASES

Table 1.1.2 depicts the number of reported cases of VPDs since the years 2012–2016 with comparative figures for the years 1980, 1990 and 2000.

Although there is a significant reduction in the total number of cases when compared to those in 1980s, it remains a matter of concern that still there are many

Table 1.1.1: Demography and vital statistics figures (1980–2016).

Development developing status		GNI/capita (US$) GDP/capita (US$)	1,590 6,089	Infant (under 12 months) mortality rate Child (under 5 years) mortality rate	38 48			
Population data in thousands								
	2016	2015	2014	2013	2012	2000	1990	1980
Total population	13,24,171	13,09,054	12,93,859	12,78,562	12,63,066	10,53,051	8,70,133	6,96,784
Live births	25,197	25,244	25,338	25,494	25,717	27,880	27,419	25,220
Surviving infants	24,277	24,291	24,348	24,461	24,635	26,057	25,021	22,372
Population less than 5 years	1,19,998	1,21,415	1,22,588	1,24,278	1,26,131	1,27,607	1,21,428	1,03,422
Population less than 15 years	3,73,356	3,75,145	3,76,631	3,78,168	3,79,513	3,65,774	3,30,036	2,73,442
Female 15–49 years	3,41,429	3,36,722	3,32,172	3,27,463	3,22,658	2,61,022	2,05,762	1,62,390

(GNI: gross national income; GDP: gross domestic product)
Source: WHO vaccine-preventable diseases: monitoring system 2017, India

Table 1.1.2: Number of reported cases of vaccine-preventable diseases in 1980, 1990, 2000 and 2012–2016.

	2016	2015	2014	2013	2012	2000	1990	1980
Diphtheria	3,380	2,365	6,094	3,133	2,525	5,125	8,425	39,231
Japanese Encephalitis	1,627	1,620	1,657	1,078	–	–	–	–
Measles	71,726	90,387	79,563	13,822	18,668	38,835	89,612	1,14,036
Mumps	–	–	–	–	–	–	–	–
Pertussis	37,274	25,206	46,706	31,089	44,154	31,431	1,12,416	3,20,109
Polio*	0	0	0	0	0	265	10,408	18,975
Rubella	8,274	3,252	4,870	3,698	1,232	–	–	–
Rubella (CRS)	25	–	–	–	–	–	–	–
Neonatal Tetanus**	227	491	492	415	588	3,287	9,313	–
Total Tetanus	3,781	2,268	5,017	2,814	2,404	8,997	23,356	45,948
Yellow Fever	–	–	–	–	–	–	–	–

*Polio refers to all polio cases (indigenous or imported), including polio cases caused by vaccine derived polio viruses (VDPV). It does not include cases of vaccine-associated paralytic polio (VAPP) and cases of non polio acute flaccid paralysis (AFP).

**Neonatal Tetanus and Total Tetanus cases equality may be the result from a lack of non-Neonatal Tetanus surveillance system.

(CRS: congenital rubella syndrome)

Source: WHO vaccine-preventable diseases: monitoring system 2017, India

preventable cases affecting children under 5 years, but this is just the "tip of the iceberg". Many cases of measles, pertussis, diphtheria, etc. may still be missing in these reports due to under-reporting.

The Magnitude

Diphtheria

Around 3380 cases of diphtheria are reported in 2016 from various parts of the country despite the existence of National Immunization Mission since 1985. It is a matter of concern for the planners as well as the implementers. In the absence of subclinical infection in most parts of the country, any new case of diphtheria is bound to cause dreaded complications like diphtheritic myocarditis/neuroparalytic complications, etc.

In India, the state of Andhra Pradesh accounted for 40–70% of diphtheria cases reported from the country during 2003–2006, most of them being reported from Hyderabad, the state capital. In Hyderabad, diphtheria rate increased from 11 per 100,000 in 2003 to 23 per 100,000 in 2006. Integrated Disease Surveillance Programme (IDSP), National Centre for Disease Control (NCDC), Delhi, reported 7 outbreaks of diphtheria in India during the year 2014.

The 2016 surveillance data, which comes from the states of Bihar, Haryana, Kerala, and Uttar Pradesh (UP), shows the importance of examining subnational surveillance data and coverage (Table 1.1.3).

The age distribution of cases for these states is very different, with Bihar having the highest proportion of cases under 5, Kerala having the highest proportion of

Table 1.1.3: Age distribution of diphtheria cases in states of India with case-based surveillance, 2016.

State	Total cases	Under 5	5–10 years	Over 10 years
Bihar	71	41%	34%	25%
Haryana	59	27%	53%	20%
Kerala	556	8%	18%	74%
Uttar Pradesh	844	25%	53%	22%
Total	1530	20%	39%	41%

cases over 10, and Haryana and UP showing the highest proportion of cases between 5 and 10 years of age. Survey data demonstrate that the coverage for both DTP3 and the fifth dose at 5 years of age is also highly variable among regions.

Pertussis Infection

Pertussis continues to be a major public health problem in both developing and developed countries. There is passive reporting of whooping cough cases from the public sector, the data is maintained by the Government of India and also shared with WHO. In India, the incidence of pertussis declined sharply after launch of Universal of Immunization Program (UIP). The shifting age group for new pertussis cases and complications in adolescents is a matter of concern. Pertussis in adolescents and adults is responsible for considerable morbidity in these age groups and also serves as a reservoir for disease transmission to unvaccinated/partially vaccinated young infants. It has become necessary to administer adolescent pertussis vaccine in areas endemic for pertussis.

Tetanus

A total of 3,781 cases of tetanus (inclusive of 227cases of neonatal tetanus) stresses the need for a high diphtheria-tetanus-pertussis (DTP) coverage of under 1 and under 5 children as well as a high coverage of two doses of Td (toxoid dose) to pregnant mothers. Since neonatal tetanus invariably has a high case fatality rate, which adds to the total infant mortality, urgent steps are needed to step up the Td two-dose coverage to nearly 100% of all pregnant mothers. This schedule appears to provide protective levels of antibody for well above 80% of newborns. Both WHO and Indian Academy of Pediatrics Committee on Immunization recommend replacement of tetanus toxoid by Td vaccine in the National Immunization Program (NIP).

Measles

Estimates of measles-related deaths have been considered a crucial indicator to evaluate the progress of any nation towards measles elimination. The global estimates for the year 2013 suggest that close to 0.14 million deaths were attributed to measles, accounting for nearly 16 deaths each hour. Study findings have indicated that more than 50% of the global measles associated deaths were reported in India alone. India has made important efforts and gains against measles in recent years. Measles deaths have declined by 51% from an estimated 100,000 in the year 2000 to 49,000 in 2015. This has been possible by significantly increasing the reach of the first dose of measles vaccine, given at the age of nine months under routine immunization programme, from 56% in 2000 to 87% in 2015. The National Family Health Survey-4 (2015–2016) has assessed it to be 81.1%. This is low compared to the 95% coverage level required for elimination. Indian Association of Pediatrics (IAP) has revised its recommendations on Measles and MMR vaccination schedule.The new schedule will have a dose of MMR at 9 months instead of measles, and another dose (2nd) at 15 months of age. The earlier recommendation of 2nd dose of MMR at 4–6 years of age has been removed.

Poliomyelitis

India has made remarkable progress in the control and elimination of poliomyelitis. From an alarming number of nearly 2,000 cases in 1998, the case count as on September 17, 2010 was just 39 cases. Since January 13, 2011 nil case of polio due to wild poliovirus has been reported.

In 2009, India had more polio cases than any other country in the world (756). In just two short years, India has taken a giant step toward eradicating polio globally forever. On January 13, 2012, India reached a major milestone in the history of polio eradication—a 12-month period without any case of polio. The WHO reported that in 2011 India had its first polio-free year and is therefore no longer considered polio-endemic. This date marks the unprecedented progress in India and an endorsement of the effectiveness of the polio eradication strategies and their implementation in India. India is now off the WHO list of polio-endemic countries, but has to remain free of polio for the next 2 years to achieve the status of polio-free country.

The Strategic Plan was developed in response to the May 2012 World Health Assembly which declared the completion of poliovirus eradication to be a programmatic emergency for global public health. Under this plan to achieve and sustain a polio-free world, the use of OPV must eventually be stopped worldwide, starting with OPV containing type 2 poliovirus (OPV type 2). At least one dose of Poliomyelitis vaccine (Inactivated) must be introduced as a risk mitigation measure and to boost population immunity.

Since 25th April 2016 the Ministry of Health and Family Welfare, Government of India (GoI) switched from tOPV to bOPV. Now in India only bOPV will be used both in routine immunization (RI) as well as polio campaigns. To provide protection against type-2 poliovirus to naive children born post-switch. IPV would be the only source of providing type-2 immunity to children after April 2016.

Mumps Infection

Although we do not have the accurate figures of reported cases, it is evident from the cases seen by pediatricians and family physicians in their office practice that the number of mumps cases is also of a significant proportion in India. With the availability of a safe, effective, indigenous and cost-effective vaccine, mumps should be immediately included in the UIP as MMR vaccine in place of MR vaccine. Further, there is an urgent need of initiating surveillance of clinical cases of mumps all over the country and it should be declared as a 'notifiable' disease in India. IAP has recently revised its recommendations on MMR vaccination with first dose at 9 months in place of standalone measles vaccine, and second at 15 months of age.

Rubella Infection

Although the total number of cases of rubella is not known, rubella is the most common and single cause of blindness in the newborns as reported by ophthalmologists in India with cases of congenital rubella syndrome (CRS). A recent study conducted in both rural and urban areas of 12 districts in Maharashtra shows that rubella virus infection is prevalent in these areas and almost 25% girls reach childbearing age without acquiring natural immunity against the disease. Studies conducted across India suggest similar baseline information on the susceptibility profile of women of childbearing age.

In order to raise the immunity against rubella and prevention of CRS, the following strategy is recommended: Administration of first dose of rubella containing vaccine, viz. MMR, at 9 months and the second dose at the age 15–18 months and conducting mass immunization campaigns targeting girls up to the age of 15 years. The Ministry of Health and Family Welfare launched Measles Rubella (MR) vaccination campaign in the country in February 2017. The campaign against these two diseases will start from five States/UTs (Karnataka, Tamil Nadu, Puducherry, Goa and Lakshadweep) covering nearly 3.6 crore target children. Following the campaign, Measles-Rubella vaccine will be introduced in routine immunization, replacing the currently given two doses of measles vaccine, at 9–12 months and 16–24 months of age.

Hepatitis B Virus Infection

India is rated to be in the intermediate zone for hepatitis-B prevalence with hepatitis B surface antigen (HBsAg) prevalence between 2% and 10% among populations studied. The fact remains that hepatitis B infection occurs during childhood and causes fatal complications like hepatocellular carcinoma, chronic active hepatitis or cirrhosis of liver and thus accounting for high morbidity and mortality. In India the prevalence of Hepatitis B surface antigen (HBsAg) is 3–4.2% with over 40 million HBV carriers. Every year over 100,000 Indians die due to Hepatitis B complications.

Hepatitis B vaccine is safe and is highly effective in preventing hepatitis B virus (HBV) infection and its serious consequences. Protection afforded by this vaccine is long lasting. Numerous studies have shown that adding hepatitis B vaccine into the expanded program of immunization is highly cost-effective, even in areas with low HBV endemicity. In 1991, the Global Advisory Group of the Expanded Program on Immunization of WHO recommended that hepatitis B vaccine should be introduced into NIPs in all countries by the year 1997. The World Health Assembly approved this in 1992. More than 100 countries have already included this vaccine in their NIPs. In countries that have implemented universal childhood hepatitis B immunization, HBV carrier rate has declined markedly and incidence rate of long-term consequences, like liver cancer, have shown a decrease.

It is a matter of satisfaction that the Government of India has since introduced hepatitis B vaccine in the National Schedule in select pilot project areas from the year 2002 onward, which is now extended to the entire country in a phased manner. As per 2015 national estimates, the hepatitis B vaccination coverage of children is 45% for the birth dose (within 24 hours after birth) and 86% Hepatitis B third dose. Figure 1.1.1 depicts the magnitude of the disease at the global level and in India.

Hepatitis A Virus Infection

A disease of children has now shifted to adolescents. Although complications are less compared to hepatitis B infection, effective vaccines are now available to be given in prime-boost schedule. The actual incidence is not known since many cases of hepatitis A are not reported. May be with the introduction of Integrated Disease Surveillance Project (IDSP) in India, we will have more number of hepatitis A cases reported. IDSP identified a substantial number of hepatitis cases and outbreaks during 2011–2013. The large number of hepatitis A and E outbreaks might be explained in part by the lack of adequate sewage and

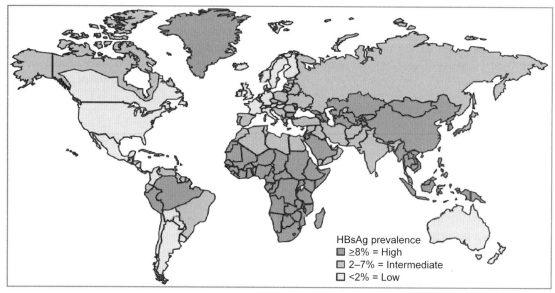

FIG. 1.1.1: Geographic pattern of global hepatitis B prevalence.

sanitation systems; defecation in open fields, which can contaminate surface drinking-water sources, remains a common practice. The large numbers of hepatitis A cases might also reflect an epidemiologic shift in the affected population in India. Hepatitis A infection during childhood often is asymptomatic and unrecognized, and typically confers lifelong immunity. With increasing age at time of infection, symptomatic cases become more common. With improved hygiene and sanitation reflecting India's improving economy, more children might escape childhood infection and remain susceptible to infection during adolescence and adulthood. The global geographic distribution is given in the Figure 1.1.2. The current recommendation is to administer hepatitis A vaccine at 12 months of age due to absence of maternal antibodies in the newborn. Killed Hep A vaccine: Start the 2-dose Hep A vaccine series for children aged 12 through 23 months; separate the 2 doses by 6–18 months. Live attenuated H_2-strain Hepatitis A vaccine: Single dose starting at 12 months and through 23 months of age.

Varicella Infection

Varicella is widely prevalent mostly in children 5–10 years of age with increasing incidence in children under 5. A vaccine with good protective efficacy is available and is being used by many pediatricians all over the country. The disease usually manifests in early summer and it is estimated that many thousands of cases are not reported to the medical facility due to traditional beliefs and customs, and because of the lesser complications attributed to the disease, *per se*. However, the available statistics reveal the magnitude to some extent.

Varicella prevalence in India

- Twenty-five million cases annually in India
- *Complications:* Secondary infection—scars, encephalitis, cerebellitis, *H. zoster*, pneumonia, congenital varicella syndrome
- *Morbidity:* School and office absenteeism
- *Mortality:* 2–25 per 100,000, immunocompromised (IC): 10–30%
- High risk groups include adults, IC host, pregnancy and neonate.
- Following breakthrough infection in 30% of children who had received a single dose of varicella vaccine, the current recommendation is to administer two doses of varicella vaccine at 15 months and 5 years simultaneously with two doses of MMR vaccine.

Human Papillomavirus (HPV) Infection

Human papillomavirus (HPV) infection is now a well-established cause of cervical cancer and there is growing evidence of HPV being a relevant factor in other anogenital cancers (anus, vulva, vagina and penis) and head and neck cancers. HPV types 16 and 18 are responsible for about 70% of all cervical cancer cases worldwide. HPV vaccines that prevent against HPV 16 and 18 infection are now available and have the potential to reduce the incidence of cervical and other anogenital cancers.

Cancer of the cervix uteri is the 4th most common cancer among women worldwide, with an estimated 5,27,624 new cases and 2,65,672 deaths in 2012. Worldwide, mortality rates of cervical cancer are substantially lower than incidence with a ratio of mortality to incidence

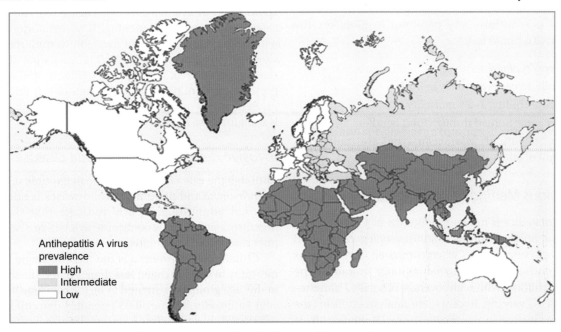

FIG. 1.1.2: Geographic distribution of hepatitis A prevalence.

to 50.3%. Current estimates indicate that every year 1,22,844 women are diagnosed with cervical cancer and 67,477 die from the disease. Cervical cancer ranks as the 2nd most frequent cancer among women in India and the 2nd most frequent cancer among women between 15 and 44 years of age. About 5.0% of women in the general population are estimated to harbour cervical HPV-16/18 infection at a given time, and 83.2% of invasive cervical cancers are attributed to HPVs 16 or 18. Prophylactic HPV vaccination has provided a powerful tool for primary prevention of cervical cancer and other HPV-related diseases. Three HPV vaccines are now available: bivalent (against HPVs 16/18), quadrivalent (against HPVs 6/11/16/18) and the recently approved 9-valent vaccine (against HPVs 6/11/16/18/31/33/45/52/58). Two doses of HPV vaccine are advised for adolescent/preadolescent girls aged 9–14 years; for girls 15 years and older, current 3 dose schedule will continue. For two-dose schedule, the minimum interval between doses should be 6 months. Human Papillomavirus (HPV) vaccination program is directed towards the prevention of cervical cancer. Delhi is now the first state to launch the Human Papillomavirus (HPV) vaccine as a public health program for school children (9–13 years).

Typhoid

The disease is prevalent throughout the year and pediatricians and pediatric hospitals get typhoid cases almost throughout the year. Although conjugated vaccine is available, the protective efficacy is around 60% and paratyphoid infection is not protected by the conjugate polysaccharide vaccine. The best ways are to adopt universal precautions and personal hygiene for the protection of typhoid fever.

Prevention of typhoid
- Five million cases annually in India
- Severe morbidity, 1–2% mortality
- *Carrier state:* Spread through food handlers
- About 50–90% of *Salmonella typhi* are multidrug-resistant of late quinolone resistance—90%.

Tuberculous Meningitis or Encephalitis

The true incidence is not known. But the fact remains that private and public institutions admit very few cases of TB meningitis or encephalitis when compared to yesteryears due to good control of hematogenous spread of the disease in children with high coverage of bacille Calmette–Guérin (BCG) vaccine. Recent meta-analysis confirms the significant decline in the incidence of TB meningitis or encephalitis, miliary TB and disseminated TB.

Meningococcal Meningitis and Disease

Meningococcal meningitis or cerebrospinal fever occurs sporadically and in small outbreaks in most parts of the world. The zone lying between 5° and 15° N of the equator in tropical Africa is called the "meningitis belt" because of the frequent epidemic waves that have been occurring in that region. During recent years, several serious outbreaks affecting numerous countries occurred, not only in the so-called meningitis belt in Africa but also in both tropical and temperate zones of other continents, viz. Americas, Asia and Europe. WHO estimates that about 500,000 cases of meningococcal disease occur every year worldwide causing 50,000 deaths. The fatality of typical untreated cases is about 80%. With early diagnosis and treatment, case fatality rates have declined.

Before 2010 and the mass preventive immunization campaigns, Group A meningococcus accounted for an estimated 80–85% of all cases in the meningitis belt, with epidemics occurring at intervals of 7–14 years. Since then, the proportion of the A serogroup has declined dramatically. During the 2014 epidemic season, 19 African countries implementing enhanced surveillance reported 11,908 suspected cases including 1146 deaths, the lowest numbers since the implementation of enhanced surveillance through a functional network.

Meningococcal disease is endemic in India. *N. meningitidis* is the third most common cause of bacterial meningitis in India in children aged <5 years, and is responsible for an estimated 1.9% of all cases regardless of age. The majority of reported cases are due to serogroup A, with rare reports of serogroups B and C. Cases of meningococcal meningitis are reported sporadically or in small clusters. During 2007, about 4,472 cases of meningococcal meningitis were reported in India with about 252 deaths. The decision to undertake mass vaccination following an outbreak is based upon the attack rate within an area. During inter epidemic and epidemic periods, immunoprophylaxis of high-risk populations is implemented and chemoprophylaxis with antimicrobials is used for close contacts.

Invasive Hemophilus Influenzae Disease

Although the exact incidence of the magnitude of invasive *H. influenzae* and pneumococcal diseases is not known, hospital admissions clearly indicate that these two organisms significantly contribute to invasive diseases like pneumonia and meningitis.

Childhood pneumonia is the leading single cause of mortality in children aged less than 5 years. The incidence in this age group is estimated to be 0.29 episode per child-year in developing and 0.05 episodes per child-year in developed countries. This translates into about 156 million new episodes each year worldwide, of which 151 million episodes are in the developing world. Most cases occur in India (43 million), China (21 million) and Pakistan (10 million), with additional high numbers in Bangladesh, Indonesia and Nigeria (6 million each). Pneumonia is responsible for about 19% of all deaths in children aged less than 5 years, of which more than 70% take place in sub-Saharan Africa and South-East Asia.

Effective vaccines are now available for their control and IAP recommends Hib vaccine for routine use preferably in combination formulation of diphtheria-tetanus-whole cell pertussis-hepatitis B/Hib (DTPw-HB-Hib) at 6, 10 and 14 weeks.

Figure 1.1.3 depicts the global disease burden including India.

Estimated invasive Hib disease in India: Based on community-based report:
- Meningitis 17 per 100,000 children per annum
- *Pneumonia 1.5 times meningitis:* 25 per 100,000 children per annum
- *Total invasive disease:* 42 per 100,000 per annum
- *Hib disease per 100,000:* 266–1,750
- Children below 5 years (15% of total population) 15, 40, 52, 287
- *Total estimates in India:* 409,640–2,695,000

Case fatality due to invasive Hib diseases
- *If CFR 2%:* 8,192–53,900 per annum
- *If CFR 10%:* 40,964–269,500 per annum

Studies reporting invasive Hib disease are limited.
Reported from all parts of India:
- *Hib pneumonia:* 2–33%
- *Hib meningitis:* 2–35%

- Almost half of the children are colonized with Hib
- Agent is present in abundance
- Risk factors for increased invasive Hib disease exist in India.

(*Source:* IAP Immunization update; 2006.)

The proposal to include pentavalent DTPw-HB-Hib vaccine formulation in NIP was recommended by National Technical Advisory Group on Immunization (NTAGI) and approved by the central cabinet to bring down the Hib disease burden in India. Government of India has successfully implemented mass immunization program with pentavalent vaccine, which is now introduced in all the states of India. The use of pentavalent vaccine automatically raises the coverage level of hepatitis B and hib vaccines. If the vaccines are given individually, the coverage of hepatitis B and hib vaccines usually lags behind DPT coverage. This gap can be filled by using pentavalent vaccine in routine immunization program.

Pneumococcal Disease

Pneumonia is the single largest infectious cause of death among under-five children worldwide, accounting for about 0.92 million deaths in 2015. It is estimated that 1 in 6 deaths in under-five children was due to pneumonia in 2015. Pneumococcal pneumonia in particular is a major public health concern for children globally. This infection accounts for 18% of all severe pneumonia cases and 33% of all pneumonia deaths worldwide. More than 80% of deaths associated with pneumonia occur in children during the first two years of life. Pneumococcal disease is also the number one vaccine-preventable cause of death in children under five, globally and in India (Fig. 1.1.4).

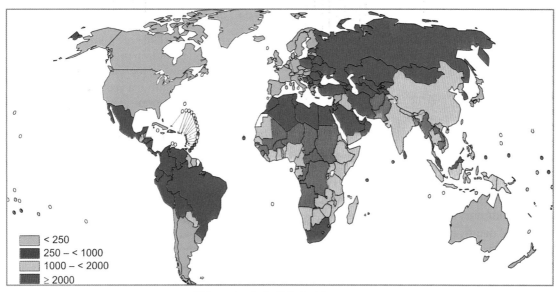

< 250
250 – < 1000
1000 – < 2000
≥ 2000

FIG. 1.1.3: Global Hib incidence rate.
Source: WHO decision-making and implementation of conjugate Hib vaccines (NUVI); 2009

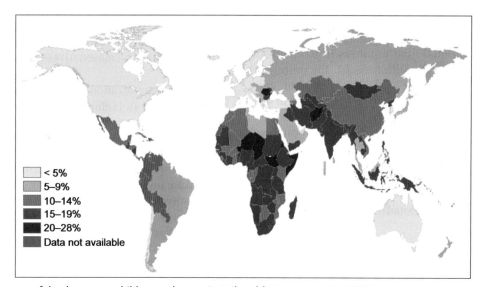

FIG. 1.1.4: Percentage of deaths among children under age 5 attributable to pneumonia, 2015.

Source: WHO and Maternal and Child Epidemiology Estimation Group (MCEE) provisional estimates 2015 http://data.unicef.org/child-health/pneumonia.html#sthash.D7850ssq.dpuf

Incidence of invasive pneumococcal diseases:

- Around 12–35% of all admissions are due to LRT in India. In 2010, 3.6 million episodes of severe pneumonia and 0.35 million all-cause pneumonia deaths occurred in children under the age of 5 years in India. Among those, 0.56 million episodes of severe pneumonia (16%) and 0.10 million deaths (30%), respectively, were caused by pneumococcal pneumonia. India has a pneumonia mortality rate of 7 per 1000 live births.
- *Streptococcus pneumococcus* is the cause for 50% of community acquired pneumonia, 20–40% of all pyogenic meningitis.
- *The rate of invasive pneumococcal disease:* 167/100,000 less than 2 years in USA (before vaccination), 224–349/100,000 less than 5 years in developing countries.

The ten countries with the highest numbers and proportions of pneumococcal cases were all in Asia and Africa; they account for 66% (44–88%) of pneumococcal cases worldwide (India 27%, China 12%, Nigeria 5%, Pakistan 5%, Bangladesh 4%, Indonesia 3%, Ethiopia 3%, Congo 3%, Kenya 2% and the Philippines 2%). Of the 14.5 million pneumococcal cases, 95.6% were cases of pneumonia, 3.7% nonpneumonia, nonmeningitis invasive pneumococcal syndromes and 0–7% meningitis.

Pneumococcal deaths in children aged 1–59 months per 100,000 children younger than 5 years (HIV-negative pneumococcal deaths only). The boundaries shown and the designations used on this map do not imply the expression of any opinion by WHO concerning the legal status of any country, territory, city or area, or of its authorities, or

concerning the delimitation of its frontiers or boundaries. Dotted lines in Figure 1.1.5 represent approximate border lines for which there may not yet be full agreement.

The new 13 valent pneumococcal vaccine, offers about 70–75% protection against the prevalent strains in India. In May 2017, Government of India decided to include pneumococcal conjugate vaccine (PCV) in UIP in a phased approach. With this phased introduction, nearly 2.1 million children in 3 states will be vaccinated with PCV in the first year. The coverage will be expanded across the entire country in the coming years.

Acute Diarrheal Diseases

Diarrhea is a leading killer of children, accounting for 9% of all deaths among children under age 5 worldwide in 2015. This translates to over 1,400 young children dying each day, or about 526,000 children a year, despite the availability of simple effective treatment.

Figure 1.1.6 depicts the global disease burden including India.

In India, diarrheal disease is a major health problem. More than 300 million episodes of acute diarrhea occur every year in children under 5 years of age. During 2005, about 1.07 million cases of acute diarrhea were reported in India with 2,040 deaths. The actual incidence must be many fold. The National Diarrhoeal Disease Control Programme has made a significant contribution in averting deaths among children under 5 years of age. Much attention has been given to acute diarrhea and its management over the last decade, which is dominated by advances in oral rehydration techniques.

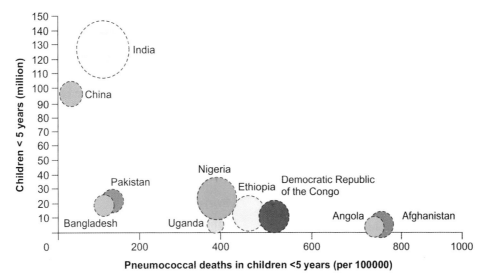

FIG. 1.1.5: Ten countries with the greatest number of pneumococcal deaths in children aged 1–59 months.

Bubble size indicates the number of pneumococcal deaths.

Country (number of deaths): India (142,000), Nigeria (86,000), Ethiopia (57,000), Democratic Republic of the Congo (51,000), Afghanistan (31,000), China (30,000), Pakistan (27,000), Bangladesh (21,000), Angola (20,000) and Uganda (19,000)

Source: Lancet. Vol 374 September 12, 2009.

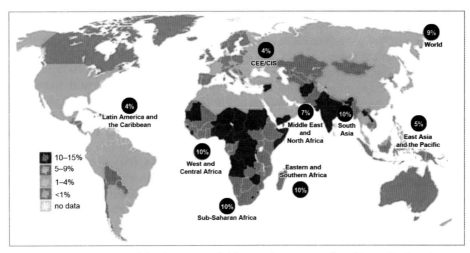

FIG. 1.1.6: Percentage of deaths among children under age 5 attributable to diarrhea, 2015.

Source: WHO and Maternal and Child Epidemiology Estimation Group (MCEE) provisional estimates 2015

The rotavirus, first discovered in 1973, has emerged as the leading cause of severe, dehydrating diarrhea in children aged under 5 years globally, with an estimated more than 25 million outpatient visits and more than 2 million hospitalizations attributable to rotavirus infections each year. In developing countries, three-quarters of children acquire their first episode of rotavirus diarrhea before the age of 12 months, whereas in developed countries the first episode is frequently delayed until the age of 2.5 years. The new rotavirus vaccines are now introduced for routine use in a number of industrialized and developing countries. The NTAGI have recommended the introduction of Rotavirus vaccine with GAVI subsidy in the NIP in a phased manner.

India has made steady progress in reducing deaths in children younger than 5 years, with total deaths declining from 2.5 million in 2001 to 1.5 million in 2012. This remarkable reduction was possible due to the inception and success of many universal programs like expanded program on immunization, program for the control of diarrheal diseases and acute respiratory infection. Even though the deaths among children under-5 years have declined, the proportional mortality accounted by diarrheal diseases still remains high. Diarrhea is the third most common cause of death in under-five children, responsible for 13% deaths in this age-group, killing an estimated 3,00,000 children in India each year.

Cholera

Cholera is an acute diarrheal infection caused by ingestion of food or water contaminated with the bacterium *Vibrio cholerae*. Cholera remains a global threat to public health and an indicator of inequity and lack of social development. Globally, the actual number of cholera cases is known to be much higher; the discrepancy is the result of under reporting and inconsistency in case definition and lack of standard vocabulary. Some countries report laboratory confirmed cases only, and so many cases are labeled as acute watery diarrhea. Researchers have estimated that every year, there are roughly 1.3 to 4.0 million cases, and 21,000 to 1,43,000 deaths worldwide due to cholera. Epidemics of cholera are frequent, striking adults as well as children.

India accounts for 675,188 cases and 20,256 deaths. In addition, an issue of concern is that 65–86% of the isolates have been found to be resistant to the commonly used antimicrobials and their prevalence is concentrated in the lowest quintile of wealth. In India, during 2005, the larger endemic foci of cholera were found in Delhi (945 cases), Tamil Nadu (724 cases and one death), West Bengal (235 cases), Andhra Pradesh (165 cases), Karnataka (214 cases and one death), Kerala (27 cases and one death) and Gujarat (82 cases and two deaths). The total number of cases reported was 3,156 with six deaths. In the year 2008, WHO has recorded 2,680 cases of cholera in India.

The most effective prophylactic measure is health education directed mainly to: (a) effectiveness and simplicity of oral rehydration therapy; (b) benefits of early reporting for prompt treatment; (c) food hygiene practices; (d) hand washing after defecation and before eating; and (e) benefits of cooked, hot foods and safe drinking water. Since cholera is a disease of the poor and ignorant, these groups should be tackled first.

Although, a parenteral cholera vaccine of Ogawa and Inaba serotypes of *V. cholerae* is available, there are still doubts about its usefulness as a preventive measure. The oral cholera vaccine now available in India is recommended for routine use in cholera endemic regions.

Diarrheal Diseases Control Program

The incidence of cholera cases and deaths has decreased in recent years. Oral rehydration therapy program was started in 1986–87 in a phased manner. The main objective of the program is to prevent diarrhea-associated deaths in children due to dehydration. The program highlights the rational management of diarrhea in children, including increased intake of home available fluids, zinc supplementation and breastfeeding. Oral rehydration solution (ORS) is being supplied as a part of subcenter kits and is promoted as a first line of treatment.

India has made steady progress in reducing deaths in children younger than 5 years, with total deaths declining from 2.5 million in 2001 to 1.5 million in 2012. This remarkable reduction was possible due to the inception and success of many universal programs like expanded program on immunization, program for the control of diarrheal diseases and acute respiratory infection. Even though the deaths among children under-5 years have declined, the proportional mortality accounted by diarrheal diseases still remains high. Diarrhea is the third most common cause of death in under-five children, responsible for 13% deaths in this age-group, killing an estimated 300,000 children in India each year.

Malaria

At present, about 109 countries in the world are considered endemic for malaria, 45 countries within WHO African region. There were an estimated 216 million episodes of malaria in 2010, with a wide uncertainty interval (5th–95th centiles) from 149 million to 274 million cases. Approximately 81%, or 174 million (113–239 million) cases, were in the African region, with the South-East Asian Region (SEAR) accounting for another 13%.

There were an estimated 655,000 (5,37,000–9,07,000) malaria deaths in 2010, of which 91% (596,000, range 4,68,000–8,37,000) were in the African Region. Approximately 86% of malaria deaths globally were of children under 5 years of age.

In the SEAR, during 2009, a total of 2.7 million confirmed malaria cases and 3,188 malaria deaths were reported whereas estimated malaria cases were around 26–36 million and malaria deaths between 42,300 and 77,300. The highest number of laboratory confirmed cases were reported from India (15,63,344) followed by Indonesia (5,44,470) and Myanmar (4,14,008) whereas the lowest number of cases was reported from Sri Lanka (558) followed by Bhutan (972) and Nepal (3,335). In case of malaria deaths, the highest number of deaths were reported from India (1,133) followed by Myanmar (972) and Indonesia (900).

In India, malaria continues to pose a major public health threat, particularly due to *plasmodium falciparum* which is prone to complications. Experts estimate that more than 1.5 million persons are infected with malaria every year. The most affected states are North-Eastern states, Chhattisgarh, Jharkhand, Madhya Pradesh, Orissa, Andhra Pradesh, Maharashtra, Gujarat, Rajasthan, West Bengal and Karnataka. However, the other states are also vulnerable with local and focal outbreaks of malaria. Much of these areas are remote and inaccessible, fore or forest fringed with operation difficulties and predominantly inhabited by tribal population.

Despite these challenges, India is working – and making progress towards the elimination of malaria. Since 2000, the country has more than halved the number of malaria cases, down from 2 million to 8,82,000 in 2013 and, the trend is continuing. To reach pre-elimination, all states in India will need to have annual parasite incidence (API) of less than 1 per 1000 and all districts within the state will also need to be less than 1. Currently, 74% of India's more than 650 districts have achieved an API of less than 1. Strong financial support, increased surveillance, more health workers, and further program integration in all levels of the health system will be needed for the country to reach elimination.

Currently, there is no vaccine available, but research is going on for a vaccine to prevent infection and/or ameliorate disease. Unlike other vaccines, a malaria vaccine even with only 50% efficacy would still be very useful in controlling the disease. The time-bound objectives set out for the Eleventh (XIth) Five-Year Plan by Ministry of Health (MoH) and Family Welfare, Government of India (GoI) is reduction of malaria mortality rate by 50% up to 2010 and an additional 10% by 2012.

Japanese Encephalitis

Japanese Encephalitis (JE) is mosquito-borne encephalitis infecting mainly animals and incidentally man. Twenty-five years ago, JE was known as an endemic disease in East Asia, especially in Japan, China and Korea but in recent years, it has spread widely in South-East Asia, and outbreaks of considerable magnitude have occurred in Thailand, Indonesia, Vietnam, India, Myanmar and Sri Lanka.

An estimated 50,000 cases of JE occur globally each year, with 10,000 deaths and nearly 15,000 disabled. About three-quarters of the cases occur in the Western Pacific countries, primarily China and adjacent countries, with the remainder occurring in South-East Asia, especially India.

In India, the states reporting repeated outbreaks are Andhra Pradesh, Assam, Bihar, Haryana, Karnataka, Kerala, Maharashtra, Manipur, Tamil Nadu, Uttar Pradesh and West Bengal. The population at risk is about 300 million. The incidence of JE in India is still increasing, and the case-fatality rate of reported cases is high, i.e. 10–30%. India currently has no national vaccination program, but the MoH has recently drawn up a plan in which children 1–12 years of age will be immunized. In Tamil Nadu and Uttar Pradesh, immunization programs are already running; thus, JE incidence might stabilize in those regions. However, overall trends for India are difficult to predict because JE endemicity is heterogeneous and because socioeconomic conditions for control differ substantially from one state to another. As per the recent figures from WHO (2008), there have been 294 cases of JE reported in India.

According to the Directorate of National Vector Borne Disease Control Programme (NVBDCP), Delhi, 1661 cases of JE were reported in the year 2014 from 15 states and union territories, out of which 293 (17.6%) died. Assam, West Bengal, Uttar Pradesh (UP) and Jharkhand reported maximum number of cases.

Following mass vaccination campaigns with live attenuated SA-14-14-2 JE vaccine among pediatric age group, adult JE cases have outnumbered pediatric cases in some JE endemic states, including Assam. This led the state government of Assam to conduct special campaigns of JE vaccines in adults (>15 years) in some most affected districts. The exact reason behind this shift in age group is not well understood. On 3rd July, 2014 the Government of India (GOI) announced the introduction of four new vaccines, including JE vaccine, in the National immunization program. Recently, NVBDCP has identified 20 high burden districts in three states—Assam, Uttar Pradesh, and West Bengal, for adult JE vaccination (>15–65 years).

Tuberculosis

It remains a worldwide public health problem. It is estimated that about one-third of the current global population is infected asymptomatically with tuberculosis (TB). Most new cases and deaths occur in developing countries where infection is often acquired in childhood. The annual risk of TB infection in high-burden countries is estimated to be 0.5–2%.

India is the highest TB burden country in the world and accounts for nearly one-fifth (20%) of global burden of TB, two-thirds of cases in SEAR. Of the 9.2 million cases of TB that occur in the world every year, nearly 1.9 million are in India. Two out of every five Indians are infected with TB bacillus. In India, almost 0.37 million people die every year.

India accounts for one fourth of the global TB burden. In 2015, an estimated 28 lakh cases occurred and 4.8 lakh people died due to TB. The table below shows the estimated figures for TB burden globally and for India reported in WHO Global TB Report for the year 2015 (Table 1.1.4).

An estimated 1.3 lakh incident multi-drug resistant TB patients emerge annually in India which includes 79000 MDR-TB patients estimates among notified pulmonary cases. India bears second highest number of estimated HIV associated TB in the world. An estimated 1.1 lakh HIV associated TB occurred in 2015 and 37,000 estimated number of patients died among them.

DOTS-Plus for the management of drug resistant TB in India had been launched in 2007. There was then very limited progress between 2007 and 2009. But by 2009, it was planned that by the end of 2011 the drug resistant

Table 1.1.4: Estimated figures for TB burden globally and for India reported in WHO Global TB Report 2015		
Estimates of TB burden (2015)	Global	India
Incidence TB cases	104 lakh	28 lakh
Mortality of TB	14 lakh	4.8 lakh
Incidence HIV TB	11.7 lakh	1.1 lakh
MDR-TB	4.8 lakh	1.3 lakh

TB services would be available across India. The DOTS-Plus services (now referred to as the "Programmatic Management of Drug Resistant TB") had been expanded across the whole country by 2012 and the service was available in all districts by 2013. By 2013 it had though been decided to decentralise the DOTS Plus services. The services were to be totally integrated into the main Revised National TB Control Programme (RNTCP) services at local level. In 2015, a total of 9,132,306 cases of suspected TB were examined by sputum smear microscopy and 1,423,181 people were diagnosed and registered for TB treatment by government's RNTCP.

The current vaccine strains are all descendants of the original *Mycobacterium bovis* isolate that Calmette and Guérin passaged through numerous cycles during the 13-year period, 1909–1921. Although, a number of BCG vaccine strains are available, in terms of efficacy, no BCG strain is demonstrably better than another, and there is no global consensus as to which strain of BCG is optimal for general use. Following closure of BCG vaccine laboratories in India, the GoI is using the BCG vaccine manufactured by Serum Institute of India Ltd., Pune, and Green Signal Bio Pharma Ltd. in its NIP.

The objective set out for TB control by MoH and Family Welfare, GoI, is to maintain 85% cure rate through entire mission period and also sustain planned case detection rate.

AIDS/HIV Infection

The acquired immunodeficiency syndrome (AIDS) is a fatal illness caused by human immunodeficiency virus (HIV) which breaks down the body's immune system, leaving the victim vulnerable to a host of life-threatening opportunistic infections, neurological disorders or unusual malignancies. Acquired immunodeficiency syndrome refers to the last stage of the HIV infection and can be called a modern pandemic affecting both industrialized and developing countries (Table 1.1.5).

Table 1.1.5: Number of people infected with human immunodeficiency virus infection and acquired immunodeficiency syndrome-related deaths.

Number of people living with HIV in 2008	*Total:* 33.4 million *Adults:* 31.3 million *Women (aged 15 and above):* 15.7 million *Children (under 15 years):* 2.1 million
People newly infected with human immunodeficiency virus in 2008	*Total:* 2.7 million *Adults:* 2.3 million *Children (under 15 years):* 4,30,000
AIDS-related deaths in 2008	*Total:* 2.0 million *Adults:* 1.7 million *Children (under 15 years):* 2,80,000

Since the beginning of the epidemic, more than 70 million people have been infected with the HIV virus and about 35 million people have died of HIV. Globally, 36.7 million [34.0–39.8 million] people were living with HIV at the end of 2015. An estimated 0.8% [0.7–0.9%] of adults aged 15–49 years worldwide are living with HIV, although the burden of the epidemic continues to vary considerably between countries and regions. Sub-Saharan Africa remains most severely affected, with nearly 1 in every 25 adults (4.4%) living with HIV and accounting for nearly 70% of the people living with HIV worldwide (Fig. 1.1.7).

In Asia, an estimated 4.9 million (4.5–5.5 million) people were living with HIV in 2009. In 2009, an estimated 300,000 (260,000–340,000) people died of AIDS-related illnesses. Asia, home to 60% of the world's population, is second only to sub-Saharan Africa in terms of people living with HIV.

As per the recently released, India HIV Estimation 2015 report, National adult (15–49 years) HIV prevalence in India is estimated at 0.26% (0.22–0.32%) in 2015. In 2015, adult HIV prevalence is estimated at 0.30% among males and at 0.22% among females. Among the States/UTs, in 2015, Manipur has shown the highest estimated adult HIV prevalence of 1.15%, followed by Mizoram (0.80%), Nagaland (0.78%), Andhra Pradesh and Telangana (0.66%), Karnataka (0.45%), Gujarat (0.42%) and Goa (0.40%). Besides these States, Maharashtra, Chandigarh, Tripura and Tamil Nadu have shown estimated adult HIV prevalence greater than the national prevalence (0.26%).

Until a vaccine or cure for AIDS is found, the only means at present available is health education to enable people to make life-saving choices. All mass media channels should be involved in educating the people on AIDS, its nature, transmission and prevention. The development of drugs (antiretrovirals) that suppress the infection rather than its complications has been an important achievement. These antiretroviral chemotherapy, while not a cure, have proved to be useful in prolonging the life of severely ill patients.

Dengue Illness

This disease is essentially a tropical one and is endemic in large parts of Latin and South America. Of late, its incidence has been on the increase in Asian countries such as India. A large number of infections may be subclinical, that is, the patients may not even be aware that they have had the disease. Treatment is usually supportive and symptomatic. Most patients will recover without any sequel. The overall mortality rate with effective treatment is close to 1% but this may be higher in children. A vaccine is in the late stages of development, but is still not available for commercial use on a large scale. Control of the mosquito population reduces the incidence of dengue, yellow fever and certain other rare fevers that are also transmitted by the same species of mosquito.

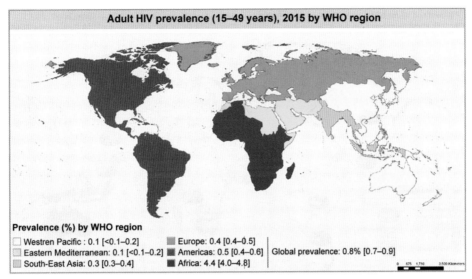

FIG. 1.1.7: A global view of human immunodeficiency virus infection.
Globally, 36.7 million [34.0–39.8 million] people were living with HIV at the end of 2015.
Source : http://www.who.int/gho/hiv/en/

As per the information from the Director, India's National Vector-borne Disease Control Programme, a total of 12,000 cases and 50 deaths have been reported in the country until October, 2010. These figures are as per the reported cases from the states/UTs and the number of actual infections is likely to be far higher.

The time-bound objectives set out for the Eleventh (XIth) Five-Year Plan by MoH and Family Welfare, GoI, is reduction of dengue mortality rate by 50% up to 2010 and sustaining at that level until 2012.

Also in 2015, Delhi, India, recorded its worst outbreak since 2006 with over 15 000 cases. In 2016, till month of September, 39,771 cases and 78 deaths were reported in India.

WHO recommends that countries should consider introduction of the dengue vaccine CYD-TDV only in geographic settings (national or subnational) where epidemiological data indicate a high burden of disease.

Chikungunya Fever

A dengue-like disease and manifested by high fever and severe excruciating articular pains in the limbs and spinal column. There was an outbreak of this disease in Kolkata in 1963–1964 and another in Chennai in 1965, which gave rise to 300,000 cases in Chennai city alone.

The disease has reappeared after 41 years. During 2006, there was a large outbreak of chikungunya in India, with 1.39 million officially reported cases spread over 16 states; attack rates were estimated at 45% in some areas. The outbreak was first noticed in Andhra Pradesh and it subsequently spread to Tamil Nadu, Kerala and Karnataka, and then northward as far as Delhi. The other states involved were Maharashtra,

Madhya Pradesh, Gujarat, Rajasthan, Puducherry, Goa, Orissa, West Bengal, Uttar Pradesh, Andaman and Nicobar Islands. During 2007, until 12th October, a further 37,683 cases had been reported by the Government of India. In the year 2010, again thousands of people have been reported to be diagnosed with the virus.

Currently in 2016, big upsurge/epidemic due to Chikungunya is going on in Delhi and cases being reported from other States/UTs too. Till, 11th September, 2016 a total of 14,656 clinically suspected cases (including 1724 in Delhi) from 18 states and 2 UT's have been reported.

Swine Flu

It is a respiratory infection and transmission is through contact with respiratory secretions from an infected person who is coughing or sneezing. The symptoms are similar to seasonal flu but with a higher intensity. The patient may present with high grade fever (≥38°C), cough, sore throat, runny or stuffy nose, body aches, lack of appetite, lethargy, headache, chills and fatigue. In addition, nausea, vomiting and diarrhea have been reported (higher rate than for seasonal flu). It was first noted in Mexico in March-April, 2009, and then rapidly spread to the US, Canada and throughout the world. More than 214 countries reported laboratory confirmed cases, including more than 18,366 deaths. In India, since 2009 until September 26, 2010, out of the total 44,350 laboratories-confirmed cases of swine flu there have been more than 2,500 deaths reported (*Source:* www.mohfw-h1n1.nic.in).

A resurgence of swine flu in several states of India has caused a considerable concern in 2012. Fresh outbreaks of the dreaded virus surfaced in Maharashtra, Rajasthan and

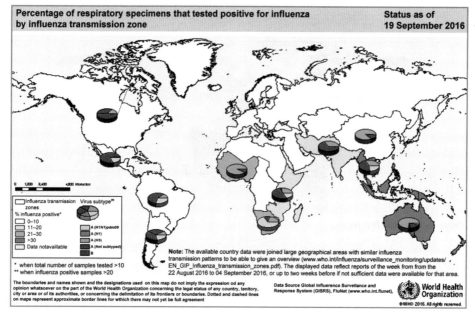

FIG. 1.1.8: Percentage of respiratory specimens that tested positive for influenza.
Source: http://www.who.int/influenza/surveillance_monitoring/updates/latest_update_GIP_surveillance/en/

some other states claiming at least 21 lives from January till March, 2012. At least 309 cases were reported in five states including Andhra Pradesh, Karnataka and Gujarat, according to the latest health ministry figures.

Of the total 21 deaths in 2012 so far, Maharashtra has reported nine deaths, followed by seven in Rajasthan and five in Andhra Pradesh. No death has taken place in Karnataka and Gujarat, which have also reported cases of H1N1 virus (Fig. 1.1.8).

In 2014, a total of 218 people died from the H1N1 flu, India recorded 837 laboratory confirmed cases in the year.

Every year, there was a rise in number of cases and deaths during winter as temperature affects virus. During 2014–15 winter, there was a spurt in cases at the end 2014. In 2015, the outbreak became widespread through India. On 12 February 2015, Rajasthan declared an epidemic.

The WHO now considers swine flu also as a seasonal epidemic and has recommended to the global and indigenous flu vaccine manufacturers to manufacture combined seasonal and swine flu vaccine. Accordingly, all WHO prequalified laboratories manufacturing flu vaccines have come out with their combined pH1N1 and the seasonal H3N2 A and B strains of the flu vaccines. For the prevention of swine flu, there are two types of vaccines which are available in the market: (1) live attenuated influenza vaccine—a nasal spray and (2) an inactivated vaccine—injection.

Statistics from sentinel centers may reveal the incidence of other infectious diseases, which are not reliable as they represent only the "tip of the iceberg". The need for establishing a Center for Disease Control, like the CDC, Atlanta and the effective monitoring of the IDSP, may help in knowing the exact disease burden in India.

FUTURE OF VACCINE PREVENTABLE DISEASES SURVEILLANCE IN INDIA

- The incidence of diphtheria, pertussis, tetanus (including neonatal tetanus), measles is still a matter of concern despite the implementation of NIP since 1985.
- A nationwide high coverage to near 100% in routine immunization is the need of the hour in India.
- The IDSP is a welcome project, but alternately the establishment of a CDC and subsequent guidelines from time-to-time for disease control are the ideal measures for activity control and elimination of infectious diseases in India.
- The updation of immunization practices by the Government and Professional agencies periodically with introduction of new vaccines like pneumococcal, HPV, etc. should also be expedited.

ACKNOWLEDGMENT

The authors are indebted to Dr Sameer Parekh and Dr Pramod Pujari, Serum Institute of India Pvt. Ltd., Pune, India, for help rendered in the preparation of this section.

BIBLIOGRAPHY

1. Annual TB Report (TB India 2017). Revised National TB Control Programme (RNTCP). Available on http://tbcindia.gov.in/WriteReadData/TB%20India%202017.pdf
2. Bavdekar S, Karande S. Elimination of measles from India: Challenges ahead and the way forward. J Postgrad Med. 2017;63(2):75-8.

3. Bitragunta S, Murhekar MV, Chakravarti A, et al. Safety and immunogenicity of single dose of tetanus–diphtheria (Td) vaccine among non/partially immune children against diphtheria and/or tetanus, Hyderabad, India, 2007. Vaccine. 2010;28(37):5934-8.

4. Borrow R, Lee JS, Vázquez JA, et al. Global Meningococcal Initiative. Meningococcal disease in the Asia-Pacific region: Findings and recommendations from the Global Meningococcal Initiative. Vaccine. 2016;34(48):5855-62.

5. Bruni L, Barrionuevo-Rosas L, Albero G, et al. ICO Information Centre on HPV and Cancer (HPV Information Centre). Human Papillomavirus and Related Diseases in India. Summary Report 19 April 2017. [Accessed on 19th July 2017]

6. Bull WHO. 1978;56(6):819-32.

7. Bull World Health Organ. 2008;86(5):408-16.

8. Dengue Cases and Deaths in the Country since 2010. National Vector Borne Disease Control Programme. Ministry of Health and family welfare, Govt of India 2016.

9. Drug resistant TB in India—Transmission, diagnosis, treatment. www.tbfacts.org

10. Garg R, Singh K. Epidemiological study of rubella outbreaks in Rajasthan, India. Int J Community Med Public Health. 2017;4(7):2417-22.

11. Government of India (2006). Health Information of India; 2005, Ministry of Health and Family Welfare, New Delhi, India.

12. Government of India (2007), NRHM Newsletter Vol. 3., No. 2, July-Aug. 2007, National Rural Health Mission, Department of Health and Family Welfare, New Delhi, India.

13. Government of India (2008), TB India 2008, RNTCP Status report, I am stopping TB, Ministry of Health and Family Welfare, New Delhi, India.

14. Government of India (2008). Annual report 2007-08, Ministry of Health and Family Welfare, New Delhi, India.

15. Gupta E, Dar L, Broor S. Seroprevalence of rubella in pregnant women in Delhi, India. Indian J Med Res. 2006;123:833-5.

16. Gupta SS, Bharati K, Sur D, et al. Why is the oral cholera vaccine not considered an option for prevention of cholera in India? Analysis of possible reasons. Indian J Med Res. 2016;143(5):545-51.

17. Hepatitis B Fact sheet 2016 India. http://www.searo.who.int/india/topics/hepatitis/factsheet_b__hepatitisday2016.pdf?ua=1.

18. Human Papillomavirus and Related Diseases Report. India HPV information Centre. Feb 2016.

19. India drives down malaria rates, sets sights on elimination April 2015. World Health Organization. http://www.who.int/features/2015/india-programme-end-malaria/en/

20. India HIV estimations 2015. Technical Report. NACO & National Institute of Medical Statistics, ICMR. Ministry of Health & Family Welfare, Government of India, New Delhi. Available from: http://www.naco.gov.in [Accessed on 19th July 2017.]

21. Influenza update – 272 19 September 2016. World Health Organization. http://www.who.int/influenza/surveillance_monitoring/updates/latest_update_GIP_surveillance/en

22. Jacobson J, Sivalenka S. Japanese encephalitis globally and in India. Indian J Public Health. 2004;48(2):49-56.

23. Khare S, Banerjee K, Padubidri V, et al. Lower immunity status of rubella virus infection in pregnant women. J Commun Dis. 1987;19(4):391-5.

24. Kristie EN Clarke. US Centers For Disease Control And Prevention. Review Of The Epidemiology Of Diphtheria – 2000-2016. Available on http://www.who.int/immunization/sage/meetings/2017/april/1_Final_report_Clarke_april3.pdf?ua=1

25. Malaria. Disease burden in SEA region. WHO regional office report for South-East Asia, 2010.

26. Meningococcal vaccines: ploysaccharide and polysaccharide conjugate vaccines, weekly epidemiological Ruord. 2002;77(40): 331-9.

27. National Guide for clinical management of Chikungunya 2016. Ministry of Health and family welfare, Gov of India.

28. O'Brien KL, Wolfson LJ, Watt JP, et al. Burden of disease caused by Streptococcus pneumoniae in children younger than 5 years: global estimates. Lancet. 2009;374(9693):893-902.

29. Parida M, Dash PK, Tripathi NK, et al. Japanese Encephalitis Outbreak, India, 2005. Emerg Infect Dis. 2006;12(9):1427-30.

30. Sachdeva A. Pneumococcal Conjugate Vaccine Introduction in India's Universal Immunization Program. Indian Pediatr. 2017;54(6):445-6.

31. Safety and immunogenicity of tetanus toxoid in pregnant women. J Obstet Gynecol India. 2009;59(3):224-7.

32. Sharma HJ, Padbidri VS, Kapre SV, et al. Seroprevalence of rubella and immunogenicity following rubella vaccination in adolescent girls in India. J Infect Dev Ctries. 2011;5(12):874-81.

33. Shrivastava S et al. Measles in India: Challenges & recent developments. Infection Ecology and Epidemiology 2015, 5:27784

34. UNICEF's global report. One is too many: Ending child deaths from pneumonia and diarrhoea. Key Findings 2016.

35. Vashishtha VM, Bansal CP, Gupta SG. Pertussis vaccines: position paper of Indian Academy of Pediatrics (IAP). Indian Pediatr. 2013;50(11):1001-9.

36. Vipin M, Vashishtha et al. IAP Position Paper on Burden of Mumps in India and Vaccination Strategies. INDIAN PEDIATRICS VOLUME 52__JUNE 15, 2015.

37. Vipin M, Vashishtha et al. Vaccination Policy for Japanese Encephalitis in India: Tread with Caution! INDIAN PEDIATRICS VOLUME 52__OCTOBER 15, 20.

38. WHO (2008), Global Tuberculosis Control, Surveillance, Planning, Financing, WHO Report, 2008.

39. WHO. Wkly Epi Rec. 2006; No. 43.

40. WHO Epi Rec. No. 13. 2010;85:117-28.

41. WHO vaccine-preventable diseases: monitoring system. 2017 global summary. Available on http://apps.who.int/immunization_monitoring/globalsummary/countries?countrycriteria%5Bcountry%5D%5B%5D=IND [Accessed on 18th Jul 2017]

42. World Health Report 1996, Report of the Director-General, WHO.

43. World Malaria Report, 2001.

1.2 INFECTIOUS DISEASES SURVEILLANCE IN INDIA

T Jacob John

INTRODUCTION

The dictionary meaning of the word surveillance is "close observation of a suspected spy or criminal". Close observation of diseases in the community—occurrence, numbers and outbreaks—provides clues about the culprits, the causative pathogens. There is thus a parallel between police intelligence in surveillance for protecting citizens against crimes and epidemiological intelligence through disease surveillance for protecting people from infectious diseases, particularly outbreaks. Epidemiological investigation after getting information about diseases through surveillance is, in fact, a form of detective work. Although diseases are kept under surveillance, their causative agents are the target of surveillance.

The World Health Organization (WHO) defines disease surveillance as: "the ongoing systematic collection, collation, analysis and interpretation of data [on diseases], followed by the dissemination of information to those who need to know in order that action may be taken". In other words, disease surveillance is required for public health action for disease prevention or control. If appropriate action does not follow, the mere collection of information is insufficient to qualify as surveillance as it may serve only the purpose of statistics for administrative understanding, but not that of public health. So, in short, surveillance is "systematic collection of information on diseases for public health action to prevent or control them." Therefore, it is often referred to as "public health surveillance". The data collected through public health surveillance will identify diseases to be prioritized for control if not already identified for control. The data will also form the basis of systematic monitoring of the degree of control being achieved year to year.

True public health surveillance has two characteristics—continuity in time and coverage in space. If there are gaps, infectious agents may cause sporadic cases or even outbreaks undetected by the designated staff. Collection of data on the incidence or prevalence of non-infectious diseases is through other methods—such as case registries, surveys of population samples, cumulating hospital statistics, etc. However, many use the term surveillance, inexactly, for other forms of data collection on health conditions, risk factors, etc. or for discontinuous collection of data on infectious diseases. In other words, the term surveillance is often loosely used for various methods of collection of data, diluting its definitional meaning. Therefore, it will be difficult now to restrict its usage strictly according to definition. In each context, it is necessary to redefine surveillance or at least understand that the term is not used according to the precise definition.

The several common usages of the term surveillance have been presented in this chapter. In most such situations the main deficiency is the lack of the requirement of public health action following data collection. As India does not have a public health infrastructure that can respond adequately to surveillance information, true surveillance as practiced in countries with public health infrastructure is not easy. Therefore, collection of data remains in many situations only for statistical purposes, as has been illustrated. Only very few diseases or their infectious agents are kept under surveillance for monitoring progress of control and for responding with public health action. They have been described in detail.

PASSIVE AND ACTIVE SURVEILLANCE

Disease surveillance is classified as passive and active. In countries with public health infrastructure, there would be a set-up for surveillance in all population units (such as districts). It is usually manned by a district officer of public health and supporting staff—epidemiologist, data management expert, laboratory personnel and field staff. The surveillance system has the afferent limb (incoming) for data receiving, a central processing unit (under the public health officer) and efferent limb (outgoing) for investigations and containment actions. This set-up is clearly separated from that which provides medical care to those who become ill. The latter is called *healthcare* and the former is called *public health*. Healthcare may be organized in the public sector or in the private sector. Many countries, such as India, have a mix of public and private sector hospitals and clinics and private practitioners, all providing healthcare services on demand. Public health infrastructure, on the other hand, is possible only in the public sector as it requires designated staff free of any responsibility for healthcare, and with legal authority for the officer and staff for enforcing disease surveillance and entering premises for disease investigations or control activities. Government funds staff salaries and all overhead expenses.

Sick people come to the attention of healthcare personnel who diagnose the diseases and treat. There would be a list of specific diseases that have been 'notified' (by the health ministry of the government) for surveillance. When a healthcare provider working in public or private sector sees a person with any notified disease, he/she is required (by law) to report that fact to the designated public health official. When all hospitals, clinics and medical practitioners report cases of notified diseases, the public health agency receives, passively so to say, continuous information on the occurrence and distribution of such cases. This method of disease reporting is called "passive surveillance". In India, every state has a list of notified diseases and the requirement for reporting on their statute books, but in the absence of public health infrastructure surveillance is not enforced. Instead, several ad hoc procedures are practiced for specific disease problems and they remain fragmented but not integrated. In many countries, passive disease surveillance is supplemented by passive reporting of laboratory evidence of specific pathogens infecting any patient.

Imagine that the local public health officer receives a few reports on cholera in a short interval of time, scattered within the community. The officer takes immediate action for searching for unreported cases in the community in order to understand the full extent of the outbreak. Public health staff may now visit all hospitals to check if unreported cases of cholera are admitted and, if any, with cholera-like illness had been seen in the outpatient service, etc. This is an active process, so to say. This is "active surveillance" in which the personnel of the public health agency go out in active search of cases. Information on all cases is required to define the geographic perimeter of the outbreak and to identify risk factors—perhaps the municipal water supply going to a few wards or another common source from which many families had drawn water was the channel of transmission of the pathogen. Further investigations on the quality of water would be done immediately and the contaminated supply would be stopped and disinfected in order to intercept the outbreak. Active surveillance is usually short-lived; once the problem is under control, the system reverts to passive surveillance, which is continuous without break. Often active surveillance is a part of the epidemiological investigations triggered by the detection of a signal from passive surveillance. When a disease is under elimination, active surveillance may become necessary to ensure no case was missed by failure of passive surveillance.

Another way to look at passive and active surveillance is to determine who generates data and how. The nodal agency for disease surveillance is local level (district or city) public health, with its personnel—the public health officer and trained staff. When they search for disease cases, the process is active—for active surveillance. When they receive reports from healthcare personnel, the nodal agency is the passive recipient—in passive surveillance. Passive surveillance *per se* costs little since healthcare workers earn their income from serving individual patients; their detecting and reporting notified diseases are incidental to their professional work and the only cost involved is postage for mailing the report or for electronic reporting. Those expenses are borne by the public health system—usually by supplying disease reporting forms and post-paid envelopes for enclosing the reports.

THE ROLE OF LABORATORY IN SURVEILLANCE

Although diseases are kept under surveillance, their causative agents are the target of surveillance. Every infectious disease has a specific etiology. In India, the demand for identifying etiology by laboratory testing in healthcare is low for two reasons: (1) patients do not usually demand information and (2) laboratory testing involves additional expenditure. Treating without arriving at etiological diagnosis is not evidence-based and may be unfair to the individual, who alone suffers the risk of diagnostic errors. It is also unfair to the community, since such errors and consequent wrong choice of drug(s) may contribute to the perpetuation of the pathogen in the community and to the development of drug-resistance in pathogens. Unnecessary antibiotics may also lead to drug resistance of normal flora that may be later transferred to pathogens through plasmids. Therefore, scientific medicine demands quality-assured diagnostic laboratory service. This cardinal requirement is not given due importance in many of India's public sector and private sector hospitals. Thus, laboratory surveillance is not practiced in India.

In public health, disease surveillance is to keep pathogens under scrutiny—hence pathogens must be identified in any clustering of cases. No error should be tolerated, as it may jeopardize the health of many in the community. For this reason, in most countries, the public health system maintains laboratories for use by its personnel. They are called public health laboratories, as distinct from clinical laboratories in hospitals. The district officer of public health must have access to public health laboratory. In India, there are public health laboratories, usually a few per state, mostly the continuation what the British had established during colonial era. Microbiology has advanced hugely since then but we have not kept our public health laboratories abreast with the times. In some countries, the central public health laboratory is very advanced and may act as referral laboratory for clinical laboratories in healthcare. In India, the National Centre for Disease Control (previously National Institute of Communicable Diseases) in Delhi is the foremost public health laboratory; it has all the advanced instrumentation and modern techniques for etiological determination of nearly all known pathogens.

THE PURPOSES OF DISEASE SURVEILLANCE

The main reason for establishing passive surveillance was (and continues to be) the early detection of any outbreak. While any one physician may see only one or two cases, collective reporting at the local or regional level will give the overall picture of an outbreak even in the beginning stage. The recognition of an outbreak is the trigger for rapid investigation and application of preventive or control measures. Surveillance of infectious diseases is thus the important link between healthcare and public health. Public health infrastructure was briefly described earlier. Public health is functionally defined as "societal actions for prevention of diseases and promotion of health". Its effective functioning requires a public health infrastructure. In other countries, it may be called ministry of public health (distinct from ministry of healthcare services), Public Health Department (under ministry of health), health protection agency or public health service. The main purpose of disease surveillance is the early detection of outbreaks in order to intercept them for the present and to pre-empt them from occurring in future. The disease surveillance system of the nation can be assessed by the successes of outbreak detection and control. The reason why many outbreaks in various parts of the country are not effectively and quickly controlled is due to the lack of public health infrastructure.

Another purpose of surveillance is to monitor, quantitatively and in real-time, the degree of decline in incidence of diseases that public health system had targeted for and funds expended for prevention and control. When a government targets a disease for control, it undertakes several activities including the application of preventive interventions and their auditing requires actual measurement of disease reduction over time. The best example in India is the surveillance for polio eradication, which has been described later. Disease control is the term applied for reducing the incidence to a predetermined acceptable level through interventions. Elimination is the extreme degree of control to zero incidence in a defined population, usually a whole country. Global level elimination is eradication. For elimination the disease, surveillance has to be efficient enough to detect even one case anywhere in the country. While control may apply to disease but not necessarily the causative pathogen (as in control of neonatal tetanus) eradication must result in removal of the pathogen from human transmission in order to maintain zero incidence (as in smallpox eradication).

A third purpose of surveillance is to discover new (emerging) diseases. In passive surveillance, physicians are instructed to report not only notified diseases, but also any undiagnosed illness that may be infectious in nature and is serious enough for public health attention. A cluster of undiagnosed illness has to be reported. In 1981, physicians in California reported a few instances of death of young men with an unusual disease. They had pneumonia due to an opportunistic pathogen, *Pneumocystis carinii* (now renamed *jerovicii*) that is always associated with severe immune suppression, usually due to malignancies and their treatments. The undiagnosed condition was provisionally named "acquired immune deficiency syndrome" (AIDS)—acquired as these adults had been without any major health problems all their lives. The United States Public Health Service swung into action and by epidemiological studies identified that the common factor among them was practicing male homosexual acts. Wearing of condoms markedly reduced risk of acquiring the putative agent—unknown then and suspected to be some chemical or an infectious agent. Eventually in 1984–85, the causative virus of AIDS was discovered. Imagine, if there was no disease surveillance, or if surveillance did not attract prompt epidemiological investigations, how much time the world would have lost in detecting this emerging

infectious disease and its causative agent(s). We now know that AIDS—causing severe unexplained loss of body weight and high case fatality, had been recognized by several physicians in African countries since the early 1970s and the disease even named locally (slim disease). If AIDS had first emerged in India, the situation would not have been much different. This incident illustrates the value of passive surveillance, the sincerity of physicians to diagnose pneumonia by its etiology, their alertness to conclude that the condition was new, their cooperation to report these cases and the efficiency of the public health system in investigating and unraveling the mystery. It also illustrates the importance of identifying risk factors for controlling further spread even before the agent is identified.

SURVEILLANCE FOR ELIMINATION OR ERADICATION

Elimination (in specified countries or cluster of neighboring countries) or eradication (globally) of diseases are examples of extreme disease control. Smallpox was eliminated in India by 1975 and so declared in 1977. Smallpox was eliminated by primary prevention with the smallpox vaccine—and by active surveillance (case-search) and vaccination of all persons who were in contact with every person with smallpox. Fortunately, smallpox did not spread widely, vaccination provided excellent protection and a fair proportion of persons in contact had been already vaccinated under the then existing practice. Immune individuals did not get infected with smallpox virus, or even if infected did not shed virus in sufficient quantity to transmit infection. Without "fever and rash" surveillance, as well as active surveillance following any rumor of fever with rash, smallpox would not have been documented to have been eradicated and eventually certified. After certification of eradication the surveillance was discontinued as the smallpox eradication staffs were reverted to their original work.

Another disease India has eliminated in the 20th century is Dracunculiasis (Guniea worm disease). In addition to human behavior modification resulting in break of the worm's transmission cycle, active surveillance was practiced in endemic geographic regions for two reasons. One was to ensure no contact between the ulcerated skin and surface water collections (to interrupt life cycle) and the second was to document its elimination.

The third major success is elimination of polio caused by natural (wild) polioviruses, as described below. Even though we speak of disease elimination or eradication, in reality what we eliminate is (in most cases) the transmission of the pathogen between humans. Therefore, in addition to clinical surveillance, every suspected case has to be investigated for the pathogen under elimination. These three examples illustrate how ad hoc and single-disease surveillance had to be established in the absence of public health surveillance. They also illustrate the non-sustainability of such efforts.

PASSIVE, ACTIVE, VIROLOGICAL AND ENVIRONMENTAL SURVEILLANCE FOR POLIO ELIMINATION

In 1988, India decided to eliminate polio to join the global polio eradication initiative of the WHO. Because India used live trivalent oral polio vaccine (tOPV) under the Universal Immunization Programme (UIP), the government expected that polio would be controlled first and then eliminated by supplementary pulse immunizations. There was need to document progress toward polio elimination; hence a polio-specific passive disease surveillance system was designed and launched under a special project—the National Polio Surveillance Project (NPSP). It established reporting of acute flaccid paralysis (AFP) by all healthcare institutions where children with AFP would be taken, both in the public and private sectors—for nationwide and continuous AFP surveillance. How does NPSP assess the completeness of AFP reporting? It was known in South America that the incidence of AFP in children under 15 years of age was about 1 per 100,000 per year. The same frequency was applied in India, but soon it was found that our AFP incidence was much greater than in South America. Therefore, surveillance quality is accepted as satisfactory if every district reported annually at least two AFP cases per 100,000 children under-15 per year. In 2011, over 35,000 healthcare institutions are on the AFP reporting network: they report only AFP, no other disease.

Since polio had to be diagnosed by etiology, a network of laboratories was established, by upgrading several existing virus laboratories. They are in Kasauli, Ahmedabad, Kolkata, Lucknow, Delhi, Mumbai, Bengaluru and Chennai. The Mumbai laboratory (Enterovirus Research Centre of Indian Council of Medical Research) has been recognized by the WHO as National Reference Laboratory and as Global Specialized Laboratory, one of seven such units in the world. Stool samples were collected from every child with AFP: the aim was to get two samples from every child to increase diagnostic sensitivity. They were tested in the polio laboratories to detect polioviruses and when detected, to differentiate between vaccine viruses from natural or wild polioviruses (WPVs). This is referred to as "virological surveillance" or "active laboratory surveillance". If laboratories passively reported the detection of agents under public health surveillance, it would supplement clinical surveillance and would qualify for "passive laboratory surveillance". Since NPSP staff collected stool samples from all children with AFP and got them tested, the process illustrates "active laboratory surveillance". In 2011, over 60,740 stool samples were collected and tested but only 1 WPV (type 1) was detected.

Wild polioviruses can circulate silently for short periods of time. For decades, sewage samples had been collected and tested for WPVs, by the Enterovirus Research Centre in Mumbai and WPVs were regularly detected. Since the year 2000, Mumbai sewage showed up imported WPVs with origins in Uttar Pradesh or Bihar. Sewage is equivalent to stools from hundreds of thousands of individuals. Yet, the testing sample comes from the environment. Therefore, in the context of polio, regular (usually weekly) sewage sample testing is referred to as "environmental poliovirus surveillance". Since 2011, environmental surveillance is conducted in Mumbai, Delhi, Patna and Kolkata. In 2012, so far, all samples have proved negative, adding supportive evidence that India has eliminated WPV transmission.

SURVEILLANCE IN AIDS CONTROL

Acquired immune deficiency syndrome control is another success story in India. While AIDS received wide global media publicity, during the early 1980s, the government lacked a mechanism to monitor its arrival in India. Had we practiced public health surveillance, we could have expected some physicians reporting suspected cases of AIDS or at least diseases or death due to undiagnosed causes. Recognizing this deficiency, the virology department of the Christian Medical College in Vellore conducted systematic search for infection, resulting in detection of infected women in sex work in Chennai, Madurai and Vellore in February 1986. The Indian Council of Medical Research established an AIDS Task Force in mid-1986 and adopted the Vellore model of testing within hospital settings both a high-risk group (male patients in STD clinics) and a low-risk group (antenatal women) for human immunodeficiency virus (HIV) infection as the parameter for monitoring time trends of epidemiology. Thus, annual repetitive sentinel hospital-based anonymous unlinked sample surveys were established—and it got a popular name as "sentinel surveillance". In 1986 itself, 62 "sentinel surveillance" sites were operative. Since then a number of sites have increased to over 1,000 in 2010, covering all cities and most districts in every State and Union Territory.

Today "sentinel surveillance" for HIV provides annually large samples of denominator-population and their HIV prevalence. This is the method of monitoring infection trends to date, a unique method designed in India. There is no other disease for which denominator-based infection prevalence data are available in India. Other countries did not resort to serological surveys to monitor time trends, as they had passive surveillance of cases of AIDS. However, the term sentinel surveillance is a misnomer as it is not based on principles of public health surveillance. It lacks continuity and has incomplete coverage. However, the objective is to monitor time trend, which it serves well.

THE STATE OF PUBLIC HEALTH SURVEILLANCE IN INDIA

During British Raj, public health surveillance was practiced in all provinces, under the Epidemics Act of 1890 and the Madras Public Health Act of 1939. Each province had established its own list of diseases for reporting. After independence the posts of Director General of Indian Medical Service, Public Health Commissioner of India and India Health Epidemiologist were abolished; thus public health surveillance was orphaned. The newly created post of Director General of Health Services was not assigned the responsibility of public health surveillance. As all emphasis was given to healthcare, the need for surveillance was not appreciated. However, when a disease was brought under control mode, special surveillance for that disease was established. Smallpox, Guinea Worm and polio surveillance activities were described above.

Malaria Surveillance

The National Malaria Control Programme was established in 1953. Two modes of surveillance were established: (1) active surveillance where malaria was hyperendemic and (2) passive surveillance everywhere else. Since passive surveillance was not enforced for any disease, malaria surveillance also fell by the wayside. For active surveillance, a worker visits every household once in 2 weeks, and blood smear is collected from anyone who had fever during the interval—smears are examined for malarial parasites. Using the data, the following indices are derived: slide positivity rate; slide falciparum rate; annual parasite incidence; annual blood examination rate; annual falciparum incidence.

Leprosy Surveillance

The National Leprosy Control Programme was established in 1955. Leprosy-specific diagnosis and treatment centers were established at key locations. The leprosy workers conducted periodic population surveys (active surveillance) for clinical evidence of leprosy—thus annual prevalence rate was calculated. After the goal of leprosy elimination was declared occasional mass surveys were conducted—and continues even now. The aim is to keep the new case detection at less than 1 per 10,000 population, which is used to define "elimination". However, epidemiologically this is not true elimination—which is zero incidence in the defined geographic community.

Other Diseases under Control Mode

The Union Ministry of Health has targeted a few other diseases for control, namely tuberculosis (TB), lymphatic filariasis, kala azar, dengue, chikungunya fever and Japanese encephalitis (the last five under National Vector-borne Diseases Control). Neither passive nor active surveillance is practiced for them and the status of control remains not properly monitored. In May 2012, the ministry of health has notified pulmonary TB as reportable. However, the modalities of reporting, data receiving agency, follow-up and actions following case reporting have not yet been clearly described. The present requirement is for reporting sputum smear-positive pulmonary TB; other forms including pediatric TB are not yet demanded for reporting.

Expanded Program on Immunization

The National Childhood and Antenatal Immunization Programme, launched in India in 1978–79, has been renamed the Universal Immunization Programme (UIP). Although the objective is to prevent vaccine-preventable diseases in individuals and control their incidence in the community, systematic surveillance of targeted diseases was not established. The numbers of cases reported through the hierarchy of government healthcare units are received and compiled by the union ministry of health; however, neither the sensitivity (what proportion of total cases was captured) nor specificity of case diagnosis (what proportion of cases had accurate diagnosis) is checked for validation. Countries practicing public health surveillance did not have to establish a polio-specific surveillance method, but India had to establish NPSP. Now measles is getting targeted for mortality elimination, followed by disease elimination itself. The responsibility for measles surveillance, including laboratory verification of outbreaks, has been entrusted with the NPSP. The network of polio laboratories have been equipped for measles diagnosis and supplied with the necessary reagents. The NPSP measles outbreak monitoring and laboratory confirmation project was begun in 2006 in Andhra Pradesh, Tamil Nadu and Karnataka; in 2007 Kerala, West Bengal and Gujarat were added; during 2009–2011 Rajasthan, Madhya Pradesh, Assam, Bihar and Chhattisgarh were added. When investigated, many outbreaks clinically named measles turned out to be rubella. Consequently, the UIP is getting ready to include rubella vaccination in India.

INTEGRATED DISEASE SURVEILLANCE PROJECT

The concept of integrated disease surveillance is to link together all existing ad hoc or single disease surveillance activities under one umbrella. Two models of integrated surveillance have been developed in India. In 1994, there was an outbreak of suspected pneumonic plague in Surat city. An expert committee examined the reasons why such an outbreak occurred and how the nation should prepare itself for any future outbreaks of emerging or re-emerging infectious diseases. It recommended the replication of a model established in one district in Tamil Nadu and all districts in Kerala for "district level disease surveillance" (DLDS) in which private sector and public sector physicians or pediatricians reported 15 notified diseases using a preformatted and postpaid post-card. Its advantages included low cost, immediate local action to prevent or control the spread of any outbreak. Feedback to reporting physicians was through a monthly bulletin which provided information on frequency of diseases, outbreaks and actions taken against them. This decentralized district-based system (with the afferent and efferent limbs and central processing unit within the district) was not aligned with the national policy that disease control and outbreak investigations belonged to the Union Government, while only healthcare and training or education of healthcare personnel belonged to State Governments. This tension led to the establishment of centrally sponsored and funded data collection mode named Integrated Disease Surveillance Project (IDSP).

Integrated Disease Surveillance Project was launched in November 2004 to detect disease outbreaks quickly. The Central Surveillance Unit is at National Center for Disease Control (NCDC), Delhi. Until 2012, it was in project mode, but currently it is nested within the National Rural Health Mission. Weekly reports are generated from primary care units (subcenters, primary health centers, community health centers) which were earlier reporting disease statistics using a format different from that supplied by IDSP. Hospitals in public and private sectors are also in the network, but their involvement is incomplete. Instead of case-reporting as in public health surveillance, disease reporting in IDSP is cumbersome—lengthy forms are to be filled in for "syndromic" diagnosis, probable cases and laboratory data. Electronic reporting is encouraged. Here "integration" is not linking all ongoing surveillance activities, but a new concept—combining reporting of non-communicable diseases along with infectious diseases. Thus, IDSP in India is yet another vertical project as the afferent and efferent limbs touch one central agency—the NCDC. It does not encompass the definitional requirements of public health surveillance. Private sector could not be linked as in the case of DLDS.

The weakness of IDSP is that it has not filled the gaps in disease surveillance for those diseases that are already targeted for control, namely vaccine-preventable disease, TB, malaria and several others discussed above. As the need arose for surveillance of outbreaks of acute neurological diseases (meningococcal meningitis, Japanese encephalitis and those of unknown etiology) and of pneumonias, rotavirus gastroenteritis, etc. more surveillance projects had to be launched as described below.

SENTINEL-BASED SURVEILLANCE OF SELECTED DISEASES

Influenza Sentinel Surveillance

The National Institute of Virology has been investigating influenza—epidemiology and viral strain identification—for a few decades. However, nationally influenza had not received much attention. In 2004, a multicenter influenza monitoring laboratory network was established: the sites are at Pune, Delhi, Kolkata and Chennai. After the 2009, pandemic influenza reached India; the network was expanded to more centers including Vellore, Mumbai and Lucknow. The information collected in these laboratories is submitted to the WHO.

Rotavirus Sentinel Surveillance

A network of four laboratories have been assigned the task of identifying and typing rotavirus isolates from ten sentinel hospitals in six States, namely Tamil Nadu, Maharashtra, Madhya Pradesh, West Bengal, Assam and Delhi. Under-5 children with acute gastroenteritis requiring rehydration will be monitored and their stool samples submitted to the designated laboratories (Vellore, Pune, Mumbai, Kolkata).

Invasive Pneumococcal, *Haemophilus influenzae* and Meningococcal Disease Surveillance

The Indian Council of Medical Research in collaboration with NCDC is in the process of developing 30 sentinel sites to develop data base to monitor the burden of invasive bacterial diseases due to pneumococci, meningococci and *Haemophilus influenzae* type b. Since vaccines are available against these diseases baseline data are important to help policy decisions on the use of these vaccines. Once vaccines are introduced, the assessment of vaccine effectiveness requires surveillance data. When pneumococcal vaccine is introduced, serotype prevalence needs to be monitored in case new serotypes replace vaccine serotypes.

Encephalitis Sentinel Surveillance

The Indian Council of Medical Research (ICMR), with the help of NPSP is in the process of developing sentinel surveillance in several districts where Japanese Encephalitis is prevalent. These sites will help in monitoring vaccine effectiveness.

CONCLUSION

If a government wants to control infectious diseases, the first step is to establish surveillance. All diseases targeted for control must be covered in surveillance. Since disease-control activities require a functional Public Health Department, the process of disease surveillance is best conducted by the local (district and city) public health officer and staff. Routine passive surveillance is, therefore, called "public health surveillance". In India, there is no unified public health surveillance, but instead there are several vertical, but nationwide disease monitoring programs including case-based surveillance for AFP, outbreak monitoring of measles and rubella, IDSP and several sentinel surveillance projects. Ideally integrated surveillance should replace all fragmentary disease monitoring projects, but unfortunately it is not possible under the present circumstances in which healthcare is under State Governments but disease prevention and outbreak control are under the Union Government. A practical redesign of Union–State relationship will help the creation of a truly integrated public health surveillance for all diseases of public health importance.

BIBLIOGRAPHY

1. Government of India, Ministry of Health and Family Welfare. Integrtaed Disease Surveillance. [online] Avaialble from http://www.idsp.nic.in/ and http://www.mohfw.nic.in/ NRHM/PIP_09_10/Delhi/IDSP_text.pdf.

1.3 ROLE OF GAVI IN THE CONTROL OF VACCINE-PREVENTABLE DISEASES IN INDIA

Naveen Thacker, Ashish Pathak

INTRODUCTION

Global Alliance for Vaccines and Immunization (GAVI, the Vaccine Alliance) is an international organization, which was created as a public–private partnership and is committed towards increasing access to immunization in poor countries. GAVI brings together United Nations Children's Fund (UNICEF), the World Bank, the vaccine manufactuers from resource-rich and resource-poor countries, donors from the resource-rich countries, and representatives from governments of the low-income countries across the world and Civil Society Organizations (CSOs).[1]

Since its inception in 2000, GAVI's support has contributed to the immunization of an additional 500 million children in low-income countries and has averted 7 million deaths due to vaccine-preventable diseases. GAVI has supported more than 200 vaccine introductions and campaigns in low-income countries during the 2011–2015 period between 2016 and 2020, GAVI will help countries to immunize another 300 million children against potentially fatal diseases, saving between 5 and 6 million lives in the long term.[2]

The mission of GAVI is "saving children's lives and protecting people's health by increasing equitable use of vaccines in lower-income countries".[3]

HOW DOES GAVI WORK?

GAVI invites applications for support from governments of those countries whose gross national income per capita is below GAVI's eligibility threshold, this threshold was US dollar 1580 in the year 2015. Based on the eligibility threshold, 73 countries are eligible for GAVI support. GAVI purchases vaccines through UNICEF, and provides them to governments whose applications are approved.[1]

GAVI'S STRATEGY

GAVI's strategy is a roadmap designed to help it respond to changes in the vaccine landscape and set five-year milestones en route to fulfilling its mission.[4] The 2016–2020 strategy is the latest in four distinct phases since GAVI's inception:

Phase IV (2016–2020)
Phase III (2011–2015)
Phase II (2007–2010)
Phase I (2000–2006)
Phase IV (2016–2020)

This section details the strategic objectives and operating principles for the current phase (2016–2020) as well as providing an overview of previous strategies.

The 2016–2020 strategy has four goals, each supporting GAVI's overall mission:[5]

1. **The vaccine goal**: Accelerate equitable uptake and coverage of vaccines.
2. **The systems goal**: Increase effectiveness and efficiency of immunization delivery as an integrated part of strengthened health systems.
3. **The sustainability goal**: Improve sustainability of national immunization programmes.
4. **The market-shaping goal**: Shape markets for vaccines and other immunization products.

PRINCIPLES

The GAVI's strategic framework includes eight principles, intended to define the Vaccine Alliance's characteristics, its business model and its aspirations, these are: country-led, community-owned, globally engaged, catalytic and sustainable, integrated, innovative, collaborative and accountable.[4]

GAVI'S HEALTH SYSTEM STRENGTHENING GRANTS

GAVI is dependent on the effectiveness of the countries health system to deliver life-saving vaccines, thus GAVI supports countries to strengthen country health system by proving health system strengthening (HSS) grants.[1] The strategic objectives under the health systems goal are to:

1. Contribute to resolving the major constraints to delivering immunization.
2. Increase equity in access to services
3. Strengthen civil society engagement in the health sector.

GAVI'S ESTIMATED IMPACT IN 2016–2020 PERIOD

The estimated impact of GAVI in its next phase can be measured by number of children that would be saved from vaccine-preventable diseases per country and thus, globally. In the 2016–2020 period, India will contribute to largest number of deaths averted globally (Fig. 1.3 1).

GAVI'S SUPPORT TO INDIA

India has always been special for GAVI. India is the largest and most populous GAVI-eligible country with a birth-

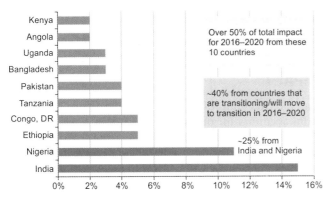

FIG. 1.3.1: Countries that will contribute to highest percentage of deaths averted through vaccine-preventable diseases through GAVI support in the period 2016–2020[6].

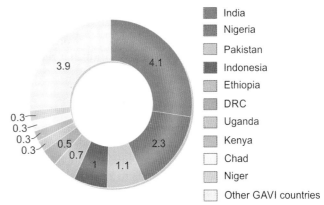

FIG. 1.3.2: Number of under-immunized children 2014 (in millions).

cohort of almost 27 million. Also, India still accounts for one-fifth of child deaths worldwide and more than a quarter of all under-immunized children in GAVI-eligible countries (please look at Figure 1.3.2 for details). India remains eligible for GAVI support based on its GNI level. But because of the large birth cohort of India, GAVI has limited its support to catalytic funding to India. Until 2011, there was a limit placed on GAVI support to India, which was removed with the condition that the GAVI Board continues to review any new support case-by-case.[7]

IPV Introduction Support

The National Technical Advisory Group on Immunization (NTAGI), the apex body for decision making on immunization related issues in India, recommended a comprehensive IPV introduction plan to the Government of India (GoI).[8] India applied for funding to GAVI in September 2014, for the period of September 2015 to 2018 at an estimated cost of US dollar 160 million. In November 2015, India launched IPV in six states and has expanded it to all states and Union Territories.[6]

HEALTH SYSTEM STRENGTHENING SUPPORT TO INDIA

As part of HSS initiative, GAVI has disbursed US dollar 30.6 million for the IPV introduction and US dollar 107 million in the year 2014–2015 to India.[1] The grant has been focused by GoI for use in 12 states and 127 underperforming districts and is synergistic to Mission Indradhanush.[10] Specifically, the grant has been used to strengthen the cold chain management. To enhance human resource capacity, national cold chain vaccine management resource center has been established in New Delhi. National cold chain training center has been strengthened in Pune. In 20 districts across UP, MP and Rajasthan, electronic vaccine intelligence network (eVIN) has been implemented to enable real time information on cold chain temperatures, vaccine stocks and flows. To increase demand for routine vaccination, National

Behavioral Change and Communication (BCC) strategy has been developed and immunization messages have been developed and broadcast through mass media. The national monitoring and evaluation plan for immunization has been drafted and monitoring and evaluation of routine immunization is currently functional in 24 of the 36 states and UTs across India. Two rounds of survey for National Immunization Coverage Evaluation have been done in 2015. This evaluation will further identify low-performing districts for routine immunization coverage. Guidelines for tagging high-risk low-coverage areas have been developed along with WHO India National Polio Surveillance Program (NPSP).[1]

Targeted Country Assistance for India for 2017

GAVI works through its incountry partners in India. They are WHO, UNICEF and the CDC. In 2017, UNICEF through GAVI support will support a) the implementation and national monitoring of Mission Indradhanush, with a focus on 12 low-performing states. The expected outcome is that improvements in immunization coverage are inclusive of the children in the most marginalized, remote and poorest communities and overall inequities within the immunization program are reduced. UNICEF will also support planning, preparedness assessment and roll out of pneumococcal and rotavirus vaccine in identified states, will support the implementation of a high-quality MR state campaigns, with a focus on social mobilization, cold-chain performance and real time monitoring and will support national electronic vial monitoring assessments. The WHO through GAVI support will address immunization equity in states with low-immunization coverage with focus on North-Eastern states. CDC, Atlanta through GAVI support will provide technical assistance to the National Institute of Cholera and Enteric Diseases (NICED), the state of West Bengal, and the Central Ministry of Health to understand the disease and economic burden of cholera in the State of West Bengal.

Impact of GAVI Initiatives in India

GAVI has been providing assistance to the Government of India since 2002. Over the past decade, India has received support in three areas:

a. Hepatitis B Monovalent Vaccine

GAVI, through its New Vaccine Support (NVS) grant, helped India to introduce the hepatitis B monovalent vaccine. Support began in 2002 with a vaccine introduction grant for $100,000. For 6 years, from 2003 to 2009 and excluding 2004, a total of $26,486,033 was disbursed for Hep B mono vaccine; funding was used to purchase the vaccine and injection supplies with the Government of India funding other immunization support.[11]

In 2002, hepatitis B was introduced in 33 districts and 10 cities in India with GAVI Phase I support. In 2007–2008, coverage was expanded to 10 states with GAVI Phase II support. In 2010, the Government of India took over funding for Hep B immunization in the 10 states, and in 2011 introduced the vaccine nationwide with its own funding.[11]

Final impact: Universal introduction of hepatitis B vaccine with Government of India supporting 100% immunization.

b. Injection Safety Support

Injection Safety Support (INS) grant helped India to introduce autodisable syringes in its immunization program. Two grants were given in 2005 and 2007 and a total of US$ 18,427,489 was disbursed.

Final impact: Autodisable syringes have become the standard for all routine Expanded Programme on Immunization (EPI), and a national policy for safe disposal of injection waste has been developed. The Government of India is now funding the purchase of auto-disable syringes 100%.[11]

c. Pentavalent (DTP-HepB-Hib) Vaccine Support

New vaccine support (NVS) to introduce pentavalent DTP-HepB-Hib (Penta) vaccine.

India's NTAGI recommended the introduction of Penta in 2008. GAVI support began in 2008 with a vaccine introduction grant for US$ 1,100,000, although 70% of this was returned when India decided on a phased introduction in 2011 instead of a nationwide introduction as was originally planned. US$ 443,500 of the grant was used to support the phased introduction. In December 2011, India introduced Penta in two states (Keral and Tamil Nadu) with GAVI support. Six additional states introduced in 2012.[12]

Final impact: Currently, all states have introduced Penta in routine immunization in India. India received a total of US $266,711,053 as of 23rd August, 2017, to support the introduction of Penta.[12]

IMMUNIZATION IN INDIA AND GAVI'S CRITICAL ROLE IN ACCELERATING GREATER ACHIEVEMENTS OF HEALTH IMPACT

With a birth cohort of 27 million children born each year, India accounts for one third of children born in GAVI-eligible countries. While India has made substantial progress in reducing the number of under-five deaths, it is still the highest in the world (1.3 million in 2013, 20% of the global total). The gravity of the problem varies significantly among states and areas of residence. Vaccine-preventable diseases are a key cause of mortality and morbidity. India has ~20% of pneumococcal, rotavirus and measles deaths worldwide, 25% of cervical cancer deaths, and 38% of the global congenital rubella syndrome (CRS) burden in terms of cases. Under India's Universal Immunisation Programme, vaccination is currently provided to prevent DTP (diphtheria, pertussis, tetanus), polio, measles, severe forms of childhood tuberculosis, hepatitis B (Hep B), *Haemophilus influenzae* type B (Hib) infections, and Japanese Encephalitis (in selected districts). GAVI provided catalytic support to accelerate the introduction of Hep B, pentavalent and inactivated polio (IPV) vaccines, as well as safe injection devices (INS) and on health systems strengthening. Under an exemption to the Alliance's co-financing policy, GAVI provides time-bound support and the government pays for introduction costs and related immunization commodities, taking on full self-financing for vaccines or devices after GAVI support ends (Fig. 1.3.3).[6]

The recent years have marked a turning point for the UIP. India's polio-free certification in 2014 and its elimination of maternal and neonatal tetanus in 2015 are landmark achievements. The political environment for immunization is also particularly strong now. In December 2014, the government launched the world's largest immunization drive, "Mission Indradhanush", aimed at increasing immunization coverage to more than 90% by 2020 by targeting districts that have the most unvaccinated or partially vaccinated children. Initial results are encouraging: 2 million children were fully immunized in the first four rounds of the mission. Mission Indradhanush builds on new approaches that are implemented through GAVI's catalytic HSS grant. The US$ 107 million grant focuses on 12 underperforming states. An innovative pilot electronic information system to manage vaccine logistics is being scaled up in three states. Regular supportive supervision of cold chain points has been initiated at primary care level, and state-level communication plans have been created. The experience and expertise gained in the vast polio infrastructure is being applied to routine immunization, contributing to India's goal of universal coverage.[6]

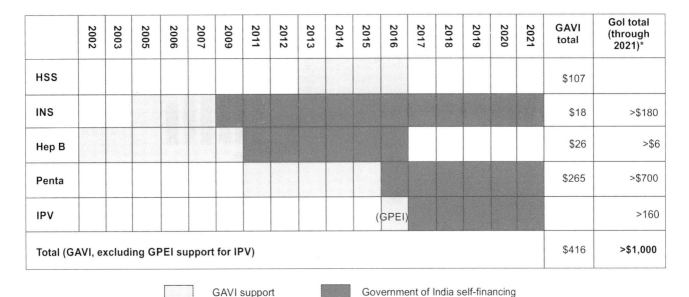

	2002	2003	2005	2006	2007	2009	2011	2012	2013	2014	2015	2016	2017	2018	2019	2020	2021	GAVI total	GoI total (through 2021)*
HSS																		$107	
INS																		$18	>$180
Hep B																		$26	>$6
Penta																		$265	>$700
IPV											(GPEI)								>160
Total (GAVI, excluding GPEI support for IPV)																		$416	>$1,000

☐ GAVI support ■ Government of India self-financing

*Projected based on current price assumptions; subject to change with future procurement conditions

FIG. 1.3.3: GAVI support to India to date, with programs sustained/to be sustained by the Government of India (US$ millions).[6]

A strengthened partnership in the coming years offers considerable benefits for both India and GAVI. GAVI's vision is that between 2016 and 2021, GAVI's targeted support will accelerate India's efforts to introduce new vaccines and achieve universal immunization coverage. Millions more children will be immunized by several vaccines in GAVI's portfolio, increasing the number of future deaths averted with GAVI support by at least half a million. India will reach a position where it can sustain a self-financed, multi-faceted and equitable immunization program. GAVI and India will both benefit by capitalizing on procurement savings and enhancing vaccine supply security, while forging a collaborative, learning-based relationship. To realize this vision, GAVI proposed a comprehensive, multi-pronged strategic alliance partnership with India. The strategy builds on the principles endorsed by the programme and policy committee (PPC), it takes India's priorities and GAVI's added value into consideration, and envisages timebound, catalytic support:

1. Increase immunization coverage and equity in India through targeted support to strengthen the routine immunization system.
2. Maximize health impact by accelerating adoption of new vaccines in India.
3. Maximize procurement savings and vaccine supply security by sharing information, coordinating tactics and building a long-term strategy that strengthens local, public and private sector manufacturers.
4. Ensure that vaccine programs in India will be sustainable beyond 2021 by supporting the government to plan for the transition and advocating for increased domestic spending on immunization.

The Coverage and Equity Opportunity

Though the UIP has been operating for more than 30 years, only 65% of children receive all vaccines during their first year. While WHO/UNICEF coverage estimates for India were revised upward this year (from 72% to 83% DTP3 coverage), India is still the country with the largest number of un- or under-vaccinated children in the world, at 4.1 million in 2014 (Fig. 1.3.1). Vaccination coverage varies significantly among geographies (Fig. 1.3.4). Some of India's states are among the largest and poorest in GAVI's portfolio. Uttar Pradesh, for example, is larger than every GAVI-eligible country except Nigeria, has gross national income per capita of only US $422, and has a DTP3 coverage of only ~60%. Coverage also varies depending on gender, area of residence, wealth and caste. Operational challenges in demand generation, cold chain and logistics management, and other areas hinder progress.

Alliance partners have work with the Government of India to develop a detailed proposal with targets and indicators and ensure that future GAVI support further addresses coverage inequity issues in the country. Cold chain and logistics management, demand generation and vaccine-preventable diseases (VPD) surveillance are some potential new areas within which GAVI is looking forward to invest.[6]

THE NEW VACCINES OPPORTUNITY

With the positive political environment, India has an ambition to eliminate measles, introduce rubella (as part of MR vaccine), rotavirus, and pneumococcal vaccines

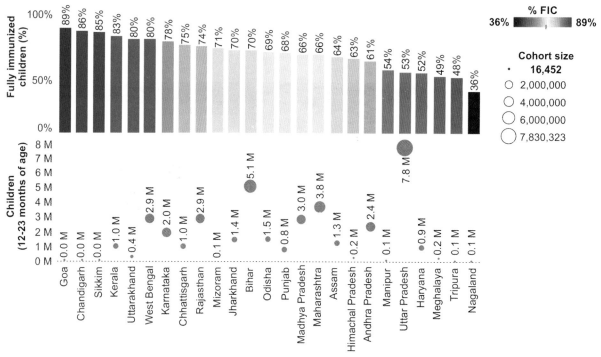

FIG. 1.3.4: Percent of fully immunized children (FIC) in large Indian states.[6]

in 2016–2017, and potentially HPV vaccine at a later time during the transition period. Rollouts of these vaccines are at different stages of planning given the status of recommendations from the National Technical Advisory Group on Immunisation (NTAGI) and political approvals for each vaccine. GAVI support will play an important role in accelerating roll-out of new vaccines, which would be critical to argue for allocation of more domestic resources in the next national Five-Year Plan and cMYP (2018–2022).

THE MARKET-SHAPING OPPORTUNITY

The strategic partnership between GAVI and the Government of India offers opportunities to optimize both short- and long-term vaccine supply security, to capture procurement cost-savings based on the increased demand, and to share information and best practices on managing vaccine markets effectively. Each vaccine market will require a specific approach. The markets with the greatest opportunities today for procurement savings are pentavalent and pneumococcal. While other markets, such as IPV, MR and rotavirus, have limited scope for procurement cost-savings, these markets will require close coordination with regard to supply. Building a strong local base of private and public vaccines and cold chain equipment that complements the global availability will be beneficial across the whole portfolio. Benefits of a well-executed partnership will extend beyond GAVI and India to include low income countries that are dependent on a

reliable supply of low-cost and high-quality vaccines and cold-chain equipment.[3]

ENSURING SUSTAINABLE PROGRAMMING

GAVI engagement in the form of senior leadership advocacy and support via communication and advocacy agencies have resulted in evidence-based policy discussions at both the national and state levels and have achieved a higher prioritization for health issues. Alliance advocacy for political commitment to increase health spending, including immunization, is paramount. A Political Forum on Child Health and Survival which includes selected Members of Parliament was recently formed in 2012. This new structure serves as a forum for political and public discourse around the need for high-quality, cost-effective public health interventions, including vaccines.

India has a successful track record in continuing the Hep B and INS programs with its domestic resources after GAVI support ended. The government has also indicated in writing to the GAVI Secretariat its commitment to sustain and further scale up rotavirus, pneumococcal and HPV programs and self-finance MR routine immunization after future catalytic support ends. However, given the magnitude of increase in resources expected with the launch of new vaccines (two to ten-fold increase by 2021 from the current ~US$ 40 million per year on vaccine costs only 25), GAVI engagement with India to ensure successful transitioning is critical.[6]

THE IMPORTANCE OF INDIA AS A MANUFACTURING BASE FOR VACCINE AND COLD CHAIN EQUIPMENT

Vaccine manufacturers in India are a key source of supply for GAVI. In 2014, they provided nearly 60% of vaccine volume, representing just over 30% of the total value of procurement. A single Indian manufacturer supplied 100% of measles-rubella (MR) and meningococcal A (MenA) conjugate vaccines and 80% of measles vaccine, while four manufacturers supplied over 80% of pentavalent vaccine.[6] Vaccine demand in India could reach nearly 30% of total demand in the 73 GAVI countries. The resulting significant increase in market volumes presents both risk and opportunity. It could disrupt supply of important vaccines if coordination is insufficient. If the increase is managed well, however, it will allow optimization of production costs and procurement savings.[6]

REFERENCES

1. Thacker N, Thacker D, Pathak A. Role of Global Alliance for Vaccines and Immunization (GAVI) in Accelerating Inactivated Polio Vaccine Introduction. Indian Pediatr. 2016;53(Suppl 1):S57-S60. PubMed PMID: 27771641.
2. GAVI 2016. Every Child Counts: The Vaccine Alliance Progress Report 2014. Available from http://www.gavi.org/progress-report/. Accessed September 11, 2017 http://www.gavi.org/results/gavi-progress-reports/
3. GAVI's strategy, Mission 2016–2020 http://www.gavi.org/about/strategy/ Accessed September 11, 2017.
4. GAVI, the Vaccine Alliance 2016-2020 Strategy http://www.gavi.org/library/publications/gavi/gavi-the-vaccine-alliance-2016-2020-strategy/ Accessed September 11, 2017.
5. GAVI's strategy, phase IV (2016-20) - GAVI, the Vaccine Alliance http://www.gavi.org/about/strategy/phase-iv-2016-20/ Accessed September 11, 2017.
6. Szeto C, Malhame M, Gehl D, et al. Report to the Board 2-3 December 2015 Alliance Partnership Strategy with India, 2016-2021.
7. GAVI 2015. Alliance Partnership Strategy with India, 2016-2021 Report to the Board 3rd December 2015. Available from http://www.gavi.org/Library/News/Press-releases/2016/Historic-partnership-between-GAVI-and-India-to-save-millions-of-lives/. Accessed September 11, 2017.
8. India's National Technical Advisory Group on Immunisation T. Jacob John. National Technical Advisory Group on Immunisation, New Delhi, India www.nitag-resource.org/.../01/6706ca25a105266e834edb78f7f81cec124420ec.pdf
9. Joint Appraisal Report India, 2015, Available from http://www.gavi.org/country/india/documents/#approvedproposal. Accessed September 11, 2017.
10. Mission Indradhanush http://www.missionindradhanush.in/about.html Accessed September 11, 2017.
11. Parthasarathy A. Textbook of Pediatric Infectious Diseases. 2013; New Delhi: Jaypee Brothers Medical Publishers.
12. Pentavalent vaccine support http://www.gavi.org/support/nvs/pentavalent/ Accessed September 11, 2017.

1.4 RATIONAL DRUG THERAPY IN PEDIATRIC INFECTIOUS DISEASES

YK Amdekar

INTRODUCTION

Rational drug therapy means "prescribing right drug for right indication, in adequate dose for optimum duration that delivers safe and appropriate benefit to the clinical needs of the patient at lowest cost". The concept of rational drug therapy is age-old, as evident by the statement made by the Alexandrian physician Herophilus, 300 BC that states "Medicines are nothing in themselves but are the very hands of God if employed with reason and prudence". The physician should always bear in mind that drugs do not cure. They may be made valuable adjuncts in our endeavor to restore normal function in an abnormal functioning organ. Improving precision and economy in prescribing drugs is a goal whose importance has much more increased with proliferation of new and potent agents and with growing economic pressures to contain health-care cost.

GENERAL PRINCIPLES OF RATIONAL DRUG SELECTION

Right Indication

Selected drug must be relevant to treatment of concerned disease. Such a drug could be either specific curative drug such as antibiotic or merely a symptomatic reliever. Specific drug therapy is possible only when there exists at least a provisional diagnosis as in case of use of antibiotic for infection. Symptomatic reliever must be used only when symptoms cause a reasonable discomfort to a child. For example, antipyretic should not be used just because of presence of fever. It should be used only if fever is high enough to make a child uncomfortable or pose danger to life as in case of hyperpyrexia. Thus, symptomatic reliever should be used as per the need (on SOS basis) and not on predetermined fixed schedule. It is also true about symptomatic therapy for cough or diarrhea. In fact, there is no cough remedy that "cures" cough. At best, it may relieve discomfort of coughing. Hence, bronchodilator or cough suppressant may be used with caution. It is now well accepted that there is no need for symptomatic control of diarrhea. Besides, stool-binding agents are harmful probiotics are not routinely indicated in diarrhea. Zinc supplement in diarrhea is rational, especially in malnourished children.

Efficacy and Safety

These are most important parameters of rationality. Safety is as much to be ensured as efficacy, more so in case of long-term therapy. It is true that every drug is likely to cause side effects and so, every attempt must be made to use non-pharmacological therapy whenever available, before prescribing a drug. For example, good ventilation, optimum room temperature and light clothing help to control fever. Similarly, hydration and propped up position help to relieve cough. Maintaining good nutrition and hydration is key to treatment of diarrhea. Control of trigger factors in treatment of asthma is vital to therapeutic success. Such measures often obviate need for a drug or can do with minimum drugs.

Risk–Benefit Ratio

It is rational to evaluate probable outcome of using or not using a drug. One must compare risk and benefit of administering the drug as well as withholding the drug. Similarly, one must choose the best drug with favorable risk–benefit ratio.

Cost

Cost is the concern to less privileged society but even to the affordable population. If alternate drug is cheap, one must not hesitate to use it. It is not true that generic drugs are inferior to branded drugs.

Quality

Unfortunately, there is no way for a doctor to assess quality of the drug. It is personal experience that dictates using a drug manufactured by a particular company. Quality of a drug is to be taken for granted although one must keep in mind the possibility of spurious drugs. Past record of the manufacturer and personal experience of a drug helps to decide the quality.

Appropriateness

Rationality cannot be considered to be fixed or rigid endpoint of drug therapy in all situations. Cotrimoxazole is a rational choice for the treatment of acute respiratory infection (ARI) in ARI control program in the community because it is cheap, safe, oral, fairly effective and available in simple dosage formulations. But, it is not necessarily the best choice for individual child as specific antibiotic can be considered better, depending upon probable bacteriological diagnosis. Appropriateness should also be decided by capability and competence of local physician to make correct diagnosis and monitor proper therapy. For example, intravenous therapy may be ideal for acute bacterial infection in an infant but may not be feasible due to physician's inability to administer intravenous drug and so intramuscular route may be an alternative, although inferior. Single dose of intramuscular injection of benzathine penicillin or aminoglycoside has been used in specific conditions.

Single Ingredient Drug

Fixed dose combination drugs are best avoided in routine practice, except in specific situations such as cotrimoxazole, anti-tuberculosis drugs or antibiotic with enzyme inhibitor. If two drugs are necessary for treatment, as in case of neonatal sepsis, they are best administered separately so that individual dosage and duration can be suitably adjusted. There are many irrational combinations in the market such as combination of quinolone and metronidazole for mixed gastrointestinal (GI) infection. Such mixed infection is rare in children.

RATIONAL ANTIBIOTIC THERAPY

Infections are common in children and fever is a common presentation. Fever does not equate with infection and not necessarily bacterial infection that may justify an antibiotic. After all, viral infections are common in the community and should not be treated with an antibiotic. Further, not all bacterial infections deserve an antibiotic prescription. However, antibiotics are prescribed for majority of children presenting with fever. In fact, they may also be prescribed for children who have no infection as in case of cough due to hyper-reactive airway disease. Thus, antibiotics are often prescribed without proper diagnosis for fear of probable bacterial infection and antibiotics are often changed or multiple antibiotics used due to fear of worsening condition. Misuse of antibiotics in this way leads to increasing drug resistance which has become a major concern today. Besides, irrational use of antibiotic may suppress but not control infection that would pose difficulty in diagnosis with increased morbidity and risk of mortality. Thus, improper antibiotic use is a threat to the community and also to an individual patient. If this trend continues, it may not be long before even a simple infection may not be amenable to drug therapy.

WHEN SHOULD AN ANTIBIOTIC BE PRESCRIBED?

Attempt a Bacteriological Diagnosis

Antibiotic is indicated only in case of bacterial infection. It is ideal to attempt bacteriological diagnosis in every child with suspected bacterial infection, although it is not practical in routine office practice. However, few conditions demand proof of bacterial infection as in case of urinary tract infection (UTI) and typhoid fever. Urinary tract infection in children is potentially a serious disease with a risk of permanent renal damage if not properly diagnosed and treated. Typhoid fever being a bacteremic infection, blood culture is often positive and technically, it is easy to culture *Salmonella typhi*. It is, therefore, expected that UTI and typhoid fever are bacteriologically diagnosed as often as possible and empirical treatment is not justified. Gastric lavage for acid-fast bacilli should be tried in the diagnosis of childhood tuberculosis. Throat swab for streptococcal infection is a routine in western countries. In case culture facilities are not available, at least, circumstantial evidence should be collected before embarking on specific antibiotic therapy.

CIRCUMSTANTIAL EVIDENCE OF BACTERIAL INFECTION

Typical clinical syndrome in an acutely febrile child may strongly suggest bacterial infection that may not need further proof for rational antibiotic prescription. Acute tonsillitis is clinically diagnosed by finding beads of pus on inflamed tonsils and tender submandibular lymph nodes. Loose stools with blood and mucus and abdominal cramps suggest acute bacillary dysentery. Localized chest findings in an acutely febrile child who develops tachypnea denotes bacterial pneumonia that may be confirmed by chest X-ray but even without chest X-ray would justify antibiotic therapy.

Laboratory evidence of bacterial infection should not be considered in isolation without clinical correlation. Neutrophilic leukocytosis and high C-reactive protein may favor bacterial infection but not adequate enough by themselves to consider antibiotic therapy. Bacteremic bacterial infections start with moderate degree of fever that becomes more severe by day 3–4 as happens typically in typhoid fever. However, bacterial infections localizing at the site of entry such as tonsillitis or UTI may start with high degree of fever.

WHEN THERE IS NO CLUE TO DIAGNOSIS

This is the most common situation in routine office practice during first few days of onset of fever. Generally, one can arrive at a reasonably correct diagnosis only after disease evolves over few days after onset of symptoms. It means that correct diagnosis is often not possible in a febrile child in first few days with exception sited above such as tonsillitis and bacillary dysentery. At such stage, it is important to assess risk of waiting without specific antibiotic in an acutely febrile child.

Following situations in acutely febrile child are considered to be at risk of serious bacterial infection that demands urgent specific action:
- Age less than 3 months
- Severe protein–energy malnutrition

- Immunosuppressed state
- Behavior abnormality—lethargy or extreme irritability
- Tachycardia and tachypnea disproportionate to degree of fever.

In such situations, laboratory tests should be ordered before starting empirical antibiotic and decision taken for need for hospitalization. Laboratory tests may be prioritized on individual merits and they include complete blood cell, urinalysis, chest X-ray, blood and urine culture and cerebrospinal fluid examination.

WHEN THERE IS NO CLUE TO DIAGNOSIS BUT IS SAFE TO WAIT

In absence of risk factors in a febrile child, it is rational to wait and observe progress without antibiotic therapy. Fever should be controlled with paracetamol. Parents must be counseled about danger symptoms such as behavioral abnormality and reduced urine output that demand reporting to medical facility. Periodic clinical examination is necessary over next few days to pick up clinical clues to diagnosis. Attempt must be made to differentiate acute bacterial infection from acute viral infection. It is possible to a reasonable extent by detailed analysis of history of fever (Table 1.4.1).

PRINCIPLE OF CHOOSING AN ANTIBIOTIC

Once need for an antibiotic is rationally decided, next step is to choose right antibiotic. Choice of antibiotic should depend upon several factors.

Site of Disease

Disease above the diaphragm is generally caused by Gram-positive cocci and is treated with penicillin, macrolide, first-generation cephalosporin. Disease below diaphragm is mostly caused by Gram-negative bacilli and is treated with aminoglycoside, third-generation cephalosporin or quinolone.

Table 1.4.1: Clue to probable cause of acute infection

	Bacterial	*Viral*	*Malaria*
Degree at onset	Moderate	High	High
Rhythm	Regular	Regular	Irregular
Response to paracetamol	Poor	Fair	Erratic
Interfebrile state	Sick	Normal	Normal
Progress on day 3–4	Persisting	Better	Variable
Contact history	None	Positive	None
Extent of disease	Localized	Generalized	—

Epidemiological Data

Antibiotic should be selected on the basis of local epidemiological data regarding drug sensitivity pattern. It may be variable in different regions and even in the same region in different institutes. It is ideal to monitor periodical changes that may occur in drug sensitivity pattern. This is important especially in critical care units wherein resistant strains may develop easily.

Source of Infection

Community-acquired infection is likely to be sensitive to first line of antibiotics, while nosocomial infection is often antibiotic resistant.

Type of Disease

Choice of antibiotic differs depending upon factors such as localized or generalized, superficial or deep, acute or chronic, mild or severe, extracellular or intracellular disease.

Drug Factors

It is always ideal to enquire about history of allergy to drugs. Drug interactions are best avoided by using as minimum number of drugs as possible. One must also keep in mind adverse effects of drugs and communicate effectively with parents so that timely action is taken.

Previous Exposure to Antibiotics

It is likely that organisms may have become resistant to previously used antibiotics in recent past. Hence, it may be rational to use an alternate drug with similar profile. Community-acquired antibiotic-resistant infections are likely to be met with and one must consider such a possibility based on local epidemiology.

DOSAGE, DURATION AND FREQUENCY OF ADMINISTRATION OF ANTIBIOTIC

Difficult Infections

Intracranial infection must be treated with higher dose for longer time due to variable concentration of drug achieved depending upon blood–brain barrier permeability. Thick wall, acid pH and presence of hydrolyzing enzymes necessitate higher dose of antibiotics. Higher dose for longer duration is required in endocarditis due to poor penetration at the site of infection. So the deep-seated infections, such as osteomyelitis, also demand long-term therapy.

Host Factors

Dosage and/or frequency of administration may vary as per age, nutrition, immune status, renal and hepatic function. Frequency of antibiotic administration depends upon plasma half-life of a drug and generally, 4–5 times plasma half-life maintains adequate serum concentration throughout treatment period.

Route of Administration

Oral route is always preferred except in neonates and young infants and, of course, in serious infections. Intramuscular route is not ideal as it is painful and also has erratic absorption. Single dose of penicillin or ceftriaxone has been tried with success. Intravenous route is most ideal as it ensures achieving adequate concentration although, at times, not practical. Antibiotics that are used systemically should not be used topically.

ANTICIPATING INITIAL RESPONSE TO ANTIBIOTIC

Generally, it depends upon doubling time of organism— greater the doubling time, longer the response time. Partial control of fever may be the first response to antibiotic often accompanied with improvement in other symptoms and general wellbeing. For many common bacterial infections, initiation of response is observed within 2–3 days. It may take 4–5 days for initial response to antibiotic in typhoid fever, while in tuberculosis, initial response may be obtained within 2–4 weeks.

WHEN ANTIBIOTIC FAILS IN SUSPECTED BACTERIAL INFECTION?

Antibiotic rarely fails in routine office practice in treatment of community-acquired infection in a normal host. One should expect response to antibiotic within 3–4 days. If there is no response, it calls for reassessment.

Firstly, confirm whether it is an infection and, if so, a bacterial infection. This may be done by repeated physical examination supported by repeat laboratory tests. Choice of antibiotic and its route of administration may be a factor responsible for poor response. If bacterial infection and choice of antibiotic are reasonably confirmed, look for complications such as empyema in case of bacterial pneumonia or subdural collection in case of meningitis. At times, poor response may be due to iatrogenic factor such as catheter-related infection or nosocomial infection in a hospitalized setting. Only when all such factors are ruled out that one may consider drug resistance. It is ideal even at this stage to send blood culture and then change to best considered empirical antibiotic. However, if this change

also fails, bacterial infection is ruled out and one must search for alternate diagnosis. It is not wise to persist with empirical antibiotic trial beyond one change.

WHEN NOT TO PRESCRIBE AN ANTIBIOTIC?

Non-bacterial infections obviously do not call for an antibiotic, and so also non-infective fevers. In routine office practice, it is possible to arrive at a provisional diagnosis by analyzing detailed history and focused physical examination. Typical viral infection starts with high fever at onset of illness that declines by day 3 or 4. Fever is rhythmic, rising every 4–6 hourly. As fever is partly controlled in 20–30 minutes after administration of paracetamol, child becomes active and does not look sick during inter-febrile period. Viral infection results in generalized affection of involved system. Thus, it may be accompanied with symptoms and physical signs of upper and lower respiratory tract involvement. There is often history of similar infection in other family members. Gastrointestinal symptoms in the form of vomiting and watery diarrhea denote involvement of upper (stomach) and lower GI tract (intestine) as a result of viral infection. Thus, viral infection is often disseminated, while bacterial infection is often localized.

Malaria presents with erratic pattern of fever that is essentially nonrhythmic. Child does not appear to be sick during interfebrile period.

Tuberculosis rarely presents as acute infection although acute onset of allergic pleural effusion may be a manifestation of tuberculosis in a healthy child. Non-infective conditions may present with fever wherein there is no localization during initial period. Disease evolves over time and at times may take even few months before being correctly labeled. Differentiation between acute bacterial infection and non-infective inflammatory disorder is, at times, difficult and in such a case, trial of antibiotic would fail to reveal correct diagnosis.

PRESENT SCENARIO OF IRRATIONAL ANTIBIOTIC USE

Antibiotics are considered to be the greatest discovery of twentieth century. In pre-antibiotic era, infectious diseases accounted for significant morbidity and mortality, and invasive procedures were fraught with risk of infection. All this changed with the use of antibiotics. But this miracle seems to be short-lived. Irresponsible and erratic use of these life-saving drugs has resulted in development of drug resistance in many organisms and death due to hospital-acquired infections is on the rise. It appears that our complacency is leading us into bigger problems in the present millennium.

Various studies conducted in developed as well as developing countries during the last few years show that irrational drug use is a global phenomenon.

WHY DO DOCTORS OVERPRESCRIBE ANTIBIOTICS?

Uncertainty of diagnosis and lack of confidence are two major reasons for irrational use of antibiotics. Faulty training of medical students, lack of effective continued medical education and poor communication between doctors and patients have compounded the problem of irrational therapy. Many doctors succumb to peer pressure and parental pressure. Ineffective drug regulation and aggressive pharmaceutical marketing practices have contributed to increasing irrationality of drug prescriptions. "Mixed" infections with bacteria and ameba are not known to occur and this "mixing" is done by drug industry to sell two drugs where none may be indicated. Fear of legal suit makes doctors overreact to patient's need of drugs because of firm belief that error of commission is acceptable but not error of omission. Even, irrational drug prescription can be a bone of contention in courts, more so, if it results in side effects. It is the negligence that is punished and not mistakes, especially if they are within realm of expected competence and scientific limitations.

RATIONAL DRUG THERAPY: RATIONAL PRESCRIBER A PRIORITY!

Although rational drug therapy is a joint responsibility of policy makers, drug manufacturers, healthcare professionals as well as patients, doctors provide final decision of use of drugs. Hence, rational prescriber is a priority to success of rational drug therapy. Rationality should ensure safety at all costs and should try to confine to the limits of acceptable standards. Rationality may have a changing concept. Paracetamol is considered to be an antipyretic of choice but even ibuprofen or mefenamic acid is an acceptable alternative. Oral rehydration solutions have undergone modifications and have been the mainstay of treatment of diarrhea. However, it is well known that not all children suffering from diarrhea accept oral rehydration solution (ORS). It is now proved that those children who do not accept ORS lose much less electrolytes in stool. So rationality demands to hydrate a child suffering from diarrhea with suitable modification but within limits. Knowing that asthma is a chronic inflammatory disease, inhaled steroids have emerged frontline drug for its treatment. Thus, rational prescriber has to learn, unlearn and relearn to keep pace with changing concept.

HOW TO PREVENT MISUSE OF ANTIBIOTICS?

It is vital to arrive at provisional working diagnosis based on clinical analysis of detailed history and focused physical examination. If doctors learn to document provisional diagnosis, drug prescription is likely to be rational. Every doctor is expected to follow standard, national or organizational guidelines and document actions taken with justifications including instructions to parents or patients. Such documentation is a proof of honesty, transparency and responsibility on the part of the doctor. This alone increases confidence in rational therapy. Restricted hospital drug formulary would inculcate ideal therapeutic practice among doctors. Education has a role but may not ensure rational behavior of doctors. There is a need for group audit but best would be self-audit. Drug regulatory authority must ban irrational drugs. Drug controller in USA banned commonly used cold and cough remedies few years ago.

In view of misuse and overuse of antibiotics, council for appropriate and rational antibiotic therapy (CARAT) was formed in USA to guide rational antibiotic therapy.

In summary, rational drug therapy and, in particular rational antibiotic therapy is the need of the hour. Empirical antibiotic therapy has a place in routine practice, but only with rational approach. It includes assessing risk of waiting, clinically evaluating probable etiology of disease, supported by relevant laboratory tests, repeated observation to monitor progress, selecting appropriate empirical drug and reassessment in case of poor response. With indiscriminate antibiotic use, there has been increasing drug resistance and time has come to change this trend lest we are defeated by simple infections.

BIBLIOGRAPHY

1. Amdekar YK. Rational drug therapy—rational prescriber a priority! Indian Pediatr. 1991;28(10):1107-9.
2. Ghai OP, Paul VK. Rational drug therapy in pediatric practice. Indian Pediatr. 1988;25(11):1095-109.
3. Mathur GP, Kushwaha KP, Mathur S. Rational drug therapy: reasons for failure and suggestions for its implementation. Indian Pediatr. 1993;30(6):815-8.
4. Piparva KG, Parmar DM, Singh AP, et al. Drug utilization study of psychotropic drugs in outdoor patients in a teaching hospital. Indian J Psychol Med. 2011;33(1):54-8.
5. Shankar PR, Jha N, Bajracharya O, et al. Feedback on and knowledge, attitude, and skills at the end of pharmacology practical sessions. J Educ Eval Health Prof. 2011;8:12. Epub 2011 Nov 30.
6. Slama TG, Amin A, Brunton SA, et al. A clinician's guide to the appropriate and accurate use of antibiotics: the council for appropriate and rational antibiotic therapy (CARAT) criteria. Am J Med. 2005;118:1S-6S.

Diagnosis and Management

Ritabrata Kundu

2.1   PRINCIPLES OF MANAGEMENT OF BACTERIAL INFECTION AND DRUG RESISTANCE

Ritabrata Kundu

INTRODUCTION

Choosing an antimicrobial agent for children is often difficult as laboratory support in our country is inadequate. Knowledge about the most prevalent organism responsible for the infection and the antibiotic susceptibility pattern is essential. Virulent organisms cause infection in both healthy and immunocompromised in contrast to low virulent organism in only immunocompromised. Bacteriostatic drugs may be adequate in most infections, but bactericidal activity is needed in children with altered immune system, infection in protected areas, e.g. meningitis or systemic infections like staphylococcal bacteremia. Most likely bacterial agents responsible for common infection are organ specific and age dependent. Skin and soft tissue infections in children are mostly due to *Staphylococcus* or B hemolytic streptococci. *Listeria* may be one of the causative organism in meningitis in neonates whereas very unlikely in meningitis in immunocompetent children.

MECHANISM OF ACTION OF ANTIBIOTICS

- Beta-lactam antibiotics (penicillins, cephalosporins, carbapenems and monobactams) inhibit bacterial cell wall synthesis, which eventually leads to cell lysis. Glycopeptides (vancomycin and teicoplanin) also have similar action.
- Aminoglycosides, macrolides, linezolid, tetracyclines and chloramphenicol inhibit protein synthesis by interacting with bacterial ribosomes.
- Sulfonamides and trimethoprim are antimetabolites leading to impaired bacterial synthesis of folic acid resulting in cessation of bacterial cell growth and at times to cell death.

- Quinolones, rifampicin and metronidazole either inhibits bacterial nucleic acid synthesis or its activity.
- Polymyxins like colistin interfere with permeability of bacterial coat leading to its death.

ANTIBIOTICS COMMONLY USED IN CHILDREN

Penicillins

Penicillins are drug of choice for spirochetes (*Treponema pallidum, Leptospira*), streptococci (groups A and B, *viridans* and susceptible strains of *Streptococcus pneumoniae*) and most *Neisseria* spp.

Semisynthetic penicillins like cloxacillin, are used for staphylococcal infection caused by susceptible organism.

Aminopenicillin (ampicillin, amoxicillin) extends the spectrum of penicillin to some gram-negative rods like *Escherichia coli* and *Haemophilus influenzae*.

Carboxy pseudomonal penicillins are also active against some *Proteus, Klebsiella* and *Serratia* spp. beside *Pseudomonas* spp. However, antipseudomonal penicillins are no longer available due to rapid emergence of resistance and are combined with beta-lactamase inhibitors like piperacillin-tazobactam.

Cephalosporins

First-generation cephalosporins include parenteral preparation like cefazolin and oral preparations like cephalexin and cefadroxil. They are used for gram-positive bacteria like methicillin-susceptible *Staphylococcus* and penicillin-susceptible to *Streptococcus*. They are also active against many isolates of *E. coli, Klebsiella pneumoniae* and *Proteus mirabilis*. However, they are ineffective against enterococci, methicillin-resistant *Staphylococcus*, *Pseudomonas* and are poorly active against *H. influenzae*.

They are commonly used for skin and soft tissue infection and as empirical therapy for community-acquired urinary tract infection.

Second-generation cephalosporins include oral preparations like cefaclor, cefuroxime axetil and parenteral form as cefuroxime. Besides having activity against gram-positive cocci they are also active against some gram-negative organism like *H. influenzae*. They are used in outpatients for management of otitis media, sinusitis and lower respiratory tract infection although cheaper agents, which are equally effective, are preferable.

Third-generation cephalosporins have injectable like cefotaxime, ceftriaxone and ceftazidime along with oral preparations as cefixime and cefpodoxime. They have broad spectrum of activity against enteric gram-negative rods including *Salmonella*. Ceftazidime is particularly active against *Pseudomonas*. Their activity against gram-positive bacteria is variable. They have poor action against methicillin-susceptible *Staphylococcus* as compared to first generation. Both cefotaxime and ceftriaxone have excellent activities against *S. pneumoniae*. They are ineffective against methicillin-resistant *Staphylococcus* and *Enterococcus*.

Carbapenems

They include imipenem, in combination with cilastatin, and meropenem and ertapenem. They are antibiotics with broadest spectrum against gram-positive, gram-negative and anaerobes covering virtually all bacterial pathogens except methicillin-resistant *Staphylococcus* and *Enterococcus*. As imipenem cilastatin causes seizure in children, meropenem is the carbapenem of choice for pediatric use.

Monobactam

Aztreonam has wide range of activity against gram-negative enteric bacilli including *Pseudomonas*. It has no action against gram-positive and anaerobic organism. It is second-line antibiotics for treatment of resistant typhoid fever.

Vancomycin

It is effective against gram-positive cocci particularly, staphylococci, streptococci and enterococci. It should be reserved for use in methicillin-resistant *Staphylococcus aureus* (MRSA) and penicillin and cephalosporin-resistant *S. pneumoniae*.

Aminoglycosides

They are rapidly bactericidal drugs, which include streptomycin, gentamicin, kanamycin, tobramycin, amikacin and netilmicin. They are active against gram-negative bacteria and staphylococci, but have no action against anaerobic bacteria. It is the drug of choice in gram-negative septicemia in neutropenic patients. Along with beta-lactam antibiotics, they exert synergistic action in treatment for staphylococcal, enterococcal and streptococcal viridans endocarditis. Their disadvantage is poor penetration in acidic environment and low-oxygen tension. They achieve poor concentration in abscesses and central nervous system infection. Toxicity of aminoglycosides includes nephrotoxicity and ototoxicity.

Macrolides

Erythromycin, clarithromycin and azithromycin are macrolides commonly used in children. They are used for treatment of gram-positive bacteria and treatment of atypical pneumonia caused by *Mycoplasma*, *Chlamydia* and *Legionella*. Their use is limited to skin and soft tissue infection, community-acquired pneumococcal pneumonia and streptococcal pharyngitis in penicillin allergic patients.

All three macrolide has similar antibacterial spectrum; however, clarithromycin and azithromycin have lesser gastrointestinal side effect as compared to erythromycin. It is important to note that bacteria resistant to erythromycin will also be resistant to the other two.

Lincosamides

Clindamycin belonging to this group is commonly used in children. It has action against gram-positive cocci, and both gram-positive and gram-negative anaerobes. It has no activity against gram-negative enteric bacilli. Its use is mainly for MRSA infection and severe invasive group A streptococcal infection.

Linezolid

Its activity is limited to gram-positive bacteria particularly streptococci, staphylococci and enterococci. As the drug has only bacteriostatic activity its use is limited in systemic or severe staphylococci infections.

PRINCIPLE OF ANTIBIOTIC SELECTION

It is important to consider the most common organisms which are responsible for infection depending upon the organ involved and the age of the patient.

Lower respiratory infection beyond neonatal period in immunocompetent child is mainly due to *E. coli* and other gram-negative organisms and *Listeria* whereas in infants and children it is *Neisseria meningitidis*, *Pneumococcus* and *H. influenzae*.

Information of use of antibiotics in recent past in infected child is also important. It might provide due to treatment failure, which by removing the susceptible flora makes infections with resistant organism more likely.

Hosts immune function is also an important consideration. As polymorphonuclear leukocytes are one of the major defenses against acute infection, patient with neutropenia should be treated aggressively with bactericidal antibiotics. Similarly, in patients with deficient humoral immunity and asplenia-encapsulated organisms like pneumococci should be an important consideration as one of the etiologic agents.

Susceptibility of the bacteria to a definite antibiotic can be measured in the laboratory by measuring the lowest concentration of the antibiotic that can inhibit the growth of the bacteria, the minimum inhibitory concentration (MIC). Bacteria are taken to be susceptible if the antibiotic can attend peak serum concentration which exceeds MIC by approximately fourfold.

In general, antibiotic effect is related directly to either the concentration attained at the site of infection or the time during which an effective concentration of the antibiotic is present at the site of infection. Thus, there are concentration-dependent antibiotics in which more increase in antibiotic concentration above MIC leads to a more rapid rate of bacterial death. On other hand, in time-dependent antibiotics, the duration during which the antibiotic concentration remains above the MIC is the crucial factor. Aminoglycosides and fluoroquinolones are examples of concentration-dependent antibiotic where high doses at infrequent interval are effective.

Beta-lactams are time-dependent antibiotics where dosing are frequent to maintain the concentration of antibiotic above MIC of the bacteria for a long time. High dose amoxicillin (80–100 mg/kg/day) in otitis media not only increases the concentration of the drug in the inner ear, but also the duration of time that concentration exceeds the MIC for *Pneumococcus*.

In general, antibiotics given parenterally results in higher serum concentration than when given orally. Serum concentration of beta-lactam antibiotics are 10–15% of that given parenterally when given orally. Quinolones and linezolids have serum concentration almost similar when given either orally or parenterally. One should be aware about antibiotic concentration in various body compartments which vary and also the elimination rates which also varies. Parenteral *ceftriaxone* achieves concentration in ear comparable to that of serum, but elimination half-life from serum is 4–6 hours, whereas in ear fluid is 24 hours. Hence, with a single dose of *ceftriaxone* concentration in the middle ear fluid is well above the MIC for *Pneumococcus* and *H. influenzae* for at least 72 hours.

All antibiotics have some toxicities with which the prescribers should be familiar. In general, beta-lactams are safer antibiotics as compared to others. Information about allergies to antibiotic must be sought and allergy testing may be done if the risk cannot be assessed merely by history taking.

MECHANISM OF RESISTANCE TO DIFFERENT ANTIBIOTICS

Bacteria become resistant to antibiotics either by mutation of its genes or by acquiring new genes. Resistant gene may pass from one bacterium to another by plasmids, transposons or bacteriophages. Irrational excessive antibiotic use kills the sensitive bacteria, but helps in survival and selections of resistant strains.

With gram-positive organism like *Staphylococcus*, which becomes resistant to penicillin by elaborating plasmid-mediated enzyme penicillinase, which disrupts the beta-lactam ring. To overcome this problem, penicillinase-resistant penicillin-like methicillin and cloxacillin was introduced. Within few years, resistance to methicillin and MRSA was found by altering the penicillin-binding proteins (PBP). Subsequently, vancomycin was antibiotic of choice for MRSA. With passage of time staphylococci also showed redness susceptibility (vancomycin-intermediate *S. aureus*) and resistance (vancomycin-resistant *S. aureus*) to vancomycin. This resistance is due to trapping of vancomycin in abnormal peptidoglycan thus denying entry to target sites.

Beta-lactams

Many gram-positive and gram-negative bacteria secrete an enzyme beta-lactamase which hydrolyzes the beta-lactam ring of the antibiotics. Third-generation cephalosporins are stable in the presence of this enzyme encoded by extrachromosomal genetic element. Some beta-lactamase of gram-negative bacteria encoded by extrachromosomal genes like *E. coli* and *K. pneumoniae* or encoded by chromosomal genes like *Enterobacter* spp. hydrolyzes all beta-lactam antibiotics. In order to avoid this problem of beta-lactamase enzyme beta-lactam antibiotic is combined with an inhibitor (clavulanic acid, tazobactam and sulbactam), which avidly binds with the hydrolyzing enzyme, thereby sparing the antibiotic. Unfortunately not all chromosomal beta-lactamase (e.g. *Enterobacter* spp.) bind with the inhibitor. Hence, no combination of beta-lactam antibiotics and inhibitors can resist all of the many beta-lactamases that have been identified.

Bacteria like *Staphylococcus*, *Streptococcus*, *Meningococcus* and *Gonococcus* become resistant to beta-lactam antibiotic by altering PBP target to which the antibiotics bind. Hence, in such circumstances combination of beta-lactam antibiotics with inhibitors are of no use.

In some gram-negative bacteria, there is decreased outer membrane permeability, which hinders entry of antibiotics along with rapid efflux of the antibiotics to the exterior of the cell. Resistance of *Pseudomonas* spp. to cephalosporin and ureidopenicillin is by this mechanism.

Vancomycin

Enterococci, some isolates of *S. aureus* and *S. epidermidis* have become resistant by altering the vancomycin binding target. This resistance is transmitted by mobile genes in plasmide from one cell to another.

Aminoglycosides

Bacteria develop resistance by altering the antibiotic by modifying enzyme so that it cannot bind properly to its target.

P. aeruginosa is resistant by decreased antibiotic uptake due to modification of its outer membrane.

Quinolones

Widespread irrational use of this antibiotic resulted in resistance in *Staphylococcus* and *Pseudomonas* spp. and also in *S. pneumoniae*. This is due to insensitivity of targets of the antibiotics.

MULTIPLE ANTIBIOTIC RESISTANCE

In recent years, single bacteria has started developing resistance to multiple unrelated antibiotics. This may be due to acquisition of multiple resistant genes or development of mutation in single gene. The former is seen in areas of high antibiotic use like in hospitals where gram-negative bacteria, enterococci and staphylococci have become resistant. In community setting salmonellae and pneumococci have developed resistance to multiple antibiotics. The later type of resistance due to mutation is seen in gram-negative bacteria to beta-lactam antibiotics, quinolones and aminoglycosides.

INDICATIONS OF ANTIBIOTIC THERAPY

Antibiotics should be used in only certain definite indications. Unnecessary use of antibiotics results in the destruction of susceptible bacteria and selective proliferation of resistant strain resulting in bacterial drug resistance.

Definitive Therapy

This is for proven bacterial infection. Every effort should be made to confirm it and susceptibility testing should be done. Based on susceptibility report narrowest effective spectrum should be used.

Empirical Therapy

Antibiotic therapy before a definite specific bacteria is identified as empirical therapy. Choice of antibiotic will depend upon the most likely pathogen in that particular site and the sensitivity pattern in that locality. Such therapy is given in life-threatening infection where appropriate sample should be collected and examined. Initially broad spectrum antibiotic or combinations are used followed by narrower spectrum when sensitivity results are available.

In some less severe community acquired infections in outpatients like upper and lower respiratory infection, throat infection and cystitis antibiotics, are prescribed without obtaining cultures. Failure of response or recurrence in such situation is an indication for culture studies.

Anatomical site of infection is a vital determinant of choice of antibiotic patients with suspected meningitis beyond neonatal period usually caused by meningococci, pneumococci and *H. influenzae*. They should receive antibiotics that can cross blood–brain barrier and should be bactericidal as there is relative paucity of natural defense as phagocytes.

Similarly, for bone and joint infection in children, *Staphylococcus*, *Pneumococcus*, *H. influenzae* and *Kingella kingae* are usual causative organisms. Vegetations in bacterial endocarditis are protected from normal most defenses; hence, they need antibiotics which are bactericidal and for a long time.

Prophylactic Therapy

Antibiotic prophylaxis is given to some susceptible patients to prevent specific infection, which is detrimental for the patient. Antirheumatic prophylaxis, antiendocarditis prophylaxis are some examples of such therapy.

Combination Antibiotic Therapy

Although single agent narrow spectrum antibiotic diminishes, alteration of normal bacterial flora reduces cost and adverse effect, but there are certain situations where antibiotics are often combined.

Prevention of Resistant Strains

Predictable mutations occur in genes encoding for resistance in certain bacteria. Treatment with single antibiotic in certain infection will kill the sensitive strains and help to select the resistant strains. Examples are rifampicin for staphylococci and imipenem for *Pseudomonas*. Addition of a second antibiotic with a different mode of action like aminoglycoside plus imipenem in systemic *Pseudomonas* infection might be helpful.

Synergistic or Additive Activity

Examples of such activity are combination of third-generation cephalosporin with aminoglycoside for enterococci, streptococci viridans and *P. aeruginosa.*

Polymicrobial Infections

In certain infection either a mixture of pathogen is suspected or the patient is severely ill. Examples are intra-abdominal infections, brain abscesses and fever in neutropenic patients, where antibiotics are given in various combinations.

Reduction of Adverse Effects

Antibiotics with low safety may be combined in lower doses provided they are synergistic to reduce adverse effects. Combination of streptomycin and penicillin in subacute bacterial endocarditis due to *S. faecalis.*

BIBLIOGRAPHY

1. Archer GL, Polk RE. Treatment and prophylaxis of bacterial infections. In: Kasper DL, Braunwald E, Fauci AS, Hauser SL, Longo DL, Jameson JL (Eds). Harrison's Principles of Internal Medicine, 16th edition. New York: McGraw-Hill; 2005. pp. 789-806.
2. Craig WA. Basic pharmacodynamics of antibacterials with clinical applications to the use of beta-lactams, glycopeptides, and linezolid. Infect Dis Clin North Am. 2003;17(3):479-501.
3. Pankey GA, Steele RW. Tigecycline: a single antibiotic for polymicrobial infection. Pediatr Infect Dis J. 2007;26(1): 77-8.
4. Pong AL, Bradley JS. Guidelines for the selection of antibacterial therapy in children. Pediatr Clin North Am. 2005;52(3):869-94.
5. Schleiss MR. Principles of antibacterial therapy. In: Kliegman RM, Jenson HB, Behrman RE, Stanton BF (Eds). Nelson Textbook of Pediatrics, 18th edition. Philadelphia: Saunders Elsevier; 2008. pp. 1110-22.

2.2 INFECTION CONTROL IN HOSPITAL AND OFFICE PRACTICE

Jaydeep Choudhury

INTRODUCTION

Infections remain a leading cause of disease in most part of the world, including India. Hence, its control is an integral part of pediatric practice in office as well as in hospitals. It is obvious that all healthcare professionals should be aware of routes of infection, transmission and ways to prevent transmission of infectious agents. Nosocomial infection or healthcare associated infections (HCAI) are essentially preventable condition. Unfortunately, due to lack of awareness, the simple methods of prevention are overlooked and attention is paid toward the costly treatment of the infections. It is imperative that simple measures of control of infection are economically cheaper than actual treatment.

Microbes cannot be confined by geographical, social or manmade boundaries. It is quite obvious that we share a single global ecosystem in terms of antibiotic resistance too. Clinically and microbiologically antibiotic resistance is a cause of great concern because detection of even a single instance of antibiotic resistance is a microcosm of a larger perspective. The emergence of a resistant microbacterium to an antibiotic at one place is an ominous sign for the whole society. Although the pattern of resistance may vary marginally from country to country and place to place, but unfortunately, there is no limiting factor for spread of antimicrobial resistance.

All the countries and infectious disease academy or society should have written policies and procedures for infection control and prevention. It should be developed, implemented and reviewed at least every 2 years.

STANDARD PRECAUTIONS IN OUTPATIENT SETTING

Important principles of infection control in an outpatient setting are as follows:

- Every clinic is a potential source of infection. Infection control should begin as soon as a child enters the office or clinic. Standard precautions should be used for all patients.
- Contact between contagious children and uninfected children should be minimized. Immunocompromised children should be kept away from people with potentially contagious infections, typically the viral infections like measles and varicella.
- Patients or their accompanying people with suspected respiratory tract infections should be motivated to use respiratory hygiene and cough etiquette.
- Hand hygiene—it should be performed by all healthcare personnel before and after each patient contact. Alcohol-based hand sanitizers are preferred for healthcare settings. Thorough soap and water wash is indicated when the hands are visibly dirty or contaminated with proteinaceous material, such as blood or other body fluids.
- Healthcare professionals should be familiar with aseptic technique. Alcohol is ideal for skin preparation before immunization or venipuncture. Skin preparation for collection of blood for culture, suture or incision requires 10% povidone iodine, 70% alcohol, alcohol tinctures of iodine or 2% chlorhexidine.
- Safe injection practice is of great importance. Needles and sharps should be handled with utmost care. Needle disposal containers should be readily available. Safe disposals of the collected needles should be done.
- Healthcare personnel should receive influenza vaccine annually and other vaccine-preventable infections that can be transmitted in ambulatory setting.
- Physicians should update themselves regularly about various guidelines regarding infection control and should be aware of the requirements of the government agencies.

INFECTION CONTROL IN HOSPITALIZED CHILDREN

Hospitals provide an environment that contains common drug sensitive as well as unique, antibiotic-resistant microorganisms and susceptible individuals. Hospital personnel are exposed to multiple agents and many patients. They may serve as vectors for disease transmission. Healthcare associated infections are a leading cause of morbidity and mortality in hospitalized children, particularly in children admitted to intensive care units. The single most important practice in prevention and control of healthcare associated infection is proper hand hygiene before and after each patient contact.

Standard Precautions for Care of Patients in Healthcare Settings

The standard precautions are simple but very effective. Adherence to these methods is the key to control of healthcare associated infection.

- Hand hygiene
- Personal protective equipment (PPE)
  - Gloves—it should be used for handling blood, body fluids and touching mucous membrane and nonintact skin.
  - Gown—it should be used during when contact of clothing or exposed skin with blood and body fluids are suspected.

- Mask, eye protection—when procedures can cause splash like endotracheal intubation and suction or for patient protection.
- Soiled patient care equipment
- Environmental control
- Safe injection practices
- Appropriate handling of waste
- Isolation of patients.

Hand Hygiene

Microorganisms can be acquired on the hands during daily duties and when there is contact with blood, body fluids, secretions, excretions and contaminated equipment or surfaces. In order to minimize infection transmission, hands should be washed in all of the above situations and also in between examination and handling of two patients. It is also important to wash hands after removing the gloves as gloves do not provide complete protection against hand contamination. Indications for hand washing with soap and water strictly for 2 minutes are the following:

- At the entry of intensive care unit (PICU, NICU)
- Before performing any invasive procedure, e.g. inserting vascular lines before wearing gloves
- When hands are visibly soiled with dirt or organic material
- After touching soiled linen or other items, mucous membranes, wounds, dressings even if the hands are not soiled
- After examining a culture proven sepsis patient
- After removing gloves.

Alcohol-based hand antiseptics are not effective on hands that are visibly dirty or contaminated with organic material, blood or if exposure to spores (*Clostridium difficile, Bacillus anthracis*) unless they are first washed with soap and water. Alcohol-based hand rubs have been shown to be superior to soap and flowing water hand washing in decreasing the bacterial colony counts. They are recommended to be used after drying hands following hand washing and also before and after every routine patient contact.

Use of Personal Protective Equipment

Personal protective equipment provides a physical barrier between microorganisms and the wearer. It offers protection by helping to prevent microorganisms from contaminating hands, eyes, clothing and other body parts, and be transmitted to other patients and personnel in the healthcare setting.

The various PPEs include the following:

- Gloves
- Mask
- Gown
- Cap
- Protective eye wear

- Apron
- Boots or shoe covers.

Personal protective equipment should be used by healthcare workers who provide direct care to patients and support staff who may have contact with patients' organic material (blood, body fluids, excretions or secretions). It should also be used by cleaners, laundry staff, laboratory staff, who handle patient specimens and family members who provide care to the patients.

Handling of Patient Care Equipment and Soiled Linen

Patient care equipment soiled with organic material should be handled with care in order to prevent exposure. All reusable equipment should be cleaned and reprocessed appropriately before being used on another patient. Used linen that is soiled with organic material should be handled with care to ensure that there is no leaking of organic fluid into the surrounding surface. The method and periodicity of decontamination of various materials depends on the equipment type and is shown in Table 2.2.1.

Table 2.2.1: Patient care equipment and linen decontamination.

Item	Activity	Periodicity
Incubators, warmers, trolleys	In use: detergent and water	In use: daily
	Not being used: 2% cidex	Not being used: dismantle weekly and clean with 2% cidex
Ventilator body	2% carbolic acid	Once daily
Infusion pumps/monitors	Clean with moist cloth	Once daily
Ambu bag and accessories	Dismantle, wash visible contamination then 2% cidex for 30 minutes	After each use
Rubber and plastic tubings	2% cidex for 6 hours	Once daily
Humidity bottles, suction bottles and oxygen hoods	Clean with detergent	Once daily
Laryngoscopes	Clean with spirit	After each use
	2% cidex for 30 minutes	Once daily
Thermometer, stethoscopes, measuring tapes	Wipe with spirit	Before and after each use
Weighing machines	Wipe with moist cloth	Once daily
Saturation probes and BP cuff	Preferably use disposable, when reusing wipe with spirit	Before and after each use
Procedure sets	Autoclave	After each use
Linen/gowns	Manually clean and then autoclave	After each use
Feeding utensils	Wash with detergent, boil for 20 minutes	Before each use

Prevention of Needle Stick or Sharps Injuries

Needles, scalpels and other sharp instruments or equipment should be used with caution. It is preferable to use sterile, single use, disposable syringe and needle for each injection. Single dose medication vials are also preferred. Used disposable syringes and needles, scalpel blades and other sharp items should be placed in a puncture-resistant container with a lid that closes. It should be located close to the area in which the item is used. Needles should never be recapped or bent. Sharps must be appropriately disinfected and/or destroyed. Proper disposal of needles and sharps should be taught to all the members of healthcare providers.

Patient Placement

Spacing between beds: In general wards, there should be adequate spacing between the beds to reduce the risk of cross infection occurring from direct or indirect contact or/and droplet transmission. Optimum spacing between beds is 1–2 meters.

Single rooms: Single rooms reduce the risk of infection transmission from the patient to others by reducing direct or indirect contact transmission.

Cohorting: Patients infected or colonized by the same organism can be cohorted.

Transportation of Patients

Shifting and transportation should be limited to reduce the opportunities for transmission of microorganisms to other areas of the hospital. If transportation is unavoidable, suitable precautions should be taken to reduce the risk of transmission of microorganisms to other patients, healthcare workers or the hospital environment.

Environmental Cleaning and Management Practices

Routine cleaning of hospital, including the waiting rooms are important to ensure a clean and dust-free hospital environment. There are usually many microorganisms present in "visible dirt" and routine cleaning helps eliminate this dirt. Patient care areas should be cleaned by wet mopping. The use of a neutral detergent solution improves the quality of cleaning. Hot water (80°C) is a useful and effective environmental cleaner.

Areas contaminated with blood or body fluids should be cleaned immediately with detergent and water. Isolation rooms and other areas that have patients with known transmissible infectious diseases should be cleaned with a detergent or disinfectant solution at least once daily. All horizontal surfaces and all toilet areas should be cleaned daily. The periodicity of housekeeping is given in Table 2.2.2.

Table 2.2.2: Housekeeping periodicity routines.

Item	Activity	Periodicity
Floors	Mop with phenyl	Thrice daily
Walls	Wipe with detergent/carbolic acid	Thrice daily
Fans	Wipe with detergent	Every 15 days
Basins	Clean with detergent	Thrice daily
Shelves	Wipe with phenyl carbolic acid	Thrice daily
Telephone	Wipe with moist cloth	Once daily

Air ventilation: Air quality is a very important factor in controlling HCAI and thus special importance is given to it. Ventilation systems should be designed and maintained to minimize microbial contamination. The air conditioning filters should be cleaned periodically and fans that can spread airborne pathogens should be avoided in high-risk areas. High-risk areas, such as operating rooms, critical care units and transplant units require special ventilation systems. Filtration systems designed to provide clean air should have high efficiency particulate air (HEPA) filters in high-risk areas. Unidirectional laminar airflow systems should be available in appropriate areas in the hospital construction.

Special air handling: For the operating room and for immunocompromised patients special air handling is needed.

Critical parameters for air quality in operation theater are as follows:
- Frequent maintenance of efficacy of filters (according to manufacturer's requirements) and pressure gradient across the filter bed.
- Minimum 15 air changes per hour.
- Temperature should be maintained between 20°C and 22°C and humidity between 30% and 60% to inhibit bacterial multiplication.
- General areas should be well ventilated if they are not air-conditioned.

Air control parameters for rooms of immunocompromised patients are as follows:
- Ultraclean unidirectional air is required in some units such as hematology or intensive care.
- To minimize airborne particles, air must be circulated into the room with a HEPA filter. The HEPA filter removes particles to a certain defined size. If particles 0.3 microns in diameter are removed, the air entering the room can be classified as being clean and free of bacterial contamination.

Other than special air handling, immunocompromised patients need other protective methods like preventing the entry of healthcare workers and visitors with infections (for example, upper respiratory tract infections or herpes simplex blisters), using strict aseptic technique for all clinical procedures, environmental cleaning, avoiding keeping flowers or plants in the room.

Handling of Waste

Hospital waste is a potential reservoir of pathogenic microorganisms and requires appropriate, safe and reliable handling. The main risk associated with infection is sharps contaminated with blood. There should be a person or persons responsible for the organization and management of waste collection, handling, storage and disposal. Waste management should be conducted in coordination with the infection control team. Waste management practices must meet national and local requirements.

Steps in the management of hospital waste include:

Segregation and collection: Infectious waste should be collected and segregated from non-infectious waste in dedicated containers at the source. This prevents contamination by infectious waste to other hospital waste.

Transportation: Waste should be transported in a dedicated trolley. The carts or trolleys used for the transport of segregated waste collection should not be used for any other purpose—they should be cleaned regularly.

Storage: Waste should be stored in specified areas with restricted access. Sharps should be stored in sharps containers. Sharps containers should be made of plastic or metal and have a lid that can be closed. They should be marked with the appropriate label or logo, e.g. a biohazard symbol for clinical (infectious) waste.

Treatment: Each healthcare facility should identify a method for the treatment of infectious waste. This may consist of transportation of infectious waste to a centralized waste treatment facility or on-site treatment of waste.

Final disposal: Sharps should be autoclaved after chemical treatment shred and landfill or microwave. Deep burial should be done in a secure area. Burial should be 2–3 meters deep and at least 1.5 meters above the groundwater level.

Anatomical parts, animal carcasses, cytotoxic drugs (residues or outdated) and toxic laboratory chemicals other than mercury should be incinerated. Patient-contaminated non-plastics and non-chlorinated plastics may be also incinerated.

Chlorinated plastics, volatile toxic wastes, such as mercury, should not be incinerated. Plastics, non-plastics contaminated with blood, body fluids, secretions and excretions and infectious laboratory wastes also should not be incinerated. Such wastes should be treated by steam sterilization in autoclavable bags or microwave

treatment. Chemical treatment with 1% hypochlorite or a similar disinfectant is recommended. However, excessive use of chemical disinfectants should be avoided as it may be a health and environmental hazard. Radioactive waste should be dealt with according to national laws. Color coding, treatment and final disposal of waste are shown in Table 2.2.3.

Transmission-based Precautions

These additional precautions are designed for patients documented or suspected to have colonization or infection with pathogens for which these precautions beyond standard precautions are recommended to prevent transmission. The three types of transmission routes on which these precautions are based are: (i) airborne, (ii) droplet and (iii) contact.

Airborne Precautions

Airborne precautions are aimed to reduce the transmission of diseases spread by the airborne route. Airborne transmission occurs when droplet nuclei (evaporated droplets) less than 5 microns in size are disseminated in the air. These droplet nuclei can remain suspended in the air for long time. Diseases which spread by this mode include open or active pulmonary tuberculosis (TB), measles,

Table 2.2.3: Color coding, treatment and final disposal of waste.

Color coding	Waste	Treatment and final disposal
Yellow (solid infectious material)	Human tissues, organs and body parts Microbiology and biotechnology waste (wastes from lab cultures, specimens, live attenuated vaccines, etc.). Waste items contaminated with blood and body fluids, including cotton dressings, soiled plaster casts, linen and other materials	Incineration
Red (solid non-infectious material)	Waste generated from disposable items other than sharps like tubings, catheters, IV sets	Disinfect by chemical treatment (1% hypochlorite) then either autoclave or later shredding
Blue (sharps)	Needles , syringes, scalpel blades, glass, etc.	Disinfect by chemical treatment (1% hypochlorite) then either autoclave or later shredding
Black (other waste)	Discarded medicines and left over foods	Taken for landfill

chickenpox, pulmonary plague and hemorrhagic fever with pneumonia.

The followings are complementary to the standard precautions:

- Patient should be placed in a single room that has a monitored negative airflow pressure. The air should be discharged to the outdoors or specially filtered before it is circulated to other areas of the healthcare facility. It is important to gain the support of engineering services to ensure that the negative airflow pressure is maintained.
- Doors should always remain closed. Anyone who enters the room must wear a special, high filtration, particulate respirator (e.g. N 95) mask.
- If transport is necessary, surgical mask should be used to the patient to minimize dispersal of droplet nuclei.

Droplet Precautions

Droplets are usually generated from infected person during coughing, sneezing, talking or when healthcare workers undertake procedures, such as tracheal suctioning. Droplet transmission occurs when there is adequate contact between the mucous membranes of the nose and mouth or conjunctivae of a susceptible person and large particle droplets (>5 microns). Diseases, which are transmitted by this route, include pneumonias and meningitis caused by various organisms like *Hemophilus influenzae* type B, *Mycoplasma pneumoneae* and *Neisseria meningitis*, pertussis, diphtheria, influenza, mumps, rhinovirus, rubella, and viral hemorrhagic fever. In these cases, patient should be placed in a single room (or in a room with another patient infected by the same pathogen). Healthcare persons should wear a surgical mask when working within 1–2 meters of the patient. A surgical mask should be placed on the patient if transport is necessary.

Contact Precautions

Contact transmission is the most common route of transmission of healthcare associated infections. It can be direct or indirect contact transmission.

Direct contact transmission: It involves direct body surface to body surface contact and physical transfer of microorganisms between a person with infection or colonization and a susceptible host. It may happen when a healthcare provider attend to an infected patient and has direct physical contact.

Indirect contact transmission: It involves contact of a susceptible host with a contaminated intermediate object such as instruments, needles, dressings, hands, etc.

Specific infections that require contact precaution are the following:

- Multidrug resistant bacteria, such as methicillin-resistant *Staphylococcus aureus* (MRSA), vancomycin-resistant enterococci (VRE), multidrug resistant gram-negative bacilli
- *C. difficile*
- *Salmonella*
- *Shigella*
- *S. aureus*
- Major abscess, cellulitis
- Herpes simplex virus
- Enteroviruses
- Respiratory syncitial virus
- Rotavirus
- Viral hemorrhagic fever
- Conjunctivitis—viral and hemorrhagic

It is ideal to place the patient in a single room (or in a room with another patient infected by the same pathogen). Clean, non-sterile gloves and gown should be used when entering the room. Limit the movement and transport of the patient from the room; patients should be moved for essential purposes only. If transportation is required, use precautions to minimize the risk of transmission. The specification for category based isolation is summarized in Table 2.2.4.

Healthcare-associated infections are a major cause of mortality and morbidity in hospitalized children, particularly in children admitted to the intensive care units. Hand hygiene before and after each patient contact remains the single most important practice in preventing and controlling healthcare-associated infections.

Adult and Sibling Visitation

Anybody with fever or contagious illness ideally should not visit sick hospitalized children. Visitors with cough who may have TB or pertussis or a person with cold visiting an immunosuppressed child should be barred. Medical and nursing staff should be vigilant, especially for oncology, neonatal intensive care units and transplant units.

Sibling visits may be beneficial for the hospitalized children, but few guidelines have to be followed:

- Children with acute illness like upper respiratory infection, gastroenteritis, dermatitis should not be allowed to visit.
- Visiting children should have received all recommended immunizations for age, including influenza vaccine during influenza season.

Table 2.2.4: Transmission-based precautions for hospitalized patients.

Category	Single-patient room	Respiratory tract/mucous membrane protection	Gowns	Gloves
Airborne	Yes	Respirators	No	No
Droplet	Yes	Surgical mask	No	No
Contact	Yes	No	Yes	Yes

- The visiting sibling should visit only his or her sibling and not allowed to play in rooms with groups of children.
- Recommended hand hygiene should be performed.
- Sibling visits should always be supervised.

PREVENTION OF ANTIBIOTIC RESISTANCE

Control of drug resistant infections is an important aspect of infection control in healthcare facility. It is obvious that the strategy to tackle a problem of such magnitude and gravity should be wide based and systematic. The whole emphasis of antibiotic policy revolves around antibiotic resistance. Antibiotic resistance can be introduced, selected, maintained and spread in health institutions by the following six mechanisms as described below:

- Introduction of a few resistant organisms into a population where resistance previously was not present, usually by transfer from another healthcare system, sometimes also from the community.
- Acquisition of resistance by a few previously susceptible strains through genetic mutation in reservoirs of high organism concentration, such as an abscess.
- Acquisition of resistance by a susceptible strain through transfer of genetic material, for example in the gut or on the skin.
- Emergence of inducible resistance that is already present in a few strains in the bacterial population, usually from direct selection by antibiotic prescribing.
- Selection of a small resistant subpopulation of organisms, again by antibiotic prescription.
- Dissemination of inherently resistant organisms locally within the specific setting due to poor infection control procedures.

Dynamics of Antimicrobial Resistance

According to the definition by Center for Disease Control, resistant bacteria are those judged by the infection control program, based on current state, regional or national recommendations, to be of special clinical and epidemiological significance.

The four interacting determinants of antibiotic resistance are: (i) the patient, (ii) the organism, (iii) the drug and (iv) the environment. It is important to understand the interplay between these four determinants, the epidemiology and the specific mechanisms of resistance in order to understand how the antibiotic policies help in controlling resistance.

- *The patient:* A person who is colonized or infected can cause common source of outbreak. Any process that lowers the drug concentration at the site of infection helps in selection of resistance and slow eradication of infection. Another major concern is the development of resistance in the normal flora, as this resistance may spread to more pathogenic flora.
- *The organism:* Bacteria can adopt a number of ways to develop resistance to antimicrobials. One of the most remarkable traits is the genetic mechanism for resistance to antimicrobials. Many times a single resistant bacterial strain found in a hospital may possess several of the resistant mechanisms simultaneously and this is a very complex situation.
- *The drug:* Rational use of antibiotics is crucial. Wherever possible the pathogen and the sensitivity should be determined in clinical practice. A narrow spectrum antibiotic is always beneficial as they have less effect on normal flora. The antibiotic dose is also an important determinant. A higher dose which achieves higher concentration at the site of infection is less likely to cause resistance. Sometimes, combination antibiotic therapy is an effective mode to tackle resistance in special situations. This has been proved effectively in the treatment of TB and HIV.
- *The environment:* The term environment covers both institution and community. It should be distinguished whether the resistant organism originates from community or from nosocomial isolates. The hospital acquired resistance may be restricted to a great extent by proper antibiotic policy. At the same time the isolates should be identified from body site and hospital location. The emerging resistance may be *de novo* or the result of clonal spread. In the later, cross-infection and environmental contamination are also important. Antibiotic restriction may not be of much effect in this situation.

The Problems

- In hospitals throughout the world, there are special problems with methicillin-resistant *S. aureus*—the nosocomial or hospital acquired methicillin-resistant *S. aureus* (HA-MRSA) as well as the new strains of community acquired methicillin-resistant *S. aureus* (CA-MRSA).
  The explosion of infections with vancomycin-resistant *Enterococci* (VRE) is remarkable.
- Resistance of gram-negative rods to quinolones and third-generation cephalosporins continues to increase.
  The emergence of strains of *S. aureus* with intermediate levels of resistance to vancomycin (VISA) has been noted in several countries.

The Issues

The etiology of antibiotic resistance are not clearly known, but surely unnecessary use of antibiotics is one of the leading causes. Such high use leads to the selection of resistant organisms. Once a patient has a resistant organism, then the possibility exists for transmission to other patients. The second issue is proper infection control. The pillars for infection control are isolation and hand washing. The third issue relates to the influx of patients harboring resistant strains on admission to the hospital. Such patients need to be quickly identified and isolated.

Surveillance for Resistant Bacterial Pathogens

The clinical microbiology laboratory plays an important role by providing the data on bacterial isolates and antimicrobial susceptibility to guide clinicians in antibiotic therapy. Susceptibility testing data acts as the pivot for therapeutic guidance and strain typing for potential infection outbreak.

There are two components of surveillance. The first is the periodic review of minimum inhibitory concentration (MIC) or the zone diameter data for changes in resistance patterns. A decrease in the mean zone diameter around antibiotic disk in susceptibility testing may be first sign of emergence of antimicrobial resistance.

The second and equally important component of surveillance is reporting of the resistance pattern to the authority, who should take the initiative in formulating appropriate policy.

Prevention of Emergence of Resistance

The two principal goals are prevention of emergence of antibiotic resistance and control of established resistance. For both these goals the approach is similar. It is quite obvious that prevention of acquisition of infection is easier than curbing the established resistance.

The following strategies have to be adopted in order to reduce antimicrobial resistance and to make an antibiotic control program effective:

- *Optimal use of all antimicrobials:* Ideally all patients should be treated with the most effective, least toxic and least costly antibiotic for the precise duration of time needed to cure or prevent an infection. Another strategy to curtail the development of antimicrobial resistance, in addition to the judicious overall use of antibiotics, is to use drugs with a narrow antimicrobial spectrum or "older" antibiotics. Several investigations suggest that some infections, such as community-acquired pneumonia and urinary tract infections, can usually be successfully treated with narrow-spectrum antibiotic agents, especially if the infections are not life-threatening. New antimicrobials should be used with caution.
- *National protocols of common infections:* It is of utmost importance to develop national guidelines and treatment algorithms. Consensus-driven recommendations should be developed for the treatment of hospital-acquired and community-acquired infections.

- *Restriction policy:* Selective removal or control of use of specific agents or classes of agents has been employed in many hospitals. But the strategy has to be determined by careful consideration of the resident flora.
- *Antibiotic cycling and scheduled antibiotic changes:* It is also known as rotation of antibiotics. A class of antibiotics or a specific antibiotic drug is withdrawn from use for a defined period and is reintroduced at a later time in an attempt to limit bacterial resistance.
- *Combination antimicrobial therapy:* It has been used successfully for *Mycobacterium tuberculosis* and HIV infections. It has been proposed as a strategy to reduce the emergence of bacterial resistance. In addition, combination antimicrobial therapy may be more effective at producing clinical and microbiological responses. This could also help to minimize antibiotic resistance by preventing the horizontal transmission of inadequately treated antibiotic-resistant pathogens. But combination antibiotic therapy should not be misused in situations which can be tackled by a single antibiotic. Injudicious use of combination antibiotics cause more harm than benefit.

Non-antimicrobial Prevention Strategies

The specific prevention strategies may not be effective if it is not complemented by the non-antimicrobial prevention strategies. The non-antimicrobial prevention strategies may be implemented at two levels: (i) primary prevention program for specific infections and (ii) use of infection control practices to prevent horizontal transmission of nosocomial infection.

Primary prevention program for specific infections:
- *Adoption of WHO strategies:* Integrated Management of Childhood Illness (IMCI), DOTS for TB, HIV/AIDS control program are some of the policies.
- *Vaccination and immunoglobulins:* It is the most effective means to contain resistance.
- *Reducing length of stay in hospital and avoidance of invasive procedures:* Prolonged hospital stay results into antibiotic use for a longer duration and exposure to circulating hospital microbes for prolonged period.

Prevention of horizontal transmission:
- *Hand-washings*
- *Gloves and gowns.*

Community Level Prevention

- *Reduction of use of antimicrobials in livestock:* Antimicrobials normally prescribed for humans should be prohibited as growth promoters or as an alternative to high quality hygiene in animals.
- *Vector control:* Proper control of vectors can prevent the vector-borne diseases.

- *Increased availability and access to antimicrobials:* Inadequate access to appropriate antimicrobials results in improper treatment which in turn hastens the development of resistance. Often cost in inhibitory, which prompts premature discontinuation of antimicrobials.
- *Education and awareness of health workers and public:* The aim is to inculcate sense of hygiene and curb the misuse of antibiotics. Proper cleanliness goes a long way in preventing infection.

Under any situation more than 20% of all hospital acquired infections can be prevented. Most of the interventions are simple, basic and related to individual healthcare worker. Careful hand washing, appropriate isolation, use of gloves when required and proper use of devices go a long way in prevention of nosocomial infections.

BIBLIOGRAPHY

1. Bennett JV, Brachman PS. Hospital Infection, 4th edition. Philadelphia: Lippincott Williams and Wilkins; 1997.
2. Choudhury J. Strategies for prevention of antibiotic resistance. In: Choudhury J, Kundu R (Eds). Pediatric Infectious Disease Update, 1st edition. New Delhi: Jaypee Brothers Medical Publishers (P) Ltd. 2012.
3. Choudhury J. Strategies to prevent antibiotic resistance. Indian J Pract Pediatr. 2007;9:47-51.
4. Communicable Diseases Network Australia. Infection Control Guidelines for the Prevention of Transmission of Infectious Diseases in the Health Care Setting, 2nd edition. Canberra: Department of Health and Aging, Commonwealth of Australia; 2002.
5. Goldman D, Larson E. Hand-washing and nosocomial infections (Editorial). Lancet. 1992;327:120-2.
6. Gould IM. A review of the role of antibiotic policies in the control of antibiotic resistance. J Antimicrob Chemother. 1999;43:459-65.
7. Health Canada, Laboratory Centre for Disease Control. Infection Control Guidelines. Routine practices and additional precautions for preventing the transmission of infection in health care. Canada Communicable Disease Report. 1999 Jul; 25 (Suppl 4): 1-155. Electronic access: http://www.hc-sc.gc.ca/hpb/lcdc/publicat/ccdr/99pdf/cdr25s4e.pdf
8. Jain RK. Antimicrobial resistance: can we overcome it? In: Ghosh TK (Ed). Infectious Diseases in Children and Newer Vaccines, 1st edition. Ahmedabad, Kolkata: IAP Infectious Diseases Chapter Publication; 2003. pp. 113-24.
9. McGowan JE, Tenover FC. Control of antimicrobial resistance in the health care system. Infect Dis Clinics North Am. 1997;11:297-311.
10. Pakyz AL, Kockler DR. Managing antibiotic resistance: what works in the hospital. In: Wenzel R, Bearman G, Brewer T, Butzler J-P (Eds). A Guide to Infection Control in the Hospital, 4th edition. Boston: International Society for Infectious Diseases; 2008. pp. 74-80.
11. Prüss A, Giroult E, Rushbrook P (Eds). Safe Management of Wastes from Health-care Activities. Geneva: World Health Organization, 1999. Electronic access: http://whqlibdoc.who.int/publiations/9241545259.pdf
12. Red Book. Report of the Committee on Infectious Diseases, American Academy of Pediatrics, 28th edition. New Delhi: Jaypee Brothers; Medical Publisher (P) Ltd. 2009.
13. Sehulster L, Chinn RY. Guidelines for environmental infection control in health-care facilities. Recommendations of CDC and the Healthcare Infection Control Practices Advisory Committee (HICPAC). MMWR Recomm Rep. 2003;52(RR-10):1-42.
14. Steele RW. Clinical Handbook of Pediatric Infectious Disease, 3rd edition. New York: Informa Healthcare; 2007. pp. 253-6.
15. World Health Organization. Prevention of Hospital Acquired Infections—A Practical Guide, 2nd edition. Geneva: WHO, 2002. Electronic access: WHO/CDS/ EPH/2002.12.

2.3 | MANAGEMENT OF LABORATORY DIAGNOSIS OF INFECTION

Sankar Sengupta

INTRODUCTION

The microbiology laboratory plays a crucial role in the diagnosis of infectious diseases. Many different types of tests are available for the detection of infection. There are several ways of making a microbiological diagnosis:

- Microscopy
- Culture isolation
- Serology
- Molecular techniques.

COLLECTION OF SPECIMENS

Body fluids, secretions and biopsy material can all be examined to detect pathogens, its products or antigens or the immune response to them. Samples from the environment, e.g. water, food or soil, may also be examined. Some samples must be collected at a particular time; for example, malaria parasites are best sought at the peak of fever and a short time afterward, whereas blood for bacterial culture should be taken as the fever begins to rise. Special precautions must often be taken to ensure survival of the pathogen and exclude contaminants, e.g. cleaning the perineum before collecting a midstream specimen of urine. Anaerobic species may die if exposed to atmospheric oxygen and survive better in samples of pus, rather than in swab specimens. Many pathogens, such as *Neisseria* and most anaerobic species, die quickly outside the body and must be transported to the laboratory without delay. *Neisseria gonorrhoeae* is susceptible to drying, so specimens likely to contain this organism should be inoculated into microbiological medium near to the patient; many genitourinary medicine clinics are equipped to do this.

UNIVERSAL PRECAUTIONS AND LABORATORY SAFETY

Specimens may contain hazardous pathogens and must be handled with care. A system of "universal precautions" is employed to reduce the risk of transmitting blood-borne defection. These are personal protective measures, taken in collecting and examining specimens irrespective of their source. The idea is to handle specimens on the assumption that they may contain a transmissible pathogen, rather than relying on clinical suspicion or written clinical details, which may be faulty or absent. For example, any sputum specimen is assumed to carry the risk of tuberculosis even if this is not the test requested.

DIRECT MICROSCOPIC EXAMINATION

Antoni van Leeuwenhoek first saw microscopic "animalcules", and Alexander Ogston, a surgeon, described the characteristic microscopical morphology of staphylococci in pus and discovered their role in pyogenic sepsis. The light microscope has since been indispensable in the study of microorganisms. The equipment required is cheap, reagent costs are low and early results can be obtained. The diagnosis of malaria or vaginal trichomoniasis, for instance, can be made while the patient waits at the clinic. The organism sought need neither multiply nor even be alive. Microscopy is especially useful for detecting organisms that are difficult or dangerous to grow.

TYPES OF MICROSCOPY FOR THE DIAGNOSIS OF INFECTIONS

Unstained preparations

- *Simple stains:* Gram and Giemsa
- *Special stains:* Ziehl–Neelsen, Gomori–Grocott, India ink
- *Immunofluorescence:* Direct and indirect
- Electron microscopy.

Microscopy of Unstained Preparations

Direct Microscopy of Unstained Preparations

- Fecal protozoa and helminths
- Vaginal discharge
- Urine for bacteria and pus cells.

Direct examination of unstained "wet" preparations is suitable for rapid diagnosis in the laboratory and the outpatient setting. Many pathogens have a characteristic appearance, e.g. parasites in the feces, or may appear in diagnostic circumstances, for instance bacteria, together with white cells, in the urine form a case of acute urinary tract infection. Viruses can also be detected directly by electron microscopy, using a negative-staining technique. The viruses are concentrated by vigorous centrifugation and are then suspended in a heavy metal solution. As it dries, the heavy metal salt fills in the spaces between the viruses, providing an electron-dense background that outlines the virus. This technique is useful for detecting viruses with distinctive morphology, such as poxviruses in scrapings from the lesions of Orf and *Molluscum contagiosum*, herpes viruses in vesicle fluid or one of the many gastrointestinal viruses such as rotavirus or calicivirus in diarrhea stool.

Microscopy of Stained Preparations with Simple Stains

Gram Stain

Dried preparations of specimens that are fixed to kill the organisms can be examined using simple stains, such as Gram stain, that dye the bacteria. This technique can demonstrate the shape of the bacteria and the capability of "gram-positive" bacteria to retain the methylene blue dye. The Gram stain provides a rapid evidence of preference of any organism. It is most useful when sterile fluids, such as cerebrospinal fluid (CSF) or pleural fluid, are examined. However, the sensitivity of Gram stain is relatively low and at least 10,000 organisms/mL of specimen must be present for its detection.

Gram stain:
- Sterile fluids (CSF, ascites, pleural fluid)
- Sputum (to exclude poor-quality specimens)
- Pus from any site
- Urethral discharge.
- Gram staining alone can rarely recognize the organism, because the morphology of bacteria is rarely diagnostic. Important exceptions to this include the finding of gram-positive or gram-negative diplococci in CSF from a patient with meningitis, or the characteristic appearances of *Borrelia* and *Fusobacterium* in Vincent's angina. Similarly, a gram stained preparation of urethral pus showing gram-negative intracellular diplococci is sufficiently characteristic to allow a presumptive diagnosis of gonorrhea.

Other Simple Stains

Other simple stains include acridine orange (which is more sensitive in demonstrating organisms than Gram stain, but more prone to confusing artifactual effects), lactophenol blue to demonstrate the morphology of fungi, or India ink, which is used to detect the presence of *Cryptococcus neoformans* in the CSF by negative staining.

Special Stains

Stains, such as Ziehl–Neelsen (ZN), are used to demonstrate specific features of organisms that simple stains will not demonstrate. Specimens are stained with carbol fuchsin, destained with an acid-alcohol solution and then counterstained with methylene blue. The lipid-rich mycobacterial cell wall retains the pink dye resistant to decoloration by acid alcohol solution and organisms are seen as pink bacilli against the blue background. The number of acid-fast species is limited, and this technique is therefore useful in the diagnosis of *Mycobacterium* infection, including tuberculosis and leprosy, and parasitic infections such as cryptosporidiosis.

A variation of this technique uses the naturally fluorescent substance auramine to stain the organisms. The specimen is processed in a similar way to the ZN method, and acid-fast organism fluorescent bright yellow under an ultraviolet light. Auramine microscopy is used for screening large numbers of specimens but, because it lacks the specificity of the ZN stain, all positive specimens must be over stained by the ZN method, and reexamined to confirm the findings (Table 2.3.1).

Romanowsky Stains

Romanowsky stains, which color cytoplasm and chromatin, are widely used to demonstrate blood cells. Stains of this type are very useful for revealing blood parasites. In malaria or filariasis Giemsa-stained smears not only demonstrate the presence of the organisms, but also permit speciation by displaying morphological details.

Special Stains Used in Microbiology

- *Ziehl–Neelsen: Mycobacterium* spp.
- *Gomori–Grocott:* Fungi, *Pneumocystis carinii*
- *Giemsa:* Malaria, filaria

Immunofluorescence

Direct immunofluorescence techniques detect organisms by their binding with fluorescence-labeled antibodies. Specimens are dried on a multiwell slide, together with positive and negative "control" specimens. A specific fluorescein-labeled antibody is then added. The slides are washed and examined microscopically under ultraviolet illumination. Where the antibody has bound to the pathogen there is an apple green fluorescence. This

Table 2.3.1: Characteristics of some important stains.

Name of the stain	Primary stain	Decoloriser	Counter stain	Purpose
Gram stain	Crystal violet	Acetone/acetone-alcohol	Safranine	For seeing gram-positive (violet) and gram-negative (pink) organisms
Ziehl–Neelsen stain	Hot carbol fuchsin	20% H_2SO_4/5% H_2SO_4	Methylene blue	For seeing *Mycobacterium tuberculosis*, MOTT, *Mycobacterium leprae*
Kinyoun method of Ziehl–Neelsen stain	Cold carbol fuchsin	1% H_2SO_4	Methylene blue	For seeing stool parasites like *Cryptosporidium*, *Cyclospora*, *Isospora*
Albert stain	Albert I	--	Albert II	For seeing Diphtheria bacilli (Chinese letter arrangement and metachromatic granules)

technique is both sensitive and specific and provides a rapid, presumptive diagnosis. It can be applied to a wide range of specimens and is used in the diagnosis of upper respiratory tract virus infections, including influenza, parainfluenza and respiratory syncytial virus, and also measles and rabies.

Some Organisms Detectable by Direct Immunofluorescence (Figs. 2.3.1 to 2.3.6)

- *Viruses:* Parainfluenza viruses, respiratory syncytial virus
- *Bacteria: Legionella, Treponema pallidum*
- *Protozoa/fungi: Giardia intestinalis, Pneumocystis jiroveci (carinii).*

CULTURE METHODS

Culture can aid diagnosis in bacterial, parasitic and viral diseases. In bacteriology, culture permits amplification of the number of bacteria. Isolating them on solid media makes identification ZN and susceptibility testing possible. Bacterial culture is made possible by the use of agar, a gelatinous substance derived from seaweed, which melts at 90°C but solidifies at 50°C. It is highly stable, is rarely affected by organisms in cultures and can be mixed with nutrients, such as blood, serum and protein digests to make solid media. Koch introduced agar to microbiology to replace gelatin, which melts at a lower temperature, near to that used for incubation.

Bacteriological culture on solid agar is usually performed in Petri dishes: these are plastic dishes, 90 mm in diameter, with a vented lid. When prolonged culture is necessary, as in the diagnosis of mycobacterial or fungal infection, it is usually performed in sealed containers to prevent desiccation and the entry of contaminating organisms. The choice of medium and the conditions of incubation depend on knowledge of the organism's requirements for optimum growth.

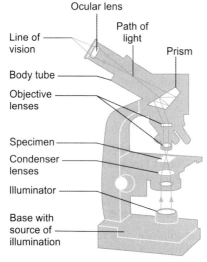

FIG. 2.3.1: Microscope showing path of light (bottom to top).

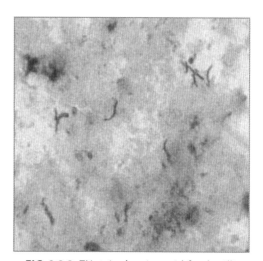

FIG. 2.3.3: ZN stain showing acid-fast bacilli.

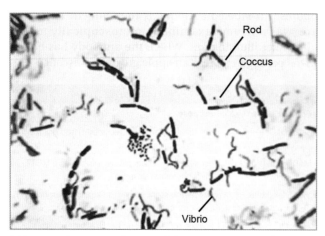

FIG. 2.3.2: Gram stain showing different morphology of bacteria.

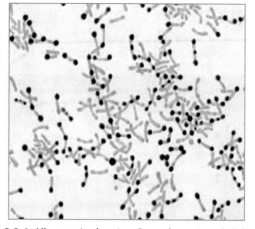

FIG. 2.3.4: Albert stain showing *Corynebacterium diphtheriae.*

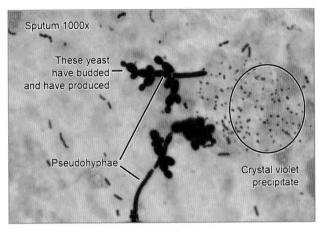

FIG. 2.3.5: Yeast.

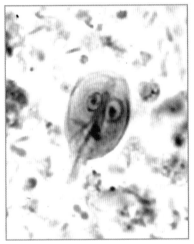

FIG. 2.3.6: *Giardia lamblia.*

MEDIA

Three types of bacteriological media are used: (i) enrichment, (ii) selective and (iii) indicator.

Enrichment Media

Enrichment media are used to ensure that small numbers of fragile pathogens that can multiply sufficiently to be detected. They are useful when seeking to identify fastidious organisms, such as *Streptococcus* spp., *Haemophilus influenzae* or *Bacteroides fragilis*. Enrichment media are made by adding blood, yeast extracts, tissue infusions, meat, etc. to simple base media. Some enrichment media include materials to neutralize toxic bacterial products that would otherwise inhibit growth. An example of this is charcoal in the enrichment medium for *Bordetella*. The media may be solid, for example blood agar, or liquid, as with Robertson's cooked meat broth. Liquid media are especially valuable for investigating body fluids that are normally sterile. Very small numbers of organisms in such fluids will multiply in the highly nutritious medium,

and they can then be subcultured on to solid media for identification and susceptibility testing.

Enrichment medium aims to amplify the organism by growth, e.g. for *Neisseria* spp., *Streptococcus* spp. or *Vibrio* spp.

Selective Media

Selective media are used to identify a pathogen existing in a mixture of organisms (Table 2.3.2). Many body sites, such as the upper respiratory tract or the gut, have normal resident flora, and pathogens must be isolated from this bacterial competition. Selective media contain compounds, such as chemicals (selenite F), dyes (crystal violet) or mixtures of antibiotics (lincomycin, amphotericin B, colistin and trimethoprim in New York City medium) that selectively inhibit the normal flora, enabling the pathogen to grow through. These complex media often require careful preparation. Although selective agents have their maximum effect on the unwanted organisms, some inhibition of the target organism inevitably occurs. Therefore, an enrichment medium should also be inoculated so that small numbers of pathogens can be detected.

Selective cultures, e.g. sputum, stool or throat-swab specimens aim to identify, for instance, *Haemophilus* spp., *Salmonella* spp. or *Streptococcus* spp. from among normal flora. Antibiotics, dyes, antiseptics, chemicals and bile salts are examples of substances used in selective bacteriological media. Culture of pathogens from sites with normal flora requires selection, and from sterile sites requires enrichment.

Indicator Media

Indicator media are used to identify colonies of pathogens among the mixture of organisms able to grow on the selective medium. Many indicator media are also selective. An example of a selective indicator medium is MacConkey's agar, which uses bile salts to select for bile-tolerant enteric organisms. It also contains lactose and the indicator neutral red. Colonies of lactose-fermenting organisms produce

Table 2.3.2: Examples of selective media for bacteriological culture from sites containing a normal flora.			
Medium	*Selective agent*	*Specimen*	*Organism/s sought*
Crystal violet-blood agar	Crystal violet	Throat swab	*Streptococcus pyogenes*
Deoxycholate citrate	Deoxycholate	Feces	*Salmonella, Shigella*
New York city medium	Lincomycin, colistin, amphotericin, trimethoprim	Urethral or cervical	*Neisseria gonorrhoeae*
Selenite broth	Selenite F	Feces	*Salmonella*
Sabouraud's agar	High dextrose content	Many	Fungi

lactic acid, and are colored red by the neutral red indicator. Some enteric pathogens, such as *Salmonella* and *Shigella*, are usually non-lactose fermenters, which produce easily identified, colorless colonies in this medium.

Indicator medium (often combined with selective function), e.g. MacConkey:
- Selects with bile salts
- Indicates lactose fermentation with pH indicator.

There are many liquid indicator media, containing different sugars or other substrates, such as urea and citrate. They also contain indicator dyes, which change color when bacterial metabolic products of the substrates alter the pH of the medium. Thus, an organism that ferments a particular sugar lowers the pH, or one that metabolizes urea produces ammonia and raises the pH. These indicator media are usually used in banks of tests that allow identification of an organism by its biochemical profile. Prepared sets of mini-culture vials are commercially available.

AUTOMATION

Bacterial culture is time-consuming and labor-intensive. Before automation of blood cultures became widely available, it was necessary to subculture each bottle manually, after 12, 24 and 48 hours, and later, as necessary. Nowadays, bacterial growth is detected by the microbial production of carbon dioxide, or changes in the electrical impedance of the medium, indicating the need for subculture. These detection systems provide continuous monitoring of blood culture bottles, allowing earlier subculture, identification and testing of pathogens. Such methods have been adapted to *Mycobacterium*, reducing the time taken to detect a positive culture from a mean of 5 weeks to 2 weeks or less. Some automated systems can analyze the results of multiple biochemical tests on duplicated isolates. The pattern of results is compared with a computer database to permit species identification. These systems usually include a battery of antibiotic susceptibility tests. All of these "intelligent" systems allow the operator to choose result profiles that, for example, permit identification of expanded spectrum beta-lactamase producers.

Automation in Blood Culture and Susceptibility Testing

A clinically suspected infection is ultimately confirmed by isolation or detection of the infectious agent. Subsequent identification of the microorganism and antibiotic susceptibility tests further guide effective antimicrobial therapy. Bloodstream infection is the most severe form of infection and is frequently life-threatening, and blood culture to detect circulating microorganisms has been the

diagnostic standard. Much of the scientific and technologic advances in blood culture were made from the 1970s to 1990s; continuous monitoring of blood cultures offers the potential for a more rapid diagnosis of septicemia.

The performance of different automated systems is influenced by several key variables, including volume of the blood sample, the use of resins, shaking to increase the recovery of aerobic microorganisms, duration of incubation and final subculture. The Bactec, BacT/Alert, BioArgos and environmental sample processor systems are recognized automated system worldwide. Oxoid automated septicemia investigation system, a new automated blood culture system, based on continuous monitoring has been introduced very recently in the clinical laboratory facility.

The sensitivity of an isolate to a particular antibiotic is measured by establishing the minimum inhibitory concentration or breakpoint, this is the lowest concentration (conventionally tested in doubling dilutions) of antibiotic at which an isolate cannot produce visible growth after overnight incubation.

For laboratories conducting a large number of assays there are fully automated systems which are widely used, these normally combine identification with sensitivity testing and as the whole test is set-up and read automatically, not only is the workload reduced but also the result is less subjective, more reproducible. Results are usually faster, with same day results possible as the instruments monitor growth by taking continuous readings and base results on growth kinetics. Whilst automated systems have many advantages, they can be less flexible in terms of the choice of antibiotics available, consumable costs are usually higher and equipment costs need to be met.

For both the semiautomated zone readers and the fully automated identification and susceptibility systems, the data collected can be assessed by expert or smart software systems for interpretation, highlighting unusual anomalous results, suggesting other possible antibiotics to try and can be exported to other laboratory information management systems for further reporting.

LIMITATIONS OF CULTURE

The main limitation of bacterial culture is the time required for incubation. For ill, infected patients requiring immediate treatment, decisions on initial therapy must be made based on the clinical features of the case, plus rapid microscopical examination and hematological or biochemical results. Culture is valuable for confirmation or rebuttal of a diagnosis, and particularly for revealing unusual or unexpected organisms, or unusual antibiotic susceptibility patterns. The initial therapy in such cases may need modification when the culture result is available. Even in dangerously ill patients, the bacterial load in easily obtained specimens may be very small. Treating the patient with antibiotics before taking cultures may lead to falsely negative culture results. The main reason for performing culture is to identify the infecting pathogen. The likely course of disease and treatment response can then be predicted from our knowledge of the organism's behavior. As antibiotic resistance is becoming more common, culture allows the susceptibility pattern of the infecting organism to be determined. However, molecular methods are now increasingly used to predict bacterial antibiotic susceptibility, and are already the standard way of predicting viral susceptibility. Culture has an important epidemiological purpose, not related to the treatment of individual patients. Most cases of acute diarrhea could be managed properly without microbial culture. The isolation of the same *Salmonella* spp. from several individuals, however, might prompt a search for a common source, such as a contaminated food. Similarly, the isolation of a toxigenic strain of *Corynebacterium diphtheriae* from a throat swab should prompt immediate surveillance and control measures among the patient's contacts.

SCREENING

Microbiological culture can be used to screen patients and healthcare workers for colonization with pathogens such as *Streptococcus pyogenes* or epidemic methicillin-resistant *Staphylococcus aureus* (MRSA). It can allow a prompt response to the presence, in a hospital setting, of dangerous or difficult-to-treat organisms, such as multiple drug resistant *Acinetobacter baumannii*.

ANTIMICROBIAL SUSCEPTIBILITY TESTING

Testing antimicrobial susceptibility is an important function of the microbiology laboratory. Apart from confirming expected results, it is valuable when infecting pathogens have unpredictable antimicrobial susceptibilities. This is especially true of Enterobacteriaceae, among which multidrug resistance easily develops and spreads in the hospital environment. In some geographical areas *Salmonella* may be resistant to most of the commonly used therapeutic agents. Strains of *Streptococcus pneumoniae*, previously sensitive to many antimicrobials, have recently developed resistance to penicillin and other drugs, making empirical therapy difficult. Almost all currently available methods of antimicrobial susceptibility testing depend on isolation of the organism, followed by reculture of the pure growth in the presence of antimicrobial agents. Minimum inhibitory concentration-based susceptibility testing is introduced either by E-test or automated systems like Vitek 2, Phoenix or Trek system. Identification of extended-spectrum beta-lactamase, New Delhi metallo-beta-lactamase, MRSA or pan-resistant pseudomonas can be done by interpretation of susceptibility toward specific antimicrobial disk or automated identification systems only.

Laboratory Aids for Selection of Antimicrobial Therapy

The antimicrobial drugs used previously on the basis of "best guess". Before administration of these drugs proper sample are obtained for proper isolation of the causative agent/s and drug susceptibility test which necessitate the selection of a different drug which is optimally effective. The commonly performed drug susceptibility test is done by disk diffusion method of Kirby Bauer. The choice of drug to be included in a routine susceptibility test battery should be based on the susceptibility pattern of isolates in the laboratory, the type of infection (community acquired or nosocomial), source of infection and the cost efficacy analysis for the patient population. Nowadays, instead of disk diffusion test, a new semiquantitative Minimum inhibitory concentration (MIC) test procedure is gaining popularity. The MIC provides better estimate of the probable amount of drug necessary to inhibit the growth of the microorganism in vivo and thus helps in gauging the dosage regimen necessary for the patient.

Clinical microbiology laboratories perform disk diffusion test and test based on determining the MIC and interpret the results using the guidelines established by Clinical Laboratory Standard Institute (CLSI) located in Wayne, Pensylvania.

TYPING MICROORGANISMS

Typing is the use of further identification methods to distinguish between strains of organisms within the same species.

For most clinical purposes, it is sufficient to identify the genus or species of an infecting organism. Further characterization is desirable when, for example, increased numbers of *Salmonella typhimurium* infections could be caused by different strains of this common pathogen. Showing that the strains are identical, by typing, proves that the cases represent an outbreak. An effective typing system divides a species of microorganism into sufficient different groups to be epidemiologically discriminating. For example, a system separating a species into only six groups would not be useful, nor would a system that placed all the common strains in the same group. Typing methods should be reproducible so that results from one laboratory can be compared with those of another. They should also be simple to perform, as delay in receiving results hinders early control of an outbreak. Finally, typing should be inexpensive. The results of typing should also be "portable" so that they can be used by anyone with access to computers.

Methods of Typing Microorganisms

Methods of typing are numerous, ranging from simple biochemical to complex genetic characterization.

Simple Laboratory Typing

Simple phenotypic markers can indicate that isolates are probably identical, but are not sufficiently discriminating to ensure certainty. There are a wide range of phenotypic typing methods, including biochemical activity, serology and phage typing, which are often used in combination. Such methods are being increasingly superseded by genetic methods.

Serological Typing

Many laboratories still type enteric pathogens, such as *Shigella flexneri* or *Salmonella* using sets of antisera *raised* in mice or guinea pigs. Serological typing is performed by suspending a pure growth of the organism in a drop of antiserum on a glass slide and mixing them with a rocking movement of the slide. The development of agglutination indicates that the organism carries the antigen specific to the antiserum used.

Phage Typing

Many bacteriophages lyse the bacteria they infect as part of their life cycle (this is known as a lytic cycle). Different strains of an organism have different sensitivities to the phages that commonly infect the species. This property is still used to type *Salmonella* spp.

Molecular Methods

Many molecular typing methods are now used in clinical and research practice, much improving our ability to follow outbreaks and to study the epidemiology of infection.

Nucleic Acid Typing

Nucleic acid typing methods use the activity of endo-nuclease enzymes to split the genome into a characteristic range of different sized fragments. Genomic or Plasmid deoxyribonucleic acid (DNA), or ribosomal ribonucleic acid (rRNA), is harvested from the test organisms and digested with restriction endonucleases. The resulting fragments are then separated by electrophoresis or pulsed-field gel electrophoresis, to produce a pattern of bands. The variation in band patterns is called restriction fragment length polymorphism. This method can be varied by using a frequently cutting enzyme, and using electrophoresis to demonstrate the presence of repetitive sequences of DNA. Many organisms have characteristic sequences, or numbers of repeats. This approach has proved to be especially valuable in typing *Mycobacterium tuberculosis*. Larger DNA fragments can be investigated by Southern blotting. In this process the DNA is bound to a membrane; after washing, a nucleic acid probe is added and if homologous sequences are present on the membrane it will bind to them. Detecting the presence of bound probe will confirm the presence of the DNA fragments from the pathogen. The problem of gel-to-gel variation is reduced by computer programs that "normalize" the gels, then store and compare the data, making it possible to build-up enormous international databases that can be used to track the transmission of organisms across the globe.

Polymerase Chain Reaction-based Methods

Polymerase chain reaction methods can be used to generate DNA, from a variable gene or genes, for RFLP typing. Genes encoding the variable outer membrane proteins of *Neisseria* may be analyzed in this way. Bacterial genomes contain many repetitive nucleotide sequences. Polymerase chain reaction method protocols can be designed to amplify parts of these, allowing organisms that possess them to be typed using PCR-based methods. Primers are designed to permit amplification of the repeated element, and characterize the organism by the number of copies that it possesses. The number of each of the identified repeating elements possessed by the strain is collated into a score (strain number) for that strain. The strain number can be compared with numbers for other known strains in a relational database.

Multilocus Sequence Typing

In multilocus sequence typing, a number of genes related to physiological bacterial functions are chosen. These genes should usually be "stable", and not under selective pressure, so their sequence changes slowly. Approximately 450 bp segments of the genes are amplified and sequenced. The sequences of the selected genes are compared with an international central database using the internet. Any single base pair change in any of the genes is defined as a new allele: only those strains with exactly the same sequence are considered identical.

Methods of Typing Bacteria

- Serotyping
- Phage typing
- Restriction fragment length polymorphism typing
- Polymerase chain reaction-based methods:
  - Outer membrane protein genes
  - Repetitive elements
  - Multilocus sequence typing

CULTURE OF PROTOZOA AND HELMINTHS

Culture of protozoa and helminths tends to be difficult and often produces no better diagnostic yield than microscopy. For many organisms, such as *Cryptosporidium parvum*, only one stage in the life cycle may be cultivable. In some, such as *Strongyloides stercoralis*, the conditions of the natural environment can be reproduced in the laboratory.

Using activated charcoal as a culture medium, larvae in fecal specimens will mature and multiply. Trophozoites of *Plasmodium falciparum* can be cultured in banked red blood cells, enabling direct testing of sensitivity to antimalarial agents. Although relatively simple, this technique is inappropriate for routine diagnosis, as direct microscopy is sufficiently sensitive to detect clinically significant parasitemia. Similarly, amebae can be cultured in solid media if certain bacteria are included, but simple microscopy provides accurate and rapid diagnosis, and culture remains a research procedure. The promastigote stage of *Leishmania* can be cultured in artificial media. To achieve culture of the amastigote, or tissue stage, material must be inoculated into isolated peripheral blood macrophages or macrophage cell lines.

TISSUE CULTURE FOR VIRUSES AND OTHER INTRACELLULAR ORGANISMS

Viruses and *Chlamydiae* are obligatory intracellular pathogens, so culture for these organisms must be performed in living cells or tissues. Cells are usually prepared as monolayer on to which the prepared specimen is inoculated. Some cells used for culture are "primary cultures", extracted directly from an organ, as with fetal lung cells. Primary cell lines can be propagated for up to 50 generations, and are essential for isolation of some viruses. Alternatively, continuous cell lines can be subcultured indefinitely. Cell cultures are maintained at 37°C in an atmosphere of increased humidity and carbon dioxide. Cultured viruses infect the cells and take over their metabolic processes as they do in the human host. The cell monolayer is inspected at intervals for the presence of viral damage to the cells [the cytopathic effect (CPE)]. Some viruses may be presumptively identified by their distinctive CPE; for example, measles virus produces multinucleated giant cells. Some viruses produce no visible CPE but growth of the virus is detected by, for example, adherence of red cells to viral hemagglutinin molecules expressed on the cells. Viral antigens can be directly demonstrated by fixing the cell monolayer and using immunofluorescence staining techniques.

Evidence of Virus Growth in Cell Cultures

- Cytopathic effect
- Hemagglutination
- Antigen detection
- Electron microscopy.

Virus Neutralization

Identification of virus isolates can be achieved by lysing the cells of the monolayer and visualizing the virus under the electron microscope. Alternatively, inhibition of subculture by specific antibodies can be used to identify the species. This is known as virus neutralization.

SEROLOGY IN THE DETECTION OF INFECTION

Serological techniques depend on the interaction between antigen and specific antibody. They are of particular value when the pathogen is difficult or impossible to culture, or is dangerous to handle in hospital laboratories. The process can be divided into two parts: (i) the antigen–antibody interaction and (ii) the demonstration of this interaction by a testing process. The antigen–antibody reaction depends on the specific binding between epitopes on the pathogen and the antigen-binding sites on the immunoglobulin molecules. The sensitivity of a serological test depends partly on the specificity and strength of the antigen–antibody reaction, but mostly on the ability of the test system to detect the reaction. In older tests antigen–antibody binding was detected by observing a natural consequence of this interaction: precipitation, agglutination or the ability of the antigen–antibody complex to bind and activate (fix) complement. Some laboratory tests based on these reactions are still in daily use. Newer tests use "labeled" immunoglobulin molecules to facilitate detection. The main methods employed are labeling with fluorescein or enzymes.

Agglutination Tests

Slide Agglutination

Agglutination tests are used to identify the species or serotype of an infecting organism, by observing the aggregation of a suspension of bacteria in the presence of specific antibody. They can be performed on glass slides and are in daily use in speciating fecal pathogens, such as *Salmonella*, *Shigella* or *S. pneumoniae*.

Tube Agglutination

In tube agglutination, particulate antigens form a lattice with specific antibody in the serum being tested, and fall to the bottom of the test vessel as a fine mat (a positive result). In a negative test, the particulate antigen falls quickly to the bottom to form a condensed button. This technique has been widely used in *Brucella* standard agglutination tests. A rapid microagglutination test is still the standard test for antibodies to *Legionella pneumophila*.

Coagglutination

Specific antibodies can be attached to uniform latex particles, or killed protein A-possessing staphylococci. These particles will be agglutinated when they attach in large numbers to antigen molecules. In this way, otherwise soluble immune complexes may be detected in an agglutination reaction. Such latex and coagglutination techniques are used to detect the presence of the polysaccharide antigens of *S. pneumoniae*, *Haemophilus influenzae* type b, *Neisseria meningitidis* and *C. neoformans* in CSF, or *S. pyogenes* in throat swabs.

Complement Fixation Tests

In a complement fixation test, defined antigen is added to a patient's serum (which has been heated to destroy naturally occurring complement) and supplemented with a measured amount of guinea pig complement. When specific antibody is present in the serum, it interacts with the antigen, which activates (or fixes) complement. Sheep red cells sensitized with rabbit anti-sheep red cell antibody are added and if complement has already been fixed, none remains to lyse the sensitized sheep cells, so no lysis will occur (a positive result). In contrast, if no antigen-antibody reaction has taken place in the first reaction, the complement is still available to lyse the red cells (a negative result). The test is technically difficult and requires careful standardization.

Indirect Fluorescent Antibody Tests

Specific antigen is fixed on to a multiwell microscope slide and patient's serum added. The slide is incubated, and then washed. Fluorescein-labeled antihuman immunoglobulin is then added, followed by further incubation. After a final wash the slides are examined under ultraviolet illumination. Where antibodies from the patient's serum have bound to the antigen, the antihuman globulin will bind, and is indicated by apple-green fluorescence. Individual positive sera may be titrated. Indirect immunofluorescence is both sensitive and specific, but rather time-consuming. It is used in the diagnosis of a number of infections, especially where the throughput of specimens is small, for instance in the diagnosis of syphilis (fluorescent treponemal antibody test) or parasitic disease, such as leishmaniasis or amoebiasis.

Enzyme-linked Immunosorbent Assay

In this technique either the antigen or antibody in the reaction is allowed to bind to a solid phase, such as the walls of microtiter wells. There are many variations of enzyme-linked immunosorbent assay (ELISA) but four will be described here.

Antibody-detecting Enzyme-linked Immunosorbent Assay Tests

In an antibody-detecting ELISA, specific antigen is coated on to the wells of a microtiter ELISA plate. The patient's serum is added and any specific antibody binds to the antigen (antibody-capture). The plates are then washed and enzyme-labeled antihuman immunoglobulin is added. Plates are washed again and substrate for the enzyme is added. The enzyme-substrate reaction generates a color, which indicates the specific antibody interaction.

The optical density of the wells is measured by an ELISA reader. A positive result can be determined by reference to control values; for example, a positive result may be defined as a well with an optical density three standard deviations above the mean of a series of negative controls. Alternatively, control positive and negative sera can be examined in parallel and a positive result is reported if the optical density is significantly higher than that of the control negative. As in other serological techniques, sera can be titrated but this is time-consuming and defeats the main advantages of ELISA, which are simplicity of performance and automation. Presence of antibody may not indicate a recent infection. If a diagnosis is to be made on a single specimen, specific immunoglobulin M (IgM) must be detected. This can be achieved by purifying an IgM fraction from the serum and retesting this in an antibody detection test. A simpler alternative is the IgM antibody-capture ELISA described below.

Immunoglobulin M Antibody-capture Enzyme-linked Immunosorbent Assay

By placing antihuman IgM antibody on the solid phase, it is possible to capture all IgM antibodies. After washing, labeled antigen is placed in the well so that if the serum contains antigen-specific IgM the labeled antigen will bind. A positive result is detected by adding substrate, when a color will be produced by the enzyme-labeled antigen.

Antigen-capture Enzyme-linked Immunosorbent Assay

Antibody to a specific antigen is bound on the solid phase. If antigen is present in the specimen, it will bind to the antibody. After washing, the bound antigen is then detected by enzyme-labeled specific antibody. The amount of antigen present can be quantified by reference to an antigen standard curve.

Competitive Enzyme-linked Immunosorbent Assay

Competitive ELISA is a technique that is particularly useful for the measurement of antigen concentrations and is also used to detect antibodies or antibiotic concentrations. Microtiter plates are coated with antibody and the patient's serum is added together with a known quantity of labeled antigen. Labeled antigen and any unlabeled antigen existing in the specimen compete for binding sites on the solid phase. The quantity of labeled antigen bound is then determined by the addition of substrate and measurement of the optical density as before. If antigen is present in the specimen, little labeled antigen will bind and there will be no color change. Results are computed in comparison with a control antigen curve. Enzyme-linked immunosorbent assay techniques utilize relatively inexpensive reagents and simple, inexpensive detection systems. They readily lend themselves to automation and the reagents have a long shelf life. Enzyme-linked immunosorbent assays are therefore widely applied in the diagnosis of bacterial, parasitic and viral infections.

WESTERN BLOTTING (IMMUNOBLOTTING)

Microbial proteins can be separated by sodium dodecyl sulfate-polyacrylamide gel electrophoresis and transferred electrophoretically to a nitrocellulose membrane. Strips of the membrane are exposed to the patient's diluted serum, so that any antibodies specific to microbial proteins are bound, and can be detected using enzyme-labeled antihuman antibodies. The pattern of antibody recognition can be used to confirm a diagnosis and to demonstrate the stage of disease by the repertoire of antibody specificities that the patient has developed. This is useful in the diagnosis of Lyme disease, in which simpler serological techniques are unreliable. It is also used in the study of human immunodeficiency virus (HIV) seroconversion illnesses.

MOLECULAR AMPLIFICATION METHODS

Polymerase Chain Reaction

In a polymerase chain reaction (PCR), a reaction mixture consists of the specimen together with a pair of primers (short sequences of nucleotides specific for a nucleic acid sequence of the pathogen sought). Nucleotides and Taq polymerase (an enzyme that catalyzes the construction of DNA but is stable at high temperatures) are added. The reaction mixture is heated, to separate all DNA strands. The primers bind to their target sequences, if they exist in the specimen, and are then annealed by cooling the mixture. The Taq polymerase adds nucleotides to make double-stranded DNA fragments. At the end of one cycle there are therefore two copies of the nucleic acid sequences bound by the primers. The cycle of temperature manipulations is repeated, allowing exponential multiplication of these sequences. In positive reactions, the amplified sequences are detected by a variety of methods including the characteristic size of the product, or by hybridization.

A range of different nucleic acid amplification tests (NAAT) have followed the development of PCR. These use different reaction procedures, which all result in amplifying the target nucleic acid DNA. Nucleic acid amplification tests methods can be modified to demonstrate viral RNA by using reverse transcriptase to make DNA, which is then amplified in the usual way. It has been applied to the diagnosis of many viral diseases, including HIV, cytomegalovirus and some, such as hepatitis C, whose agent cannot be cultivated. Nucleic acid amplification test methods have transformed viral diagnosis, allowing rapid detection of many pathogens. It is also transforming other disciplines in microbiology.

A most important development has been the introduction of "real time" NAAT. This uses an amplification process that incorporates labeled primers that, although varying between different test platforms, permit measurement of the product as it forms. Once the signal level passes a preset threshold the test is positive. The specificity can be checked by testing the "melting point" of the product. As well as significantly increasing the speed of testing, the time at which the specimen signals positive is directly proportional to the bacterial or viral number in the original specimen. This allows rapid, accurate monitoring of antiretroviral therapy and is helpful in deciding the significance of positive viral NAAT. For many pathogens NAAT are significantly more sensitive than conventional culture methods, improving the diagnostic rate. An example of this is Chlamydia diagnosis, where the increased sensitivity of NAAT allows effective screening, using noninvasive specimens such as urine. Rapid positive detection could be used to select specimens for culture, and also allowing the microbiologist to determine susceptibility of the organism. Other advantages are the availability of a rapid negative for many specimens, and species identification for many positive samples.

Applications of Molecular Amplification Methods

Detection of Pathogens that Grow Slowly or that cannot be Cultured

A major advantage of NAAT is that they avoid the need to await growth of the organism in culture. This is especially important for virology where tissue culture is complex, expensive and slow and many common viruses cannot readily be cultured. *Tropheryma whippelei*, the causative bacterium of Whipple's disease, was first identified by the use of 16S rRNA gene NAAT, which remains the diagnostic method of choice. Tuberculosis can be reliably diagnosed by NAAT in one day, compared to the many weeks required for culture. Nucleic acid amplification tests methods obviate the need for culture of dangerous organisms in the diagnosis of Lassa fever or anthrax. They have also been adapted for detection of bioterrorist attacks by allowing workers to detect suspected organisms in minutes using hand-held devices.

Use of Nucleic Acid Amplification Tests in Routine Bacteriology

One of the disadvantages of NAAT is that it only detects the organisms that match the chosen test. In clinical practice, one of the ranges of organisms may be causing the patient's illness, and it would be impractical to apply numerous specific NAAT to search for them all. Ribosomal RNA genes (16S in bacteria, 18S in fungi) are highly conserved with stretches of variability. Primers designed for the constant regions can allow amplification of segments, including the interspersed variable regions. Sequencing the resulting products and comparing them with databases allows the infecting species to be identified. However, if more than one organism is present, the mixed sequence is jumbled and unreadable. When this happens the initial reaction products can be cloned and the "nonsense" rRNA gene inserted into an *E. coli* vector. The *E. coli* will "sort out" any functional rRNA sequences. On culturing the *E. coli*, random colonies can be picked for re-examination of the rRNA, and the new PCR products can be sequenced for comparison with the rRNA database.

SUSCEPTIBILITY TESTING

The molecular basis of drug resistance is now becoming understood. For some organisms the presence of a particular gene is associated with resistance to antimicrobial agents, for example the Pfmdr gene in multidrug-resistant *P. falciparum*. HIV readily mutates to resistance, and the nucleotide sequence of the affected genes (protease and reverse transcriptase genes) can confirm the resistance and indicate which other drugs may also be affected. High density DNA "arrays" can identify patterns of relevant genes in a microorganism, in a single procedure.

Several research groups are studying their use for detecting an organism's range of drug-resistance genes.

Response to Treatment

Amplification techniques can be useful in showing the early response to treatment. Examples include their use in measuring the response to antituberculosis therapy; the number of organisms in a respiratory sample can be estimated, using limiting-dilution PCR (as the number of organisms falls, negative results are obtained after fewer dilutions). A quicker alternative is to detect bacterial mRNA, which is short-lived and only present in viable bacteria. The presence of specific mRNA implies the presence of viable organisms allowing the success or failure of therapy to be judged. In managing HIV and hepatitis C infections, PCR is used to quantify the number of viral genome copies in the serum (viral load). The progress of treatment can be followed by serial measurements.

CONCLUSION

An important skill in clinical infectious diseases and microbiology is the choosing of appropriate diagnostic investigations. Molecular diagnostic techniques now provide microbiologists with the possibility of providing a diagnosis more rapidly than was possible with culture-based methods. It must be remembered that timely and accurate diagnosis depends on obtaining the correct specimen, at the optimum time of collection. Specimens must be transported to the laboratory quickly and in conditions that maintain the viability of the organisms present or the integrity of the antigen or DNA sought. In the laboratory the correct diagnostic method must be used and the results effectively communicated to the doctor managing the case. This process depends on close cooperation between clinician, microbiologist and laboratory scientists.

BIBLIOGRAPHY

1. Australian Medicines Handbook Pvt Ltd. (In): Ryan KJ, Ray CG (Eds). Sherris Medical Microbiology, 4th edition. New York: McGraw Hill; 2004. pp.556;566-9.
2. Cheesbrough M. Medical Laboratory Manual for Tropical Countries., Microbiology and AIDS Supplement. Tropical Health Technology. 1991;2:479.
3. Cimolai N. Laboratory Diagnosis of Bacterial Infections, 1st edition. 2001.
4. Courcol RJ, Duhamel M, Decoster A. BioArgos: a fully automated blood culture system. J Clin Microbiol. 1992;30(8):1995-8.
5. Forbes BA, Sahm DF, Weissfeld AS. Immunochemical methods used for organism detection. In: Forbes BA, Sahm DF, Weissfeld AS (Eds). Bailey and Scott's Diagnostic Microbiology, 10th edition. St. Louis, MO: Mosby; 1998. pp.208-19.
6. Greer S, Alexander GJ. Viral serology and detection. Baillieres Clin Gastroenterol. 1995;9(4):689-721.
7. Hawkins BL, Peterson EM, de la Maza LM. Improvement of positive blood culture detection by agitation. Diagn Microbiol Infect Dis. 1986;5(3):207-13.
8. Jones RN. Laboratory diagnosis of viral infections. J Antimicrob Chemother. 2000;46(4).
9. Lee M. Basic skills in interpreting laboratory data, 4th edition. 2009.
10. Lennette EH. Laboratory Diagnosis of Viral Infection, 2nd edition. 1991.
11. Monget D, Villeval F, Couturier C. A new automated blood culture system, abstr. P62. Abstr. 5th Eur Congr Clin Microbiol Infect Dis. 1991.
12. Nolte FS, Williams JM, Jerris RC. Multicenter clinical evaluation of a continuous monitoring blood culture system using fluorescent-sensor technology (BACTEC 9240). J Clin Microbiol. 1993;31(3):552-7.
13. Sawhney D, Hinder S, Swaine D, et al. Novel method for detecting micro-organisms in blood cultures. J Clin Pathol. 1986;39(11):1259-63.
14. Thorpe TC, Wilson ML, Turner JE, et al. BacT/Alert: an automated colorimetric microbial detection system. J Clin Microbiol. 1990;28(7):1608-12.
15. WHO Library Cataloging in Publication Data. Basic laboratory methods in medical parasitology. World Health Organization. 1991.
16. Jawetz, Melnick & Adelberg, Medical Microbiology. 25th edition, USA; McGraw Hill; 2010.

2.4 METHICILLIN-RESISTANCE *STAPHYLOCOCCUS AUREUS*: PREVALENCE AND CHALLENGES

Dhanya Dharmapalan, Vijay N Yewale

INTRODUCTION

The threat of methicillin-resistance *Staphylococcus aureus* (MRSA) has been looming large since more than a half century, and continues to be a growing concern in both healthcare and community settings. The disease spectrum ranges from colonization with MRSA without clinical evidence of disease to death. It leads to increased morbidity and mortality apart from added costs of long-term hospitalization and expensive treatment. Although lots of work have been done to understand the genetic component, virulence, pathogenesis, transmission, treatment and eradication aspects, the rising prevalence of this disease both globally and in India suggests the herculean challenges yet to be met for its control.

Evolution of MRSA Strains

Methicillin-resistant *Staphylococcus aureus* was first identified in 1960s. The myth that MRSA is a nosocomial pathogen affecting individuals in healthcare setting was broken by the reports of MRSA from the US in 1997. It was found affecting immunocompetent individuals from the community without the identified risk factors. These cases, labeled as community-acquired MRSA (CAMRSA), differed from the hospital-acquired MRSA (HAMRSA) in terms of epidemiology, antimicrobial susceptibility and virulence. CAMRSA proved to be highly virulent with striking similarity to other clonal MRSA strains. Different staphylococcal chromosome cassette (SCC) mec types are associated with hospital-acquired (HA)-MRSA (SCC mecA I-III) and community-acquired (CA)-MRSA (type SCC mecA IV-V).

Hospital-acquired MRSA are resistant to all beta-lactamase resistant beta-lactam and cephalosporins because the SCC harbors more resistant determinants. These infections are predisposed by hospitalization within the previous year, antimicrobial use in recent three months, prolonged hospital stay, presence of intravascular or peritoneal catheters and tracheal tubes, increased number of surgical procedures or frequent contact with person with one or more preceding risk factors.

Community-acquired MRSA although resistant to all beta-lactam antimicrobial agents are susceptible to drugs like trimethoprim-sulfamethoxazole, gentamicin and doxycycline. Crowded settings and poor personal hygiene have been identified as risk factors for CAMRSA. Skin and soft tissue infections are the most common manifestations of CAMRSA.

PREVALENCE

International

There is an increasing trend in the prevalence of MRSA globally. CAMRSA shows an alarming rise compared to HAMRSA which seem to remain at a stagnant level in many countries.

US and Canada

A recent study from New York in patients greater than one year reported a sharp rise from 1.47 to 10.65 per 10,000 people from 1997 to 2006. A similar trend was observed in a 12-year national surveillance in hospitalized pediatric patients in Canada on MRSA, which showed that the HAMRSA figures had relatively remained stable while there was a sharp rise in the rate of CAMRSA per 10,000 patient days increased from 0.08 to 3.88.

UK and Other European Countries

The proportion of *S. aureus* bacteremia due to MRSA rose steadily from 0.9% in 1990 to 13% in 2000; the proportion being higher in infants. The proportion of MRSA in various European countries ranged from less than 0.5% in Denmark and Sweden to more than 30% in Spain, France and Italy. A recent prospective surveillance study on children in the UK and Republic of Ireland, concluded that the overall incidence rate of MRSA isolated from cases was 1.1 per 100,000 child population per year, 61% of the children were aged less than 1 year (a rate of 9.7 cases per 100,000 population per year).

Southeast Asian Countries

Methicillin-resistance *Staphylococcus aureus* was the most frequent causative pathogen for severe sepsis in children as per the national pediatric care registry of Japan for the period of 2007–2009.

Nepal reported a very high prevalence MRSA prevalence of 45%. MRSA prevalence was 42.6% in skin infection, 82.3% in lower respiratory tract infection and 30.8% in urinary tract infection.

India

An extensive literature review was conducted on the blood culture isolates reported from hospitalized children across India over past 15 years. Of the 50,454 positive blood cultures , majority of which were reported from the neonatal intensive care units (78.7%), it was found that *Staphylococcus aureus* was the most commonly isolated gram-positive pathogen (14.7%) of which half the isolates were methicillin resistant. Around 30–70% incidence of MRSA has been reported from hospitals in various parts in India although there is paucity of data on CAMRSA. The prevalence rate may vary not only from region to region, but also between institutions in the same region.

Northern India

A multicenter study done in three tertiary hospitals in Delhi showed a prevalence of 20.6% of MRSA in children below 15 years with variation in the prevalence rate and genetic type from institution to institution. The study concluded that the dissemination of multidrug-resistant MRSA clones warrants continuous tracking of resistant genotypes in the Indian subcontinent.

S. aureus nasal carriage rate in healthy children below 5 years attending outpatient clinics of two hospitals in Ujjain was 6.3% of healthy children out of which 16.3% were MRSA.

Chatterjee et al. studied nasal colonization of 489 school children (5–15 years of age) belonging to rural, urban and semi-urban areas of Haryana using enriched culture media and PCR assay for mecA gene, colonization was found in 256 (52.5%) children. Out of these, an alarming 3.9% were MRSA.

Southern India

In 2010, emergence of MRSA gene, Panton-Valentine-Leukocidin was reported among both CAMRSA and HAMRSA from Chennai in a study population added between 12 years and 80 years. Around 57% were positive for the mecA gene which codes for methicillin resisance.

Ramana et al. reported a prevalence of 16% for *S. aureus*, 19% of which were MRSA among school going children (5–15 years) in Narketpally, Andhra Pradesh.

A microbiological study from Mangaluru showed that of the total of 83 strains of CAMRSA isolated from abscess and folliculitis, 20 were from age group 11–20 years and 18 were from 0–10 years indicating a high prevalence in the younger age groups. The rate of inducible clindamycin resistance was 15.65%.

Another study in the same year from a different institution in Mangalore reported MRSA prevalence of 29% in the pediatric intensive care unit.

CAMRSA prevalence of 16.6% was reported from Bengaluru, with highest incidence (58%) in the age group 1–5 years. Vancomycin resistance was observed in 1.4% of the *S. aureus* isolates.

Western India

In Maharashtra, the nasopharyngeal carriage of *S. aureus* was detected in 7.38% school going children aged 6–10

years, residing in urban community of Nagpur, of which 4.16% was MRSA. Colonization rate of MRSA in the pediatric population in the community was detected to be 0.31%.

Eastern India

Sikkim reported a high prevalence of MRSA with 38.14%. Of the 291 staphylococcal isolates out of 821 samples, 111 isolates were MRSA. Of these 111 MRSA, 84.68% belonged to patients younger than 30 years of age. Alarmingly, high vancomycin resistance has been reported in this study to the tune of 20.27% but the resistance was not substantiated by MIC testing.

CHALLENGES

Uncertainty of Virulence and Pathogenesis of MRSA

The role of Panton-Valentine leukocidin (PVL) most frequently associated with soft tissue infection and necrotizing pneumonia caused by CAMRSA is controversial. Uncommonly it has also been found in methicillin-sensitive *Staphylococcus aureus* (MSSA) also. The pore forming alpha-hemolysin, phenol soluble modulins (PSMs), arginine catabolic mobile element (ACME), and accessory gene regulator (AGR) have been implicated in the virulence of MRSA; however, their exact roles are still uncertain.

Diagnostic Challenge: Clinical Differentiation between MSSA and MRSA (Not Simple)

Predisposing factors for HAMRSA as mentioned earlier can give a clue to suspect MRSA in the patients in a hospital settings. But diagnosing CAMRSA and clinically differentiating from CAMSSA is a greater challenge.

Both CAMRSA and CAMSSA produce a similar spectrum of disease—furuncles, carbuncles, abscesses. Typical MRSA cutaneous lesions have been described as spontaneous tender-red lesions which progress to develop necrotic center. However, they are not pathognomic and can occur with PVL positive MSSA strains. Similarly the severe complications, like extensive cellulitis, necrotizing fasciitis, purpura fulminans, septic thrombophlebitis, pyomyositis, septic arthritis and osteomyelitis, necrotizing pneumonia, again have no particular pattern to be called the hallmark of MRSA. Recurrent (two or more in 6 months) furuncles or abscesses, or clusters of infections within a household may indicate PVL-positive CAMRSA. Also if there is poor response to beta-lactam antibiotics or use of multiple antibiotics in past one year especially macrolides and fluoroquinolone, then MRSA may be considered.

Challenge of Surveillance: Should the Approach be Universal or Targeted Population?

The increasing trend in the MRSA prevalence warrants a continuous ongoing surveillance. Universal screening although ideal is difficult in resource limited settings and passive surveillance along with targeted nasal screening of at risk groups has yielded adequate information. This approach, however, is likely to underestimate the prevalence of CAMRSA.

Challenge of Surveillance: Which Site to Sample?

The anterior nares are the most common site for MRSA carriage; sampling multiple anatomical sites increases sensitivity. *S. aureus* decolonization strategies may need to address extranasal colonization. This was brought to light by a cross-sectional study of adults and children with *S. aureus* skin infections and their household contacts in Los Angeles and Chicago, where the subjects were surveyed for *S. aureus* colonization of the nares, oropharynx, and inguinal region and risk factors for *S. aureus* disease. Here it was found that survey of only anterior nares would have missed 51% of MRSA colonized persons. Moreover 26% of MRSA isolates in household contacts were discordant with the index patients' infecting MRSA strain type. The inguinal fold may be an important consideration for active surveillance programs in hospitals.

Diagnostic Test Dilemma: Culture versus PCR?

Rapid culture methods that utilize chromogenic agar allow detection of MRSA from active surveillance specimens at 24 hours with high specificity, but lower sensitivity than conventional culture. A novel assay, the KeyPath MRSA/MSSA blood culture test, uses bacteriophages that replicate only in the presence of *S. aureus* to detect and distinguish between MRSA and MSSA in blood cultures with gram-positive cocci in approximately 5 hours. Phage amplification, in both the presence and absence of cefoxitin, indicates the presence of MRSA. But this test has limitations of low sensitivity for immediately reporting negative results. Pulsed-field gel electrophoresis is an excellent method for typing MRS PCR typing methods also differentiate MRSA strains adequately in many situations and are more rapid. Nucleic acid amplification tests, such as the polymerase chain reaction (PCR), can be used to detect the mecA gene, is the most common gene that mediates oxacillin resistance in staphylococci.

In the choice between culture method and PCR method for screening MRSA, although rapid tests saves time and allows for early detection and treatment, it also adds to cost. Hence, it has been suggested that rapid tests may be economical only in settings with high rate of prevalence or in patients with high risk of infection.

Therapeutic Challenge: Limited Number of Drugs against MRSA and the Increasing Emergence of Multidrug-resistant Strains

Resistance to clindamycin may emerge during therapy in strains of MRSA with the inducible macrolide-lincosamide-streptogramin B (MLS)-resistance mechanism. D-test which helps identify such strains is helpful in these situations. A study from India has reported 15.65% inducible clindamycin resistance, indicating B (MLS) resistance cannot be ignored and clindamycin should be avoided in these patients.

Vancomycin is the treatment of choice for invasive MRSA infections in children. Its pharmakokinetic variability, renal toxicity and treatment failures due to resistance limit its use

There are report's of vancomycin intermediate sensitive strains (VISA) and vancomycin-resistant strains (VRSA). The following definition are used for vancomycin susceptible—less than or equal to 2 μg/mL (≤4 μg/mL), vancomycin intermediate (VISA)—4–8 μg/mL (8–16 μg/mL), vancomycin resistant (VRSA)—greater than or equal to 16 μg/mL (≥32 μg/mL). Therapeutic dilemma arises with the increasing identification of *S. aureus* isolates that do not respond to vancomycin therapy *in vivo,* but are not vancomycin resistant by MIC determinations. Teicoplanin, another glycopeptide has similar spectrum of activity and is less nephrotoxic, teicoplanin resistant strains have also been reported.

Linezolid has the advantage of being available in both intravenous and oral formulations. As a bacteriostatic, linezolid is not approved for endovascular infections. Its prolonged use is associated with myelosuppression, peripheral and optical neuropathy, and hyperlactatemia. There is evidence that modification of binding site on ribosome and mediated by the *cfr* gene localized on transferable elements can explain linezolid resistance. Though presently reports of linezolid resistance are rare but there exists a dreadful potential to disseminate considering its irrational and prolonged use.

Daptomycin though not FDA approved for use in pediatrics due to limited data, there is evidence to suggest it as an effective alternative to treat MRSA bacteremia, endocarditis, skin and bone infections.

Recently ceftaroline fosamil, a novel cephalosporin, has recently received FDA approval for use in complicated MRSA skin infections in children. Only strict regulations for its use can help control development of resistance developing to this latest antibiotic.

Challenges for Control: Poor Compliance to the Most Simple and Effective Measure of Strict Handwash among the Healthcare Workers Blamed for Failure of Control of HAMRSA

Unless the healthcare workers are educated and made compliant to the infection control measures like routine hand washing with soap or alcohol disinfectant, disinfection of equipment required to be shared among patients, it will be impossible to keep nosocomial infections under check. Use of isolation method is dependent on the infrastructural capacity of the institution as well as cost factors.

Mupirocin Resistance: Another Setback for Decolonization

Decolonization therapy includes application of mupirocin ointment in the anterior nares two to three times per day for 3–5 days. The patient should be recultured following treatment to confirm that MRSA carriage has been eradicated. However, the prevalence of mupirocin resistance is alarmingly high at 6.9% as per a study from Delhi. Such a scenario will make infection control all the more difficult.

Challenges for Robust Strategies and Policy Making

Although education and infection control seem to be the best possible measures for the control and prevention of community-associated MRSA infection, the strategies have not yet been optimally developed.

Other Challenges

CAMRSA and HAMRSA: Losing their Individual Identities

There appears to be a dissemination of the MRSA infection from (or to) a hospital or community setting. A study on CAMRSA found out that three of the five MRSA isolates had features pertinent to nosocomial strains, such as SCCmec types 1 and 2 along with multidrug resistance. Due to these reasons the terms HAMRSA and CAMRSA are gradually losing its significance.

Vaccine against *Staphylococcus aureus* is still an ongoing research.

CONCLUSION

The prevalence of MRSA is high and still on the rise globally, including India. There are diagnostic and therapeutic challenges especially with the emergence of multidrug resistant strains. Robust strategies need to be designed to tackle not only the HAMRSA, but, also the growing menace of CAMRSA. The epidemiological data of the disease can vary from institutions in the same region. Policies for effective surveillance and eradication have cost limitations.

BIBLIOGRAPHY

1. Chande CA, Shrikhande SN, Jain DL, et al. Prevalence of methicillin-resistant *staphylococcus aureus* nasopharyngeal carriage in children from urban community at Nagpur. Indian J Public Health. 2009;53(3):196-8.
2. Chatterjee SS, Ray P, Aggarwal A, et al. A community-based study on nasal carriage of *Staphylococcus aureus*. Indian J Med Res. 2009;130:742-8.
3. Cosseron-Zerbib M, Roque Afonso AM, Naas T, et al. Control programme for MRSA (methicillin-resistant *Staphylococcus aureus*) containment in a paediatric intensive care unit: evaluation and impact on infections caused by other micro-organisms. J Hosp Infect. 1998;40(3):225-35.
4. Dharmapalan D, Shet A, Yewale V, Sharland M. High Reported Rates of Antimicrobial Resistance in Indian Neonatal and Pediatric Blood Stream Infections. J Pediatric Infect Dis Soc. 2017 Feb 18.
5. Farr AM, Aden B, Weiss D, et al. Trends in hospitalization for community-associated Methicillin-Resistant *Staphylococcus aureus* in New York City, 1997-2006: data from New York State's Statewide Planning and Research Cooperative System. Infect Control Hosp Epidemiol. 2012;33(7):725-31. Epub 2012 May 14.
6. Fernandoa AMR, McQueen S, Sharland M. Coping with MRSA. Current Paediatrics. 2005;15(5):7-42.
7. Fritz SA, Hogan PG, Hayek G, et al. *Staphylococcus aureus* colonization in children with community-associated *Staphylococcus aureus* skin infections and their household contacts *Staphylococcus aureus* colonization in children. Arch Pediatr Adolesc Med. 2012;166(6):551-7.
8. Gadepalli R, Dhawan B, Kapil A, et al. Clinical and molecular characteristics of nosocomial meticillin-resistant *Staphylococcus aureus* skin and soft tissue isolates from three Indian hospitals. J Hosp Infect. 2009;73(3):253-63. Epub 2009 Sep 25.
9. Goud R, Gupta S, Neogi U, et al. Community prevalence of methicillin and vancomycin resistant *Staphylococcus aureus* in and around Bangalore, Southern India. Rev Soc Bras Med Trop. 2011;44(3):309-12.
10. Harbartha S, Hawkeyb PM, Tenoverc F, et al. Update on screening and clinical diagnosis of meticillin-resistant *Staphylococcus aureus* (MRSA). International Journal of Antimicrobial Agents. 2011;37(2):110-7.
11. Johnson AP, Sharland M, Goodall C, et al. Enhanced surveillance of methicillin-resistant *Staphylococcus aureus* (MRSA) bacteraemia in children in the UK and Ireland. Arch Dis Child. 2010;95(10)781-5.
12. Matlow A, Forgie S, Pelude L, et al. The Canadian Nosocomial Infection Surveillance Program. National Surveillance of Methicillin-Resistant *Staphylococcus aureus* among Hospitalized Pediatric Patients in Canadian Acute Care Facilities, 1995-2007. Pediatr Infect Dis J. 2012 [Epub ahead of print].

13. Miller LG, Eells SJ, Taylor AR, et al. *Staphylococcus aureus* colonization among household contacts of patients with skin infections: risk factors, strain discordance, and complex ecology. Clin Infect Dis. 2012;54(11):1523-35. Epub 2012 Apr 3.

14. Nagarajana A, Ananthia M, Krishnana P, et al. Emergence of panton-valentine leucocidin among community- and hospital-associated meticillin-resistant *Staphylococcus aureus* in Chennai, South India. Journal of Hospital Infection. 2010;76(3):269-71.

15. Nathwani D, Morgan M, Masterton RG, et al. Guidelines for UK practice for the diagnosis and management of methicillin-resistant *Staphylococcus aureus* (MRSA) infections presenting in the community. J Antimicrob Chemother. 2008;61(5): 976-94.

16. Pathak A, Marothi Y, Iyer RV, et al. Nasal carriage and antimicrobial susceptibility of *Staphylococcus aureus* in healthy preschool children in Ujjain, India. BMC Pediatr. 2010;10:100.

17. Patra PK, Jayashree M, Singhi S, et al. *Nosocomial pneumonia* in a pediatric intensive care unit. Indian Pediatr. 2007;44(7):511-8.

18. Prabhu K, Bhat S, Rao S. Bacteriologic profile and antibiogram of blood culture isolates in a pediatric care unit. J Lab Physicians. 2010;2(2):85-8.

19. Ramana KV, Mohanty SK, Wilson CG. *Staphylococcus aureus* colonization of anterior nares of school going children. Indian J Pediatr. 2009;76(8):813-6. Epub 2009 Jun 26.

20. Rebollo-Perez J, Ordoñez-Tapia C, Herazo-Herazo C, et al. Nasal carriage of panton valentine leukocidin-positive methicillin-resistant *Staphylococcus aureus* in healthy preschool children. Rev. Salud Pública, Bogotá. 2011;13(5):824-32.

21. Shenoy MS, Bhat GK, Kishore A, et al. Significance of MRSA strains in community associated skin and soft tissue infections. Indian J Medical Microbiol. 2010;28(2):152-4.

22. Shime N, Kawasaki T, Saito O, et al. Incidence and risk factors for mortality in paediatric severe sepsis: results from the national paediatric intensive care registry in Japan. Intensive Care Med. 2012;38(7):1191-7. Epub 2012 Apr 18.

23. Shrestha B, Pokhrel B, Mohapatra T. Study of nosocomial isolates of *Staphylococcus aureus* with special reference to methicillin resistant *S. aureus* in a tertiary care hospital in Nepal. Nepal Med Coll J. 2009;11(2):123-6.

24. Singhi S, Ray P, Mathew JL, et al. Nosocomial bloodstream infection in a pediatric intensive care unit. Indian J Pediatr. 2008;75(1):25-30.

25. Tsering Dechen C, Pal R, Kar S. Methicillin-resistant *Staphylococcus aureus:* prevalence and current susceptibility pattern in Sikkim. J Glob Infect Dis. 2011;3(1):9-13.

2.5 EXTENDED-SPECTRUM BETA-LACTAMASE INFECTIONS

Anuradha De

INTRODUCTION

Drug-resistant pathogens are a major concern, as they carry a higher morbidity and mortality and are more difficult to identify by routine laboratory assays, which can lead to a delay in diagnosis and institution of appropriate antimicrobial therapy. There is also a growing concern regarding the lack of new antibiotics especially for multidrug-resistant gram-negative bacteria which produces extended-spectrum beta-lactamases (ESBLs). ESBLs are primarily produced by the *Enterobacteriaceae* family of gram-negative bacilli, e.g. *Klebsiella pneumonia, Escherichia coli, Enterobacter, Citrobacter, Proteus* spp., etc. They are also produced by nonfermentative gram-negative bacteria, such as *Acinetobacter baumannii* and *Pseudomonas aeruginosa.*

Extended-spectrum beta-lactamases have been reported worldwide. They have become a major cause of hospital-associated infection, particularly in the intensive care units (ICUs), neonatal units and hematology-oncology units, with the majority of ESBL-producers being isolated from critical care patients.

Overuse of broad spectrum antibiotics, especially third generation cephalosporins play an important role in the development of ESBL infections. The ESBL-producers pose a threat to treatment failure because of high resistance to other non-β-lactam antibiotics. They are also difficult to detect because of different levels of activity against various cephalosporins. Moreover, under-reporting by microbiology laboratories has led to widespread lack of awareness by clinicians.

Therefore, in June 2010, the Infectious Diseases Society of America gave testimony before the House Committee on Energy and Commerce Subcommittee on Health, on the critical need for stewardship of antimicrobials and the urgent necessity of research and development into newer therapies.

DEFINITION

Beta-lactamases are hydrolytic enzymes which cleave the β-lactam ring and are the primary mechanisms of conferring bacterial resistance to β-lactam antibiotics, such as penicillins and cephalosporins. The original method of β-lactamase categorization is the Ambler classification which divides the enzymes into four classes (A, B, C and D) based on molecular structure. In 1995, Bush et al. devised a classification of β-lactamases based upon their functional characteristics and substrate profile, a classification which is widely used now. The enzymes are divided into three major groups: Group 1: cephalosporinases which are not inhibited by clavulanic acid, the larger Group 2: broad spectrum enzymes which are generally inhibited by clavulanic acid (except for the 2d and 2f groups) and the Group 3: metallo-β-lactamases. Table 2.5.1 shows the classification of β-lactamases.

Extended-spectrum beta-lactamases are Class A β-lactamases and may be defined as plasmid-mediated enzymes that hydrolyze oxyimino-cephalosporins and monobactams but not cephamycins or carbapenems. ESBLs belong to Group 2 in the Bush-Medeiros-Jacoby system and to class A in the Ambler system.

Table 2.5.1: Classification of beta-lactamases.

Bush-Jacoby-Medeiros system	Major subgroups	Ambler system	Main attributes
Group 1 cephalosporinases	–	C (cephalosporinases)	Usually chromosomal; resistance to all β-lactams except carbapenems; not inhibited by clavulanate
Group 2 penicillinases (clavulanic acid susceptible)	2a	A (serine β-lactamases)	Staphylococcal penicillinases
	2b	A	Broad-spectrum—TEM-1, TEM-2, SHV-1
	2be	A	Extended-spectrum—TEM-3–160, SHV-2–101
	2br	A	Inhibitor resistant TEM (IRT)
	2c	A	Carbenicillin-hydrolyzing
	2e	A	Cephalosporinases inhibited by clavulanate
	2f	A	Carbapenemases inhibited by clavulanate
	2d	D (oxacillin-hydrolyzing)	Cloxacillin-hydrolyzing (OXA)
Group 3 Metallo-β-lactamase	3a	B (metalloenzymes)	Zinc-dependent carbapenemases
	3b	B	
	3c	B	
Group 4		Not classified	Miscellaneous enzymes, most not yet sequenced

Table 2.5.2: The major types of extended-spectrum beta-lactamases (ESBLs).

Types	First discovered	Characteristics
TEM (Temoniera)	In 1965 in Enterobacteriaceae but has since spread to *Haemophilus, Neisseria* and *Vibrio* species. Possibly first TEM-ESBL was isolated in Liverpool in 1982	Over 100 TEM-type β-lactamases have been described, of which the majority are ESBLs
SHV (Sulfhydryl variable)	SHV-1 was discovered in 1979 and commonly occurs in *K. pneumoniae*. In 1983, a *K. ozaenae* isolate from Germany was discovered to possess a β-lactamase that hydrolyzed cefotaxime. Differed from SHV-1 by replacement of glycine by serine at the 238 position	To date, the majority of SHV-type derivatives possess ESBL phenotype. This mutation alone accounted for its extended-spectrum properties and was designated as SHV-2
CTX-M	The first CTX-M ESBL was found as recently as 2,000 in Europe, in a solitary isolate of *K. oxytoca*. It was first reported in India from Lucknow in 2006	Mainly seen in *E. coli*, now over 50 types have been described, the most common being CTX-M 15. Most of the latter are multiresistant to aminoglycosides, fluoroquinolones and trimethoprim as well as all β-lactams, except carbapenems and temocillin

They hydrolyze penicillins, cephalosporins and monobactams, and are inhibited *in vitro* by clavulanic acid. Organisms producing ESBLs also have the capacity to acquire resistance to other antimicrobial classes such as the quinolones (ciprofloxacin), tetracyclines, trimethoprim-sulfamethoxazole and aminoglycosides (gentamicin and tobramycin), which further limits therapeutic options. Many ESBL genes also have the propensity to jump between organisms, thus leading to outbreaks of infection if this occurs in an easily transmissible pathogen.

There are now more than 150 ESBLs identified worldwide. Of these, the most common are the sulfhydryl variable (SHV), temoniera (TEM) and CTX-M types. Group 2 enzymes include the commonly encountered TEM enzymes and SHV enzymes. Other clinically important types include VEB, PER, BEL-1, BES-1, SFO-1, TLA and IBC. Table 2.5.2 shows the major types of ESBLs.

EPIDEMIOLOGY

The prevalence of bacteria producing ESBLs varies worldwide, with reports from North America, South America, Europe, Africa and Asia. Data from the tigecycline evaluation and surveillance trial (TEST) global surveillance database shows the rate of ESBL production was the highest among the *K. pneumoniae* isolates collected in Latin America, followed by Asia/Pacific region, Europe and North America (44.0%, 22.4%, 13.3% and 7.5% respectively).

Extended-spectrum beta-lactamases were first recognized in the early 1980s in the United States of America. In the late 1980s, the major enzymes appear to be the TEM and SHV types, with a minimal appearance of CTX-M types, which resulted in resistance to the β-lactam class of antibiotics. However, since 2006, outbreaks of CTX-M producing *K. pneumoniae* is being reported from Canada, including other parts of the world.

First case of ESBL in the United States was detected in 1987. The SENTRY study of US pediatric institutions in 2004 showed that 1.9% of *E. coli* and 1.1–3.2% of *K. pneumoniae* were ESBL-producers. Prevalence of ESBL-producing organisms in pediatric bloodstream infections in the United States and Korea is between 7–17.9% for *E. coli* and 18–52.9% for *Klebsiella* spp. The National Nosocomial Infections Surveillance Systems report issued in October 2004 from the centers for disease control and prevention (CDC) compared data on nosocomial infections from several centers across the United States.

First reported in 1983 in Europe, the numbers of resistant isolates appear to be rising. The striking proliferation of the CTX-M enzymes has resulted in a change in the distribution of ESBL types across Europe. Currently, CTX-M and TEM are the main types. Since 2012, community-acquired ESBL producing organisms causing urinary tract infections (UTI), especially *E. coli*, are showing a worrying rise in numbers. It has been consistently shown that rate of ESBLs in Europe is higher of that in the United States of America but lower than in Latin America and Asia.

The high rate of ESBL producers in the developing world is of grave concern. The lack of funds for effective infection control and limited access to effective antimicrobials has clear implications with regards to curbing the morbidity and mortality associated with these infections. In Asia, high rates of ESBL producing Enterobacteriaceae are seen. This was first highlighted by the SENTRY antimicrobial surveillance programme 1998–1999. A large variation is seen in prevalence rates and genotype of ESBLs. In the West, ESBL production in Enterobacteriaceae varies 5–52% and in Asian countries other than India varies 5–60%. Table 2.5.3 shows the prevalence of ESBLs in some Asian countries.

In India, 55–61% of *E. coli* and *K. pneumoniae* are ESBL-producers in the pediatric age group, and 63.6–86.6% of *E. coli* and *K. pneumoniae* are ESBL-producers amongst neonates. Table 2.5.4 shows the prevalence of ESBLs in some Indian states.

RISK FACTORS

Infections that occurred in patients who had never been hospitalized, or occurred less than 48 hours after

Table 2.5.3: Prevalence of extended-spectrum beta-lactamase (ESBL) organisms in some Asian countries.

Country	Klebsiella species (%)	Escherichia coli (%)
China	20–60	13–16
Taiwan	21.7	16.7
Philippines	31.3	13.3
Malaysia/Singapore	38.0	5.6
Indonesia	33.3	23.0
Japan	5.0	8.1

Table 2.5.4: Prevalence of extended-spectrum beta-lactamase (ESBL) organisms in some Indian states.

Place	Year	Prevalence	Population screened
Chennai	2001	6.67% in *Klebsiella* species	In children <5 years of age
Karnataka	2004	74% in *K. pneumoniae*	In intensive care areas
Chennai	2004	41% in *E. coli* and 40% in *K. pneumoniae* in urinary isolates	In a tertiary care hospital
Andhra Pradesh	2007	9% in *K. pneumoniae*	In children <5 years of age
New Delhi	2007	97.1% in multidrug resistant (MDR)-*K. pneumoniae*	In a tertiary care hospital
Aligarh	2007	34.42% in *E. coli* and 27.3% in *K. pneumoniae* in urinary isolates	Outpatient setting
Lucknow	2009	63.6% in *E. coli* and 66.7% in *K. pneumoniae*	In a tertiary care hospital
Mumbai	2011	33.3% in cases of sepsis	In neonates

Table 2.5.5: Characteristics of community onset and hospital onset of extended-spectrum beta-lactamase (ESBL) infections.

Characteristics	Community onset	Hospital onset
Organism	*E. coli*, usually sensitive to gentamicin	*Klebsiella* species
Type of ESBL	CTX-M	SHV, TEM
Type of infection	Usually UTIs, but also bacteremia and GI infection	Bacteremia, intra-abdominal, and respiratory and urinary infection
Molecular epidemiology	Isolates not always related	Isolates usually related, e.g. an outbreak
Risk factors	Recurrent UTI, diabetes mellitus, household contact of a patient with ESBL infection, previous ESBL/*E. coli* colonization, antibiotic intake within 3 months, recent exposure to third generation cephalosporins/fluoroquinolones, prior instrumentation to urinary tract. Age ≥ 65 years, male sex and travel to ESBL-endemic areas	*In neonates*—prematurity, very low birth weight, antibiotic exposure and prolonged stay in NICU. *In children*—chronic medical conditions, anatomic abnormalities, frequent hospitalizations and neutropenic patients. *In adults*—ICU admissions, renal failure, burns, chronic medical conditions, use of third generation cephalosporins, frequent hospitalizations, neutropenic patients, on prolonged and extensive antibiotic therapy, on long-term urinary catheters, have undergone organ transplantation/gastrointestinal surgery and older persons

Abbreviations: UTI, urinary tract infections; NICU, neonatal intensive care unit

hospitalization in a patient without a history of hospital admission in the last 30 days is defined as community onset of ESBL infection. Table 2.5.5 shows the characteristics of community and hospital onset of ESBL infections.

Spectrum of Clinical Disease with ESBL-producing Bacteria

Clinical disease ranges from colonization to infection. Colonization implies that microorganisms are present in the host but do not invade or cause a specific immune response or infection. Infection and colonization should be distinguished clearly.
- Urinary tract infection
- Bacteremia—primary or secondary
- Respiratory tract infection—nosocomial pneumonia or ventilator associated pneumonia
- Gastrointestinal tract infection—intra-abdominal abscess, peritonitis and cholangitis
- Skin and soft tissue infection
- Catheter or device related infection
- Neutropenic patients
- Sinusitis
- Neurosurgical meningitis, related to ventricular drainage catheters.

Risk Factors for Infection or Colonization with ESBL-producing Organisms

- *Device related*: Arterial catheters, central venous catheters, urinary tract catheters, gastrostomy or jejunostomy tube, umbilical catheters
- *Surgical related*: Abdominal surgery and emergency laparotomy
- *Antibiotic exposure*: Prior use of third-generation cephalosporins (especially ceftazidime) within 2 weeks of presentation, prior use of fluoroquinolones and trimetroprim-sulfamethoxazole.

- Reliance on ampicillin and third-generation cephalosporins for initial therapy in pediatric outpatient settings.
- Intubation and mechanical ventilation
- Previous stay in nursing home
- Prolonged duration of hospital or ICU stay (2 weeks or longer). Longer stay is associated with more severe underlying disease, with invasive procedures and with antibiotic administration
- Renal insufficiency
- Severity of illness acute physiology and chronic health evaluation (APACHE III score).

ESBL Detection Methods

Both screening and confirming the presence of an ESBL producer can be technically difficult, as well as time consuming. This can be a significant clinical problem, as time to appropriate antibiotic is crucial in the management of a septic patient.

ESBL Screening Methods

Standard disk diffusion method: *In vitro* sensitivity testing using established CLSI guidelines is carried out with ceftazidime (30 µg), cefotaxime (30 µg), ceftriaxone (30 µg), aztreonam (30 µg) and cefpodoxime (10 µg). Zone diameters are read according to the CLSI guidelines as shown in Table 2.5.6. Any zone diameter within the "gray zone" must be considered as a probable ESBL producing strain requiring phenotypic confirmatory testing.

Double disk synergy (DDS)/disk approximation method: This method uses multiple target disk with clavulanic acid disk or a single cefpodoxime disk with clavulanic acid disk. Mueller–Hinton agar (MHA) plate is inoculated with a suspension made from an overnight agar plate of the test strain, adjusted to 0.5 McFarland turbidity standard. Disk containing the standard ceftazidime, ceftriaxone, aztreonam or cefpodoxime are placed 15–20 mm (edge to edge) from an amoxicillin–clavulanic acid disk. Plates are then incubated overnight at 35°C. Enhancement of zone of inhibition is indicative of presence of an ESBL. Proper storage of antibiotic disks, bringing disks to room temperature together with regular performance of quality control (QC) on the antibiotic disks are critical to the sensitivity of the disk approximation test.

Phenotypic Confirmatory Methods

- *Disk diffusion method*: Ceftazidime (30 µg) versus ceftazidime/clavulanic (30/10 µg) and cefotaxime (30 µg)versus (cefotaxime/clavulanic acid (30/10 µg) are placed onto a MHA plate lawned with the test organism and incubated as described above. Regardless ofthe zone diameters, a greater than 5 mm increase in the zone diameter for an antimicrobial agent tested in

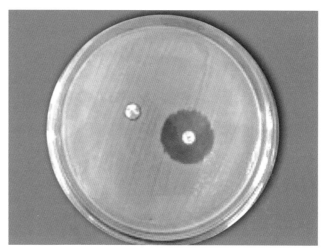

FIG. 2.5.1: Disk diffusion method—a phenotypic confirmatory test for extended-spectrum beta-lactamases (ESBL).

combination with clavulanic acid versus its zone size when tested alone, indicates probable ESBL production (Fig. 2.5.1).

- *Agar supplemented with clavulanate:* The disks of third generation cephalosporins and aztreonam are placed on MHA supplemented with 4 µg/mL clavulanate and on clavulanate free MHA plate. A difference in β-lactam zone width of greater than or equal to 10 mm on the two media is considered positive for ESBL production.
- *Minimum inhibitory concentration(MIC) method:* By ESBL E-test strips (AB Biodisk, Sweden). Two E-test combination strips, e.g. ceftazidime/ceftazidime-clavulanic acid and cefotaxime/cefotaxime-clavulanate are employed to perform the phenotypic confirmatory testing. These strips are inoculated on the surface of the agar plate and incubated overnight. Any reduction of greater than 3 log 2 (doubling) dilution is considered as positive. MIC of ESBL-producing strains to cefotaxime and ceftazidime can also be determined by agar dilution method.
- *Triple ESBL detection MIC strip:* A single strip is coated with three different antibiotics mixture (ceftazidime, cefotaxime and cefepime) with or without clavulanic acid in the upper and lower half respectively in a concentration gradient manner. When the ratio of the value obtained for MIX/the value of MIX in combination with clavulanic acid is greater than or equal to 8 µg/mL or no zone in MIX and zone obtained in MIX combination, it is considered to be ESBL positive strain (Fig. 2.5.2).
- *Three-dimensional test:* It gives phenotypic evidence of ESBL-induced inactivation of extended-spectrum cephalosporins or aztreonam without relying on the demonstration of inactivation of the β-lactamases by a β-lactamase inhibitor. The test depends on the ability of a culture of the test organism to distort the zone of inhibition around an oxyimino—beta-lactam

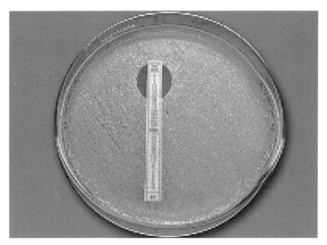

FIG. 2.5.2: Triple extended-spectrum beta-lactamases (ESBL) detection minimum inhibitory concentration (MIC) strip.

disk. This test was determined to be sensitive, but it is more technically challenging and labor intensive than other methods.

- *Vitek ESBL test:* This utilizes cefotaxime and ceftazidime alone and in combination. A predetermined reduction in the growth of the cefotaxime or ceftazidime wells containing clavulanate, compared with the level of growth in the well with cephalosporin alone indicates a positive test.
- *10-disk test:* It is done to confirm presence of ESBL in the following instances:
  - Any *E. coli* or *Klebsiella,* when the phenotype does not agree with ESBL confirmation test on Vitek or other automated susceptibility system (e.g. ceftazidime is I or R but ESBL confirmatory test is negative).
  - Any Enterobacteriaceae resistant to all drugs, except imipenem.

Antibiotic disks used are aztreonam, ceftazidime, ceftazidime + clavulante, cefotaxime, cefotaxime + clavulante, cefoxitin, ceftriaxone, cefepime, ertapenem (10 μg) and imipenem.

Interpretation is as follows:

- If the zone size increases 5 mm or more when clavulanate is added compared to the drug alone, the isolate is considered an ESBL. Only one antibiotic must be "reversed" by the clavulanate to be an ESBL.
- If an "enhancement" or extension of the zone of inhibition is seen between any of the cephalosporin antibiotics and the clavulanate containing disks, the presence of an ESBL can be predicted. This phenomenon is often referred to as the "keyhole" effect or "clavulanic" effect and is indicative of ESBL production.

- *Broth microdilution assay:* Using ceftazidime (0.25–128 μg/mL), ceftazidime plus clavulanicacid (0.25/4–128/4 μg/mL), cefotaxime (0.25–64 μg/mL) and cefotaxime plus clavulanic acid (0.25/4–64/4 μg/mL). The use of both antibiotics is recommended. The test is done using standard methods. Phenotypic confirmation is considered as 3-twofold-serial-dilution decrease in MIC of either cephalosporin in the presence of clavulanic acid to its MIC when used alone.

Minimum inhibitory concentration and inhibition zone criteria for the detection of ESBLs in *K. pneumoniae* and *E. coli* are shown in Table 2.5.6. The advantages and disadvantages of the phenotypic detection methods are shown in Table 2.5.7.

QUALITY CONTROL STRAINS RECOMMENDED

- *Klebsiella pneumoniae* ATCC 700603 is used as a positive control for ESBL tests.
- *Escherichia coli* ATCC 25922 is used as a negative control for ESBL tests.

Screening for ESBL-producing Organisms from Carriage Sites

In event of an outbreak, patients may be screened for ESBL producing organisms. Selective media for screening ESBL producing Enterobacteriaceae is by using MacConkey agar containing ceftazidime 4 mg/L. Any lactose-fermenting colonies growing on the above selective media will be confirmed as an ESBL producer by using double disk technique.

Table 2.5 6: MIC and inhibition zone criteria for the detection of ESBLs in *K. pneumoniae* and *E. coli.*

Antibiotics/disk concentration	Zone diameter for susceptible strains (mm)	Zone diameter for possible ESBL-producing strains (mm)	MIC for susceptible strains (mg/L)	MIC for possible ESBL-producing strains (mg/L)
Aztreonam (30 μg)	>17	≤27	≤1	≥2
Cefotaxime (30 μg)	≥25	≤27	≤1	≥2
Cefpodoxime (10 μg)	≥16	≤22	≤4	≥8
Ceftazidime (30 μg)	≥18	≤22	≤1	≥2
Ceftriaxone (30 μg)	≥24	≤25	≤1	≥2

Abbreviations: MCI, minimum inhibitory concentration; ESBLs, extended-spectrum beta-lactamases
Source: Adapted from Clinical and Laboratory Standards Institute (CLSI). 2011;M100–S21.

Table 2.5.7: Phenotypic extended-spectrum beta-lactamase (ESBL) detection methods.

Test	Advantages	Disadvantages	Sensitivity (%)	Specificity (%)
Standard CLSI interpretive criteria	Easy to use, performed in every lab	ESBLs not always "resistant"	NA	NA
CLSI ESBL confirmatory test	Easy to and interpret	Sensitivity depends on choice of oxyiminocephalosporin	NA	NA
Double-disk approximation test	Easy to use, easy to interpret	Distance of disk placement for optimal sensitivity not standardized	79–97	94–100
Agar supplemented with clavulanate	Easy to use, easy to interpret	Need to freshly prepare clavulanate containing media	93–96	100
Three-dimensional test	Sensitive, easy to interpret	Not specific for ESBLs, labor intensive	NA	NA
E-test ESBL strips	Easy to use	Not always easy to interpret, not as sensitive as double-disk test	87–100	95–100
Vitek ESBL test	Easy to use, easy to interpret	Reduced sensitivity	>90	>90

Abbreviations: NA, not available; CLSI, Clinical and Laboratory Standards Institute

Reporting

For all confirmed ESBL-producing strains:

- If laboratories have not yet implemented the new cephalosporin and aztreonam interpretive criteria, the test interpretation should be reported as resistant for all penicillins, cephalosporins and aztreonam.
- If the laboratory has implemented the new cephalosporin and aztreonam interpretive criteria, then test interpretations for these agents do not need to be changed.

Patients' report must state that the isolate is a suspected or proven ESBL-producer. ESBL production may predict therapeutic failure with β-lactam antibiotics.

MOLECULAR METHODS

Reference laboratories can test for genes encoding ESBLs by molecular analysis, primarily polymerase chain reaction (PCR) amplification with oligonucleotide primers specific for TEM and SHV enzymes. Amplification of the gene by PCR followed by restriction enzyme analysis indicates the presence of specific TEM/SHV derived ESBLs. PCR of specific sequences are done by using $bla_{TEM/SHV/CTX-M}$ (OPERON Biotechnologics, Germany) specific primers. Nucleotide sequencing of the PCR products can be done using fluorescent label dye terminator technique. These are usually reserved for epidemiological purposes, as it identifies the particular genotype of ESBL. Molecular analysis also allows the clones to be identified, thereby helping in controlling hospital outbreaks at both the individual and institutional level. Combination of PCR-single strand confirmation polymorphism (SSCP) with PCR-restriction fragment length polymorphism (RFLP) can be done for newer SHV variants and CTX-M subtypes. Ligase chain reaction (LCR) is used for the identification of SHV genes.

Newer technologies like modifications of mass spectrometry [matrix-assisted light desorption ionization time-of-flight (MALDITOF)] ESBLs are being mooted as quicker alternatives to conventional laboratory diagnosis. However, these technologies are still relatively new in development and are not for use in most clinical institutions.

MANAGEMENT

Carbapenems: These are regarded as the antibiotic of choice and mainstay against severe infections caused by ESBLs. They are rapidly bactericidal and demonstrate time-dependant killing. They are stable against the hydrolytic activity of the enzyme. Imipenem, meropenem and ertapenem are the major drugs available in this class and generally have equal efficacy against most bacteria. However, ertapenem is more resistant than the other two. Imipenem/cilastatin appears to be the best choice for empiric antibiotic therapy for bloodstream infections and other non-CNS infections in the Indian setting—from 4 weeks to 3 months of age, 25 mg/kg of body weight 6 hourly and above 3 months of age and 15 mg/kg 6 hourly are recommended for 10 days. It is not recommended in pediatric patients less than 30 kg with impaired renal function and in cerebrospinal fluid (CSF) infections.

Meropenem is the most active agent in Indian setting against ESBLs. Meropenem monotherapy (10–20 mg/kg of body weight 8 hourly for 14–21 days) is effective when given empirically to infants and children hospitalized with non-CNS infections, particularly sepsis and nosocomial pneumonia. It is also effective in febrile neutropenia. In meningitis, the dose should be 40 mg/kg of body weight 8 hourly.

Doripenem is a newer carbapenem and is licensed for use in several countries (including Japan, United States of America and in Europe) for the treatment of severe bacterial sepsis. It is considered to have greater efficacy against *P. aeruginosa*.

Resistance to carbapenems has been seen in some strains of *Klebsiella* and *E. coli* species, in the form of carbapenemases [*Klebsiella* producing carbapenemases (KPC) and New Delhi metallo (NDM)-β-lactamases] and there is an increasing concern on the overreliance on carbapenem therapy.

- *Quinolones:* If the ESBL producing organism is sensitive to ciprofloxacin *in vitro*, a good clinical outcome can be achieved using quinolones. In UTIs caused by susceptible ESBLs, quinolones may be regarded as an excellent treatment option. However, the empirical use of fluoroquinolones is generally not recommended in serious infections.
- *Aminoglycosides:* It can be a useful adjunct due to their rapidly bactericidal activity, provided the ESBL-producer has a MIC appreciably lower than susceptibility breakpoints. However, their use as monotherapy should be avoided, particularly in serious infections.
- *Fosfomycin:* It has excellent *in vitro* activity against ESBL-producing *Enterobacteriaceae* and can be administered orally. It is effective against susceptible ESBL-producing isolates causing cystitis and UTI and also for nonurinary and gastrointestinal tract infections.
- *Tigecycline:* It is a derivative of minocycline with a broad spectrum of activity. It has excellent in vitro activity against ESBL-producers, especially *E. coli* isolates. It should never be used against serious infections, particularly against hospital acquired pneumonia (HAP) or ventilator associated pneumonia (VAP). Reports are there of increased mortality in tigecycline treated patients as compared with other antibiotics, possibly due to its bacteriostatic mode of action.
- *Cephalosporins:* These are not recommended treatment for ESBL infections as these enzymes inactivate the drug even if *in vitro* antibiotic testing reports a susceptible organism. Indeed, such isolates should be reported as resistant. Cefepime therapy (minimum 2 g/day) has high failure rates as compared to carbapenem therapy. Cefepime resistance is more frequent in strains producing CTX-M type ESBLs.
- *Beta-lactamase inhibitor combinations:* This may be active against organisms possessing a single ESBL. While it should never be used for serious infections, amoxycillin/clavulanate may be effective in community acquired UTIs caused by susceptible ESBLs. Tazobactam has been shown to be more effective against CTX-M ESBLs compared with clavulanate, while both appear superior to sulbactam against SHV and TEM types. Clinical data on the use of these drugs against ESBLs is lacking and so using these agents would not be appropriate in serious infections.

- *Polymyxins (Colistin and polymyxin B):* Colistin is often used to combat multidrug-resistant organisms, particularly *A. baumannii* and *P. aeruginosa*. It has excellent efficacy against ESBL-producers and carbapenem-resistant organisms (KPCs).
- *Nitrofurantoin:* This can be effective in uncomplicated UTIs caused by ESBL-producers.
- *Temocillin:* It is a derivative of ticarcillin and is licensed for use in the United Kingdom and Belgium for serious infections. It is active against all SHV, TEM and CTX-M ESBLs, making it an excellent alternative to carbapenem in sensitive bacteria. It is also well tolerated. It is especially effective in serious infections, especially hospital acquired pneumonia caused by susceptible ESBL-producers. The major drawback of temocillin is its lack of activity against Gram-positive organisms, anaerobes and *P. aeruginosa*. However, in the battle against ESBL-producing infections, there is ample evidence to suggest that temocillin is an extremely useful agent.

Table 2.5.8 shows the treatment of ESBL infections.

Table 2.5.8: Treatment of extended-spectrum beta-lactamase (ESBL) infections.

Infections	Drug of choice	Second-line treatment
Bacteremia	Carbapenems	Fluoroquinolones
Nosocomial pneumonia (The diagnosis of nosocomial pneumonia can be problematic. The isolation of an ESBL-producing organism from a sputum sample or an endotracheal aspirate does not necessarily indicate that it is the cause of the pneumonia. In the absence of clinical signs such as fever, signs of consolidation or radiological changes, a positive culture may indicate colonization and may not require any antibiotic therapy)	Carbapenems	Fluoroquinolones
Intra-abdominal infection	Carbapenems	Fluoroquinolones
Urinary tract infections (Isolation of an ESBL-producing organism from urine, in the absence of clinical symptoms or signs does not require treatment)	Fluoroquinolones	Amoxycillin-clavulanate
Nosocomial meningitis	Meropenem	Intrathecal polymyxin B in CSF shunt infections

Abbreviation: CSF, cerebrospinal fluid

Management of Infections by ESBL-producing Organisms in the Intensive Care Unit

Multi-resistant infections in ICU patients are a major cause of morbidity, increased length of ICU stay and mortality. Rates of ICU infection with ESBL-producing *K. pneumoniae* have ranged from 11% to 59%, of which 84% are hospital-acquired. They are associated with high mortality (46%). Therefore, a critically ill patient with a high possibility of ESBL-*K. pneumoniae* infection should be treated empirically with a carbapenem (imipenem/meropenem). If culture results confirm ESBL-bacterial infection, carbapenem treatment should continue along with an aminoglycoside. Flowchart 2.5.1 shows the algorithm for the management of critically ill patient with evidence of sepsis criteria.

Management of Infections Caused by ESBL-producing Organisms in Neonates

Rates of ESBL-production among *K. pneumoniae* and *E. coli* in neonates vary between countries, ranging from 11.8% to 100%. Infections caused by ESBL-producing organisms in neonates are usually hospital acquired and these may involve the bloodstream, lungs, central nervous system and urinary tract. Carbapenems (imipenem/meropenem) are recommended in treatment of infections caused by both ESBL and non-ESBL producing gram-negative bacteria in neonates. Meropenem is preferred when these infections involve the central nervous system due to its lower seizurogenic potential.

Although there is in vitro activity of quinolones against ESBL-producing isolates causing infections in neonates, there is a lack of clinical data to guide treatment. Sporadic case reports suggest clinical efficacy with ciprofloxacin for nosocomial sepsis and meningitis. Side effects are limited to dental dyschromia. Ciprofloxacin should only be considered for therapy when there are no other alternative antibiotics that are active in vitro or there are severe adverse reactions with carbapenems.

Management of ESBL-producing Bacterial Infections in Neutropenic Patients

The screening for ESBL colonizers and identification of risk factors for ESBL colonization/infection should be performed upon admission for all patients prior to administration of cytotoxic chemotherapy.

Neutropenic patients are at high risk for various infections even if cultures of clinical specimens are not positive. Between 48% and 60% of neutropenic patients who become febrile have an established or occult infection, and about 16% of patients with neutrophil counts of less than 100/mm³ have bacteremia. Bacteremia due to aerobic

FLOWCHART 2.5.1: Algorithm for the management of critically ill patient with evidence of sepsis *criteria.

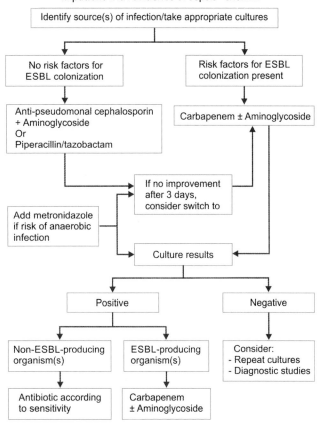

- *Risk factors for gram-positive infection present? Suspect MRSA? Add vancomycin*
- *Risk factors for fungal infection present? Add antifungal*

Criteria: Fever, leukocytosis, tachycardia, tachypnea, hypotension, organ impairment.

Important practice issues:

- *Regular clinical review*
- *Therapeutic drug monitoring*
- *Dose modification in hepatic, renal impairment*
- *Optimal duration of antimicrobial therapy*
- *Institute further diagnostic interventions*
- *Repeat cultures for unresolved sepsis *criteria.*

Abbreviations: ESBL, extended-spectrum beta-lactamase; MRSA, Methicillin-resistant *Staphylococcus aureus*

gram-negative bacilli is the leading cause of death in febrile neutropenic patients, accounting up to 30%.

Pediatric oncology patients show relatively high incidence of ESBL-producing bacteremia—about 50–56% of all *K. pneumoniae* blood isolates and about 18% of *E. coli* isolates. The mortality due to resistant organisms shows a higher trend in neutropenic patients, as well as in patients with ESBL-producing *K. pneumoniae*. Flowchart 2.5.2 shows the algorithm for the management of neutropenic patients with infections caused by ESBL-producing organisms.

FLOWCHART 2.5.2: Algorithm for the management of neutropenic patients with infections caused by ESBL-producing organisms.

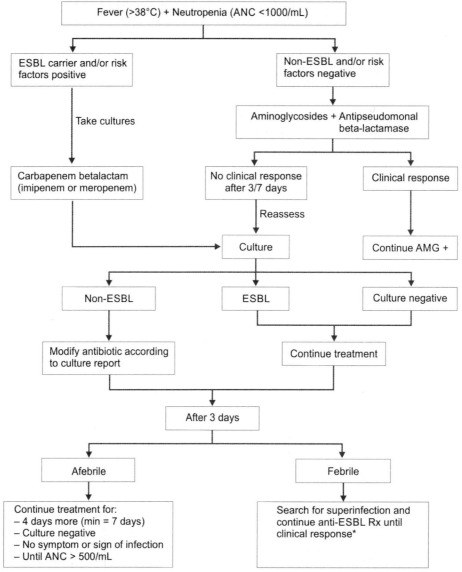

Clinical response includes afebrile, stable vital signs, no new clinical signs.

Abbreviations: ANC, absolute neutrophil count; ESBL, extended-spectrum beta-lactamase; AMG, aminoglycosides

PREVENTION AND CONTROL

Extended-spectrum beta-lactamases producing organisms can spread easily within the hospital environment. Most commonly, the transient carriage of organism on the hands of healthcare workers are implicated in patient-to-patient spread. Environmental contamination is also a potential source with sinks, baths and medical equipment such as bronchoscopes, blood pressure cuffs and ultrasound gel—all being reported as sources of infection. Small hospital outbreaks tend to be caused by a single clone and usually occur in high-risk areas, such as the ICU, neonatal units and hematology-oncology units. Large outbreaks usually involve several circulating strains of organism at one time and affect several areas in a healthcare setting.

Effective infection control requires a multidisciplinary approach and the principles are the same as with tackling any multidrug resistant organism.

- Correct hand hygiene and an adequate level of nursing staff are crucial in order to reduce the risk of spread between patients.
- Antimicrobial stewardship is of paramount importance, especially in this era of increasingly resistant organisms, coupled with a lack of antimicrobial options. Selection pressure must be avoided by judicial and prudent use of antibiotics. Although limiting widespread use of third

generation cephalosporins is effective in limiting ESBL infections, β-lactams, cephalosporins and a variety of antibiotic classes must also be considered a risk for inducing selective pressure.

- Certain medical procedures increase the risk of infection by promoting translocation of these organisms from colonizing areas. Gastrointestinal surgery, intubation and urinary catheterization are all associated with this occurrence.

Infection Control Measures in Managing Infections Caused by ESBL-producing Bacteria Surveillance

Laboratory-based surveillance should be conducted on a continuous basis to detect ESBL-producing gram-negative bacteria among patients who had cultures obtained for clinical reasons. If ESBL gram-negative bacteria are isolated from any sample, the ward should be informed promptly. Known ESBL cases at the time of readmission are identified via ESBL labels. Screening of patients in high-risk units (ICUs, neonatology and hematology-oncology wards) is optional after discussion with the microbiologist.

Preventing Cross-infection

Some degree of physical separation of patients infected with resistant gram-negative bacteria will definitely decrease the risk of transmission of the resistant organisms. Therefore, isolation precautions are recommended for both colonized and infected patients.

Controlling Antimicrobial Pressure

Antimicrobial committee should be set-up in each hospital which will provide guidelines for the use of appropriate antimicrobial agents in that hospital, thus minimizing the pressure for emergence of resistant bacteria among patients.

Education

Awareness programs should be set-up for hospital personnel and visitors about the use of proper precautions and their responsibility for adhering to them.

For Patients Infected/Colonized by ESBL-producers:
- If possible, patient should be attended last after dealing with all noninfected patients.
- Hand wash and barrier precautions should be used when handling or nursing the patient.
- Disposal of all clinical wastes in a color-coded bag for incineration.
- Aseptic procedure should be used for insertion of urinary catheters. Patients should not be catheterized repeatedly.

- Transfer/transport to other hospital departments should be limited for essential purpose only and the receiving unit should be informed.
- Patients should be discharged early (if possible) provided there is no medical contraindication.

CONTROL OF AN OUTBREAK

In an outbreak situation, it is important to establish whether the infection is caused by the same clone (oligoclonal) or by multiple clones (polyclonal) of the organism. Oligoclonal outbreaks imply horizontal transfer, i.e. person-to-person spread of the same bacteria, whereas polyclonal outbreaks may be caused by selective antibiotic pressure. This allows the institute to focus its control measures appropriately. Monitoring prevalence can control endemic situations as well as arrest outbreaks.

In the event of an outbreak—Action Group should be formed comprising of ward nurse, ward sister and patient's doctor—the infection control team (ICT).
- The group should review the ward procedures, ingested nasogastric feeds, disinfectants and moist equipments that come in contact with the patients.
- Should inspect the bedpan washer, medical equipments, gel and liquid, treatment room facilities.
- Surveillance of infected and high risk patients to monitor the outbreak (if possible), otherwise all patients in the affected unit are assumed to be colonized. Rectal swabs on selective media are used for screening.
- Patients should be nursed in a single room, or cohorting may be necessary if such isolation facilities are limited.
- The current nursing arrangement and hand hygiene practices should be reviewed.
- Unnecessary procedures, including central venous catheterization should be avoided.
- New admissions should be restricted, unless unavoidable.
- Screening of stool and urine for patients being admitted or transferred from other institutions, including nursing and residential homes.
- Review of antibiotic policy of the affected ward by restricting the use of broad spectrum agents (especially third generation cephalosporins) is advocable. The switch of cephalosporins to imipenem or piperacillin-tazobactam might curb the rising rates of ESBL-producers.
- On an institutional level, screening and isolating all infected patients with appropriate infection control practices, restricting the use of broad spectrum cephalosporin across the hospital and investigating environmental contamination are important.
- For community outbreaks due to CTX-M producing *E. coli*, frequently encountered in UTI—thorough investigation and termination of food sources (raw meats commonly), scrutinizing any ongoing environmental

risks and screening of high-risk admissions to healthcare facilities are all important in preventing spread. A word of caution here by remembering that CTX-M types are increasingly associated with other resistance mechanisms, which further limits antibiotic options.
- Infection control team meet regularly with the ward staff to review the outbreak and results of screening.
- It may be important to review the overall use of all β-lactam antibiotics and the empirical use of these antibiotics should be reviewed.

CONCLUSION

- There is no doubt that ESBL-producing infections are of grave concern to the medical fraternity, especially in ICU areas, neonatology and hematology–oncology units. They are associated with an increased morbidity and mortality and can be difficult and time consuming to identify. Coupled with the fact that prevalence rates are rising globally, including in nonhospital settings and the dire lack of effective antimicrobial therapy, the future is tremendously disheartening.
- The prevalence of ESBL-producing organisms in India also appears to be on the rise. Since ESBL-producing organisms often acquire additional mechanisms of resistance they can become resistant to many classes of antibiotics, thus posing a formidable clinical challenge to the clinicians.
- Extended-spectrum beta-lactamases-producing organisms are increasingly isolated in children. Therefore, pediatricians must be vigilant about the possibility of ESBL infection in children, especially if they fail to respond to standard antibiotic therapy.
- Presently, the carbapenems appear to be the most reliable β-lactam antibiotics for the treatment of ESBL-producing organisms. There is a dearth of new anti-gram-negative antimicrobials, although some new fluroquinolones and carbapenems (including oral agents) are in the pipeline. The use of new antibiotics is particularly an issue for children, as safety and FDA approval typically lag years behind that for adults.
- Selective decontamination of the digestive tract (SDD) using nonabsorbable antibiotics like polymyxin has been used to eliminate gut carriage of aerobic gram-negative bacilli. However, SDD is an expensive option and not without its drawbacks.
- Quicker, cost-effective and reliable diagnostic tools are urgently required.

- An effective antimicrobial policy in every hospital is the need of the hour.
- There is also a need to improve on infection control methods. Education and behavior modification are the cornerstones of improving compliance with infection control measures.
- A "magic bullet" is indeed hard to find. The future development of novel β-lactams resistant to hydrolysis by these enzymes and discovery of highly potent second generation β-lactamase inhibitors are eagerly awaited.

Therefore, screening for ESBLs in microbiology laboratories should be mandatory. Infection control measures and reduction in the use of third generation cephalosporins are critical for limiting ESBLs in institutions. Finally, it is essential to develop containment strategies to prevent ESBL-producers from becoming a common problem in hospitals and the community.

BIBLIOGRAPHY

1. Al-Jasser AM. Extended-Spectrum Beta-Lactamases (ESBLs): a global problem. Kuwait Med J. 2006;38:171-85.
2. Ambler RP, Coulson AF, Frère JM, et al. A standard numbering scheme for the class A beta-lactamases. Biochem J. 1991;276:269-70.
3. Boucher HW, Talbot GH, Bradley JS, et al. Bad bugs, no drugs: no ESKAPE! An update from the Infectious Diseases Society of America. Clin Infect Dis. 2009;48:1-12.
4. Bush K, Jacoby GA, Medeiros AA. A functional classification scheme for beta-lactamases and its correlation with molecular structure. Antimicrob Agents Chemother. 1995;39:1211-33.
5. Bush K. New beta-lactamases in Gram-negative bacteria: diversity and impact on selection of antimicrobial therapy. Clin Infect Dis. 2001;32:1085-9.
6. Clinical Laboratory Standards Institute. Performance standards for antimicrobial susceptibility testing; Twenty-second informational supplement. M100-S22. 2012;32:50-1.
7. Consensus guidelines for the management of infections by ESBL-producing bacteria—Year 2001. Ministry of Health Malaysia, Academy of Medicine of Malaysia, Malaysian Society of Infectious Diseases and Chemotherapy.
8. Dhillon RH, Clark J. ESBLs: A Clear and Present Danger? Crit Care Res Pract. 2012;2012:625170. Epub 2011.
9. Hawser SP, Bouchillon SK, Hoban DJ, et al. Emergence of high levels extended-spectrum-beta-lactamase-producing Gram-negative bacilli in the Asia-Pacific region: data from the study for monitoring antimicrobial resistance trends (SMART) program, 2007. Antimicrob Agents Chemother. 2009;53:3280-4.
10. Paterson DL, Bonomo RA. Extended-spectrum β-lactamases: a clinical update. Clin Microbiol Rev. 2005;18:657-86.

2.6 FEVER WITHOUT FOCUS

Upendra Kinjawadekar

INTRODUCTION

Fever is a common symptom in childhood, usually but not always indicating an infection. The vast majority of young children with fever and no apparent focus of infection have self-limited viral infections that resolve without treatment and are not associated with significant sequelae. However, a small proportion of young children with fever who do not appear to be seriously ill may be seen early in the course of serious bacterial illnesses or may have occult bacteremia. A very small proportion of these children may subsequently develop a serious illness, such as meningitis. Despite numerous studies that attempted to identify the febrile child who appears well, but who actually has a serious infection and to assess potential interventions, no clear answers have emerged. The best approach to the management of the febrile child combines informed estimates of risks, careful clinical evaluation and follow-up of the child, and judicious use of diagnostic tests.

Routine antimicrobial treatment of febrile children for possible occult bacteremia is not without risk. In addition to substantial financial costs, antimicrobial agents have predictable as well as idiopathic adverse side effects. Widespread use of antibiotics selects for resistant organisms. Loss of clinical improvements as a marker of natural history of infection in a partially treated child, difficulty in interpreting mildly abnormal cerebrospinal fluid (CSF) at follow-up and frequent contaminated blood cultures all lead to increased frequency of unnecessary hospitalization and increased use of laboratory tests and of antimicrobial therapy. Perhaps most important, thoughtful assessment, individualized managements and close follow-up of the febrile child may be forgotten.

ETIOLOGIC AGENTS

The list of microbes that cause fever in children is extensive. Relative importance of specific agents varies with age, season and associated symptoms (Table 2.6.1). The focus of this chapter is the febrile child with occult bacterial infection.

Table 2.6.1 shows the most common causes of serious bacterial infection in children younger than 3 months. The division at 1 month is not absolute; considerable overlap exists. It is also important to remember that certain viruses, notably herpes simplex and enteroviruses, can cause serious infections in neonates, mimicking septicemia and beginning as fever with no apparent focus of infection.

In children older than 3 months, most bacterial infections with no apparent focus are caused by *Streptococcus pneumoniae* (in unimmunized children),

Table 2.6.1: Causes of bacteremia and meningitis in young children.

Under 1 month old:
• *Escherichia coli* (and other enteric gram-negative bacilli)
• *Streptococcus pneumoniae*
• *Haemophilus influenzae*
• *Staphylococcus aureus*
• *Neisseria meningitidis*
• *Listeria monocytogenes*
• *Salmonella* spp.
• Group B *Streptococcus*
1–3 months old:
• *Streptococcus pneumoniae*
• Group B *Streptococcus*
• *Neisseria meningitidis*
• *Salmonella* spp.
• *Haemophilus influenzae*
• *Listeria monocytogenes*
Over 3 months old:
• *Streptococcus pneumoniae*
• *Haemophilus influenzae*
• *Neisseria meningitidis*
• *Salmonella* spp.

Neisseria meningitidis, or *Salmonella* spp. (the latter often occurring in association with symptoms of gastroenteritis). *Haemophilus influenzae* type b, formerly an important cause of occult bacteremia, has become rare in developed countries. Other common causes of invasive bacterial infections in children, such as *Staphylococcus aureus*, are usually associated with identifiable focal infections.

OTHER CONSIDERATIONS

Human herpes virus (HSV) 6 (and, to a lesser extent, human herpes virus 7) has been implicated as a common cause of fever in young children. Although other serious illnesses, such as autoimmune diseases and inflammatory bowel disease, can manifest as fever without a focus, they are rare and come to attention because of persistence or recurrence of fever.

MECHANISMS OF INFECTION

Newborn infants are at a greater risk of systemic infection. Hematogenous spread of infection is very common in this age group and in immunocompromised patients. However, most young children who develop bacteremia are immunologically intact. The process is initiated by nasopharyngeal colonization and followed by bacterial invasion of the blood and rare systemic dissemination. Both colonization and bacteremia are often associated with a preceding viral respiratory tract infection.

In neonates, modes of pathogenesis that need to be considered include *in utero* infections, infections acquired at delivery, infections acquired in the nursery, infections acquired in the household and infections acquired due to underlying anatomic or physiological abnormalities.

EVALUATION OF FEVER WITHOUT IDENTIFIABLE SOURCE IN A PREVIOUSLY HEALTHY CHILD LESS THAN 3 YEARS OF AGE

General Points

- Fever is generally defined as a rectal temperature greater than 38°C (100.4°F). Typically oral and axillary temperatures are about 0.6°C (1.0°F) and 1.1°C (2.0°F) lower than rectal, respectively.
- Of major importance is to identify the children with serious bacterial infections, i.e. SBI [bacteremia, urinary tract infection (UTI), meningitis, bacterial gastroenteritis or pneumonia] or serious viral illness for which treatment is available (i.e. herpes simplex infection in neonates).
- Approximately 13% of infants less than 28 days with a temperature above 38.1°C will have a SBI.
- Among children over 3 months, SBI is usually associated with a temperature above 39.0°C. In children 3–24 months who are nontoxic, temperature greater than 39.4°C (103°F) and without an identifiable focus of infection, about 3% will be bacteremic.

General Approach

During the early 1990s, specific practice guidelines were published by American Academy of Pediatrics to facilitate the initial management of febrile infants and children without an obvious source of infection. Although these guidelines remain controversial, many primary care physicians have found them to be helpful and have changed the way they evaluate young children with fever. Nevertheless, each patient continues to require individual assessment, with application of the recommendations as appropriate to the individual context of the patient. Considerations of the inconvenience, discomfort, and cost of laboratory testing and the increasing resistance to antibiotics in the community must be weighed carefully against the risk of missing a serious bacterial infection, with its subsequent morbidity and mortality. Therefore,

physicians must make the best decisions possible in an environment of incomplete certainty about the presence of serious disease. Parents need to be part of these discussions, and adequate follow-up of all patients is crucial, no matter what is decided in the initial visit. Fever during the first 28 days of life has been associated with a high incidence of bacterial disease. A temperature above 98.6°F (37°C) occurs in 1% of all newborns; of these children, 10% have a bacterial infection, usually caused by gram-negative enteric pathogens. A full work-up is indicated in these children, including a complete blood count and differential count, a urine analysis, and cultures of the blood, urine and CSF; antibiotics if administered should be started after thorough investigations including a CSF examination and until the results of culture are known.

Low-risk criteria, such as the Rochester criteria (Table 2.6.2), may not be consistently reliable to differentiate young patients with serious bacterial infection from those who have more benign disease. Although some studies have demonstrated only a 0.2% incidence of bacteremia or meningitis in neonates satisfying the low-risk criteria; others have found that up to 6% of neonates who satisfy low-risk criteria have a serious bacterial infection. Of note is that neonates with respiratory syncytial virus infection do not have a lower incidence of serious bacterial infection when they have fever. Concomitant UTIs are especially common, occurring in 5–7% of patients.

Clinical judgment and febrile infant protocols do not work in neonates. Therefore, every neonate with fever is considered to have SBI until proved otherwise.

Fever above or equal to 100.4°F (38.0°C) in infants between 28 days and 60 days of age is associated with a 5–10% incidence of serious bacterial infection. *Unfortunately, neither height of fever nor apparent degree of toxicity has been a reliable predictor by itself of bacteremia or*

Table 2.6.2: Rochester criteria.	
1	Infant appears generally well
2	• Infant has been previously healthy • Born at term (≥37 weeks of gestation) • Did not receive perinatal antimicrobial therapy • Was not treated for unexplained hyperbilirubinemia • Had not received and was not receiving antimicrobial agents • Had not been previously hospitalized • Was not hospitalized longer than mother
3	No evidence of skin, soft tissue, bone, joint or ear infection
4	Laboratory values: • Peripheral blood white blood counts 5.0–15.0 × 10⁹ cells/L (5,000–15,000/mm³) • Absolute band form count ≤1.5 × 10⁹ cells/L (≤1,500/mm³) • Less than or equal to 10 white blood count per high-power field (× 40) on microscopic examination of a spun urine sediment • Less than or equal to 5 white blood count per high-power field (× 40) on microscopic examination of a stool smear (only for infants with diarrhea)

serious bacterial infection. Instead of using single predictors, a combination of clinical and laboratory criteria appears to be more useful in identifying infants who are at low risk for having a bacterial infection. The most wellknown of these combinations are the Rochester criteria.

The management of febrile young children without apparent source of infection remains controversial, because there has been no test available with adequate sensitivity and specificity required to distinguish children with occult bacterial infection from nonbacterial illness. Blood culture is the gold standard to detect occult bacteremia; however, results are not quickly available. In children having fever without obvious focus, measurement of C-reactive protein (CRP) may suggest (but not confirm) the presence of bacteremia (bacterial infection). The critically appraised evidence is relevant, current and extendible to the Indian context.

Reactive thrombocytosis was a frequent finding in young infants with SBI. Thrombocytosis 450,000 cells/mm^3, in combination with leukocytosis, elevated CRP and pyuria, may help in early recognition of febrile young infants at risk for SBI.

A urine culture is especially important because UTIs are common bacterial infections in this age group, even in the absence of pyuria.

If the infant appears nontoxic and meets the low-risk criteria, then examination and culture of the CSF and blood might reasonably be avoided as long as good observation and follow-up can be made within 24 hours and antibiotics are not administered. If antibiotics are to be administered, then a full work-up, including blood and CSF cultures, should always be performed.

Pediatricians often use a term, "toxicity" or talk about a "toxic child", to describe febrile children who are non-specifically unwell, based on assessment of the child's level of activity, responsiveness, feeding and peripheral perfusion. The sensitivity of an assessment that an infant less than 3 months old was toxic varied from 11% to 100% in four studies. This variation may reflect the experience of the clinicians and thus be measuring their clinical acumen. Various researchers have attempted to define and quantify the signs and symptoms for clinical scoring systems to predict the likelihood of serious infection. The Yale observation score, the young infant observation scale and a Melbourne scoring system have all been evaluated. Studies have shown that febrile children who are judged as being toxic are more likely to have SBI. Large prospective studies show that scoring systems identify only 33–76% of infants under 3 months old with SBI. For older children, clinical scoring systems are even less sensitive, and there is a group of children with high fever and so-called occult bacteremia who are not judged as being toxic by any criteria. Most of these children had occult pneumococcal bacteremia.

If a young febrile child under 36 months old is judged as toxic, the risk of their having SBI is increased to the extent that it would seem wise to admit them to hospital for empiric antibiotics, pending the results of cultures. The signs of toxicity described in the infant observation scales are one or more of the following decreased alertness and arousal, altered breathing blue lips, cold peripheries, weak, high-pitched cry, and decreased fluid intake and/or urine output. These signs are summarized in Box 2.6.1.

Children older than 3 years are more likely to have signs and symptoms consistent with a recognizable illness. If they have nonspecific symptoms, an urgent consultation with a physician is probably unnecessary; however, regardless of age, all febrile children with localized signs and symptoms, such as swollen joints, meningismus, labored respirations, chest pain, dysuria, petechiae, alteration of consciousness and severe abdominal pain, should be examined immediately.

Although many febrile children do not have signs and symptoms pointing to an obvious cause, a complete physical examination may reveal important clues to the origin of the fever. As most infections involve the respiratory tract, this area must be examined carefully from tympanic membranes, pharynx, nose and lungs. Conjunctivae, skin, musculoskeletal system and lymph nodes may provide a clue for the cause of fever and usefulness of careful and repeated complete physical examination cannot be overemphasized. In India, malaria and dengue fever should always be considered at every stage in evaluating fever without focus and careful physical examination and necessary investigations should be done to rule them out.

Focus of Infection

If there is clinically apparent focus of infection, this will direct investigations and specific therapy and also alters the likelihood of bacteremia. For example, a child with high fever who has acute otitis media or acute tonsillopharyngitis is less likely to be bacteremic than a child with no focus of infection. Some children with a focus can be treated with oral antibiotics without further investigation and sent home, e.g. acute otitis media. A child who is toxic should be assessed carefully, even if there is a focus of infection, because a child with acute otitis media, for example, may also have systemic sepsis.

Box 2.6.1

Signs of toxicity in febrile young children aged 0–36 months.
Toxicity: ABCD
The signs of toxicity in infants are:
A. Arousal, alertness and activity (decreased in a toxic child)
B. Breathing difficulties (tachypnea or labored breathing)
C. Color (pale) and/or circulation (cold peripheries) and/or cry (weak, high-pitched)
D. Decreased fluid intake (<half normal) and decreased urine output (<4 wet nappies a day)
- Abnormality of any of these signs places the child at increased risk of serious illness
- The presence of more than one sign increases the risk
- The toxic child may appear drowsy, lethargic or irritable, pale mottled and tachycardic.

FLOWCHART 2.6.1: Algorithm of febrile patients with apparent focus.

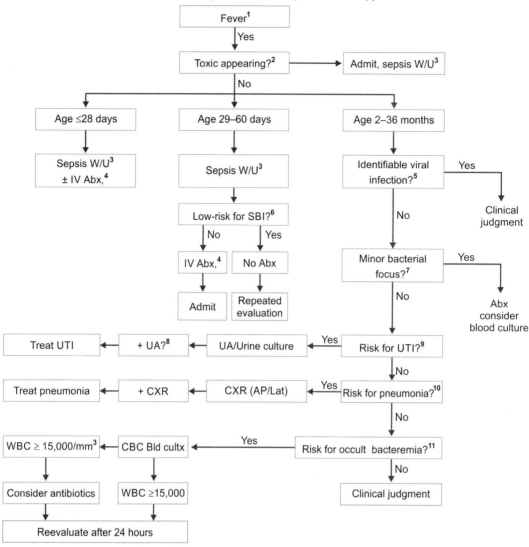

1. *Fever:* Rectal temperature greater than or equal to 38°C/100.4°F.
2. *Toxicity:* Altered mental status, poor eye contact, inappropriate response to stimuli, abnormal vital signs, poor skin perfusion, cyanosis, grunting.
3. *Sepsis W/U includes:* CBC/diff: bld cultx; cath urinalysis (UA)/urine cx; LP (CSF Gram stain/cx/protein/glucose/cell count/consider HSV or enteroviral PCR); chest X-ray (CXR) (AP/Lat) for resp. signs/sx.
4. *IV Antibiotics:* cefotaxime/ceftriaxone ± gentamicin/amikacin.
5. *Identifiable viral infection includes:* Bronchiolitis, croup, *varicella zoster* virus, herpangina, hand-foot-mouth disease, *HSV* gingivostomatitis; adenovirus (Note: URI or viral gastroenteritis have not been identified as a fever "source" in infants 0–36 months of age).
6. *Low-risk criteria for serious bacterial illness:* No bacterial focus on physical examination (excludes otitis media); CSF less than 8 WBC/mm³ in non-bloody specimen, negative CSF Gram stain; peripheral WBC less than 15,000/mm³; band to neutrophil ratio less than 0.2, normal UA (negative nitrite and/or <10 WBC/hpf), no infiltrate on CXR; when diarrhea present no heme and few or no stool WBC/hpf; reliable and easily contacted caretaker.
7. *Minor bacterial focus:* Otitis media, pharyngitis, sinusitis.
8. *+UA = (any of the following):* + nitrite; ≥ mod LE, + Gram stain, ≥10 WBC/hpf (spun specimen), ≥10 WBC/mm³ (unspun specimen, "enhanced UA").
9. *Risk for UTI (any of the following):* Female (particularly aged ≤24 months); male aged ≤6 months or uncircumcised; malodorous urine; hematuria; abdominal or suprapubic tenderness; hx UTI, genitourinary (GU) abnormality.
10. *Risk for pneumonia (any of the following):* Increased work of breathing (e.g. tachypnea, retractions), focal auscultatory findings; $SaO_2 < 97\%$ (room air), WBC≥20,000/mm³.
11. *Risk for occult bacteremia (both should be present):*
    - Less than 2 doses of HIB and pneumococcal 13-valent conjugate vaccine
    - Temperature ≥39°C/102.2°F (age 2–24 months) or ≥39.5°C/103°F (age 24–36 months).
    - Malaria and dengue should always be considered while evaluating a child with fever without focus.

CONCLUSION

Febrile children younger than 3 years without a clear source of infection have a small but important risk of sepsis and meningitis. These infections are associated with potential morbidity and mortality, even with prompt recognition and appropriate treatment. Although the risk of serious bacterial infections has decreased in countries where vaccination for *S. pneumoniae* and *H. influenzae* has been introduced, in absence of such mass scale vaccination program, our country needs vigilance and thorough evaluation of each febrile child followed by proper antimicrobial treatment when appropriate. As more data accumulate on the efficacy of vaccination, new modalities of management for fever with no focus of infection will emerge. An algorithm of a febrile patient with apparent focus has been discussed in Flowchart 2.6.1.

BIBLIOGRAPHY

1. Brook I. Unexplained fever in young children: how to manage severe bacterial infection. BMJ. 2003;327(7423):1094-7.
2. David Isaacs D. Fever: Evidence Based Pediatric Infectious Diseases. BMJ Book Blackwell Publishing; 2007.
3. Digant D. Shastri. Approach to fever in office practice. IAP Textbook of Pediatrics, 4th edition. 2009.
4. Fever without source. An evidence based approach family medicine forum November 4, David Mcgillivray Montreal Childrens Hospital, Mcgill University.
5. Jhaveri R, Byington CL, Klein JO, et al. Management of non-toxic-appearing acutely febrile child: a 21st century approach. J Pediatr. 2011;159(2):181-5.
6. Mathew JL. Can CRP predict bacterial infection in children with fever?. Indian Pediatr. 2008;45(2):129-33.
7. Nield L, Kamat D. Fever without a focus. Nelson Textbook of Pediatrics, 19th edition.

2.7 FEVER WITH RASH

M Indra Shekhar Rao, S Venkat Reddy

INTRODUCTION

An exanthem is any eruptive skin rash that may be associated with fever or other systemic symptoms. Diseases that present with fever and rash are usually classified according to the morphology of rash (maculopapular, pustular, vesiculobullous, diffuse/erythematous, or petechial/purpuric). The differential diagnosis is extensive, ranging from self-limiting conditions (e.g. roseola) to life-threatening illnesses, such as meningococcal septicemia. In children, exanthems are most often related to infection and, of these, viral infections are the most common.

- **Macule**: A flat skin lesion <0.5 cm in greatest diameter. When a macular lesion extends beyond 0.5 cm, the appropriate term is a **patch.**
- **Papule**: A raised skin lesion <0.5 cm in diameter. When papular lesions are >0.5 cm in size, the appropriate term is a **plaque** (palpable lesions elevated above the skin surface) or a **nodule** (a larger, firm papule with a significant vertical dimension).
- **Vesicle**: A papule containing clear serous fluid.
- **Bulla**: A larger vesicle >1 cm.
- **Pustule**: A raised blister containing purulent fluid.
- **Urticaria**: A wheal or hive.
- **Morbilliform eruption**: Rash that resembles that of measles.
- **Petechiae**: Small hemorrhages of skin capillaries.
- **Purpura**: Larger areas of bleeding into the skin.
- **Erythema marginatum**: A fleeting pink rash typically involving the trunk and proximal extremities.
- **Erythema nodosum**: A hypersensitivity reaction involving the subcutaneous fat, presenting as red, tender nodules most commonly over shins, calves, and buttocks.
- **Target lesions**: Annular erythematous rings with an outer erythematous zone and central blistering sandwiching a zone of normal skin tone.
- **Targetoid lesions**: Similar to target lesions but without central blistering.

HISTORY AND CLINICAL EXAMINATION

History and detailed examination will give diagnosis in most of the children. Initial evaluation includes morphology, duration, and distribution of rash and then age, family history, medications, and known allergies. A full history should include current and previous medications, existing systemic conditions, possible exposure to infection, Contact with people with existing conditions, such as impetigo or scabies, and viral infections such as chickenpox, Epstein-Barr virus (EBV), erythema infectiosum (fifth disease), roseola infantum (sixth disease), and hand-foot-and-mouth disease. History of pharyngitis (as a source of streptococcal infection)

Examination of the primary lesion should include type of rash, its extent, distribution and involvement (or sparing) of the mucous membranes.

A full systemic examination should record any associated features, such as pyrexia, pruritus, lymphadenopathy, or hepatosplenomegaly.

Generally, rash in the absence of fever or systemic symptoms is not an emergency.

For many childhood rashes, diagnosis is clinical, and tests are not routinely recommended. However, laboratory investigations may be appropriate in patients in whom the cause is not clear.

In a rash suspected to be caused by a drug, no laboratory tests to determine or confirm the responsible drug are readily available.

Few common conditions in children are discussed below based on the morphology of rash (Flowchart 2.7.1).

Some clinical conditions in children with type of rash and other features to differentiate are mentioned in Table 2.7.1.

MACULOPAPULAR RASHES

This is the most common type of rash in a viral infection, but can also occur with immune-mediated diseases, drug rashes, and systemic bacterial infections. Systemic rashes mostly appear centrally rather than peripherally. Representative viral diseases include measles, rubella and infectious erythema. In contrast, among bacterial infections, scarlet fever shows a typical systemic rash. Systemic rashes are also found in other bacterial infections, including leptospirosis, *Mycoplasma* infection, and disseminated gonococcal infection. In addition, systemic rashes are found in tinea versicolor, a fungal infection caused by *Pityrosporum orbiculare*. These rashes can also be found regionally in rickettsial infections like tsutsugamushi fever. Erythema multiforme is the most representative disease with a peripheral maculopapular rash, and is mostly seen in 20–30 years olds.

Scarlet Fever

It is most common in young children and usually occurs in the seasons between autumn and spring. A positive contact history may be reported. Caused by group A streptococcal pyrogenic exotoxin.

A 'sandpaper-like' generalized erythematous rash with discrete skin-colored papules, Strawberry tongue, pharyngeal erythema with exudates, palatal petechiae, tender cervical adenopathy. It may involve linear petechial streaks (Pastia lines) in skinfolds, particularly in the axillary, inguinal, and antecubital fossae.

FLOWCHART 2.7.1: An approach to the child with fever and rash.

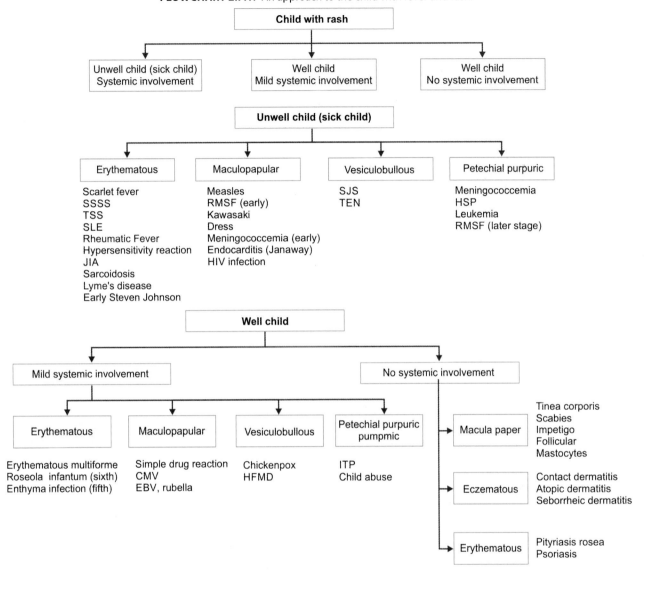

Serological investigations include rapid strep test (pharyngeal swab) or anti-streptolysin O titer to confirm scarlet fever.

Measles

Measles is caused by a virus belonging to the Paramyxoviridae family, genus *Morbillivirus*. Incubation period is approximately 10–12 days, and usually presents with symptoms of fever, conjunctivitis, rhinorrhea, sore throat and a dry cough. **Koplik spots** (gray–white papules on the buccal mucosa) may be seen during this prodromal phase. Typical exanthem of coalescing erythematous macules and papules erupts 3–4 days after the prodromal symptoms. Rash usually starts behind the ears and in the hairline area, and spreads over the rest of the skin over a period of a few days. The eruption typically resolves in the same order as its appearance, and will often desquamate.

Diagnosis is based on clinical presentation with laboratory confirmation, if necessary. Measles IgM can usually be detectable after the first 3 days of the exanthem. Currently, there is no specific antiviral therapy for measles and treatment is symptomatic. The measles vaccine makes the disease easily preventable.

Complications of measles include transient immunosuppression, acute postinfectious encephalitis and subacute sclerosing panencephalitis (SSPE). Transient immunosuppression occurs during the illness and lasts for approximately 6 weeks. During this time, an infected individual is at risk for secondary bacterial infections, such as otitis media, pneumonia or gastroenteritis. Postinfectious encephalitis occurs in approximately one in 1000 patients, and manifests approximately 1 week after the onset of the exanthema. A lesser-known entity, known as measles inclusion-body encephalitis, can affect

Table 2.7.1: Rashes in children.

Condition	Incubation period (days)	Prodrome	Rash	Laboratory tests	Comments, other diagnostic features
Adenovirus	4–5	URI; cough; fever	Morbilliform (may be petechial)	Normal; may see leukopenia or lymphocytosis	Upper or lower respiratory symptoms are prominent. No Koplik spots. No desquamation.
Drug allergy	—	None, or fever alone, or with myalgia, pruritus	Macular, maculopapular, urticarial, or erythroderma	Leukopenia, eosinophilia	Rash variable. Severe reactions may resemble measles, scarlet fever; Kawasaki disease; marked toxicity possible.
Enterovirus	2–7	Variable fever, chills, myalgia, sore throat	Usually macular, maculopapular on trunk or palms, soles; vesicles or petechiae also seen	Variable	Varied rashes may resemble those of many other infections. Pharyngeal or hand-foot-mouth vesicles may occur.
Erythema multiforme	—	Usually none or related to underlying cause	Discrete, red maculopapular lesions; symmetrical, distal, palms and soles; target lesions classic	Normal or eosinophilia	Reaction to drugs (especially sulfonamides), or infectious agents (*Mycoplasma*; herpes simplex virus). Urticaria, arthralgia also seen.
Kawasaki disease	Unknown	Fever, cervical adenopathy, irritability	Polymorphous (may be erythroderma) on trunk and extremities; red palms and soles, conjunctiva, lips, tongue, pharynx. Desquamation is common.	Leukocytosis, thrombocytosis, elevated ESR or C-reactive protein; pyuria; decreased albumin; negative cultures and streptococcal serology; resting tachycardia	Swollen hands, feet; prolonged illness; uveitis; aseptic meningitis; no response to antibiotics. Vasculitis and aneurysms of coronary and other arteries occur (cardiac ultrasound).
Leptospirosis	4–19	Fever (biphasic), myalgia, chills	Variable erythroderma	Leukocytosis; hematuria, proteinuria; hyperbilirubinemia	Conjunctivitis; hepatitis, aseptic meningitis may be seen. Rodent, dog contact.
Measles	9–14	Cough, rhinitis, conjunctivitis	Maculopapular; face to trunk; lasts 7–10 d; Koplik spots in mouth	Leukopenia	Toxic. Bright red rash becomes confluent, may desquamate. Fever falls after rash appears. Inadequate measles vaccination.
Parvovirus (erythema infectiosum)	10–17 (rash)	Mild (flulike)	Maculopapular on cheeks ("slapped cheek"), forehead, chin; then down limbs, trunk, buttocks; may fade and reappear for several weeks	IgM-EIA; PCR	Purpuric stocking-glove rash is rare, but distinctive; aplastic crisis in patients with chronic hemolytic anemia. May cause arthritis or arthralgia.
Rocky mountain spotted fever	3–12	Headache (retro-orbital); toxic; GI symptoms; high fever; flulike	Onset 2–6 d after fever; palpable maculopapular on palms, soles, extremities, with spread centrally; petechial	Leukopenia; thrombocytopenia; abnormal liver function; CSF pleocytosis; Serology positive at 7–10 d of rash; biopsy will give earlier diagnosis	Eastern seaboard and southeastern United States; April–September; tick exposure.
Roseola (exanthem subitum) (HHV-6)	10–14	Fever (3–4 d)	Pink, macular rash occurs at end of febrile period; transient	Normal	Fever often high; disappears when rash develops; child appears well. Usually occurs in children 6 mo–3 y of age. Seizures may complicate.

Contd...

Contd...

Condition	Incubation Period (days)	Prodrome	Rash	Laboratory Tests	Comments, Other Diagnostic Features
Rubella	14–21	Usually none	Mild maculopapular; rapid spread face to extremities; gone by day 4	Normal or leukopenia	Postauricular, occipital adenopathy common. Polyarthralgia in some older girls. Mild clinical illness. Inadequate rubella vaccination.
Staphylococcal scalded skin	Variable	Irritability, absent to low fever	Painful erythroderma, followed in 1–2 d by cracking around eyes, mouth; bullae form with friction (Nikolsky sign)	Normal if only colonized by staphylococci; leukocytosis and sometimes bacteremia if infected	Normal pharynx. Look for focal staphylococcal infection. Usually occurs in infants.
Staphylococcal scarlet fever	1–7	Variable fever	Diffuse erythroderma; resembles streptococcal scarlet fever except eyes may be hyperemic, no "strawberry" tongue, pharynx spared	Leukocytosis is common because of infected focus	Focal infection usually present.
Stevens-Johnson syndrome	—	Pharyngitis, conjunctivitis, fever, malaise	Bullous erythema multiforme; may slough in large areas; hemorrhagic lips; purulent conjunctivitis	Leukocytosis	Classic precipitants are drugs (especially sulfonamides), *Mycoplasma pneumoniae* and herpes simplex infections. Pneumonitis and urethritis also seen.
Streptococcal scarlet fever	1–7	Fever, abdominal pain, headache, sore throat	Diffuse erythema, "sandpaper" texture; neck, axillae, inguinal areas; spreads to rest of body; desquamates 7–14 d	Leukocytosis; positive group A *Streptococcus* culture of throat or wound; positive streptococcal antigen test in pharynx	Strawberry tongue, red pharynx with or without exudate. Eyes, perioral and periorbital area, palms, and soles spared. Pastia lines. Cervical adenopathy. Usually occurs in children 2–10 y of age.
Toxic shock syndrome	Variable	Fever, myalgia, headache, diarrhea, vomiting	Nontender erythroderma; red eyes, palms, soles, pharynx, lips	Leukocytosis; abnormal liver enzymes and coagulation tests; proteinuria	*Staphylococcus aureus* infection; toxin-mediated multiorgan involvement. Swollen hands, feet. Hypotension or shock.

Abbreviations: CSF, cerebrospinal fluid; EIA, enzyme immunoassay; ESR, erythrocyte sedimentation rate; GI, gastrointestinal; HHV-6, human herpesvirus 6; IFA, immunofluorescent assay; PCR, polymerase chain reaction; URI, upper respiratory infection.

immunocompromised patients from weeks to months after acute infection. SSPE affects approximately one in 100,000 patients, and manifests as a slow, progressive disease, which can present months or even years after resolution of the acute infection. The onset of SSPE is insidious, and psychiatric manifestations are prominent. Subsequently, myoclonic seizures usually lead to a final stage of akinetic mutism. In total, 95% of individuals with SSPE die within 5 years of diagnosis. SSPE is caused by a persistent infection of the CNS with the virus, and early childhood infection with measles is a risk factor for SSPE.

DENGUE FEVER

Dengue is an arthropod-borne viral illness. It is transmitted by mosquitoes of the genus *Aedes*. The incidence of dengue has increased dramatically in recent decades, with estimates of 40%–50% of the world's population at risk for the disease in tropical, subtropical, and, most recently, more temperate areas. Dengue fever is typically a self-limited disease with a mortality rate of less than 1% when detected early and with access to proper medical care. When treated, severe dengue has a mortality rate of 2%–5%, but, when left untreated, the mortality rate is as high as 20%.

Dengue fever is an acute febrile illness of 2–7 days duration associated with 2 or more of the following:
- Severe and generalized headache
- Retro-orbital pain
- Severe myalgias, especially of the lower back, arms, and legs
- Arthralgias, usually of the knees and shoulders
- Characteristic rash
- Hemorrhagic manifestations
- Leukopenia

Facial flushing, a sensitive and specific predictor of dengue infection.

The rash is variable and may be maculopapular or macular. Petechiae and purpura may develop as hemorrhagic manifestations. Hemorrhagic manifestations most commonly include petechiae and bleeding at venipuncture sites.

Diagnosis can be made in early febrile phase by Ns1-Ag and later by dengue IgM.

Treatment is mainly supportive care with, frequent monitoring, antipyretics, oral and/or intravenous fluid.

ERYTHEMA INFECTIOSUM (FIFTH DISEASE)

Erythema infectiosum (EI) is a childhood exanthematous illness caused by parvovirus B19—a virus belonging to the Parvoviridae family. The name B19 comes from the blood bank code, where the original positive serum sample was labeled (i.e. Row B, Sample 19). It is the only parvovirus that has been linked directly to disease in humans. Erythema infectiosum manifests in three overlapping stages. Incubation period is 1–2 weeks.

Parovirus B19 infection can have different clinical manifestations but erythema infectiosum is the most commonly recognized. A history of exposure to an infected person may be given. Erythema infectiosum is particularly seen in children aged 4–10 years during the winter and spring. In first stage, patients present with fiery-red facial erythema, which has been described as having a 'slapped cheeks' appearance. 1–4 days later, the second stage develops as a reticulate macular or urticarial exanthem and is mainly seen over the proximal extremities. In the third stage, the exanthem recurs intermittently in response to stimuli, such as local irritation, high temperatures and emotional stress. In children, approximately 10% of children have joint symptoms and affects larger joints, such as the knees, wrists and ankles, and in an asymmetric pattern.

The diagnosis of erythema infectiosum is usually made clinically. An ELISA is commercially available with high sensitivity, although false-positive results may recur owing to crossreaction to other viruses or the rheumatoid factor. PCR can detect viral DNA in clinical samples of urine, respiratory secretions, body tissues and serum.

ROSEOLA INFANTUM (SIXTH DISEASE)

Roseola infantum is caused by human herpesvirus (HHV) types 6 and 7, and belongs to the *Roseolovirus* genus in the subfamily of Betaherpesvirinae. Approximately 24% of all children with HHV-6 infection will manifest clinical symptoms of roseola. Incubation period is 5–15 days.

A high fever for 3–5 days (with the appearance of rash during defervescence), mild upper respiratory symptoms, and seizures may be reported. A generalized rose-pink rash on the trunk and proximal extremities is seen. Red papules and erosions at the soft palate and uvula (Nagayama spots) are characteristic. Cervical or occipital lymphadenopathy may be present. Occasionally, encephalopathy and aseptic meningitis develop.

Both HHV-6 and 7 are highly prevalent in the healthy population, and establish latency in macrophages and T lymphocytes. They are frequently shed in saliva of healthy donors, and the pathogenic potential of reactivated virus ranges from asymptomatic infection to severe diseases in transplant recipients.

The diagnosis of roseola is made clinically. Roseola infection can cause leukopenia and rarely, thrombocytopenia and hepatitis. Patients generally recover without sequelae. However, approximately 22% of patients with roseola may develop febrile seizures. Laboratory diagnosis of HHV-6 and -7 infections is difficult owing to the limited availability of antibody tests, problems with antigenic cross reaction and lack of understanding of the clinical relevance and epidemiology of these two viruses.

SIMPLE DRUG REACTION

A drug reaction should be suspected when a rash presents within 4–12 days of beginning a new medication.

A pruritic maculopapular eruption on the trunk and extremities may be seen. In patients undergoing chemotherapy, a maculopapular rash characterized by monomorphic erythematous papules may be seen.

Antibiotics and anticonvulsants are most commonly implicated in cutaneous drug reactions, although other drugs and herbal/nutritional products may also be responsible. Patients may have a history of medication allergy.

EBV INFECTION

Epstein–Barr virus (EBV) is a member of the Herpesvirus family, belonging to the genus *Lymphocryptovirus*. While only approximately 5–10% of children infected with EBV manifest an exanthema, if amoxicillin or ampicillin is administered, a characteristic bright-red morbilliform eruption almost always occurs. This eruption begins 5–9 days after exposure to the medication, starting on the trunk before becoming generalized as confluent macules and papules. The eruption most likely results from ampicillin–antibody immune complexes as a consequence of polyclonal B-cell activation. This consistently occurs in adolescents and adults with infectious mononucleosis administered ampicillin, but resolves without specific measures. This reaction is not considered a 'true' drug allergy and, in most children, re-exposure to the antibiotic after the EBV infection will not trigger a similar response. However, since antimicrobial therapy is not necessary for infectious mononucleosis, the antibiotic should be discontinued during the acute EBV infection.

Although approximately 7% of mononucleosis-like illnesses are caused by cytomegalovirus (CMV), CMV does not appear to give this drug-related exanthem.

CYTOMEGALOVIRUS INFECTION

In healthy people, cytomegalovirus (CMV) infection is often asymptomatic or manifests as an infectious mononucleosis like syndrome, where pharyngitis, fever, malaise, headache, lymphadenopathy (cervical, submandibular, or generalised) and hepatosplenomegaly are common. A maculopapular rash, with petechiae is seen.

In immunocompromised patients, severe CMV disease with signs of sepsis may be seen.

RUBELLA INFECTION

Rubella, or German measles, is caused by an RNA virus in the *Togaviridae* family. Incubation period is 2–3 weeks. Approximately 50% of infected individuals become symptomatic. Rubella is responsible for a mild, self-limiting illness in children. Clinical disease is more common in unimmunized or immunodeficient patients. A prodrome, including fever, headache, upper respiratory symptoms, arthralgia and tender lymphadenopathy is seen. Petechial macules on the soft palate (Forschheimer spots) are characteristic of rubella infection.

A characteristic eruption of rose-pink macules is seen. This begins on the face and extends cephalocaudally, lasting 2–3 days before fading in the same order. The typical progression is more helpful in suspecting this diagnosis than is the apparently rather nonspecific eruption.

The most serious complication of rubella is congenital rubella syndrome, which classically presents with the triad of deafness, cataracts and cardiac disease.

The diagnosis of rubella can be made with IgM antibody titers. Patients are contagious 1 week prior to the eruption of the rash until a week after the rash resolves. The treatment of rubella is supportive.

PAPULAR ACRODERMATITIS OF CHILDHOOD

Papular acrodermatitis of childhood (PAC), also known as Gianotti–Crosti syndrome (GCS), is a unique cutaneous disorder characterized by the abrupt onset of an erythematous papular exanthem found on the extremities, buttocks and face. It is a relatively common dermatosis, seen worldwide, primarily affecting children between 2 and 6 years of age.

Papular acrodermatitis of childhood was first described by Gianotti in 1953, in a young child with a monomorphous erythematous papular rash confined to the extensor surfaces of the arms and legs. After finding hepatitis B surface antigen in the serum of affected children, it was believed that PAC was solely a manifestation of hepatitis

B infection. However, subsequently, EBV has become recognized as the most common viral agent associated with GCS. However, many other viruses and infectious agents have been associated with PAC, and these include hepatitis A virus, CMV, human herpesvirus, Coxsackie virus A16, B4 and B5, rotavirus, parvovirus B19, molluscum contagiosum (MC), respiratory syncytial virus, mumps virus, and parainfluenza virus types 1 and 2.

Clinically, PAC usually presents with symmetrical monomorphous papular or papulovesicular exanthem over the cheeks, extensor aspects of the extremities and gluteal areas. Occasionally, the papules coalesce into larger plaques and become hemorrhagic or form scales. The trunk, elbows and knees are usually spared; lesions typically fade within 3–4 weeks.

Treatment is usually unnecessary as the disease is self-limiting.

SYSTEMIC LUPUS ERYTHEMATOSUS

Systemic lupus erythematosus (SLE) is a chronic inflammatory disease that has protean manifestations and follows a relapsing and remitting course. More than 90% of cases of SLE occur in women, frequently starting at childbearing age. A malar erythematous butterfly rash suggests SLE, but a discoid or photosensitive rash may also be seen.

Sysytemic Lupus International Collaborating Clinics (SLICC) classification criteria of SLE helps in diagnosing SLE.

Classify a patient as having SLE if:

The patient has biopsy-proven lupus nephritis with ANA or anti-dsDNA OR the patient satisfies four of the criteria, including at least one clinical and one immunologic criterion.

CLINICAL CRITERIA

- Acute or subacute cutaneous lupus
- Chronic cutaneous lupus
- Oral/nasal ulcers
- Nonscarring alopecia
- Inflammatory synovitis with physician-observed swelling of two or more joints OR tender joints with morning stiffness
- Serositis
- Renal: Urine protein/creatinine (or 24 hours urine protein) representing at least 500 mg of protein/24 hours or red blood cell casts
- Neurologic: seizures, psychosis, mononeuritis multiplex, myelitis, peripheral or cranial neuropathy, cerebritis (acute confusional state)
- Hemolytic anemia
- Leukopenia (<4000/mm³ at least once)
OR
Lymphopenia (<1000/mm³ at least once)
- Thrombocytopenia (<100,000/mm³) at least once

Immunologic Criteria

- ANA above laboratory reference range
- Anti-dsDNA above laboratory reference range (except ELISA: twice above laboratory reference range)
- Anti-Sm
- Antiphospholipid antibody
  - Positive test for lupus anticoagulant
  - False-positive test for syphilis
  - Anticardiolipin—at least twice normal or medium-high titer
  - Positive for anti-beta 2 glycoprotein 1
- Low complement
  - Low C3
  - Low C4
  - Low CH50
- Direct Coombs test in absence of hemolytic anemia.

KAWASAKI DISEASE

Kawasaki disease (KD) is an acute febrile vasculitic syndrome of early childhood that, although it has a good prognosis with treatment, can lead to death from coronary artery aneurysm (CAA) in a very small percentage of patients.

It typically affects children aged <5 years, with a seasonal bias (winter to late spring). A polymorphous maculopapular rash on the trunk may be seen. The rash is typically generalized and exanthematous without petechiae. In the febrile phase, perineal erythema and desquamation may be noted.

Diagnosis is by clinical criteria

Fever for five or more days, together with any four of five:

- Bilateral, nonexudative, painless bulbar conjunctival injection
- **Polymorphous rash** (not vesicular): Usually generalized but may be limited to the groin or lower extremities
- **Oropharyngeal changes**: Erythema, fissuring, and crusting of the lips; strawberry tongue; diffuse mucosal injection of the oropharynx.
- **Changes in the peripheral extremities**: Initial reddening or edema of the palms and soles, followed by membranous desquamation of the finger and toe tips or transverse grooves across the fingernails and toenails (Beau lines).
- Acute nonpurulent cervical lymphadenopathy with lymph node diameter greater than 1.5 cm, usually unilateral.

ROCKY MOUNTAIN SPOTTED FEVER

Rocky Mountain spotted fever (RMSF) is a tick-borne disease caused by the organism *Rickettsia rickettsii*. RMSF is the most common rickettsial infection. Because of its diverse clinical features, RMSF is often confused with other infections. The hallmark of RMSF is a petechial rash beginning on the palms of the hands and soles of the feet.

Outdoor activities and possible exposure in tick-endemic areas may be reported. Actual antecedent tick bite or tick attachment is made in 45%–60% of cases.

Clinical symptoms include headache, confusion, malaise, nausea, vomiting, myalgia, abdominal pain, and diarrhea. Seizures are uncommon. In 90% of cases a rash develops 2–4 days later. A macular eruption on the wrists, ankles, palms, and soles, and spreading centrally, generally sparing the face, is a feature of RMSF secondary to a tick bite. This may become petechial as the rash progresses. Intense inflammation or ecchymoses may be present at the site of the tick bite. Conjunctivitis, altered mental status, lymphadenopathy, peripheral oedema, and hepatomegaly may be present.

Diagnosis is confirmed based on indirect immuno-fluorescent antibody (IFA) test results, latex agglutination, or enzyme immunoassay. Serology specific for *R. rickettsii* infection develops within 6–8 weeks. Serologic test results are negative prior to convalescence.

ERYTHEMA MULTIFORME

A self-limiting generalized exfoliative dermatitis, often considered a milder variant of the SJS/TEN spectrum. Presentation is rapid and lesions are painful. A recent medication history of sulfonamides, penicillin, anti-malarials, or anticonvulsants, or a history of recent infection with *Mycoplasma*, herpes, EBV, or CMV may be reported.

Target lesions (annular erythematous rings with an outer erythematous zone and central blistering sandwiching a zone of normal skin tone) with symmetrical distribution on the extremities is seen in erythema multiforme.

Atypical targetoid papules (no central blistering) may also be present. Oral/genital mucosal erosions may be seen.

VESICULAR RASHES

A representative disease with a systemic vesicular rash is chickenpox, whereas local vesicular rashes are seen in diseases including herpes simplex and herpes zoster. Moreover, vesicular rashes can occur in children with impetigo caused by staphylococcal skin infection in the summer.

VARICELLA-ZOSTER INFECTION (CHICKENPOX)

Varicella is caused by varicella-zoster virus (VZV), responsible for varicella (chickenpox) and herpes zoster (shingles). Primary infection causes varicella, after which, the virus becomes latent.

The transmission of VZV, is more commonly transmitted by respiratory secretions via an aerosol route and also by skin-to-skin contact.

When a susceptible individual is exposed to VZV, the virus initially undergoes primary replication, beginning 3–4 days after exposure, and occurring in the oropharynx and regional lymph nodes. This is followed by a primary viremia. A secondary viremia occurs 10–21 days after exposure and, during this time period, patients manifest with prodromal symptoms, fever, malaise and myalgias. The exanthem begins soon after as erythematous pruritic macules, which develop into papules and fluid-filled vesicles, described as 'dewdrops on a rose petal'. The lesions usually begin in the hairline and spread in a cephalocaudal pattern, involving the scalp and mucous membranes. The vesicles crust over, typically within 4–5 days of the onset of the initial lesion. Older lesions crust over as newer lesions form, and so giving a polymorphous appearance to the exanthem. Lesions may heal with hypopigmentation and scarring.

Neurological complications can also occur, and these include meningitis, meningoencephalitis, cerebellar ataxia, transverse myelitis and Guillain–Barré syndrome. Other complications include arthritis, glomerulonephritis, myocarditis, thrombocytopenia and purpura fulminans. Immunocompromised patients are at risk for severe and protracted varicella, multiorgan involvement and hemorrhagic varicella.

The other common clinical manifestation of VZV infection is herpes zoster (shingles). VZV becomes latent in dorsal root ganglia cells until reactivation, at which time, the virus travels back to the skin along the sensory nerve, manifesting as a unilateral vesicular skin eruption involving one to three dermatomes. Skin vesicles may be painful or pruritic, especially in adults. Zoster generally is a milder disease in children than in adults. Reactivation is probably due to declining cell-mediated immunity, which explains the increased incidence in the elderly and in immunocompromised patients.

Varicella is usually a benign, mild, self-limiting disease in most immunocompetent individuals. Oral acyclovir (ACV) is not routinely recommended. However, since adolescents and young adults are at a moderately high risk for developing severe illness, oral ACV should be administered for 5 days, ideally starting within 24 hours of the development of a varicella rash.

Intravenous ACV is used for patients at serious risk for, or who have, a severe or potentially severe VZV infection, such as immunocompromised patients. The recommended duration of ACV therapy is 7 days, or until no new lesions have appeared for 48 hours Ideally, therapy should be started within 24 hours of onset, but ACV can still be effective up to 72 hours after the appearance of the skin lesions.

Individuals should be vaccinated twice, once at an age of 12–15 months and again at 4–6 years.

The diagnosis of VZV infection is usually made by history and clinical findings. Laboratory confirmation can be conducted by demonstrating the presence of specific viral antigens in skin scrapings by immunofluorescence using a commercial monoclonal antibody to VZV conjugated to fluorescein, or by PCR.

HERPES ZOSTER

Herpes zoster is a clinical skin disease caused by secondary infection by the varicella zoster virus, and does not commonly occur in children. Invasion of this virus into the peripheral nerves causes vesicular rashes in that region of skin. However, children, unlike adults, rarely have severe pain; invasion into the facial nerve can be accompanied by paralysis, and invasion into the trigeminal or auditory nerve can also be accompanied by dizziness or hearing loss. These skin lesions persist for 5 days or longer.

HERPES SIMPLEX VIRAL FOCAL INFECTION

Herpes simplex virus mostly presents with focal skin lesions on the skin around the lips. A macular rash suddenly evolves into a papular rash at first, and painful vesicles occur almost simultaneously. As these vesicles burst, findings of secondary infection and eschars occur, followed by natural healing. Herpes simplex viral focal infection can occur on any part of the skin.

HAND, FOOT AND MOUTH DISEASE

Hand, foot and mouth disease (HFMD) is a distinct monomorphous exanthem caused by viruses of the Picornaviridae family in the Enterovirus genus. Although the enteroviruses can cause an assortment of virus-mediated exanthems, HFMD is a recognizable and common clinical manifestation. The most common pathogen is the Coxsackie A16 virus, but other Coxsackie viruses and enteroviruses have been implicated as well. In particular, human enterovirus 71 appears to be responsible for recent epidemics of HFMD.

The infection has a typical incubation period of 3–7 days. The main manifestations are fever, lymphadenopathy, followed by the appearance of 2–8 mm painful oval, gray vesicles on the palmar and plantar skin, buccal mucosa and tongue after 1–2 days. Papular and vesicular lesions can also occur on other parts of the body, and the buttocks may often exhibit a nonspecific eruption prior to the onset of the vesicular exanthem. In the oral cavity, the hard palate, tongue and buccal mucosa are most commonly affected.

Most HFMD cases are self-limiting, and only required supportive treatment. Rarely, there may be a neurological or cardiopulmonary complication, such as meningoencephalitis or myocarditis. Uncomplicated HFMD usually resolves in 5–7 days.

The diagnosis of HFMD is usually made on clinical grounds. Confirmation is possible via isolating the virus from the vesicles, nasopharyngeal secretions, cerebrospinal fluid, blood or biopsy materials.

VESICULAR IMPETIGO

A systemic vesicular rash occurs in this disease, and purulent changes appear sequentially. These rashes have a characteristic distribution, mostly appearing in the inguinal area and the abdominal region, and are absent from the palms and soles. Staphylococcus is detected in these skin lesions.

HEMORRHAGIC RASH (PETECHIAE AND PURPURA)

Systemic symptoms were significantly associated with petechiae or purpura both cutaneous and mucosal. This probably depended on the infectious etiology of the hemorrhagic pattern. In fact, since petechial and purpuric rashes appear as terminal symptoms in diseases, such as meningococcemia, encephalomeningitis, or sepsis caused by pathogens, such as bacteria, viruses, and fungi, patients with these rashes who also show acute and severe clinical symptoms must undergo proactive diagnosis in the early stages, followed by appropriate treatments. Although *Meningococcus* infection is most common among bacterial diseases with these rashes, they can also be caused by *Pneumococcus* and *Staphylococcus*.

MENINGOCOCCAL SEPTICEMIA

A generalized macular rash may be the initial presenting feature of meningococcemia. This may progress to a more purpuric rash. Fever, malaise, and nuchal rigidity are generally present. Signs of sepsis such as cool peripheries, pallor or mottled skin, drowsiness, and respiratory distress may be seen.

Although most cases of meningococcemia are sporadic, a history of contact with an infected person may be reported. Immunocompromise (e.g., secondary to asplenia or HIV infection) is a predisposing factor for meningococcal disease.

SEVERE CUTANEOUS ADVERSE DRUG REACTIONS

Stevens-Johnson Syndrome/Toxic Epidermal Necrolysis

This is a spectrum of epidermal necrosis with designation dependent on the extent of involvement of body surface area.

In Stevens-Johnson Syndrome (SJS) <10% of body surface area is affected (typically the palms, soles, and extensor surfaces).

In toxic epidermal necrolysis (TEN) >30% of the skin surface is involved, with widespread cutaneous involvement.

A recent medication history (e.g. anticonvulsants, sulfonamides, NSAIDs, allopurinol, antihelminthics, antimalarials, corticosteroids, nevirapine, selective COX-2 inhibitors, and lamotrigine) may be reported. Other historical aspects include recent URI, infection with *Mycoplasma*, or viral infection (e.g. herpes, EBV, or CMV).

Skin lesions are initially targetoid and often become confluent. Bullous lesions develop, and a positive Nikolsky sign may be seen in involved areas. Pain is prominent. Mucosal surfaces (oral, conjunctival, anogenital) are also affected, with erosive lesions. Most patients appear acutely unwell, and evidence of secondary infection may be seen.

Acute Generalized Exanthematous Pustulosis

Acute generalized exanthematous pustulosis (AGEP) is an acute febrile drug eruption characterized by numerous small, primarily nonfollicular, sterile pustules, arising within large areas of edematous erythema. In AGEP drug-specific T cells produce interleukin-8/CXCL8, leading to neutrophil recruitment resulting in acute widespread edematous erythema followed by a sterile pustular eruption. The onset of disease is typically rapid and often within 1–3 days of drug initiation. The condition is also characterised by fever and possible eosinophilia. Beta-lactam antibiotics, quinolones, hydroxychoroquine, pristinamycin, sulfonamides, diltiazem, and terbinafine are all known to cause AGEP. AGEP has been rarely associated with infections, nondrug antigens and viral reactivation. The prognosis is usually good, with resolution occurring within 15 days.

DRESS or Systemic Hypersensitivity Syndrome

DRESS/DIHS/HSS by definition is associated with fever, rash, eosinophilia and/or atypical lymphocytosis, cutaneous involvement and hepatitis typically occurring 2 or more weeks after first drug initiation.

Patients may have a recent history of anticonvulsants and sulfonamide use. Other drugs (including lamotrigine, allopurinol, NSAIDs, captopril, calcium-channel blockers, mexiletine, fluoxetine, dapsone, terbinafine, metronidazole, minocycline, and antiretroviral drugs) have also been linked to this syndrome.

The time interval between intake of the offending medication and symptoms may be up to 8 weeks.

A morbilliform (measles-like) eruption, initially involving the face, upper trunk, and upper extremities, with later involvement of lower extremities may suggest DRESS or systemic hypersensitivity syndrome.

Fever, lymphadenopathy, and clinical features of severe visceral involvement (e.g. right upper quadrant tenderness/hepatomegaly with hepatitis, crackles/wheezes/tachypnea with pneumonitis) may be seen.

The diagnosis is made if the following criteria are met:
- Drug-induced generalized eruption,
- Associated systemic involvement (lymph node or visceral), and
- Presence of eosinophilia (eosinophil count ≥1500/microliter and/or circulating atypical lymphocytes).

DIFFUSE ERYTHEMA WITH DESQUAMATION

Staphylococcal-scalded Skin Syndrome

This usually occurs in infants and toddlers and is caused by coagulase-positive staphylococci. The characteristic skin lesions of this disease have sudden-onset, and are generalized, diffusely erythematous rashes accompanied by edema around the eyes, with associated pain, and with gradual progression to a vesicular rash. Thereafter, skin lesions show Nikolsky's sign, in which the uppermost layer of skin is removed by even mild pressure or injury; tissue fluid leaks from the exposed skin, causing severe dehydration and electrolyte imbalance, and even aggravates nutritional deficiencies. In addition, the skin around the eyes and mouth is severely distorted. These skin lesions start to improve and recover after 1 week, when the systemic erythema disappears. Drug-induced toxic epithelial dermal necrolysis also shows similar findings, including systemic erythema and desquamation. However, while staphylococcal-scalded skin syndrome (SSSS) shows desquamation of only the superficial, epithelial granular layer, all the epithelial layers peel off in drug-induced toxic epithelial dermal necrolysis, which allows for differentiation.

TOXIC SHOCK SYNDROME

The symptoms of this syndrome include fever, hypotension, muscular pain, and syncope. It is caused by *Staphylococcus aureus*, with inflammatory findings in the mucosa, edematous erythema in the hands and feet, and scarlet fever-like rashes over the curved areas of the extremities. The most notable characteristic skin lesion in this syndrome is nonpitting systemic edema. Thick skin desquamation appears on the hands and feet at around 7–14 days of disease progression, and might be followed by hair desquamation or shedding of fingernails and toenails after 2–3 months.

SOME COMMON CONDITIONS OF RASHES IN CHILDREN (FIGS. 2.7.1 TO 2.7.6)

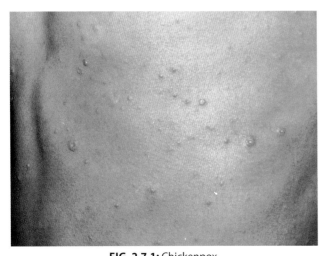

FIG. 2.7.1: Chickenpox.
Source: Dr D Ranganath, Professor, Department of Pediatrics, Malla Reddy, Medical Sciences, Hyderabad, Telangana, India

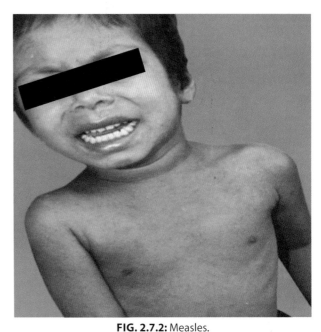

FIG. 2.7.2: Measles.
Source: Dr D Ranganath, Professor, Department of Pediatrics, Malla Reddy, Medical Sciences, Hyderabad, Telangana, India

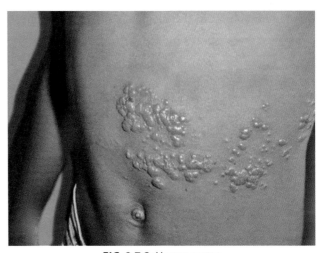

FIG. 2.7.3: Herpes zoster.
Source: Dr D Ranganath, Professor, Department of Pediatrics, Malla Reddy, Medical Sciences, Hyderabad, Telangana, India

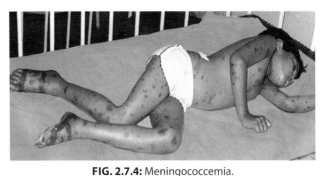

FIG. 2.7.4: Meningococcemia.
Source: Dr D Ranganath, Professor, Department of Pediatrics, Malla Reddy, Medical Sciences, Hyderabad, Telangana, India

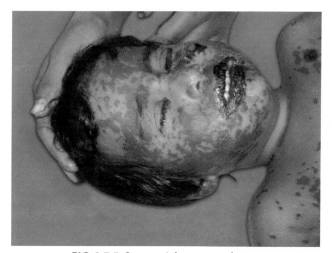

FIG. 2.7.5: Stevens-Johnsons syndrome.

Source: Dr D Ranganath, Professor, Department of Pediatrics, Malla Reddy, Medical Sciences, Hyderabad, Telangana, India

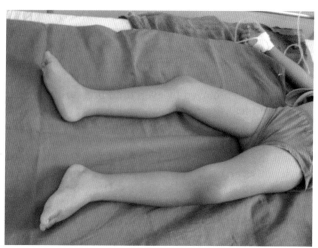

FIG. 2.7.6: Dengue fever.

Source: Dr D Ranganath, Professor, Department of Pediatrics, Malla Reddy, Medical Sciences, Hyderabad, Telangana, India

INVESTIGATIONS IN FEVER WITH RASH

For many viral exanthems, diagnosis is clinical, and tests are not routinely recommended (Table 2.7.2):
- CBC, ESR, CRP, biochemical studies, and urinalysis may be helpful in the diagnosis of systemic illness.

These include meningococcal disease, DRESS, systemic hypersensitivity syndrome, Kawasaki disease, SLE, Henoch–Schönlein purpura, and juvenile arthritis. Bone marrow biopsy should be considered if leukemia is suspected.

Table 2.7.2: Diagnostic tests for viral infections.

Agent	Rapid antigen detection (Specimen)	Tissue culture mean days to positive (Range)	Serology			Comments
			Acute	Paired	PCR[a]	
Cytomegalovirus	+ (tissue biopsy, urine, blood, respiratory secretions)	2 (2–28)	+	+	+	Diagnosis by presence of IgM antibody
Epstein-Barr virus	–	–	+	+	+	Single serologic panel defines infection status; heterophil antibodies less sensitive
Hantavirus	–	–	+	ND	RL	Diagnosis by presence of IgM antibody
Hepatitis B virus	+ (blood)	–	+	ND	+	Diagnosis by presence of surface antigen or anti-core IgM antibody
Hepatitis C virus	–	–	+	ND	+	Positive serology suggests that hepatitis C may be the causative agent. PCR is confirmatory.
Herpes simplex virus	+ (mucosa, tissue biopsy, respiratory secretions, skin)	1 (1–7)	+	+	+	Serology rarely used for herpes simplex. IgM antibody used in selected cases.
Human herpesvirus-6 and 7	–	2	+	+	+	Roseola agent
Human immunodeficiency virus	+ (blood) (acid dissociation of immune complexes)	15 (5–28)	+	ND	+	Antibody proves infection unless passively acquired (age <15 months); culture not widely available; PCR definitive for early diagnosis in infant
Measles virus	+ (respiratory secretions)	–	+	+	+	Difficult to grow; IgM serology diagnostic
Parvovirus B19	–	–	+	ND	+	Erythema infectiosum agent
Rubella virus	–	> 10	+	+	+	Recommended that paired sera be tested simultaneously
Varicella-zoster virus	+ (skin scraping)	3 (3–21) RL	+	+	+	

[a]Useful only when performed on selected specimens by qualified laboratories.

Key:
- Plus signs signify commercially or widely available; minus signs signify not commercially available. Note: Results from some commercial laboratories are unreliable.
- RL, CDC: Specific antibody titers or PCR available by arrangement with individual research laboratories or the Centers for Disease Control and Prevention.
- ND: Not done.

Abbreviations: ELISA, enzyme-linked immunosorbent assay; PCR, polymerase chain reaction; RBC, red blood cell.

- Skin prick testing, patch testing or radioallergosorbent test (RAST), serum IgE levels, may be helpful in allergic contact or atopic dermatitis and wide spread urticaria.
- Serological investigations may include rapid strep test (pharyngeal swab) or anti-streptolysin O titer to confirm scarlet fever; enzyme-linked immunosorbent assay (ELISA) or immunofluorescence assay, and IgM and IgG immunoblot (Western blot) assays in suspected Lyme disease; indirect immunofluorescent antibody serology and convalescent serology in RMSF; rapid streptococcal antigen test and streptococcal antibody titre if rheumatic fever is suspected; ELISA for *Staphylococcus aureus* toxin in SSSS; and rheumatoid factor in suspected juvenile arthritis. Assays for HIV, HBV, and HCV infection should be considered.
- Blood cultures should be ordered if meningococcal septicemia, TSS, bacterial endocarditis, or SJS/TEN is suspected. Lumbar puncture with CSF analysis should be ordered if meningococcemia is suspected.
- Echocardiography should be ordered if rheumatic fever, bacterial endocarditis, or Kawasaki disease is suspected.
- A chest X-ray should be ordered if rheumatic fever or sarcoidosis is suspected.
- Skin biopsy may be considered in SSSS, SJS/TEN, DRESS, psoriasis, pityriasis rosea, or mastocytosis and Henoch–Schönlein purpura.

- In suspected infectious etiologies, Gram stain and/or culture of lesional fluid may be prudent when the diagnosis is in doubt or if the patient does not respond to appropriate empirical therapy.

BIBLIOGRAPHY

1. Evaluation of rash in children, BMJ best practice.
2. IAP Textbook of Pediatrics, 5th edition; 2013.
3. Kang JH. Febrile Illness with Skin Rashes. Current diagnosis and treatment: pediatrics, 19th edition. Infect Chemother. 2015;47(3):155-66. CURRENT Pediatrics > Chapter 38. Infections: Viral & Rickettsial > Viral Infections >http://bestpractice.bmj.com/best-practice/monograph/857/diagnosis/
4. Mckinnon HD Jr, Howard T. Dewitt Army Community Hospital, Fort Belvoir, Virginia. Am Fam Physician. 2000;62(4):804-16.
5. Nelson Textbook of Pediatrics, 17th edition, Behrman, Kliegman, Jenson; 2004.
6. Pavlos R, Mallal S, Ostrov D, et al. Fever, rash and systemic symptoms: understanding the role of virus and HLA in severe cutaneous drug allergy. J Allergy Clin Immunol Pract. 2014;2(1):21-33.
7. Petri M, Orbai AM, Alarcon GS, et al. Derivation and validation of the Systemic Lupus International Collaborating Clinics classification criteria for systemic lupus erythematosus. Arthritis Rheum; 2012.
8. Textbook of Pediatrics Infectious Diseases, ID chapter publication; 2013.
9. Textbook of Pediatrics Infectious Diseases; 2014.

2.8 SEPSIS AND SEPTIC SHOCK IN CHILDREN

Tanu Singhal

INTRODUCTION

Sepsis accounts for about 6 million neonatal and childhood deaths a year, accounting for 60–80% of annual child mortality. It also accounts for a significant proportion of health care utilization. This chapter attempts to provide a comprehensive account of *severe sepsis and septic shock* focusing primarily on the infectious/microbiologic/antibiotic aspects.

DEFINITIONS

The terms systemic inflammatory response syndrome (SIRS), infection, sepsis, severe sepsis, septic shock and multiple organ dysfunction syndrome (MODS) are commonly used in literature and clinical practice. Definitions for the same have been laid out in the International Pediatric Sepsis Consensus Conference, 2005. These are detailed in Tables 2.8.1 to 2.8.3. The term SIRS is used when a patient has a systemic inflammatory response in form of fever or hypothermia, tachycardia, tachypnea or abnormal white cell count. SIRS can be caused by infectious or noninfectious factors such as trauma, injury, surgery. The term sepsis is used when SIRS results from a suspected or proven infection. If sepsis is associated with organ dysfunction the term severe sepsis is used. The term septic shock is employed if there is circulatory impairment and MODS is used when several organs are dysfunctional.

The recently published Sepsis 3 guidelines have revised the definition of sepsis in adults which are no longer based on the SIRS criteria. The pediatric guidelines have not been modified as the evidence for change remains weak. But this may change in future.

EPIDEMIOLOGY

Incidence and prevalence data on paediatric sepsis is scanty from India. But broadly speaking, sepsis is the leading cause of under five mortality in India.

A point prevalence study to determine the global epidemiology of pediatric sepsis (the SPROUT study) recruited 6,925 patients from 128 PICU's in 26 countries (2 sites from India). The prevalence of severe sepsis was 8.2%; median age was 3 years; the respiratory tract was the commonest site and 65% of all cases were culture positive. Gram positive and gram negative pathogens contributed to a quarter each of severe sepsis while fungi were isolated in 13%. *Staphylococcus aureus* was the commonest pathogen. The mortality rate was 25%.

In another recently published observational cohort study by Saha et al. the epidemiology of possible serious bacterial infections (pSBI) in infants aged less than 60 days was studied at 5 sites in Pakistan, India and Bangladesh between 2011–2014. The incidence of pSBI was 95.4 per 1000 live births. Causes were established in 28% of the

Table 2.8.1: Definitions of sepsis (International Pediatric Sepsis Consensus Conference).

A. Systemic inflammatory response syndrome (SIRS)	The presence of at least two of the following four criteria, one of which must be abnormal temperature or leukocyte count: Core (oral or rectal) temperature of > 38.5°C or <36°C; Tachycardia, in the absence of external stimulus, chronic drugs or painful stimuli; or otherwise unexplained persistent elevation over a 0.5 hour time period or for children < 1-year-old: bradycardia, in absence of external vagal stimulus, β blocker drugs or congenital heart disease or persistent depression over a 0.5 hour time period; Tachypnea for an acute process not related to underlying neuromuscular disease; Leukocyte count elevated or depressed for age (not secondary to chemotherapy-induced leukopenia) or>10% immature neutrophils
B. Infection	A suspected or proven infection caused by any pathogen or a clinical syndrome associated with a high probability of infection. Evidence of infection includes positive findings on clinical examination, imaging, or laboratory tests (e.g. leukocytes in a normally sterile body fluid, perforated viscus, chest radiograph consistent with pneumonia, petechial or purpuric rash, or purpura fulminans) or a positive culture, tissue stain or polymerase chain reaction test
C. Sepsis	SIRS in the presence of or as a result of suspected or proven infection
D. Severe sepsis	Sepsis plus one of the following: cardiovascular dysfunction or acute respiratory distress syndrome or two or more other organ dysfunctions. Organ dysfunctions are defined in Table 2.8.2
E. Septic shock	In a child with sepsis presence of: hypotension (systolic BP <70 mm Hg in infant; <70 + 2 X age after 1 year of age) or need for vasoactive drug to maintain BP above fifth centile range (dopamine 5 µg/kg/minute or dobutamine, epinephrine or norepinephrine at any dose) or signs of hypoperfusion—any three of the following: decreased pulse volume (weak or absent dorsalis pedis pulse), capillary refilling time >3 sec tachycardia heart rate as defined in Table 2.8.4, core (rectal/oral) to peripheral (skin-toe) temperature gap >3°C and urine output <1 mL/kg/hour (<20 mL/hour in > 20 kg child) or sepsis and cardiovascular organ dysfunction as defined in Table 2.8.3
F. Multiple organ dysfunction	The detection of altered organ functions in the acutely ill patient constitutes multiple organ dysfunction syndrome (MODS; two or more organ involvement).

Table 2.8.2: Age-specific upper and/or lower limits of heart rate to define tachycardia and bradycardia, respiratory rate to define tachypnea and systolic blood pressure to define hypotension.

Age group	HR (bpm) mean (range)	RR (bpm)	Systolic BP (mm Hg)	MAP-CVP (mm Hg)
Up to 1 month	140 (100–190)	> 60	< 60	55
2 months–1 year	130 (80–180)	> 50	< 70	60
1–5 years	80 (60–140)	> 40	< 70 + (2 × age in years)	65
6–10 years	80 (60–130)	> 30	< 70 + (2 × age in years)	65
>10 years	75 (60–100)	> 30	< 90	65

Abbreviations: HR, heart rate; RR, respiratory rate

Table 2.8.3: Organ dysfunction criteria.

Cardiovascular dysfunction

- Hypotension (systolic BP <70 mm Hg in infant; < 70 + 2 × age after 1 year of age) or
- Need for vasoactive drug to maintain BP above fifth centile range (dopamine >5 µg/kg/minute or dobutamine, epinephrine or norepinephrine at any dose) or
- Signs of hypoperfusion—any three of the following: decreased pulse volume (weak or absent dorsalis pedis pulse), capillary refilling time >3 seconds, tachycardia (heart rate as defined in Table 2.8.2), core (rectal/oral) to peripheral (skin-toe) temperature gap >3°C and urine output <1 mL/kg/hour (20 mL/hour in >20 kg child)
- In early stage there is an increase in heart rate and poor peripheral perfusion in form of weak pulse and prolonged capillary refill time. Hypotension occurs late, and may lead to precipitous cardiac arrest

Respiratory dysfunction*

- Proven need for supplemental oxygen** or > 50% FiO_2 to maintain saturation > 92% or
- Need for nonelective mechanical ventilation*** or
- PaO_2/FiO_2 < 300 in absence of cyanotic heart disease or pre-existent lung disease or
- $PaCO_2$ >65 torr or 20 mm Hg over baseline $PaCO_2$

Neurologic dysfunction

- Glasgow coma score <11 or
- Acute change in mental status with decrease in Glasgow coma score >3 points from abnormal baseline

Hematologic dysfunction

- Platelet count <80,000/mm³ or a decline of 50% in platelet count from highest value recorded over the past 3 days (for chronic hematology/oncology patients) or
- International normalized ratio >2

Renal dysfunction

- Serum creatinine >1 mg/dL

Hepatic dysfunction

- Total bilirubin >4 mg/dL (not applicable for newborn) or alanine transaminase two times the upper limit of normal for age

*Acute respiratory distress syndrome must include a PaO_2/FIO_2 ratio <200 mm Hg, bilateral infiltrates, acute onset, and no evidence of left heart failure. Acute lung injury is defined identically except that the PaO_2/FiO_2 ratio should be less than <300 mm Hg.

**Proven need assumes that oxygen requirement was tested by decreasing the flow with subsequent increase in flow if required.

***In postoperative patients the requirement can be met if the patient has developed an acute inflammatory or infectious process in the lung that prevents him or her from being extubated.

episodes of which 16% were bacterial and 12% viral. Respiratory syncytial virus followed by Ureaplasma were the most common pathogens. The most common bacterial pathogens were *Klebsiella, E. coli, S. aureus* and group A *Streptococcus* in that order.

ETIOLOGY

Sepsis can result from any infection with bacteria, viruses, fungi and protozoa or their products and toxins. The etiology of sepsis depends on many factors including age, whether infection is community or hospital acquired, local epidemiology, season, site of infection and presence of any host predisposing factors, such as immunodeficiency. Etiology is discussed with respect to age since it is most clinically relevant and of practical utility.

Neonates and Young Infants (0–3 Months)

The common organisms responsible for neonatal sepsis in India are predominantly gram-negative bacteria, such as *Klebsiella* and *Escherichia coli*. Other pathogens include *Staphylococcus aureus, Enterococcus, Candida* and less commonly Hib and *Pneumococcus. Listeria monocytogenes* and group B *Streptococcus* are infrequently encountered in the Indian setting. Nosocomially acquired infections and many community acquired infections are often resistant to the third generation cephalosporins by virtue of production of extended spectrum beta lactamases. Some nosocomially acquired infections are even carbapenem resistant.

Post Neonatal Period

Etiologic agents again vary with age and site of infection.

Bacteremia/Viremia/Parasitemia/Toxemia

- Bacteremia due to *Streptococcus pneumoniae, Haemophilus influenzae* and *Meningococcus*, particularly in children below 36 months of age.
- *Salmonella typhi* and *paratyphi* are very important causes of sepsis in Indian children; the incidence rising with age. However, being of relatively lower virulence, they are rarely associated with severe sepsis and septic shock.
- Dengue and malaria (predominantly falciparum) in Indian children of all ages particularly in the monsoon season.
- Leptospirosis, rickettsial infections, such as scrub typhus and spotted fever, brucellosis in particular epidemiologic settings.
- Toxic shock syndromes due to infection with toxigenic strains of staphylococci and streptococci.

Site-specific Infections

- Acute bacterial meningitis is usually due to *S. pneumoniae, H. influenzae* and *Meningococcus*.

- Lower respiratory infections and pneumonia are due to viruses (influenza, parainfluenza, RSV, adenovirus, *human metapneumovirus*), bacteria including *S. pneumoniae, H. influenzae* and *S. aureus* and atypical organisms such as *Mycoplasma*.
- Urinary tract infections are most commonly due to *E. coli* and less often due to *Klebsiella pneumoniae* and *Proteus*. There is a rising incidence of cephalosporin-resistant Enterobacteriaceae due to extended-spectrum beta lactamase (ESBL) production even in community acquired infections.
- Gastrointestinal (GI) and intra-abdominal infections include acute gastroenteritis, bacillary dysentery, appendicitis, cholecystitis, liver abscess and peritonitis. Common etiologic agents of intra-abdominal infections are *E. coli*, anaerobes and enterococci.
- Skin and soft tissue infections, such as cellulitis and pyomyositis are usually due to *S. aureus* or *Streptococcus pyogenes*. Necrotizing fasciitis common causes of which include *S. aureus, S. pyogenes*, anaerobes or less commonly gram-negative organisms results in refractory septic shock and is associated with high mortality unless extensive surgical debridement is done. Rising incidence of community acquired methicillin-resistant *S. aureus* is being now reported.
- Bone and joint infections most commonly due to *S. aureus*; *Pneumococcus* and *H. influenzae b* (Hib) may cause some of these infections in children below 5 years of age.

Nosocomial Infections

Nosocomial or healthcare-associated infections are an increasing cause of pediatric sepsis in today's era with increasing penetration of intensive care. These infections are more common in children admitted to the intensive care unit (ICU) particularly the neonatal ICU. They include bloodstream infections, healthcare associated pneumonia, urinary tract infections and surgical site infections. The most common etiologic agents in the Indian setting are gram-negative pathogens, such as *E. coli, Klebsiella, Pseudomonas* and *Acinetobacter*. Most of these are multidrug resistant due to production of ESBLs, Amp C or now even carbapenem destroying enzymes. Next in the list are gram-positive pathogens, such as *Enterococcus*, methicillin sensitive and resistant *S. aureus*. *Candida* predominantly non-*albicans* species, such as *Candida tropicalis* has also become an increasingly common cause of nosocomial infections.

Infections in the Immunocompromised Host

Sepsis is the most common cause of morbidity and mortality in immunocompromised patients. This group includes children with cancer, transplant recipients, those on immunosuppressive drugs, such as corticosteroids, children with anatomic or functional asplenia, burns patients, children with chronic illnesses (e.g. diabetes) and those with congenital and acquired immunodeficiency. The etiologic agents differ based on severity and type of immunocompromise. In patients with humoral immunodeficiency capsulated pathogens, such as *Pneumococcus*, Hib and *Meningococcus* are implicated. Those with cellular immunodeficiency are susceptible to intracellular pathogens, such as viruses, *Mycobacterium tuberculosis, Salmonella* and *Pneumocystis carinii*. Those with phagocytic defects are particularly susceptible to gram-negative bacteria, *Nocardia, S. aureus* and fungi, such as *Aspergillus*.

PATHOGENESIS

The pathophysiology of sepsis can be initiated by the outer membrane component of gram-negative organisms [e.g. lipopolysaccharide (LPS), lipid A, endotoxin] or gram-positive organisms (e.g. lipoteichoic acid, peptidoglycan), as well as fungal, viral and parasitic components. These components activate monocytes via a family of transmembrane receptors known as Toll-like receptors. The activated monocytes and macrophages then produce proinflammatory cytokines, such as tumor necrosis factor-α (TNF-α), and interleukin-1 (IL-1). TNF-α and IL-1 lead to the production of toxic downstream mediators, including prostaglandins, leukotrienes, platelet-activating factor and phospholipase A2. These mediators damage the endothelial lining, leading to increased capillary leakage. Furthermore, these cytokines lead to the production of adhesion molecules on endothelial cells and neutrophils. Neutrophilic endothelial interaction leads to further endothelial injury through the release of the neutrophil components. Finally, activated neutrophils release nitric oxide, a potent vasodilator that leads to septic shock.

Interleukin-1 and TNF-α also have direct effects on the endothelial surface and cause expression of tissue factor (the first step in the extrinsic pathway of coagulation) on the surfaces of the endothelium and of monocytes. Tissue factor leads to the production of thrombin, which itself is a proinflammatory substance. Thrombin results in fibrin clots in the microvasculature, a sequela most easily recognized in meningococcal septic shock with purpura fulminans. Fibrinolysis is also impaired during the septic process. IL-1 and TNF-α lead to the production of plasminogen activator inhibitor-1, a potent inhibitor of fibrinolysis. The proinflammatory cytokines also inhibit the naturally occurring anticoagulants (activated protein C and antithrombin) thus preventing limitation of the coagulation cascade. Understanding of the key role of activated protein C in the pathogenesis of sepsis (Flowchart 2.8.1) that leads to its commercial development as a novel treatment of

FLOWCHART 2.8.1: Pathogenesis of sepsis.

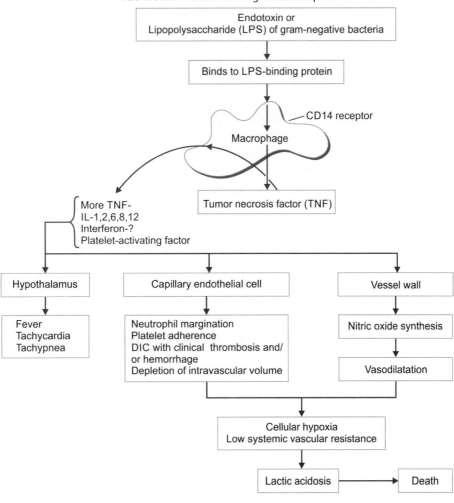

sepsis a decade back (Xigris). However, it has been recently withdrawn as new trials failed to show benefit in reducing sepsis mortality.

CD4 lymphocytes play a key role in the inflammatory response seen in sepsis. Early in the sepsis process, these cells assume a Th1 phenotype, where they produce large amounts of the proinflammatory mediators, including interferon gamma, TNF-α and IL-2. CD4 lymphocytes may evolve over time to a Th2 phenotype, whereby the CD4 lymphocytes produce anti-inflammatory cytokines, including IL-10, IL-4 and IL-13. This is often driven by the release of stress hormones, such as catecholamines and corticosteroids. These cytokines dampen the immune response and can lead to the deactivation of monocytes. Additionally, TNF released early can cause apoptosis of lymphocytes in the gut, leading to further immunosuppression.

As a result of the vicious cycle of inflammation and coagulation, cardiovascular insufficiency and multiple organ failure occur, and often lead to death. Cardiovascular insufficiency can occur at the level of the myocardium as a result of the myocardial depressant effects of TNF or at the level of the vessel, caused by vasodilation and capillary leak.

CLINICAL FEATURES

The most common manifestation of sepsis is fever; however, sepsis in neonates may not be associated with fever and may present as hypothermia. Conversely, not all fevers are due to infection; autoimmune disorders and malignancies may be misdiagnosed as sepsis and treated as such. This is particularly true about autoimmune disorders, like Kawasaki disease and systemic onset of juvenile rheumatoid arthritis, which are also associated with leukocytosis, high erythrocyte sedimentation rate (ESR) and C-reactive protein (CRP). Apart from fever, there are symptoms unique to each etiology and to the affected organ system, such as rash, central nervous system (CNS)/respiratory/abdominal/musculoskeletal/urinary symptoms and signs. With severe sepsis, septic shock and MODS, symptoms and signs of organ dysfunction appear (Table 2.8.1).

DIAGNOSIS

All children with suspected sepsis should be evaluated first for evidence of organ dysfunction (mental, respiratory, circulatory status) such that those with severe sepsis or septic shock can be identified and appropriate resuscitation started. Search for etiology should follow later. Etiologic diagnosis is established by careful history and examination supported by investigations. Common investigations in suspected sepsis are discussed below and summarized in Table 2.8.4.

Complete Blood Count with Platelet Count and Peripheral Smear

This is perhaps one of the most important investigations in sepsis. The white cell count is as per definition of SIRS is either elevated or depressed. An elevated white cell count may be seen in both viral and bacterial infections, but extreme elevations with neutrophilic predominance and immature neutrophils (band cells) make bacterial etiology more likely. Similarly, while a depressed white cell count is more common in viral infections, it may also be present in certain bacterial infections, such as enteric fever, and due to consumption in overwhelming bacterial infections and septic neonates. It is important to understand that a normal white cell count does not rule out sepsis. Presence of atypical lymphocytes in the smear is indicative of viral infections. Platelet counts are generally low in sepsis due to bone marrow suppression or consumptive coagulopathy and can be very low in infections such as malaria and

dengue. The Hemoglobin can be low in infections, such as malaria. Serial complete blood counts rather than a single count can sometimes be more useful in tracking the etiology of and recovery from sepsis (e.g. in dengue). The total white cell count, absolute neutrophil count and band cell count are an integral component of the septic screen in neonates.

Smear for Malarial Parasite or Rapid Malarial Antigen Tests

Testing a child with suspected sepsis in the Indian setting for malaria irrespective of the season is strongly recommended. The thick smear is the gold standard as it has the highest sensitivity, gives information on the parasite load, prognosis and response to therapy. However, if reliable microscopy is not available, the rapid malaria antigen tests based on parasite antigen can also be used. Tests should be repeated every 6–8 hourly in those patients with negative results on the preliminary test, but strong suspicion of malaria.

Blood Culture

Blood cultures should be sent for all patients with suspected sepsis before the administration of antibiotics but even if antibiotics have been already administered. Cultures should be collected by peripheral venipuncture after cleaning the skin with 2% alcoholic chlorhexidine. If a patient has a central line, simultaneous cultures from a peripheral site and the central line (all lumens) should be drawn. Greater the amount of blood collected, higher is the sensitivity. The sensitivity is highest (around 95%) with three sets of blood cultures where one set is one bottle each of aerobic and anaerobic media. In children at least 1% of the circulating blood volume should be collected (e.g. a 10 kg child with an 80 mL/kg circulating blood volume should have 8 mL blood collected for culture. The blood and media ratio should be optimal around 1–5 to ensure good recovery (excess blood reduces recovery due to the bacterial inhibitors in the blood). Hence, in a pediatric bottle that usually has 20 mL of media 3–4 mL of blood should be added. In neonates, bacterial density is high and studies show that even 0.5–1 mL of blood is sufficient for pathogen recovery. Automated blood culture systems, such as BACTEC and BACT ALERT, are preferable over conventional systems since the recovery is faster and better. If conventional media are used then attention should be paid to media quality, e.g. use of sheep blood for media preparation enhances recovery of pneumococci and Hib. The results of the cultures should be interpreted carefully. Isolation of coagulase-negative *Staphylococcus* (CONS) in a single culture may be due to contamination during collection. CONS should be considered a pathogen only if it is repeatedly isolated; if the patient has an indwelling central line or in very low-birth-weight babies. Growth in

Table 2.8.4: Laboratory investigations in child with severe sepsis or septic shock.

Essential investigations

- CBC with platelet count
- Smear for malarial parasite or rapid malaria antigen test
- At least 1 set of blood cultures
- Urine routine and urine culture
- CXR
- US abdomen
- CRP and, if available, PCT

Other investigations (depending on clinical suspicion/preliminary investigations)

- LP and CSF analysis
- Dengue serology
- Tests for leptospira and rickettsia
- CT chest and abdomen
- Pus or tissue cultures

Investigations that help in supportive care

- Liver and renal functions
- Arterial and venous blood gas
- Serum lactate
- Coagulation profile

Abbreviations: CBC, complete blood count; CXR, chest X-ray; CRP, C-reactive protein; CSF, cerebrospinal fluid; CT, computed tomography; LP, lumbar puncture; PCT, procalcitonin; US, ultrasound

the central line culture with a negative peripheral blood culture can also be due to colonization. If the central line culture flags positive 120 minutes earlier than the peripheral culture, infection is considered related to the central venous device and removal of such a device should be considered. If the initial sets of cultures are negative, cultures should be repeated if sepsis is not resolving and especially before changing antibiotics. New methods such as MALDI TOF and film array panels are now available for quicker identification of bacteria than those by automated systems such as VITEK. Appropriate antimicrobial susceptibility testing is important in the current era of drug resistance. Automated testing by VITEK and E strip is rapidly replacing conventional disc diffusion testing.

Urine Analysis and Culture

These are mandatory investigations in children with suspected sepsis. The urine routine specimen should be processed for cell count, Gram stain and rapid tests like leukocyte esterase and nitrite. All of them individually have sensitivities and specificities ranging around 80%, but combined sensitivity (either leukocyte esterase or nitrite or microscopy) is as high as 99% with specificity of 80%. This means that if none of the parameters are positive a urine infection is highly unlikely. Specimen for urine culture should be collected by the clean catch method in younger children and midstream method in older children. Bag samples are not recommended. Suprapubic puncture or catheter samples may be needed if suspicion of urinary tract infection is high and urine cannot be collected by noninvasive methods. Since many children with severe sepsis or septic shock will need catheterization for assessment of urine output, a sample for culture can be sent immediately after catheterization. The sample for culture should be processed within 1 hour of collection and if the same cannot be done it should be refrigerated. A colony count of more than 50,000/mL is significant [recently proposed by American Academy of Pediatrics (AAP) as significant bacteriuria in children as opposed to 100,000/mL in adults]. The result of the urine culture should be interpreted carefully in conjunction with the routine. Significant bacteriuria in the absence of pyuria may just indicate colonization/contamination.

Biomarkers (Acute Phase Reactants (ESR/CRP/Procalcitonin)

The acute phase reactants are estimated in patients with suspected sepsis to help differentiate between non-infectious SIRS and sepsis, viral and bacterial causes of sepsis and also to assess severity and follow response to therapy. ESR was the first of the acute phase reactants to be evaluated, is cheap and widely available but unfortunately of limited sensitivity and specificity. A high ESR may be

seen in anemia and other non-infectious conditions while the ESR may be normal in full blown sepsis. The micro ESR, a component of neonatal septic screen in the past, has been largely supplanted by CRP. A very high ESR in three digits may indicate an inflammatory etiology such as systemic onset juvenile rheumatoid arthritis and Kawasaki's disease.

The CRP is an acute phase reactant produced by the liver in response to IL-6, TNF-α and other cytokines. It rises in 6 hours, peaks within 48 hours and has a half-life of 8 hours. A level of more than 6 mg/L is considered positive. It rises and falls more quickly than ESR. A rise of CRP may be seen in any SIRS, including infections, trauma, necrosis and inflammation. Hence, it does not distinguish infectious from noninfectious causes of SIRS. It rises in both viral and bacterial infections although the rise is more in bacterial than viral. There is no accurate cut-off that distinguishes viral from bacterial infections; however, if the CRP is very high (>100 mg/L) bacterial etiology is more likely. The CRP is an important component of neonatal septic screen (where a level more than 10 mg/L is considered positive) and in evaluation of fever without focus. Serial CRPs help in tracking the progress of infections especially in patients with bone and joint infections.

Procalcitonin (PCT) is a newly evaluated acute phase reactant; it is produced by most cells of the body in response to injury and infection. It rises and falls earlier than CRP and does not rise in many inflammatory and neoplastic conditions. Studies have shown that it is more reliable than CRP in differentiating viral from bacterial infections. A level of more than 2 ng/mL is specific for serious bacterial infection. Moreover its levels correlate with severity of infection and prognosis. Very high PCT levels at onset and failure of PCT to decline with treatment have been associated with poor outcome. PCT estimation is however more expensive than CRP. It is not superior to CRP in evaluating neonatal sepsis or fever without focus. Unlike what was believed earlier, PCT levels can be high even in non-infective SIRS such as pancreatitis, burns and surgery.

Interleukin-18 and CD64 are other biomarkers being evaluated. At present serum PCT is the best biomarker for diagnosis and prognosis of pediatric sepsis.

Imaging

A chest X-ray (CXR) is indicated in all children with suspected sepsis. Even in the absence of respiratory symptoms, one may find a "opacity" picking up an occult pneumonia. The CXR is not reliable in distinguishing between viral, atypical and bacterial pneumonia. Serial CXRs may help in tracking disease severity and development of complications. In patients with septic shock of nonrespiratory etiology, the CXR may be abnormal due to development of acute respiratory distress syndrome.

An ultrasonography (USG) of abdomen helps diagnose intra-abdominal problems, such as appendicitis, liver abscesses, cholecystitis and pyelonephritis. A contrast-enhanced computed tomography (CT) scan is sensitive than an USG to pick up intra-abdominal sepsis but is more expensive, not always available and not always possible if the child is critically sick.

Other imaging modalities include cranial CT scan/magnetic resonance imaging (MRI) for picking up intracranial infections, chest CT scan, and in patients with suspected musculoskeletal infections, skeletal X-ray and USG/MRI of joints.

Lumbar Puncture and CSF Analysis

This is indicated in all neonates with culture proven sepsis even in the absence of neurological symptoms and in all children with sepsis when an intracranial focus is suspected. It may have to be deferred in children with signs of raised intracranial pressure, severe thrombocytopenia and those with hemodynamic or respiratory instability. The CSF should be evaluated within 30 minutes of collection and must never be refrigerated. It should be processed for cell count, sugar and protein content, Gram stain, latex agglutination tests and culture. Other tests including lactate may be done if so indicated. Random blood sugar estimation prior to the lumbar puncture is mandatory to enable accurate estimation of CSF: blood sugar ratio.

Serologic Tests

Testing for dengue is indicated in pediatric sepsis with clinical features/complete blood count suggestive of dengue in the appropriate epidemiologic setting. The dengue NS1 antigen detects a highly conserved secretory glycoprotein of the dengue virus. It is positive in early dengue (sensitivity 90% in the first 4 days) with sensitivity dropping as disease advances and in secondary dengue due to early appearance of antibodies (sensitivity 70%). The specificity is very high (>95%). The importance of dengue IgM and IgG has declined since the NS1 antigen has become available. IgM antibodies are detectable by the 5th day in 70% of patients and 10th day in 99% and persist for up to 1 year. They may be absent in 20% of patients with secondary dengue. Low level IgG antibodies appear in primary dengue infection and persist for life whereas high levels of IgG antibodies are seen in secondary dengue. Dengue antibody detection is useful only for retrospective diagnosis and rarely helps in patient management. The best sensitivity is achieved by sending NS1 antigen, IgM and IgG in a single sample at the time of presentation. ELISA is superior to rapid immunochromatic test.

The Widal test is a commonly used test for diagnosis of enteric fever although very inferior to blood cultures. It has limited sensitivity and specificity and results need to be carefully interpreted. It should be sent only after the 1st week of fever and a level of both O and H of more than 1:160 is considered significant. The typhidot IgM is not superior to the WIDAL test in diagnosis of typhoid fever.

Immunoglobulin M *Leptospira* is a commonly ordered test in a febrile illness in endemic areas and during the monsoon. However, it is positive only after the first 5 days and false-positive results abound. The gold standard test for diagnosis of leptospirosis is MAT, which is available only in reference labs. The diagnosis of infectious mononucleosis is best established by EBV VCA IgM, which is a more accurate test as compared to Paul Bunnel or monospot test. For diagnosis of rickettsial infections, the Weil Felix is available, but not very sensitive or specific. IgM enzyme-linked immunosorbent assay (ELISA) for scrub typhus and spotted fever are more accurate, but less easily available.

Tissue/Pus Cultures

Pus at any site should be promptly drained and sent for culture and susceptibility testing.

Molecular Tests in Diagnosis of Sepsis

The molecular tests have revolutionized the diagnosis of sepsis. Multiplex PCR in blood is available to detect common tropical fevers such as dengue, leptospira, chikungunya and rickettsia. Multiplex PCR panels for detecting bacterial, viral and fungal infections are also available for CNS infections, respiratory infections and GI infections. The cost and availability of these tests limits their use.

Investigations that Aid Supportive Care

Certain laboratory investigations aid in supportive care in patients with pediatric sepsis and often need frequent estimation. These include liver functions tests, renal function tests, including serum electrolytes, arterial blood gases, serum lactate and coagulation profile.

ANTIMICROBIAL MANAGEMENT

Empirical Antimicrobial Therapy

Appropriate antibiotics must be initiated at the earliest in suspected pediatric sepsis since delaying antibiotics or inappropriate choice of antibiotics increase mortality. The choice of initial antibiotic depends on various factors that include:
- Likely pathogen
- Likely antimicrobial susceptibility
- *Prior antibiotic exposure:* Receipt of antibiotics in the past particularly in the last 3 months increases the risk of infection with drug-resistant pathogens, such as drug-resistant *S. pneumoniae* and ESBL producing gram-negative organisms.

- *Severity of illness:* More severe the illness, more important to get the right antibiotic at first opportunity as upgrading antibiotics in case of nonresponse is limited.
- *Host comorbidities:* If the host is immunocompromised, broader spectrum and more potent drugs may be needed. If there is associated renal impairment, nephrotoxic drugs should be avoided.
- *Site of infection:* If there is CNS infection, drugs with good meningeal penetration must be used.

Neonates

In antibiotic naïve community acquired neonatal sepsis initial antibiotic therapy with a third generation cephalosporin, such as cefotaxime with an aminoglycoside or a *beta-lactam beta-lactamase* inhibitor combination such as piperacillin tazobactam/cefoperazone sulbactam should be initiated. In very sick neonates with septic shock or suspected CNS involvement meropenem may have to be used upfront.

Infants and Children

In children beyond the neonatal period who have severe sepsis with no localizable focus, a combination of ceftriaxone with aminoglycoside is recommended as it adequately covers common bacterial pathogens, such as *Pneumococcus*, Hib, *Salmonella* and gram-negative pathogens, causing urinary tract infections and intra-abdominal infections. If malaria is suspected, IV artesunate should be initiated till smear reports are available. In areas endemic for rickettsia, doxycycline should be added to the empiric regime when there is clinical suspicion for rickettsial disease.

In children with suspected bacterial meningitis empiric therapy with ceftriaxone alone is considered adequate. However, with increasing prevalence of ceftriaxone resistance in pneumococcus (reported from Vellore recently as 15%) guidelines may change to include the addition of vancomycin in the regime.

Empirical monotherapy with ceftriaxone is indicated in most children with community-acquired pneumonia. In children with severe/very severe CAP due to suspected atypical pathogens addition of macrolide to ceftriaxone is recommended. If there are features of staphylococcal infection such as extreme toxicity, necrosis and pneumatocele formation empiric addition of vancomycin/linezolid may be considered. With increasing incidence of community-acquired urinary tract infections due to ESBL producing gram-negative pathogens, addition of an aminoglycoside to ceftriaxone or use of a beta-lactam–beta-lactamase inhibitor combination in children with suspected severe UTI who have received prior antibiotics is advisable. Children with suspected intra-abdominal sepsis should receive a combination of metronidazole

and ceftriaxone or a monotherapy with a beta-lactam–beta-lactamase inhibitor (BL-BLI) combination, such as piperacillin tazobactam/cefoperazone sulbactam or cefepime tazobactam. Children with skin, soft tissue and musculoskeletal infections where the usual culprit is methicillin sensitive *S. aureus* or *Streptococcus pyogenes* can be treated with cloxacillin/cefazolin monotherapy. An increasing incidence of community acquired methicillin-resistant *Staphylococcus aureus* (MRSA) has been noted; infections due to CA MRSA are characterized by severe toxicity, necrosis and leucopenia. If CA MRSA is suspected then addition of an anti-MRSA agent, such as vancomycin/teicoplanin/linezolid to cloxacillin is recommended. It is notable that for methicillin-sensitive *Staphylococcus aureus* (MSSA) cloxacillin/cefazolin are more efficacious than any anti-MRSA agent. For children with necrotizing fasciitis/toxic shock syndrome a toxin-inhibiting drug, such as clindamycin should be added to cloxacillin/cefazolin.

Nosocomial Infections

In children with nosocomial infections, choice of antibiotic therapy depends on the local flora, antibiogram, severity of infection previous antibiotic therapy, host comorbidities and the site of infection. For children with non-severe nosocomial sepsis treatment with BL-BLI combination (piperacillin tazobactam/cefoperazone sulbactam/cefepime tazobactam) with or without an aminoglycoside can be initiated. In patients with severe sepsis where the inoculum size is likely to be higher, BL-BLI combination therapy is inappropriate and here group 2 carbapenems, such as meropenem/imipenem or doripenem should be used. If the unit has a high incidence of MRSA infections, empirical therapy should also include an anti-MRSA drug preferably vancomycin. In the current day scenario where carbapenem resistance is increasing, some children with nosocomial sepsis and previous carbapenem exposure may require treatment with colistin/polymyxin B. Presence of risk factors for fungal infections, such as prolonged ICU stay, receipt of broad spectrum antibiotics, presence of central line, use of intralipids, dialysis, renal failure, use of corticosteroids, abdominal surgery merits addition of antifungal agent, such as fluconazole to the treatment regime. In some units where there is high incidence of fluconazole resistant *Candida* infections, echinocandins or amphotericin B may be required.

Infections in the Immunocompromised

Empirical antimicrobial therapy is complex and depends on the type and severity of the immunocompromised state and hence the likely etiologic agents. Broadly speaking, treatment should be initiated with a potent gram-negative cover such as BL-BLI combination or carbapenems with or without aminoglycoside. Additional anti-MRSA, broad spectrum antifungal therapy (echinocandins/

voriconazole/amphotericin B), antiviral therapy and therapy for pneumocystis carinii may be considered on a case by case basis. All efforts should be made to establish an etiologic diagnosis.

Dosing of Antimicrobial Drugs

In patients with severe sepsis, the highest recommended doses should be used as per recommended dosing interval. Attention should be paid to pharmacokinetic and pharmacodynamic parameters. Loading doses are needed for antibiotics such as colistin, polymyxin, tigecycline and vancomycin. Antibiotics which have time dependent action like beta lactams can be given as prolonged infusions over 3–4 hours to treat resistant infections. For BL-BLI combinations dosing should be on the basis of the parent beta lactam and not the whole combination. Since patients with severe sepsis are on several other drugs, the prescription should be checked for any drug interactions. Renal function should be monitored and doses of antibiotics adjusted if needed. The first dose in a patient with impairment of renal function is always the full dose.

Modification of Further Antibiotic Therapy

The empirical antibiotic therapy should be reviewed at 24–48 hours. If a diagnosis of a nonbacterial infection is made, antibiotics can be stopped. If cultures are positive, then therapy should be optimized as per cultures. The culture and susceptibility reports should be interpreted carefully and attention given to MIC (minimum inhibitory concentration) data if available. If an anti-MRSA drug has started at the outset and cultures are negative for MRSA the drug can be stopped. It is important to remember that many patients with community acquired severe sepsis and septic shock are likely to have a prolonged ICU stay and hence are at risk of drug-resistant nosocomial infections. If high end antibiotics are used at the outset, antibiotic options for future infections become limited. Therefore, if de escalation is possible, it should be practiced.

If cultures are negative, but patient is improving then the same antibiotics may be continued. If cultures are negative and the child is not improving or worsening, upgradation of antibiotics can be considered. Before upgrading antibiotics, fresh cultures should be sent and other causes of poor response should be considered. These include non-drainage of pus, non-removal of an infected central venous catheter, or a different pathogen, which will not respond to the current antimicrobial regime (e.g. rickettsial infections and atypical organisms will not respond to beta lactams).

Duration of Antibiotic Therapy

Duration of antibiotic therapy depends on the microbial etiology and site of infection. In neonates, culture negative sepsis needs to be treated for 7 days, culture positive sepsis for 2 weeks and meningitis for 3 weeks. In older children most infections can be adequately treated in 10–14 days, staphylococcal infections, bone and joint infections and endocarditis need longer treatment for 4–6 weeks. There has been a trend towards reducing the duration of antibiotics for most infections. Uncomplicated community acquired pneumonia can be adequately treated with 5–7 days therapy. Primary bacterial peritonitis, acute cholecystitis and appendicitis may be treated for as short as 5 days. Stopping treatment when the procalcitonin becomes normal is being increasing practised and evaluated in adult patients.

SOURCE CONTROL

The importance of source control in management of pediatric sepsis cannot be understated. This includes removal of infected central lines, drainage of pus and relief of urinary tract obstruction. If patients are sick for operative intervention, radiology (CT/USG) guided drains/pigtails can be inserted till the patient is stabilized.

SUPPORTIVE CARE IN SEVERE SEPSIS AND SEPTIC SHOCK

Supportive care includes the ABC of resuscitation, i.e. airway, breathing and circulation. Resuscitation guidelines as proposed by the Indian Academy of Pediatrics (IAP) intensive care chapter are detailed in Flowchart 2.8.2. Respiratory support, aggressive and early fluid therapy and optimum use of inotropes are the cornerstones of successful management. The guidelines for hemodynamic support have been very dynamic; the American College of Critical Care Medicine has recently in 2017 published guidelines on management of pediatric and neonatal septic shock.

Additional strategies include source control, use of corticosteroids in patients with catecholamine resistant shock and suspected or proven adrenal insufficiency, use of blood and blood products where needed, correction of hypoglycemia/hypocalcemia, avoidance of hyperglycemia and renal replacement therapy where indicated. Deep vein thrombosis (DVT) prophylaxis should be given in postpubertal children with severe sepsis. The role of intravenous immunoglobulins and G-CSF in severe sepsis/septic shock is controversial. Activated protein C (drotrecogin alpha) has been withdrawn from the market when randomized controlled trials failed to show its benefit on 28 day mortality.

PROGNOSIS

Severe pediatric sepsis is a disease with hospital mortality ranging 10–30%. Mortality is higher in resource limited

FLOWCHART 2.8.2: Supportive management in pediatric sepsis.

IAP intensive care chapter pediatric sepsis guidelines for resource-limited countries

0 min: Recognize depressed mental status and poor perfusion in a febrile child with or without focus of infection

Step I
O_2 by non-rebreathing mask if effortless tachypnea and septic shock
Flow inflating bag if grunt, retractions, abdominal respiration
Bag valve mask (BVM) ventilation if airway unstable, if bradypnea, apnea: plan early intubation

5 minutes: Establish intravenous/intraosseous access

Step II
Start normal saline/ringers 20 mL/kg over 15–20 minutes if BP normal; Rapidly by pull push 20 mL/kg if BP low, first dose of antibiotics (after drawing appropriate cultures)
Correct documented hypoglycemia and hypocalcemia

Monitor for clinical therapeutic goals after each bolus till all goal achieved: Respiratory rate, work of breathing, heart rate, capillary refill, BP, peripheral temperature, urine output, sensorium, liver span

| Therapeutic goals attained. No pulmonary edema/hepatomegaly | Goals not attained, No pulmonary edema/hepatomegaly | Therapeutic goals not attained, pulmonary edema/hepatomegaly |

2nd bolus 20 mL/kg at the rate of 15–20 minutes
3rd bolus 20 mL/kg at the rate of 15–20 minutes, if needed, assess the response after each

Goals not attained after 60 mL/kg
No pulmonary edema/hepatomegaly
Fluid refractory shock

Goals not attained pulm edema/hepatomegaly

Start inotrope, interrupt fluids briefly, intubate, catheterize. Start positive pressure bag ventilation

Pulmonary edema and hepatomegaly resolve goals not attained

*Dopamine at the rate of 10 μg/kg/min, add
Dobutamine 10 μg/kg/min: Titrate, intubate, catheterize for urine output monitoring,
Continue fluids in smaller aliquots, till goals attained

Titrate fluids 10–20 mL/kg at the rate of 10–20 minutes until goals achieved

Step III   40 minutes

Goals achieved

Pulmonary edema/hepatomegaly recur/not resolved:
no further fluids

60 minutes

Continue monitoring

Fluid refractory dopamine resistant shock

*Dopamine may be started after 2nd bolus

Shift to ICU

Plan epinephrine infusion early if bradycardia, BP remains low or falls with cold shock at any step.
Relief of tamponade, such as pneumothorax, or pericardial tamponade, increased intra-abdominal pressure due to fluid should be considered at any point.

countries. The mortality of severe pediatric sepsis as reported in the United States is 10.3% (lower than adults). A retrospective chart review revealed that apart from the in-hospital mortality which was 6.8%, follow-up mortality in the survivors in the following year was also 6.5% with half of the survivors requiring admission at least once during the following year. Rates of readmission were higher in children who had coexisting diseases and who had cardiovascular and hematologic dysfunction in the sentinel admission. The Sepsis Prevalence, Outcomes, and Therapies (SPROUT) study on pediatric sepsis reported mortality rates of 25%.

PREVENTION

Streptococcus pneumoniae, Hib, *Salmonella*, measles, *Rotavirus,* chicken pox are common causes of pediatric sepsis that are preventable by immunization. Malaria and dengue can be controlled to a large extent by appropriate vector control strategies. Dengue vaccines have recently become available. Asepsis during delivery, promotion of breast feeding, avoidance of malnutrition and vitamin A supplementation are other important strategies to reduce the burden of pediatric sepsis and its attendant morbidity and mortality. Prevention of nosocomial sepsis involves strict adherence to infection control policies in ICUs. Efforts should be made to reduce the incidence of antimicrobial resistance especially in gram-negative organisms by rational antimicrobial prescribing practices and antibiotic stewardship so that treatment options for these infections continue to exist.

SUMMARY

Pediatric sepsis, particularly severe sepsis is a very common cause of morbidity and mortality in children. It is important to recognize severe sepsis early, institute early appropriate antimicrobial treatment, initiate supportive care particularly volume resuscitation to improve outcomes. At the same time immunization, hand hygiene, asepsis, promotion of nutrition, adherence to infection control strategies are other primary prevention measures. Rising antimicrobial resistance especially with advent of carbapenem destroying beta lactamases is seriously compromising treatment options for severe pediatric sepsis in our country.

BIBLIOGRAPHY

1. Bone RC. The pathogenesis of sepsis. Ann Intern Med. 1991;115:457-69.
2. Davis AL, Carcillo JA, Aneja RK, Deymann AJ, Lin JC, Nguyen TC, et al. American College of Critical Care Medicine Clinical Practice Parameters for Hemodynamic Support of Pediatric and Neonatal Septic Shock. Crit Care Med. 2017;45:1061-93.
3. Goldstein B, Giroir B, Randolph A. International Consensus Conference on Pediatric Sepsis. International pediatric sepsis consensus conference: definitions for sepsis and organ dysfunction in pediatrics. Pediatr Crit Care Med. 2005;6:2-8.
4. Gupta A, Kapil A, Lodha R, et al. Burden of healthcare-associated infections in a paediatric intensive care unit of a developing country: a single centre experience using active surveillance. J Hosp Infect. 2011;78:323-6.
5. Ismail J, Jayashree M. Advances in the Management of Pediatric Septic Shock: Old Questions, New Answers. Indian Pediatr. 2018; 55:319-25.
6. Khilnani P, Singhi S, Lodha R, et al. Pediatric sepsis guidelines: summary for resource-limited countries. Indian J Crit Care Med. 2010;14:41-52.
7. Kumar A, Roberts D, Wood KE, et al. Duration of hypotension prior to antimicrobial administration is the critical determinant of survival in human septic shock. Crit Care Med. 2006;34:1589-96.
8. Patel D, Nimbalkar A, Sethi A, et al. Blood culture isolates in neonatal sepsis and their sensitivity in Anand District of India. Indian J Pediatr. 2014;81:785-90.
9. Saha SK, Schrag SJ, El Arifeen S, Mullany LC, Shahidul Islam M, Shang N, et al. Causes and incidence of community-acquired serious infections among young children in South Asia (ANISA): an observational cohort study. Lancet. 2018;392:145-59.
10. Standage SW, Wong HR. Biomarkers for pediatric sepsis and septic shock. Expert Rev Anti Infect Ther. 2011;9:71-9.
11. Weiss SL, Fitzgerald JC, Pappachan J, Wheeler D, Jaramillo-Bustamante JC, Salloo A, et al. Sepsis Prevalence, Outcomes, and Therapies (SPROUT) Study Investigators and Pediatric Acute Lung Injury and Sepsis Investigators (PALISI) Network. Global epidemiology of pediatric severe sepsis: the sepsis prevalence, outcomes, and therapies study. Am J Respir Crit Care Med. 2015;191:1147-57.

2.9 INFECTIONS IN IMMUNOCOMPROMISED CHILDREN

Rakesh Kumar

INTRODUCTION

A child is said to be immunocompromised when his immune system is not able to fight infections appropriately. Infective organisms which do not cause disease in normal children may cause serious disease in immunocompromised children. A child may be immunocompromised due to number of congenital or acquired immune-deficiencies. A number of nonimmune barriers to infection are also there in our body (e.g. skin and mucous membranes) and they assume even more importance in a host who has weak immune system to fight infections. A child should be suspected to be immunocompromised if he/she has more than usual frequency of common infections, unusual organisms causing infections, infections at unusual sites or common infections having unusual severity. Treatment of infections in immunocompromised host is not so different than an immunocompetent host but it is very important to suspect, confirm and label a patient to be immunocompromised so that timely and aggressive treatment for specific infections can be initiated. It is easy to suspect and confirm acquired immunodeficiencies, like HIV, malnutrition, diabetes, neutropenia, etc. but it is primary immune deficiencies which are not usually suspected and confirmed. A high index of suspicion and good laboratory set-up is important to confirm primary immune deficiencies.

ETIOPATHOGENESIS

Barriers against Infection

A healthy child is protected against infections by a number of immunological and nonimmunological barriers. Non-immune barriers are even more important in children who have underlying immune deficiencies. Breach in any of these protective barriers can predispose children to severe infections. Skin is the most important nonimmune protective barrier. Its outer (horny) layer is impermeable and dry which forbids entry of microorganisms. Conjunctiva and mucous membranes are other two important non-immune barriers against infections. Barriers along with their active components which protect against infection are listed in Table 2.9.1.

Breakage of specific barrier may have risk of specific infections as shown in Table 2.9.2. Knowledge of these causative organisms in particular barrier defect is important to start empirical antibiotic therapy awaiting the culture reports, e.g. a child coming with suspected cerebrospinal fluid (CSF) shunt infection has to be empirically started on antibiotic with good activity against *Staphylococcus* spp.

Table 2.9.3 enlists common congenital and acquired immune-deficiency conditions in children which can make them prone to infections. Most common of these conditions and specific types of infections associated with these conditions will be discussed further.

Table 2.9.1: Nonimmunologic barriers against infections.

Barrier	Specific glands/ mechanisms	Active components
Skin	Outer horny layer Sebaceous glands Normal skin flora	Impermeability and desquamation Fatty acids Inhibits growth of pathogenic organisms (microbial interference)
Mucous membranes	Mucus	Microbial interference and desquamation
Gastrointestinal tract	Salivary glands, gastric mucosa, bile, peristalsis	Lysozyme, gastric acid, bile salts
Respiratory tract Urinary tract	Goblet cells Mucosal ciliated cells, coughing reflex	Mucus, mucociliary elevator activity
Vagina	Periodic voiding Acidic pH	Hydrokinetic forces and flushing action
Conjunctiva	Lacrimal glands Tears	Lysozyme and lactoferrin Flush away foreign material

Table 2.9.2: Defects in nonimmunological barriers and organisms causing infection.

Defects	Barrier affected	Organisms commonly isolated
Intravenous catheters	Skin	*Staphylococcus epidermidis, Bacteroides, Pseudomonas, Candida, Cryptococcus*
Urinary catheters	Mucosa	*Pseudomonas, Serratia, S. epidermidis, Candida*
Cerebrospinal fluid shunts	Skin	*S. epidermidis, Staphylococcus aureus, Bacillus* spp., *Diphtheroids,* enteric bacteria
Surgical wounds	Skin	*S. epidermidis, S. aureus, Pseudomonas, Alcaligenes faecalis, Candida*
Burns	Skin	*Pseudomonas, Serratia, Staphylococcus, Candida, Mucor*
Inhalation therapy	Mucosa	*Pseudomonas, Serratia*
Impacted foreign body under skin	Skin	*S. aureus,* enteric organisms, *Mycobacteria Spp., Nocardia, Vibrio* spp.
Dermal sinus	Skin	*S. epidermidis, Diphtheroids*

Table 2.9.3: Common immune deficiencies—congenital and acquired.

Congenital immunodeficiencies					Acquired immunodeficiencies
T-cell defects	Combined B- and T-cell defects	B-cell defects	Phagocyte defects	Disorders of the complement system	
Thymic dysplasia (DiGeorge syndrome)	Severe combined immunodeficiency	X-linked agammaglobulinemia	Leukocyte adhesion deficiency	Congenital asplenia	HIV
Defective T-cell receptor	Combined immunodeficiency	Common variable immunodeficiency	Chédiak–Higashi syndrome	Splenic dysfunction (hemoglobinopathies)	Malignancies (and cancer chemotherapy)
Defective cytokine production	Omenn syndrome	Selective immunoglobulin A (IgA) deficiency	Myeloperoxidase deficiency		Transplantation • Bone marrow and stem cell • Solid organ
T-cell activation defects	Thrombocytopenia and eczema (Wiskott–Aldrich syndrome)	IgG subclass deficiencies	Chronic granulomatous disease		
CD8 lymphocytopenia	Ataxia-telangiectasia	Hyper-IgM syndrome	Leukopenia		
	Hyper-IgE syndrome		Congenital neutropenia (Kostmann syndrome)		Burns
			Shwachman–Diamond syndrome		Sickle cell disease
					Cystic fibrosis
					Immunosuppressive drugs
					Asplenia
					Implanted foreign body
					Malnutrition

INFECTIONS ASSOCIATED WITH COMMON CONGENITAL IMMUNE DEFICIENCIES

Disorders of Phagocyte System

After the physical barriers of skin and mucous membranes are breached, phagocyte system is the first line of defence against the invading microorganisms. Polymorphonuclear phagocytes are neutrophils, eosinophils, and basophils. Mononuclear phagocytes constituting monocytes and macrophages are relatively less in number but are also critical in maintaining defence against the microorganisms as highlighted by diseases resulting because of their deficiencies. Phagocyte system may be defective owing either to deficiency in number of cells or qualitative functional defects in cells. Neutropenic patients irrespective of the cause are thus prone to infections. Acquired neutropenia is caused by suppression of bone marrow by infections or drugs. Congenital neutropenia also called Kostmann syndrome is not very common. It is characterized by early onset of pyogenic infections (in infancy usually) like cellulitis and perirectal abscesses

caused by *S. aureus* and *Pseudomonas aeruginosa*. Cyclic neutropenia is a condition with neutropenia occurring in cyclical manner every 3–4 weeks and lasting for 3–6 days leaving the patient prone to infections particularly with *Clostridium perfringens* for such periods. Patient clinically presents with cyclical fever, aphthous ulcers and stomatitis and occasionally severe necrotizing cellulitis.

Defects of function (neutrophil count high or normal) can further be of two types, including defects of cells migration and defects of microbicidal activity. Leucocyte adhesion deficiency (LAD) is a prototype disorder of defects in cell migration resulting from defect in beta chain of integrin (CD18), which is required for process of neutrophil aggregation and attachment to endothelial surfaces. These patients usually present with infection of skin and mucosal surfaces without pus formation like gingivitis, periodontitis and mucosal candidiasis. Children with severe defect may present in neonatal period with delayed cord separation. Ecthyma gangrenosum and pyoderma gangrenosum may also occur. Common organisms causing infections in LAD are *S. aureus*, *Candida albicans* and gram-negative bacilli. Chronic granulomatous disorder (CGD) is a prototype entity for defects in microbicidal activity of the phagocytes.

It is inherited in an autosomal recessive or X-linked pattern having defective neutrophil NADPH oxidase function with defective superoxide generation and intracellular killing of microorganisms. Children usually present with chronic or recurrent infections of lymph nodes and internal organs commonly lungs, liver and bone. Common organisms isolated are *S. aureus, Serratia, Burkholderia cepacia* and *Aspergillus*. Myeloperoxidase deficiency resulting from mutation in gene encoding for this enzyme in neutrophils leads to absent killing of *C. albicans* and *Aspergillus fumigatus* apart from common infections as seen in CGD. Chediak–Higashi Syndrome, a rare autosomal recessive disorder is characterized by partial oculocutaneous albinism, recurrent pyogenic infections, peripheral neuropathy and neutropenia. *S. aureus* is responsible for 70% of infections in these children.

Defects in Complement System

Recurrent infections in these defects are due to defective opsonization by macrophages. It occurs in group of children who have asplenia, are splenectomized or have splenic dysfunction due to sickle cell anemia or other hemoglobinopathies. Common organisms causing infections in these children are encapsulated organisms like *Streptococcus pneumoniae, H. influenzae, N. meningitidis, Salmonella* presenting as sepsis pneumonia, meningitis and osteomyelitis. Children with C3 deficiencies tend have more serious infections than in children with deficiencies of C5 to C9.

B-cell Defects

Humoral deficiency is produced by decreased production of protective antibodies by the B-type lymphocytes. There is large spectrum of antibody deficiencies depending on type and degree of deficiency. X-linked agammaglobulinemia is prototype disorder in this group in which there is virtual absence of all classes of antibodies, absence of plasma cells from the circulation and no antibody formation after antigenic stimulation. Children with these defects commonly present with recurrent pyogenic infections starting after 6 months with encapsulated organisms such as *S. pneumoniae and H. influenzae* type b. Viruses and fungi are not of major concern in these children, with some exceptions. Rotavirus infections in these children can atypically present as persistent diarrhea rather than acute self-limiting infection. Enteroviruses can disseminate to cause chronic meningoencephalitis. They have more risk of vaccine-associated paralytic polio after live oral polio vaccination. Children with selective IgA deficiency commonly have mucosal infections like sinopulmonary and gastrointestinal infections. Hyper-IgM syndrome is characterized by deficiency of IgG and IgA and excess of IgM and patients are at risk to *Pneumocystis*

jiroveci and *Cryptosporidium* infections apart from other sinopulmonary infections.

T-cell Defects

Isolated T-cell defects are rare compared to combined B-cell and T-cell defects. T-cell defects can be primary or secondary to malnutrition, immunosuppressive drugs, HIV, etc. Children with combined or isolated T-cell defects usually present early in life with chronic diarrhea, mucocutaneous candidiasis, pneumonia, rhinitis and otitis media. Children with DiGeorge syndrome have thymic dysplasia with hypocalcemia and cardiac anomalies. Chronic mucocutaneous candidiasis (CMC) is another rare disorder associated with primary T-cell dysfunction usually associated with multiple endocrinopathies. Children with CMC lack delayed hypersensitivity skin test to *Candida* antigen despite chronic infection.

Combined B-cell and T-cell Defects

Children with these defects have variable propensity to infections depending on degree of defect. Severe combined immunodeficiency syndrome (SCID) is the severest form of immunodeficiency in this group. These children present within 6 months of age with failure to thrive, disseminated candidiasis, chronic diarrhea, *P. jiroveci* pneumonitis and cytomegalovirus (CMV) infection. After 6 months they are also prone to both gram-positive and gram-negative bacterial infections and live virus vaccination can also cause dissemination and disease. Partial deficiency of combined B-cell and T-cell defects is seen in ataxia-telangiectasia, Wiskott–Aldrich syndrome, hyper-IgE syndrome and X-linked immunodeficiency syndrome. Wiskott–Aldrich syndrome is an X-linked recessive disease associated with thrombocytopenia, eczema and impaired antibody response to polysaccharide antigens. Infections with *S. pneumoniae, H. influenzae* type b and *P. jiroveci* are common. Children with hyper-IgE syndrome (Job syndrome) have elevated levels of IgE and present with recurrent episodes of *S. aureus* abscesses of the skin, lungs and musculoskeletal system. They also have increased chances of fungal infections.

INFECTIONS ASSOCIATED WITH SECONDARY IMMUNODEFICIENCIES

Common conditions leading to secondary immune deficiencies are listed in Table 2.9.3. Most of these conditions affect T-cell arm of immune system and lead to a state of T-cell deficiency in the host.

Malnutrition

Malnutrition has greatest effect on T cells and antibody response is typically good. These children are more prone to infections by common environment pathogens, e.g. measles and tuberculosis. The risk of infection increases with increasing severity of malnutrition. It is recommended to give broad-spectrum antibiotics to all children with grades 3 and 4 malnutrition admitted in hospital for any condition.

HIV Infection

It primarily affects CD4+ T cells. Spectrum of infections occurring in HIV-infected children is thus same as seen in primary T-cell deficiencies. Recommendations regarding prophylaxis and treatment of opportunistic infections in children with HIV can be seen in detail in pediatric guidelines issued by *National AIDS Control Organization* (NACO) and Indian Academy of Paediatrics (Website: www.nacoonline.org).

Malignancies and Cancer Chemotherapy

Children with malignancies are prone to infections due to following factors:
- Malignant cells release tumor-induced factors and directly affect the immune system, primarily T cells.
- Drugs used for treatment cause excessive bone marrow suppression and decrease in all cell lines. However, it is deficiency of WBCs which make these patients prone to infections. Lesser the WBC count more is the chance of serious infections.
- Malnutrition induced by the malignancy.
- Frequent hospitalizations and interventions done for treatment.
- Long-term antibiotic treatment altering normal body flora.

Specific organisms commonly causing infections in these children are *Enterobacter* spp., *S aureus*, *S. pneumoniae*, *H. influenzae*, Salmonella, group D streptococci, *Serratia*, *Candida*, *Toxoplasma*, CMV, herpes simplex viruses and papovaviruses. Hepatitis and varicella infections are also commonly seen. Necrotizing enteropathy caused by gram-negative organisms is also common. Some general rules which can be followed in such children are: fever in acute leukemia is usually caused by gram-negative septicemia, persistent fever in relapse is usually caused by fungal infections, intracellular organisms like *M. tuberculosis*, *P. jirovecii*, *Listeria*, *Brucella*, etc. are common cause of infections in Hodgkin disease, gram-positive organisms commonly cause infections in chronic leukemia and febrile neutropenia in these patients should be considered a medical emergency.

Neutropenia in these patients is major cause of infections. Degree of neutropenia is directly proportional to risk of infections in these children. Children are at very high risk if absolute neutrophil count is less than 500/mm³. At such low counts children may not have inflammatory response and can present with only fever without other symptoms and signs of infection. Common organisms isolated from febrile neutropenic patients are gram-positive cocci, followed by *P. aeruginosa*, *E. coli*, *Klebsiella*, *Enterobacter* and *Acinetobacter*. Patients who receive prolonged broad-spectrum antimicrobial therapy are prone to develop opportunistic fungal infections with *Candida* and *Aspergillus*.

Immunosuppressive Drugs

Different types of immunosuppressive drugs are used for diseases like collagen vascular disorders, malignancies and for transplantation. Commonly used drugs are corticosteroids, cyclosporine and cancer cytotoxic drugs. Steroids are known to cause transient decrease in number of T cells. Cyclosporine causes inhibition of synthesis of cytokines. Cytotoxic cancer chemotherapeutic agents usually affect both T and B cells. Common bacterial infections in these children are caused by *P. aeruginosa*, *E. coli*, *Klebsiella*, *Proteus* spp., *Herellea* and *Serratia* spp. Common viral infections in these children are herpes simplex, varicella-zoster, CMV, Epstein-Barr virus and measles.

Transplantation

Different organ transplants are being done in children more recently in India. Patients who have undergone transplant have specific problems related to infections because of number of factors. Immunosuppressive therapy instituted to these patients is major cause of infections in these children. Moreover they are already immunocompromised by the chronic diseases. They have like chronic kidney disease, chronic liver disease and chronic problems requiring bone marrow transplant.

Bone marrow transplant patients have majority (around half) of infections in 1st month after transplant when there is intense granulocytopenia. Bacterial infections caused by aerobic gram-negative bacilli and gram-positive cocci form bulk of infections in 1st month after transplant. *Aspergillus, Fusarium* and *Pseudallescheria boydii* are common fungal infections in this period. After this period, develops depression of both humoral and cellular immunity leading to viral and protozoal infections. Common among these are CMV, adenoviruses, *P. carinii* and varicella zoster.

In solid organ transplants the need for strong immunosuppressive therapy used is the main reason for infections. Infections occurring in abdominal transplants (kidney, liver, etc.) in 1st month are usually caused by enteric gram-negative bacteria, *Enterococcus* and *Candida*. After thoracic transplants (heart and lung) common pathogens expected are *S. aureus* and gram-negative bacteria. Viral infections in these patients are more common after a month of transplantation. Common viruses causing infections are CMV, *Epstein–Barr virus* (EBV) and varicella-zoster virus.

MODALITIES OF DIAGNOSIS

Following practical points should be kept in mind regarding diagnosis while managing such children:

- As a rule threshold for investigating and treating infections in such children should be kept very low.
- Any organism isolated from such patients should be considered as having potential to cause serious infection and its complications.
- A detailed history of any exposure to infections in the family or setting in which patient is residing is important.
- Baseline cultures of throat and stool should be obtained to determine bacterial flora and their antibacterial sensitivity.
- Cultures from all possible sites should be taken to actively make a search for focus of infection when there is no obvious focus of infection on history and clinical examination.
- Special consideration has to be given to diagnose unusual pathogens as well. Sputum examination for *P. jiroveci* should also be done in patient with pneumonia apart from search for common bacteria and *M. tuberculosis*.
- In patients with severe immune deficiencies antibodies assay against *Toxoplasma*, CMV, EBV, varicella zoster and measles should be done.
- Stool cultures should also be sent for atypical organisms like *Cryptosporidium*.
- Repeated cultures from different sites, particularly when such patient is hospitalized and has number of indwelling catheters in situ, have to be performed to monitor for opportunistic infections.

TREATMENT

General principles in treatment of infections in immunocompromised children are as under:

- Basic principles of treatment of infections in such children are actually no different than normal children when we know the causative organisms. Appropriate antibiotics in adequate doses are to be given as per sensitivity patterns for the causative organisms.
- Initial empiric antibiotics need to be started after cultures and serologic tests for establishing etiology have been obtained. We need to give empirical broad-spectrum antibiotics which are known to be effective against the expected organism in particular immunocompromised condition. Antimicrobial agents chosen should be broad spectrum, synergistic and microbicidal.
- Every effort should be made to isolate the organism from every possible site and specific antibiotic therapy given as early as possible.
- Some viruses have been particularly associated with serious infections in immunocompromised children,

like herpes simplex, varicella, influenza, CMV, Rous sarcoma virus (RSV), and specific antiviral treatment is available for them provided we recognize these in time.
- Fungi and parasitic infections should be particularly suspected in following situations: prolonged immunosuppressive therapy, culture negative febrile neutropenic patients, intensive and prolonged antibacterial treatment without any response, culture negative and antimicrobial resistant diarrhea and chronic mucositis. So, patients with these risk factors should be aggressively evaluated for fungal and parasitic infections and treated promptly.
- Immunoglobulin therapy may be helpful in a subset of patients particularly with humoral and combined immunodeficiencies.

Treatment of Febrile Neutropenia

Febrile neutropenia is defined as a single oral temperature of above or equal to 38.3°C (≥101°F) or a temperature of above or equal to 38°C (≥100.4°F) for greater than or equal to 1 hour in a patient with a neutrophil count of less than 500 cells/mm^3, or a count of less than 1,000 cells/mm^3 with a predicted decrease to less than 500 cells/mm^3. Causes of neutropenia have already been discussed and most common cause in clinical practice is neutropenia resulting from cancer chemotherapy.

Treatment of febrile neutropenia is considered a medical emergency and prompt broad-spectrum empirical antibiotics are given to cover both gram-positive and gram-negative organisms. Infectious diseases society of America (IDSA) has come out with guidelines for management of febrile neutropenia in 1997 and which were last updated in 2010. It has been shown that, at least one-half of neutropenic patients who become febrile have an established or occult infection, and at least one-fifth of patients with neutrophil counts of less than 100 cells/mm^3 have bacteremia. The common sites of infection often include the alimentary tract, where cancer chemotherapy-induced mucosal damage allows invasion of opportunistic organisms. Breach of skin by invasive procedures, such as placement of vascular access devices, often provides portals of entry for infectious organisms. In these patients symptoms and signs of inflammation may be minimal or absent, especially if they have anemia in addition to neutropenia. Therefore, a search should be undertaken for subtle symptoms and signs, including pain at the sites that are most commonly infected. These sites are the periodontium, pharynx, lower esophagus, lung, perineum (including the anus), eye (fundus), and the skin, including bone-marrow aspiration sites, vascular catheter access sites, and tissue around the nails.

Gram-positive bacteria now account for 60–70% of microbiologically documented infections, although the rate of gram-negative infections is increasing in some places. Some of the gram-positive organisms may be methicillin resistant and, therefore, are susceptible only to vancomycin and teicoplanin. As per IDSA guidelines, patients with febrile neutropenia are divided into high and low risk for developing severe infections and management is often decided by the risk status a patient is admitted with. Patients with high risk are those with absolute neutrophil count of less than 100 cells/mm^3, absolute monocyte count of less than 100 cells/mm^3, normal chest radiograph, normal results of hepatic and renal function tests, neutropenia of less than 7 days, resolution of neutropenia expected in less than 10 days, no intravenous catheter-site infection, early evidence of bone marrow recovery, malignancy in remission, peak temperature of less than 39°C, no neurological or mental changes, no appearance of illness, no abdominal pain, no comorbidity or complications, no hypotension, no chronic obstructive pulmonary disease, solid tumor or no fungal infection, no dehydration and outpatient at onset of fever.

For deciding initial empiric antibiotic regimen, following approach has been recommended. First, determine whether the patient is at low or high risk for serious life-threatening infection on the basis of the criteria observed at the time of presentation. If the risk is high, intravenous antibiotics must be used; if risk is low, the patient may be treated with either intravenous or oral antibiotics. High-risk patients who require hospitalization for IV empirical antibiotic therapy; single drug antipseudomonal beta-lactam agent, such as cefepime, meropenem or imipenem-cilastatin, or piperacillin-tazobactam, is recommended. Second, decide whether the patient qualifies for vancomycin therapy. If the patient qualifies, begin treatment with a two- or three-drug combination with vancomycin plus cefepime, ceftazidime, or a carbapenem, with or without an aminoglycoside. Inclusion of vancomycin in initial empirical therapy may be appropriate for selected patients with the following clinical findings: (a) clinically suspected serious catheter-related infections (e.g. bacteremia, cellulitis), (b) known colonization with penicillin- and cephalosporin-resistant pneumococci or methicillin-resistant *S. aureus*, (c) positive results of blood culture for gram-positive bacteria before final identification and susceptibility testing, or (d) hypotension or other evidence of cardiovascular impairment. Two-drug combinations may be used for management of complicated cases or if antimicrobial resistance is a problem. Adults selected for oral therapy may receive ciprofloxacin plus amoxicillin-clavulanate. Initial therapy with oral antibiotics alone is not recommended for children. In the selection of the initial antibiotic regimen, one should consider the type, frequency of occurrence, and antibiotic susceptibility of bacterial isolates recovered from other patients at the same hospital. The use of certain antibiotics may be limited by special circumstances, such as drug allergy or

organ (e.g. renal or hepatic) dysfunction. Such drugs as cisplatin, amphotericin B, cyclosporine, vancomycin, and aminoglycosides should be avoided in combination, if possible, because of their additive renal toxicity. Patient has to be reassessed after 3–5 days after starting initial empiric antibiotics. Some patients deteriorating fast may warrant change of empirical therapy even within 48–72 hours. *If patient becomes afebrile after 3–5 days of initial antibiotic*s modify antibiotic therapy for specific organisms, if identified, and continue use of broad-spectrum antibiotics for at least 7 days, until cultures are sterile and the patient has clinically recovered. If the causative organism is not found and the patient is receiving drugs intravenously and was at low risk at the onset of treatment, treatment may be changed to oral ciprofloxacin plus amoxicillin-clavulanate for adults or cefixime for children after 48 hours, if clinically preferable. The same intravenous antibiotics should be continued for high-risk patients. If patient continues to be febrile after 3–5 days of less than 500/mm^3 on day 7 and patient was initially grouped as high risk antibiotics have to continue till absolute neutrophil count (ANC) improves. If patient does not become afebrile after 3–5 days and ANC is greater than or equal to 500/mm^3 one can stop antibiotics after 4–5 days and reassess. If ANC is less than 500/mm^3 one has to continue antibiotics for 2 weeks and reassess. *Empirical antifungal treatment* and investigation for invasive fungal infections should be planned for patients with persistent fever after 4–7 days of antibiotics and whose duration of neutropenia is expected to be more than 7 days.

Antiviral drugs: They are indicated only if there is clinical or laboratory evidence of viral disease.

Granulocyte transfusions and colony stimulating factors: There are no specific indications for these agents and are better avoided as they are costly and do not alter mortality in these patients.

PREVENTION OF INFECTIONS IN IMMUNOCOMPROMISED CHILDREN

Many of the immunocompromised conditions leave the host at continuous threat to acquire infections which can be minimized to some extent by giving prophylactic antibiotics, vaccination, supplementing deficient immunoglobulins (antibody deficiencies). Apart from these, basic measures like isolating such patients when they are hospitalized, proper hygiene, good orodental and skin care and avoiding undue exposure to common infections at home and locality should also be taken care. Combination of all these measures will be more helpful rather than laying stress on just antibiotic prophylaxis. Common conditions requiring prophylaxis and antibiotics used are given in Table 2.9.4. To remember this we again need to keep in mind common organisms causing infections in each condition.

Table 2.9.4: Recommended prophylaxis for common immunodeficiency states to prevent infections.

Immunodeficiency condition	Prophylaxis
Malignancy	Co-trimoxazole (TMP-5 mg/kg/day bid) at least 3 times a week during periods of neutropenia Ketoconazole/miconazole during neutropenia Pneumococcal vaccine
Immunosuppressive therapy	Cotrimoxazole as above Isoniazid, 10 mg/kg od (in Mantoux positive and chest X-ray negative patients) during prolonged immunosuppressive therapy Pneumococcal vaccine Varicella Zoster immune globulin within 5 days of exposure
Transplant patients	Cotrimoxazole as above Acyclovir 15–45 mg/kg/day q8h in bone marrow recipients seropositive for herpes simplex virus
T- and B-cell combined immunodeficiencies	Cotrimoxazole (2 mg/kg/day bid TMP) Isoniazid, 10 mg/kg od (in Mantoux positive or exposure to tuberculosis) Varicella Zoster immune globulin within 5 days of exposure Measles immunoglobulin within 6 days after exposure Maintenance intravenous immunoglobulin monthly (400 mg/m²) in severe combined immunodeficient
B-cell defects	Maintenance intravenous immunoglobulin monthly (400 mg/m²) Penicillin, if recurrent respiratory infections
Complement deficiency	Penicillin V 250 mg bid Vaccinations for *Pneumococcus* and *Meningococcus*
Job syndrome	Dicloxacillin 25 mg/kg/day q 12 hours
Chronic granulomatous disease	Sulfisoxazole 50 mg/kg/day bid
Chediak–Higashi syndrome	Dicloxacillin 25 mg/kg/day q 12 hours
Sickle cell anemia	Penicillin V 250 mg bid/amoxicillin 20 mg/kg/day bid Vaccinations for Pneumococcus, *H. influenzae type* b, *Salmonella typhi*

BIBLIOGRAPHY

1. American Academy of Pediatrics. Passive and active immunization. In: Pickering LK (Ed). Red Book 2006: Report of the Committee on Infectious Diseases, 27th edition. Elk Grove Village, IL: American Academy of Pediatrics; 2006. pp. 1-103.
2. Chinen J, Kline MW, Shearer WT. Primary immunodeficiencies. In: Feigin RD, Cherry JD, Demmler GJ, Kaplan SL (Eds). Textbook of Pediatric Infectious Diseases, 6th edition. Philadelphia, PA: Saunders Elsevier; 2009. pp. 1021-36.
3. Freifeld AG, Bow EJ, Sepkowitz KA, et al. Infectious Diseases Society of Americaa. Clinical practice guideline for the use of antimicrobial agents in neutropenicpatients with cancer: 2010 Update by the Infectious Diseases Society of America. Clin Infect Dis. 2011;52(4):427-31.
4. Kesson AM, Kakakios A. Immunocompromised children: conditions and infectious agents. Paediatr Respir Rev. 2007;8(3):231-9.
5. Lekstrom-Himes JA, Gallin JI. Immunodeficiency diseases caused by defects in phagocytes. N Engl J Med. 2000;343(23):1703-14.
6. Michaels MG, Green M. Infections in immunocompromised persons. In: Kliegman RM, Stanton BF, St. Geme III JW, Schorr NF, Behrman RE (Eds). Nelson Textbook of Pediatrics, 19th edition. Philadelphia PA: Saunders Elsevier; 2011. pp. 902-3.
7. Stiehm ER, Ochs HD, Winkelstein JA. Immunodeficiency disorders: general considerations. In: Stiehm ER, Ochs HD, Winkelstein JA (Eds). Immunologic Disorders in Infants and Children, 5th edition. Philadelphia, PA: Elsevier Science; 2004. pp. 289-355.
8. Weber DJ, Rutala WA. Immunization of immunocompromised persons. Immunol Allergy Clin North Am. 2003;23(4):605-34.
9. Wood P, Stanworth S, Burton J, et al. Recognition, clinical diagnosis and management of patients with primary antibody deficiencies: a systematic review. Clin ExpImmunol. 2007; 149(3):410-23.

Agni Sekhar Saha

2.10 **HEALTHCARE-ASSOCIATED INFECTIONS**

INTRODUCTION

Healthcare-associated infection (HCAI) has become a major issue with increasing complexity all over the world with the Indian subcontinent providing some of the most difficult challenges. HCAI has important outcome, resource and quality implications. The different nomenclatures used in literature are confusing which should be clarified first.

Nosocomial Infection

Nosocomial infection (NI) as defined by Centers for Diseases Control and Prevention (CDC), USA, is a localized or systemic condition (1) that results from adverse reaction to the presence of an infectious agent(s) or its toxin(s) and (2) that was not present or incubating at the time of admission to the hospital. For all practical purpose—this means new infections that occur at least 48 hours after hospital admission. Patient may develop HAI even after discharge from the hospital. Infection in a neonate as the result of passage through the birth canal is considered a NI unlike congenital infections due to transplacental transmission.

Hospital-acquired Infection

This term is interchangeable with "nosocomial infection".

Healthcare-associated Infection

This is a relatively new term which is used to denote any infection that arises because of contact with the healthcare system in its widest sense. It emphasizes two factors: (1) healthcare is now delivered not only in hospitals, but also in varied settings like outdoor clinics or even patient's own home, and HCAI may occur in any of these settings and (2) it may affect the patient as well as others like care givers or even visitors.

Colonization

Colonization as defined by CDC is the presence of microorganisms on skin, on mucous membranes, in open wounds or in excretions or secretions which are not causing adverse clinical signs or symptoms.

Healthcare-associated infections can affect many organ systems. However, ventilator-associated pneumonia (VAP), catheter-related bloodstream infection (CRBSI) and catheter-associated urinary tract infection (CAUTI) are other major issues. Other HCAIs include surgical site infection, skin and soft tissue infection, gastrointestinal infection including *Clostridium difficile* colitis, etc. HCAIs are iatrogenic and should be considered as system failures,

so most of the focus should be given on preventing them rather than treating.

EPIDEMIOLOGY

Prevalence of HCAI would vary depending on the patient population, area of the hospital—higher on pediatric intensive care units (PICU) and neonatal intensive care units (NICU) than general wards, geographical location of the hospital, diagnostic criteria, method of surveillance and other factors. Hence there is a wide variation in reported prevalence. An often quoted overall figure from the National Nosocomial Infections Surveillance System (NNIS), USA, is 6.1/100 patients with an incidence density of 14.1 infections/1,000 patient days. A cross-sectional pediatric study also quoted similar overall figure of 7.7/100 patients. Younger age, prematurity, longer duration of hospital stay, admission to NICU or PICU, presence of invasive devices, immune-suppression and recent surgery, all are associated with HCAI. In a multicenter study of 43 children's hospitals—median overall incidence density per 1,000 patient days were 8.9 in NICUs and 13.9 in PICUs.

Unlike adults where CAUTI is the most common—CRBSI is the most common HCAI in most pediatric studies followed by VAP with CAUTI being the third commonest. Most of the infections are associated with invasive devices, for example, NNIS data showed 91% BSIs are associated with central venous lines, 95% hospital-acquired pneumonia occurred in ventilated children and 77% hospital-acquired UTI happened in children with urinary catheter.

MICROBIOLOGY AND ANTIBIOTICS

Multiple drug resistance (MDR) is the single most important factor in HCAI making their management difficult. The situation is changing very rapidly all over the world and is now one of the most important and difficult issues in medicine.

Methicillin-resistant *Staphylococcus aureus* (MRSA) is possibly the most important pathogen globally; especially in the Western world, where consistently more than 50% of all HCAIs are attributed to MRSA. In India and the subcontinent, the situation is slightly different. In recent studies done on clinical samples, among *S. aureus* strains 29.1%, 46% and 51.8% were MRSA in three different studies in tertiary centers from South India, North India and Central India respectively. Very importantly, 100% of them in all three studies were sensitive to vancomycin and also linezolid, when tested. Although it is not possible to interpret how many of them are community acquired and how many are HCAIs and what percentage of HCAIs they represent—it seems reasonable to conclude that MRSA is a significant issue all over India. However, the situation is possibly not as worrying as in the Western world because:

- Vancomycin-resistance is not an issue as yet
- MRSA contributes less percentage of over-all HCAIs.

However, gram-negative organisms, i.e. *Enterobacteriaceae* (*mainly Escherichia coli, Klebsiella*), *Pseudomonas* and *Acinetobacter* are posing a much larger and more serious threat in India. Gram-negative organisms are known for relentlessly developing resistant mechanisms. Production of extended-spectrum beta-lactamases (ESBL) is one such mechanism. These are enzymes that can hydrolyze cephalosporins with an oxyimino side-chain like cefotaxime, ceftriaxone and ceftazidime as well as the oxyimino-monobactams like aztreonam but not cephamycins—namely cefoxitin and cefotetan. They are often encoded in plasmids, which also carry resistance to other groups like aminoglycosides or quinolones and could be easily transferred even between different species. Organisms carrying ESBLs usually remain sensitive to carbapenems which are the drug of choice for ESBL producers. ESBLs are now rampant, especially in tertiary centers in India. As for example, in a single tertiary center South Indian study, 85.4% of nosocomial *E. coli* and *Klebsiella* isolates were ESBL producers as opposed to 53% of community-acquired isolates. In another study, 42.8% of *E. coli* and *Klebsiella* were ESBL positive even in a rural Indian hospital. A high degree of co-resistance to other classes of antibiotics was also universally noted, but they usually remained sensitive to carbapenems. This has a major impact on the empiric selection of antibiotics in HCAI.

The situation has been further complicated recently by the arrival of zinc-based metallo-beta-lactamases (MBL) and serine-based carbapenemase—both are capable of hydrolyzing penicillins, cephalosporins as well as carbapenems. In addition, new chromosomally coded Amp-C type ESBLs are also reported which confer resistance to cephamycins and sometimes even to carbapenems. Among the MBLs New Delhi metallo-beta-lactamase-1 (NDM-l) is relatively new being first reported in 2009. Although it has been subsequently detected in places as diverse as Africa, Europe, America and Japan there is evidence to suggest that it is widely prevalent in India. As for example, in the worldwide salmeterol multicenter asthma research trial (SMART) study (2009)—among 235 ertapenem-resistant *Enterobacteriaceae*, 33 isolates (5 different species) carried NDM-1 and all of them were from India. In the global SENTRY study—15 out of 39 carbapenem-resistant strains of *Enterobacteriaceae* from India carried NDM-1 as early as 2006–2007. In a single center Indian study—25% of *Pseudomonas* isolates were carbapenem-resistant and 20% were MBL producers. Particularly worrying is the fact that most of these strains also carry resistance to other groups of antibiotics. We are now regularly coming across isolates, often *Acinetobactor*, *Klebsiella* and *Pseudomonas* that are resistant to all groups

of antibiotics except colistin, polymixin-B and tigecycline; fosfomycin, the only other antibiotic likely to be effective in such situation not being tested routinely. The exact prevalence of these organisms is still unknown, but we know they are definitely there and possibly increasing in frequency.

In view of this, the initial empiric choice of antibiotic has become a vexing problem. Although standard recommendations for initial empiric therapy are there, and they are presented in the relevant sections, utility of such recommendations are reducing. Indeed, all such guidelines recommend to be *guided by local culture isolates and sensitivities* and that is now the most important factor. This is even more relevant for critically-ill patients, where the initial choice of antibiotic is of paramount importance as it is well-known to significantly affect mortality. As for example, in a study of adult ICU patients with sepsis, mortality was 61.9% in the group receiving inappropriate initial antibiotic as opposed to 28.4% in the group receiving appropriate antibiotics. In the absence of a centralized database, it is now essential for all hospitals to have their own database of culture and sensitivity (C/S) to inform choice of antibiotics for HCAIs. This database needs to be updated and circulated at least quarterly if not monthly.

While it is important to make sure that the initial antibiotic(s) cover the organisms causing HCAI especially in critically-ill patients, it is equally important to rationalize and downgrade antibiotics once sensitivities are known to prevent future resistance.

The problem of antibiotic resistance is at least partly iatrogenic. Guidelines are there for effective stewardship. Essentially, we need to make sure that appropriate antibiotics are given at the right dose (under-dosing being more dangerous), at right intervals (OD dosing for aminoglycosides, more frequent dosing or even infusions for beta-lactams and carbapenems), through right route and for right duration (both shorter and longer courses than optimal being detrimental). Above all, unnecessary use of antibiotics must be discouraged.

Several strategies have been tried to improve antibiotic use. They include prescription reviews, antibiotic cycling or switching, antibiotic restriction, education of staff, etc. While some strategies like education, antibiotic restriction, etc. seems to be more effective than antibiotic cycling or prescription review in reducing antibiotic use and cost, the evidence for any of these measures actually reducing resistance is rather weak.

PREVENTION

Prevention of HCAI is a multidisciplinary task involving at least the hospital management, clinicians, nurses, microbiology department, pharmacy, patient handlers, food handlers, sterilization service, laundry service and housekeeping service. So any intervention that does not involve all these services is not going to be effective.

There are many instances in the literature of successful implementation of an infection control program in a hospital with impressive effectiveness. Detailed discussion of such a program is outside the scope of this chapter. However, key structures of such a program are the following:

- *Hospital administration:* Responsible for resource allocation and review of performance.
- *Infection control committee:* It is a multidisciplinary committee with representation from all clinical departments and services related to infection control. The committee would report to the administration and is primarily responsible for policy making and making annual reports and business plan.
- *Infection control team:* They would be responsible for implementation of policies, surveillance and investigation of outbreaks, as well as taking decision on day-to-day infection control issues. It would consist of at least one physician—the infection control officer and at least one nurse—the infection control nurse.
- *Infection control manual:* This is a written document containing all relevant policies and guidelines and should be widely and easily available.

Specific prevention measures for individual HCAIs are discussed in the relevant section.

HAND HYGIENE

Any discussion on prevention of HCAI will remain incomplete without "hand hygiene". Most HCAIs are transmitted horizontally from health-workers, other patients, fomites, medical equipment, etc. and hands of the caregiver are the final common link. There is plenty of good quality evidence of its effectiveness. In a neonatal study, as compliance of hand hygiene increased from 40% to nearly 60% following a campaign, HCAI decreased from 11.3 to 6.2/1,000 patient days, i.e. greater than 45% reduction. This is a low-cost, low-technology measure which works. However, compliance has typically been around 50–60% even after awareness programs and doctors often fare worse than nurses.

The recommendations are simple. Hands must be disinfected using alcohol-based hand rubs:

Before and after:

Each patient contact, or contact with wounds, catheters or drains.

Before: Invasive procedures (even if using gloves), procedure with potential for contamination (preparing infusions, drawing up syringes, etc.).

After: Contact with biological fluids (secretions, blood, urine, etc.), removal of gloves. There is a high probability of contamination of hands while removing gloves which explains why hands should be disinfected after removing gloves. In a study on vancomycin-resistant *Enterococcus*, it was found in the hands of staff in 30% cases even after wearing gloves.

Alcohol-based hand-rubs are very effective for all clinically relevant organisms except the spores (not the vegetative forms) of spore-forming bacteria like *C. difficile*. Enough must be taken to cover every part of both hands, especially the fingertips and thumbs. They must be allowed to air-dry which usually takes around 30 seconds. Dispensers must be easily and widely accessible.

Protective gloves should be used while examining incontinent patients, patients positive for MRSA or *C. difficile*, handling biological fluids, removal of drains or bandages and sampling blood.

Hands should be washed with soap and water only sparingly. Hand-rubs are much more effective than washing with soap even for 3 minutes in reducing contaminating flora. Frequent hand-washing leads to hand eczema which may actually hinder hand hygiene. Hands should be definitely washed if they are visibly soiled, after using toilets and before performing sterile procedures. It is vitally important to do it properly using the right technique (Fig. 2.10.1).

DIAGNOSIS AND TREATMENT

Diagnosis involves establishing clinical features and getting microbiological confirmation from culture of appropriate sample. It is very important to send samples for reasons that are discussed later. Treatment involves appropriate antibiotics. In critically-ill patients, it is often not possible and actually harmful to withhold antibiotics while awaiting culture results. However, in clinically stable patients and where likelihood of infection is low, it may be prudent to wait. Diagnostic criteria for individual HCAIs and specific treatment aspects are discussed in relevant sections.

2.10.1 HEALTHCARE-ASSOCIATED PNEUMONIA/VENTILATOR-ASSOCIATED PNEUMONIA

DEFINITION

Healthcare-associated pneumonia (HCAP) includes any patient who was hospitalized in an acute care hospital for two or more days within past 90 days; resided in a nursing home or long-term care facility; received recent intravenous antibiotic therapy, chemotherapy or wound care within the past 30 days of the current infection; or attended a hospital or hemodialysis clinic.

Hospital-acquired pneumonia (HAP) is defined as pneumonia that occurs 48 hours or more after admission to a hospital, which was not incubating at the time of admission.

Ventilator-associated pneumonia (VAP) refers to pneumonia that arises more than 48 hours after endotracheal intubation (all CDC definitions).

Early HAP/VAP occurs within the first 4 days of hospitalization/intubation and late HAP/VAP occurs after that.

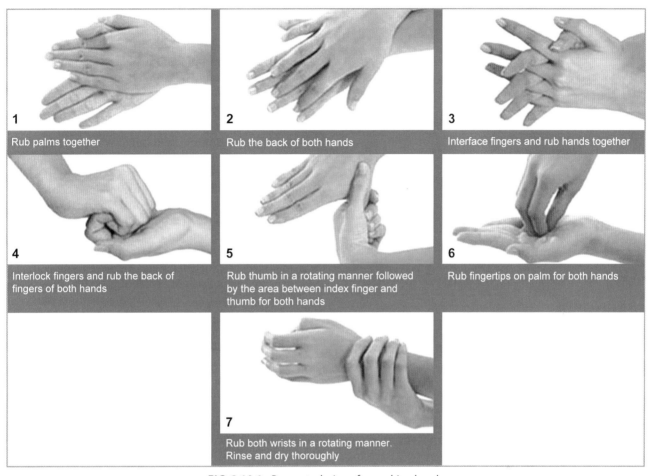

1. Rub palms together
2. Rub the back of both hands
3. Interface fingers and rub hands together
4. Interlock fingers and rub the back of fingers of both hands
5. Rub thumb in a rotating manner followed by the area between index finger and thumb for both hands
6. Rub fingertips on palm for both hands
7. Rub both wrists in a rotating manner. Rinse and dry thoroughly

FIG. 2.10.1: Proper technique for washing hands.

As stated earlier most HAPs are VAPs. Most of the evidence on the subject is related to VAP and are extrapolated to HAP.

EPIDEMIOLOGY

Ventilator-associated pneumonia is the second commonest NI on PICU and NICU and is the leading cause of death among all HCAIs. Incidence varies widely, which is partly explained by the non-uniformity of diagnostic criteria and surveillance. VAP occurs in 3–30% of ventilated PICU patients. In terms of device days among PICU patients NNIS reported rates of 2.9–8.1/1,000 ventilation days. In NICU, VAP rates as wide as 2.4–52/1,000 ventilation days has been reported. Case fatality varies 20–70%. Late-onset VAP has a higher crude mortality and associated with MDR organisms than early-onset VAP.

PATHOPHYSIOLOGY

The most important factor contributing to VAP is the presence of the endotracheal tube (ET). Noninvasive ventilation has a much lesser incidence of pneumonia. As the ET stents the vocal cords, microaspirations of oral secretions and any regurgitated gastric content can lead to VAP. ET also provides a direct access to the bronchial tree during ET suction.

ETIOLOGY

This essentially represents the nosocomial flora of the unit/hospital. Most studies have shown a preponderance of Gram-negative rods (*Pseudomonas*, *Klebsiella*, *Enterobacter*, *Acinetobacter*, etc.) followed by gram-positive Cocci (*S. aureus* including MRSA, *Pneumococcus*, etc.). Being nosocomial antibiotic resistance is common. Anaerobic organisms, which contribute as much as 25% of adult cases, are rare in the pediatric population. Fungal VAP is very rare unless patient has suppressed immunity. It must also be noted that not all VAPs are bacterial. It could also be due to viruses, respiratory syncytial virus being the most common in pediatric population.

Following factors have been associated with VAP in different studies—prematurity, longer duration of ventilation, longer ICU stay, use of H_2 blockers, re-intubation, transfer out of ICU while ventilated, manipulation of ventilator circuit, use of muscle relaxants, etc. Factors associated with MDR organisms are given in Table 2.10.1.

Table 2.10.1: Risk factors for MDR pathogens causing HAP, HCAP and VAP.

- Antimicrobial therapy in preceding 90 d
- Current hospitalization of 5 d or more
- High frequency of antibiotic resistance in the community or in the specific hospital unit
- Presence of risk factors for HCAP:
  - Hospitalization for 2 d or more in the preceding 90 d
  - Residence in a nursing home or extended care facility
  - Home infusion therapy (including antibiotics)
  - Chronic dialysis within 30 d
  - Home wound care
  - Family member with multidrug-resistant pathogen
- Immunosuppressive disease and/or therapy

Abbreviations: MDR, multidrug-resistant; HAP, hospital-acquired (or nosocomial) pneumonia; VAP, ventilator-associated pneumonia; HCAP, healthcare-associated pneumonia

Source: Adapted from the ATS and IDSA guidelines for management of HAP, VAP and HCAP. Am J Resp Crit Care Med. 2005;171:388-416

DIAGNOSIS

Clinical Diagnosis

Clinical diagnosis of pneumonia itself is difficult and VAP is even more so mainly because of the frequency of pre-existing pulmonary pathology. The CDC criteria (Table 2.10.2) are now widely accepted. However, even such combination of clinical features cannot avoid either false positive or false negative diagnosis. For example, a European task force concluded chest X-ray (CXR) changes plus two of three features (fever, purulent tracheal aspirate and leukocytosis) have 69% sensitivity and 75% specificity, which was the best combination. Using all three features reduced sensitivity while using one of three features reduced specificity to unacceptable levels.

Clinical pulmonary infection score (CPIS) was devised to diagnose VAP. However, it does not perform better than conventional systems. It might be useful in monitoring response to therapy and identifying a group of patients in whom antibiotics could be stopped early.

Invasive Diagnostic Tests

In a study of 132 patients, in the BAL positive group, mortality was 38% if initial empiric antibiotic was appropriate while it was 89% when initial antibiotic was inappropriate. Moreover, even when therapy was changed after C/S report became available, mortality remained comparable to those who continued with the inappropriate antibiotic. In another study of 107 patients with VAP, mortality was 69.7% if appropriate antibiotic was delayed for greater than or equal to 24 hours whereas it was only 28.4% when there was no such delay. Such delay also increased length of stay. So, as in the case of severe sepsis, it is vital to "guess the antibiotic right first time" and start them without delay.

In spite of the above considerations, it is absolutely essential to send some sample before adding or modifying antibiotics. This is for the following reasons:

- If C/S is positive, it would allow to rationalize antibiotics thereby limiting use of broad spectrum antibiotics. This information is also vital to create the database, which would allow to correctly "guess" empiric antibiotic(s) in first place. This would also "confirm" diagnosis of VAP and limit investigations to exclude differentials.
- If C/S is negative, it has a high negative predictive value making VAP very unlikely provided no change in antibiotics were done in the previous 72 hours before obtaining the sample. Depending on the clinical situation, this may lead to stopping antibiotics or at least direct investigations to other sources of sepsis.

Table 2.10.2: Criteria for diagnosis of VAP, ventilator-associated pneumonia VAP in pediatric population.

Age	≥13 years of age	1–12 years of age	<1 year of age
Essential criteria	≥ 2* serial chest X-ray with new or progressive and persistent infiltration or consolidation or cavitation developing ≥48 hours after starting mechanical ventilation		
Additional criteria	Criteria A and/or B and at least two of criteria C, D, E, F	At least 3 of the criteria below	Criteria D and at least 3 of the other criteria
A. Temperature	>38°C without other recognized cause	>38.4°C or <37°C without other recognized cause	Temperature instability without other recognized cause
B. WBC count	<4000/mm³ OR >12,000/mm³	<4000/mm³ >15,000/mm³	<4000/mm³ OR >15,000/mm³ and band forms >10%
C. Sputum or secretions	New onset purulent sputum or change in character of sputum or increased secretions, or increased need for suctioning		
D. Worsening oxygenation	Worsening gas exchange (O₂ desaturations), increasing requirement for supplemental O₂ or increased need for ventilation		
E. Respiratory symptoms	New onset or worsening of cough, dyspnea or tachypnea		Apnea, tachypnea, nasal flaring with retraction of chest wall or grunting
F. Auscultation findings	Rales or bronchial breath sounds		Wheezing, rales or rhonchi
G. Cough	N/A		Present
H. Heart rate	N/A		<100 beats/min OR >170 beats/min

Purulent sputum is defined as secretions from the lungs, bronchi or trachea that contain ≥25 neutrophils and ≤10 squamous epithelial cells per low power field (X100). Change in character of sputum refers to the color, consistency, odor, and quantity.

*In patients who do not have underlying pulmonary or cardiac disease, one definitive chest radiograph is acceptable.

However, there is considerable controversy over which sample to send. The most easily obtained and most commonly used sample is an endotracheal-tube aspirate (EA). But the problem is both contamination and colonization of upper airway, which makes this sample less specific but adequately sensitive. Other alternatives are bronchoscopically obtained samples either protected brush sample (PSB) or bronchoalveolar lavage (BAL). PSB possibly has best specificity. However, it is rarely used in pediatric population because of the need and size of the bronchoscope involved. The sensitivity and specificity of both PSB and BAL are mostly in the 70s–80s depending on the study quoted with a cut-off of greater than 10^4 CFU/mL. In pediatrics, another sample is very commonly used the nonbronchoscopic alveolar lavage (NBAL). After pre-oxygenation a suitable sized catheter is inserted all the way down until it wedges with the patient's head turned to left to access right bronchus. Then 1 mL/kg (Max 10 mL) of normal saline is injected through the catheter. Ideally, patient is bagged a few times with the catheter in following which the sample is aspirated. Recovery of 40–60% of the instilled volume with bubbles (from Surfactant) suggests an adequate sample. Once sample is drawn it should be incubated as soon as possible to obtain optimum result. Many studies showed sensitivity and specificity of NBAL to be comparable to BAL with good safety profile which explains the popularity of this sample.

Quantitative culture of samples is another issue. Cut-off points for different sample types are: PSB—10^3 CFU/mL, BAL—10^4 CFU/mL, NBAL—10^5 CFU/mL, EA—10^6 CFU/mL. Quantitative cultures at least theoretically address the issue of colonization/contamination. A problem is that very few laboratories provide quantitative reports although it does not require any special infrastructure.

Main advantage of other samples compared to EA is the higher specificity, which does translate to lesser antibiotic use especially when combined with quantitative culture and this has been proved in many studies. However, any survival advantage is doubtful. So far, only one large, multicenter French study involving 413 patients have shown higher 14 days mortality in the conventional group using EA sample compared to the group using bronchoscopic sample and quantitative culture. However, this effect was lost at 28 days. Moreover, several others, albeit smaller, studies have failed to demonstrate even any initial survival advantage. In view of this and the higher resource need to obtain bronchoscopic samples, it is difficult to recommend routine use of such samples. The 2008 UK Health Protection Agency (UK HPA) guideline does not support either invasive sampling or quantitative culture, and also does not clearly favor any particular sample type. Possibly NBAL would be the optimal sample in most Indian centers.

Gram stain of samples to identify the organism is a simple and quick method to guide empiric therapy. Quantification of neutrophils with intracellular organism (ICO) is another quick method. Cut-offs from 1 to 10% has been used. Generally, it is considered to be highly specific but less sensitive. In the absence of standardization, it is still not very useful. Moreover, hardly any laboratory report ICO although this does not need any additional equipment.

PREVENTION

Naturally for an iatrogenic condition like VAP most emphasis should be on prevention. Following are the principal strategies:

Suctioning endotracheal tube: ET suction is not mentioned in any research paper as a factor associated with VAP. But papers are published from established centers. Common sense dictates that it could be a factor leading to at least contamination of upper airway and conceivably to subsequent VAP in a new unit where practice for proper suctioning is no yet established. Although suctioning is essentially a nursing procedure—physician supervision would be advisable until the skill level is reached. Tracheal toileting is a two person job irrespective of the skill level of the personnel unless using a closed system. Tip of the suction catheter must be treated like a sterile device. Even in resource-poor settings reuse of an open suction catheter is counterproductive and unacceptable. By preventing VAP much more resources would be saved than what would be spend for the suction catheters. Each ET suctioning, repositioning of patient and ET handling should be preceded by oropharyngeal suction to prevent possible aspiration. Using a separate catheter (can be reused), tubing and canister for oral suction has also been suggested.

There is no fixed routine for suctioning. Frequency will depend on the clinical need of the patient. Both unnecessary suction and too infrequent suction are bad.

Adult evidence for any reduction of VAP rate by using in-line suction is not consistent and pediatric studies have shown no benefit.

Regular subglottic suction using ET with a separate dorsal channel does prevent VAP in adults and is recommended. Pediatric studies are awaited.

Endotracheal tube and intubation: ET cuff pressure should be maintained at 25–30 cm water and regularly checked to prevent microaspiration and injury to tracheal mucosa. Using polyurethane cuff and tapering cuff showed promise. But none are still regularly used.

Nasal intubation is consistently associated with maxillary sinusitis although association with VAP is less clear. Oral intubation should be the default unless there is specific reason to use the nasal route. Reintubation is associated with increased VAP and should be avoided.

Oral care: Dental plaques develop surprisingly quickly in ventilated patients (within 48 hours) with a preponderance of gram-negative bacteria. There is good evidence in adult literature showing protective effect of maintenance of oral hygiene in reducing both colonization and VAP rate. The study showing the largest effect size was a good quality, prospective, placebo-controlled, double blind study with an absolute risk reduction of 20% giving a number needed to treat (NNT) as low as 5. Unfortunately, pediatric data are sparse. In infants and small children (<6 years) the oral flora might be different. However, given the simplicity and low-cost of the intervention, it is sensible to incorporate this at least in older children. Using chlorhexidine mouthwash with an applicator and brushing teeth twice daily coupled with 2 hourly oral rinsing by normal saline is the simplest solution.

Ventilator-circuit-related issues: Initially, it was common practice to change the circuit twice every week. However, many studies have shown no difference in VAP rate between changing the circuit once every week and twice weekly. Subsequent studies showed no difference between changing weekly and not changing at all. Indeed, the current CDC guideline suggests change of circuit only if it is visibly contaminated or malfunctioning and this is now standard practice. Use of a heated humidifier is unique to pediatric and neonatal ventilation. There is some evidence to suggest that using a heated humidifier is associated with increased VAP rate compared to a heat and moisture exchange (HME) filter, but the evidence is not consistent. In older children, HME filters could be considered because active humidification is not so important. Humidifiers or HME filters must be changed as per the manufacturer's advice.

It is important to make sure that there is no accumulation of condensate and it does not get aspirated. Check for this every 2–4 hours and every time before changing the position of the patient. Modification of the circuit has been associated with VAP and should be discouraged.

Use of H$_2$-blockers/Proton-pump inhibitors/Sucralfate: Critically-ill patients almost routinely receive either H$_2$-blockers or proton-pump inhibitors (PPI). There is good evidence that they reduce gastric hemorrhage and possibly even save lives. Gastric acidity normally reduce bacterial flora of gastric content. As gastric acidity decreases due to such therapy, there is concern that it may increase VAP. Sucralfate is thought to be a better alternative as it acts without changing the pH. In adult literature, many studies and meta-analyses have been done on this issue and there is a consistent trend toward increased VAP rate with H$_2$-blockers, which often reached statistical significance. In many studies, sucralfate is associated with lower VAP rates than H$_2$ blockers, although this is not consistent. At the same time, sucralfate compared to ranitidine has been associated with increased risk of clinically important gastrointestinal bleeding. There are very few studies in the pediatric population and none of these studies have found any significant relation between such therapy and VAP, let alone the superiority of sucralfate. This might either mean that such relation does not exist in pediatric population or the studies are not powerful enough to find the effect. While we wait for further evidence—the sensible approach might be to start some therapy while the patient is very sick and nil-by-mouth. As of now, the choice of therapy would be a matter of personal preference. Enteral feeding should always be tried early for its numerous benefits and once established, therapy should be stopped.

Elevation of Head of the Bed

Elevating the head-end by 30–45° is thought to reduce gastric reflux and thus reduce aspiration and VAP. One adult study has shown a remarkable effect of semirecumbent positioning with an absolute risk reduction of 18% (from 23 to 5%) giving an NNT of near 5. The effect size has been somewhat less in other studies. Still, there is meta-analysis level evidence showing beneficial effect of this intervention. This is recommended in standard guidelines and is now standard practice in adults. There is very little pediatric evidence and they do not show any benefit. In infants and small children, logistically also it is often difficult or impossible to raise only the head end. Using reverse-Trendelenburg position works on the same principle, but it is difficult to obtain 30–45° elevation and studies have indicated elevation may not be effective if it is less than 30°. However, given the adult evidence, the simplicity of the intervention and the fact that it does not involve any cost or harm, it should be practiced provided there is no contraindication like cardiovascular instability.

Hand Hygiene

The importance of proper hand-washing practices in reducing all horizontal transmission of infection in hospital setting is well documented and cannot be over-emphasized. This obviously also applies to VAP. Although study focusing only on VAP and hand hygiene is relatively scarce, but there are many studies showing significant association of hand-washing practice and rate of HCAI, where VAP is a part of the infections studied.

Early Extubation

Although this is not really a separate intervention, length of ventilation is a consistent risk factor for VAP even in centers with a low VAP rate. Conceivably it would be an even more important factor in situations where VAP rate is high. Current adult guidelines suggest a daily "fitness to extubate" trial. Such practice has been tried for pediatric patients, but has proved to be either ineffective or even counterproductive in a recent trial. However, early extubation is always desirable and the clinician should be actively looking for opportunities to wean and limit the duration of ventilation.

Managing sedation and muscle relaxants are also important factors here. Neuromuscular blockers are associated with many complications and they should be used only when it is absolutely necessary, used as boluses rather than continuous infusion and stopped as early as possible. In adults, standard recommendation is to stop sedation at least for an hour every day. In pediatrics, it is difficult to do so in all patients because of the concern for accidental extubation. However, it should be tried whenever possible and heavy sedation should be avoided unless the clinical condition warrants this.

Selective Decontamination of the Digestive Tract

The idea is to deliver antibiotics to gut that are not absorbed but reduce the gut flora, like vancomycin, gentamicin, etc. so that microaspirations would not lead to VAP. It is often also combined with systemic prophylaxis. This has been extensively tried in adults and the result has been remarkably consistent in showing a reduction of VAP both at individual study level as well as meta-analysis or systematic review level, although sometimes not reaching statistical significance. The situation is somewhat less clear in terms of survival benefit. Studies with a systemic prophylactic antibiotic component have shown mortality benefit unlike studies using only topical SDD. The effect size is high and consistent giving an NNT of five to prevent one VAP in both a Cochrane review of 36 randomized controlled trials (RCT) and another meta-analysis of 33 RCTs while NNT to prevent one death is 21 and 23 respectively. The obvious concern has been emergence of resistance, but all studies have consistently shown no increase in resistance except some occasional reports. Indeed, SDD has been recommended in the latest UK guideline. However, in spite of this, SDD is still not widely practiced, either in adults or pediatric patients. One issue is that the studies have used different combination of antibiotics in varied doses and choosing one would be essentially arbitrary. There is very few data on Indian context and the issue of emergence of resistance would depend on local sensitivity, which is very different in India compared to the Western world. In view of this, it is difficult to recommend routine use of SDD. However, SDD needs consideration if the local VAP rate is high as there is no doubt about its effectiveness.

Other Measures

There are some strategies which have been tried to reduce VAP rate. They include continuous lateral rotation therapy using continuous-motion bed-frames, use of a low-sodium solution for tracheal toilcting, novel positioning of patient and even use of probiotics. However, none is established yet as standard practice.

Education and the Bundle Approach

A look at the risk factors for VAP makes it apparent that preventing VAP needs a multipronged approach, which involves the entire medical team rather than only the physicians or the nurses. Up-to-date knowledge of a few selected members of the team or having an excellent protocol alone is unlikely to be effective. What is needed is education and awareness of the entire medical team. There are many studies showing the effectiveness of such interventions. It is also important to continue such

Table 2.10.3: Commonly utilized pediatric VAP bundle items.

- Items to prevent iatrogenic spread of infection
  - Adherence to good hand hygiene practices
  - Use of universal precautions
- Items to prevent aspiration of gastric contents
  - Elevate the head of the bed between 30 and 45 degrees
  - Monitor/drain gastric contents
- Items to improve oral hygiene
  - Oral rinsing/cleaning with chlorhexidine (0.12%)
  - Use of toothbrush and oral swabs in daily oral care
- Items to decrease endotracheal tube risk factors
  - Use of in-line suction equipment where appropriate and available
  - Suction of the hypopharynx prior to endotracheal suctioning and repositioning
- Items to avoid contamination of respiratory equipment
  - Dedicated oropharyngeal suction equipment
  - Prevention of accumulation of respiratory circuit condensates
  - Prevention of contamination of ventilation equipment
- Items to decrease the duration of mechanical ventilation
  - Daily readiness for extubation trials
  - Neuromuscular blockade holidays

Abbreviation: VAP, ventilator-associated pneumonia.

Source: Curley MA, Schwalenstocker E, Deshpande JK, et al. Tailoring the Institute for Health Care Improvement 1,00,000 Lives Campaign to pediatric settings: The example of ventilator-associated pneumonia. Pediatr Clin North Am. 2006;53(6):1231-51.

programs rather than do a one-off program to maintain and enhance the effectiveness.

Bundle approach is a collection of effective measures which, when performed together, leads to even greater effectiveness. It has been successfully adopted in many scenarios in adult practice. As for example, one study reported 44.5% reduction in VAP rates across 35 facilities. A VAP bundle is rather well-established in adult practice. There is also evidence of remarkable success of a bundle approach for VAP in PICU. However, they are still not widely used but this would probably change. Table 2.10.3 is an example of a pediatric VAP bundle.

TREATMENT

Please refer to the "Microbiology and Antibiotics" part of the General section first.

Treatment essentially consists of initial intravenous (IV) empiric antibiotics. As already stated, it is of paramount importance to ensure appropriate antibiotics are started without delay once microbiology samples are collected if VAP is clinically suspected (note "invasive diagnostic tests" in this section). Initial coverage has to be broad-spectrum covering nosocomial Gram-negative and Gram-positive organisms guided by the local sensitivity pattern and possibility of MDR organisms and a universal recommendation are difficult. However, the latest American Thoracic Society (ATS) and Infectious Disease Society of America (IDSA) guideline are given below for reference (Tables 2.10.1, 2.10.4 and 2.10.5).

As already stated, it is very important to *rationalize and de-escalate* antibiotics if possible once C/S results are known.

Table 2.10.4: Initial empiric antibiotic therapy for HAP, HCAP and VAP in patients with no known risk factors for MDR, early onset and any disease severity.

Potential pathogen	Recommended antibiotic
Streptococcus pneumoniae[†]	Ceftriaxone
Haemophilus influenzae	or
Methicillin-sensitive Staphylococcus aureus	Levofloxacin, moxifloxacin, or ciprofloxacin
Antibiotic-sensitive enteric gram-negative bacilli	or
Escherichia coli	Ampicillin/sulbactam
Klebsiella pneumoniae	or
Enterobacter species	Ertapenem
Proteus species	
Serratia marcescens	

[†]The frequency of penicillin-resistant S. pneumoniae and multidrug-resistant S. pneumoniae is increasing; levofloxacin or moxifloxacin are preferred to ciprofloxacin and the role of other new quinolones, such as gatifloxacin, has not been established.

Abbreviations: MDR, multidrug-resistant; HAP, hospital-acquired (or nosocomial) pneumonia; VAP, ventilator-associated pneumonia; HCAP, healthcare-associated pneumonia.

Source: The ATS and IDSA guidelines for management of HAP, VAP and HCAP. Am J Resp Crit Care Med. 2005;171:388–416.

Table 2.10.5: Initial empiric therapy for HAP, HCAP and VAP in patients with late-onset disease or risk factors for MDR pathogens and all disease severity.

Potential pathogens	Combination antibiotic therapy
Pathogens listed in Table 2.10.3 and MDR pathogens	Antipseudomonal cephalosporin (cefepime, ceftazidime)
Pseudomonas aeruginosa	or
Klebsiella pneumoniae (ESBL+)[†]	Antipseudomonal carbapenem
Acinetobacter species[†]	(Imipenem or meropenem) or β-Lactam/β-lactamase inhibitor (piperacillin–tazobactam) plus Antipseudomonal fluoroquinolone[†] (ciprofloxacin or levofloxacin) or Aminoglycoside (amikacin, gentamicin, or tobramycin) plus
Methicillin-resistant Staphylococcus aureus (MRSA)	Linezolid or vancomycin[‡]
Legionella pneumophila[†]	

[†]If an ESBL+ strain, such as K. pneumoniae, or an Acinetobacter species is suspected, a carlbapenem is a reliable choice. If L. pneumophila is suspected, the combination antibiotic regimen should include a macrolide (e.g. azithromycin) or a fluoroquinolone (e.g. ciprofloxacin or levofloxacin) should be used rather than an aminoglycoside.

[‡]If MRSA risk factors are present or there is a high incidence locally.

Abbreviations: MDR, multidrug-resistant; HAP, hospital-acquired (or nosocomial) pneumonia; VAP, ventilator-associated pneumonia; HCAP, healthcare-associated pneumonia.

Source: The ATS and IDSA guidelines for management of HAP, VAP and HCAP. Am J Resp Crit Care Med. 2005;171:388-416.

As for duration of therapy, an 8-day course is adequate in most cases and unnecessary prolongation of antibiotic should be avoided. The only exception is gram-negative non-Lactose fermenters (*Pseudomonas* and *Acinetobacter* being the two most important genus) where an 8-day course have shown significantly increased rate of recurrence compared to a 15-day course. In such cases, the optimum duration is not known and probably lies somewhere between 10 and 15 days. For *Acinetobacter* needing colistin, a useful choice would be to change to nebulized colistin after the initial IV therapy, which produces enough local drug concentration but obviates the concern for nephrotoxicity.

2.10.2 CATHETER-RELATED BLOODSTREAM INFECTION

INTRODUCTION

A range of devices are used for intravascular access depending on the clinical need. All such device is a potential source of BSI, but different devices have different risks. Devices with the highest risk are those used to access central veins. They are of three major types:

- *Non-tunneled central venous catheters (CVC):* This is the most common type and mostly used in intensive care setting.
- *Peripherally inserted central catheter (PICC):* This is frequently used in neonates, often for parenteral nutrition (PN). It is also used in older children, usually in subacute setting—when the access is needed for few weeks, as for example, to complete a 3-week course of antibiotics for gram-negative meningitis.
- *Surgically inserted, tunneled and often cuffed lines:* These are for long-term use—months to years—as for example, for chemotherapy of leukemia or blood transfusion in a child with thalassemia. Examples include portacath, broviac or hickman line.

Umbilical arterial catheter (UAC) and umbilical venous catheters (UVC) are unique in neonatal practice.

Tunneled lines are associated with the least chance of infection and they are not considered in this chapter. This chapter mostly deals with non-tunneled CVCs.

EPIDEMIOLOGY

Central line related bloodstream infection (CLABSI) is the most common HCAI in the pediatric age group. The reported incidence density for CVCs has been anything between 3.5 and 11.5/1,000 catheter days depending on the study quoted. One Indian study quoted infection in 25% of central lines, but it was mostly for cancer patients having long-term lines. Factors affecting this rate are—types of catheter—as already stated, duration of catheter use, number of lumens, patient population (premature neonates and burns patients being more vulnerable), patient characteristic (severity of illness, immune-suppression), situation of insertion (lines sited during an emergency having higher rates than those done in controlled situation), and location in the hospital (cardiothoracic units having the lowest rates compared to medical or trauma units). Infusion of lipids are associated with both coagulase negative *Staphylococcus* (CONS) and Candida infection, especially in very low-birth-weight (VLBW) infants. Central line infections definitely lengthen length of stay as well as cost. Many studies have also shown increased mortality but it is not consistent. Especially once severity of illness is controlled there is usually no significant difference in mortality. So, attributable mortality is possibly not high.

PATHOPHYSIOLOGY

Infection can be introduced through four possible routes:
- Migration of pathogens from skin through the entry site along the tract.
- Colonization of hubs during handling the lines and subsequent infection.
- Hematogenous seeding of the catheter from other sources of BSI.
- Rarely, the infusate itself can be contaminated.

The first two mechanisms are the most common and important targets for preventive measures.

Certain strains like CONS have increased ability to adhere to the catheter and produce a "Biofilm", made of extracellular polysaccharides, which then act as a protective barrier against host defense as well as antibiotics. Some *Candida* species also have this ability, especially in presence of glucose.

ETIOLOGY

It is important to differentiate between colonization and infection (Note "Diagnosis" section). Colonization is very common especially as the catheter becomes older. As for example— in an Indian study on PICU patients—all CVCs were colonized after 11 days. CONS have always been very common. Among other Gram-positive organisms *S. aureus* and *Enterococcus* are important in Western literature. According to NNIS data (1992–99) CONS was responsible for 37% whereas *S. aureus* and Enterococci each caused 13% of CLABSI. Gram-negative bacilli caused 14% cases. *Candida* is the other important pathogen responsible for 8% of cases. *Candida* is even more important in premature neonates. There is not much Indian data, but it seems that the overall profile is the same except that Gram-negatives are more common in India. As for example—in an Indian study on PICU patients—33.3% of isolates were *Pseudomonas* and 29.6% were CONS.

DIAGNOSIS AND DEFINITION

Clinical diagnosis is often difficult and a high degree of suspicion is the key. The only specific feature is local change over the catheter site in the form of pain, erythema which might be spreading over the length of the catheter,

so-called "tracking", swelling, induration or frank pus. Another clinical indication is rigor and/or fever every time a specific lumen of the catheter is accessed.

It is important to understand the difference between CLABSI and CRBSI. CLABSI as defined by the CDC is a primary BSI in a patient who had a central line at least for the last 48-hour period before the development of the BSI and is not related to an infection at another site. This definition is operationally very easy and is actually a surveillance definition. However, it is obviously not specific and would lead to over-diagnosis.

Catheter-related bloodstream infection on the other hand is a clinical definition and much more precise. The CDC definition of CRBSI is slightly complex. As for CLABSI, patient must have a central access at least for the preceding 48 hours and have new-onset unexplained fever. Additional criteria vary depending on whether the catheter is removed and sent for C/S or kept *in situ*.

- If catheter is removed then 5 cm from its tip should be cultured either by roll-plate method or by quantitative broth culture after sonication. If there is growth of greater than 15 CFU/plate in roll-plate method or greater than 10^2 CFU/mL in broth culture and the same organism is also grown from a peripheral venipuncture sample that establish the diagnosis of CRBSI. Growth of less than 15 CFU/plate has good negative predictive value and effectively rules CRBSI out and is diagnostic of colonization. Qualitative broth culture of a catheter tip does not provide any useful information although it is still widely done.

- If the catheter is kept *in situ* then blood culture should be sent from the catheter as well as a peripheral sample. Although the guideline is not very clear in a multilumen catheter, ideally, sample should be sent from all lumens. It is very important to mark the samples correctly and also mark the lumens and culture reports also must mention these. In addition, it is also important to send correct and identical volume of blood for each sample. If culture is done quantitatively then at least one lumen sample must have colony counts (of the same organism) greater than or equal to 3 times that from the peripheral sample. If culture is done in an automated continuous monitoring system then CRBSI is diagnosed if catheter sample detects growth at least 120 minutes before the peripheral sample. This is the differential time to positivity (DTP) criteria. If a peripheral sample could not be sent then greater than or equal to five fold difference between samples sent from different lumens would also diagnose CRBSI. As per CDC guideline DTP criteria in such situation is an unresolved issue although some studies have used 180 minutes as the cut-off in such situation.

There are many practical issues which make this definition less useful. Firstly, in pediatric practice—vascular access can often be difficult and often it might not be wise to take the line out—especially when the suspicion is not very strong as studies have shown that in most such cases,

CRBSI is ultimately not proven. Secondly, laboratories doing quantitative blood culture is vanishingly rare making the quantitative criteria not useful. Thirdly, although automated culture systems are now more popular, but they are still not used by most laboratories. Even if it is available DTP has to be specifically asked for as this does not form a part of usual reporting. Fourthly, if a triple lumen catheter, which is the most popular CVC, is involved then four sets of culture need to be sent including the peripheral sample. The cost incurred might be difficult to justify. Sometimes, a lumen might not sample but still work especially with the narrow 4.5F catheters.

Because of these reasons—in practice, we often settle with a diagnosis of CLABSI rather than CRBSI—especially in the pediatric population.

PREVENTION

As with VAP, much more emphasis is given on prevention than on treatment. There is a good body of literature on different aspects of prevention, but most of it is from adult literature, which is extrapolated in pediatric practice. Measures that are proven to be effective are mentioned in a temporal fashion.

Before Putting a Line

- A checklist for inserting CVCs should be available and completed for each CVC insertion attempt.
- Catheter cart/kit: A cart/tray must be readily accessible containing all materials needed for aseptic insertion of CVCs in all areas of the hospital where CVCs are used.
- All healthcare personnel inserting and managing CVCs must go through an educational program and their knowledge and adherence to standard practice should be periodically audited.
- Indication for any central line should be clear-cut and mentioned in the checklist and the notes.

Inserting a Central Line

- *Site of insertion:* Although there is some conflict of results among studies, it would be reasonable to state that subclavian route is associated with least infection rate compared with either internal jugular or femoral route in adults. Femoral catheters also carry the additional risk of deep vein thrombosis. However, subclavian is also the site with highest mechanical complication rates like pneumothorax, etc. and is hazardous in a patient with bleeding tendency because direct pressure could not be applied over the insertion site in case of active bleeding. Subclavian route should also be avoided in patients who might need long-term hemodialysis as this might lead to stenosis of the vein making future fistula development difficult. However, many pediatric studies have consistently shown no difference in CLABSI rates between femoral and nonfemoral routes. As for example—in an Indian study—subclavian catheters

had a higher rate (68.2%) of colonization in comparison to femoral catheters (40%). Hence, unlike adults, no site is preferable over the other and is a matter of personal preference. Actually femoral route is still popular and is possibly the mostly used route.

- *Ultrasound probe:* Use of ultrasound guide to identify the vessel and determine its patency does reduce mechanical complication rate and number of attempts and many guidelines recommend their routine use. However, it also depends on resource availability and skill of the operator. Ideally, it should be available and once available its use should be encouraged if not made mandatory.
- *Maximal sterile barrier precaution:* This is vitally important and has proved to significantly reduce infection rates. This includes proper hand-washing, sterile gloves, sterile full gown, cap, mask and a large sterile drape covering most of the patient. This might not be possible in emergencies in which case catheter should be replaced within 48 hours.
- *Skin preparation:* Skin preparation with alcohol based 2% chlorhexidine solution significantly reduce infection rate compared to either 10% povidone-iodine or 70% alcohol. This is a low-cost evidence-based measure with proven efficacy. The solution should be allowed to completely air dry which usually takes around two minutes. Use of 2% chlorhexidine is not licensed in patients less than 2 months old as is often the case with so many other agents. Using a chlorhexidine impregnated dressing system has resulted in dermatitis in as many as 15% of VLBW babies in contrast to only 1.5% of babies weighing more than 1,000 g. In view of this, 10% povidone-iodine is recommended for VLBW babies. Tincture iodine is to be avoided for its possible effect on neonatal thyroids. For patients who had reacted to chlorhexidine 10% povidone iodine could be used.

Type of Catheter

- *Catheter material:* Polyvinyl or polyethylene catheters are associated with higher infection rates compared with either teflon or polyurethane catheters. Polyurethane catheters are widely available and used.
- *Antibiotic coated catheters:* Catheters impregnated with different antibiotic preparations like chlorhexidine-silver sulfadiazine or minocycline-rifampicin significantly reduce infection rates. However, benefit would last only in the initial days (definitely ≤30 days). They cost considerably more. Favorable cost benefit analysis has been published, but their relevance to Indian setting is near zero. Emergence of resistance is a theoretical risk. They may be considered in situations where prevention of infection is paramount as in an immune-compromised patient. Their routine use is suggested only after more basic steps to reduce CLABSI rate has failed to bring down the rate to a certain figure, which is often taken as 5 per 1,000 catheter days.

- *Number of lumens:* Common sense as well as clinical evidence dictates that higher the number of lumens higher is the chance of CLABSI. So, rather than automatically choosing a three lumen catheter, careful consideration should be given to the possibility of reducing the number of lumens without affecting the effectiveness of the catheter.
- *Asepsis during procedure:* The importance of this is obvious and cannot be over-emphasized. Many CLABSI happens very early after the insertion and the most likely mechanism is contamination during the procedure. So, every care should be taken to maintain asepsis. If a catheter is replaced over guidewire then a new pair of gloves must be used before handling the new catheter.
- *Use of topical antibiotic at insertion site:* Routine prophylactic use of povidone-iodine ointment at the insertion site of hemodialysis catheters reduced catheter tip colonization and sepsis in many studies and is recommended. Similar use of mupirocin in CVCs has also shown modest decrease in infection rate. However, such use is also proven to cause emergence of resistance and can cause mechanical failure of polyurethane catheters. Studies with other topical preparations also shown increased colonization with *Candida*. In view of these issues topical antibiotic preparations should not be used prophylactically.
- *Dressing for CVCs:* There is no significant difference in infection rate between traditional gauze dressing and transparent polyurethane-based dressing. However, transparent dressing is preferred as it has an advantage of direct inspection of insertion site which is important for monitoring and needs to be changed less often. However, if the insertion site remains soaked then gauze dressing should be used as transparent dressing does not work.

Management of CVCs after Insertion

- *Accessing a CVC:* Proper hand hygiene, which means either washing with soap and water (especially if the hand is visibly soiled) or using an alcohol-based solution, is an absolute must before accessing the catheter, changing dressing or doing any sort of manipulation. In addition, the operator must also use sterile gloves if the operator is going to touch the sterile dressing or manipulate the catheter. Otherwise clean nonsterile gloves would be acceptable.
- All access procedures must be done by the "no touch" technique (Fig. 2.10.2).

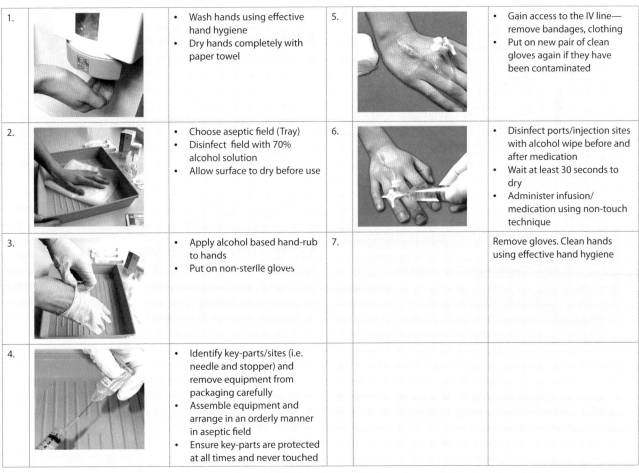

1.		• Wash hands using effective hand hygiene • Dry hands completely with paper towel
2.		• Choose aseptic field (Tray) • Disinfect field with 70% alcohol solution • Allow surface to dry before use
3.		• Apply alcohol based hand-rub to hands • Put on non-sterile gloves
4.		• Identify key-parts/sites (i.e. needle and stopper) and remove equipment from packaging carefully • Assemble equipment and arrange in an orderly manner in aseptic field • Ensure key-parts are protected at all times and never touched
5.		• Gain access to the IV line—remove bandages, clothing • Put on new pair of clean gloves again if they have been contaminated
6.		• Disinfect ports/injection sites with alcohol wipe before and after medication • Wait at least 30 seconds to dry • Administer infusion/medication using non-touch technique
7.		Remove gloves. Clean hands using effective hand hygiene

FIG. 2.10.2: Accessing IV cannula and administering medication using aseptic non-touch technique.

- Always clean all ports and hubs with 70% alcohol wipes *before* and *after* accessing them.
- Cap all stopcocks with *sterile* bungs when not in use. If sterile bungs are not available, bungs may be recycled using 70% alcohol. Although this is not evidence based, but it works well and saves cost.
- The more frequently a CVC is accessed the higher is the CLABSI rate. In addition, administering medication through a CVC involves much higher nursing input that administering through a peripheral cannula. Hence, CVCs should not replace or be used as a substitute of peripheral cannula as most bolus injections could be given through a peripheral cannula.
- *Active removal of nonessential catheters:* The default position for a CVC is to be out. Any catheter should earn its right to remain in. Reviewing the CVC management is an integral part of daily round and whether the line needs to stay should be reviewed daily.
- *Dressing regimen:* Traditional gauze dressings should be routinely changed every 2nd day and polyurethane transparent dressings should be routinely changed every 7th day. In addition, all visibly soiled dressing should also be changed. All dressing changes must be aseptic. However, because of the very nature of pediatric patients, change of dressing carries a higher chance of accidental removal. There is no definite evidence on optimal dressing change regime for pediatric patients and decision to change dressing should be taken on a case-by-case basis.
- *Changing administration sets:* Infusion sets that are continuously used should be changed no more frequently than every 96 hours and no less frequently than every 7 days unless transfusing lipid emulsions or blood products which warrants change every 24 hours or less. The situation is less clear for sets that are used intermittently. Possibly they could be safely changed every 72–96 hours.
- *Parenteral nutrition:* Trying to keep a separate clean lumen that has never been used before for PN has been practiced for some time. However, in practice, it is often not possible to achieve and there is no evidence base to support this practice.
- *Use of multidose/single-dose vials:* Single-dose vials do not contain any preservative and once contaminated, organisms might grow significantly. Therefore, any leftover ideally should be discarded unlike a multidose vial. However, we all face the dilemma of cost-implications of discarding the leftover, especially while treating a neonate or a small child. If reuse of the leftover cannot be avoided due to cost then the vial must be refrigerated to reduce any possible bacterial growth and utmost care should be taken while drawing from the vial as that is the time when contamination occurs. Only sterile needles should be used to access and "no touch technique" must be employed. The diaphragm of the vial must be wiped with 70% alcohol before and after each access.

- *Use of antibiotic lock:* This involves routinely leaving a supraphysiologic dose of antibiotic solution in the hub to prevent CLABSI. The most commonly studied antibiotic is vancomycin, which has been shown to be effective in multiple studies. However, all such studies are done on patients having long-term lines and therefore are not considered here.

Surveillance of CVCs for CLABSI

- Catheter sites should be monitored daily by palpation and/or visually through the intact dressing for tenderness, erythema, swelling, induration or purulence. If patients have any unusual sign, fever without focus or other manifestations suggesting local or BSI, the dressing should be completely removed and the site thoroughly examined and a clinical decision taken whether to remove the CVC or not.
- Patients should be encouraged to report anything unusual/new about the CVC site.
- Routine culture of catheter tips is not recommended and should be done only if CLABSI is suspected.
- A clinical decision should be made about whether an episode should be called a CLABSI or not and this should be clearly documented both in the notes and the CVC checklist.

Replacement of CVCs

- CVC should be replaced only if it is malfunctioning or suspected to cause CLABSI.
- Routine replacement of CVCs after 7 days or exchange over a guidewire has not reduced CRBSI and is not recommended. This approach can only lead to increased cost and mechanical complications as the number of attempted CVC insertion increases.
- Exchange of a malfunctioning CVC over a guidewire is acceptable and preferred than using a new site as this is associated with lesser patient discomfort and mechanical complications.

Considerations for Arterial Lines

Infection rate for arterial lines is lower than CVCs. However, they are being used more frequently as invasive blood pressure monitoring gets popular and may contribute significantly to overall CLABSI incidence.

- In pediatric population—radial, posterior tibial and dorsalis pedis can be used. Brachial artery should not be used, especially in small children although they could be used in adults. Femoral or axillary artery can also be used but is not preferred. There is some adult evidence to suggest higher infection rate associated with femoral arterial lines.
- Full barrier precaution is needed for femoral arterial lines. Otherwise cap, mask, sterile gloves and sterile drape should suffice.

- There have been many reports of infective complications from reusable pressure transducer systems. Therefore, disposable transducers are preferred, although they cost more.
- Disposable or reusable pressure transducers should be changed with all tubing every 96 hours.
- Sterility of the entire pressure monitoring system should be maintained. The system should be accessed as sparingly as possible.
- As for CVC arterial lines should be removed as soon as possible and should be replaced only if malfunctioning.

Considerations for Umbilical Lines

Umbilical venous catheters and umbilical arterial catheter are unique and popular in neonatal practice. Both are associated with similar CLABSI rates.

- Full barrier precaution must be maintained while placing an UAC/UVC.
- They should be treated just as CVCs and all points listed under CVC should be observed.
- Low-dose Heparin (0.25–1.0 U/mL) should be added to the fluid infused through UACs to avoid thrombotic complications and prolong the patency of the catheter.
- While using UAC lower limbs should be monitored for any sign of vascular insufficiency. If any such sign develops the catheter must be removed.
- A UAC should not be kept in situ for more than 5 days.
- A UVC could be used up to 14 days. However, like any other central access they too should be removed as soon as they are not needed.

TREATMENT

Treatment of suspected CLABSI varies depending on the clinical situation. The most common scenario is a patient with short-term CVC developing new fever for which no focus could be found. Studies have shown that most such cases turn out not to be CRBSI. The other scenario is new-onset fever with local changes over insertion site, making line infection likely. In both situations relevant cultures must be sent and antibiotics started unless the patient is very stable. Initial empiric antibiotics should be broad-spectrum and the choice should be guided by local flora and sensitivities. For gram-positive coverage vancomycin is often used unless MRSA is known to be rare in the hospital in which case cloxacillin can be used to cover CONS. For gram-negative coverage either β-lactam/β-lactamase inhibitor combinations, carbapenems or fourth generation cephalosporins are used (consider the prevalence of ESBL producing organisms). An aminoglycoside is often added in critically-ill patients. Antifungals are indicated in patients receiving PN, prolonged broad-spectrum antibiotics and previous colonization with *Candida*, hematological malignancy, bone-marrow or solid organ transplant. Initial choice could be fluconazole unless patient received azoles in last 3 months in which case an echinocandin like caspofungin

can be used. Antibiotics should be rotated through different lumens unless the infected lumen is identified.

The big decision is whether to remove the line or not. The safest option (but not necessarily the wisest) is to remove the catheter for C/S. However, as already stated, most of the "new fever without focus" are not CRBSI. In pediatric patients getting another access can be very difficult or impossible and the central line might be crucial for ongoing management. In addition, in case of long-term lines in stable patients, antibiotics are always tried first with the catheter in situ and up to 75–90% catheters could be salvaged and evidence of line salvage is accumulating even in acute scenarios. Another factor affecting the decision is the status of the patient. We would be more likely to keep the catheter in situ in a stable patient than in a patient with severe sepsis. Although not ideal, another option is to replace the catheter over guidewire and then replace again if C/S is positive, but patient has clinically improved. So, it is a decision which involves many issues, which would vary case-to-case and no universal recommendation is possible. If catheter is kept then patient must be monitored closely. Any clinical deterioration should prompt removal. Daily C/S should be sent (ideally paired, i.e. catheter and peripheral sample) and if C/S is positive 72 hours after starting antibiotics then also catheter is removed.

Ideally repeat C/S should be sent even if catheter is removed and duration of therapy is counted from the day of first positive blood culture. Usual duration is 10–14 days. For *S. aureus* longer duration of 4–6 weeks is recommended if the catheter is kept, C/S is positive after 72 hours, in immunosuppressed patients including patients on steroids, diabetics and patients with other intravascular prosthetic devices. Catheter should be removed in case of *S. aureus* and especially *Candida*. Although, there are some case reports of catheter salvage even in *Candida* CRBSI in unusual circumstances, but they are not recommended for routine practice.

There is a volume of work on antibiotic lock solutions to treat CRBSI, but nearly all of them are for long-term catheters. In acute setting, it is usually not possible to achieve the dwell-time as the catheter is used frequently. However, one recent retrospective study on PICU patients described 70% ethanol lock salvaging 77% of 26 catheters using dwell time of just a few hours. Organisms included both *S. aureus* and *Candida*. More such studies are needed before they could be considered standard practice in acute setting.

2.10.3 CATHETER-ASSOCIATED URINARY TRACT INFECTION

INTRODUCTION

Compared to VAP or CLABSI, the evidence base for CAUTI is weak. Pediatric evidence is very sparse. There is a good deal of confusion regarding nomenclature and definitions of CAUTI and catheter-associated asymptomatic bacteriuria (CA-ASB). However, relatively clear recommendations for prevention are available which should be the focus.

EPIDEMIOLOGY

Catheter-associated urinary tract infection is the most common HAI among adults occurring in 15–25% of patients, but is the third most common among pediatric patients. Incidence density ranged 3.1–7.5 per 1,000 catheter days. A multicenter PICU study reported rate of 4.0 per 1,000 catheter days.

Catheter-associated urinary tract infection increase length of stay and therefore cost. Mean increase have been around 2 days in many studies. Whether CAUTI increases mortality or not is less clear. In one big study of nearly 1,500 patients excess mortality was noted, but many subsequent studies did not replicate this. In order to affect mortality, CAUTI must lead to sepsis. 1–4% of CAUTI develops bacteremia and mortality of this group has been reported to be between 10% and 15%.

PATHOPHYSIOLOGY

The organism can access urinary tract either by extraluminal ascension or intraluminally. Extraluminal ascension is more common in one study accounting for two-thirds of the cases. However, contamination of even closed collection system also happens frequently. CA-USB is very common and the most important factor is duration of catheter. By 30 days nearly all patients develop CA-USB, but not CAUTI (note "diagnosis and definition"). Biofilm generation is also almost universal by 30 days, which acts as a protector against both host-immunity and antibiotics.

ETIOLOGY

E. coli is the most common organism. Other Gram-negative organisms like *Klebsiella*, *Pseudomonas*, etc. are also common. Gram-positives include *Enterococcus* and CONS. Candid is the most common fungus with a wide prevalence range of 3–30% depending on the study quoted. Most CAUTI are caused by a single pathogen except in long-term catheters where polymicrobial infections are common. In most Indian studies, gram-negative organisms accounted for vast majority of cases. As in other situations ESBL is very common. As for example, in a study from South India, 96% of *Klebsiella* isolates from urine were ESBL positive. Most Indian studies reported ESBL in 50–75% of gram-negative isolates. MDR organisms are also a big issue (Please note "Microbiology and Antibiotics" in General section).

DIAGNOSIS AND DEFINITION

This is an area of considerable uncertainty even more so for pediatric patients. Various definitions have been used

which add to the confusion. The CDC and IDSA definitions are often accepted and are discussed here.

Catheter-associated asymptomatic bacteriuria is defined by CDC as well as IDSA as a urine sample growing more than or equal to 10^5 CFU/mL of less than or equal to two species in an asymptomatic patient with indwelling catheter. Latest CDC surveillance criteria actually removed CA-ASB as a separate infection.

Catheter-associated urinary tract infection is defined by IDSA as urine growing more than or equal to 10^3 CFU/mL of more than or equal to one species in a patient with indwelling catheter or whose catheter has been removed in the last 48 hours who also has signs or symptoms of UTI. Signs or symptoms include new onset or worsening of fever, rigors, altered mental status, malaise or lethargy with no other identified cause; flank pain; costovertebral angle tenderness; acute hematuria; pelvic discomfort; and in those whose catheters have been removed, dysuria, urgency, frequency or suprapubic pain or tenderness.

On the other hand, CDC defines CAUTI as clinical features of UTI in a patient who has been catheterized for at least past 48 hours or whose catheter has been removed in the last 48 hours and whose urine sample either:
- Grown greater than or equal to 10^5 CFU/mL of less than or equal to two species
- Grown greater than or equal to 10^3 to smaller than 10^5 CFU/mL of less than or equal to two species and has a positive urine analysis, i.e. positive dipstick for leukocytes/nitrite, pyuria [$\geq$10 white blood cells (WBC)/ mm^3 or $\geq$3 WBC/HPF] or microorganisms on Gram stain.

Features of UTI is at least one of unexplained fever (>38°C), costovertebral/suprapubic pain/tenderness, and in those whose catheters have been removed, dysuria, urgency and frequency. For patients below or of 1 year, they are at least one of fever (> 38°C), hypothermia (<36°C), apnea, bradycardia, dysuria, lethargy or vomiting.

CATHETER-ASSOCIATED BACTERIURIA INCLUDES BOTH CA-ASB AND CAUTI

Catheter-associated asymptomatic bacteriuria is common and does not necessarily lead to CAUTI. As for example, in a study of nosocomial CA-bacteriuria, 90% patients were afebrile and asymptomatic. Symptomatic UTI was equally likely among patients with/without CA-bacteriuria. In another study of more than 500 patients, neither fever nor leukocytosis was associated with CA-bacteriuria. It is thought that about 25% patients with CA-ASB might eventually develop CAUTI. Previously, CA-ASB was routinely treated and there is good evidence that this practice is still continuing. In view of this, much emphasis is now given to differentiate between CAUTI and CA-ASB and not to either monitor or treat CA-ASB as this is unnecessary and more importantly leads to excessive use of antibiotics which might have implications on emergence of resistance.

Differentiating CAUTI from CA-ASB is entirely dependent on presence or absence of clinical features. The problem with critically ill and/or small children is the unreliability of signs/symptoms of UTI in this age group. However, in a patient with indwelling catheter who develops new onset fever without focus, it is perfectly justified to send urine for C/S as this does not amount to monitoring for CA-ASB. If C/S is positive, the fever itself would make it CAUTI rather than CA-ASB.

Collecting urine sample has always been an issue in pediatric UTI. Urine should never be collected from the bag. In a catheterized patient fresh sample should be collected from the catheter before starting or changing antibiotics. If decision is taken to replace the catheter then sample should be drawn from the new catheter rather than the old one. In patients without catheter, mid-stream voided sample should be taken. CDC clearly stated that there is insufficient data to give any cut-off for condom-catheter sample. IDSA has not even mentioned anything about condom-catheter or bagged sample.

PREVENTION

Just like the other two HAIs; here also prevention is most important. However, the evidence base on this aspect is also weaker for CAUTI than VAP or CLABSI. Standard recommendations are given below:

Before Inserting a Catheter

- *Reduce inappropriate use of catheters:* Catheters should not be used just for incontinence or as a substitute for nursing care. In a recent CDC publication, valid indications were as follows:
  - Acute retention or bladder neck obstruction
  - Need of accurate output measurement, as in critically-ill patients
  - Patient needing prolonged immobilization, e.g. unstable spinal fracture, pelvic fracture, etc.
  - Selected perioperative uses in urologic or genitourinary surgery, prolonged surgery, need to transfuse large volume of fluids or diuretics or closely monitor output intraoperatively. Most postoperative catheters could be removed within 24 hours.
  - Improve comfort in patients on palliative care.
- *Consider alternatives to indwelling catheters:* Condom-catheters are commonly used and widely recommended although it does not have strong evidence base. Intermittently weighing diapers is also often practiced, and reliability has been tested by many studies—mostly in neonates. There would always be some evaporation of urine, depending on use of warmers or incubators or ambient temperature. In incubators humidity is another factor and may even lead to false weight-gain of diapers. The percentage loss by evaporation becomes less as the urine output increase. Overall, it seems to be a reasonable alternative unless very close monitoring of output is paramount as in a cardiovascular or renal unstable patient. Keeping the warmer output as low as clinically safe, weighing or changing frequently, keeping the diaper closed and using a sensitive digital balance would minimize errors.

Intermittent catheterization is better than indwelling catheters in patients with bladder neck obstruction like myelomeningocele.

- *Catheter material:* Antibiotic coated catheters have been studied, but results are not uniform and any possible benefit is likely to be short lasting (<1 week). They may be considered in situations where preventing CAUTI is crucial, as in immunocompromised patients. They are not widely available. Silicone catheters may be preferable in patients with long-term catheters having recurrent catheter obstruction due to encrustation.

Inserting a Urinary Catheter

This should be done only by adequately trained staff. Hand hygiene is must before and after any insertion or manipulation or removal of catheter. Intermittent catheterization is a clean procedure. In contrast, placing an indwelling catheter in acute setting is a sterile procedure involving sterile gloves, drape, gauze and lubricant jelly (preferably single use). Whether cleaning with antiseptic solution is better than cleaning with sterile water or normal saline is not clear. It is possibly wiser to use antiseptic solution until more evidence become available.

Managing Urinary Catheter after Insertion

- Once inserted, catheter should be connected to a closed collection system and it should be disconnected as little as possible. The bag should always be kept at a level lower than the patient and tubes must not be kinked. The bag should be regularly drained making sure spout of the bag does not touch the container.
- The catheter or collection system should not be changed routinely at any interval unless it is malfunctioning or CAUTI suspected.
- There is no role of routine irrigation, prophylactic systemic antibiotic, meatal care with topical antibiotic or placing antiseptic solution in the bag.
- Surveillance urine C/S should not be done.

Removing a Urinary Catheter

- *Indwelling catheters should be removed at the earliest and whether the catheter is still needed should be actively questioned on daily rounds.* Many interventions have been tried like nurse-driven protocols, electronic automated reminders, reminders by the nurse, etc. and have been shown to be effective. Institutions should determine what mechanism would be best suited to their circumstances, but it is advisable to have some system to encourage early removal of catheters.

- Routine clamping of catheter before removal is not indicated. Clamping makes no difference to re-catheterization but may increase bacteriuria.
- One good quality study among adult females has shown significant benefit of monitoring for and treating CA-ASB that is persistent 48 hours after removal of catheter. However, no such recommendation could be made for either adult males or pediatric patients based on current evidence.

TREATMENT

Again, surprisingly little evidence is available, even in adult literature. An important question is whether existing catheters should be removed or not. There is some evidence to support changing catheter in a suspected CAUTI if the catheter is more than 2 weeks old. In such case, sample should be sent from the new catheter (or voided sample if catheter is not replaced) for more reliable C/S results. If C/S is positive and the catheter had not been replaced; then although there is not much evidence, but it seems prudent to replace the catheter.

Choice of antibiotic should be guided by the pattern and sensitivity of local flora. Monotherapy is sufficient unless patient is very ill and other differentials could not be excluded. As always, antibiotic must be rationalized once C/S is available.

Duration of therapy will depend on severity of the CAUTI and response to treatment. CAUTI includes uncomplicated lower UTI, pyelonephritis, pyelonephritis with abscess and UTI with secondary bacteremia. Naturally duration would vary. Aim should be to keep duration as short as possible to reduce antibiotic resistance without reducing efficacy of therapy. It seems reasonable to treat for 7 days in patients with good response and 10–14 days in others. There is some evidence that a shorter course (even a single dose) may be effective in uncomplicated lower UTI if the catheter is removed and in such situation a short course of 3 days may be considered.

BIBLIOGRAPHY

1. American Thoracic Society Documents. Guidelines for the Management of Adults with Hospital-acquired, Ventilator-associated, and Healthcare-associated Pneumonia. Am J Respir Crit Care Med. 2005;171:388-416.
2. Gould CV, Umscheid CA, Agarwal RK, et al. Guideline for prevention of catheter-associated urinary tract infections 2009. HICPAC, CDC Guidelines.
3. Hooton TM, Bradley SF, Cardenas DD, et al. Diagnosis, prevention, and treatment of catheter-associated urinary tract infection in adults: 2009 International Clinical Practice Guidelines from the Infectious Diseases Society of America. Clin Infect Dis. 2010;50:625-63.
4. Masterton RG, Galloway A, French G, et al. Guidelines for the management of hospital-acquired pneumonia in the UK: Report of the Working Party on Hospital-Acquired Pneumonia of the British Society for Antimicrobial Chemotherapy. J. Antimicrob. Chemother. 2008;62:5-34.
5. Mello MJ, Albuquerque Mde F, Lacerda HR, et al. Risk factors for healthcare-associated infection in pediatric intensive care units: a systematic review. Cad Saude Publica. 2009;25(Suppl 3):S373-91.
6. Mermel LA, Allon M, Bouza E, et al. Clinical practice guidelines for the diagnosis and management of intravascular catheter-related infection: 2009 Update by the Infectious Diseases Society of America. Clin Infect Dis. 2009;49:1-45.
7. O'Grady NP, Alexander M, Burns LA, et al. Guidelines for the prevention of intravascular catheter-related infections. CDC Guideline. 2011.
8. Prevention of hospital-acquired infections. A practical guide, 2nd edition. WHO, Dept. of Communicable Disease, Surveillance and Response. 2002.
9. Randolph AG, Brun-Buisson C, Goldmann D. Identification of central venous catheter-related infections in infants and children. Pediatr Crit Care Med. 2005;6(3 Suppl):S19-24.
10. Venkatachalam V, Hendley JO, Willson DF. The diagnostic dilemma of ventilator-associated pneumonia in critically ill children. Pediatr Crit Care Med. 2011;12:286-96.

2.11 FEBRILE NEUTROPENIA

Priyankar Pal

INTRODUCTION

Febrile neutropenia is defined as an axillary temperature above 38.5°C lasting more than 1 hour in the context of an absolute neutrophil count (ANC) less than 500 cells/mm³. Fever has also been defined as a single oral temperature of 38.3°C (101°F) or a temperature of 38°C (100.4°F) for more than 1 hour.

Normal neutrophil count is 1,500–8,000 cells/mm³. Neutropenia is defined as neutrophil count less than 1,500 cells/mm³ and is graded as follows:

- *Mild neutropenia:* 1,000–1,500 cells/mm³
- *Moderate neutropenia:* 500–999 cells/mm³
- *Severe neutropenia:* <500 cells/mm³
- *Profound neutropenia:* <100 cells/mm³

Febrile neutropenia is a *medical emergency* typically encountered in oncologic patients undergoing chemotherapy. In a neutropenic patient fever may be the only manifestation of a serious underlying infection, as inflammatory signs and symptoms are typically attenuated.

The management guidelines were thus formulated for oncologic neutropenic patients. However, the same principles can be extrapolated while managing a nononcologic neutropenic (congenital or acquired) child presenting with fever.

INITIAL ASSESSMENT AND INVESTIGATION

As already mentioned this is a medical emergency and success depends on prompt recognition and institution of therapy. Different centers experience different patterns of principal causative pathogens and the underlying guidelines are based on the Infectious Diseases Society of America (IDSA) 2010 updated guidelines and the European Society Medical Oncology (ESMO) recommendations. They are intended for use alongside local antimicrobial policies.

Initial evaluation should categorize the patient as low or high risk and determine whether vancomycin therapy is needed.

A number of instruments have been developed in attempts to predict those high-risk cases where complications are more likely. The most widely used instrument, the multinational association for supportive care in cancer (MASCC) index allows the clinician to rapidly assess risk before access to the neutrophil count and without knowledge of the burden of underlying cancer, and has been prospectively validated. The criteria and weighting scores are listed in Table 2.11.1. Low-risk cases are those scoring greater than or equal to 21.

Table 2.11.1: Multinational association for supportive care in cancer (MASCC) scoring index.

Characteristic	Score
Burden of illness: no or mild symptoms	5
No hypotension	5
No chronic obstructive pulmonary disease	4
Solid tumor or no previous fungal infection	4
No dehydration	3
Burden of illness: moderate symptoms	3
Outpatient status (at onset of fever)	3
Age < 20 years	2

High risk patients are those children with any of the following criteria:

- Profound neutropenia (ANC < 100/cmm) anticipated to last more than 7 days.
- Presence of any associated comorbid medical problems:
  - Hemodynamic instability
  - Oral or gastrointestinal mucositis
  - Abdominal symptoms like pain, nausea, vomiting or diarrhea
  - Neurological or mental status changes of new onset
  - Intravenous (IV) catheter infection especially catheter tunnel infection
  - New pulmonary infiltrate or hypoxemia, or underlying chronic lung disease
  - Hepatic insufficiency [serum glutamic-oxaloacetic transaminase (SGPT) > 5X normal values] or renal insufficiency (creatinine clearance <30 mL/minute).
  - Multinational association for supportive care in cancer index less than 21.

While initially evaluating a patient one should note for presence of any indwelling IV catheter and look for symptoms or signs suggesting any obvious infective focus. This entails a thorough systematic examination including respiratory, gastrointestinal, genitourinary, skin and perineal regions and central nervous system.

Initial investigations are enumerated in Box 2.11.1.

Blood cultures—at least two sets of blood culture specimens should be obtained prior to initiation of antibiotics. Most centers limit blood draws to not more than 1% of patients total blood volume (usually 3–5 mL in children). Blood culture sets from all central venous catheter lumens as well as one set from a peripheral vein are advocated.

Initial investigations.
- Routine blood testing to assess bone marrow, renal and liver function
- Coagulation screen
- C-reactive protein
- Blood cultures (minimum two sets) including cultures from iv catheter
- Urinalysis and culture
- Sputum microscopy and culture
- Stool microscopy and culture (if diarrhea present)
- Skin lesions (aspirate/biopsy/swab)
- Chest radiograph (if respiratory symptoms present or outpatient therapy considered)

MANAGEMENT

High risk patients should be admitted for IV empirical antibiotic therapy; monotherapy with an antipseudomonal agent, like ceftazidime, a carbapenem (meropenem or imipenem-cilastatin) or piperacillin-tazobactam, is recommended. Other antibiotics (aminoglycosides or fluoroquinolones and/or vancomycin) may be added if antibiotic resistance is suspected or proven.

Indications of Vancomycin Therapy

- Severe mucositis
- Obvious catheter-related infection
- Colonization with methicillin-resistant *Staphylococcus aureus* (MRSA)
- Hypotension
- Patient on quinolone prophylaxis
- Skin or soft tissue infection/pneumonia.

If the patient has associated diarrhea, assess for clostridium difficile and add metronidazole.

Low risk patients may initially receive oral antibiotics instead of IV medications, or may be initiated with IV and converted to outpatient oral treatment at the earliest. Ciprofloxacin plus co-amoxiclav is commonly recommended for oral treatment. Others like levofloxacin or ciprofloxacin alone or ciprofloxacin plus clindamycin are also commonly used. Patients on fluoroquinolone prophylaxis should not receive empirical oral therapy with fluoroquinolone. Hospital admission is required for persistent fever or signs of worsening infection.

Daily Follow-up and Assessment of Response

The frequency of clinical assessment is determined by severity of symptoms, but may be required every 2–4 hours in cases of needing resuscitation. Daily assessment of fever trends, blood counts and renal function is indicated until the patient is apyrexial and ANC greater than or equal to 500/cmm.

Modifications to initial antibiotic therapy are recommended if the patient's condition is unstable or if initial blood culture results suggest a resistant organism. Patients who remain hemodynamically unstable after initial doses with standard agents should have their regimen broadened to include resistant gram-positive, Gram-negative and anaerobic bacteria. Persistant fever after 4–7 days in a high risk patient warrants addition of an antifungal agent.

However, unexplained persistent fever in a patient who is otherwise stable rarely requires an empirical change in antibiotics.

Role of Antifungals

Choice for empirical therapy depends on likely fungal pathogens, toxicity and cost. If patient was not receiving antifungal prophylaxis, then candidemia is initially the greatest concern. For patients on fluconazole, then fluconazole resistant candida or an invasive mold infection is more likely. Traditionally amphotericin B (deoxycholate, lipid formulation or liposomal) is the drug of choice. Reliable alternatives include itraconazole, voriconazole and caspofungin.

Every attempt should be made to identify a fungal infection by serum tests for fungal antigens or deoxyribonucleic acid (DNA) or high resolution computed tomography (CT) of chest and sinuses. Pre-emptive management, although attractive is largely experimental; and presumptive therapy remains the standard.

Duration of Empiric Antibiotic Therapy

Duration of therapy will depend on particular organism and site of infection and should continue till marrow recovery (ANC > 500/cmm). Alternatively, if therapy has been completed and patient is afebrile and stable but remains neutropenic, oral fluoroquinolone prophylaxis may be initiated till marrow recovery.

Role of Antivirals

- Herpes simplex virus (HSV)-seropositive patients undergoing allogeneic hematopoietic stem-cell transplantation (HSCT) or leukemia induction should receive acyclovir.
- Treatment for HSV or varicella-zoster virus (VZV) is indicated only if there is evidence of active viral disease.
- Influenza infection should be treated if the infecting strain is susceptible and during influenza outbreaks all symptomatic neutropenic patients should receive empirical treatment.
- All patients undergoing cancer chemotherapy should receive yearly inactivated influenza vaccine.

- Respiratory syncytial virus (RSV) treatment should not be given to patients who present with upper respiratory tract symptoms.

Role of Hematopoietic Growth Factors [G-Cerebrospinal Fluid (CSF) or GM-CSF] in Management

Prophylactic use is recommended in patients with anticipated risk of neutropenia. For treatment of established fever and neutropenia, they are usually not recommended.

Role of Prophylactic Antibiotics Following Recovery from Fever

Fluoroquinolone (levofloxacin or ciprofloxacin) prophylaxis should be given to patients with expected prolonged (more than 7 days) and severe neutropenia (ANC <100/cmm).

Addition of a gram-positive agent is generally not required. Low risk patients with expected short (<7 days) duration of neutropenia are generally not put on antibiotic prophylaxis.

Role of Prophylactic Antifungals

Prophylaxis against *Candida* infections is recommended in high risk groups like allogeneic HSCT recipients, or those undergoing intensive remission induction chemotherapy for acute leukemia. Fluconazole, itraconazole, voriconazole, posaconazole and caspofungin are all acceptable alternatives.

Prophylaxis against invasive aspergillus with posaconazole should be considered for selected patients more than 13 years, undergoing intensive chemotherapy for acute myeloid leukemia or myelodysplastic syndrome.

Environmental Precautions

- Hand hygiene is the single most effective way of preventing transmission of infections.
- Follow standard barrier protection for all patients.
- Allogeneic HSCT recipients should be placed in rooms with more than 12 air exchanges/hour and high efficiency particulate air (HEPA) filtration.

- Do not allow plants or fresh or dried flowers in rooms of neutropenic patients.
- Healthcare workers should be encouraged to report their illnesses.
- All close contacts should receive measles, mumps, rubella, varicella and annual influenza vaccines.

Skin and Oral Care

- Patients should take daily showers or baths.
- Regular inspection of skin sites likely to be portal of infections (IV access sites/perineum).
- Rectal thermometers, enemas, suppositories and rectal examinations are contraindicated. Menstruating females should not use tampons because of the risk of skin abrasion.
- With ongoing mucositis, oral rinses 4–6 times/day with sterile water, normal saline or soda bicarbonate solutions. Teeth should be brushed at least twice daily.

Patient Education and Local Policies

Success in management requires prompt recognition of, and reaction to, potential infection. Vital to this is educating outpatients to monitor symptoms including body temperature, and clear written instructions on when and how to contact the appropriate service in the event of concerns.

BIBLIOGRAPHY

1. Guideline for the Management of Fever and Neutropenia in Children with Cancer and/or Undergoing Hematopoietic Stem-Cell Transplantation. Children's Oncology Group Supportive Care Endorsed Guidelines. Version date: September 25, 2015. http://www.sickkids.ca/Haematology Oncology/IPFNG/index.htm.
2. Robinson PD, Lehrnbecher T, Phillips R, et al. Strategies for Empiric Management of Pediatric Fever and Neutropenia in Patients With Cancer and Hematopoietic Stem-Cell Transplantation Recipients: A Systematic Review of Randomized Trials. J Clin Oncol. 2016;34(17):2054-60.

2.12   PROPHYLACTIC ANTIMICROBIALS

Rohit Agrawal, Rajesh G Patel

INTRODUCTION

Antimicrobial prophylaxis is a modality of antimicrobial therapy which is being initiated in anticipation or belief to prevent serious bacterial illness or serious outcome of the present bacterial infection or at times to prevent the recurrence [e.g. for urinary tract infection (UTI)] or relapses (in case of malaria). Antibiotic therapy can be categorized in four categories like (1) presumptive, (2) empirical, (3) definitive and (4) prophylactic.

- *Presumptive:* When the clinical occurrence is convinced or presumed beyond doubts.
- *Empirical:* When the diagnosis is certain and the disease warrants the need of antibiotic. Classical example being pneumonia.
- *Definitive:* When the pathogen is either isolated or confirmed with various laboratory diagnostics.

The clinician must remember that antibiotics means anti-bio, which is anti-life. While killing an organism it may damage the host. Microbe is supposed to be 3 billion year old in this universe and probably by the virtue of this, they are equipped with a very strong and a prolific genetic engineering mechanism by which they can quickly develop "drug resistance" and can transfer the technology to other species of organism. Unfortunately due to irrational use and abuse of antibiotics, microbial resistance is always a looming threat and a medical catastrophe is awaiting in the wings to occur, should this abuse not be stopped. The commonest misused weapons are prophylactic antibiotics in viral infections or prophylactic antibiotics to neonate in nursery, so-called precious baby or at risk babies.

PRINCIPLES IN THE CHOICE OF ANTIBIOTIC PROPHYLAXIS

- The chosen antibiotic should be effective, at the same time be nontoxic with fever or no side effects. The benefits should outweigh the risks of side effects.
- It should not damage the indigenous bacterial flora.
- It should not induce bacterial resistance.
- The antimicrobial prophylaxis should ideally be initiated as soon as possible after the contact to a susceptible individual (e.g. meningococcal prophylaxis or varicella prophylaxis) and for shortest possible time (e.g. surgical prophylaxis).
- One must always remember that extensive prophylactic antibiotics use may enhance emergence or re-emergence of resistant organism in the community (e.g. abuse of third generation cephalosporins may lead to emergence of enterococci resistance to vancomycin). Also the benefit of prophylactic antibiotic is limited when there is high prevalence of antibiotic resistant organism in the community.

Antimicrobial prophylaxis is targeted at three sites:

- Prevention of infection or disease by a specific pathogen
- Prevention of infection or disease at infection from body tissue/site
- Generalized protection of a susceptible or vulnerable host.

Antibiotic prophylaxis is either short term (e.g. surgical prophylaxis), long term (e.g. UTI) or lifelong (e.g. rheumatic disease).

Antimicrobial prophylaxis can be divided into three major groups:

- Prophylaxis for specific pathogens: Following pathogens, warrants prophylaxis for prevention of long-term sequelae:
  - Group A *Streptococcus* (GABHS)
  - Group B *Streptococcus* (GBS)
  - *Streptococcus viridans*
  - *Streptococcus pneumoniae*
  - *Neisseria meningitidis*
  - *Meningococcus.*

Pertussis

Diphtheriae

- *Mycobacterium tuberculosis*
- *P. vivax/P. falciparum*
- *Herpes simplex*
- Varicella
- Influenza
- Leprosy
- *Pneumocystis carinii*
- Plague

Prophylaxis for infection prone sites and systems:

- Cardiovascular system:
  i. Rheumatic heart disease
  ii. Infective endocarditis
- Urinary tract infection
- Surgical
- Human immunodeficiency virus (HIV)

Prophylaxis for nosocomial infections.

Specific Pathogen

Group A Streptococcus: It is known to cause acute rheumatic fever and heart disease and acute glomerulonephritis. However, this condition may be well prevented if appropriate antibiotic therapy is instituted up to 9 days of onset of symptoms of true bacterial streptococcal pharyngotonsillitis. However, 30% of patients which may go undetected as subclinical streptococcal pharyngotonsillitis, may develop rheumatic fever or streptococcal glomerulonephritis.

Prophylactic antibiotic for primary prevention:
- Drug of choice is oral penicillin V 250 mg BID/TID (<30 kg—250 mg BID, >30 kg—250 mg TID)
- Benzathine penicillin (0.6–1.2 million IU) intramuscular (IM) single dose
- In case of allergy to penicillin, erythromycin (40 mg/kg/day) 3–4 doses/day x 10 days
- First generation cephalosporin (30–40 mg/kg/day) x 10 days.

The patient who has already suffered one or more attacks of rheumatic fever or has rheumatic heart disease (RHD) or valvulitis must receive long course of prophylactic antibiotics for at least 2–25 years or at least 5 years after the last attack of rheumatic fever or in certain high-risk case, lifelong.

The drug of choice is injection benzathine penicillin G (0.6–1.2 million IU) every 21 days.

Penicillin can be used as an antimicrobial prophylaxis orally if the patient is complying, but is usually of inferior choice.

Group B Beta Hemolytic Streptococcus (GBS)

Group B beta hemolytic *Streptococcus* (GBS) disease fortunately is very uncommon in India; hence routine screening for neonatal GBS disease is not needed in pregnant Indian women.

According to Western protocol, maternal prophylaxis to prevent early maternal disease is given based on vaginorectal screening which is routinely performed for all pregnant women from 35–37 weeks of gestation.

In Indian circumstances
- Prolonged rupture of membrane more than 18 hours
- Maternal intrapartum fever higher than 38°C
- Foul smelling liquor
- Premature delivery less than 37 weeks, warrants routine intrapartum prophylaxis.

Drug of choice
- Penicillin G 5 million IU IV every 6 hourly.
- Ampicillin 2 g IV loading followed by 1–2 g every 4–6 hourly.

Fortunately, there is no GBS drug resistance being reported for penicillin and ampicillin. For penicillin allergic patient, clindamycin or erythromycin can be used. For penicillin intolerant patient, cefazolin (50 mg/kg/dose) can be used. In case of multiple drug resistance, vancomycin may be used.

The above prophylaxis is continued until the baby is delivered. In case of proven GBS infection in mother, the baby should be put on ampicillin (100 mg/kg/day) in 3–4 divided doses for 7–10 days.

Streptococcus pneumoniae: Chemoprophylaxis for prevention of invasive pneumococcal disease, although of importance are not routinely practiced in view of developing resistance to penicillin (amoxicillin, erythromycin, TMP-SMX).

The advent of newer generation conjugate vaccine has almost replaced the role of chemoprophylaxis. However, the group of children who are at high risk are patients with HIV, hematological malignancy, sickle cell disease, functional or anatomical asplenia, humoral and complement immunodeficiency, chronic heart, lung, liver or renal disease, nephrotic syndrome, diabetes mellitus and cerebrospinal fluid (CSF) leak may have to be provided with chemoprophylaxis in addition to conjugate vaccine since the vaccine do not provide 100% coverage for the invasive pneumococcal diseases.

Drug of choice:
- Oral amoxicillin (125 mg BID <3-year-old child, 250 mg BID >3-year-old child). The studies have shown that the use of this prophylaxis regime have substantial effect in reducing the incidence of pneumococcal sepsis in children at high risk.
- Intramuscular benzathine penicillin may be an alternative. However, in community with high incidence of penicillin resistance, alternate antibiotics like cefotaxime may be necessary.

The duration of prophylaxis is controversial in children with asplenia and sickle cell disease. At least, it should be continued for 5 years or according to the some experts, throughout the childhood.

Neisseria Meningitidis

Meningococcal infection is potentially very serious in nature and can be fatal; hence, an appropriate prophylaxis should be initiated as soon as possible for the close contacts like those in households, day care, nursery, etc. or those who have had the close contact with patient during the 7 days prior to the onset of illness.

Drug of choice
- Rifampin (10 mg/kg) maximum 600 mg/day orally every 12 hours for 4 doses (5 mg/kg) for infants less than 1 month of age, OR
- Ceftriaxone 125 mg for children less than 12 years old, and 250 mg greater than 12 years old, as single IM injection, OR
- Ciprofloxacin 500 mg orally as single dose in individual greater than 18 years of age.

Corynebacterium Diphtheriae

Antibiotics are recommended in all close contacts irrespective of the immunity status. Single dose IM benzathine penicillin 6 million IU (<6 years) and 12 million IU (>6 years) or 7–10 days of oral erythromycin (40 mg/kg/day, max 1 g/day) is adequate.

Unimmunized contact should complete immunization schedule. Those contacts who have received primary immunization but no toxoid in the past 5 years should receive a booster dose of the vaccine [diphtheria-tetanus (DT) in those <7 years and tetanus-diphtheria (Td) in those >7 years].

Bordetella Pertussis

Pertussis is highly transmissible illness with secondary attack rate up to 80% in susceptible household contacts who are exposed to the index case during the period of infectiousness (First 4 weeks of the illness, maximum 1st week).

Postexposure prophylaxis of contacts has however not been shown to reduce the incidence of culture confirmed cases or clinical symptoms and has additional problems of costs, drug side effects and adherence. Also in most clinical instances, the diagnosis of pertussis in the index case is only presumptive.

All other contacts should be placed on surveillance and antibiotics started at the first respiratory symptom. The same regime as used for therapy is effective for prophylaxis.

Three doses of trivalent vaccines diphtheria, tetanus and pertussis (DTP)/diphtheria, tetanus and acellular pertussis (DTaP) at 6, 10 and 14 weeks and a booster at 18 months and at 4–6 years is recommended in view of waning immunity as the age progresses, additional doses of vaccination are recommended in adolescents to prevent the breakthrough of the disease.

Mycobacterium Tuberculosis

Contact—Defined as any child who lives in a household with an adult taking antituberculosis therapy or have taken antitubercular therapy in the past 2 years.

World Health Organization (WHO) recommends tuberculosis (TB) chemoprophylaxis for:
- Neonate born to mother with TB.
- Close household contact less than 3 years with asymptomatic positive Mantoux test.
- Close household contacts less than 5 years with Grade 3 or 4 malnutrition and for asymptomatic positive Mantoux test.
- Severe immunocompromised condition and HIV.
- Asymptomatic recent tuberculin converts.

Close surveillance is necessary for 5–12-years-old contact.
- *Baby born to mother with TB:* Breastfeeding should be continued, prophylaxis isoniazid [INH (5 mg/kg/day)] has been found to be efficacious. Suppression of baby from mother should occur only if mother is seriously ill/hospitalized/nonadherent to her treatment/infected with MDR strain of microbacterial TB.
- Isoniazid should be given for a total of 6 months or up to 3 months after mother becomes culture negative.

- *TB chemoprophylaxis in patients with HIV infection:* According to the current WHO guidelines, INH preventive therapy is recommended for HIV-infected children, if living in high TB prevalence areas or who are in household contacts of TB patients. The current recommendations from RNTCP and IAP are 6 months INH (10 mg/kg/day). However, there is a non-definitive data of optimal duration of INH preventive therapy for children in TB endemic developing countries.

There is no evidence of bacillus Calmette-Guérin (BCG)- induced protective effect in HIV-infected children; however, on the contrary, studies have documented that BCG vaccination poses a risk of developing disseminated TB in perinatally infected infants with HIV and other primary immunodeficiency children. Global Advisory Committee on Vaccine Safety (GACVS) and strategic advisory group of experts (SAGE) recommend a contraindication for BCG vaccination in such cases.

Note: No chemoprophylaxis is required for BCG adenitis.

Malaria Prophylaxis

Frequent infection of malaria unfortunately neither confers any protective immunity nor there is any vaccine available at present for prevention. Hence, chemoprophylaxis becomes prudent for personal protection whenever physical, particularly for those who are traveling in high-endemic areas. Most parts of India have a high transmission of *P. vivax* and chloroquine resistant *P. falciparum* malaria (Table 2.12.1).

Chemoprophylaxis for relapse in malaria: After optimal and recommended chemotherapy of *P. vivax*, a course of primaquine (0.3 mg/kg) should be initiated for 14 days as prophylaxis of further relapse.

Viral Infections

- *Herpes simplex:* Antiviral drug for the prophylaxis of the herpes infection are usually used in immunocompromised host or in individuals with frequent recurrent oral or genital herpes infections.
  The drug of choice—Acyclovir 200 mg—4 times a day for 6–12 months, valacyclovir and famciclovir are other drugs which are being used, with refrain due to high cost constraints and are inferior choices.
- *Varicella:* Antiviral chemoprophylaxis is indicated in only immunocompromised patient as postexposure prophylaxis.
- The drug of choice—Acyclovir 10–20 mg/kg/dose, 4 times a day starting from 7th day of exposure for next 7 days.
- *Influenza:* Although influenza is correlated to common cold and is seasonal viral infection, it is prevalent throughout the year. Although relatively benign, it may be severe with severe outcomes, may be fatal at times in persons at risks like asthma,

Table 2.12.1: Dosage of drugs for different types of malaria transmission.

Types of malaria transmission	Drugs	Dosage
Areas with chloroquine sensitive *P. falciparum*	Chloroquine (start 1 week before exposure, continue during exposure and for 4 weeks thereafter)	5 mg of base/kg once weekly (up to 300 mg of base)
Areas with chloroquine resistant *P. falciparum* (low degree, not widespread)	Chloroquine (same as above) + Proguanil (Start 1–2 days before, continue during exposure and for 4 weeks thereafter)	5 mg/kg of base once weekly <2 years: 50 mg/day 2–6 years: 100 mg/day 7–9 years: 150 mg/day >9 years: 200 mg/day
Areas with chloroquine resistant *P. falciparum* (high degree, widespread)	Mefloquine (start 2–3 weeks before, continue during exposure and for 4 weeks thereafter) or Chloroquine + Proguanil or Doxycycline (start 1 week before, continue during exposure and for 4 weeks thereafter)	<15 kg: 5 mg of salt/kg 15–19 kg: ¼ tab/week 20–30 kg: ½ tab/week 31–45 kg: ¾ tab/week >45 kg: 1 tab/week As above >7 years: 2 mg/kg up to adult dose

cardiopulmonary disease, immunocompromised conditions, bronchopulmonary dysplasia (BPD), cardiomyopathies, congenital and acquired valvular diseases and neuromuscular disorders. Unvaccinated healthcare providers and laboratory technicians, particularly who are in close contact of the index case or specimens especially during the community influenza outbreak are ideal candidates for chemoprophylaxis. The drug of choice—Amantadine

Rimantadine (5 mg/kg/day) BID for 5 days

In novel H1N1 influenza infection with a shifted genetic subtype, oseltamivir is found to be very effective.

Leprosy

Dapsone (1–4 mg/kg/week) per os (PO) for 3 years or till the index case becomes bacteriologically negative, for all the household child contacts with a leprosy patient.

Plague

Chemoprophylaxis with either tetracycline or sulfonamides is highly recommended for all the contacts and healthcare workers during an epidemic.

Systemic Infections

Urinary tract infection: Infections of urinary tract are common in childhood. Most often the patients have an underlying urinary tract anomaly, mostly vesicoureteral reflux (VUR). Early detection of urinary tract anomaly and treatment of urinary tract infection prevents from developing of chronic kidney diseases and its sequelae.

In spite of proper treatment, recurrence of urinary tract infection after the first episode is observed in 30–50% of children, commonly infants. *E. coli* being the most common organism isolated.

Risk factors for recurrent UTI
- Female gender
- Age below 6 months
- Obstructive uropathy

Table 2.12.2: Dosage of different antibiotics used as prophylaxis.

Drug	Dosage (mg/kg/day)	Comments
Cotrimoxazole	1–2 of trimethoprim	Avoid in infants <6 weeks, in G6PD deficiency
Nitrofurantoin	1–2	Contraindicated in G6PD deficiency, renal insufficiency
Nalidixic acid	15–20	Given in two divided doses
Cephalexin	10	Useful in neonate and infants
Cefadroxil	3–5	—
Cefaclor	5–10	1–2 divided doses
Cefixime	2	Sustained bactericidal effect
Ampicillin/Amoxicillin	10–20	In newborn and young infants where cotrimoxazole and nitrofurantoin are contraindicated

- Severe (Grade 3–5) VUR
- Repeated pyelonephritis
- Voiding dysfunction
- Constipation
- Repeated catheterization in neurogenic bladder.

Antibiotic prophylaxis is recommended in:
- Infants with UTI pending completion of evaluation
- Children with VUR
- Children with recurrent febrile UTI even if the urinary tract is normal
- Children with recurrent UTI (>3 episodes/year)
- Following surgical correction of VUR for 6 months
- Dosage of different antibiotics used as prophylaxis in Table 2.12.2.

Infective endocarditis

Infective endocarditis (IE) is a life-threatening infection of endocardium which is caused by a wide variety of organisms and requires a proper antimicrobial prophylaxis to prevent cardiac complications and any fatal eventualities (Table 2.12.3).

Table 2.12.3: Antibiotics with dosage used in prophylaxis for infective endocarditis before procedure.

Drugs	Dosage	Route	Timing with procedure	Comments
Amoxicillin	50 mg/kg, maximum 2 g	Oral	1 hour before procedure	Majority of patients
Ampicillin	50 mg/kg, maximum 2 g	IM/IV	½ hour before procedure	Patient unable to take oral ABx
Clindamycin or Cephalexin or Cefadroxil or Azithromycin or Clarithromycin	20 mg/kg, maximum 600 mg 50 mg/kg, maximum 2 g 15 mg/kg, maximum 500 mg	Oral	1 hour before procedure	Patient allergic to penicillin
Cefazolin or Clindamycin	25 mg/kg, maximum 1 g 20 mg/kg, maximum 600 mg	IV/IM IV	30 minutes before procedure	Allergic to penicillin and unable to take oral ABx

Bacterial agents in pediatric IE:
- Native valve or other cardiac lesions:
  - Viridans group streptococci (*S. mutans, S. sanguis, S. mitis*)
  - *Staphylococcus aureus*
  - Group D *Streptococcus* [*Enterococcus* (*S. bovis, S. faecalis*)]
- Prosthetic valve
  - *Staphylococcus epidermidis*
  - *Staphylococcus aureus*
  - *Viridans group Streptococcus*
  - *Pseudomonas aeruginosa*
  - *Serratia marcescens*
  - Diphtheroids
  - *Legionella* species
  - *Haemophilus, Actinobacillus, Cardiobacterium hominis, Eikenella corrodens, Kingella* (HACEK) group
  - *Fungi.*

Serious sequelae can result from IE if antimicrobial prophylaxis is not initiated on time. Heart failure, pericarditis, myocardial abscess, rupture of chordate, systemic thromboembolic episodes and systemic sepsis are some of those.

Antimicrobial prophylaxis before various procedures reduces the incidence of IE in susceptible patients. Ensuring dental and oral hygiene is most important measure in preventive IE. The IE prophylaxis is broadly divided in two groups (Table 2.12.4):

Cardiac conditions

High-risk categories:
- Prosthetic cardiac valves including bioprosthetic and homograft valves
- Previous bacterial endocarditis
- Complex cyanotic congenital heart disease [tetralogy of Fallot (TOF), transposition of great arteries]
- Surgically constructed systemic pulmonary shunts or conduits

Moderate-risk categories: Most other congenital cardiac malformations except isolated secundum atrial septal defect
- Acquired valvular dysfunctions (RHD)
- Hypertrophic cardiomyopathy
- Mitral valve prolapsed without valvular dysfunction.

Noncardiac conditions associated with procedures: Dental procedures known to induce gingival/mucosal bleeding including dental cleaning, filling cavities and dental replacement
- Tonsillectomy/Adenoidectomy
- Surgical operation involving intestinal/respiratory mucosal
- Rigid bronchoscopy
- Sclerotherapy for esophageal varices
- Esophageal dilation
- Gallbladder surgery
- Cystoscopy or urethral dilation
- Urethral catheterization or urinary tract surgery if UTI is present.

Rheumatic Heart Diseases

In a proven rheumatic fever poststreptococcal chances of relapses are very high for at least 5 years and may lead to RHD (Carditis and valvular lesions). It is strongly recommended by American Heart Association (AHA) to give a prophylaxis to prevent relapse in a normal healthy child with benzathine penicillin (0.6 million units for <30 kg and 1.2 million units for >30 kg) as IM injection for every 21 days ideally up to 21–25 years of age or at least for 5 years after the first episode.

Benzathine penicillin may be replaced by oral penicillin V 250 mg twice daily. In case of penicillin allergy erythromycin may be used in a dose of 250 mg twice daily. In case the patient is already having RHD, longer prophylaxis is needed lifelong to prevent IE, valvular vegetations and thromboembolic episodes.

Table 2.12.4: Antibiotics with dosage used as prophylaxis for infective endocardium in high and moderate risk patient before procedure.

Drugs	Regimens	Situations
Ampicillin + Gentamycin	Ampicillin—50 m/kg, maximum 2 g IV/IM; Gentamycin—1.5 mg/kg, 30 minutes before procedure, 6 hours later ampicillin 25 mg/kg IM/IV	High-risk patient
Vancomycin + Gentamycin	Vancomycin—20 mg/kg IV over 1–2 hours + Gentamycin—1.5 mg/kg, 30 minutes before procedure	High-risk patient allergic to penicillin
Amoxicillin/Ampicillin	Amoxicillin—50 mg/kg orally, 1 hour before procedure, or ampicillin—50 mg/kg IV/IM, 30 minutes before procedure	Moderate risk patient
Vancomycin	20 mg/kg IV over 1–2 hours 30 minutes prior to procedure	Moderate risk patient allergic to penicillin

Abbreviations: IM, intramuscular; IV, intravenous.

Surgical Prophylaxis

Many surgeons prefer an antimicrobial prophylaxis prior to surgeries, particularly abdominal, urogenital and thoracic. It can be categorized into the following categories:
- *Clean cases:* First or second generation injection cephalosporin single dose—2 hours prior to surgery.
- *Clean contaminated cases* like appendectomy, cholecystectomy, etc., where the abdomen is explored but not the bowels. The antibiotic should cover both gram-positive and gram-negative organisms like third-generation cephalosporins or co-amoxiclav. They should be started 2 hours prior to surgery and should be continued for at least 48 hours postsurgery.
- *Infected contaminated cases* like peritonitis, perforated aspirations or fear of aspirations, antibiotics should be started 2 hours prior to surgeries and should be continued for at least 5–7 days and aminoglycosides with IV metronidazole should be added to the third generation cephalosporin to take care of gram-negative bugs and anaerobes.
- *Prostheses or implants:* In clean cases, when prosthesis is implanted, antibiotic prophylaxis with a third generation cephalosporin is recommended for 7 days.

Human Immunodeficiency Virus

- Prophylaxis for prevention against opportunistic infections (OI) in HIV-infected child refers to an infection by a microorganism that normally does not cause disease, but becomes pathogenic when the body's immune system is impaired. HIV is one of the most common conditions when the cellular immunity of the body is compromised, not only cellular but humoral and innate immunity defect also increases the susceptibility to many infectious diseases.

Opportunistic infections can be acquired either vertical from mother, or horizontally from the environment, from food, water and animals that they interact. The risk of developing OI in HIV-infected child is inversely proportionate to CD-4 count, i.e. as the risk of an OI increases the CD-4 count declines. However, OI is not uncommon in child with normal CD-4 count as well.

Indications of P. carinii Pneumonia (PCP) Prophylaxis:
- All HIV-exposed newborns
- All HIV-exposed exclusive formula feeding (EFF) children
- All HIV-exposed breastfeeding children
- HIV-infected infants less than 12 months old
- For HIV-infected children 1–5 years with/without antiretroviral therapy (ART)
- HIV-infected children older than 6 years of age with or without ART
- Any HIV-infected child with high risk for bacterial infections, e.g. severe malnutrition, on oncological drugs or corticosteroids or at the risk of malaria
- HIV-infected child with previous PCP infection.

The drug of choice for prophylaxis is cotrimoxazole at the different doses (Table 2.12.5 and 2.12.6).

Fungal infections
- *Candidiasis: Candida albicans* is the most common fungal infections among HIV-infected children which can be local or systemic. Children with recurrent oropharyngeal or esophageal disease should be given daily prophylaxis with oral fluconazole (3–6 mg/kg/day).
- *Cryptococcal disease: Cryptococcus* is a fungus which is commonly found in the soil. HIV-infected children with fever and headache should be thought of having cryptococcal disease. Primary prophylaxis is not usually recommended. Lifelong secondary prophylaxis is recommended with fluconazole 3–6 mg/kg/day maximum 200 mg/day PO. Alternatively, itraconazole 2–5 mg/kg/day PO single dose, maximum 400 mg/day or amphotericin B 1 mg/kg weekly IV may be used.

Viral infections
- *Herpes simplex 1 and 2 infections:* Oral acyclovir 80 mg/kg/day in 3–4 divided doses are given for prophylaxis in HIV patients with frequent or severe relapses or if they have severe and slowly healing lesion.
- *Herpes zoster:* Daily acyclovir is recommended if patients have recurrent episodes of zoster.
- *Cytomegalovirus (CMV):* Lifelong prophylaxis with ganciclovir 5 mg/kg/day IV daily is initiated after an episode of end organ disease.

Table 2.12.5: Doses of cotrimoxazole as per age/weight.

Age or weight of child	Dose	Suspension (200 mg SMX/40 mg TMP/5 mL)	Single strength tablet (400 mg SMX/80 mg TMP)	Double strength tablet (800 mg SMX/160 mg TMP)
<6 months/<5 kg	100 mg SMX/20 mg TMP	2.5 mL	¼ tablet	—
6 months to 5 years/5–15 kg	200 mg SMX/40 mg TMP	5 mL	½ tablet	—
6–14 years/15–30 kg	400 mg SMX/80 mg TMP	10 mL	1 tablet	½ tablet
>14 years/30 kg	800 mg SMX/160 mg TMP	—	2 tablet	1 tablet

Abbreviations: SMX, sulfamethoxazole; TMP, trimethoprim.

Table 2.12.6: Other drugs for *P. carinii* pneumonia (PCP) prophylaxis.

Dapsone	2 mg/kg/day PO, maximum 100 mg daily or 4 mg/kg, maximum 200 mg weekly
Pentamidine	Inhaled 300 mg pentamidine isethionate inhaler every 28 days for more than 5 years

Perinatal HIV and TB

In the developing world that is affected by HIV, TB acts as one of the major infections in this immunocompromised individual. While pregnant HIV mother with TB holds a high-risk factor to its offsprings compared to a pregnant woman suffering from TB but not immunocompromised.

Prophylaxis for newborn exposed to TB:

- *Asymptomatic newborn:* INH (10 mg/kg/day) + Rifampin (10 mg/kg/day) are given for 3 months. BCG vaccination is withheld during this period and following 3 months child is screened for other coinfections like CMV, herpes simplex and Herpes Zoster and X-ray chest. If the child shows signs suggesting TB or cultures are positive, then full anti-TB therapy is given to child for 6 months.
- *Symptomatic newborn:* Treated as a standard TB regime.
- *Multidrug resistant TB:* Baby is given a high dose of INH (15 mg/kg/day), ethionamide and quinolone.

Prophylaxis for prevention of HIV transmission from HIV positive mother to child (Table 2.12.7):

- A management plan for the delivery should be documented between 34 and 36 weeks for all pregnant HIV positive women. ARV reduces the viral replications and thus reduces mother to child transmission of HIV by lowering the plasma viral load and also act as a postexposure prophylaxis in newborn.

Postexposure prophylaxis (PEP) following occupational exposure to HIV:

- Health personnel (employee, student, doctors and worker/volunteers) those in contact with patient or with blood or body fluids are on an average exposed to a risk of 0.3%.
  Significant exposure is defined as:
  - Needle stick or cut with a sharp instrument
  - Contact of mucus membrane or nonintact membrane

Table 2.12.7: Regimes for prevention of mother to child transmission of HIV.

Trial	Prophylaxis for mother	Breast-feeding	Prophylaxis for child
Thailand, 1998	Initiation of HAART from 36 weeks, oral ZDV 300 mg x 2 doses. Intrapartum oral ZDV 300 mg/3 hourly till baby delivers	No	ZDV 2 mg/kg BID for 4 weeks
NACO (India)	Antipartum—nil. Intrapartum—NVP 200 mg at onset of labor, postpartum—no medication	Yes	NVP 2 mg/kg to the baby within 72 hours after birth
BHIVA (United Kingdom)	Antipartum—ART started in first trimester, ZDV and 3TC. Intrapartum—continue ART + ZDV infusion 2 mg/kg/hour over 1 hour followed by 1 mg/kg/hour till delivery. Postpartum—discontinue ART and can be stopped	No	ZDV 2 mg/kg BID for 4 weeks
DHHS	Antipartum—HAART started after first trimester, ZDV and 3TC to be included. Intrapartum—continue ART + ZDV infusion 2 mg/kg/hour over 1 hour followed by 1 mg/kg/hour till delivery. Postpartum—discontinue ART and can be stopped	No	ZDV 2 mg/kg BID for 4 weeks

Abbreviations: HAART, highly active antiretroviral therapy; ZDV, zidovudine; NACO, National AIDS Control Organization; NVP, nevirapine; BHIVA, British HIV Association; 3TC, lamivudine; ART, antiretroviral therapy; DHHS, Department of Health and Human Services.

- Body fluids that is infectious like blood, semen, vaginal secretions, etc.

If the HIV status of the source is unknown then the sample must be sent and PEP is started and discontinued if results are negative (Tables 2.12.8 and 2.12.9).

Table 2.12.8: Drugs used in PEP.

Basic regimen	Zidovudine (AZT/ZDV) 300 mg twice daily + Lamivudine 150 mg twice daily for 4 weeks
Expanded regimen	Basic regimen (ZDV + 3TC) + Indinavir 800 mg thrice a day for 4 weeks. Instead of indinavir, abacavir, efavirenz and nelfinavir may be used

Table 2.12.9: Exposure and HIV status of source patient.

Exposure type	HIV status of source patient		
	HIV positive Class 1	HIV positive Class 2	HIV status unknown
Percutaneous injury			
Less severe	Basic PEP	Expanded PEP	No PEP
More severe	Expanded PEP	Expanded PEP	No PEP
Mucous membrane/nonintact skin exposure			
Small volume	Basic PEP	Basic PEP	No PEP
Large volume	Basic PEP	Expanded PEP	No PEP

Table 2.12.10: Drugs for *Mycobacterium avium* complex infections.

Drug	Dose and schedule
Clarithromycin	15 mg/kg/day, maximum 1 g PO in two divided doses
Azithromycin	10 mg/kg/day PO single dose max 500 mg/day or 20 mg/kg/week maximum 1.2 g. Weekly dose only for primary prophylaxis and not for secondary
Rifabutin	5–10 mg/kg/day PO single dose, maximum 300 mg
Ethambutol	15 mg/kg/day, maximum 900 mg

Less severe: Superficial injury and solid needle.

More severe: Large bore hollow needle, deep puncture, visible blood or needles used for patient's artery/vein.

Small volume: Few drops.

Large volume: Major splash.

Mycobacterium avium Complex Infections

Mycobacterium avium complex (MAC) consists of two species *M. avium* and *M. intracellulare*. These organisms are responsible for disseminated infections in immune compromised patients with low CD4 counts. The incidence of this infection is very less in India.

Primary prophylaxis with either azithromycin, clarithromycin or rifabutin is given to patients with low CD4 count before the development of disease (Table 2.12.10).

Secondary prophylaxis is indicated in patients who have suffered from MAC and it is given lifelong.

Toxoplasmosis

Children with severe immune suppression (CD4 count <15%) should be screened for immunoglobulin (Ig) G antibodies against toxoplasma and prophylaxis initiated in positive cases against *Toxoplasma gondii*. Children who receive TMX-SMX for PCP (on daily basis) are protected against this disease. Patient sensitive to cotrimoxazole should be given Dapsone—2 mg/kg maximum 25 mg PO daily with pyrimethamine 1 mg/kg PO daily + leucovorin 5 mg PO every 3 days.

Following an episode of CNS toxoplasmosis, lifelong suppressive therapy is given with sulfadiazine 100 mg/kg/day in 2–4 divided doses + pyrimethamine 1 mg/kg maximum 25 mg daily + leucovorin 5 mg PO every 3 days.

Prophylaxis for Nosocomial Infections

Nosocomial infections are significant challenges in pediatric intensive care units (PICUs) particularly when the child is on ventilator. Hand washing, judicious and minimal use of intraventions and proper asepsis during the procedures are the most important practices for the prevention of nosocomial infection. Usually the spectrum of pathogens is polymicrobes including at times, anaerobes and fungus. The other common pathogens are Gram-negative pathogens and ELBS producers like *E. coli, Enterobacteriaceae, Klebsiella, Acinetobacter, Pseudomonas*, etc.

Although there are no clear cut guidelines and there are insignificant evidences to support the use of prophylactic antimicrobial in intensive care settings, a BLBLI combinations, like piperacillin—tazobactam, ceftazidime, vancomycin, may be used to prevent nosocomial pneumonia following prolonged ventilation. Most of the nosocomial invasive infections in children occur due to central venous lines; mupirocin ointment may reduce bacterial colonization of catheters, but may increase colonization rates of fungi. Prophylaxis with fluconazole/ketoconazole in critically ill patients reduces invasive fungal infections.

Common Systemic Infections

Jaydeep Choudhury

3.1   CONGENITAL INFECTIONS

Naveen Jain

INTRODUCTION

Congenital infections contracted by the baby during pregnancy or peripartum period can have devastating effects like mortality and long-term disability. The mother may have no specific signs and the baby may be asymptomatic or the clinical signs at birth may not be specific. The available laboratory tests and management of the infections in mother and baby are not mostly evidence based. The timing of infection in pregnancy and immune state of the mother before infection (due to natural infection or immunization) determines the infant's outcome. Some infections have been known for a long time, some are newer health concerns—this chapter tries to cover each of the relevant infections (Box 3.1.1).

Cytomegalovirus (CMV) toxoplasmosis, rubella, herpes, syphilis, hepatitis-B and C, parvo-B, varicella, virus, H1N1, chikungunya, malaria, tuberculosis, *Enterovirus*, human immunodeficiency virus (HIV), prematurity and EONS (GBS): not covered.

TORCH SCREENING FOR ALL NEONATES IN INDIA

In a prospective study from Delhi, 1302 infants cord samples were screened for total immunoglobulin M (IgM), if greater than 20 mg/dL, specific IgM for CMV, rubella, toxoplasma were performed and babies followed for ophthalmic, hearing and developmental assessment. Raised IgM was found in 20%, specific IgM for rubella was positive in 8 (0.6%), of these three had symptomatic rubella, IgM CMV was positive in 23 (1.8%), only two had symptomatic disease. None were positive for toxoplasma. There was no difference in prematurity and low-birth-weight (LBW) rate in the babies with high and low IgM.

Box 3.1.1

General principles: Congenital infections may be prevented by following strategies.

- Vaccinate girls against rubella, varicella and all neonates against hepatitis-B at birth
- Syphilis is completely curable and maternal screening and treatment are crucial
- Fetal hydrops due to parvovirus has good outcome following intrauterine therapy 'mother to baby transmission' of HIV can be reduced significantly by mother and baby therapy
- HIV and tuberculosis can be coinfections and early diagnosis and treatment are associated with good outcome
- Hepatitis-B vaccination and hepatitis-B immunoglobulin are very effective in preventing carrier state in children
- Hand hygiene (especially in women in contact with saliva of children) and food hygiene (under cooked animal products/poorly washed vegetables) in pregnancy
- Fever, rash, arthralgia or contact with such illness may be only pointers to risk of congenital infections and ideally should be investigated
- Screening of all mothers may be a strategy if the congenital infection is very prevalent
- Antenatal scans suggesting central nervous system malformations may be due to congenital infections
- Immunoglobulin M (IgM) in mother is not a good single test as it remains positive for long duration and does not necessarily suggest primary infection in mother; in most cases paired sera of immunoglobulin G (IgG) done 2 weeks apart is more useful. Polymerase chain reaction is also emerging as a useful modality in diagnosing infection in fetus/newborn
- Congenital cytomegalovirus infection may be ameliorated by use of antiviral drugs
- Postnatal treatment of toxoplasma is likely to be beneficial although antenatal therapy to prevent infection of fetus is not proven
- In India, nonavailability of reliable laboratory tests readily has limited the understanding of prevalence and magnitude of various congenital infections.

TORCH SCREENING FOR ALL LOW-BIRTH-WEIGHT NEONATES

In a study retrospective published from Netherlands, 6 years data of 112 small for gestational age babies who had a Toxoplasmosis, Rubella, Cytomegalovirus, and Herpis (TORCH) work-up in mother/baby and/or urine CMV tested, none had any of the TORCH serology positive, two had urine CMV positive but did not confirm IgM CMV.

ROLE FOR TORCH SCREENING IN CATARACT

In a study from a referral eye hospital in India, 600 infants with cataract from 10 days to 12 months age were screened with TORCH serology. IgM was positive for CMV in 17.8%, rubella 8.4%, herpes simplex virus (HSV) 5.1%, toxoplasma 1.7% and none for *Treponema pallidum* hemagglutination assay [TPHA (syphilis)]. Any one IgM was positive in 20% babies.

HUMAN CYTOMEGALOVIRUS INFECTION

Cytomegalovirus is the most common perinatal viral infection in developed countries. It is the most common nongenetic cause of hearing impairment.

Epidemiology

Prevalence

Very high prevalence of infection, 0.15–2% of all births in developed world. As girls are unexposed they are at risk of primary infection when pregnant (lower chance in low-resource countries like India).

Infection in pregnant mother

The followings are the Infection in pregnant mother:
- Prevalent in developed world. In geographic areas with poor hygiene most children are infected and immune, and fewer girls are susceptible when pregnant. In higher socioeconomic settings, pregnant girls may have never been exposed previously and may still be susceptible
- "Saliva sharing"/sex partners, close contact—saliva, urine, semen, cervical secretions, breast milk, etc. It is not commonly spread by droplets. Infected children secrete virus for long, adults are noninfectious in months
- Mother could have a latent CMV infection that is reactivated and new CMV infections can occur in infected mothers (heterogeneous strains)
- Virus is easily disinfected by soap, detergent, disinfectant and heating.

Mother to child infection
- Fetus is infected in the first weeks of pregnancy (placental transfer from mothers with primary infection, rarely reactivation)—teratogenic—brain migration disorders result
- Infection after brain structure is complete (myelination stage)—inflammatory changes noted on MRI
- Infections later in gestation or spread through cervical secretions or breast milk has no neurological problems associated
- Postnatal CMV can occur in extreme preterm babies through milk, blood, transplant—produce sepsis like picture.

Clinical Presentation in Mother: When to Suspect and How to Diagnose

- Maternal infections are silent, rarely mononucleosis like syndrome (< 5%)
- Maternal IgM is indicative of recent or ongoing infection. Low avidity anti-CMV IgG helps to identify a primary infection in mother (high-risk of fetal transmission)
- Fetal infection can be identified by amniotic fluid (AF) assay for viral presence
- Placenta enlarged, fetal anomalies may suggest infection.

Clinical Presentation in the Newborn and Child

- Prenatal pointers may be oligohydramnios or polyhydramnios, periventricular calcification or hyperechoic bowel
- Around 90% of the babies are asymptomatic at birth—even asymptomatic babies are at risk of neuro-developmental problems as they grow up
- Symptomatic babies at birth—babies may be intrauterine growth restriction (IUGR) and have hepatosplenomegaly, petechiae, jaundice (conjugated hyperbilirubinemia and elevated transaminase) and neurological involvement—(microcephaly, seizures, lethargy, hypotonia), ocular and auditory involvement may or may not be there
- Microcephaly and CT changes predict poor outcome, and those with good head growth and normal CT are likely to be normal. CT changes in anterior part of temporal lobe point to CMV infection; other areas that can be involved are deep parietal areas, ventriculomegaly, calcification and migration disorders. Clinical disability in children can be CP, severe MR, deafness, blindness, epilepsy, learning disability and autism. MRI—polymicrogyria (migration problems), white matter involvement—ventriculomegaly, calcification, hippocampal dysplasia
- Cytomegalovirus is one of the most common causes of hearing impairment manifesting in late childhood and can occur in children who were asymptomatic neonates. Visual impairment, strabismus due to chorioretinitis, optic atrophy and cortical involvement may occur. These are less likely in children who were asymptomatic neonates. Severe forms may have hepatic dysfunction

and disseminated intravascular coagulation (DIC) as cause of death. Inguinal hernia and defective enamel of deciduous teeth are rare manifestation.

Diagnosis: Fetus and Newborn

Neuroimaging (Ultrasonography, Computed Tomography, Magnetic Resonance Imaging)

Calcification or other findings, like ventriculomegaly, white matter changes, may be visible only in 70% of infected babies. A few babies with calcification may have normal outcome. Calcification is present in 35–70%; it may be periventricular, in basal ganglia (BG) and in parenchyma. The BG calcifications are faint and punctuate—this helps to differentiate from other conditions causing BG calcification. Migrational abnormalities are seen in 10%—lissencephaly, pachygyria, polymicrogyria. Lissencephaly with calcification or diffuse nodular cortical surface (polymicrogyria) points to CMV and inherited conditions are less likely. White matter involvement is mostly focal involvement in parietal and occipital area with a rim in subcortical and periventricular area spared. Diffuse white matter disease or anterior temporal white matter disease and temporal cysts are seen more often with CMV infection. Cerebellar hypoplasias are other findings.

Serology

Congenital CMV can be diagnosed by CMV IgM from fetal blood or isolation of virus from AF (after 21 weeks, when kidneys mature and excrete virus). IgM may not be positive in all infected neonates (sensitivity 70%). Tests after 3 weeks may not differentiate congenital CMV from CMV acquired after birth.

Isolation of Virus

The gold standard used to diagnose within 3 weeks of birth are viral culture from urine or viral deoxyribonucleic acid by polymerase chain reaction (PCR) amplification in saliva (more feasible).

Polymerase chain reaction may be done in dried blood spot/urine/cerebrospinal fluid (CSF) or antigen in blood or IgM in baby's blood in first 3 weeks of life. Diagnosis can be made within 24 hours by shell vial assay, where the virus is identified by immunofluorescence against nucleotides of infected cells.

Management of Mother: Prevention and Treatment

High dose of CMV hyperimmune globulin of 200 mg/kg and monthly 100 IU/kg showed reduction in transmission.

Antiviral agents have teratogenic risk in animals, recent studies have shown no teratogenic effect in early trimester, but recommendations on use are not still published. Vaccines are under development.

Management of the Baby

Decision to Treat

The decision depends on the following:
- Severe focal organ disease (severe hepatitis, bone marrow suppression, colitis or pneumonitis) or
- Symptomatic central nervous system (CNS) disease [microcephaly, radiological abnormalities on MRI/ultrasound, abnormal CSF parameters or a positive CMV PCR in CSF, chorioretinitis or sensorineural hearing loss diagnosed by brain stem audiometry (BERA)].

Infants with congenital CMV and CNS involvement were treated with ganciclovir (GCV) with 6 mg/kg/dose IV 12 hourly for 6 weeks. The incidence of hearing impairment was decreased in treated babies, head circumference, development and growth at 1 year was slightly better in treated group. But, viral excretion returned after cessation of therapy.

Valganciclovir (VGCV) at 15 mg/kg twice for 6 weeks seems to be equally effective. Oral syrup should be used and crushed tablets are unreliable. If IV access is a problem and neonate is improving well, one may shift from GCV after 2–3 weeks to VGCV. Currently trials of 6–12 months treatment with VGCV have shown benefit. Longer therapy should be used with caution due to risk of toxicity.

Foscarnet has also shown to be effective and have lower toxicity.

Monitoring Safety

When neutrophil count is less than 0.5×10^9/L, then stop medication till count returns to 1×10^9/L and platelet stop medication less than 50×10^9/L. Monitor liver and renal function. If real function drops, the dose may have to be adjusted to once a day. Viral counts and drug levels are monitored weekly.

In animal studies, high doses of GCV inhibited sperm production and it was associated with carcinogenic potential.

Follow-up

Symptomatic CMV babies: Hearing by BERA 3–6 monthly till 3 years and yearly for 6 years.

Asymptomatic CMV babies: No follow-up examination is required.

Prognosis

Around 80–90% babies with congenital CMV are normal as children, one-third of symptomatic neonates are also normal. Head circumference and neuroimaging, if normal, predict good outcome (Box 3.1.2).

TORCH screening for all neonates in India.
- Human cytomegalovirus (HCHV) is common. Risk of congenital HCHV is more in developed world
- It accounts for most of nongenetic sensorineural hearing loss and many other central nervous system malformations
- Preventive strategies include hygiene advice to pregnant mothers exposed to saliva of children
- Maternal IgM and low avidity IgG HCHV suggest primary infection
- Treatment of neonates with ganciclovir, valganciclovir seems to reduce hearing loss.

TOXOPLASMOSIS

If mother gets primary toxoplasma infection in pregnancy, baby has risk of inflammatory damage to brain, with or without hydrocephalus (and calcification) and risk of recurrent chorioretinitis and visual impairment. Most infants are asymptomatic at birth, but 80% can have problems later. Some of the manifestations of congenital toxoplasmosis may manifest as late as 2nd to 3rd decade as seizures, mental retardation, learning and visual problems. Mothers can protect themselves by avoiding uncooked meat or vegetables and fruits not washed properly. Domestic cats, especially kitten, excrete oocysts.

Etiopathogenesis

The toxoplasma is a parasite that is present in cats or kittens intestines and is excreted to soil, consumed by intermediate hosts and reaches their muscle (meat) pork or other. Uncooked meat, or vegetables or fruits contaminated and improperly washed or soiled hands carry infections to humans.

Epidemiology

Prevalence

Most Indian mothers (45% in one study) are seropositive (protected) in contrast to only 15–25% in the USA.

Route of Maternal Infection

Feco-oral route—eating under cooked raw meat or unwashed vegetables and fruits or unpasteurized goats milk, contact soil contaminated with cat litter (less common than ingestion).

Infection of the Fetus

Transplacental transfer—chance of transfer of primary infection in pregnancy is higher in 2nd and 3rd trimester, although the effect on fetus is more severe in 1st trimester. Reactivation of previously infected mother (e.g. immunocompromised HIV) is less likely a cause for fetal infection.

Clinical Presentation in Mother

Most mothers may be asymptomatic or have nonspecific flu-like symptoms with lymphadenopathy. Sometimes mothers are screened for TORCH serology. If toxoplasma IgM is positive, repeat the test on a different kit, or do serial IgG, IgA or IgG avidity.

Screening of Mothers

In some countries like France, all women are screened preconception and monthly through pregnancy to suspect a new onset infection.

The USA recommends screening only of high-risk women whose antenatal ultrasound shows hydrocephalus, calcification, microcephaly, hepatosplenomegaly, ascites and fetal growth restriction. Women with HIV also should be screened.

It appears in a country like India with high seroprevalence in mothers before pregnancy, universal screening may have very low yield in preventing congenital toxoplasmosis.

Clinical Presentation in the Newborn and in Children

Most neonates (up to 90%) are asymptomatic at birth and develop mental retardation, learning and visual problems later. Preterm infants may develop symptoms in first 3 months of life.

Eye—heavily pigmented chorioretinal scar (mistaken for coloboma), punched out lesion due to full thickness necrosis, multiple chorioretinal lesions especially in macular area (in absence of serologic evidence in mother or baby, one must be careful in making a diagnosis based on eye findings).

A recently published population study enrolling prospectively all mothers from France over a period of 16 years, 127 babies were enrolled. Around 19% of babies had ocular involvement, only 6% had visual impairment of one or both eyes. Eye lesions at birth had higher risk of macular involvement and those that appeared later involved more the periphery. A new eye lesion could appear for the first time as late as 12 years (in spite of treatment). Around 9% children developed CNS lesions in form of calcification, white matter changes on MRI, microabscess, ventricular dilatation and language delay.

The profile of illness seems to be more severe in the USA than Europe. In a study recently published from the USA where consecutive confirmed cases from laboratories over 15 years were described. Clinical profile of 164 confirmed cases of congenital toxoplasmosis showed clinical signs in 85% in eye, brain, one-third had hepatosplenomegaly, thrombocytopenia, fewer had jaundice and skin rash.

Diagnosis in Mother

Immunoglobulin M may remain positive for long time after acute infection, and therefore does not indicate

FLOWCHART 3.1.1: Test serum for presence of toxoplasma-specific IgG antibodies.

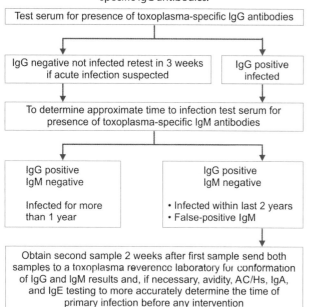

Neonate

Demonstration of clinical picture consistent with toxoplasmosis and/or serology when mother is proven to have primary infection is as following:

Immunoglobulin M is valuable in neonatal toxoplasma identification, but has limitations (false positive and negative). IgA and IgE drop faster than IgM and may suggest recent infection. Serial rise in IgG titer is a better indicator.

Microscopy or PCR demonstration of toxoplasma or inoculation into mice may be the other option.

In the USA the diagnostic criteria is IgG positive by Sabin-Feldman dye test (DT) and one of the following:

- Presence of IgM or IgA toxoplasma antibodies after 10 days of life (placental leak in first 10 days possible)
- Persistence of IgG antibodies on DT by 12 months age
- Presence of IgM antibodies in CSF
- Polymerase chain reaction or isolation from AF, CSF blood or PCR from urine.

Fundus of eye examination, CT brain, blood counts and liver function tests should be done.

recent infection. IgG avidity test also lacks the specificity to make a definitive diagnosis of recent infection (Flowchart 3.1.1).

Guide to general interpretation of *Toxoplasma gondii* serology results obtained with commercial assays has been given in Table 3.1.1.

Diagnosis

Fetus

Polymerase chain reaction from AF is safer in fetus than cord sampling, but false results are possible.

Management of Mother and the Fetus

Most studies (meta-analysis) found no benefit in maternal screening and treatment with spiramycin or combination of drugs. The hypothesis is that the infection to fetus happens very early after infection (< 3 weeks) and hence, periodic screening for serology in mothers may not be a useful strategy. Preventive treatment within 3 weeks of serological diagnosis in mother reduces risk of transmission. If mother have primary toxoplasmosis spiramycin 9 million SI units per day till delivery should be given.

If AF-PCR is positive, i.e. fetal infection, spiramycin is stopped and sulfadoxine and pyrimethamine started.

Table 3.1.1: Guide to general interpretation of *Toxoplasma gondii* serology results obtained with commercial assays.

Result		Report/Interpretation for humans (except infants)
Negative	Negative	No serological evidence of infection with toxoplasma
Negative	Equivocal	Possible early acute infection or false-positive IgM reaction. Obtain a new specimen for IgG and IgM testing. If results for the second specimen remain the same, the patient is probably not infected with toxoplasma
Negative	Positive	Possible acute infection or false-positive IgM result. Obtain a new specimen for IgG and IgM testing. If results for the second specimen remain the same, the IgM reaction is probably a false positive
Equivocal	Negative	Indeterminate—obtain a new specimen for testing or retest this specimen for IgG in a different assay
Equivocal	Equivocal	Indeterminate—obtain a new specimen for both IgG and IgM testing
Equivocal	Positive	Possible acute infection with Toxoplasma. Obtain a new specimen for IgG and IgM testing. If results for the second specimen remain the same for if the IgG becomes positive, both specimens should be sent to a reference laboratory with experience in the diagnosis of toxoplasmosis for further testing
Positive	Negative	Infected with Toxoplasma for > 1 year
Positive	Equivocal	Infected with Toxoplasma for probably > 1 year, or false-positive IgM reaction. Obtain a new specimen for IgM testing. If results with the second specimen remain the same, both specimens should be sent to a reference laboratory with experience in the diagnosis of toxoplasmosis for further testing
Positive	Positive	Possible recent infection within the last 12 months, or false-positive IgM reaction. Send the specimen to a reference laboratory with experience in the diagnosis of toxoplasmosis for further testing

After 30 weeks of pregnancy (European guidelines) or 18 weeks (American guidelines) pyrimethamine 1 gm and sulfadoxine 50 mg every 10 days along with folinic acid 50 mg should be given. Cotrimoxazole and folinic acid with spiramycin have also been tried in pregnancy.

Fetus

If mother's infection has been diagnosed before 16 weeks or if the fetus has hydrocephalus, termination of pregnancy may be advised.

Treatment of Confirmed Congenital Toxoplasmosis in Neonate

Side effects of treatment such as neutropenia, anemia and vomiting were described in only 5 of the 120 treated children in a recent series in France.

Alternate therapy of four cycles of 21 days pyrimethamine-sulfadoxine and folinic acid each with 30 days interruption with spiramycin have been tried in children with serious side effects (Box 3.1.3).

Prognosis

In France, prognosis of babies treated for 1 year after birth, born to periodically screened and treated mothers was not bad with only 6% having visual impairment and 9% CNS involvement. Although antenatal treatment did not alter the course hugely, the postnatal treatment seems to reduce problems. The study has cautioned reader against using this information outside Europe to predict outcomes. American studies have published poorer outcomes (Box 3.1.4).

RUBELLA

Infection in the first 12 weeks of pregnancy results in 80% babies with devastating congenital anomalies. As many as 100,000 cases of congenital rubella syndrome are reported every year worldwide. Rubella has been almost eliminated from countries with effective vaccination. About 57,000 cases of congenital rubella were reported per year before 1969 (before vaccination) from the USA, and currently with 90% vaccine coverage, the number is less than 10 per year.

World Health Organization (WHO) has set targets for rubella eradication. As of 2009, 130 countries had introduced rubella containing vaccines in their national program. Women of childbearing age group especially healthcare workers must be protected against rubella by vaccination.

Epidemiology

Infection of the Mother

Only human beings harbor the virus. Infection is spread by droplet. It is not very infectious and close contact is required for transmission. Detergents and heat easily destroy the virus.

Infection of the Fetus

Transplacental transfer, less dangerous if mother has primary infection after 17–18 weeks.

Clinical Presentation in Mother

Most mothers with rubella infections are subclinical:
- Rash—maculopapular, not confluent, start on face and spreads to limbs and trunk
- Arthralgia
- Lymphadenopathy—occipital, cervical, submandibular
- Fever, pharyngitis
- The virus is excreted from 7 days before rash to 7–10 days after rash.

Without laboratory tests it is not possible to differentiate from parvovirus and chikungunya that also presenting with fever, rash and arthralgia.

Box 3.1.3

Treatment of confirmed congenital toxoplasmosis in neonate.
- Pyrimethamine 1.25 mg/kg and sulfadoxine 25 mg/kg and folinic acid 50 mg/kg every week for 12 months. But the optimum duration of treatment is not determined. Three months is being evaluated against 1-year and 2-year treatment did not seem to reduce risk
- Fortnightly monitoring of complete blood counts and liver function tests should be done
- Add prednisolone 1 g/kg if cerebrospinal protein is high > 1 g and if vision is threatened.

Box 3.1.4

Key points for practice: Congenital toxoplasmosis.
- Congenital toxoplasmosis may occur in babies born to mothers with no/nonspecific symptoms and babies also may be asymptomatic at birth and manifest as eye and central nervous system lesions later, as late as adulthood. Neonatal toxoplasmosis may be indistinguishable from other congenital infections: hepatosplenomegaly, jaundice, thrombocytopenia, LBW, etc. Cerebral calcification, hydrocephalus and chorioretinitis occur more often
- Although universal screening appears the only strategy to suspect and treat timely, cost effectiveness and debated benefits of prenatal treatment have not allowed implementation except in few European countries (may not be cost-effective in India)
- Education of pregnant women seems to be the only strategy feasible for prevention
- Diagnosis can be confirmed by demonstration by mice inoculation, direct smear or polymerase chain reaction or serology (persistent IgG at 12 months)
- Maternal and neonatal diagnosis based on serology has many false positives, and treatment for 1 year with drugs that are potentially harmful must be initiated after confirmation of diagnosis
- Benefit of spiramycin antenatal is debated, most agree on treatment with sulfadoxine and pyrimethamine after birth for 12 months.

Management of a Mother Exposed to or Having Clinical Signs of Rubella-like Illness

The gestation (accurate pregnancy dating) and immune status of the mother are crucial for counseling. Even vaccinated or previously infected women should be evaluated (although risk is low). Brief exposures have low-risk (prolonged close contact like at home or workplace), but, if exposure is suspected, the pregnant woman must be investigated.

Rubella IgM and IgG should be tested immediately and IgG repeated 2–3 weeks later (paired sera).

Gestation less than 16 weeks:

- Positive IgG in less than 12 days of exposure indicates that the pregnant woman is protected, if seronegative, weekly testing for a month is required
- In mothers with symptoms of rubella and positive IgM, repeat test within 5–10 days and demonstrate rise of IgG. Positive IgM only and exposure to rash alone should not form basis for termination of pregnancy
- If more than 4 weeks elapsed after exposure, serology is not useful.

Gestation 16–20 weeks: Risk low, deafness possible.

If mother is greater than 20 weeks of pregnant—No risk to fetus.

Clinical Presentation in the Newborn and Children

Severe congenital malformations are less likely after 12 weeks of gestational age and not described after 18 weeks. Abortions can occur.

Low-birth-weight babies with purpuric rash, cataract, heart disease [pulmonary artery hypoplasia and patent ductus arteriosus (PDA)] and sensorineural deafness is the classical congenital rubella. They may also have lymphadenopathy, meningoencephalitis, thrombocytopenia, hepatitis and lytic lesions (radiolucent) in bone.

Few may not manifest at birth, but have neurological symptoms later. Some of the manifestations may present as late as 2 years.

Deafness may sometimes be the only finding, especially if infection occurred after 12 weeks.

WHO case definition for congenital rubella syndrome.

Confirmed Congenital Rubella Syndrome Case

Clinical

Two complications from section A or one from section A and one from section B:

- Cataracts, congenital glaucoma, congenital heart disease, hearing impairment, pigmentary retinopathy

- Purpura, microcephaly, splenomegaly, mental retardation, meningoencephalitis, radiolucent bone disease, jaundice with onset within 24 hours after birth and laboratory confirmation.

Diagnosis: Fetus and Newborn

- Polymerase chain reaction from AF (preferred) or IgM cord blood, taken 7–8 weeks after presumed infection (after 21 weeks of gestational age, excreted in urine of fetus)
- IgM capture enzyme immunoassay on serum or oral fluid is very useful diagnostic test in newborn. A negative test in first 3 months excludes possibility of congenital rubella. Beyond 3 months sensitivity decreases. If rubella vaccination has been taken, serology cannot be used to diagnose
- *Examine affected organs:* Complete blood count (CBC) for anemia and thrombocytopenia, liver function test (LFT), renal function test, electrolytes, lumbar puncture, cranial, renal ultrasound, ECHO chest and long bone X-rays, eye and hearing exam periodically for first few years. Screen for endocrine problems like diabetes and hypothyroidism.

Management of Mother: Prevention and Treatment

Rubella Vaccination

Two doses of measles-mumps-rubella vaccine at an interval of 4–8 weeks for all children above 15 months of age. Catch up vaccine may be given at any age.

Vaccinations must be avoided in pregnancy, within 3 months of blood transfusion or immunoglobulin, within 3 weeks of another live vaccine.

Accidental vaccination of pregnant women or pregnancy within 3 months of vaccine has not been associated with anomalies and termination of pregnancy must not be advised, HIV with mild-moderate immunosuppression may be vaccinated.

Management of the Fetus and Neonate

Neonates with congenital rubella excrete high concentrations of virus and hence isolation from other babies is necessary. Children with rubella have problems pertaining to eye, hearing, heart, etc. and will need multidisciplinary team effort. Long-term follow-up is required as some can show evidence of progressive disease even in 2nd decade.

Prognosis

Congenital heart defects are correctible surgically. But, CNS effects may be permanent and progressive (Box 3.1.5).

HERPES

If a neonate presents with seizure or encephalopathy or sepsis like syndrome at 1–3 weeks of gestation (sometimes up to 6 weeks), a possibility of HSV encephalitis must be considered and treated.

Epidemiology

Babies are infected mostly if mother gets primary genital herpes ulcers at the time of labor and delivery. Intrauterine and postpartum infection are rare, also mothers who are already immune seldom infect the baby. Infection occurs when baby passes through birth canal or through ruptured membranes. Most mothers of babies with HSV infection cannot recall genital ulcers.

Clinical Manifestations in Neonate

Usually presents within 1–3 weeks of birth, but should be considered up to 46 weeks.

Localized lesions like zoster present on skin, eye and mouth.

If localized herpes is left untreated, 70% cases can progress to disseminated disease that mimics sepsis. Some of the babies (40%) develop disseminated disease without skin lesions. Mortality with disseminated disease is high in spite of treatment—hemorrhagic pneumonitis, meningoencephalitis, hepatic failure and DIC are poor prognostic markers.

Central nervous system herpes—lethargy, irritability, poor feeding, bulging fontanel, apnea and seizures; seizures indicate poor prognosis.

Rare cases (2%) of intrauterine infections can present with active or scarred skin lesion, microcephaly, microphthalmia, retinal dysplasia and hydranencephaly.

Management

Prevention of Mother to Baby Infection

Cesarean section before rupture of membranes (within 6 hours) if mother has genital ulcers or prodrome nearing term. Avoid forceps or vacuum extraction. Antiviral suppression in mothers decreases risk (400 mg tds per oral), in mothers with genital ulcers, but identifying suitable mothers with active infection is difficult.

Management of Neonate

Mothers may not show signs of genital ulcer, babies with disseminated or CNS herpes are indistinguishable from other ill babies. High index of suspicion is required in a neonate who is sick in 1–3 weeks of life. Blood PCR, CSF-PCR are useful, but, negative test does not rule out infection. Electroencephalogram and MRI are useful adjuncts. Liver function and coagulation profile must be studied. Viral cultures from surface swabs after 48 hours of life—eye, mouth, nasopharynx, etc.

Skin, eye and mouth diseases: IV acyclovir 20 mg/kg/dose 8 hourly (infuse over 1–2 hours) for 14 days. For disseminated disease, 21 days treatment and for CNS infection, 21 days till CSF PCR becomes negative. Recurrences in skin, eye and CNS can occur. Trials of suppressive therapy with acyclovir have been tried, but, high-risk of neutropenia (in 50%) does not allow routine recommendation.

Topical ophthalmic drugs are useful. Monitor twice weekly for neutropenia while on therapy.

Prognosis

Central nervous system involvement results in poor outcome in most despite treatment (Box 3.1.6).

VARICELLA

The risk of disseminated varicella infection is the highest if mother is infected just before or after delivery and can be prevented with passive antibody and antiviral therapy. The risk of congenital varicella syndrome is less than 1% if mother gets infected in first or second trimester. In third trimester, there is no risk of congenital varicella; a few infants can develop zoster in the first 2 years of life. Maternal zoster is of no risk to child.

Epidemiology

Varicella is highly infectious—90% of family members may be infected. Infectious period is highest in the 24–48 hour period before the onset of rash to crusting or rashes (5–7 days after first rash); both respiratory droplets and rashes are infectious. The virus can remain latent in sensory nerve ganglia after primary infection.

Clinical Presentation

Varicella is characterized by a pruritic vesicular rash that appears on scalp, face and trunk. Mostly varicella has a short uncomplicated course in pregnancy and neonates. Rarely, the illness continues as a disseminated infection and involves the lungs, liver and CNS.

Congenital varicella syndrome is rare incidence of CVS 0.5% in first trimester and 1.5% in second, 0% in 3rd trimester. Congenital varicella syndrome is characterized by CNS involvement (62%)—cortical atrophy, seizures, mental retardation; eye involvement (52%)—chorioretinitis, cataract, microphthalmia; skeletal problems (44%)—limb hypoplasia and scarred skin in dermatomal pattern (72%). Prognosis is poor with severe swallowing problems (bulbar palsy), gastroesophageal reflux and aspiration pneumonia and respiratory failure with death in infancy.

Complications of perinatal varicella are pneumonia, bacterial infections of skin: necrotizing fasciitis and toxic shock syndrome.

If mothers develop varicella infection in third trimester, 1% infants can develop zoster in the first 2 years of life.

Diagnosis

Clinical—vesicular pruritic rash and often history of affected family member.

Serology is not useful and viral culture is also not sensitive. Direct antigen fluorescent staining of scrapings from the rash is rapid and accurate test. Fetal IgM and AF PCR cannot diagnose whether the fetus is infected.

Treatment

Mother with Varicella

- Both acyclovir and valacyclovir (prodrug, better drug levels when given orally) are category B drugs in pregnancy and are advised only in late pregnancy when risk to mother is higher and baby lower. In mothers with severe varicella, like pneumonia, benefit to mother allows use of acyclovir (no teratogenic effect described)
- Congenital varicella—no definite guideline on need for treatment with acyclovir
- Herpes zoster in baby is self-limiting mostly, but acyclovir may be used, if recurrent or severe pain.

Prevention

Varicella zoster immune globulin (VZIG) can be given to pregnant-susceptible mothers exposed to infection. Post-exposure vaccine and acyclovir are not safe in pregnancy.

Varicella zoster immune globulin or intravenous immunoglobulin (IVIG) should be given to neonate

Box 3.1.7

Key points for practice: Varicella.
- Perinatal varicella infection of neonate (manifests in first 10 days) that occurs if the mother is infected from 5 days before to 2 days after delivery, if not appropriately managed, case fatality in past has been described to be as high as 30%
- Congenital varicella syndrome is rare, only 1% of fetuses of infected mothers develop congenital varicella syndrome. No anomalies are described if the mother is infected after 20 weeks.

exposed to mother with rash 5 days before or 2 days after delivery, also to preterm neonates, 28 weeks of gestation. The infants may be asymptomatic at birth and develop disseminated disease after a few days and require close monitoring. The use of IVIG has shown to decrease severe neonatal illness. The neonate must be isolated (respiratory and contact till 21 days age and for 28 days if they have received VZIG). Acyclovir may be started if baby is symptomatic and continues till 48 hours after last rash (usually 7 days).

Milder form of disease occurs in neonate delivered a week after maternal infection. Symptomatic neonate must be treated with acyclovir.

Maternal zoster does not risk fetus or infant.

Universal varicella immunization is an effective strategy to decrease disease incidence across all ages. Vaccinated children were benefited most, but 75% decrease in adults was recorded although only 3% adults were immunized, possibly due to herd effect (Box 3.1.7).

CONGENITAL SYPHILIS

Syphilis responds well to penicillin and should have been eradicated. Yet, WHO estimates 1 million pregnancies are affected worldwide, 40% fetuses die and 50% survive with physical or mental disability.

Epidemiology—syphilis occurs mainly in under-privileged population, exposure to sexually transmitted infections, teenage pregnancy, sexual promiscuity, drug abuse, etc.

Clinical Manifestation in Mother

Mother develops a painless genital ulcer (chancre) in primary syphilis on labia, vagina or cervix and may be missed. Around 4–10 weeks later cutaneous and mucosal lesions develop with systemic signs of fever, poor appetite, weight loss, arthralgia in secondary phase, and then progresses to latent phase. Mother is capable of transmission of infection to fetus in all stages. Mothers have a 70% chance of transmitting infection to fetus for about 4 year's infection. About 40% pregnancy wastage occurs.

Clinical Manifestation in Neonate

Important cause of still birth (40%) of all infected fetuses. They may have nonimmune hydrops.

Asymptomatic at Birth

About 75% of live born are asymptomatic at birth.

Early Congenital Syphilis

Before 2 years age, symptoms may appear between 3 and 14 weeks—snuffles, IUGR, hepatosplenomegaly, jaundice, pseudoparalysis (pain), edema (nephritic syndrome). Hepatomegaly is a constant feature. The nasal secretions are highly infectious. Skin lesions—pink oval, brown discoloration—desquamate. Vesiculobullous lesions of palms and soles.

Coombs negative hemolytic anemia, thrombocytopenia, nephritic syndrome can occur by 2–3 months age. CNS involvement (seizures, hydrocephalus). Bone involvement by 8 months long bones, ribs, (Wimberger's sign—bilateral destruction of medial tibial metaphysis).

Late Congenital Syphilis

Noninfectious scars from primary phase are: Hutchison teeth, mulberry molars, saddle nose, interstitial keratitis, corneal clouding, chorioretinitis, glaucoma defect in hard palate and rhagades, nerve deafness, intellectual disability, epilepsy and optic atrophy.

Diagnosis in Mother

Serological testing is mainstay of screening for syphilis in mothers—venereal disease research laboratory (VDRL) and rapid plasma reagin (RPR). False positive can occur following viral infections like hepatitis and measles. Placenta: triad of enlarged hypercellular villi, necrotizing funisitis, acute or chronic villitis. Confirmed diagnosis: demonstration of treponema on dark-field microscopy. RPR or VDRL must be confirmed with treponemal: TPHA, fluorescent treponemal antibody absorption (FTA-ABS).

Serodiagnosis of infant born to mother is not useful due to passive transfer of antibodies. If the baby's antibodies are fourfold more than mothers, then the diagnosis of neonatal infection can be made.

If mother has a nontreponemal titer rising fourfold, positive treponemal test without treatment with penicillin or treated less than a month before delivery, or baby has signs of congenital syphilis, the baby should be investigated. Quantitative VDRL, CBC, long-bone X-rays, CSF examination should be done. If infection in neonate is suspected strongly—fundus exam, BERA, neuroimaging, LFT should be performed.

HIV coinfection must be excluded.

Treatment

If maternal treatment is incomplete, neonate must be treated.

One time IM 50,000 U/kg of Benzathine penicillin, or 10 days IV or IM penicillin G.

Box 3.1.8

Key points for practice: Congenital syphilis.
- Universal screening of all pregnancies with syphilis serology at early perinatal period and repeat if necessary
- Treatment with penicillin completely cures
- Still remains a major cause of congenital infections

Prevention

Early detection of maternal infection and complete treatment should be performed at least 30 days before delivery. Testing serology at initial perinatal visit. In high-risk areas/sexual history: repeat testing at 28 weeks and at delivery (Box 3.1.8).

HEPATITIS-B

Prevalence rate of HBsAg positivity in pregnant women is just under 1% in India. If maternal viral load is high, the risk of transmission to fetus is high, 80–90% and risk of chronic infection in baby is high, and 25% of them develop malignancy. Transplacental transmission is rare; most are infected during blood exposure at delivery (Box 3.1.9).

Box 3.1.9

Recommendations.
- All pregnant women should be screened for hepatitis-B virus (HBV) infection.
- Pregnant women found to be HBsAg positive should be investigated:
  - To rule out chronic liver disease and cirrhosis which might require special care during pregnancy and delivery
  - To determine how much is the risk of mother-to-child transmission (MTCT) so that if required measures can be taken to reduce the risk
- Maternal high HBV DNA and HBeAg positivity are important risk factors for MTCT. Women having these risk factors may be considered for one or more of the following measures to reduce the risk of MTCT:
  - Use of antiviral therapy (lamivudine, telbivudine or tenofovir) in 3rd trimester
  - Use of three doses of HBIG in pregnancy (200 IU at 28, 32 and 36 weeks)
  - Use of elective cesarean section before the onset of labor
- All babies should receive both HBIG and HBV vaccine within 12 hours of birth. This initial vaccine administration should be followed by at least two more injections of HBV vaccine within the first 6 months of life.
- After completion of the vaccine series, testing for HBsAg and anti-HBs should be performed by 9 months of age. HBsAg-negative infants with anti-HBs levels greater than 10 mIU/mL are considered protected and no further medical managment is required. Those with anti-HBs levels less than 10 mIU/mL are not protected and should be revaccinated with a second three-dose series followed by retesting 1–2 months after the final dose. Those with HBsAg-positive status should be referred to specialized centers.
- Breastfeeding of infants is recommended, however, mother should stop antiviral therapy to limit the exposure of infants to these drugs.

TUBERCULOSIS

Tuberculosis (TB) in pregnant women is not uncommon, but, congenital tuberculosis is rare.

Etiopathogenesis

Congenital infection occurs through two ways:
1. Hematogenous through umbilical vein—primary lesion is in the lung/liver
2. Ingestion or aspiration of infected AF—leading to pulmonary or gastrointestinal tuberculosis.

Clinical Features in Mother

Many times, the mother is asymptomatic and her infection is diagnosed because the baby is diagnosed to have tuberculosis. Mother with miliary, meningeal TB, pulmonary with sputum positive and poor compliance to therapy is more likely to transmit to baby.

Clinical Features in Baby

Babies usually become symptomatic in 1–3 weeks, but need to be monitored at least for a year. Initial presentation of neonate may be nonspecific with LBW, lethargy, poor feeding and poor-weight gain, unresolving pneumonia. Later (2–3 weeks after), baby may develop hepatosplenomegaly, jaundice, skin lesions, ear discharge, paravertebral abscess (pulmonary, military or meningeal TB). CNS involvement is less common. The baby can present with only hepatic dysfunction with no respiratory symptoms.

Definition of Congenital Tuberculosis

Proven tuberculous lesion in an infant plus any one of the following:
- Lesion occurring in the 1st week after birth
- Primary hepatic complex or caseating granuloma
- Maternal genital tract or placenta tuberculosis
- Exclusion of postnatal tuberculosis through contact screening.

Investigation of Neonate

A baby should be investigated if:
- Mother has infection
- Baby has unresponsive pneumonia
- Fever and hepatosplenomegaly
- Cerebrospinal fluid with lymphocytes elevated and no bacterial growth
- Coexisting HIV
- Chest X-ray show infiltrates in more than 50%, but are nonspecific.

Tuberculin skin tests (Mantoux) are mostly negative in congenital tuberculosis.

Gastric aspirate acid-fast bacilli (AFB)—first morning sample before feeding the infant for three consecutive days has good sensitivity and positive predictive value, sputum from ventilated baby (placed in 1% soda-bicarb for transport), CSF culture and blood culture in special bottles. Skin and ear discharge may be cultured. Repeated testing from different sites may be required for AFB and culture (12 weeks). Polymerase chain reaction in bronchoalveolar lavage may be useful. Liver, lymph node and lung biopsy may be required.

Prognosis

Risk higher if mother infected in third trimester, advanced disease or noncompliance to therapy.

Treatment

Outcome of mother and baby depends on timely therapy. Treatment of pregnant and nonpregnant person for tuberculosis is the same. Coexisting HIV has to be treated. The TB treatment should start 2 weeks prior to antiretroviral (ARV) therapy. Caution is required to monitor for drug interactions. Pyridoxine should be given to all pregnant women receiving isonicotinylhydrazine (INH).

Risk of fetus getting infection depends on maternal compliance, start of therapy at least 3 months prior to delivery. Smear positive for AFB, multidrug resistant TB increases risk of transmission to baby.

Asymptomatic Baby

Mother not having multidrug resistance TB: Start on prophylaxis INH 10 mg/kg/day for 6 months. Screen for clinical and radiological signs every 2 months. In this period, if baby has signs of TB or laboratory positive, full treatment for 6 months must be started.

Symptomatic Baby

Congenital tuberculosis is indistinguishable from other congenital infections—hepatosplenomegaly, jaundice, lymph nodes and investigations will be required for other coinfections. Accepted treatment includes INH (10 mg/kg/day), rifampicin (10 mg/kg/day), pyrazinamide (20 mg/kg/day) and either streptomycin or ethambutol (15–25 mg/kg/day) for 2 months followed by INH and rifampicin of 4–10 months.

Steroids should be used in CNS, pericardial and pleural lesions.

Therapeutic Response

Resolution of clinical signs, improvement in appetite, weight gain and radiological resolution.

Key points for practice: Tuberculosis.
- Tuberculosis in pregnant women is not uncommon, but congenital tuberculosis is rare
- Indian studies have shown increase in perinatal mortality and low-birth weight due to maternal TB
- HIV infections can coexist and complicate the management.

Coexisting HIV

Coexisting HIV should be treated. Hepatotoxicity should be watched for. In resource limited settings breastfeeding should continue (Box 3.1.10).

CONGENITAL PARVOVIRUS INFECTION

Parvovirus invades P antigen of RBC and can cause anemia and hydrops fetalis.

Epidemiology

Parvovirus causes erythema infectiosum, an infection in children characterized by fever and rash predominantly on face. The infection is spread only from humans—respiratory droplet or hand to mouth. The mothers exposed to infectious children at home is at highest risk followed by daycare teachers and other teachers. Parvovirus infections can occur as epidemics.

Clinical Presentation in Mother

Most mothers will be asymptomatic:
- *Arthropathy*: Around 80% of adults with the infection develop symmetric arthoral of hands, wrist, knee and ankles that lasts for weeks to months. Parvovirus infection cannot be differentiated without investigation from rubella, chikungunya
- *Anemia*: Bone marrow involvement causes hemolysis and transient aplasia: 7–10 days. Previously anemic, or with hemoglobinopathies are at higher risk. Immune deficient can have chronic aplasia. Such patients may only present with fever followed by anemia and no rash
- *Thrombocytopenia*: Parvovirus mostly affects red cell lines, but, rarely platelet and leukocyte counts may also drop
- *Rash*: Children develop fever, flu like symptoms and rash on face (slapped cheek) and a week later rash on body and trunk. Appearance of rash coincides with IgM antibody rise, indicating that the rash may be immune mediated. Adults are less likely to present with rash.
- *Myocarditis and heart failure*: Rare.

Infection of the Fetus

If mother has primary parvovirus infection, 17–33% risk is there for fetal infection. Fortunately most have a self-limiting course. Mostly they not associated with any congenital anomalies. Only rare case reports of congenital anomalies—CNS and craniofacial. Increased risk of abortion (before 20 weeks) and still birth is there.

Anemia and myocardial involvement can cause hydrops—parvovirus has been reported to be responsible for 8–33% of nonimmune hydrops in various series.

Management of Fetus

Polymerase chain reaction of AF or demonstration on histology of intranuclear inclusions and virus particles by electron microscopy. Fetal IgM is not detectable till 22 weeks, and may be false negative even thereafter and is not a reliable test. Maternal serum AFP levels have been associated with parvo B19 infection, but some studies have shown poor correlation.

Hydrops Fetalis

Cordocentesis is used for the assessment of hemoglobin, reticulocyte count and intrauterine therapy. Doppler of umbilical and middle cerebral arteries may be helpful in evaluation of fetal anemia. Intravascular transfusions decreased mortality by seven times against expectant management in a case series of parvovirus infections.

Antenatal steroid can be used if preterm delivery is anticipated. If baby is nearing term, early delivery may be considered.

Neonatal Outcome

Long-term neonatal outcome of over 100 mothers, who were immune, were compared to those infected, and no difference in neonatal outcomes were noted. Only rare cases of hepatitis, myocarditis and malformations have been reported (Box 3.1.11).

Key points for practice: Congenital parvovirus infection.
- If a mother is exposed to or develops symptoms suggestive of parvovirus infection she must be investigated for immune status (previous infection) or primary infection:
  - If IgG is positive and IgM is negative, she can be reassured that she is immune and safe, the tests should be repeated after 2–4 weeks
  - If both are negative and the incubation period has passed, then she is not infected and not immune either. She may consider leaving the workplace, to minimize further exposure (although evidence shows no decrease in risk of infection in mothers who left work)
  - If she is IgM positive, and rising IgG is demonstrated she is infected
- If recent infection is diagnosed, periodic scans (1–2 weekly for amniotic fluid and hydrops) will be required for 8–12 weeks. The mothers should be advised to monitor fetal movements as hydropic fetuses move less. The risk of fetal loss and hydrops must be explained. If hydrops occurs intrauterine transfusion must be considered.

LISTERIA

It is a food borne disease; outbreaks have been described, particularly in mothers who consumed a type of cheese, particular brand of pasteurized milk or raw vegetables. First and second trimester infections are associated with high mortality. It can also present as late onset sepsis with transmission within nursery.

Clinical Manifestations in Mother

Flu like illness—fever, headache, gastrointestinal symptoms are found in most mothers. In early trimester abortion, still birth or preterm labor can result.

Clinical Manifestations in Baby

Baby may pass through meconium stained/green/tainted AF (in preterm). Within 2–3 days baby presents with sepsis/pneumonia like picture and granulomatosis infantisepticum. Microabscesses and granulomas filled with organism are found throughout the body, especially liver, spleen and lungs. Purulent conjunctivitis may be prevented.

Late onset sepsis is associated with meningitis that does not respond to third generation cephalosporins.

Diagnosis

Mother with flu like illness—blood cultures/genital swab and cultures/consider AF cultures.

Isolation of organism from gastric aspirate (Gram stain), skin biopsy, CSF, joint or pleural space.

Treatment

Ampicillin and aminoglycoside for 10–14 days and 21 days, if meningitis is present. Baby must be isolated.

Prevention

Mothers must not consume soft cheese, unpasteurized milk; undercooked meats and knives, boards, etc. must be washed.

Pregnant mother with infection must be treated with ampicillin/amoxicillin for 14 days (Box 3.1.12).

Box 3.1.12

> **Key points for practice: Listeria.**
> - Food and hygiene safety in mothers
> - Preterm with meconium stained liquor or baby with abscesses and granulomas.

BIBLIOGRAPHY

1. Best JM. Rubella. Semin Fetal Neonatal Med. 2007;12(3):182-92.
2. Crane J. Parvovirus B19 infection in pregnancy. J Obstet Gynaecol Can. 2002;24(9):727-34.
3. Faucher B, Garcia-Meric P, Franck J, et al. Long-term ocular outcome in congenital toxoplasmosis: a prospective cohort of treated children. J Infect. 2012;64:104-9.
4. Fink KR, Thapa MM, Ishak GE, et al. Neuroimaging of pediatric central nervous system cytomegalovirus infection. RSNA. 2010;30(7):1779-96.
5. Kadambari S, Williams EJ, Luck S, et al. Evidence based management guidelines for the detection and treatment of congenital CMV. Early Hum Dev. 2011;87(11):723-8.
6. Kumar A. Hepatitis B virus infection in pregnancy: a practical approach. Indian J Gastroenterol. DOI10.1007/S-12664-012-0174-4.
7. Malm G, Engman ML. Congenital cytomegalovirus infections. Semin Fetal Neonatal Med. 2007;12(3):154-9.
8. Olariu TR, Remington JS, McLeod R, et al. Severe congenital toxoplasmosis in United States. Pediatr Infect Dis. 2011;30(12):1056-61.
9. Palasanthiran P, Starr M, Jones C. Australian society for infectious diseases. Published by Australasian society for infectious diseases.
10. Petersen E. Toxoplasmosis. Semin Fetal Neonatal Med. 2007;12(3):214-23.
11. Pinon JM, Dumon H, Chemla C, et al. Strategy for diagnosis of congenital toxoplasmosis: evaluation of methods comparing mothers and newborns and standard methods for postnatal detection of immunoglobulin G, M, and A antibodies. J Clin Microbiol. 2001;39(6):2267-71.
12. Plosa EJ, Esbenshade JC, Fuller MP, et al. Cytomegalovirus infections. Pediatr Rev. 2012;33(4):156-63.
13. Rubella in pregnancy SOGC clinical practice guidelines. JOGC. 2008;203:152-8.
14. Satti KF, Ali SA, Weitkamp JH. Congenital infections, part 2: parvovirus, listeria, tuberculosis, syphilis and varicella. Neoreviews. 2010;11:e681-95.
15. Tian C, Ali SA, Weitkamp JH. Congenital infections, Part I: Cytomegalovirus, Toxoplasma, rubella and herpes simplex. Neoreviews. 2010;11:2-436.

3.2 NEONATAL INFECTIONS

Sailesh Gupta

INTRODUCTION

With approximately a million deaths annually, neonatal infections remain a significant cause of death in developing countries (over 12% of all under-five child deaths) with Sub-Saharan Africa and South Asian countries experiencing the greatest burden. Neonatal infections range from local pathology, such as pneumonia, to fulminant sepsis, and symptoms and signs overlap with other neonatal conditions, such as prematurity, asphyxia and intracranial hemorrhage. These facts are compounded by inadequate training of medical and nursing personnel, the reluctance of caretakers to seek timely medical assistance and the resource poor settings in several pockets in developing nations, making it imperative to provide special attention to this cause of childhood mortality, and mortality to be able to achieve global millennium development goal 4 (MDG4).

DEFINITION

Neonatal sepsis is defined as bacteremia accompanied by hemodynamic compromise and systemic signs of infection. It can be classified according to the time of onset into early-onset sepsis (EOS), presenting in the first 72 hours of life and generally related to acquisition of infections from the maternal birth canal and late-onset sepsis (LOS), presenting after 72 hours of life, with increased risk of acquisition of microbes from the home or hospital environment. These classifications do not always hold true in developing countries, in which unhygienic birth practices and poor quality of newborn care can expose newborns to environmental pathogens both during and immediately after birth.

DISEASE BURDEN

Population-based studies from developing countries have reported clinical sepsis rate ranging from 49 to 170 per 1,000 live births. The median incidence of blood culture confirmed sepsis was 16 per 1,000 live births in developing countries, among 18 studies reviewed. This contrasts with neonatal culture confirmed sepsis rate of 1–3 per 1,000 live births reported from industrialized countries. A collaborative study from eight Asian neonatal units published in Archives of diseases of the child in 2009 indicates 453 episodes of sepsis in 394 babies. Mortality was 10.4%, with an incidence of 0.69 deaths per 1,000 live births. Group *B Streptococcus* (GBS) was the most common early-onset organism causing 38% of episodes of early-onset (< 48 hour old) sepsis. Gram-negative bacillary EOS occurred at a rate of 0.15 episodes per 1,000 live births with a mortality of 12%. There were 406 episodes of LOS. The incidence

was high at 11.6 per 1,000 live births, and mortality was 8.9%. Coagulase negative *Staphylococcus* caused 34.1% of episodes, whereas *Staphylococcus aureus* caused only 5.4%. Gram-negative bacilli caused 189 episodes (46.6%). Only 44% of Gram-negative bacilli were sensitive to both gentamicin and a third generation cephalosporin, whereas 30% were resistant to both antibiotics. Meningitis occurred in 17.2% of episodes of late sepsis, with a mortality of 20%.

PATHOGENESIS AND RISK FACTORS

Neonates are highly susceptible to infectious diseases because of the following:
- Immature immune systems and poorly developed skin barrier
- A compromised innate immunity, which forms the first line of defense against infections, is compromised in neonates and results in decreased production of proinflammatory cytokines
- Deficits in pathogen recognition, activation after stimulation, phagocytic function, and bactericidal function by monocytes, macrophages and dendritic cells
- Decreased levels of complement proteins and complement-mediated opsonic capabilities compared with adults
- Low levels of immunoglobulins at birth except for immunoglobulin G to specific antigens that are transferred across the placenta during the last trimester of pregnancy
- Impaired synthesis of fresh immunoglobulins because of constraints in the VH gene repertoire of newborns.

Neonates in developing countries are further vulnerable to infections because of exposure to external risk factors such as unsafe birthing practices. World Health Organization (WHO) estimates that only 68% of women in developing countries receive some form of antenatal care and only 35% of mothers in the least developed countries have access to skilled health personnel at delivery. Unhygienic birthing practices during childbirth and the postnatal period include, birth on floor, cord cutting with unsterile instruments, poor skin and cord care, and application of cow-dung on the umbilical stump. On the flip side, beneficial practices, such as use of colostrum and exclusive breastfeeding, are ignored or discouraged. Absence of skilled health workers at the time of delivery translates into an inability to detect high-risk neonates and decide their appropriate management. Socioeconomic and cultural factors, such as poverty, illiteracy, low social standing of women, cultural beliefs regarding confinement of mother and baby at home, resulting in delays in care seeking, absence of sanitation and clean water supply, and lack of access to healthcare facilities contribute to the high incidence of neonatal infections. Interventions during the antenatal period, such as regular visits by a healthcare worker, tetanus toxoid vaccination, and treatment of malaria and sexually transmitted diseases, such as syphilis, *Chlamydia trachomatis* and *Neisseria gonorrhoeae* can decrease neonatal morbidity and mortality. Infants born in hospitals are also at a significant risk of neonatal infections because of an absence of infection control policy in hospital delivery rooms and newborn nurseries.

Before birth, the fetus optimally is maintained in a sterile environment. Organisms causing EOS ascend from the birth canal either when the amniotic membranes rupture or leak before or during the course of labor, resulting in intra-amniotic infection. Commonly referred to as "chorioamnionitis," intra-amniotic infection indicates infection of the amniotic fluid, membranes, placenta and/or decidua. Chorioamnionitis is a major risk factor for neonatal sepsis. Sepsis can begin in utero when the fetus inhales or swallows infected amniotic fluid. The neonate can also develop sepsis in the hours or days after birth when colonized skin or mucosal surfaces are compromised. The essential criterion for the clinical diagnosis of chorioamnionitis is maternal fever. Other criteria are relatively insensitive. When defining intra-amniotic infection (chorioamnionitis) for clinical research studies, the diagnosis is typically based on the presence of maternal fever of greater than 38°C (100.4°F) and at least two of the following criteria: maternal leukocytosis (>15,000 cells/mm^3), maternal tachycardia (>100 beats/minute), fetal tachycardia (>160 beats/minute), uterine tenderness, and/or foul odor of the amniotic fluid. These thresholds are associated with higher rate of neonatal and maternal morbidity. The major risk factors for chorioamnionitis include low parity, spontaneous labor, longer length of labor and membrane rupture, multiple digital vaginal examinations (especially with ruptured membranes), meconium-stained amniotic fluid, internal fetal or uterine monitoring, and presence of genital tract microorganisms (e.g. *Mycoplasma hominis*). The major risk factors for early-onset neonatal sepsis are preterm birth, rupture of membranes more than 18 hours and maternal signs or symptoms of intra-amniotic infection. Other variables include low socioeconomic status, male sex and low Apgar scores.

COMMON ORGANISMS IN DEVELOPING COUNTRIES

The spectrum of organisms responsible for sepsis in developing countries has evolved over time, and knowledge of this spectrum is essential to plan empiric therapy, while culture reports are awaited or absent. The etiology of community acquired neonatal sepsis as per data from Zaidi et al. is shown in Table 3.2.1.

Information on the etiologic agents of neonatal sepsis from developing nations, with a high proportion of home

Table 3.2.1: Etiology of community acquired neonatal sepsis (0–28 days) in South Asia.

Staphylococcus aureus	9.86%
Streptococcus pyogenes	0.82%
Group B streptococci	7.12%
Group D streptococci/*Enterococcus*	6.03%
Group G streptococci	
Streptococcus pneumoniae	1.92%
Other *Streptococcus* species/unspecified	11.78%
Other gram-positives	0.55%
All gram-positives	38.08%
Klebsiella species	23.29%
Escherichia coli	12.05%
Pseudomonas species	10.14%
Enterobacter species	4.11%
Serratia species	
Proteus species	0.24%
Salmonella species	0.55%
Citrobacter species	1.10%
Haemophilus influenzae	0.27%
Neisseria meningitidis	
Acinetobacter species	3.56%
Other gram-negatives	5.48%
All gram-negatives	60.82%
Others	**1.10%**

births is limited. Studies conducted in hospitals, may not accurately reflect etiology of sepsis among home-born babies. Reports from hospital neonatal intensive care nurseries indicate a significant proportion of nosocomial infections. Gram-negative organisms predominate and three organisms *S. aureus*, *Escherichia coli*, and *Klebsiella* spp. are the most dominant, causing 44% of all cases of sepsis. This pattern is noted in Asia Pacific, Middle East and Central Asia, and South Asia, although with some variations. The data available showed that *Klebsiella* was the predominant pathogen, responsible for 25% of all cases, followed by *S. aureus* and *E. coli*. GBS was reported in only 7% of EOS, in contrast to it being the predominant pathogen in developed countries.

Major sources of nosocomial neonatal infections for hospital-born infants are the healthcare facilities in developing countries. Hospital delivery rooms and newborn nurseries are without basic sanitary requirements, such as gloves, washbasins, soap and running water, and hospital staff may be inadequately trained in infection control. Lack of asepsis during invasive procedures, inadequate sterilization of instruments and overcrowded nurseries contribute to neonatal infections. Unhygienic conditions in developing countries predispose newborns to infections from the environment even in the early neonatal period. Premature newborns admitted to intensive care nurseries suffer excessively high rate of nosocomial sepsis, often due to highly resistant bacteria, such as the recently described carbapenem-resistant *E. coli* and *Klebsiella pneumoniae* in India.

DIAGNOSIS

The clinical diagnosis of sepsis in the neonate is difficult, because many of the signs of sepsis are nonspecific and are observed with other noninfectious conditions. Although a normal physical examination is evidence that sepsis is not present, bacteremia can occur in the absence of clinical signs. No single symptom, sign or laboratory parameter can diagnose neonatal sepsis. A mixture of clinical acumen and intelligent interpretation of laboratory reports is required to diagnose neonatal sepsis. The Young Infants Clinical Signs Study Group recently conducted a large multi-country study to identify clinical signs with high sensitivity and specificity for predicting requirement for newborn referral. Seven clinical signs that are identified could be easily recognized by health workers. WHO has developed guidelines for the Integrated Management of Neonatal Childhood Illnesses (IMNCI) for resource-limited countries that have now been extended to include the young infant period (0–59 days of life) and the diagnostic component is based on the findings of the Young Infant Clinical Signs Study.

Criteria Used for Clinical Diagnosis of Neonatal Sepsis in Developing Countries

Definition of Clinical Sepsis: As used by Bang et al.

Presence of two or more of the following signs:
- Weak or absent cry
- Weak or reduced suckling
- Drowsy or unconscious infant
- Temperature above 37.2°C or below 35°C
- Diarrhea or persistent vomiting or abdominal distension
- Grunting or severe chest in-drawing
- Respiratory rate of 60 breaths/minute or more
- Pus in skin or umbilicus.

Definition of Clinical Sepsis: As used by Baqui et al.

Presence of one or more of the following signs:
- Convulsions
- Unconsciousness
- Fever above 38.3°C
- Breathing more than 60/minute
- Many or severe skin pustules or blisters on single large area, or pus or redness with swelling
- Severe chest in-drawing
- Body temperature below 35.3°C.

Definition of Serious Illness, Including Sepsis: Young Infant Clinical Signs Study Group

Presence of one or more of the following signs:
- Difficulty in feeding
- Convulsions
- Movement only when stimulated

- Respiratory rate of 60 or more
- Severe chest in-drawing
- Temperature above 37.5°C
- Temperature below 35.5°C.

Specific features related to various systems:
- *Central nervous system (CNS)*: Bulging anterior fontanel, vacant stare, high-pitched cry, excess irritability, stupor/coma, seizures, neck retraction. Presence of these features should raise a clinical suspicion of meningitis
- *Cardiac*: Hypotension, poor perfusion, shock
- *Gastrointestinal*: Feed intolerance, vomiting, diarrhea, abdominal distension, paralytic ileus and necrotizing enterocolitis (NEC)
- *Hepatic*: Hepatomegaly and direct hyperbilirubinemia (especially with urinary tract infections)
- *Renal*: Acute renal failure
- *Hematological*: Bleeding, petechiae and purpura
- *Skin changes*: Multiple pustules, abscess, sclerema, mottling, umbilical redness and discharge.

Laboratory Investigations

A single blood culture in a volume of 1 mL for each culture bottle is required for all neonates with suspected sepsis. *In vitro* data from Schelonka et al. demonstrated that 0.5 mL would not reliably detect low-level bacteremia. A study by Connell et al. indicated that blood cultures with an adequate volume were twice as likely to yield a positive result.

A urine culture should not be part of the sepsis workup in an infant with suspected EOS. Gastric aspirate, body surface and tracheal aspirate examination and culture may be of little value in diagnosis of early neonatal sepsis.

In bacteremic infants, the incidence of meningitis may be as high as 23%. The lumbar puncture should be performed in any infant with a positive blood culture, infants whose clinical course or laboratory data strongly suggest bacterial sepsis and infants who initially worsen with antimicrobial therapy. Cerebrospinal fluid (CSF) values indicative of neonatal meningitis are controversial. The mean number of white blood cells in uninfected preterm or term infants is consistently less than 10 cells/mm^3. The median number of white blood cells in infants who are born at greater than 34 weeks of gestation and have bacterial meningitis is 477/mm^3. In contrast, the median number of white blood cells in infants who are born at less than 34 weeks of gestation and have meningitis is 110/mm^3. In addition, the number of bands in a CSF specimen does not predict meningitis. Protein concentrations in uninfected, term newborn infants are less than 100 mg/dL. Preterm infants have CSF protein concentrations that vary inversely with gestational age. In the normoglycemic newborn infant, glucose concentrations in CSF are similar to those in older infants and children (70–80% of a simultaneously obtained blood specimen). A low glucose concentration is the CSF variable with the greatest specificity for the diagnosis of meningitis. However, meningitis occurs in infants with normal CSF values, and some of these infants have high bacterial inocula.

Total white blood cell counts have little value in the diagnosis of EOS and have a poor positive predictive accuracy. Neutropenia may be a better marker for neonatal sepsis and has better specificity than an elevated neutrophil count, because few conditions besides sepsis depress the neutrophil count of neonates. The in late preterm and term infants, the definition for neutropenia most commonly used is that suggested by Manroe et al. ($< 1,800/mm^3$ at birth and $< 7,800/mm^3$ at 12–14 hours of age). The immature to total neutrophil (I/T) ratio has the best sensitivity of any of the neutrophil indices. However, with manual counts, there are wide inter-reader differences in band neutrophil identification. The I/T ratio is less than 0.22 in 96% of healthy preterm infants born at less than 32 weeks of gestational age. Unlike the absolute neutrophil count and the absolute band count, maximum normal values for the I/T ratio occur at birth (0.16) and decline with increasing postnatal age to a minimum value of 0.12. A single determination of the I/T ratio has a poor positive predictive accuracy (approximately 25%), but a very high negative predictive accuracy (99%). The I/T ratio may be elevated in 25–50% of uninfected infants.

Despite the frequency of low platelet counts in infected infants, they are a nonspecific, insensitive and late indicator of sepsis. CRP concentration increases within 6–8 hours of an infectious episode in neonates and peaks at 24 hours. The sensitivity of a CRP determination is low at birth, because it requires an inflammatory response (with release of interleukin-6) to increase CRP concentrations. The sensitivity improves dramatically if the first determination is made 6–12 hours after birth. Benitz et al. have demonstrated that excluding a value at birth, two normal CRP determinations (8–24 hours after birth and 24 hours later) have a negative predictive accuracy of 99.7% and a negative likelihood ratio of 0.15 for proven neonatal sepsis. If CRP determinations remain persistently normal, it is strong evidence that bacterial sepsis is unlikely, and antimicrobial agents can be safely discontinued. Procalcitonin concentration has a modestly better sensitivity than does CRP concentration but is less specific.

Sepsis screening panels commonly include neutrophil indices and acute-phase reactants (usually CRP concentration). The positive predictive value of the sepsis screen in neonates is poor (< 30%); however, the negative predictive accuracy has been high (> 99%) in small clinical studies. Sepsis screening tests might be of value in deciding which "high-risk" healthy-appearing neonates do not need antimicrobial agents or whether therapy can be safely discontinued. Chest X-ray should be considered in the presence of respiratory distress or

apnea. An abdominal X-ray is indicated in the presence of abdominal signs suggestive of NEC. Neurosonogram and computed tomography (CT) scan should be performed in all patients diagnosed to have meningitis.

MANIFESTATIONS

Neonatal Pneumonia

The incidence of pneumonia ranges from 0.4 to 12.6 per 1,000 live births in developing countries. Clinical pneumonia definitions overestimate the true incidence of pneumonia, whereas culture proven pneumonia is a very small subset of all neonatal pneumonia. Neonatal pneumonia is diagnosed when a newborn presents with tachypnea, retractions, grunting or hypoxemia, and is supported by radiological or blood culture data. WHO has identified a respiratory rate of more than 60 breaths per minute in a neonate as a strong indicator of the possibility of pneumonia and also included this as a danger sign in the Integrated Management of Childhood Illnesses algorithm. Primary pathogens of neonatal pneumonia are similar to those responsible for neonatal sepsis, and the treatment guidelines are similar to those for sepsis and involve administration of parenteral antibiotics and supportive care, including oxygen therapy if needed, delivered in hospital settings. Community case management for neonatal pneumonia, with oral antibiotics decreases overall neonatal mortality by 27%, and pneumonia-specific neonatal mortality by 42%.

Neonatal Meningitis

Meningitis is more common in the neonatal period than any other time in life. Mortality from neonatal meningitis in developing countries is estimated to be 40–58%, against 10% in developed countries. Around 20–58% of survivors will have serious neurological sequelae, such as deafness. Neonatal risk factors for developing meningitis include low-birth-weight (LBW) and prematurity; maternal risk factors include premature ruptures of membranes, prolonged rupture of membranes (>18 hours), maternal colonization with GBS, maternal chorioamnionitis and low socioeconomic status. Risk factors for poor outcome include LBW, prematurity and infections caused by gram-negative organisms. The microorganism spectrum responsible for neonatal meningitis in developing countries is different from the developed world. Reasons for this difference may include population differences in colonization, genetic differences in immune response and possibly geographic differences in laboratory techniques for pathogen isolation and reporting. Also, reports from large hospitals may not accurately reflect the causative organisms in the community. Gram-negative bacilli (excluding *E. coli*) appear to be more important pathogens than in the developed world, and *Streptococcus pneumoniae* are commonly reported in some centers, with increasing incidence with age. *S. aureus* and *H. influenzae* are also more frequently reported. The diagnosis of neonatal meningitis remains problematic and depends on a high index of suspicion. Clinical presentation is often subtle and indistinguishable from that of sepsis without meningitis. The most commonly reported symptoms include fever, irritability, poor feeding and seizures. Nuchal rigidity and a bulging fontanel are inconsistent and late findings. Predictors of severe disease lack adequate sensitivity and specificity. Positive culture of CSF remains the gold standard for diagnosis and should be performed on all neonates where sepsis is suspected unless a contraindication exists. Gram stains of CSF may also provide useful information, even if CSF culture is not available. Blood cultures are positive in 40–60% of cases. Meningitis can be present even in the absence of CSF pleocytosis, and CSF protein and glucose levels are age-related in the neonatal period. Empirical antibiotic therapy must be effective against common causative pathogens and must achieve adequate bactericidal activity without toxicity in the CSF.

Neonatal Tetanus

According to WHO estimates, 59,000 neonates died of neonatal tetanus in 2008, and in 2010, 40 countries had yet to eliminate neonatal tetanus. Neonatal tetanus presents with inability to suckle starting between 3 and 10 days of age, along with muscle rigidity and spasms, convulsions, and eventually death. Mortality from neonatal tetanus can be reduced by 94% with the immunization of pregnant women and women of childbearing age with at least two doses of tetanus toxoid vaccine. Educating birth attendants and mothers about clean cutting of the cord with sterile instruments and adequate cord care in the neonatal period is also essential.

Omphalitis

In many developing countries, where traditional birth attendants conduct labor at home, the burden of omphalitis is still high. The umbilical stump is easily colonized from the maternal genital tract and unhygienic environments. Cultural practices, such as application of cow dung to umbilical stump predispose neonates to risk of omphalitis. Researchers have reported incidence rate as high as 55–197 per 1,000 live births. Case fatality from omphalitis has been reported to be as high as 15%. *S. aureus* is the major pathogen, but many infections are polymicrobial. A Cochrane review in 2004 from high-income settings found dry cord care to be equally effective as cord care with antiseptics. These findings may not be applicable to low-income settings and WHO suggests use of chlorhexidine cord antisepsis in areas where unsterile applications to the cord stump are common. Invasion of the bloodstream through an infected or colonized umbilical stump may play a major role in neonatal sepsis and mortality in home-delivered infants.

Ophthalmia Neonatorum

Purulent conjunctivitis occurring during the neonatal period is called ophthalmia neonatorum. It can cause blindness among children in developing countries. Its prevalence varies from as low as 1.6 to as high as 12%. Several organisms are responsible for neonatal ophthalmia, *C. trachomatis* and *N. gonorrhoeae* being the most common. Gonococcal ophthalmitis, if untreated, can progress to corneal ulceration, perforation and blindness. Chlamydial ophthalmitis is relatively milder. All neonates with ophthalmia need prompt treatment with antibiotics and eye irrigation at regular intervals until the discharge is eliminated. A single dose of either ceftriaxone or cefotaxime is effective therapy for gonococcal ophthalmia, whereas neonates with chlamydial conjunctivitis should receive a 2-week course of oral erythromycin (50 mg/kg of body weight/day in four divided doses). Cleaning of the eyelids and prophylaxis with topical antibiotics soon after birth will prevention ophthalmia. Silver nitrate 1% solution has been very effective in reducing the burden of ophthalmia neonatorum in industrialized countries. However, major problems with silver nitrate are its limited activity against chlamydia and the tendency to cause chemical conjunctivitis in up to 50% of cases.

MANAGEMENT

The identification of neonates at risk for EOS is based on a combination of perinatal risk factors that are neither sensitive nor specific. Diagnostic tests for neonatal sepsis have a poor positive predictive value. As a result, clinicians often treat well-appearing infants for long periods of time, even when bacterial cultures are negative. The challenges for clinicians are threefold: (1) identifying neonates with a high likelihood of sepsis promptly and initiating antimicrobial therapy, (2) distinguishing "high risk" healthy-appearing infants or infants with clinical signs who do not require treatment, and (3) discontinuing antimicrobial therapy once sepsis is deemed unlikely.

The optimal treatment of infants with suspected EOS is broad-spectrum antimicrobial agents (ampicillin and an aminoglycoside). Once a pathogen is identified, antimicrobial therapy should be narrowed (unless synergism is needed). Recent data suggest an association between prolonged empirical treatment of preterm infants (≥ 5 days) with broad-spectrum antibiotics and higher risks of LOS, NEC, and mortality. To reduce these risks, antimicrobial therapy should be discontinued at 48 hours in clinical situations in which the probability of sepsis is low.

Neonatal sepsis requires intensive care inpatient management and supportive therapy along with the use of parenteral antibiotics. Antibiotic therapy is decided on reports of blood and tissue culture. However, empirical antibiotics are given as per the policy of the intensive care unit until the reports are available. Broad spectrum

Table 3.2.2: Preferred parenteral regimens for treatment of neonatal sepsis in developing country community settings.

	Dose	Route	Interval (hour)
First line regimen Penicillin G Procaine	50,000 units/kg	IM	24
Gentamicin	13.5 mg (for 2:2,500 g)	IV, IM	24
	10 mg (for 2,000–2,499 g)	IV, IM	24
	10 mg (for <2,000 g)	IV, IM	48
Alternative regimen Ceftriaxone	50 mg/kg (for ? 2,000 g or ? 7 day old)	IV, IM	24
		IV, IM	24
	75 mg/kg (for >2,000 g and >7 day old)		

coverage should be provided and considering the predominance of gram-negative sepsis, an aminoglycoside should be an essential component of the antibiogram. Third generation cephalosporins (e.g. cefotaxime and ceftriaxone) along with gentamicin or amikacin provide adequate coverage. Some units may still start empiric therapy with ampicillin and gentamicin. In developing nations with a high proportion of home births, antibiotics are not available due to lack of healthcare facilities in rural areas. However, community-based case management for neonatal sepsis with once daily procaine penicillin and gentamicin given intramuscularly may be a feasible and effective option where hospital-based therapy is not possible. The preferred regimen of treatment of neonatal sepsis is shown in Table 3.2.2.

Alternative Regimen

Resistance to antibiotics is developing rapidly in hospital care settings. A recent review on antimicrobial resistance has highlighted the need for active surveillance and resistance monitoring in developing countries. Methicillin resistant *S. aureus* is a major pathogen of neonatal sepsis in hospital settings. *E. coli* resistance to cephalosporins and resistance of other pathogens to gentamicin is much lower in community settings compared with hospital settings. Resistance to cotrimoxazole, a drug widely used in National Pneumonia Programs, is significant. Almost 60% of all *Klebsiella* isolates are resistant to gentamicin, rendering the common regimen of ampicillin and gentamicin ineffective against most strains of *Klebsiella*.

Adjunctive Therapy

Exchange transfusion (ET): Sadana et al. have evaluated the role of double volume exchange transfusion in septic neonates with sclerema and demonstrated a 50% reduction in sepsis related mortality in the treated group. Double volume exchange transfusion is performed with cross-matched fresh whole blood as adjunctive therapy in septic neonates with sclerema. Intravenous immunoglobulin has not been found to be useful. Use of granulocyte-macrophage colony stimulating factor (GM-CSF) is still experimental. Two trials have examined the use of adjunctive steroids in neonatal meningitis. Two nonrandomized studies have suggested benefit, but a small randomized controlled trial in Jordan (*n* = 52) showed no significant difference in morbidity or mortality. It is concluded, despite that adjunctive steroids have no role in neonatal meningitis.

PREVENTION

Preventive strategies are essential to reduce the global burden of neonatal sepsis. Antenatal care should be delivered through visits in rural areas to educate mothers about clean birth practices and about maternal and neonatal risk factors for sepsis. Provision of skilled birth attendants can significantly reduce neonatal sepsis in developing countries. Administration of antibiotics to women with preterm premature rupture of membranes can reduce incidence of all neonatal infections by one-third. The benefits of use of intrapartum prophylactic antibiotics and vaginal chlorhexidine are yet to be proven in developing countries. Chlorhexidine application to the newborn umbilical stump for antisepsis appears to be a promising intervention. Early and exclusive breastfeeding is an important intervention to prevent neonatal sepsis. Breast milk contains lysozymes, lactoferrin and secretory immunoglobulin A, which inhibit *E. coli* and other pathogens. Hygienic care of the newborn is important and includes hand washing by care providers, sanitary disposal of waste and clean water supply in homes. Sunflower oil skin massage is under investigation for its impact in prevention of neonatal mortality in community settings. Kangaroo mother care (KMC) is an effective intervention to prevent neonatal sepsis. A recent meta-analysis found that KMC led to significant reductions in neonatal mortality among preterm babies in hospital settings and produced a 66% reduction in serious morbidities, including neonatal infections.

CONCLUSION

Infections are a major cause of neonatal morbidity and mortality in the developing world and simple preventive and treatment strategies can significantly reduce the burden. Resource constraints pose major problems in developing countries, but low cost-effective interventions are available and can be scaled up. Promotion of female literacy, good antenatal care and skilled birth attendants are interventions that should be scaled up by incorporating them in national public health programs. Community health workers should visit mothers at home and educate

Common Systemic Infections

them about healthy practices, and identify neonatal danger signs and provide treatment or referral. National and international collaborative efforts are needed to make this a reality. Diagnostic tests for EOS (other than blood or CSF cultures) are useful for identifying infants with a low probability of sepsis, but not at identifying infants likely to be infected. In conclusion, available evidence suggests that antibiotics have a clear role in reducing neonatal mortality in low income areas and can be effectively administered in homes via trained health workers. However, issues surrounding sustainability and acceptability on the part of families, healthcare workers, and policy makers, as well as selection and implementation of packages of care integrated across the continuum of care—with appropriate preventive as well as therapeutic interventions for scaling up—are areas needing further development. The optimal treatment of infants with suspected EOS is broad-spectrum antimicrobial agents (ampicillin and an aminoglycoside). Once the pathogen is identified, antimicrobial therapy should be narrowed (unless synergism is needed). Antimicrobial therapy should be discontinued at 48 hours in clinical situations in which the probability of sepsis is low. Data from developed countries suggests that serious neonatal bacterial infections are best managed using parenteral antibiotics, and this standard of care should be provided whenever feasible in developing countries. For many families, however, facility-based care or injectable antibiotic therapy is not within their reach. Thus, alternative strategies are needed for managing serious bacterial infections in many developing country communities. Available data indicate that a case management approach that emphasizes essential newborn care along with prompt recognition of serious bacterial infections and treatment with oral antibiotics is superior to no case management.

BIBLIOGRAPHY

1. Adejuyigbe EA, Adeodu OO, ko-Nai KA, et al. Septicaemia in high risk neonates at a teaching hospital in Ile-Ife, Nigeria. East Afr Med J. 2001;78:540-3.

2. Ali Z. Neonatal bacterial septicemia at the Mount Hope Women's Hospital, Trinidad. Ann Trop Paediatr. 2004;24:41-4.

3. Al-Zwaini EJ. Neonatal septicemia in the neonatal care unit, Al-Anbar governorate, Iraq. East Mediterr Health J. 2002;8:509-14.

4. Anyebuno M, Newman M. Common causes of neonatal bacteraemia in Accra, Ghana. East Afr Med J. 1995;72:805-8.

5. Aurangzeb B, Hameed A. Neonatal sepsis in hospital-born babies: bacterial isolates and antibiotic susceptibility patterns. J Coll Physicians SurgPak. 2003;13:629-32.

6. Bang AT, Bang RA, Baitule SB, et al. Effect of home-based neonatal care and management of sepsis on neonatal mortality: field trial in rural India. Lancet. 1999;354:1955-61.

7. Baqui AH, Arifeen SE, Rosen HE, et al. Community-based validation of assessment of newborn illnesses by trained community health workers in Sylhet district of Bangladesh. Trop Med Int Health. 2009;14:1448-56.

8. Baqui AH, El-Arifeen S, Darmstadt GL, et al. Effect of community based newborn-care intervention package implemented through two service-delivery strategies in Sylhet district, Bangladesh: a cluster randomised controlled trial. Lancet. 2008;371:1936-44.

9. Bauer K, Zemlin M, Hummel M, et al. Diversification of Ig heavy chain genes in human preterm neonates prematurely exposed to environmental antigens. J Immunol. 2002;169:1349-56.

10. Berkley JA, Lowe BS, Mwangi I, et al. Bacteremia among children admitted to a rural hospital in Kenya. N Engl J Med. 2005;352:39-47.

11. Bhutta ZA, Zaidi AK, Thaver D, et al. Management of newborn infections in primary care settings: a review of the evidence and implications for policy? Pediatr Infect Dis J. 2009;28(Suppl): S22-30.

12. Bizzarro MJ, Raskind C, Baltimore RS, et al. Seventy-five years of neonatal sepsis at Yale: 1928-2003. Pediatrics. 2005;116:595-602.

13. Black RE, Cousens S, Johnson HL, et al. Global, regional, and national causes of child mortality in 2008: a systematic analysis. Lancet. 2010;375:1969-87.

14. Chacko B, Sohi I. Early onset neonatal sepsis. Indian J Pediatr. 2005;72:23-6.

15. Country Classification Data: The World Bank. [online] Available from website http://data.worldbank.org/about/country-classifications [Accessed September, 2010].

16. Darmstadt GL, Batra M, Zaidi AK. Parenteral antibiotics for the treatment of serious neonatal bacterial infections in developing country settings. Pediatr Infect Dis J. 2009;28(Suppl):S37-42.

17. Darmstadt GL, Bhutta ZA, Cousens S, et al. Evidence-based, cost-effective interventions: how many newborn babies can we save? Lancet. 2005;365:977-88.

18. Darmstadt GL, Saha SK, Choi Y, et al. Population-based incidence and etiology of community-acquired neonatal bacteremia in Mirzapur, Bangladesh: an observational study. J Infect Dis. 2009;200:906-15.

19. Darmstadt GL, Zaidi AK, Stoll B. Neonatal infections: a global perspective. In: Remington JS, et al. (Eds). Infectious Diseases of the Fetus and Newborn Infant; 7th edition. Philadelphia, PA: Saunders/Elsevier 2010.pp.24-51.

20. Das PK, Basu K, Chakraborty P, et al. Clinical and bacteriological profile of neonatal infections in metropolitan city based medical college nursery. J Indian Med Assoc. 1999;97:3-5.

21. Das PK, Basu K, Chakraborty S, et al. Early neonatal morbidity and mortality in a city based medical college nursery. Indian J Public Health. 1998;42:9-14.

22. Edwards MS, Baker CJ. Bacterial infections in the neonate. In: Long SS, Pickering LK, Prober CG, (Eds). Principles and Practice of Pediatric Infectious Disease, 2nd edition. New York: Churchill Livingstone, 2003.

23. Escobar GJ, Li DK, Armstrong MA, et al. Neonatal sepsis workups in infants 2000 grams at birth: a population-based study. Pediatrics. 2000;106:256-63.

24. Ganatra HA, Stoll BJ, Zaidi AK. International perspective on early onset neonatal sepsis. Clin Perinatol. 2010;37:501-23.

25. Ghiorghis B. Neonatal sepsis in Addis Ababa, Ethiopia: a review of 151 bacteremic neonates. Ethiop Med J. 1997;35:169-76.

26. Gupta P, Murali MV, Faridi MM, et al. Clinical profile of Klebsiella septicemia in neonates. Indian J Pediatr. 1993;60:565-72.

27. Johnson CE, Whitwell JK, Pethe K, et al. Term newborns who are at risk for sepsis: are lumbar punctures necessary? Pediatrics. 1997;99:E10.

28. Karthikeyan G, Premkumar K. Neonatal sepsis: *Staphylococcus aureus* as the predominant pathogen. Indian J Pediatr. 2001;68:715-7.

29. Kaushik SL, Parmar VR, Grover N, et al. Neonatal sepsis in hospital born babies. J Commun Disord. 1998;30:147-52.

30. Klein JO. Bacterial sepsis and meningitis. In: Remington JS, Klein JO, (Eds). Infectious Diseases of the Fetus and Newborn Infant, 6th edition. Philadelphia, PA: W B Saunders, 2006.

31. Kuruvilla KA, Pillai S, Jesudason M, et al. Bacterial profile of sepsis in a neonatal unit in south India. Indian Pediatr. 1998;35:851-8.

32. Lawn JE, Cousens S, Zupan J. Four million neonatal deaths: when? where? why? Lancet. 2005;365:891-900.

33. Levy O. Innate immunity of the newborn: basic mechanisms and clinical correlates. Nat Rev Immunol. 2007;7:379-90.

34. Mokuolu AO, Jiya N, Adesiyun OO. Neonatal septicaemia in Ilorin: bacterial pathogens and antibiotic sensitivity pattern. Afr J Med Med Sci. 2002;31:127-30.

35. Morken NH, Kallen K, Jacobsson B. Outcomes of preterm children according to type of delivery onset: a nationwide population-based study. Paediatr Perinat Epidemiol. 2007;21:458-64.

36. Neonatal morbidity and mortality: report of the national neonatal perinatal database. Indian Pediatr. 1997;34:1039-42.

37. Owais A, Sultana S, Stein AD, et al. Why do families of sick newborns accept hospital care? A community based cohort study in Karachi, Pakistan. J Perinatol. 2011;31(9):586-92.

38. Saez-Llorens X, McCracken GH. Clinical pharmacology of antimicrobial agents. In: Remington JS, Klein JO, (Eds). Infectious Diseases of the Fetus and Newborn Infant, 6th edition. Philadelphia, PA: WB Saunders 2006.pp.1223-67.

39. Stiehm ER, Fudenberg HH. Serum levels of immune globulins in health and disease: a survey. Pediatrics. 1996;37:715-27.

40. Stoll BJ, Schuchat A. Maternal carriage of group B streptococci in developing countries. Pediatr Infect Dis J. 1998;17:499-503.

41. Stoll BJ. Neonatal infections: a global perspective. In: Remington JS, Klein JO (Eds). Infectious diseases of the fetus and newborn infant, 6th edition. Philadelphia, PA: WB Saunders; 2006.

42. Tallur SS, Kasturi AV, Nadgir SD, et al. Clinico-bacteriological study of neonatal septicemia in Hubli. Indian J Pediatr. 2000;67:169-74.

43. Thaver D, Ali SA, Zaidi AK. Antimicrobial resistance among neonatal pathogens in developing countries. Pediatr Infect Dis J. 2009;28(Suppl):S19-21.

44. Thaver D, Zaidi AK. Burden of neonatal infections in developing countries: a review of evidence from community-based studies. Pediatr Infect Dis J. 2009;28(Suppl):S3-S9.

45. Thaver D, Zaidi AK. Neonatal infections in South Aisa. In: Bhutta ZE (Ed). Perinatal and Newborn Care in South Asia: Priorities for Action. Oxford: Oxford University Press; 2007.

46. The World Bank: DEP web: beyond economic growth, glossary. [online] Available from: website http://www.worldbank.org/depweb/english/beyond/global/glossary. [Accessed September, 2010].

47. Verani JR, Schrag SJ. Group B streptococcal disease in infants: progress in prevention and continued challenges. Clin Perinatol. 2010;37:375-92.

48. WHO. Integrated management of childhood illness (IMCI). [online] Available from website http://www.who.int/child_adolescent_health/topics/prevention_care/child/imci/en/index.html. [Accessed September, 2010].

49. WHO. Integrated management of childhood illnesses chart booklet 2008. [online] Available from website http://whqlibdoc.who.int/publications/2008/9789241597289_eng.pdf. [Accessed September, 2010].

50. World Health Organization Department of Reproductive Health and Research. Proportion of births attended by a skilled health worker. Geneva: World health Organization; 2008.

51. World Health Organization: Antenatal Care in Developing Countries: Promises, achievements and missed opportunities: an analysis of trends, levels and differentials, 1990–2001. Geneva: World Health Organization, 2003.

52. Wynn JL, Levy O. Role of innate host defences in susceptibility to early-onset neonatal sepsis. Clin Perinatol. 2010;37:307-37.

53. Young Infants Clinical Signs Study Group. Clinical signs that predict severe illness in children under age 2 months: a multicentre study. Lancet. 2008;371:135-42.

54. Zaidi AK, Huskins WC, Thaver D, et al. Hospital-acquired neonatal infections in developing countries. Lancet. 2005;365:1175-88.

55. Zaidi AK, Thaver D, Ali SA, et al. Pathogens associated with sepsis in newborns and young infants in developing countries. Pediatr Infect Dis J. 2009;28(Suppl):S10-8.

3.3 UPPER RESPIRATORY TRACT INFECTIONS

A Balachandran

ACUTE RESPIRATORY INFECTION

Acute respiratory infection is defined as infection of respiratory system from nose to alveoli, caused by an infective organism, for duration of less than 1 month. Upper respiratory tract infections (URTIs) are the most common presentation especially in children below 5 years. In this age group on an average they get about 6–8 episodes per year. Upper respiratory tract infections are mostly viral in origin and are mild and self-limiting.

However, viral URTIs can cause:
- Locally ENT complications like acute sinusitis/otitis media, pharyngitis, stomatitis or tonsillitis
- Spread to lower respiratory tract like bronchiolitis/bronchitis, bronchopneumonia or Croup syndrome
- Trigger acute exacerbations of asthma
- At times have secondary bacterial super infection.

Upper respiratory tract infections in children presents with several signs and symptoms of which at least one of the following should be present—cold, cough, throat pain, tenderness over sinuses, swelling of the face, ear pain, otorrhea, mastoid swelling. On the other hand children with lower respiratory tract infection (LRTI) usually have tachypnea, chest retractions, crepitations or wheezing. Other serious conditions, such as croup, epiglottitis and retropharyngeal abscess (RPA), do not find a place in either URTI or LRTI. But it is wise to include them under URTI because of the lack of lung signs and absence of chest X-ray findings, which are the hallmark of LRTI excluding asthma. Stridor and suprasternal retractions are indicative of upper respiratory obstruction. Respiratory infection should be further classified as severe and nonsevere infections. Nonsevere infection can be treated on outpatient basis, whereas severe infections need to be hospitalized and monitored.

Upper Respiratory Tract Infection

Upper respiratory tract infection can be classified into three groups:
1. *Benign URI:* Common cold.
2. *Potentially serious URI:* Group-A beta hemolytic streptococcal pharyngitis, sinusitis and otitis media.
3. *Serious URI:* Acute laryngotracheobronchitis (ALTB), epiglottitis, retropharyngeal, lateral pharyngeal and peritonsillar abscess. Respiratory distress, dysphagia, drooling of saliva, hoarse voice, stridor, high grade fever, cyanosis, systemic toxicity, altered consciousness are the features suggestive of serious URI.

COMMON COLD

The common cold is an acute, self-limited viral infection of the upper respiratory tract. The infection may have variable degrees of manifestations as sneezing, nasal congestion and discharge (rhinorrhea), sore throat, cough, low grade fever, headache and malaise. The common cold can be caused by a variety of viruses. Rhinovirus, respiratory syncytial virus (RSV), influenza virus, parainfluenza virus and adenovirus are commonly responsible for cold in preschool children.

Cold symptoms can also be caused by corona virus, nonpolio enteroviruses (echoviruses and coxsackieviruses) and human metapneumovirus.

Some of the viruses that cause cold may also present as characteristic clinical syndromes in children (Table 3.3.1).

Epidemiology

The common cold may occur at any time of year, but there is typically a high prevalence during the winter months. These viruses are highly infectious and spread via inhalation of small particle aerosols (sneezing) or direct transfer via hand-to-hand contact (clothing, handkerchief). The cold inducing viruses may remain viable on human skin for at least 2 hours and on inanimate surfaces for a day.

Clinical Features

The presentation of the common cold in children is distinctly different from the illness seen in adults. On an average adults have 2–4 episodes of colds per year, with average symptom duration of 5–7 days. Nasal congestion is the prominent symptom and fever is usually absent. Children under the age of 6 years have an average of 6–8 episodes of cold per year with symptom duration longer than adults. The symptoms are nasal (stuffiness, sneezing and rhinorrhea), sore throat, conjunctival irritation (red, watery eyes) with or without fever. Young children in day care appear to be more susceptible to these infections than those vulnerable when they enter primary school. Colored

Table 3.3.1: Common cold-associated with clinical syndromes.

Viruses	Clinical syndromes
Respiratory syncytial virus	Bronchiolitis in younger children less than 2 years of age
Influenza viruses	Influenza, pneumonia and croup
Parainfluenza viruses	Croup
Coxsackievirus A (an *Enterovirus*)	Herpangina (fever and ulcerated papules on the posterior oropharynx)
Other nonpolio enteroviruses	Aseptic meningitis
Adenoviruses	Pharyngoconjunctival fever (palpebral conjunctivitis, watery eye discharge, and pharyngeal erythema)
Human metapneumovirus	Pneumonia and bronchiolitis

nasal discharge is characteristic and fever is common in children during the first 3 days of the illness. Other symptoms in children may include sore throat, cough, and irritability, difficulty in sleeping and decreased appetite. Physical signs are nonspecific, but may include erythema and swelling of the nasal mucosa. The wide range of overlapping manifestations of various viral agents causing cold make it impossible to identify causative virus without laboratory testing.

Common cold is usually associated with wheezing in susceptible children and in some bacterial pneumonia may follow viral respiratory infection. Other complications of common cold in children are otitis media, sinusitis, epistaxis, conjunctivitis and pharyngitis. The differential diagnosis of the common cold includes other causes of rhinitis (allergic, seasonal, vasomotor, rhinitis medicamentosa), acute bacterial sinusitis (ABS), nasal foreign body and pertussis, structural abnormalities of nose/sinuses, influenza and bacterial pharyngotonsillitis. These conditions can be differentiated from cold by the history and physical examination.

Treatment

The common cold is usually a mild and self-limiting illness. Parental guidance and supportive care are the mainstays of management. There is no role for antibiotics in the absence of bacterial superinfection. Antiviral therapy is not available for most of the viruses that cause the common cold. Over-the-counter cough and cold medications have no proven efficacy and potential for serious adverse effects. There is no definitive evidence to indicate that treatment with zinc, *Echinacea purpurea* or vitamin C is beneficial in the treatment of the common cold in children.

Ideal supportive interventions include maintaining adequate fluid intake; ingestion of warm liquids, suctioning the nose and upright positioning (small infants), saline nasal irrigation or sprays (for older children), and the use of cool mist humidifiers or vaporizers. These interventions are relatively inexpensive and unlikely to be harmful. The topical rubs containing aromatic agents (e.g. camphor, menthol, eucalyptus) for the treatment of nasal congestion in children with the common cold, only increased the perception of nasal patency but did not affect spirometry.

Over the counter medications—these include anti-histamines, decongestants, antitussives, expectorants, mucolytics, antipyretics and combinations of these medications. Various studies have shown they have no proven efficacy than placebo and have serious side effects in children.

Symptomatic therapy may be warranted if the symptoms bother the child (e.g. interrupting sleep, interfering with drinking, causing discomfort) or other family members. Cough is a physiologic response to airway irritation and functions to clear secretions from the respiratory tract. Suppression of cough may result in retention of secretions in the respiratory tract leading to potential airway obstruction.

PHARYNGITIS

Acute pharyngitis is an inflammatory condition of the pharynx and/or tonsils. Clinically if children present with nasal symptoms it is nasopharyngitis and is mostly viral (rhinovirus). If there are no nasal symptoms it is tonsillopharyngitis and it could be bacterial or viral. The major complaint is acute sore throat and/or discomfort on swallowing (dysphagia).

Etiology

Acute infectious pharyngitis is caused by a variety of agents in children and adolescents. Viruses are the most common cause of acute pharyngitis. Most of the viruses do not directly infect the throat but can cause sore throat as part of nasopharyngitis, e.g. rhinoviruses, corona viruses, RSV, influenza and parainfluenza viruses. Throat discomfort is caused by dryness due to mouth breathing or mechanical irritation due to severe cough. Some of the viruses may directly infect the pharynx and produce severe inflammation, e.g. Epstein Barr virus (EBV), cytomegalovirus, adenoviruses, herpes simplex virus (HSV), influenza viruses and enteroviruses.

Viral agents: Rhinovirus, adenovirus, *Enterovirus*, influenza virus, parainfluenza virus, etc.

Bacterial agents: Streptococcus pyogenes (Group A streptococci: GAS), *Haemophilus influenzae, N. meningitidis, C. diphtheriae, Neisseria gonorrhoeae, Mycoplasma pneumoniae* (in adolescents) and pneumococci, *Staphylococcus aureus.*

Clinical Features

It is important to distinguish viral pharyngitis from *S. pyogenes* (GAS) pharyngitis. Possible differentiating points between viral and bacterial pharyngotonsillitis are discussed in the Table 3.3.2. Although clinically difficult, if three or more of the following: (1) fever, (2) tonsillar exudates, (3) tender and enlarged anterior cervical node, (4) absence of cough, are present this favors a streptococcal pharyngitis.

The following conditions mimic streptococcal pharyngitis:
- Ulcerative pharyngotonsillitis, herpangina and hand, foot and mouth disease mainly caused by enteroviruses (*coxsackievirus* and echovirus)
- Epstein-Barr virus pharyngitis/tonsillitis
- Primary HSV stomatitis.

The other causes for membranous pharyngitis are; diphtheria, infectious mononucleosis, agranulocytosis, oral thrush and Vincent's angina (caused by B Vincent/

Table 3.3.2: Differentiation between bacterial and viral infection.

Points	Viral	Bacterial
Suspicion	• Acute onset, red eyes, rhinorrhea, exanthema, diarrhea, hoarseness, cough+++ • Pharyngeal exudates and cervical lymphadenopathy less often	• Explosive onset • Pain in throat • Rapid progression • Usually little coryza or cough • Pharyngeal congestion+++ • Thick exudates, ulcers and vesicles • Purulent, patchy tonsils • Tender lymphadenopathy (often) • Toxicity+++
Diagnosis	Clinical	Culture for GAS: Before starting antibiotics
Clinical course and management	Usually self-limiting symptomatic management for 3–4 days	Antibiotics, symptomatic

Spirochete denticola). Oral hygiene is important in the management of all these conditions. In acute presentation of unilateral enlarged tonsil one should always suspect a peritonsillar abscess. Persistent unilateral enlarged tonsils even though asymptomatic requires close follow-up and it is always worthwhile to rule out lymphoma (malignancy).

Diagnosis

The diagnostic approach to acute infectious pharyngitis in children and adolescents focuses on identification of pathogens that require treatment to prevent complications or transmission of disease. This strategy helps to minimize the unnecessary use of antibiotics in children and adolescents who have viral infections. The majority of cases of acute pharyngitis in children and adolescents are caused by viruses. It is important to determine which cases are caused by Group A *Streptococcus* GAS, since GAS is the most common pathogen that requires antimicrobial therapy.

Most clinicians prescribe symptomatic measures for children with pharyngitis that is not caused by GAS. Symptoms usually resolve promptly, and the infection is presumed to be virus. In the occasional child with acute onset with severe symptoms and rapid progression or with epidemiologic clues to specific etiologies, specific diagnostic testing may be necessary.

Throat Swab Culture

Throat swab culture is considered the gold standard for diagnosing streptococcal pharyngitis. A positive result does not reliably distinguish acute streptococcal pharyngitis from asymptomatic carriage. The false-negative rate for a properly performed throat swab culture is 5–10%, and many patients

with this result are thought to be chronic GAS carriers, anyway not needing treatment. Therefore, a negative throat swab culture result has a very high negative predictive value for GAS pharyngitis. The major drawback of throat swab culture is the 18–48 hours required for results. This delay does not decrease the ability to prevent rheumatic fever, but it can make convincing the patients of the wisdom of withholding antibiotics difficult for the physician.

Rapid Antigen Detection Tests or Rapid Streptococcal Antigen Test

Rapid antigen detection tests (RADTs) detect the presence of the Lancefield group, a carbohydrate antigen. Reported sensitivities of RADTs are 65–91% and specificities of greater than 95%. A negative RADT do not rule out GAS, hence a throat swab culture is performed in all negative RADT.

Serology

Streptococcal antibody testing has no role in the diagnosis of acute streptococcal pharyngitis as it takes several weeks to become positive. Elevated titers for both antistreptolysin-O and antideoxyribonuclease B can persist for several weeks or even months.

Pathogens other than GAS that may require specific therapy are listed below:
- Non-GAS if the patient remains symptomatic when the results of the culture are confirmed
- Epstein-Barr virus mononucleosis (activity restriction may be necessary to prevent splenic rupture in patients with splenic enlargement)
- *Neisseria gonorrhoeae*
- Influenza virus—antiviral therapy may be provided if the diagnosis is made early in the course of illness and the symptoms are severe, in children at increased risk of severe or complicated influenza infection, or in children who live with someone at increased risk for complications.
- Primary human immunodeficiency virus infection.
- *Corynebacterium diphtheriae*
- Tularemia.

Complications

The potential complications of GAS tonsillopharyngitis are discribed below.

Suppurative Complications (Early)

Tonsil pharyngeal cellulitis or abscess, otitis media, sinusitis are the common complications. Necrotizing fasciitis although rare can follow acute varicella or after trauma. Streptococcal bacteremia, meningitis or brain abscess are rare suppurative complications of streptococcal tonsillopharyngitis in the era of antibiotic therapy.

Nonsuppurative Complications (Late)

Acute rheumatic fever, scarlet fever, acute glomerulone-phritis, streptococcal toxic shock syndrome and pediatric autoimmune neuropsychiatric disorder associated with GAS are the nonsuppurative complications of GAS tonsillopharyngitis.

Management

General Management

It includes rest, oral fluids and warm saline gargling (for soothing effects) are the main supportive measures. Analgesics and antipyretics may be used for relief of pain or pyrexia. Acetaminophen is the drug of choice. Normal saline nasal drops may help in young children (1–3 years) but oxymetazoline and xylometazoline may be sparingly used in older children as short-term nasal relievers. Anesthetic gargles and lozenges, such as benzocaine, may be used for symptomatic relief (Flowchart 3.3.1).

Rhinorrhea: The first generation antihistamines may relieve rhinorrhea by 25–30% due to their anticholinergic action. Second generation antihistamines are poorer in efficacy.

Cough: Antihistamines may help by reducing secretions and preventing postnasal drips. Cough suppressants (dextromethorphan, codeine) and expectorants (guaifenesin, ammonium citrate, ambroxol, etc.) have not proved to be effective in meta-analysis. Use of cough medication should be predicted by severity of symptoms.

Specific Treatment of Bacterial Pharyngitis

Antimicrobial Treatment

Group A *Streptococcus* pharyngotonsillitis is a self-limiting disease recovering within 3–4 days. The goals of

Table 3.3.3: Antibiotic therapy for bacterial pharyngitis.

In children with no penicillin allergy		
Antibiotic (route)	Children (30 kg) (days)	Children (> 30 kg) (days)
Penicillin V (oral)	250 mg BID x 10 days	500 mg BID x 10 days
Amoxicillin (oral)	40 mg/kg/day x 10 days	250 mg TID, can be given BID
Benzathine penicillin G (1M)	600,000 units (single dose)	1200,000 Lakh Units (single dose)
In children with penicillin allergy		
Antibiotic (route) (days)	Children (< 27 kg)	
Erythromycin ethylsuccinate (oral) (10 days)	40–50 mg/kg/day TID	
Azithromycin (oral) (5 days)	12 mg/kg OD	
First generation cephalo-sporin (oral) (10 days)	Cephalexin/Cefaclor* in usual doses	
Clindamycin (oral) (10 days)	10–20 mg/kg	

*Early second generation
Source: RTI-GEM: IAP Action Plan; 2006

pharmacotherapy are to reduce morbidity and to prevent complications. Ten days of treatment with penicillin, is the drug of choice. While penicillin is the drug of choice amoxicillin is a good alternative and used widely. The drug of choice for GAS pharyngitis is penicillin (< 30 kg 250 mg BD > 30 kg 500 mg BD) or amoxicillin (40 mg/kg/day TDS or BD) for 10 days. Alternative therapy is with oral first generation cephalosporin or erythromycin ethylsuccinate (40–50 mg/kg/day BD or TDS) for 10 days or with oral azithromycin (12 mg/kg/day) for 5 days (Table 3.3.3).

Surgical Intervention

Tonsillectomy is advised in children with recurrent culture proven streptococcal pharyngitis, i.e. more than 7 episodes per year or more than 5 episodes in each of the preceding 2 years or peritonsillar abscess and enlarged tonsils that cause severe airway obstruction.

ACUTE SINUSITIS

Sinusitis is defined as inflammation of the paranasal sinuses. Paranasal sinuses are an extension of the upper respiratory tract and sinusitis is a usual complication of URI and hence it is commonly called rhinosinusitis. Uncomplicated acute viral sinusitis normally resolves without specific treatment in 7–10 days and if it continues beyond 10 days a possibility of secondary bacterial sinusitis should be considered. Based on the duration of

FLOWCHART 3.3.1: Management protocol of acute pharyngitis.

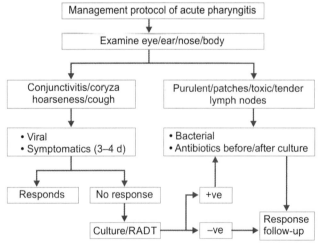

Source: RTI-GEM: IAP Action Plan; 2006

illness, sinusitis is divided into acute (< 30 days), recurrent acute (at least 10 days symptom free interval in between), subacute (30–90 days) and chronic (> 90 days of low-grade persistent signs and or symptoms).

Etiology

The sinuses are an extension of the upper respiratory tract and hence the causative organisms of sinusitis are similar to the ones responsible for URTIs. It typically begins as a viral infection with rhinoviruses, adenoviruses or parainfluenza and as the disease enters the 2nd week secondary bacterial superinfection develops.

The common organisms in acute and subacute sinusitis are *Streptococcus pneumoniae,* nontypeable *H. influenzae, Moraxella catarrhalis* and *S. pyogenes* (GAS).

Whereas, in chronic sinusitis, bacterial pathogens are not well-defined and usually polymicrobial infections are found. The commonly implicated bugs are alpha-hemolytic streptococci, *S. aureus*, coagulase-negative staphylococci, nontypeable *H. influenzae* (more common than in acute sinusitis), *Moraxella catarrhalis,* anaerobic bacteria, including *Peptostreptococcus, Prevotella, Bacteroides*, and *Fusobacterium* species.

Clinical Anatomy and Pathology

The four paranasal sinuses (maxillary, frontal, ethmoid and sphenoid) develop as out pouch of the nasopharynx. The maxillary and ethmoid sinuses start developing in the 10th week of gestation and are fully formed at birth. The sphenoid sinuses develop around 3 years and complete development occurs by 7–8 years. The frontal sinuses are the last to develop and start development at 7–8 years and do not complete developments till the early teens. The posterior ethmoid sinuses drain into the superior meatus and all other sinuses drain into the ostiomeatal complex in the middle meatus.

The valveless veins passing through the posterior walls of the frontal sinuses may allow intracranial spread of frontal sinus infection. The sphenoid sinuses cradle the pituitary gland, and the optic nerve traverses over the lateral and superior aspects of the sinus. The sphenoid sinus is in close proximity to the cavernous sinus, the carotid artery as well as the dura of both the middle and anterior cranial fossa. Infection of these sinuses can therefore be dangerous.

Predisposing Factors

Nasal: Allergic rhinitis, polyps, foreign body (including nasogastric/endotracheal tube).

Oral: Cleft palate, dental infections, adenoidal hypertrophy.

Others: Ciliary dysfunction, cystic fibrosis, immunodeficiency.

Clinical Features

Clinically there can be profuse mucopurulent nasal discharge with or without nasal obstruction. The other clinical manifestations are fever, cough, headache, facial pain, anosmia and irritability in young infants and children. The clinical signs of acute severe infection are purulent rhinorrhea, high-grade fever and facial pain or tenderness. On clinical examination, nasal mucosa may be erythematous. Presence of purulent discharge at the middle meatus may be a strong pointer and periorbital edema can be a sign of ethmoidal sinusitis. Tenderness on percussion of the maxillary or frontal sinuses may be present. Transillumination of the sinuses is not helpful for the diagnosis. There may be effusion in the ear as acute otitis media (AOM) is commonly seen in young children.

Diagnosis

The diagnosis of acute sinusitis is essentially clinical. In patients with recurrent sinusitis, persistent symptoms or chronic sinusitis investigations may be required. It is mainly radiological. X-ray paranasal sinuses or CT/MRI of paranasal sinuses and osteomeatal complex are usually done. Investigations are not required for the management of acute sinusitis as the diagnosis is essentially clinical. However, investigations are necessary to identify associated conditions and complications.

Laboratory tests are not very useful in diagnosis although they can help in detecting presence of associated conditions, e.g. allergic rhinitis, cystic fibrosis or immunodeficiency.

Radiology

X-rays

In children with persistent symptoms, the prediction based on history is so high, routine X-rays may not be useful. Involved sinuses show complete opacification, mucosal thickening of at least 4 mm, or an air-fluid level. Usually X-rays are reserved for patients who do not recover or worsen on appropriate antimicrobial therapy or have complications or unclear diagnosis. In general, Waters, Caldwell and lateral views are obtained to visualize the sinuses.

CT Scans/MRI

Those with complications, persistent or recurrent infections that are not responsive and to plan surgical intervention, including sinus aspiration CT scan/MRI are done. MRI is generally reserved for complicated case or suspected fungal cases.

Microbiological Diagnosis

Although sinus aspiration is the gold standard for the diagnosis of ABS, it is an invasive, time-consuming, and potentially painful procedure not routinely recommended in children. Sinus aspirate should only be performed by a person trained in it and is not recommended for the routine diagnosis of bacterial sinus infections in children. However, recovery of bacteria from the cavity of a paranasal sinus is diagnostic and correlate with clinical and radiographic findings in children with acute respiratory symptoms.

Complications

Children with untreated bacterial sinusitis are at risk for serious complications, which may be the presenting manifestations. Complications may result from intraorbital or intracranial extension. Findings that should prompt consideration of intracranial extension include the combination of eye swelling with persistent headache and vomiting. Vomiting and headache that requires hospital admission, particularly in older children with altered level of consciousness, focal neurological deficits with signs of meningeal irritation arouse suspicion of intracranial complications of acute sinusitis. Systemic complications are toxic shock syndrome, systemic sepsis and triggering of asthma.

Treatment

Any child with persistent rhinorrhea (character of discharge is not important) with or without cough for more than 10 days or earlier if there is clinical deterioration or with signs and symptoms of severe URTI (fever 39°C, facial swelling, facial pain) need treatment with antibiotics. Approximately 6–13% of viral rhinosinusitis in children is complicated by ABS.

Antibiotic Therapy

Antibiotics that are used to treat ABS must provide antibacterial coverage for *S. pneumoniae, H. influenzae* and *Moraxella catarrhalis*. Additional factors to be considered include the severity of clinical illness, recent exposure to antibiotics and other factors that increase the likelihood of infection with a resistant bacterial species. Drug of choice is amoxicillin 40–50 mg/kg/day BD or TDS. High or double dose of amoxicillin is advised in the West in view of strains of drug-resistant *Streptococcus pneumoniae* (DRSP) showing intermediate and high level of resistance to penicillin, which is circumvented by increase in drug dosage. As the incidence of DRSP is currently low in India, a high dose of amoxicillin is not warranted. In a child, attending day care or with a history of recent antibiotics (in the last 4 weeks) with penicillin group of drugs are at a risk of having resistant strains and high dose of amoxicillin (80–90 mg/kg/day) may be advised. The duration of antibiotics is for 10–14 days or for 7 days beyond the resolution of symptoms whichever is later. The other drugs that could be used are co-amoxiclav, macrolide, cephalosporins (cephalexin, cefuroxime, cefdinir, cefpodoxime and parenteral ceftriaxone/cefotaxime).

Surgical Interventions

Surgical option like functional endoscopic sinus surgery, antrostomy, adenoidectomy, polypectomy and ethmoidectomy are reserved for chronic sinusitis. Adjuvants like decongestants, antihistamines, nasal saline irrigation and topical steroids have been tried with varied results. There are limited data regarding the efficacy of these therapies in children with ABS.

ACUTE OTITIS MEDIA

Otitis media is defined as inflammation of the middle ear. It is classified as:
- *Acute otitis media (AOM):* Acute onset of signs and symptoms of middle ear inflammation with presence of fluid in the middle ear.
- *Recurrent otitis media:* Defined as three episodes of AOM in 6 months or four episodes/year.
- *Otitis media with effusion:* It is presence of fluid in the middle ear following an episode of AOM with no signs and symptoms of inflammation.
- *Chronic suppurative otitis media:* It is chronic discharge from middle ear through the perforated ear drum following an AOM.

Causative Organisms

Colonization of the upper respiratory tract precedes infection. In the developing countries more than 50% of children are colonized with pathogens by 6 months compared to a slower rate in developed countries. Common organisms implicated in the infection of the middle ear are viruses like RSV, influenza, rhinovirus, bacterial trinity of *S. pneumoniae,* nontypeable *H. influenzae, M. catarrhalis*; rarely bacteria like other streptococci, staphylococci and *Pseudomonas* are also known to cause AOM in children.

Clinical Features and Diagnosis

History of earache, ear discharge, dizziness and fever, usually accompanied by URI is common. In younger age nonspecific symptoms like irritability, lethargy and disturbed sleep are seen. The diagnosis is by history and otoscopic examination. Otoscopy may reveal red inflamed drum, perforation, bulging or retracted tympanic membrane and air-fluid level behind the drum.

Distinguishing AOM from otitis media with effusion in clinical practice is important. The effusion can be confirmed by the existence of an air-fluid level, air bubbles behind the tympanic membrane or reduced mobility when pneumo-otoscopy or a type B tympanogram is performed. In addition to middle ear effusion, diagnosis of AOM requires the recent onset of signs and symptoms of acute inflammation, such as earache, ear tugging or a bulging tympanic membrane.

Treatment

Antibiotic usage depends on age and severity of illness. Antibiotic is commenced immediately in children less than

2 years of age and in others with severe disease such as children with temperature above 102°F with toxemia and substantial otalgia. In nontoxic children older than 2 years watchful waiting for 48 hours and commencing antibiotics if clinical deterioration occurs is advisable. Initial therapy for severe cases is with amoxicillin-clavulanate (45 mg/kg/day BD) or IV ceftriaxone (50 mg/kg/day) and for non-severe cases is with oral amoxicillin (45 mg/kg/day BD). The duration of therapy is for 10 days and in children above 5 years, 7 days treatment is sufficient. In a child, attending day care or with a history of recent antibiotics (in the last 4 weeks) with penicillin group of drugs are at risk of having resistant strains and high dose of (80–90 mg/kg/day) amoxicillin may be advised. Other drugs like macrolides (clarithromycin, azithromycin), cefaclor, cefuroxime, cefdinir and cefpodoxime can be used for treatment of AOM (Flowchart 3.3.2).

In otherwise healthy children, the primary intervention is tympanostomy tube insertion (grommet). The indications being persistent hearing loss of 40 decibels or greater or symptomatic disease (balance difficulties or sleep disturbance associated with intermittent ear pain, fullness or popping). Antihistamines and decongestants are ineffective and therapy with antimicrobials or corticosteroids does not result in lasting benefit. The risk with antibiotic prophylaxis is the emergence of drug-resistant strains in the community.

In recurrent otitis media the options available are antibiotic prophylaxis (amoxicillin/erythromycin/cotrimoxazole with half the therapeutic dose as once or twice a day dose), tympanostomy tube insertion, adenoidectomy and vaccination against pneumococcus and *H. influenzae*. Antibiotic prophylaxis may have the risk of relapse on stopping medication.

For earache oral paracetamol should be given in AOM. Topical agents like antimicrobial, anti-inflammatory or steroids play no role in intact tympanic membrane.

In children with severe pain, myringotomy is an effective method to attain relief.

Risk group for AOM are early in the 1st year of life, male gender, family history of frequent recurrent infections and day care attendance. Breastfeeding for the first 6 months of life seems to delay the age of onset of AOM.

Complications

Acute mastoiditis, facial nerve paralysis, labrynthitis, temporal bone osteomyelitis, intracranial abscess can occur after AOM.

CROUP SYNDROME

Introduction

Croup is a respiratory illness characterized by inspiratory stridor, cough and hoarseness. These symptoms result from inflammation in the larynx and subglottic airway. A barking cough is the hallmark of croup among infants and young children, whereas hoarseness predominates in older children and adults. Although croup usually is a mild and self-limited illness, significant upper airway obstruction (UAO), respiratory distress and rarely mortality can occur. The term croup has been used to describe a variety of upper respiratory conditions in children, including laryngitis, laryngotracheitis, laryngotracheobronchitis, bacterial tracheitis or spasmodic croup.

Pathophysiology

Stridor is a harsh high-pitched sound produced by vibration of upper airway structures at or near the larynx mostly during inspiration. Stridor is due to extrathoracic airflow limitation/obstruction (i.e. UAO). Upper airway obstruction is defined as blockage of any portion of the airway above the thoracic inlet. Stridor is more during inspiration as the

FLOWCHART 3.3.2: Management protocol for acute otitis media.

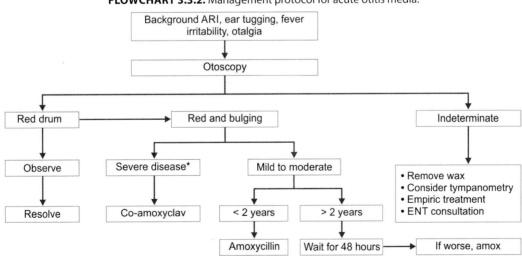

*Severe disease – explosive onset, severe otalgia, toxicity and high grade fever 102° F⁺
Source: RIT-GEM: IAP Action Plan; 2006

pressure within the upper airway is negative relative to the atmosphere causing collapse of the upper airway. There can be an expiratory component in severe obstruction producing flow limitation during expiration as well or when the lesion extends into intrathoracic level. Upper airway obstruction can range from nose block to life threatening obstruction of the larynx/upper trachea. Stridor is minimal during sleep as the inspiratory flow rate is minimal. Hoarseness is suggestive of vocal cord involvement. Upper airway obstruction results in some degree of suprasternal retraction as a result of pressure gradient between the trachea and the atmosphere.

In supraglottic etiology, the stridor changes with position of the head and neck. Usually supraglottic lesions exhibit less stridor on crying as the surrounding muscle tone increases, whereas in contrast obstructive lesion below glottis causes more stridor in view of increased inspiratory flow of air. Positional stridor always suggests anatomical origin.

Lower airway obstruction, i.e. below thoracic inlet produces more symptoms during expiration as intrathoracic pressure is more relative to atmospheric pressure during exhalation. Intrathoracic airway can cause inspiratory symptom when associated with severe lesion or fixed lesion or with increased airway secretions.

Viral Croup

Viral ALTB or croup is the most common UAO in childhood with peak incidence at 2 years (range 6 months to 6 years). The most common cause for croup is parainfluenza virus; other organisms implicated are influenza virus, RSV and rhinovirus. Rarely mycoplasma, measles and adenovirus are also implicated.

Clinical Features

Croup has an insidious onset. It usually follows a prodrome of mild fever, rhinorrhea and sore throat either in the child or family members. Acute laryngotracheobronchitis has a triad of stridor, barking cough and retraction (suprasternal) in a nontoxic child. A small number of patients may get recurrent croup. Croup tends to be worse at late night and early morning. On chest auscultation the breath sounds are usually normal. There can be wheeze suggestive of bronchitis. In croup, routine throat examination and laryngoscopy may precipitate complete obstruction and must be performed only when required by those with expertise in intubation with necessary equipment on standby.

Differential Diagnosis

Upper airway obstruction can be classified as supraglottic and subglottic obstruction. In supraglottic obstruction like epiglottitis, peritonsillar/RPA the stridor is mild and the voice is muffled. The child is usually toxic with high fever, drooling

of saliva, trismus, dysphagia and usually assumes a sitting up or arching posture to compensate for the airway patency. In subglottic obstruction like croup, angioedema, foreign body or tracheitis the stridor is loud with hoarse voice. The child is usually not toxic except in tracheitis and there can be facial edema in angioedema. Other differentials for croup include foreign body, laryngitis and neurogenic stridor.

Epiglottitis

Common in 2–6 years of age and the most common organism is *H. influenzae* type B. The onset is rapid with short prodrome (Table 3.3.4). The child is usually toxic, has a tripod sitting posture, i.e. leaning forward and looks agitated. Lateral neck X-ray can show thumb sign (thickened epiglottis). Treatment is usually with parenteral ceftriaxone and endotracheal intubation by a trained intensivist to maintain airway patency when there is an impending risk of obstruction in severe cases. Prevention is by vaccination against *H. influenzae* type B.

Peritonsillar Abscess

It has usually a biphasic illness with sudden deterioration following sore throat and is common in older children above 10 years of age. The causative organisms are usually GAS and anaerobes. It is a toxic condition. The management is by surgical drainage and antimicrobials, IV penicillin or 3rd generation cephalosporin with metronidazole or clindamycin. It can be usually prevented by early treatment of GAS sore throat with antibiotics.

Retropharyngeal Abscess/Lateral or Parapharyngeal Abscess

Retropharyngeal abscess has an insidious to sudden onset of toxic manifestation involving the posterior pharynx. It is common in boys younger than 3–4 years, the retropharyngeal node involutes after 5 years making RPA in older children and adolescents uncommon. In RPA and lateral pharyngeal abscess the causative organisms are usually polymicrobial, the usual pathogens being GAS, *Staphylococcus* and oropharyngeal anaerobes.

Table 3.3.4: Clinical difference between epiglottitis and viral croup.

	Epiglottitis	*Croup*
Stridor	Quiet	Loud
Voice alteration	Aphonic, muffled	Hoarse
Dysphagia	+	–
Postural preference	+	–
Barky cough	–	+
Fever	+++	+
Toxicity	++	–
X-ray neck	Thumb sign	Steeple sign

The presentation of RPA depends upon the stage of illness. The disease in the early stages may be indistinguishable from those of pharyngitis. As disease progresses the symptoms are related to inflammation and obstruction of the upper aerodigestive tract. In severe cases, RPA can present as neck stiffness or torticollis and lateral pharyngeal abscess can also cause dysphagia.

In lateral neck X-ray, the anteroposterior diameter of the prevertebral soft-tissue space in children should not exceed that of the contiguous vertebral bodies. CT scan of the neck with IV contrast generally differentiates RPA from cellulitis.

Management of RPA or lateral pharyngeal abscess is intravenous antibiotics with or without surgical drainage. Surgical intervention is required if they have sign of UAO or fail to respond medically. Most of them respond well to medical management. Clindamycin or IV penicillin or third generation cephalosporin and IV metronidazole or ampicillin with sulbactam are the antibiotics commonly used.

Membranous Croup (Bacterial Tracheitis)

It is a biphasic illness following a croup or influenza virus infection with secondary bacterial infection. *S. aureus* is the most common offending agent, whereas *S. pneumoniae*, Moraxella and *H. influenzae* are also implicated. It is a severe toxic condition which can manifest as toxic shock syndrome. Lateral radiograph of the chest may reveal ragged irregular tracheal borders and nonspecific edema or intraluminal membranes of tracheal wall. Therapy with cloxacillin and aminoglycoside is preferred. Alternative drugs like cefazolin/cefuroxime/vancomycin can be used.

Spasmodic and Recurrent Croup

It has a sudden onset of symptom similar to viral croup. It is common in the age group of 3 months to 3 years of age. They are not toxic with no associated signs and symptoms. The attacks are usually at night, but seldom life-threatening and are common in children with atopic tendency. Diagnosis is mainly based on clinical background; however, it is difficult to ascertain the diagnosis from initial attacks. A striking feature of spasmodic croup is its recurrent nature; hence the alternate descriptive term "frequently recurrent croup" is used. Cool mist may be of benefit in these children and in rare scenarios management like a viral croup may be required.

Classification of Viral Croup Severity

Croup severity is based on general features and degree of respiratory distress (Table 3.3.5). Score above 7 needs ICU admission, intense monitoring, corticosteroids and nebulized adrenaline.

Danger signs of impending airway obstruction are: Agitation, fatigue, drowsiness, decreased air entry, tachypnea with severe retractions and tachycardia.

Table 3.3.5: Croup severity based on scoring system.

Features	Score		
	0	1	2
Stridor	None	Inspiratory	Inspiratory and expiratory
Air entry	Normal	Decreased	Minimal to absent
Retractions	None to minimal	Suprasternal	Suprasternal, sternal, subcostal
Color	Normal	Cyanosis in room air	Cyanosis in 40% oxygen
Consciousness	Alert	Irritable, consolable by parents	Drowsy

Investigations

Diagnosis is mainly clinical and investigations are required when the diagnosis is uncertain. Unnecessarily disturbing the child may worsen the distress and obstruction. In viral croup the X-ray anteroposterior or posterior anterior view of the soft tissue of the neck reveals a tapered narrowing (steeple sign) of the subglottic trachea instead of the normal shouldered appearance. The radiological finding does not reflect the severity of airway obstruction.

Management

In mild croup, (i.e. barking cough in an otherwise normal child with stridor only on crying or coughing and no stridor at rest, with minimal or no increase in work of breathing) there is no need for specific therapy. Regular observation for worsening of clinical features should be reinforced. Humidification with saline nebulization or steam inhalation is sufficient to moisturize the airway and provide symptomatic relief.

In moderate to severe croup that can be life-threatening, an aggressive therapy with oxygen, steroids and inhaled adrenaline with minimal handling of patient is beneficial. Humidified oxygen is the initial management of moderate to severe croup if SaO_2 is less than 92%. Then nebulized racemic adrenaline (1 in 1,000 dilutions at a dose of 0.5 mL/kg to a maximum dose of 5 mL) can be given. The mode of action being topical vasoconstriction. Croup score improves within 30 minutes and the effect lasts for 2–4 hours and, if needed, it can be repeated accordingly.

Oral prednisolone (1–2 mg/kg/day) or oral/IV/IM dexamethasone (0.6 mg/kg/day) or nebulized budesonide (2 mg every 12 hours) are all found to be effective and can be continued for 48–72 hours. Systemic steroids have been found to decrease the number of adrenaline nebulization, length of hospital stay and the need for intubation.

In severe UAO associated with signs of impending airway obstruction endotracheal intubation with one-half smaller size tube should be done by an expert with adequate backup.

Always watch for development of air leak around the tube which indicates resolution of edema. Ventilation is usually not required as the lungs are normal and intubation is only to bypass the obstruction. Tracheostomy should be reserved only when all other measures fail. Antibiotics have no role in viral croup. If croup not responding well for treatment an alternative diagnosis should always be considered.

BIBLIOGRAPHY

1. Agrawal R, Singh V, Yewale V. RTI facts; bugs, drugs and you. IAP Consensus Guidelines on Rational Management of Respiratory Tract Infection in Children. IAP Action Plan, 2006.
2. Cherry JD, Shapiro NL. Sinusitis. In: Feigin RD, Cherry J, Demmler-Harrison GJ, Kaplan SL (Eds). Feign and Cherry's Textbook of Pediatric Infectious Diseases, 6th edition. Philadelphia: Saunders, 2009.p.201.
3. Cherry JD. Clinical practice. Croup. N Engl J Med. 2008;358(4): 384-91.
4. Kliegman RM, Stanton BF, St Geme JW, et al. The respiratory system. In: Nelson Textbook of Pediatrics, 19th edition. Philadelphia: Elsevier Saunders; 2012.pp.1429-53.
5. Singh M, Singh M. Heated, humidified air for the common cold. Cochrane Database Syst Rev. 2011;5:CD001728.
6. Subramanyam L, Sivabalan So, Gowrishankar NC, et al. Upper respiratory tract infection. Essentials of Pediatric Pulmonology, 3rd edition. Chennai: Pediatric Pulmonology Foundation of India; 2008.pp.149-57.
7. Wald ER. Acute bacterial sinusitis in children: clinical features and diagnosis. In: Kaplan SL, Friedman EM, Wood RA (Eds). Waltham MA, 2012.
8. Wald ER. Approach to diagnosis of acute infectious pharyngitis in children and adolescents. In: Edwards MS, Friedman EM (Eds). Up To Date. Waltham MA, 2012.

3.4 COMMUNITY-ACQUIRED PNEUMONIA

Sushil Kumar Kabra

INTRODUCTION

Pneumonia is an acute inflammation of the lung parenchyma usually caused by infections. There is no universally accepted definition of pneumonia. Some define pneumonia based on history of respiratory symptoms and clinical findings while others look at chest X-ray (CXR) for the infiltrates to define pneumonia. World Health Organization (WHO) has defined pneumonia solely based on clinical findings, looking for the respiratory rate and presence of chest retractions.

EPIDEMIOLOGY

The incidence of pneumonia in children below 5 years is estimated to be 0.29 episodes per child-year in developing countries and 0.05 episodes per child-year in developed countries. There are about 156 million new episodes each year worldwide of which 151 million episodes are in the developing world accounting for more than 95% of all new cases worldwide. Among the developing world, India shares the largest burden with 43 million new episodes of pneumonia every year followed by China, Pakistan, Bangladesh and Indonesia. Among all community cases 7–13% are severe enough to be life-threatening and require hospitalization, killing more than 2 million children every year.

ETIOLOGY

Pneumonia can be caused by infectious or noninfectious agents. Most cases of pneumonia are caused by microorganisms (bacteria, virus, fungi and occasionally parasites). The noninfectious causes include aspiration of food or gastric acid, foreign bodies, hydrocarbons, lipid substances, hypersensitivity reactions and drug or radiation-induced pneumonitis.

The infective etiology depends on age of patient. In neonatal period gram-negative enteric bacteria are the most common pathogens and are transmitted via vertical transmission from the mother during birth. Group B β-hemolytic streptococci, commonly reported as etiological agents in this group from industrialized country are rarely reported from India.

In children between ages 2 months and 5 years, in developing countries, bacterial infections are the most common cause of pneumonia in less than 5 years of age. Based on lung aspirates 62% of pneumonia were due to bacterial infections. The common bacterial pathogens identified were *Streptococcus pneumoniae* and *Haemophilus influenzae* in 27% patients each. Other pathogens were *Staphylococcus* and gram-negative bacilli. Viral pathogens have been isolated in nasopharyngeal aspirates of children below 5 years of age with pneumonia in 44–49% cases and respiratory syncytial virus is the most common virus isolated. Atypical organisms like *Mycoplasma pneumoniae* and *Chlamydia pneumoniae* are emerging pathogens for community-acquired pneumonia (CAP) in preschool-aged children and are common causes of CAP in older children and adolescents. There are very few studies that have looked in for all possible etiological agents in children. Table 3.4.1 gives summary of etiological agents based on all the published studies in literature. Mixed infections due to bacteria and viruses may be seen in 10–40% in hospitalized children.

In children with HIV infection, bacterial infection remains the major cause of pneumonia, but additional pathogens like *Pneumocystis jirovecii* should be considered particularly in infants and children with low CD4 counts. Other causes of pneumonia in such children include mycobacterial infections, fungal infections and viral infections.

Pertussis should be considered in all children with CAP, especially if immunizations are not complete. *Mycobacterium tuberculosis* may cause CAP in children who have been exposed to adult patient with sputum *acid-fast bacillus* positive tuberculosis.

CLINICAL FEATURES

Children with pneumonia may present with fever with or without chills, cough, fast breathing and in severe cases chest retractions, nasal flaring, lethargy or irritability, inability to feed. Very severe cases of pneumonia may present with cyanosis and respiratory failure. Among these the fever and fast breathing are the most consistent symptoms. The atypical manifestations include vomiting, diarrhea, abdominal distention, neck retraction in infants and small children, and chest pain, shoulder pain, abdominal pain in older children.

Children with bacterial pneumonia may have high grade fever, chills, productive cough and systemic manifestations including that of sepsis. Rapid progression is characteristic of more severe cases of bacterial pneumonia. Wheezing is not a feature of bacterial pneumonia. Children with viral pneumonia may have the prodrome with symptoms of upper respiratory tract illness including cough and rhinitis later developing fast breathing and low to moderate grade fever and wheezing. Children with pneumonia due to mycoplasma and chlamydia infection (called atypical pneumonia) may have gradual onset with headache, malaise, nonproductive cough, low grade fever and rhonchi.

During physical examination, one should assess the general well-being of the child, count the respiratory rate

Table 3.4.1: Etiological agents of acute lower respiratory infection in children.

Age group	Common causes of pneumonia	Less common causes of pneumonia
Neonates and infants:	**Bacteria:**	**Bacteria:**
< 2 months	*Klebsiella pneumoniae,*	Pneumococci
	E. coli	*H. influenzae*
	Other gram-negative bacteria	Anaerobic organisms
	Staphylococcal infections	*Ureaplasma urealyticum*
		Viruses:
		Cytomegalovirus
		Herpes simplex virus
2 months to 5 years	**Bacteria:**	**Bacteria:**
	Pneumococci	Pertussis
	H. influenzae	*M. tuberculosis*
	S. aureus	*N. meningitidis*
	Klebsiella pneumoniae	
	Chlamydia	**Viruses:**
	Mycoplasma	Measles
		Varicella zoster
	Viruses:	
	Respiratory syncytial virus	
	Parainfluenza virus	
	Influenza virus	
	Human metapneumovirus	
	Adenovirus	
	Rhinovirus	
More than 5 years	**Bacteria:**	**Bacteria:**
	Pneumococci	*H. influenzae*
	Mycoplasma	*S. aureus*
	Chlamydia	*M. tuberculosis*
		Viruses:
		Adenovirus
		Epstein-Barr virus
		Influenza virus
		Parainfluenza virus
		Respiratory syncytial virus
		Rhinovirus

for full 1 minute when the child is not crying, assess the hydration status and examine the respiratory system for physical abnormality. Review of other system should also be done to look for the associated infections or complications.

The physical examination findings depend on the severity, stage of pneumonia and associated complications. Some time, there may not be any abnormality on auscultation. Early in the course of illness decreased breath sounds and crackles and rhonchi may be present on the affected lung field. With increasing consolidation or development of pleural effusion, pyothorax or pyopneumothorax there will be dull note on percussion and diminished or absent breath sounds on affected side. Other physical abnormalities include abdominal distension due to paralytic ileus, neck rigidity which may be due to associated meningitis or apical lobe pneumonia, severe gastroesophageal reflux disease which may have aspiration pneumonia.

DIAGNOSIS

Pneumonia is usually a clinical diagnosis. The utility of various clinical features in making the diagnosis of pneumonia has been studied. Tachypnea is the consistent useful sign of pneumonia with sensitivity of 64–81% and specificity of 54–70%. It has the advantage of high reproducibility, very less interperson variability, does not need high expertize and hence it can be used at community level by health worker in making the diagnosis of pneumonia. However, tachypnea alone may occur with other conditions like fever, reactive airway disease, nasal blockade which may be associated with pneumonia or upper respiratory illness. This may lead to unnecessary antibiotic therapy that is not desirable. Therefore presence of tachypnea may be a starting point not a diagnostic criterion for making a diagnosis of pneumonia in children under care of pediatricians.

Chest in-drawing has sensitivity of 17–35% and specificity of 82–84% in identifying pneumonia. Auscultatory signs have lower specificity and poor reproducibility between observers. Crackles are 43–57% sensitive and 75–80% specific in identifying pneumonia in the community. These criteria may not be as sensitive in malnourished children.

Fall in oxygen saturation or cyanosis is generally a late sign and may not help in making the diagnosis of pneumonia when present, it indicates severe pneumonia. Normoxia does not necessarily correlate with mild disease.

In developing world, the diagnosis of pneumonia is made based on the WHO's age-specific criteria for tachypnea which can also be used at community level for making diagnosis and referral. The criteria for diagnosis and the assessment of severity of CAP in children are listed in Table 3.4.2.

Chest X-ray is done to confirm the diagnosis of pneumonia. The CXR in viral pneumonia is characterized by hyperinflation, bronchial wall thickening and focal areas of atelectasis. Confluent lobar consolidation indicates pneumococcal pneumonia. Chest X-ray may be normal if it is taken early in the course of pneumonia. Chest X-ray does not differentiate causative agents of pneumonia. Since CXR does not change the outcome of pneumonia, it is not

Table 3.4.2: Diagnosis and assessment of severity of pneumonia in children aged 2 months to 5 years with cough or difficult breathing.

Clinical category	Essential features
Very severe pneumonia	Central cyanosis, or not able to breastfeed or drink, or convulsions, or lethargy or unconsciousness, or severe respiratory distress (e.g. head nodding)
Severe pneumonia	Lower chest in drawing, or nasal flaring, and no signs of very severe pneumonia
Pneumonia	Fast breathing, e.g. Age RR/min • 2 months up to 12 months ≥ 50 • 12 months up to 5 years ≥ 40 and no indicators of severe or very severe pneumonia
No pneumonia	No fast breathing and no indicators of severe or very severe pneumonia

recommended for making a diagnosis of pneumonia. It should be reserved for only those children with ambiguous clinical findings, persistent pneumonia, pneumonia that is unresponsive to antibiotic therapy and for those with suspected complications of pneumonia such as pleural effusions.

For rational treatment of pneumonia it is desirable that etiological agent is identified by clinical features or rapid and less expensive laboratory tests. It is not easy to distinguish bacterial and viral pneumonias based on clinical features or CXR findings. Bacterial pneumonia in children is associated with moderate to high grade fever, polymorphonuclear response in blood, increased levels of acute phase reactants like C-reactive proteins and procalcitonin in blood and alveolar consolidation on radiograph of chest. Viral pneumonia is more commonly associated with young age, breathlessness and wheezing. However, all the clinical features and laboratory test do not have desirable sensitivity and specificity to use them in clinical practice.

The common methods used for identification of the etiologic agents include blood culture, lung puncture, nasopharyngeal aspirates, immunoassays of blood and urine. All these methods have their own drawbacks. The blood culture is not a reliable investigation because of its low yield (ranging from 5% to 30% in various studies) in bacterial pneumonias. Lung puncture is an invasive procedure associated with high incidence of pneumothorax and pulmonary hemorrhage and hence cannot be performed routinely in all cases. Nasopharyngeal aspirates can be used for isolation of viruses, *Chlamydia* and *Mycoplasma*, but a possibility of concomitant bacterial pneumonia cannot be ruled out with confidence. There are various immunoassays for identifying bacteria, viruses, mycoplasma, *Chlamydia* and *P. jirovecii* but are expensive and need standardization in community studies. In view of difficulties faced with identification of organisms, the high cost and lack of availability of the investigations, the laboratory tests are not

ordered routinely for the diagnosis of CAP. Most of the cases are diagnosed on clinical grounds and treated accordingly. In children with poor response, underlying systemic disease and immunocompromised hosts, an aggressive attempt should be made to identify etiological agents.

MANAGEMENT

In developing world, in view of very high incidence of pneumonia it is recommended to make the diagnosis of pneumonia at community level based on clinical features alone. The diagnostic criteria suggested by WHO are very cost-effective for CAP. There is no indication for any test in a child with suspected CAP. Children with nonsevere CAP with no danger signs should be treated on outpatient basis with oral antibiotics and antipyretics.

Indications for Hospitalization

Children with danger signs should be hospitalized. Factors determining the need for hospital admission in children with CAP are listed in Box 3.4.1.

Indications for Intensive Care Unit Admission

Children with very severe pneumonia may need intensive care. Indications for shifting the child with severe pneumonia to intensive care unit are listed in Box 3.4.2.

Box 3.4.1

Indications for admission in hospital.
- Age younger than 2 months
- Toxic appearance
- Hypoxemia
- Oxygen saturation <92%
- Cyanosis
- Respiratory difficulty
- Apnea
- Grunting
- Flaring of the nostrils
- Dehydration, vomiting or poor feeding
- Immunocompromised status
- Failure to respond to oral antibiotics
- Inadequate observation or supervision by family

Box 3.4.2

Indications for intensive care unit admission.
- PaO_2/FiO_2 <250
- Mechanical ventilation
- Chest X-ray showing bilateral, multilobar pneumonia with increase in the size of the opacity >50% in 48 hours prior to admission
- Hypotension
- Vasopressors requirement
- Acute renal failure

Selection of Antibiotic

Administration of appropriate antibiotics in the early course of pneumonia alters the outcome of illness particularly when the causative agent is a bacterium. Antibiotics may not have any role in pneumonia caused by viruses. Unnecessary antibiotics administration in children may lead to selection of resistant organism and thus promotes drug resistance and serious illness in the future. However, in view of the public health implications of better outcome of pneumonia by early administration of antibiotics and lack of reliable laboratory test in identification of causative agents, antibiotics are administered empirically in most instances. Treatment decisions are based on the child's age and clinical and epidemiologic factors. Factors that may help in selection of appropriate antibiotics include: knowledge of etiological agents, sensitivity of pathogens to antibiotics, severity of the disease, immune status, nutritional status, previous antimicrobial usages in the recent past, history of hospitalization, duration of illness, associated complications and cost and safety of antibiotics.

Likely etiological agents: The common etiological agents of CAP in infants below 2 months include gram-negative bacilli. In children from 2 months to 5 years, it is commonly caused by *S. pneumoniae, H. influenzae, Staphylococcus aureus* and atypical organisms and in children above 5 years of age *S. pneumoniae, S. aureus* and *Mycoplasma.*

Sensitivity of pathogen: Common etiological agents including *S. pneumoniae* and *H. influenzae*, are sensitive to wide range of antibiotics including semisynthetic penicillin (amoxicillin, ampicillin), cephalosporins (cephalexin, cefaclor, cefuroxime), macrolides (erythromycin, roxithromycin, azithromycin and clarithromycin), cotrimoxazole and chloramphenicol. Gram-negative bacilli are sensitive to ampicillin, third-generation cephalosporins and aminoglycosides.

Atypical organisms such as *Chlamydia* and *Mycoplasma* are sensitive to macrolides and tetracycline. The latter is not used in children below 8 years of age due to dental staining later in life. Thus macrolides are the drug of choice for treatment of pneumonia due to atypical organisms.

Newer quinolones such as gatifloxacin and levofloxacin have an advantage of good coverage for *S. pneumoniae, H. influenzae* and atypical organisms. However, the experience of these antimicrobials in children is limited and need more studies before they can be used as first-line drug in CAP.

Severity of illness: In most circumstances microbial etiology of pneumonia remains similar despite varying degree of severity of illness. However, it is logical to select the most appropriate antibiotics that have lesser chance of failure due to possible resistant organisms in more severe disease.

Underlying disease: Knowledge about the underlying disease (pulmonary or extrapulmonary) is essential in selecting antibiotic as many chronic diseases have special predisposition to particular organisms. Children with hemoglobinopathies or nephrotic syndrome are more susceptible to pneumococcal infections. A child with cystic fibrosis is more likely to have infections with *Staphylococcus, H. influenzae* or *Pseudomonas.* Immunodeficiency whether primary or secondary predisposes a child to opportunistic infections. Pneumonia in HIV infection may be due to Gram-negative bacilli, *P. jirovecii* and fungi in addition to usual pathogens. The progression of disease is rapid in this group of patients due to immunodeficiency and hence most efficient antibiotic combinations are used as first-line treatment. Children with neutropenia should be treated with antibiotics that are effective against Gram-negative bacilli, *Staphylococcus* along with common pathogens like *S. pneumoniae* and *H. influenzae.* Hence the drug of choice may be ceftazidime with aminoglycosides with/without cloxacillin or vancomycin. If patient does not respond over 2–3 days the next may be to consider antifungal antibiotics and treatment of *P. jirovecii* pneumonia.

Nutritional status: Malnourished children are predisposed to more frequent and severe episodes of pneumonia. The etiology of pneumonia in malnourished children is generally similar to that in well nourished, with an added predisposition for gram-negative organisms. Pneumonia in malnourished children may progress to severe disease rapidly. The symptoms of pneumonia may be masked in severely malnourished children possibly due to a blunted inflammatory response.

Previous antibiotics: History of antibiotics for the current episode or in the recent past (previous 2–4 weeks) may give an idea about possible resistant organisms. If a patient had received repeated course of antibiotics patient's microbial flora may be resistant to those antibiotics. If a patient has already received cotrimoxazole or amoxicillin, it is better to give amoxicillin-clavulanic acid, cefuroxime or cefpodoxime rather than giving same antibiotics.

History of hospitalization: After hospitalization the microbial flora of a patient changes to gram-negative bacilli. Hence, pneumonia in hospitalized child or hospitalized in recent past is more likely to be due to gram-negative bacilli. The staphylococcal infection in hospital setting is likely to be resistant to penicillin and needs vancomycin or linezolid. In such situations, cefuroxime or amoxicillin-clavulanic acid may be used as primary drugs in nonsevere illness and combination of quinolone or third-generation cephalosporins with vancomycin may be used in severe pneumonia.

Duration of illness: A short duration of the illness suggests a possible bacterial etiology. Prolonged illness of more than 2 weeks may be due to infection with *M. tuberculosis*, atypical organism or certain viral infections like adenovirus.

Indications for intravenous antibiotic therapy: Intravenous antibiotic therapy is warranted if the child has severe

Table 3.4.3: The choice of antibiotics in pneumonia for children.

| | Community-acquired pneumonia | | Pneumonia with high risk factors | |
	Nonsevere	*Severe*	*Nonsevere*	*Severe*
First line	Amoxicillin	Penicillin/Ampicillin + Gentamicin	Amoxicillin-clavulanic acid	Third-generation cephalosporin+ aminoglycosides
Alternative	Cefaclor, Cephalexin, Macrolides, Cotrimoxazole	Cefuroxime, Amoxicillin-clavulanic acid	Cefuroxime	Amoxicillin-clavulanic acid + Aminoglycoside, Cefuroxime + Aminoglycoside
Second line	Cefuroxime, Amoxicillin-clavulanic acid, Cefpodoxime, Cefdinir	Amoxicillin-clavulanic acid + Aminoglycoside, Cefuroxime + Aminoglycoside	Cotrimoxazole + Macrolide Amoxicillin-clavulanic acid + Macrolide	Third-generation cephalosporin + Aminoglycoside + Cloxacillin/ vancomycin
Alternative	Amoxicillin-clavulanic acid		Third-generation Cephalosporin + Cloxacillin	Quinolones + Vancomycin + Aminoglycosides

pneumonia, disturbed consciousness, improper swallowing, frequent vomiting and suspected drug malabsorption. Switch to oral when the child starts accepting orally and shows significant clinical improvement. Complete intravenous therapy is needed if the patient is newborn.

TREATMENT OF PNEUMONIA

Most cases of CAP respond well to antimicrobials. The case fatality is increased with presence of risk factors. To decrease the case fatality due to pneumonia, patients can be stratified into children with or without risk factors.

Community-acquired Pneumonia with no Risk Factors

Nonsevere pneumonia: Nonsevere pneumonia can be managed on ambulatory basis. Antimicrobials commonly used are amoxicillin, cotrimoxazole and oral cephalosporins. The usual duration of therapy is 5 days. Recent meta-analysis have demonstrated that a short course of antibiotic therapy given for 3 days is as effective as a 5 days therapy for nonsevere pneumonia in children under 5 years of age. Three days of antibiotics may be used only in WHO-defined CAP where follow-up of these patients is possible. Children being treated on outpatient basis should be reassessed after 3 days. Mother or caregiver should be alarmed about the danger signs which include lethargy, unable to drink, chest in-drawing, cyanosis and seizures. The attending pediatrician may assess the child by asking the parents about the general condition, feeding, fever, vomiting, sleep, etc. The child may be examined for tachypnea, air entry in chest, chest in-drawing, crepitations or rhonchi and bronchial breathing. If the assessment suggests deterioration, child may be treated with second-line oral drugs if there is no indication for hospital admission. If the child's condition is same, the primary drug may be continued for another 2 days and then reassessed. Deterioration in clinical conditions at any time

or no response even on day 4 of antibiotic therapy should be managed with second-line drugs as listed in Table 3.4.3. A CXR is warranted in such situation to look for the cause of poor or no response to antibiotic therapy.

Severe or very severe disease pneumonia: Children with severe or very severe disease need hospitalization. The first-line antibiotics include penicillin, cefuroxime or amoxicillin-clavulanic acid given by intravenous route. Recent meta-analysis comparing various antibiotics has shown that penicillin is better than chloramphenicol in children hospitalized for pneumonia. Once the child shows significant clinical improvement and starts accepting orally, the antibiotic should be shifted to oral route. A recent study has demonstrated improvement of severe pneumonia with oral amoxicillin. It is not advocated to generalize the same till large scale randomized studies are available. The optimal duration of antibiotics for severe pneumonia is unclear. Conventionally antibiotics are continued for a total of 7–10 days.

Community-acquired Pneumonia with Risk Factors

Nonsevere pneumonia: The antibiotics are selected based on the risk factors and severity of pneumonia. A child with nonsevere pneumonia should be treated with oral cefuroxime or amoxicillin-clavulanic acid for a period of 5–7 days. Monitoring, follow-up and assessment remain similar to CAP. In case of deterioration or failure of therapy the second-line antibiotic for these patients may be third-generation cephalosporins.

Severe pneumonia: Severe pneumonia with risk factors may be treated with third-generation cephalosporin with aminoglycoside with or without cloxacillin or vancomycin. The alternative antibiotics in such situations may be cefuroxime or amoxicillin-clavulanic acid with aminoglycosides. In selected cases, a combination of quinolones with cloxacillin or vancomycin may be required.

Community-acquired Pneumonia in Children above 5 Years of Age

The causes of pneumonia in children above 5 years of age are similar to that of adults including pneumococci and mycoplasma. There are no large studies documenting etiology of pneumonia in children above 5 years of age from India. Till we have more studies that document burden of pneumonia due to mycoplasma, treatment of pneumonia for this age group may be similar to that of children below 5 years of age. If a patient does not improve with antibiotics or there are clinical features pointing toward infections due to atypical organism a course of macrolide antibiotics may be given to these patients.

Monitoring for Response

Clinical improvement may take up to 48–96 hours; fever can last 2–4 days, leukocytosis usually resolves by day 4, abnormal physical findings may persist for more than 7 days. Most nonsevere CAP shows clinical resolution of symptoms in 2–3 days. Radiographs may worsen even though clinical picture is improving and CXR usually returns to normal within 6 weeks in patients and hence there is no role of follow-up CXR to look for the recovery.

Causes of Failure to Improve

The possible causes of failure to respond adequately are inadequate therapy which may be due to inappropriate antibiotic selection, inappropriate dosing and poor compliance. It can also be due to development of complications like empyema or lung abscess. If there is impaired host defense mechanism or there is development of drug resistance in the community, there may be delayed response or poor response. Nonbacterial CAP have longer course than expected. Bronchial obstruction due to endobronchial lesions, foreign body or mucus plug and pre-existing lung diseases like cystic fibrosis, ciliary dyskinesia or bronchiectasis may take longer than usual course to improve.

Supportive Therapy

Although antibiotic is the mainstay of therapy, children should be given supportive therapy for the associated problems. Children with pneumonia may have fever, poor oral intake, vomiting, electrolyte abnormalities, hypoxia and respiratory failure. It takes some time for the antibiotics to act.

Fever should be treated with paracetamol in doses of 10–15 mg/kg/dose. It can be repeated every 4–6 hourly.

Cough is common symptom associated with pneumonia. Cough suppressants should be avoided. Common household remedies, like tulsi, ginger and honey, may be given to the child. If there is bronchospasm, inhaled bronchodilators like salbutamol can be prescribed.

Vomiting in children with pneumonia often follows cough which do not require any treatment. If there is persistent vomiting, it should be managed with antiemetics after ruling out other causes of vomiting including central nervous system infection, acidosis or intestinal problems.

Associated comorbid conditions, like diarrhea, malnutrition, congenital heart diseases, immunodeficiencies, increase the case fatality in children with pneumonia. Children with congenital heart disease require careful monitoring for fluid and electrolyte balance as they are at risk of developing congestive heart failure. Children with diarrhea may need more fluids for correction of dehydration and ongoing losses apart from maintenance fluids.

In malaria endemic areas possibility of malarial infection presenting as pneumonia or malaria as comorbid condition should be kept in mind.

There may be hyponatremia due to syndrome of inappropriate antidiuretic hormone secretion. A careful monitoring and restriction of fluid is the intervention required in most cases.

Hypoxia may be present in children with severe pneumonia. Hypoxia if untreated may be associated with increased case fatality rates. Since it is difficult to identify hypoxia by clinical features alone, oxygen should be administered to all children with severe tachypnea (respiratory rate >70/minute), chest in-drawing, poor feeding or cyanosis. Oxygen may be administered by nasal prongs, nasopharyngeal tubes (Low flow, i.e. 1–2 L/min), oxygen hood or face mask (high flow 4–8 L/min). Small children tolerate oxygen with hood better than nasal or nasopharyngeal cannula or face mask. Nasal cannula after cutting the prongs is also well tolerated by children. Noninvasive monitoring of hypoxia by saturation monitoring is well-accepted method. However, it should be kept in mind that oxygen saturation gives idea about oxygenation and does not give any idea about CO_2. Even with respiratory failure the saturation may be normal with high flow oxygen inhalation. Therefore, it is advised that in critically sick children, a baseline arterial blood gas should be done and subsequently monitored with oxygen saturation. With clinical deterioration a repeat arterial blood gas for documentation of rising CO_2 is desirable.

PREVENTION OF PNEUMONIA

Routine immunization against pertussis, measles have decreased significant number of deaths due to CAP. The common pathogens like *H. influenzae* and pneumococci causing pneumonia are also vaccine preventable. In western countries with routine use of *H. influenzae* type B vaccine, the pneumonia and related deaths due to

H. influenzae have dropped significantly. Vaccines against pneumococci are also effective in preventing invasive diseases due to pneumococci. Therefore, these vaccines should be administered preferably to all children.

BIBLIOGRAPHY

1. Agarwal G, Awasthi S, Kabra SK, et al. Three day versus five day treatment with amoxicillin for non-severe pneumonia in young children: a multicentre randomised controlled trial. BMJ. 2004;328(7443):791-6.
2. Arora NK, Awasthi S, Gupta P, et al. India Clinical Epidemiology Network (IndiaCLEN) Task Force on Pneumonia Rational use of antibiotics for pneumonia. Indian Pediatr. 2010;47:11-8.
3. Berman S. Epidemiology of acute respiratory infection in children of developing countries. Rev Infect Dis. 1991;13(Suppl 6):S454-62.
4. Broor S, Pandey RM, Ghosh M, et al. Risk factors for severe acute lower respiratory tract infection in under-five children. Indian Pediatr. 2001;38(12):1361-9.
5. Chaudhry R, Nazima N, Dhawan B, et al. Prevalence of mycoplasma pneumoniae and chlamydia pneumoniae in children with community acquired pneumonia. Indian J Pediatr. 1998;65(5):717-21.
6. John TJ, Cherian T, Steinhoff MC, et al. Etiology of acute respiratory infections in children in tropical southern India. Rev Infect Dis. 1990;13(Suppl 6):S463-9.
7. Kabra SK, Broor S, Lodha R, et al. Can we identify acute severe viral lower respiratory tract infection clinically? Indian Pediatr. 2004;41(3):245-9.
8. Kabra SK, Lodha R, Broor S, et al. Etiology of acute lower respiratory tract infection. Indian J Pediatr. 2003;70(1):33-6.
9. Kabra SK, Lodha R, Pandey RM. Antibiotics for community-acquired pneumonia in children. Cochrane Database Syst Rev. 2010;3:CD004874.
10. Kabra SK, Singhal T, Lodha R. Pneumionia. Indian J Pediatr. 2001;68(Suppl 3):S19-23.
11. Kabra SK, Singhal T, Verma IC. The introduction of antibiotics in 1940"s revolutionized the practice of medicine. Indian J Pediatr. 2001;68(Suppl 3): S5-7.
12. Kabra SK, Verma IC. Acute respiratory tract infection: the forgotten pandemic. Indian J Pediatr. 1999;66(6):873-5.
13. Kumar RM, Kabra SK, Singh M. Efficacy and acceptability of different modes of oxygen administration in children: implications for a community Hospital. J Trop Pediatr. 1997;43(1):47-9.
14. Lodha R, Bhadauria PS, Kuttikat AV, et al. Can clinical symptoms or signs accurately predict hypoxemia in children with acute lower respiratory tract infections? Indian Pediatr. 2004;41(2):129-36.
15. Maitreyi RS, Broor S, Kabra SK, et al. Rapid detection methods for diagnosis of acute lower respiratory tract infection in children due to respiratory syncytial virus. Indian J Med Microbiol. 1999;17:10-3.
16. Maitreyi RS, Broor S, Kabra SK, et al. Rapid detection of respiratory viruses by centrifugation enhanced cultures from children with acute lower respiratory tract infections. J Clin Virol. 2000;16(1):41-7.
17. Pandey A, Chaudhry R, Kapoor L, et al. Acute lower respiratory tract infection due to chlamydia species in children under five years of age. Indian J Chest Dis Allied Sci. 2005;47(2):97-101.
18. Pandey A, Choudhry R, Nisar N, et al. Acute respiratory tract infections in Indian children with special reference to mycoplasma pneumoniae. J Trop Pediatr. 2000;46(6):371-4.
19. Rudan I, Boschi-Pinto C, Biloglav Z, et al. Epidemiology and etiology of childhood pneumonia. Bull World Health Organ. 2008;86(5):408-16.
20. Rudan I, Tomaskovic L, Cynthia Boschi-Pinot, et al. Global estimates of the incidence of clinical pneumonia among children under five years of age. Bulletin of the World Health Organisation. 2004;82(12):895-903.
21. Sarthi M, Lodha R, Kabra SK. Pneumonia. In: Kabra SK, Lodha R (Eds). Essential Pediatric Pulmonology, 2nd edition. New Delhi: Nobel Vision; 2010.pp.64-79.

3.5 BACTERIAL MENINGITIS

Jaydeep Choudhury, K Pandian

INTRODUCTION

Bacterial meningitis is an inflammation of the leptomeninges triggered by bacteria present in the subarachnoid space. It is one of the most serious infections in pediatric age group. The outcome of bacterial meningitis is not primarily dependent on the organism, but the inflammatory reaction that it produces. Deficient local host defences, cerebral blood flow alterations secondary to infection, effects of raised intracranial pressure (ICP), destruction and poor repair of damaged neurological tissue all make the brain tissue most vulnerable.

Bacterial meningitis occurs in all age groups with manifestations depending on the age, immunological status and other coexistent morbidities. Most of the cases occur between 1 month and 5 years of age. The organisms vary with age group and geographical location.

ETIOLOGY

Many organisms may cause bacterial meningitis. The most common organisms responsible are *Streptococcus pneumoniae*, *Neisseria meningitidis* and *Haemophilus influenzae* type b *(Hib)*. This triad is responsible for more than 80% of all cases. Gram-negative bacteria, particularly *Escherichia coli*, streptococci (Group B streptococci), *Listeria monocytogenes* and staphylococci may also cause bacterial meningitis particularly in neonates.

The etiological agent of bacterial meningitis is dependent on the age of the child, underlying diseases and immunological status of the child. Among children in the postneonatal age group *S. pneumoniae* and Hib are the most common pathogenic pathogen causing acute bacterial meningitis. Mixed bacterial infections with more than one agent is seen among children who are immunocompromised have a parameningeal source of infection such as sinusitis skull fracture or previous neurosurgery.

In India, the burden of invasive *H. influenzae* (Hib) is substantial, with the incidence of Hib meningitis estimated to be 50–60 cases per 100,000 children less than 5 years of age. Serogroups A, B, C, Y and W135 are responsible for almost all meningococcal disease. Serogroup A is responsible for epidemic disease in sub-Saharan Africa and in other developing countries, serogroups B and C are responsible for most of the infections in developed countries, as well as in developing regions.

Prospective multicentric hospital surveillance of *S. pneumoniae* disease in India was conducted by the invasive bacterial infection surveillance group and International Clinical Epidemiology Network. The most common serotypes were 6, 1, 19, 14, 4, 5, 45, 12 and 7.

Table 3.5.1: Age-related etiology of acute bacterial meningitis in pediatric age group.

Age	Bacteriology
Neonate (0–1 month) Early-onset	*S. agalactiae, E. coli, K. pneumoniae, L. monocytogenes*
Late-onset	Gram-negative enteric bacilli, (*E. coli, K. pneumoniae*, enterobacter, *Salmonella*), *S. aureus*, or same as early onset in neonate
Age: 1–3 months	Same as in neonate + *S. pneumoniae, N. meningitidis* and *H. influenzae* type b
Age: 3 months to 5 years	*S. pneumoniae*, Hib and *N. meningitidis*
Age: > 4 years children and adults	*S. pneumoniae* and *N. meningitidis*

Serotypes 1 and 5 accounted for 29% of disease. Penicillin resistance was infrequently present with intermediate resistance to penicillin noted in only 1.3% isolates; however, resistance to cotrimoxazole and chloramphenicol was seen in 56% and 17% isolates respectively. Age-related etiology of acute bacterial meningitis in pediatric age group is shown in Table 3.5.1.

PATHOGENESIS

Most cases of bacterial meningitis result from bacteremia and mostly after colonization of nasopharyngeal mucosa by pathogens. Transmission of respiratory pathogen is from person to person and in neonates by vertical transmission, during delivery, after delivery or following intravenous lines and ventilation. The bacteria gain entry into the meninges through various routes like, hematogenous, contiguous, direct implantation and malformations with communication to the CSF space. Hematogenous route is the commonest which follows blood stream infection occurring as a part of septicemia or blood stream infection. Non-hematogenous infection occurs from structures around the brain like otitis media, mastoiditis, sinusitis, trauma, VP shunts. Pathogens reaching the cerebrospinal fluid (CSF) are likely to survive because of paucity of resident macrophages and deficient opsonization caused by low concentration of capsule-specific immunoglobulin and complement in CSF fluid. Exudation occurs in the subarachnoid spaces and cisterns. This may obstruct CSF flow and vascular flow is compromised by perivascular reaction (Fig. 3.5.1).

CLINICAL FEATURES

A high index of suspicion is essential to reduce morbidity and mortality in bacterial meningitis. Bacterial meningitis

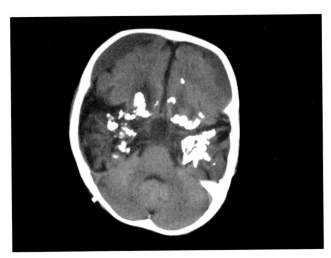

FIG. 3.5.1: CT scan showing exudates in cisternal spaces.

usually presents with fever, seizures, vomiting and abnormal behavior. In neonates, symptoms may be subtle with irregular fever, incessant cry, lethargy, refusal of feeds, persistent vomiting with no focus of sepsis on clinical examination. Sometimes altered sensorium with a bulging fontanelle may be present. A bulging fontanelle in a child not crying is suggestive of raised ICP.

In older children fever, headache, pain in the neck, altered sensorium, vomiting, seizures with irritability, photophobia and focal deficit may be present. Signs of meningeal irritation include neck stiffness, Kernig or Brudzinski sign. Associated cranial nerve palsies may be present. Hemorrhagic rash on the skin and features of shock suggest meningococcal meningitis.

Signs of intracranial hypertension are headache, vomiting, 3rd, 4th, 6th cranial nerve palsy, papilledema and seizures. Focal neurological deficits are sometimes seen. Meningococcal infection may present with shock.

DIAGNOSIS

Initial diagnosis of meningitis requires prompt hospitalization for examination and culture of CSF. However, evidence of impending brain herniation, cardiopulmonary instability and infection of skin overlying the site of lumbar puncture (LP) is a contraindication for LP. Features of imminent herniation include abnormal respiration from hyperventilation, apnea, respiratory arrest, ataxic breathing and Cheyne-Stokes respiration. Fixed deviation of the eyes, abnormal pupil size and reflex and absent oculocephalic response are also ominous signs. Other signs include generalized seizures and decorticate or decerebrate postures. Thrombocytopenia with platelet count below 20,000/cmm is a relative contraindication of LP. In such cases neuroimaging may be done.

Blood culture should be sent always and empiric antibiotic therapy should be started immediately when there is any possible delay in imaging. It is recommended to collect the CSF before initiation of antibiotic therapy; however, treatment must not be delayed pending LP.

Cerebrospinal fluid is the gold standard for diagnosis of meningitis performed properly. Blood sugar should be taken before performing LP as it corresponds to the CSF sugar level.

Cerebrospinal Fluid Transport

Cerebrospinal fluid should be sent to the laboratory as early as possible preferably while still warm. In case of delay during transport or examination, CSF should be divided into two containers. One for making smear for staining and biochemical tests and the other in a bottle containing few drops of glucose broth for culture. A delay can cause the cells in the CSF to disintegrate which will not reflect the true picture. Smear and culture should be done as early as possible. The specimen should be stored at 37°C (room temperature) till microscopy and bacterial cultures are done.

Cerebrospinal Fluid Examination

Macroscopic Examination

Normal CSF is clear and colorless. In case of pyogenic meningitis it can be turbid due to high cell count or protein content. It may be yellowish or blood stained due to hemorrhage.

Traumatic tap invalidates the CSF cell count. In case of traumatic LP with blood in the spinal fluid interpretation of the CSF cell count is difficult. Several methods are used to distinguish peripheral blood WBC but none is accurate.

Microscopic Examination

Cerebrospinal fluid should be transferred in a sterile centrifuge tube and should be centrifuged at 3,000 rpm for 5 minutes. The supernatant fluid is transferred to a clean container for chemical examination, whereas the pellet should be stained with Gram stain and examined. Presence of lanceolate gram-positive diplococci or in short chains is suggestive of *S. pneumoniae*.

Gram-negative plano convex diplococci indicate *N. meningitidis*. Gram-positive cocci in chains are suggestive of streptococci. The likelihood for visualization of bacteria on Gram stain depends upon the CSF concentration of the bacteria. The Gram stain is positive in 97% of cases when the CSF concentration of bacteria is more than 10^5 CFU/mL. However, the yield of Gram stain may be approximately 20% lower for patients who have received previous antibiotic therapy.

Cytological examination is done on a white cell counting chamber and stained with Giemsa stain for identifying polymorphonuclear and other cells. In untreated bacterial meningitis, the WBC count is elevated usually in the range of 500–5,000 cells/cmm with a polymorphonuclear leukocytic predominance between 80% and 90%. The CSF-white blood cell (WBC) count generally remains abnormal for several days despite using antibiotic. Thus, LP and CSF study should be done in suspected meningitis even if the child is on antibiotics.

Biochemical Test for Protein and Glucose

The CSF glucose concentration is usually less than 40 mg/dL but a ratio of CSF to serum glucose of 0.4 or less is more specific and sensitive for the diagnosis of bacterial meningitis in children above 2 months of age. In neonates and in children under 2 months of age a ratio less than or equal to 0.6 is considered to be suggestive of bacterial meningitis.

Cerebrospinal fluid protein concentration is usually elevated (100–500 mg/100 mL) in patients with bacterial meningitis. The glucose and protein concentration are not altered for several days in spite of antibiotic administration.

Culture for Suspected Pathogens

The culture should be done as rapidly as possible. Specimen should be stored at 37°C till bacterial culture is performed. The yield of bacterial CSF culture decreases by previous antibiotic with the exception of those caused by gram-negative enteric bacilli.

Other Tests

The basis of other tests is detection of bacterial antigens or antibodies against the bacteria. It is sometimes indicated in those who have received prior antibiotics which reduces the yield of both CSF Gram stain and culture. Latex agglutination is rapid, sensitive and easy to perform under field condition. Commercially available kits for detecting antigens of *N. meningitidis* A, B and C, *S. pneumoniae* and *H. influenzae* type b are available. However, a negative bacterial antigen test results does not rule out bacterial meningitis.

Polymerase chain reaction may be an important tool in the diagnosis of meningitis particularly on those patients reporting with previous antibiotic. These tests are not recommended at present for routine use. In partially treated meningitis the cell type may change from polymorphonuclear leukocytes to lymphocytes as early as 24 hours. The protein shows no major change but CSF glucose to blood glucose ratio is altered.

Repeat Lumbar Puncture

In patient who has adequately responded to antibiotic therapy does not require repeat LP to document CSF sterilization. Repeat LP is indicated under the following circumstances:
- No clinical improvement after 48 hours of appropriate antibiotic therapy
- Highly resistant pneumococcal meningitis, particularly who have also received adjunctive dexamethasone therapy
- Neonatal meningitis

- Meningitis caused by gram-negative organism
- Meningitis complicating CSF shunt.

Blood Culture

Blood should be collected under aseptic condition and inoculated in blood culture media.

Petechial Fluid

This sample may be utilized for diagnosis of meningococcal disease. Petechial lesions are gently irrigated by injecting 0.2 mL of sterile saline solution and the fluid is collected for Gram stain and culture.

Neuroimaging

It is sometimes useful in follow-up. Ventricular size and presence of debris can be detected. Serial evaluation can be done by ultrasound scanning in infants and neonates. In patients with no clinical response worsening status focal deficits CT scan or MRI brain is useful to exclude subdural effusion, brain abscess, hydrocephalus and infarcts.

MANAGEMENT

Empirical treatment can be initiated based on the most likely pathogen and prevalence while awaiting culture reports or when LP is deferred.

Empirical Antibiotic Therapy

The choice of antibiotics in infants and children depends upon the causative organism in that particular age group. Most common organism in the postnatal age group includes *S. pneumoniae, N. meningitidis* and Hib. As *S. pneumoniae* has developed resistance to penicillin, the choice of antibiotic depends on the grade of resistance. The National Committee for Clinical Laboratory Standards defines *S. pneumoniae* as susceptible, intermediate or highly resistant to penicillin when the isolate has a penicillin MIC of less than or equal to 0.06 µg/mL, 0.1–1 µg/mL or more than 2 µg/mL respectively. Data from our country are few with studies showing intermediate resistance to penicillin in 1.3–7.8% of isolates. In contrast developed countries report penicillin resistance as high as 50%. Resistance to cefotaxime and ceftriaxone are rarely reported in our country. Most strains of *N. meningitidis* are sensitive to both penicillin and cephalosporin. *H. influenzae* type b is sensitive to third generation cephalosporin with reports of their resistance to penicillin and ampicillin. Recommended practice of initial therapy with penicillin and chloramphenicol is not upheld because of its poorer CSF sterilization, side effects and higher cost. In case of irrefutable evidence of meningococcal infection like petechiae and purpuric rash one can start with penicillin.

Antimicrobial agent will be able to clear bacteria from the CSF only if it can cross the blood-brain barrier and achieve optimum CSF concentration. Parenteral therapy is recommended in treatment of meningitis.

In children more than 1 month of age, third generation cephalosporin, ceftriaxone or cefotaxime are recommended for initial therapy. Cefotaxime 200 mg/kg/24 hours given every 6 hour or ceftriaxone 100 mg/kg/24 hour given every 12 hour is currently recommended. As India has started showing intermediate resistant pneumococci penicillin is no longer recommended. Vancomycin has role in therapy of penicillin or cephalospori-resistant meningitis in combination with cephalosporin. Monotherapy with vancomycin is not recommended because of unpredictable CSF penetration and reports of clinical failure. The combination of vancomycin plus third generation cephalosporin has an additive or synergistic effect in children with bacterial meningitis. Vancomycin is used in the dose of 60 mg/kg/24 hours given every 6 hours. In patients who are immunocompromised and where Gram-negative bacterial meningitis is suspected empiric therapy may start with ceftazidime and aminoglycosides. In patients with CSF shunt empiric therapy can be initiative with vancomycin and meropenem. Combination of third generation cephalosporin plus beta lactamase inhibitor has no role in the treatment of pyogenic meningitis.

Pathogen-specific Antimicrobial Therapy

S. pneumoniae or *N. meningitidis* which are susceptible to penicillin or ampicillin (MIC <0.6 μg/mL) should be treated with penicillin G or ampicillin. If they are not susceptible to penicillin but susceptible to cephalosporin third generation cephalosporins like ceftriaxone or cefotaxime must be used. Isolates that are not susceptible to penicillin and have a MIC of more than 1 mcg/mL to third generation cephalosporin should be treated with vancomycin plus cefotaxime or ceftriaxone. For *S. pneumoniae* with intermediate resistance to penicillin cefepime and meropenem may be considered as alternative therapy. However, trails with cefepime are not adequate but may be tried in patients who fail with other antibiotic courses. The other organism which might be responsible for bacterial meningitis in children should be treated with antibiotics as summarized in Table 3.5.2. The dosage of commonly used antibiotics is shown in Table 3.5.3.

Duration of Therapy

Duration of therapy depends upon the causative pathogen and clinical course. For complicated cases longer course may be needed. For *S. pneumoniae* 10–14 days therapy is required, whereas *N. meningitidis* and Hib meningitis should be treated for 5–7 days and 7–10 days respectively. If the CSF reports are suggestive of acute bacterial meningitis without any identifiable pathogen patients should continue to receive therapy for 7–10 days. Gram-negative bacillary meningitis should be treated for 3 weeks or at least 2 weeks after CSF sterilization. In case of 7 days non-responders try to determine the cause by clinical examination, CSF and imaging studies modify duration of treatment accordingly.

Corticosteroids in Bacterial Meningitis

Corticosteroid therapy has been found to ameliorate inflammation. In pediatric patients, adjunctive dexamethasone in childhood bacterial meningitis showed beneficial effects in *H. influenzae* meningitis with regard to hearing outcome and *S. pneumoniae* meningitis also demonstrated benefit.

Dexamethasone therapy should be started intravenously at the same time as, or slightly before, the first dose of antibiotic, at a dose of 0.15 mg per kilogram of body weight every 6 hours for 2–4 days. However, there are concerns following steroid therapy about the antibiotic penetration, CSF sterilization and side effects of dexamethasone like gastrointestinal hemorrhage.

Table 3.5.2: Summary of treatment with antibiotics in bacterial meningitis in children.

Bacteria	Antibiotic of choice
Listeria	Ampicillin ± Gentamicin
E. coli	Ceftriaxone or cefotaxime ± aminoglycoside
Pseudomonas aeruginosa	Ceftazidime or cefepime ± aminoglycoside
S. aureus	
Methicillin-sensitive (MSSA)	Cloxacillin or oxacillin or nafcillin
Methicillin-resistant (MRSA)	Vancomycin ± Rifampicin
Streptococcus agalactiae	Penicillin G or Ampicillin ± Gentamicin
Enterococcus	
Ampicillin-sensitive	Ampicillin + Gentamicin
Ampicillin-resistant	Vancomycin + Gentamicin

Table 3.5.3: Dosages of commonly administered antibiotics for bacterial meningitis in infants and children.

Antibiotics	Total daily dose	Dosing interval in hours
Ampicillin	200–300 mg/kg	6
Cefepime	150 mg/kg	8
Cefotaxime	200–300 mg/kg	6–8
Ceftazidime	150 mg/kg	8
Ceftriaxone	100 mg/kg	12–24
Gentamicin	7.5 mg/kg	8
Meropenem	120 mg/kg	8
Penicillin G	400,000 units/kg	4–6
Rifampicin	10–12 mg/kg	12–24
Linezolid	10 mg/kg	12

Supportive Therapy

Usually the life-threatening complication of the disease occurs in this initial period. Hence supportive care is crucial in the initial period. The most important supportive care is as follows:

- Proper monitoring
- Control of increased intracranial tension, seizures if any
- Adequate feeding.

The various aspects of supportive care are the following:

- Vital parameters like pulse rate, blood pressure and respiratory rate is to be recorded frequently. It should be preferably done hourly for the 1st hour and thereafter 3 hourly for first 24 hours. Daily recording of weight and serial measurements of head circumference is also recommended.
- Patients with shock or systemic hypotension calls for urgent intervention with fluid and inotropic support and intensive monitoring with central lines in an intensive care unit setup because it may otherwise compromise central nervous system (CNS) circulation and cause CNS ischemia. Shock must be treated aggressively to prevent brain and other organ dysfunction like acute tubular necrosis and acute respiratory distress syndrome. Normal saline is the fluid of choice in shock. Fluid restriction is not needed in all patients of meningitis but they should be given maintenance fluid as per their age.
- Patients with syndrome of inappropriate antidiuretic hormone secretion with hyponatremia need intervention. In patients with serum sodium in between 120 mEq/L and 130 mEq/L, needs fluid restriction. Patients who have serum sodium less than 120 mEq/L or are symptomatic need treatment with hypertonic saline.
- Blood urea, sugar, serum electrolytes, urine output and fluid input/output chart should be maintained meticulously. Complete blood count (CBC) and particularly in presence of petechiae, purpura and signs of bleeding, platelet count and prothrombin time, activated partial thromboplastin time and fibrinogen should be measured.
- Neurological assessment includes pupillary reflexes, level of consciousness, motor function, cranial nerve examination and evaluation for seizures.
- Systemic hypotension calls for urgent intervention with fluid and inotropic support and intensive as it may compromise CNS circulation and cause CNS ischemia.
- Neurological complication includes raised intracranial temperature (ICT). If ICP is not controlled, the patient can develop cerebral herniation that presents with widely dilated or unequal pupils, impaired ocular movements, bradycardia, hypertension, decerebrate/decorticate posture or apnea. In such cases start with rapid IV, 20% mannitol infusion, 5 mL/kg over 20 minutes. It can be repeated with smaller dose 2.5 mL/kg up to 3–6 doses. Prolonged use can cause dyselectrolytemia and hence not recommended.

- Uncontrolled raised ICT can also be treated emergently with endotracheal intubation and controlled hyperventilation to maintain the PCO_2 at approximately 25 mm Hg.
- Subdural effusion develops in approximately 10–30% cases more in infants but is usually asymptomatic. Symptomatic effusion should be aspirated through the open fontanel. Fever alone is not an indication of aspiration.
- Seizures occurring within 48 hours are common in bacterial meningitis which merits a brief course (≤ 7 days of anticonvulsants). In contrast, late onset seizures required anticonvulsant therapy for a longer period. For immediate control of seizures diazepam, lorazepam or midazolam may be used. Adequate airway and oxygenation should be maintained during the episodes of seizures apart from the treatment with anticonvulsants. Serum glucose, calcium and sodium should be measured to rule out metabolic etiology. After initial control patient should be put on phenytoin or fosphenytoin to prevent further recurrence. Phenytoin is preferred over phenobarbitone as it is less sedative and thus does not interfere with the assessment of level of consciousness. In nonresponsive convulsion midazolam infusion may be used but one has to investigate for its cause.
- Audiological screening is recommended for all cases of meningitis 6 weeks after discharge.

COMPLICATIONS

Acute complications are persistent fever and meningeal signs, subdural effusion, abscess, infarcts, ventriculomegaly, hydrocephalus (Fig. 3.5.2), ventriculitis, focal neurological deficit and hearing impairment.

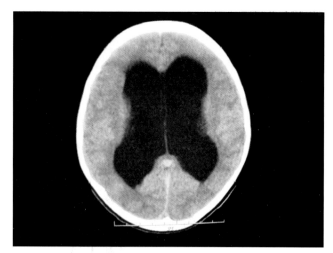

FIG. 3.5.2: Hydrocephalus following meningitis.

Sequelae include regression and delay in milestones, mental retardation, motor deficit hemiplegia, spasticity, cranial nerve palsies, seizures, hearing loss, behavioral problems.

PREVENTION

Prophylaxis for prevetion of development of Hib meningitis in household contacts is with rifampicin 20 mg/kg/day for 4 days. Persons in close contact with *Meningococcus* may be given rifampicin 10 mg/kg/dose twice daily for 2 days. Vaccines against Hib, *S. pneumoniae* and *N. meningitidis* are available and should be given as per recommendation.

BIBLIOGRAPHY

1. Agrawal S, Nadel S. Acute bacterial meningitis in infants and children: epidemiology and management. Pediatr Drugs 2011;13:385-400.
2. Chavez-Bueno S, McCracken GH J. Bacterial meningitis in children. PediatrClin North Am. 2005;52(3):795-810.
3. John TJ, Cherian T, Raghupathy P. *Haemophilus influenzae* disease in children in India: a hospital perspective. Pediatr Infect Dis J. 1998;17(9 Suppl):S161-71.
4. Kanegaye JT, Soliemanzadeh P, Bradley JS. Lumbar puncture in pediatric bacterial meningitis: defining the time interval for recovery of cerebrospinal fluid pathogens after parenteral antibiotic pretreatment. Pediatrics. 2001;108(5): 1169-74.
5. Prober CG. Central nervous system infections. In: Behrman RE, Kliegman RM, Jenson HB (Eds). Nelsons. Textbook of Pediatrics, 17th edition. Philadelphia: Saunders; 2004.pp.2038-47.
6. Prospective multicentre hospital surveillance of streptococcus pneumonia disease in India. Invasive Bacterial Infection Surveillance (IBIS) Group, International Clinical Epidemiology Network (INCLEN). Lancet. 1999;353(9160):1216-21.
7. Pyogenic Meningitis. IAP Infectious Diseases Chapter Protocol for Diagnosis and Management of Pyogenic Meningitis in Children. IAP Infectious Diseases Chapter Publicatio, 2008.
8. Saez-Llorens X, McCracken GH Jr. Antimicrobial and anti-inflammatory treatment of bacterial meningitis. Infect Dis Clin North Am. 1999;13(3):619-36.
9. Sinner SW, Tunkel AR. Antimicrobial agents in the treatment of bacterial meningitis. Infect Dis Clii North Am. 2004;18(3):581-602.
10. Tunkel AR, Hartman BJ, Kaplan SM, et al. Practice Guidelines for the management of bacterial meningitis. Clin Infect Dis. 2004;39(9):1267-84.

Apurba Ghosh

INTRODUCTION

Encephalitis is inflammation of the parenchyma of brain. It may be associated with variable degree of inflammation of the meninges (meningitis), spinal cord (myelitis) and nerve roots (radiculitis). Encephalitis can be caused by viruses, bacteria, mycobacteria, fungi, parasites and prions. Encephalitis can be classified as primary or postinfectious/ parainfectious. Primary encephalitis results from direct invasion and replication of the infectious agent in central nervous system (CNS), whereas postinfectious encephalitis is an immune-mediated process following a febrile illness or vaccination.

The clinical case definition, applied to suspected cases of acute encephalitis syndrome (AES) is recommended by WHO and is currently used for Japanese encephalitis surveillance in India. Clinically, a case of AES is defined as a person of any age, at any time of year with the acute onset of fever and a change in mental status (including symptoms such as confusion, disorientation, coma or inability to talk) and/or new onset of seizures (excluding simple febrile seizures). Other early clinical findings may include an increase in irritability, somnolence or abnormal behavior greater than that seen with usual febrile illness.

EPIDEMIOLOGY

The epidemiology of viral encephalitis (VE) depends on the prevalence of virus in that area, seasonal and climatic condition, geography and animal exposure. Enterovirus encephalitis occurs mainly in summer in temperate climates. Geographically restricted encephalitis are found prevalent in those areas of the world, e.g. West Nile fever in America and Africa and some areas of Europe.

Herpes simplex virus (HSV) encephalitis is the most common cause of VE in developed countries, both among adults and children with an incidence of 1 in 250,000–500,000.

Japanese encephalitis virus (JEV) is the most common vaccine-preventable cause of encephalitis in Asia, occurring throughout most of Asia and parts of the Western Pacific. Local transmission of JEV has not been detected in Africa, Europe, or the Americas. In India, the highly affected states are Andhra Pradesh, Assam, Bihar, Goa, Karnataka, Manipur, Tamil Nadu, Uttar Pradesh and West Bengal.

Transmission principally occurs in rural agricultural areas, often associated with rice cultivation and flooding irrigation. In some areas of Asia, these ecologic conditions may occur near or occasionally within urban centers. In temperate areas of Asia, transmission is seasonal, and human disease usually peaks in summer and fall. In the subtropics and tropics, seasonal transmission varies with monsoon rains and irrigation practices and may be extended or even occur year round.

In endemic countries, Japanese encephalitis (JE) is primarily a disease of children. However, travel-associated JE can occur among people of any age.

The overall incidence of JE among people from non-endemic countries traveling to Asia is estimated to be less than one case per one million travelers. However, expatriates and travelers who stay for prolonged periods in rural areas with active JEV transmission are likely at similar risk as the susceptible resident population (5–50 cases per 100,000 children per year). Short-term (< 1 month) travelers whose visits are restricted to major urban areas are at minimal risk for JE. In endemic areas there are few human cases among residents because of vaccination or natural immunity. Japanese encephalitis virus is often still maintained in an enzootic cycle between animal and mosquitoes. Therefore, susceptible visitors may be at risk for infection.

Nipah virus is an emerging disease endemic in Southeast Asia. Nipah virus encephalitis was first recognized among pig farmers in Malaysia between 1998 and 1999 and subsequently documented among the abattoir workers in Singapore. There have been several outbreaks between 2001 and 2008 in Malaysia, Bangladesh and Northern India and case fatality ranges from 40 to 70%.

ETIOLOGY

In more than 70% of cases of VE the etiological agent remains unidentified in spite of extensive laboratory workup. Herpes simplex virus is the most common cause of sporadic non-epidemic VE. About 90% of herpes simplex encephalitis (HSE) is due to HSV-1; 10% is due to HSV-2. Herpes simplex virus-2 usually causes encephalitis in immunocompromised adults and neonates. Other viruses most commonly associated with VE are measles, mumps virus, rubella, and varicella zoster virus (VZV), enteroviruses, influenza viruses, rabies and arboviruses.

Arthropod-borne viruses (arboviruses) are important causes of encephalitis worldwide. More than 20 arboviruses that can cause encephalitis have been identified. Common agents are: alphaviruses (Eastern equine virus, Western equine virus, Venezuelan equine encephalitis virus), flaviviruses [St. Louis encephalitis virus, JEV, West Nile virus (WNV)] and bunyaviruses (La Crosse virus).

Japanese encephalitis is the most widespread of the arboviral encephalitides, affecting China, Japan, India, Pakistan, Eastern Russia, and the Philippines. Japanese encephalitis is caused by a mosquito-borne flavivirus carried by *Culex* species mosquitoes. Pigs and wild birds are reservoir of infection and often called amplifier hosts in the transmission cycle, while man and horse are dead-end hosts.

Enteroviral encephalitis is the third most common cause of all encephalitis, after HSV and arboviruses. Enteroviruses commonly associated with encephalitis: are coxsackie A2, 4–7, 9, 10, 16 and B1–5, echoviruses 1–9, 11–25, 27, 30, 33 and enterovirus 71. Polioviruses may rarely cause encephalitis. Enteroviruses generally cause aseptic meningitis and usually have a benign course. Enteroviral infections are seasonal with peak in summer and fall with a higher incidence in children than in adults. Enterovirus 71 appears to have a particular propensity for the CNS, producing aseptic meningitis, acute flaccid paralysis or brainstem encephalitis.

The Nipah virus is a paramyxovirus related to Hendra virus. Fruit bats of the genus *Pteropus* have been identified as natural reservoirs of Nipah virus. The probable mode of transmission is close contact with infected pigs. Majority of cases occur in adult males. The Nipah virus causes severe encephalitis characterized by fever, headache, reduced consciousness and brainstem dysfunction. There is high mortality, morbidity and there may be persistent neurological deficits in survivors.

Encephalitis caused by vaccine-preventable viruses such as measles and mumps is less common in industrialized nations. Mumps virus can cause acute VE, or a delayed immune-mediated encephalitis. Measles virus causes a postinfectious encephalitis, which can sometimes have a severe hemorrhagic component (acute hemorrhagic leukoencephalitis). Finland became the first country to be free of indigenous mumps and rubella with national immunization program with two doses of measles, mumps, and rubella (MMR) vaccine. However, in India the national program does not use MMR, but only measles. Mumps continue to occur in epidemics every 5–10 years.

It is now well-known that dengue infections can also result in encephalopathy and neurological complications. These could be due to direct viral invasion and not only multisystem derangement as previously thought.

Immunocompromised patients are at risk of encephalitis caused by cytomegalovirus (CMV), Epstein-Barr virus (EBV) and human herpes virus (HHV)-6.

Mycobacterium pneumoniae is also a major cause of infectious encephalitis in children. Symptoms may be very similar to those of VE and may not be readily suspected.

PATHOLOGY

Viral encephalitis is a parenchymal infection of the brain almost invariably associated with meningeal inflammation (meningoencephalitis) and sometimes with simultaneous involvement of the spinal cord (encephalomyelitis).

Some viruses infect specific cell types (such as oligodendrocytes), while others preferentially involve particular areas of the brain (such as medial temporal lobes or the limbic system). Latency is an important facet of several viral infections of the CNS (e.g. herpes zoster, progressive multifocal leukoencephalopathy). Systemic viral infections in the absence of direct evidence of viral penetration into the CNS may be followed by an immuno-mediated disease, such as perivenous demyelination causing acute disseminated encephalomyelitis (ADEM) and acute necrotizing hemorrhagic encephalomyelitis.

Clinical manifestations of encephalitis can result from a direct or an indirect effect of an infectious agent on the brain. Rabies, arbovirus, herpes simplex and enteroviral encephalitides are examples in which the viral infections directly involve tissue cells within the brain. In contrast, encephalitic symptoms in bacterial meningitidis and in rickettsial infections may be caused by the vasculitis and liberated toxins of the surrounding infection.

The arboviruses infection causes lymphocytic meningoencephalitis (sometimes with neutrophils), and a tendency for inflammatory cells to accumulate perivascularly. Multiple foci of necrosis of gray and white matter are found in particular, there is evidence of single-cell neuronal necrosis with phagocytosis of the debris (neuronophagia). Microglial cells form small aggregates around foci of necrosis, called microglial nodules. In severe cases there may be a necrotizing vasculitis with associated focal hemorrhages, while some viruses reveal their presence by inclusion bodies.

Herpes simplex virus most severely involves the inferior and medial regions of the temporal lobes and the orbital gyri of the frontal lobes. The infection is necrotizing and often hemorrhagic in the most severely affected regions. Perivascular inflammatory infiltrates are usually present, and Cowdry type A intranuclear viral inclusion bodies may be found in both neurons and glia.

After virus is introduced by a mosquito bite, replication locally and within regional lymphatic tissue leads to a secondary amplified viremia and infection of various organs and the brain. Neuroinvasion is thought to occur through cerebral capillaries, infection crosses from the vascular side of the endothelial cell to the perivascular space, with subsequent neuronal infection. Neurons show evidence of viral antigen in the cell body, axons, and dendrites, suggesting a mechanism of viral spread within the brain from cell to cell. Cerebrospinal fluid (CSF) levels of catecholamines and their metabolites are acutely lowered. Infiltrating T cells elicit a broad inflammatory response, with B and T cells and macrophages found in perivascular cuffs and macrophages and T cells in the parenchyma. Neuronophagia proceeds with the formation of microglial nodules and the eventual disappearance of neurons, leaving ghost-like remnants with antigen accumulated within macrophages.

The rapidity of the neutralizing antibody response is thought to be a principal determinant of outcome. Most fatal cases occurring within approximately 5 days after the onset of illness have no detectable CSF-antibody response while virus is recoverable from the CSF, a finding indicative of unimpeded viral replication. In experimentally infected animals, passive immunization reduces mortality, even when it is given 4–5 days after inoculation. However, other studies have found that antigen persists in neurons for extensive periods in the presence of intrathecal antibody and immune complexes, thus suggesting a failure of antibody-mediated viral clearance. A role for immunopathological mechanisms, including the development of anti-neurofilament antibodies, has been proposed as an alternative correlation of outcome. Cerebrospinal fluid interleukin-8 levels remain elevated for a longer interval in patients with severe prolonged illness.

Why most JE virus infections are subclinical or lead to no signs of infection in the CNS is unclear. Epidemiologic observations indicate an elevated risk for JE in the elderly and increased severity in young children, but the biologic basis for this increased susceptibility has not been defined. Cross-reactive flaviviral immunity as a result of previous dengue virus infection may modulate the severity of JE in some cases. Pathologic observations have shown a higher prevalence of neurocysticercosis in fatal JE cases than in deaths from other causes, which suggests that physical or physiologic disruption of the brain architecture by infection or other mechanisms could facilitate neuroinvasion. Experimental dual infection of animals with JE virus and other agents supports this hypothesis. In experimental animals, other host factors associated with a risk of acquiring illness and having a poor outcome include a specific gene defining resistance, age, levels of sex hormones, and cold and stress responses.

CLINICAL FEATURES

The history should be reviewed carefully, questioning specifically for symptoms of neurologic problems that manifested in the days or weeks before the acute disorder occurred. The physical examination must be performed with special attention given to focal neurologic abnormalities, cerebellar signs and evidence of increased intracranial pressure (ICP). Conducting a careful fundus examination is important but may be impossible in an agitated patient or young child. The presence of papilledema indicates that neuroimaging should be performed before doing the lumbar puncture (LP). If spontaneous venous pulsations are noted on fundus examination, ICP is not increased, and the LP can be done without imaging the patient.

There is a wide range and severity of clinical manifestations. Most commonly children present with fever, headache, nausea, vomiting and altered consciousness. Cerebral dysfunction manifests as behavioral changes, cognitive dysfunction, seizures and focal neurological deficits (hemiparesis, cranial nerve palsies, speech disturbance, etc.). Generalized seizures are common. Mental dullness may progress to stupor and coma. There may be neck rigidity which is not as pronounced as in meningitis. Viral encephalitis may be preceded by mild upper respiratory symptoms as in influenza and HSE.

Focal seizures and focal neurological deficits are more common in HSE. Neonatal HSE characteristically presents with features of disseminated viral infection, notably liver involvement. Cerebellar signs may indicate a postinfectious cerebellitis often associated with VZV infection. The presence of multifocal lower motor neuron signs in a febrile patient might indicate poliomyelitis. Children with rhombencephalitis or basal meningoencephalitis present with lower cranial nerve palsies.

In JE most of the people are asymptomatic and less than 1% develop clinical disease. Acute encephalitis is the most commonly recognized clinical manifestation of JEV infection. Milder forms of disease, such as aseptic meningitis or undifferentiated febrile illness, can also occur. The incubation period is 5–15 days. Illness usually begins with sudden onset of fever, headache, and vomiting and seizures. Mental status changes, focal neurologic deficits, generalized weakness and movement disorders may develop over the next few days.

A subacute presentation with more subtle features may be seen in immunocompromised children.

DIFFERENTIAL DIAGNOSIS

When confronted with a child with fever, headache and altered mental status, the clinician must distinguish between encephalitis and encephalopathy and next determine whether it is the result of direct viral invasion or a postinfectious immune-mediated process (e.g. ADEM). In children presenting with acute febrile encephalopathy (fever, altered sensorium, acute onset illness), VE is the most common cause followed by pyogenic meningitis, tuberculous meningitis and cerebral malaria. The common differential diagnosis are:

- Metabolic encephalopathy (diabetic ketoacidosis, hypoglycemia, mitochondrial, hepatic)
- Toxic encephalopathy (drugs Reye's syndrome)
- Central nervous system infections
- Postinfectious encephalopathy (ADEN)
- Mass lesions
- Central nervous system vasculitis.

Encephalitis versus Encephalopathy

The main feature which distinguishes encephalopathy from encephalitis is that it usually results from noninfectious processes and there is focal or generalized dysfunction of neurons without inflammation. It is mediated via metabolic processes and can be caused by intoxications, drugs, systemic organ dysfunction (e.g. liver, pancreas) or systemic infection that spares the brain. Hence, there is absence of CSF pleocytosis and focal changes on MRI or electroencephalography (EEG). Usually there is generalized slowing without focal features on EEG and nonfocal changes in neuroimaging studies.

Central Nervous System Infections

It is often difficult to distinguish between VE and other CNS infections because of similar presentations. In acute meningitis, symptoms of meningeal irritation, like intense headache, neck stiffness and photophobia, appear early. It is important to recognize acute meningitis and to distinguish between bacterial, partly treated bacterial and viral meningitis. Cerebrospinal fluid shows high white cell count usually greater than 500×10^6 cells/L, high protein, and low glucose levels.

Tubercular Meningitis

It is the most important cause of chronic meningitis in developing countries and may mimic encephalopathy. It has a subacute onset with low grade fever, irritability, apathy progressing to obtundation, focal neurodeficits and seizures. Cerebrospinal fluid shows 25–500 cells/mm³ with predominantly lymphocytes, very high protein and low glucose levels.

Mycoplasma Pneumoniae

It can cause CNS manifestations like aseptic meningitis, encephalitis and ADEM. Controversy exists as to whether encephalitis is the result of direct invasion of brain parenchyma or the result of an immune process. Positive serum immunoglobulin M (IgM) or rising immunoglobulin G antibodies to *M. pneumoniae* may help in diagnosis. Polymerase chain reaction (PCR) is available for detection of the *Mycoplasma* genome in CSF.

Lyme Disease

It is caused by *Borrelia burgdorferi*, which is associated with subacute and late CNS and peripheral nervous system complications, including cranial neuropathies, aseptic meningitis and encephalitis. Serologic detection of CSF Lyme-specific IgM is routinely used as the diagnostic test of choice.

Cerebral Malaria

It is considered to be an example of infective encephalopathy rather than true encephalitis since the neurological symptoms of cerebral malaria result from brain hypoxemia and metabolic complications (hypoglycemia and acidosis) due to the heavy parasitemia of the red blood cells by *Plasmodium falciparum* leading to capillary occlusion.

Parainfectious or Postinfectious Causes

Acute disseminated encephalomyelitis is a multifocal inflammatory demyelinating process that can involve cerebrum as well as cranial nerves, brainstem and spinal cord. It is an immune-mediated process which may be precipitated by respiratory tract infection, vaccination or other illnesses. Fever is usually absent. MRI in ADEM shows multifocal lesions involving white matter, whereas acute encephalitis usually produces lesions that involve both gray and white matter. Acute disseminated encephalomyelitis in contrast to VE requires treatment with steroids.

Mass Lesions

Mass lesions, such as tumor or abscess, may produce signs of raised ICP and focal neurodeficit mimicking VE. Central nervous system vasculitis may be primary CNS angiitis or a part of systemic vasculitis. Systemic symptoms, aseptic meningitis and focal neurological deficit may occasionally simulate VE. Diagnosis is made by serological and immunological tests and angiographic appearances of CNS vasculitis.

DIAGNOSIS

Encephalitis is a pathological diagnosis which can be confirmed only by brain biopsy and the etiology ascertained by recovery of infectious agents from the brain tissue. But this is not practical, so ultimately the diagnosis is based on neurologic manifestations, inflammatory cells in CSF, inflammation shown on neuroimaging and evidence of infection by serology or isolation of infectious organisms and exclusion of the common differential diagnosis. It is essential to take a meticulous history and do a detailed general and neurological examination.

Investigations

Baseline Investigations

Peripheral smear: Relative lymphocytosis in the peripheral blood is common in VE. Leukopenia and thrombocytopenia are characteristic of rickettsial infections and viral hemorrhagic fevers. The most sensitive and specific test for cerebral malaria is the peripheral blood film; both thick and thin peripheral smears are necessary. Peripheral blood monocytes may reveal the characteristic cytoplasmic inclusions in patients with human monocytic ehrlichiosis, 10% of whom are known to develop a meningoencephalitic syndrome.

Renal and liver function tests: To exclude metabolic and toxic causes of encephalopathy, liver enzymes may be elevated in EBV and CMV infections.

Electrolytes: Hyponatremia due to SIADH (syndrome of inappropriate antidiuretic hormone) may be seen in encephalitis. Blood culture should be done to exclude bacterial meningitis and brain abscess.

Chest radiography: It is also advisable in all patients with acute encephalitis. Characteristic changes on chest radiography may point to the possibility of mycoplasma, legionella or tuberculous infections.

Cerebrospinal Fluid Analysis

Lumbar puncture should be performed in all cases of suspected CNS infection unless there are contraindications. It helps to identify if there is an infection and helps to distinguish between bacterial and viral infection and to guide subsequent management.

Conducting a careful funduscopic examination is important but may be impossible in an agitated patient or young child. If spontaneous venous pulsations are noted on funduscopic examination, ICP is not increased, and LP can be done without imaging the patient.

In VE, CSF is usually clear, with a mild to moderate CSF pleocytosis of 5–1,000 cells/mm^3, mainly lymphocytes. Tubercular meningitis and partially treated bacterial meningitis can give a similar CSF picture. The CSF red cell count is usually normal or mildly elevated, but it may be markedly raised in HSV encephalitis or in acute necrotizing hemorrhagic leukoencephalitis. Glucose is usually normal, although it may be low in mumps. Protein is mildly elevated (between 0.5 and 1.0 g/L). It is important to remember that early in the disease process CSF findings can be normal and may require a repeat testing.

Routine CSF studies rarely help in identification of a specific agent. Polymerase chain reaction is the most common method used for CSF analysis, with specificity 94%, and 98% sensitivity. In HSV encephalitis, PCR remains positive in about 80% of patients even 1 week after starting antiviral therapy.

It is important to distinguish a bloody tap from hemorrhagic fluid in HSV encephalitic or acute hemorrhagic leukoencephalitis. A bloody tap will falsely elevate the CSF white cell count and protein. To correct for a bloody tap, subtract one white cell for every 700 red blood cells/mm^3 in the CSF, and 0.1 g/dL of protein for every 1,000 red blood cells.

Neuroimaging

Brain imaging is now an established practice in patients with suspected acute encephalitis and usually precedes any other specific investigations. Magnetic resonance imaging is the cranial imaging of choice in acute encephalitis, although it may be simpler to obtain a computed tomogram quickly and easily in restless patients.

Most CNS infections appear on neuroimaging areas of decreased densities on CT scan or as hypointense signal on T1 and hyperintense signal on T2 and fluid-attenuation inversion recovery in MRI. MRI has been shown to be more sensitive than CT in detection of VE. Fluid-attenuation inversion recovery sequence in MRI is extremely sensitive in detecting early changes. Diffusion-weighted MRI and magnetic resonance spectroscopy are newer techniques that are more sensitive. Another imaging technique that

has proved to be helpful in establishing the diagnosis of encephalitis is single photon emission computed tomography. It can provide information about brain chemistry, cerebral neurotransmitters and brain function.

Neuroimaging changes in VE are asymmetric and involve both white and gray matter structures. In most cases of VE, CT and MRI yield normal results or only nonspecific changes, such as swelling or edema. The characteristics MRI finding of some of the VE are enumerated below:

- Magnetic resonance imaging of brain is the investigation of choice in HSE. Bilateral temporal lobe involvement is pathognomonic of HSE but it does involve the inferior frontal cortex and insula. The localization of HSE in the temporal lobes and orbitofrontal cortex may, in part, reflect the route of entry of the virus into the host, entering along the olfactory route, through the cribriform plate into the olfactory bulbs. In neonatal HSE, widespread changes occur in the periventricular white matter, often sparing the medial temporal and inferior frontal lobes. Human herpes virus-6 can mimic HSE in immunocompromised patients with exclusive involvement of the medial temporal lobes on MR imaging.
- In VZV encephalitis, vasculitis is a major pathogenic process producing large vessel arteritis and ischemic, hemorrhagic infarctions or small infarcts mixed with demyelinating lesions on MRI and magnetic resonance angiogram.
- In Eastern equine encephalitis, JE and tick-borne encephalitis abnormalities in basal ganglia and thalamus are seen.
- Enterovirus rhombencephalitis causes hyperintense signals in the brainstem on T2-weighted MRI.
- In Nipah virus encephalitis discrete focal lesions can be seen throughout the brain but mainly in subcortical and deep white matter of the cerebral hemispheres.

Electroencephalography

Electroencephalography results are generally normal or show nonspecific, diffuse, high amplitude slow waves. The presence of periodic lateralized epileptiform discharges on EEG were once thought to be diagnostic of HSE but are nonspecific. Periodic lateralized epileptiform discharges can be seen in stroke, infectious mononucleosis encephalitis, etc. The EEG in subacute sclerosing panencephalitis also shows a typical generalized periodic EEG pattern.

SPECIFIC DIAGNOSIS

In a patient with suspected VE, CSF, blood, feces and throat swabs should be sent to a laboratory offering viral diagnostic services. Polymerase chain reaction has been widely used for detection of both DNA and RNA viruses in CSF, whereas culture may take a minimum of 1–28 days, and give negative results after initiation of antiviral drugs; PCR is a rapid diagnostic technique, with a turnaround time of 24 hours or less and remains sensitive even after short courses of antiviral therapy. Polymerase chain reaction is also preferable to serology, which often requires 2–4 weeks after acute infection for rise in antibody titers. Polymerase chain reaction has high sensitivity and specificity (both >95%) and rapid and noninvasive; however, it may be negative in the first few days of the illness or after about 10 days.

Previously considered as the gold standard for diagnosis of HSV-1 encephalitis, brain biopsy has been replaced by PCR as the investigation of choice.

In JE detection of IgM antibody in serum and/or CSF by either capture of enzyme-linked immunosorbent assay (ELISA) or particle agglutination assay is the mainstay of diagnosis. Antigen detection tests such as reverse passive hemagglutination, immunofluorescence (IF) and PCR detection are also available.

Polymerase chain reaction may also aid in the detection of VZV, enteroviruses (coxsackievirus types A and B, echoviruses, enterovirus types such as EV71) and mycoplasma. In an immunocompromised patient, CSF PCR is performed for detection of EBV and CMV. Polymerase chain reaction may be false negative early in the illness or with low viral load. It may be false-positive in cases in which a breakdown of the blood-brain barrier has occurred (e.g. in severe bacterial meningitis) or contamination of the CSF with blood.

Serological Tests

Serological tests can also be an option to detect antibodies to HSV, VZV, CMV, EBV, HIV and others can be measured from serum and CSF by using enzyme immunoassay (EIA) tests.

Antigens of RSV, influenza viruses, parainfluenza and adenoviruses can be studied from throat specimens with IF test or EIA and may provide a possible etiology for encephalitis.

Polymerase chain reaction, electron microscopy from vesicular fluid in chickenpox (VZV), hand, foot and mouth disease (EV71), genital herpes (HSV-2) can also be done.

Viral culture is rarely useful and has a low diagnostic yield (positive in <5% cases).

MANAGEMENT

Viral encephalitis is a devastating condition and early recognition and management can change the outcome. Management comprises of:
- Stabilization of the patient
- General supportive treatment
- Specific treatment
- Treatment of immediate complications
- Prevention of secondary complications
- Rehabilitation.

General Management

All patients with severe VE should be treated in an intensive care setting. Make an assessment of level of coma using the modified Glasgow coma score. Careful monitoring of cardiorespiratory status, fluids and electrolytes is essential. Intubation and ventilation may be required in deeply comatose patients or in those with refractory seizures requiring high doses of sedative anticonvulsants. Periodic evaluation of neurological status for focal neurodeficits and signs of raised ICP should be done. An ICP monitor may need to be placed with the aim of maintaining ICP at less than 15 mm Hg. Intravenous fluids and electrolytes must be given initially. Nutrition must be maintained. Care of the bowel, bladder and back is necessary.

Treatment of Immediate Complications

Control of raised intracranial pressure
- Nurse the patient with head elevated to 30°
- Intravenous dexamethasone, mannitol or oral glycerol may be used to reduce cerebral edema.

Control of convulsions
- Generalized seizures are common in VE and even focal seizures may occur
- Seizures may be refractory to the usual therapy
- Lorazepam is the preferred initial anticonvulsant
- Intravenous phenytoin (or preferably fosphenytoin) is the next drug of choice. Midazolam infusion or propofol may be required in refractory seizures.

Prevention of Secondary Complications

Secondary complications, like cerebral infarction, cerebral venous thrombosis, SIADH, aspiration pneumonia, upper gastrointestinal bleeding, urinary tract infections and disseminated intravascular coagulation, may arise in the course of VE.

Bed sores can be prevented by regular turning in bed and appropriate mattresses. Compression stockings and prophylactic heparin can be used to reduce the risk of deep vein thrombi and pulmonary embolism. Physiotherapy of limbs is required to prevent joint contractures.

Specific Treatment
- Parenteral antibiotics, preferably a cephalosporin, should be administered until bacterial meningitis or brain abscess have been excluded.
- *Antiviral therapy:* For most forms of VE (except HSV and few others) there is no specific treatment. Acyclovir should be given as soon as there is a suspicion of VE even before an etiological diagnosis is made.
- *Acyclovir:* When started early in HSE, acyclovir reduces both mortality and morbidity and has been proved to

be more effective than vidarabine. It is excreted mainly in urine and hence renal function should be monitored closely, and adequate hydration maintained. Dose should be adjusted according to renal clearance. Oral acyclovir should not be used in HSV encephalitis, because the levels achieved in the CSF are not high enough. Neonatal HSE and infants less than 3 months: 20 mg/kg every 8 hours by intravenous infusion for 21 days; children from 3 months to 12 years: 500 mg/m^2 8 hourly for 14–21 days, children 12–18 years: 10 mg/kg 8 hourly for 14–21 days. Acyclovir might also be effective for VZV encephalitis.

- Valacyclovir is a prodrug of acyclovir. Valacyclovir may be used if intravenous treatment is proving difficult, but only after the first 10 days of intravenous treatment. Role of valacyclovir in HSE needs further evaluation. Ganciclovir and foscarnet are used for CMV encephalitis and severe HHV-6 disease in immunocompromised patients. Pleconaril is used for enteroviral encephalitis.
- Interferon-alpha has been used in WNV and other flavivirus infections, but a randomized controlled *trial* in JEV showed that it was not effective. Antiretroviral therapy must be added or continued in HIV-infected patients.

Role of Steroids

Use of corticosteroids in VE is controversial. It is probably effective in VZV encephalitis because of the strong vasculitic component of the disease and in case of cerebral edema. Treatment with high dose of steroids is required in ADEM and hence it is important to distinguish VE from ADEM.

REHABILITATION

After recovery, supportive and rehabilitative efforts are required. Assessment of cognition, memory, speech, vision, hearing and motor impairment should be made at discharge and at follow-up visits to judge the extent of damage. Long-term sequelae like memory, cognitive and speech problems, behavior and personality changes and epilepsy are common. Rehabilitation will require the joint efforts of a pediatrician, pediatric neurologist, physiotherapist, speech therapist and a psychiatrist.

PROGNOSIS

The spectrum of brain involvement and prognosis depend mainly on the age, immune status and specific pathogen. Although specific therapy is limited to few viral agents, early diagnosis and symptomatic and specific treatment improve survival and reduce the extent of permanent brain injury in survivors. Herpes simplex encephalitis is the most important cause of encephalitis in the developed world and has a high rate of morbidity and mortality. Prompt treatment with intravenous acyclovir improves outcomes and therefore it is imperative to have a high index of suspicion in any child presenting with the relevant features. Mortality rate in untreated HSE is around 70%. Two-thirds of survivors have significant neuropsychiatric sequelae, including memory impairment, personality and behavioral change, dysphasia and epilepsy.

In JE the case-fatality ratio is approximately 20–30%. Among survivors, 30–50% have significant neurologic, cognitive or psychiatric sequelae.

PREVENTION

Japanese encephalitis has epidemic potential in India and has a high case fatality and disease control will be impossible without a surveillance system. Surveillance is important to detect actual disease burden and early warning signals for predicting JE outbreak and to initiate timely effective control measures. Till 2005, JE was reported as suspected JE; however, as per the revised guidelines prepared by *National Vector Borne Disease Control Programme*, JE is being reported under the umbrella of AES. For surveillance of AES, the case definition recommended by WHO is used. Japanese encephalitis surveillance system collects the information on epidemiologic, clinical, laboratory and entomological parameters from the identified sites on a regular basis. In the sentinel surveillance network, AES/JE will be diagnosed by IgM Capture ELISA, and virus isolation will be done in National Reference Laboratory. It is very important to report all the suspected cases of AES or JE to the appropriate health authorities to prevent further spread of disease. Blood (serum) and CSF specimen are to be collected and transported to reference laboratories as per the guidelines.

Vaccination

Some VE may be prevented by immunization (e.g. MMR, JE and rabies). Universal immunization is recommended against MMR and poliovirus. Adequate vector control and environmental sanitation are essential to prevent large outbreaks of arboviral encephalitis such as JE. A sentinel surveillance system is operational in India to monitor disease burden of acute encephalitis including JE in India. Travellers to specific geographical destinations should receive advice regarding vaccination against rabies and JE. Vaccination and vector control measures are useful preventive strategies in arboviral encephalitis.

Three types of vaccine against JE are used worldwide: inactivated mouse brain, inactivated and live-attenuated primary hamster kidney cells. In India, inactivated mouse brain vaccine produced from the Nakayama strain manufactured at Central Research Institute, Kasauli, Himachal Pradesh, is used. In the past, JE vaccination in India was carried out in small geographic areas, but following massive outbreaks in Uttar Pradesh and Bihar in 2005, vaccination campaigns were intensified. Indian Academy of Pediatrics Committee on Immunization recommends that the government should implement universal immunization with this vaccine in all children in JE endemic states.

BIBLIOGRAPHY

1. Chaudhuri A, Kennedy PG. Diagnosis and treatment of viral encephalitis. Postgrad Med J. 2002;78(924):575-83.

2. Christie LJ, Honarmand S, Talkington DF, et al. Pediatric encephalitis: what is the role of Mycoplasma pneumoniae? Pediatrics. 2007;120(2):305-13.

3. Clinical management of acute encephalitis syndrome including japanese encephalitis. Government of India. Directorate of National Vector Borne Disease Control Programme (2009). [online] Available from www.nvbdcp. gov.in/Doc/Revised%20guidelines%20on%20AES_JE.pdf.

4. Coyle PK. Post-infectious encephalomyelitis. In: Davis LE, Kennedy PGE (Eds). Infectious Diseases of the Nervous System. Oxford: Butterworth-Heinemann; 2000. pp. 83-108.

5. Domenech C, Leveque N, Lina B, et al. Role of mycoplasma pneumoniae in pediatric encephalitis. Eur J Clin Microbiol Dis. 2009;28(1):91-4.

6. Feigin RD, Cherry JD, Demmler-Harrison GJ, et al. (Eds). Feigin and Cherry's Textbook of Pediatric Infectious Diseases, Encephalitis and Meningoencephalitis, 6th edition. Philadelphia: Saunders; 2009.

7. Guidelines for Prevention and Control of Japanese Encephalitis. World Health Organization: Geneva. Available from www.whoindia.org/LinkFiles/Communicable_ Diseases_Guidelines_for_Prevention_and_Control_ Japanese_Encephalitis.pdf.

8. Karmarkar SA, Aneja S, Khare S, et al. A study of acute febrile encephalopathy with special reference to viral etiology. Indian J Pediatr. 2008;75(8):801-5.

9. Kneen R, Solomon T. Management and outcome of viral encephalitis in children. Paediatr and Child Health. 2007;18:1.

10. Koelfen W, Freund M, Gückel F, et al. MRI of encephalitis in children: comparison of CT and MRI in the acute stage with long-term follow-up. Neuroradiology. 1996;38(1):73-9.

11. Solomon T, Hart IJ, Beeching NJ. Viral encephalitis: a clinician's guide. Pract Neurol. 2007;7(5):288-305.

12. Steiner I, Budka H, Chaudhuri A, et al. Viral encephalitis: a review of diagnostic methods and guidelines for management. Eur J Neurol. 2005;12(5):331-43.

13. Varatharaj A. Encephalitis in the clinical spectrum of dengue infection. Neurol India. 2010;58(4):585-91.

14. Whitley RJ. Herpes simplex virus infection. Semin Pediatr Infect Dis. 2002;13(1):6-11.

15. Worldwide Distribution of Major Arboviral Encephalitides. Centres for Disease Control: New York. Available from www. cdc.gov/ncidod/dvbid/arbor/worldist.pdf.

Savitri Shrivastava, Ashutosh Marwah

3.7 INFECTIVE ENDOCARDITIS

INTRODUCTION

Infective endocarditis (IE) is a microbial infection of the endocardial (endothelial) surface of the heart. Native or prosthetic heart valves are the most frequently involved sites. Endocarditis also can involve septal defects, the mural endocardium, or intravascular foreign devices such as intracardiac patches, surgically constructed shunts, and intravenous catheters.

Infective endocarditis continues to remain a serious disease despite advances in its recognition and treatment modalities. It is uncommon in pediatric population; however, the incidence may be on rise. In a review of several published studies between 1986 and 1995, the estimated incidence in children was 0.3 per 100,000 children per year with a mortality of 11.6%. In the western world, the epidemiology of heart disease has changed over past few decades. There has been a decline in population with rheumatic heart disease and a gradual increase in the survivors of children with congenital heart defects (CHD). Congenital heart defects now constitute the predominant underlying cause in developed countries. The situation in India is even worse; there is a huge load of rheumatic heart disease and also a growing population of patients with CHD. To complicate the issues further there is a rampant use of antibiotics and lack of laboratory facilities for proper identification of cases.

Incidence of IE in developed countries has been reported to be around 1.7–6.2 cases per 100,000 patient years, accounting for 1 out of 1,280 pediatric admission per year. The exact incidence of endocarditis remains unknown. In various published series rheumatic heart disease still contributes to greater number of patients. The blood cultures are more often negative and there is higher mortality and morbidity due to delay in diagnosis.

PATHOGENESIS

Two important factors in the pathogenesis of IE are:
1. Structural abnormalities of the heart or great arteries, with significant pressure gradient or turbulence, resulting in endothelial damage and platelet and fibrin aggregation.
2. Presence of bacteria in blood stream, even if transiently.

Most patients who develop IE have an underlying CHD or acquired heart disease such as rheumatic heart disease. All CHDs with exception of a fossa ovalis atrial septal defect (ASD) can be risk factors for endocarditis. Most frequently encountered lesions include small ventricular defects, tetralogy of Fallot, patent ductus arteriosus (PDA), bicuspid aortic valve, mitral valve, etc. In developed world there has been a decline in cases of rheumatic heart disease, children with congenital cardiac defects have emerged as major group developing endocarditis. Most of these have had previous corrective or palliative surgery for CHD, with or without implanted vascular grafts, patches or prosthetic cardiac valves often associated with indwelling central lines or catheters. In 8–10% of pediatric population endocarditis develops without any structural heart disease or identifiable risk factor and usually involves aortic or mitral valve secondary to *Staphylococcus aureus* bacteremia. Children with immune deficiencies but without an identifiable risk factor do not seem to have an increased risk for endocarditis. Intravenous drug abuse and degenerative heart disease are not common predisposing factors in children.

In children with cardiac defects high velocity jet stream of blood predisposes to formation of nonbacterial thrombotic endocarditis, the lesions are sterile clumps of platelets and fibrin. Presence of bacteria in the bloodstream in sufficient numbers may lead to colonization and proliferation of bacteria. The organisms trapped within the vegetation are protected from phagocytes and host defense mechanisms. Bacterial load in these vegetations may reach as high as 10^7 colony forming units/gram of tissue.

PATHOLOGY

Vegetations of IE are found on the low pressure side of the defect or either around the defect or on opposite surface of the defect. Vegetations are found in the pulmonary artery in PDA, or on the atrial surface of mitral valve in mitral regurgitation and on mitral valve chordae in patients with acute regurgitation. Surgical correction of CHDs with exception of ASD and PDA may not completely eliminate the risk of endocarditis.

Microorganisms

The majority of cases of IE are caused by relatively small number of organisms. These organisms display propensity for adherence to human and canine valves. In most series of adult patients, gram-positive cocci account for about 90% of cases. Similar trends have been reported in children. Alpha hemolytic streptococci are responsible for most cases of endocarditis in all age groups. Gram-negative organisms cause less than 10% of endocarditis in children. Neonates, immunocompromised patients and intravenous drug abusers are at an increased risk for Gram-negative infection. Among the HACEK group *Haemophilus* species are more common in children.

In instances of prosthetic valve endocarditis the infective organism differ, depending on whether endocarditis occurs early (<3 months) or late after surgery. Early onset endocarditis is caused by possible contamination during the surgery or through occult bacteremia occurring during hospital stay. Most often these organisms are multidrug resistant. In contrast late onset endocarditis is caused by coagulase negative streptococci or staphylococci.

Fungal endocarditis is the most dreaded form of endocarditis. *Candida albicans, Aspergillus* species and *Torulopsis glabrata* are the frequent organisms. Fungal endocarditis is often found in drug addicts or after cardiac surgery. In neonates fungal endocarditis may occur following prolonged use of broad spectrum antibiotic and indwelling catheters. The mortality rate with fungal endocarditis is high even with intensive medical and surgical therapy.

According to western data approximately 5% of patients with endocarditis have negative blood cultures. This could be due to fastidious organisms or prior treatment with antibiotics. Consultation with the clinical microbiologists is invaluable in looking for fastidious organisms.

CLINICAL FEATURES

Presentation in children is usually indolent, with prolonged fever, weight loss, diaphoresis and myalgia. The manifestation is secondary to ongoing bacteremia, valvulitis, embolic and immunological phenomenon.

The cardiac involvement may result in new or changing murmur, ECG abnormalities and congestive failure. The peripheral manifestations, such as Roth spots, Janeway lesions, Osler's nodes and renal abnormalities, are caused by circulating immune complexes. The vegetations may embolize and produce symptoms of ischemia or hemorrhage of the organ involved. There may be metastatic abscess secondary to septic emboli and mycotic aneurysms may be seen in the brain.

On occasion endocarditis may present as acute illness with spiking temperatures and rapid worsening of patient's condition due to cardiac decompensation secondary to cardiac lesion. These children often require urgent surgical interventions. In patients with palliated CHDs there may not be much change in the murmurs but declining oxygen saturation and congestive cardiac failure may be indirect pointers toward endocarditis.

DIAGNOSTIC CRITERIA

The diagnosis of endocarditis may be straight forward in patients with classical manifestations: valvulitis, bacteremia peripheral emboli and immune phenomenon. In many, the classical manifestations may be few or absent. Variability in clinical presentation of endocarditis requires diagnostic criteria that are both sensitive and specific. Duke's criteria enable the identification of a high proportion of definite cases, are flexible and are an accurate reflection of current clinical practice. These criteria have been validated in large series of both adults and children.

Box 3.7.1

Definitions of terms used in the Duke's criteria for the diagnosis of infective endocarditis.

Major criteria
- Positive blood culture for IE:
  - Typical microorganism consistent with IE from two separate blood cultures as noted below:
    - *Viridans streptococci**, *Streptococcus bovis* or HACEK group or
    - Community-acquired *S. aureus* or enterococci, in the absence of a primary focus or
  - Microorganisms consistent with IE from persistently positive blood cultures defined as:
    - Greater than or equal to 2 positive cultures of blood samples drawn > 12 hours apart or
    - All of three or a majority of ≥ 4 separate cultures of blood (with first and last sample drawn ≥ 1 hour apart)
- Evidence of endocardial involvement:
  - Positive echocardiogram for IE defined as:
    - Oscillating intracardiac mass on valve or supporting structures, in the path of regurgitant jets, or on implanted material in the absence of an alternative anatomic explanation, or
    - Abscess, or
    - New partial dehiscence of prosthetic valve or
- New valvular regurgitation (worsening or changing of pre-existing murmur not sufficient)

Minor criteria
- *Predisposition:* Predisposing heart condition or IV drug use
- *Fever:* Temperature ≥ 38.0°C
- *Vascular phenomena:* Major arterial emboli, septic pulmonary infarcts, mycotic aneurysm, intracranial hemorrhage, conjunctival hemorrhages and Janeway lesions
- *Immunologic phenomena:* Glomerulonephritis, Osler nodes, Roth's spots and rheumatoid factor
- *Microbiological evidence:* Positive blood culture but does not meet a major criterion as noted above or serological evidence of active infection with organism consistent with IE
- *Echocardiographic findings:* Consistent with IE but do not meet a major criterion as noted above

Abbreviations: HACEK, hemophilus species, Actinobacillus (Hemophilis) actinomycetemcomitans, *Cardiobacterium hominis*, *Eikenella* species and *Kingella kingae*; IE, infective endocarditis; IV, intravenous.

*Includes nutritionally variant strains (*Abiotrophia* species).

Excludes single positive cultures for coagulase-negative staphylococci and organisms that do not cause endocarditis.

Recently proposed modified criteria have been shown to be superior to previous criteria in adult population and are outlined in the Boxes 3.7.1 and 3.7.2. The sensitivity of these criteria in Indian population remains to be tested. In absence of positive blood cultures and limited availability of echocardiography a large number of patients may be missed.

LABORATORY ASSESSMENT

Blood Culture

In patients with known cardiac lesion blood cultures are indicated in all patients with fever of unexplained origin. The bacteremia is usually continuous, it is not necessary to obtain cultures only during fever, but it is important to send

Duke's clinical criteria for diagnosis of infective endocarditis.

Definite IE:

Pathological criteria:

- *Microorganisms:* Demonstrated by culture or histology in a vegetation, a vegetation that has embolized, or an intracardiac abscess, or
- *Pathological lesions:* Vegetation or intracardiac abscess present, confirmed by histology showing active endocarditis

Clinical criteria as defined in Box 3.7.1:

- Two major criteria, or
- One major criterion and three minor criteria, or
- Five minor criteria

Possible IE:

- Findings consistent with IE that fall short of "definite" but not "rejected"

Rejected:

- Firm alternative diagnosis for manifestations of endocarditis, or
- Resolution of manifestations of endocarditis with antibiotic therapy for ≤ 4 days or
- No pathological evidence of IE at surgery or autopsy, after antibiotic therapy for ≤ 4 days

Abbreviation: IE, infective endocarditis.

adequate volumes of blood (1–3 mL in infants and 5–7 mL in older children). At least three blood cultures are obtained by separate venipuncture on 1st day and two more cultures may be obtained if there has been no growth by 48 hours. According to ACC guidelines, it is not necessary to send anaerobic cultures as it is rare to have anaerobes as the etiological agent.

A large number of patients in our country receive antibiotics before they present at tertiary care centers. This results in more number of negative cultures. Sometimes withholding antibiotics for 3–4 days before sending blood culture helps in improving the yield, but such a practice is hard to follow even at best of institutes. In published series from India the blood culture positivity has been reported to be between 47% and 67%. Fastidious organism, such as Coxiella, HACEK group, *Chlamydia*, etc., may not grow on routine cultures and require special serological tests for exact diagnosis.

A false-positive blood culture is also not so uncommon in clinical setting. Blood samples should be taken with strict aseptic technique to avoid contamination by normal skin commensals such as coagulase negative staphylococci and prevent overtreatment. Bacteremia in hospitalized patients does not always result in endocarditis; however, any persistent and unexplained bacteremia should be investigated properly. Approximately 12% patients with staphylococcal bacteremia develop endocarditis, whereas almost 50% patients with prosthetic valves with associated staphylococcal bacteremia develop endocarditis. Recent guidelines have included staphylococcal bacteremia as major criterion.

Echocardiography

Cross-sectional echocardiography has become an essential tool for diagnosing and management of endocarditis.

Echocardiographic findings have been included as major criteria in recent Duke's criteria. Echocardiography can detect the site of infection, the extent of cardiac involvement and cardiac function and the size of vegetation, large vegetation being suggestive of fungal or staphylococcal endocarditis. Associated problems such as pericardial effusion, abscess formation, valve or patch dehiscence can also be detected. Large mobile vegetation on left-sided structures may need early surgery to prevent embolization. Transthoracic echo (TTE) has been reported to have sensitivity of 81% in pediatric population. It remains the investigation of choice in most clinical setting. However, a transesophageal echocardiography has been shown to be superior to TTE in adults for detection of vegetations on native and prosthetic valves. No similar comparisons are available in children. Transesophageal echocardiography may be used in patients with poor imaging windows or patients already on ventilators.

Echocardiography may also be used to monitor the progress of the patients. Cardiac size, worsening of valve incompetence, increase in size of vegetation or development of myocardial abscess can all be monitored. Although echocardiography may be able to pick up vegetations in culture negative endocarditis, absence of vegetation does not exclude the diagnosis of endocarditis. Also one must remember old vegetations, sterile mass, ruptured chordae or a normal anatomical variation may be confused for active endocarditis.

Molecular Techniques

Fastidious organisms, such as *Coxiella*, *Legionella*, *Chlamydia*, etc. are often difficult to culture by routine methods. Techniques such as polymerase chain reaction (PCR) with signal amplification alone or in combination with sequence analysis allow a rapid and reliable identification of the causative agent. Polymerase chain reaction may also help in differentiating commensals after isolating different bacteria in different samples. Although the technique offers a great advantage over the routine cultures but it has its limitations. It is not able to give any antimicrobial sensitivity pattern. There is risk of contamination leading to false-positive results. Presence of PCR inhibitors may lead to false-negative results. Another disadvantage in our country is the cost and nonavailability of these tests for routine use.

Histological and Immunological Methods

Demonstration of microbial organism on a pathological specimen (resected valve or vegetation) remains the reference standard for diagnosis of endocarditis. It may be possible to culture the organism from the vegetation or identify the agent using immunohistological techniques. *Coxiella burnetii* may be easily identified by serological testing with enzyme linked immunosorbent assay.

Miscellaneous Investigations

Other investigations include a hemogram showing polymorphic response and anemia of chronic illness. There may be raised erythrocyte sedimentation rate, and C-reactive protein. Urine microscopy may show red blood cell casts and proteinuria.

ANTIBIOTIC TREATMENT

Recommendations for antibiotic treatment in adults have been made by American Heart Association (AHA). Tables 3.7.1 to 3.7.3 give guidelines for children based on the AHA recommendations.

Streptococcal Infective Endocarditis on Native Cardiac Valves or Prosthetic Material

Viridans group of streptococci remain the most common cause of IE in community. In patients with organisms susceptible to penicillin [minimum inhibitory concentration (MIC) < 0.1 µg] a 4-week regime of crystalline penicillin G achieves a high cure rate. In adults ceftriaxone given for 4 weeks has been recommended but experience in pediatric population is limited. A 2 week course of penicillin or ceftriaxone in combination with gentamicin also results 98% cure rate in adults. This regimen is recommended for children with uncomplicated endocarditis of less than 3 months duration. It is also inappropriate for children at risk of adverse effects caused by gentamicin therapy. Once daily use of gentamicin is popular in adults; however, such a practice is not recommended for children with IE.

In patients with streptococci relatively resistant to penicillin (MIC >0.5 mg/mL) use of penicillin or ampicillin or ceftriaxone in combination with gentamicin for first 2 weeks has been recommended. For patients sensitive to penicillin vancomycin has been recommended.

Patients with endocarditis of prosthetic cardiac valves with penicillin-susceptible strains should be treated for 6 weeks. Patients sensitive to penicillin should receive vancomycin for 6 weeks along with gentamicin for first 2 weeks.

Table 3.7.1: Regimens for therapy of native valve, i.e. caused by viridans group streptococci, *Streptococcus bovis* or enterococci.*

Organism	Antimicrobial agent	Dosage (per kg per 24 hours)	Frequency of administration	Duration, week
Penicillin-susceptible streptococci (MIC ≤ 0.1 µg/mL)[†]	Penicillin G[†]	200,000 U IV	q 4–6 hours	4
	or			
	Ceftriaxone	100 mg IV	q 24 hours	4
	Penicillin G[†]	200,000 U IV	q 4–6 hours	2
	or			
	Ceftriaxone	100 mg IV	q 24 hours	2
	plus			
	Gentamicin	3 mg IM or IV	q 8 hours[‡]	2
Streptococci relatively resistant to penicillin (MIC >0.1–0.5 µg/mL)	Penicillin G[†]	300,000 IV	q 4–6 hours	4
	or			
	Ceftriaxone	100 mg IV	q 24 hours	4
	plus			
	Gentamicin	3 mg IM or IV	q 8 hours[†]	2
Enterococci,¶ nutritionally variant viridans Streptococci or high-level penicillin-resistant Streptococci (MIC >0.5 µg/mL)	Penicillin G[†]	300,000 U IV	q 4–6 hours	4–6[§]
	Plus gentamicin	3 mg IM or IV	q 8 hours[‖]	4–6[§]

For treatment of patients with prosthetic cardiac valves or other prosthetic materials, see text. MIC indicates minimum inhibitory concentration of penicillin.

* Dosages suggested are for patients with normal renal and hepatic function. Maximum dosages per 24 hours: penicillin 18 million units; ampicillin 12 g; ceftriaxone 4 g; gentamicin 240 mg. The 2-week regimens are not recommended for patients with symptoms of infection >3 months in duration, those with extracardiac focus of infection, myocardial abscess, mycotic aneurysm or infection with nutritionally variant viridans streptococci (*Abiotrophia* spp.).

[†] Ampicillin 300 mg/kg per 24 hours in 4–6 divided dosages may be used as an alternative to penicillin.

[‡] Studies in adults suggest gentamicin dosage may be administered in single daily dose. If gentamicin is administered in three equally divided doses per 24 hours, adjust dosage to achieve peak and trough concentrations in serum of ≈3.0 and <1.0 µg of gentamicin per mL respectively.

[§] Studies in adults suggest that 4 weeks of therapy is sufficient for patients with enterococcal IE with symptoms of infection of <3 months' duration; 6 weeks of therapy is recommended for patients with symptoms of infection of >3 months' duration.

[‖] Adjust gentamicin dosage to achieve peak and trough concentrations in serum of ≈3.0 and <1.0 µg of gentamicin per mL respectively.

¶ For enterococci resistant to penicillin, vancomycin, or aminoglycosides, treatment should be guided by consultation with specialist in infectious diseases (cephalosporins should not be used to treat enterococcal endocarditis regardless of *in vitro* susceptibility).

Table 3.7.2: Treatment regimens for therapy of infective endocarditis caused by viridans group streptococci, *Streptococcus bovis* or enterococci in patients unable to tolerate β-lactam.[*]

Organism	Antimicrobial agent	Dosage (per kg per 24 hours)	Frequency of administration	Duration, week
Native valve (no prosthetic material)				
Streptococci	Vancomycin	40 mg IV	q 6–12 hours	4–6
Enterococci[†] or nutritionally variant viridans streptococci	Vancomycin plus	40 mg IV	q 6–12 hours	6
	Gentamicin	3 mg IM or IV	q 8 hours[‡]	6
Prosthetic devices				
Streptococci	Vancomycin plus	40 mg IV	q 6–12 hours	6
	Gentamicin	3 mg IM or IV	q 8 hours[‡]	2
Enterococci[†] or nutritionally variant viridans streptococci	Vancomycin plus	40 mg IV	q 6–12 hours	6
	Gentamicin	3 mg IM or IV	q 8 hours[‡]	6

[*]Dosages suggested are for patients with normal renal function. Maximum daily dose per 24 hours of gentamicin is 240 mg.

[†]For enterococci resistant to vancomycin or aminoglycosides, treatment should be guided by consultation with specialist in infectious diseases.

[‡]Dosage of gentamicin should be adjusted to achieve peak and trough concentration in serum of ≈3.0 and <1.0 µg of gentamicin per mL respectively.

Table 3.7.3: Treatment regimens for endocarditis caused by staphylococci.[*]

Organism	Antimicrobial agent	Dosage (per kg per 24 hours)	Frequency of administration	Duration
Native valve (no prosthetic materials)				
Methicillin-susceptible	Nafcillin or oxacillin	200 mg IV	q 4–6 hours	6 weeks
	With or without gentamicin[†]	3 mg IM or IV[#]	q 8 hours	3–5 days
β-Lactam allergic	Cefazolin[§] with or without	100 mg IV	q 6–8 hours	6 weeks
	Gentamicin[†]	3 mg IM or IV[#]	q 8 hours	3–5 days
	or			
	Vancomycin	40 mg IV	q 6–12 hours	6 weeks
Methicillin-resistant	Vancomycin	40 mg IV	q 6–12 hours	6 weeks
Prosthetic device or other prosthetic materials				
Methicillin-susceptible	Nafcillin or oxacillin	200 mg IV	q 4–6 hours	≥6 weeks
	or			
	Cefazolin[§]	100 mg IV	q 6–8 hours	≥6 weeks
	Plus rifampin[‖]	20 mg po	q 8 hours	≥6 weeks
	Plus gentamicin[†]	3 mg IM or IV[#]	q 8 hours	2 weeks
Methicillin-resistant	Vancomycin	40 mg IV	q 6–12 hours	≥6 weeks
	Plus rifampin[‖]	20 mg po	q 8 hours	≥6 weeks
	Plus gentamicin[†]	3 mg IM or IV[#]	q 8 hours	2 weeks

[*]Dosages suggested are for patients with normal renal and hepatic function. Maximum daily doses per 24 hours: oxacillin or nafcillin 12 g; cefazolin 6; gentamicin 240 mg; rifampin 900 mg.

[†]Gentamicin therapy should be used only with gentamicin-susceptible strains.

[#]Dosage of gentamicin should be adjusted to achieve peak and trough concentrations in serum of ≈ 3.0 and <1.0 µg of gentamicin per mL respectively.

[§]Cefazolin or other first-generation cephalosporin in equivalent dosages may be used in patients who do not have a history of immediate type hypersensitivity (urticaria, angioedema and anaphylaxis) to penicillin or ampicillin.

[‖]Dosages suggested for rifampins are based upon results of studies conducted in adults and should be used only with rifampin-susceptible strains.

Enterococcal Endocarditis

Enterococcal endocarditis is rare in children. The treatment for native valve endocarditis is penicillin plus gentamicin for 6 weeks or vancomycin plus gentamicin for 6 weeks in patients sensitive to penicillin. The aminoglycoside should be given for entire 6 weeks and in patients with normal renal function aminoglycoside should be administered in two or three divided doses rather than single daily dose. Enterococci are resistant to cephalosporin and these drugs are not recommended for treatment of enterococcal endocarditis. Vancomycin-resistant isolates of enterococci are often multidrug resistant and difficult to treat. Linezolid has resulted in cure rate of about 77% in patients with vancomycin-resistant enterococcal infections. Use of double-beta lactam antibiotic combinations such as imipenem and ampicillin or cephalosporin plus ampicillin has also been recommended for treating high-level resistant strains. Surgery may offer the best cure for some of these patients.

Staphylococcal Endocarditis

Both coagulase-positive and coagulase-negative staphylococci can cause IE in susceptible patient. Most staphylococci are resistant to beta-lactam antibiotics. Endocarditis due to staphylococci susceptible to beta-lactamase resistant penicillin (the methicillin-susceptible staphylococci) should be treated for 6 weeks using oxacillin or nafcillin. Gentamicin may be added for 3–5 weeks to achieve rapid cure. First-generation cephalosporin such as cefazolin can be used as an alternative for first 3–5 days of the therapy. Patients not able to tolerate penicillin should receive vancomycin for minimum of 6 weeks.

Methicillin-resistant *Staphylococcus* is seen often in community. Patient with endocarditis due to methicillin-resistant strains should be treated with combination of vancomycin and gentamicin for minimum of 6 weeks.

Prosthetic-valve Endocarditis

Treatment of prosthetic-valve endocarditis is often difficult. In patients with early onset of staphylococcal or fungal endocarditis one should always consider replacement of the infected material. The timing of surgery should be individualized. Experience in adults shows lower mortality if infected valves are replaced early.

Infection caused by gram-negative organisms requires treatment for 6–8 weeks based on *in vitro* culture sensitivity, whereas diphtheroids are best treated with penicillin gentamicin or vancomycin and gentamicin for at least 6 weeks.

Prosthetic-valve endocarditis caused by streptococci, enterococci should be treated on the guidelines discussed earlier.

Culture-negative Endocarditis

A lot of patients in our country receive or self-medicate themselves before presenting to a tertiary care center. If cultures are negative after careful evaluation therapy should be initiated with ceftriaxone and gentamicin. Beta-lactamase resistant penicillin should be added to the regimen if staphylococcal infection is suspected. Vancomycin should be added if methicillin-resistant staphylococcal infection is suspected. A team approach in consultation with infectious disease specialist is helpful in optimizing the treatment of culture-negative endocarditis.

ROLE OF SURGERY

Patients with IE with congestive heart failure (CHF) should be evaluated for surgery. Despite higher surgical mortality rate in patients with CHF the mortality is lower in patients undergoing timely surgery, as compared to those managed on medical therapy alone. The incidence of reinfection of implanted valves is about 2–3% as compared to mortality without surgery, which can approach 51% on medical management alone.

Surgery is also indicated in cases of valve dehiscence, periannular abscess formation, or a fistulous tract into pericardium. Other indication for surgery is presence of large vegetation greater than or equal to 10 mm, which are at the risk of systemic embolization. The greatest risk of embolization is in first 2 weeks of therapy. Fungal infection or infection with aggressive antibiotic-resistant bacteria, persistent culture positivity after 1 week of antibiotics or one or more embolic events during first 2 weeks may also warrant surgery. In children with endocarditis of shunts or prosthetic conduits likelihood of cure with antibiotics alone is low and surgical intervention is often needed.

Care at Completion of Treatment

In patients completing the treatment an echocardiogram should be obtained to establish a new baseline for subsequent comparisons. A thorough dental referral should be done to remove any infected teeth and proper dental hygiene advised all indwelling catheters should be removed. A relapse may occur despite successful treatment. Fresh cultures should be obtained before initiating treatment of relapse. Every effort should be made to identify and treat the cause of relapse. Congestive heart failure may worsen during follow-up and may need aggressive decongestive therapy or valve replacement. Late onset complications of antibiotic toxicity should be looked into and treated.

BIBLIOGRAPHY

1. Baddour LM, Sullam PM, Bayer AS. The pathogenesis of infective endocarditis. In: Sussman M (Ed). Molecular Medical Microbiology. San Diego, California: Academic Press; 2001. pp. 999-1020.

2. Baddour LM, Wilson WR, Bayer AS, et al. Infective endocarditis: diagnosis, antimicrobial therapy, and management of complications: a statement for healthcare professionals from the Committee on Rheumatic Fever, Endocarditis, and Kawasaki Disease, Council on Cardiovascular Disease in the Young, and the Councils on Clinical Cardiology, Stroke, and Cardiovascular Surgery and Anesthesia, American Heart Association: endorsed by the Infectious Diseases Society of America. Circulation. 2005;111(23):e394-434.

3. Baltimore RS. Infective endocarditis. In: Jenson HB, Baltimore RS (Eds). Pediatric Infectious Diseases: Principles and Practice. Norwalk, CT: Appleton and Lange; 1995.

4. Berkowitz FE. Infective Endocarditis in Childhood. St Louis: CV Mosby; 1995. pp. 961-86.

5. Caviness AC, Cantor SB, Allen CH, et al. A cost-effectiveness analysis of bacterial endocarditis prophylaxis for febrile children who have cardiac lesions and undergo urinary catheterization in the emergency department. Pediatrics. 2004;113(5):1291-6.

6. Choudhury R, Grover A, Varma J, et al. Active infective endocarditis observed in an Indian hospital 1981–1991. Am J Cardiol. 1992;70(18):1453-8.

7. Citak M, Rees A, Mavroudis C. Surgical management of infective endocarditis in children. Ann Thorac Surg. 1992;54(4):755-60.

8. Coward K, Tucker N, Darville T. Infective endocarditis in Arkansan children from 1990 through 2002. Pediatr infect Dis J. 2003;22(12):1048-52.

9. Daniel WG, Mugge A, Grote J, et al. Comparison of transthoracic and transesophageal echocardiography for detection of abnormalities of prosthetic and bioprosthetic valves in the mitral and aortic positions. Am J Cardiol. 1993;71(2):210-5.

10. Durack DT, Lukes AS, Bright DK. New criteria for diagnosis of infective endocarditis: utilization of specific echocardiographic findings. Duke Endocarditis Service. Am J Med. 1994;96(3):200-9.

11. Durack DT. Prevention of infective endocarditis. N Engl J Med. 1995;332(1):38-44.

12. Ferrieri P, Gewitz MH, Gerber MA, et al. Unique features of infective endocarditis in childhood. Circulation. 2002;105(17):2115-26.

13. Francioli P, Etienne J, Hoigne R, et al. Treatment of streptococcal endocarditis with a single daily dose of ceftriaxone sodium for 4 weeks: efficacy and outpatient feasibility. JAMA. 1992;267(2):264-7.

14. Gavalda J, Torres C, Tenorio C, et al. Efficacy of ampicillin plus ceftriaxone in treatment of experimental endocarditis due to Enterococcus faecalis strains highly resistant to aminoglycosides. Antimicrob Agents Chemother. 1999;43(3):639-46.

15. John MD, Hibberd PL, Karchmer AW, et al. Staphylococcus aureus prosthetic valve endocarditis: optimal management and risk factors for death. Clin Infect Dis. 1998;26(6):1302-9.

16. Karchmer AW, Gibbons GW. Infection of prosthetic heart valves and vascular grafts. In: Bisno AL, Waldvogel FA (Eds). Infections Associated with Indwelling Medical Devices, 2nd edition. Washington, DC: American Society for Microbiology; 1994. pp. 213-49.

17. Kavey RE, Frank DM, Byrum CJ, et al. Two-dimensional echocardiographic assessment of infective endocarditis in children. Am J Dis Child. 1983;137(9):851-6.

18. Martin JM, Neches WH, Wald ER. Infective endocarditis: 35 years of experience at a children's hospital. Clin Infect Dis. 1997;24(4):669-75.

19. Mugge A, Daniel WG, Frank G, et al. Echocardiography in infective endocarditis: reassessment of prognostic implication of vegetation size determined by transthoracic and transesophageal approach. J Am Coll Cardiol. 1989;14(3):631-8.

20. Olaison L, Pettersson G. Current best practices and guidelines indications for surgical intervention in infective endocarditis. Infect Dis Clin North Am. 2002;16(2):453-75.

21. Saiman L, Prince A, Gersony WM. Pediatric infective endocarditis in the modern era. J Pediatr. 1993;122(6):847-53.

22. Sexton DJ, Spelman D. Current best practices and guidelines. Assessment and management of complications of infective endocarditis. Cardiol Clin. 2003;21(2):273-82.

23. Sexton DJ, Spelman D. Current practices and guidelines. Assessment and management of complications in infective endocarditis. Infect Dis Clin North Am. 2002;16(2):507-21.

24. Stockheim JA, Chadwick EG, Kessler S, et al. Are the Duke criteria superior to the Beth Israel criteria for the diagnosis of infective endocarditis in children? Clin Infect Dis. 1998;27(6):1451-6.

25. Tissieres P, Gervaix A, Beghetti M, et al. Value and limitations of the von Reyn, Duke, and modified Duke criteria for the diagnosis of infective endocarditis in children. Pediatrics. 2003;112(6 Pt 1):e471.

26. Tissieres P, Jaeggi ET, Beghetti M, et al. Increase in fungal endocarditis in children. Infection. 2005;33(4):267-72.

27. Tolan RW, Kleiman MB, Frank M, et al. Operative intervention in active endocarditis in children: report of a series of cases and review. Clin Infect Dis. 1992;14(4):852-62.

28. Van Hare GF, Ben-Shachar G, Liebman J, et al. Infective endocarditis in infants and children during the past 10 years: a decade of change. Am Heart J. 1984;107(6):1235-40.

29. Vuille C, Nidorf M, Weyman AE, et al. Natural history of vegetations during successful treatment of endocarditis. Am Heart J. 1994;128(6 Pt 1):1200-9.

30. Wilson WR, Karchmer AW, Dajani AS, et al. Antibiotic treatment of adults with infective endocarditis due to streptococci, enterococci, staphylococci, and HACEK microorganisms. American Heart Association. JAMA. 1995;274(21):1706-13.

31. Wilson WR, Thompson RL, Wilkowske CJ, et al. Short-term therapy for streptococcal infective endocarditis. Combined intramuscular administration of penicillin and streptomycin. JAMA. 1981;245(4):360-3.

3.8 URINARY TRACT INFECTION AND PYELONEPHRITIS

M Vijayakumar

INTRODUCTION

Urinary tract infection (UTI) is a common bacterial infection in children with variable symptomatology. In neonatal period UTI manifests usually as septicemia and is of acute nature. In infants and older children, UTI can present as either acute or chronic infection. High recurrence is common. Urinary tract infection can be associated with various urinary anomalies and voiding dysfunctions (VDs), which aids in chronicity. In chronic UTI high morbidity is usual with renal scarring, calculi disorder, hypertension and chronic renal failure. The diagnostic evaluation of childhood UTI has undergone useful changes, and noninvasive methods, such as ultrasonography and radioisotope imaging, have become very useful and reliable investigatory tools. Infancy and young age, delayed, inadequate and improper antibacterial treatment, recurrent UTI, VD and associated high grades of vesicoureteral reflux (VUR) are risk factors for renal scarring in a growing kidney of young children. Revised statement on management of UTI from Indian Society of Pediatric Nephrology (ISPN) is also available at present.

EPIDEMIOLOGY

The risk of UTI occurring before 14 years is around 1% in boys and 3–5% in girls. In infancy the male to female ratio is 3–5:1. Male to female ratio of 1:10 beyond this time with female preponderance is noted. About 50% of the children with symptomatic UTI have recurrences. Asymptomatic bacteriuria (ABU) is usually benign and studies had shown that it was not a significant risk factor for renal scarring even without treatment. Hospital-acquired infection should be always kept in mind, especially with indwelling urinary catheter.

DEFINITIONS

Presence of pyuria and bacteriuria in an appropriately collected urine sample are diagnostic of UTI. Infection of the urinary tract is identified by growth of a single species in the urine, in the presence of symptoms. The diagnosis of UTI should be made only in children with a positive urine culture, since this has implications for detailed evaluation and follow-up. With midstream urine sample, infection is likely if the colony count is greater than 10^4 in a boy and the probability of infection is 95% in a girl with three consecutive specimens showing greater than 10^5 colony count. If urine is collected by suprapubic aspiration, the probability of infection is more than 99% even with any growth. If catheterized sample is used, the probability is 95% if colony count is greater than 10^5 colony forming unit/mL and infection is likely if it is between 10^4 and 10^5.

Significant bacteriuria in the absence of symptoms of UTI is called ABU and is commonly seen in school going and adolescent girls and documented usually on screening. A child is considered to have symptomatic UTI if child has significant bacteriuria with symptoms like dysuria, frequency and urgency with or without fever and renal or flank pain.

For a complicated UTI, the child should have fever greater than 39°C, systemic toxicity, persistent vomiting, and dehydration, renal angle tenderness with or without raised serum creatinine. In simple UTI, children will have dysuria, frequency, urgency, with or without fever and none of the symptoms of complicated UTI.

Urinary tract infection with lower tract symptoms like urgency, dysuria and frequency due to inflammation of bladder mucosa is called lower tract UTI or cystitis and is being described as dysuria-frequency syndrome. Usually fever is not the rule. Lower tract infection is common in females and can be benign with less chance of associated anomalies.

On the contrary, features of UTI include fever, flank pain and systemic symptoms. Upper tract infection is a significant infection of renal parenchyma and is termed as acute pyelonephritis (APN). Upper tract infection should be always considered as a serious infection and most of the time is associated with urinary tract anomalies.

Second attack of UTI is usually termed as recurrent UTI. It is the recurrence of symptoms and significant bacteriuria in a child who had previously recovered clinically with appropriate treatment. A relapse is recurrence of UTI within 2 weeks and reinfection if it is later than 2 weeks.

ETIOLOGY

Majority of UTI is due to gram-negative bacteria, the normal inhabitant of large bowel. About 90% of acute infections and 70% of chronic infection are due to *Escherichia coli*. *Klebsiella*, *Proteus*, *Pseudomonas* and enterococci are the other gram-negative organisms encountered in childhood UTI. Staphylococci and streptococci are relatively less common. In recurrent and chronic UTI and UTI associated with instrumentation, foreign body in the tract, immunocompromised host and in nosocomial infections, *Proteus* and *Pseudomonas* are usually seen. *Candida albicans*, *Cryptococcus*, adenovirus and schistosomiasis are uncommon pathogens.

PATHOGENESIS

Pathogenesis of UTI is complex involving interaction of several factors in the host, the child and many factors of the parasite, the bacteria. Route of infection, host factors and virulence factors of the bacteria are important. The route of entry by hematogenous route is possible in neonates. Well-documented bacteremia in 30% of neonates and infants less than 3 months substantiate the point. It is intraurethral ascent in infants and children facilitated by the bacterial adhesions, VUR and obstruction of the urinary tract either anatomical or functional. The mechanism by which the invading organisms ascend from periurethral and vaginal region into the urinary bladder is not fully understood. The organisms, essentially from the bowel flora with emergence of uropathogenic strains, are colonized in the perineal and anterior urethral regions. Vaginal colonization can occur in females. The useful normal mucosal defense barriers have to be crossed for these organisms to induce pathogenetic effect. The interaction between the pathogens with bacterial virulence and the host with various host factors play a major role. The host factors include enhanced uroepithelial adherence, VUR, intrarenal reflux, obstructed urinary tract and foreign body commonly urinary catheter. If interaction is positive the mucosal barrier is broken and urinary bladder is involved with cystitis. If conditions are further favorable APN ending in urosepsis or in renal scarring occurs. Bacteremia developing from a primary focus of infection within the urinary tract is called as urosepsis. Several experimental data is available to show that bacteria can ascend from the urinary bladder into the kidneys and cause acute parenchymal infection. But obstruction of the urinary tract is considered an important prerequisite for this ascent. Vesicoureteral reflux and intrarenal reflux are known factors in the conduction of bacteria and hence the ascent.

Host factors like VUR, intrarenal reflux, urinary tract obstruction, urinary catheter as a foreign body and ureterocele are anatomical issues in UTI. Increased uroepithelial cell adherence is an important host factor predisposing to UTI. Bacterial washout during voiding and various local and mucosal defense mechanisms are other important host factors in the prevention of bacterial adherence to the uroepithelium. Interference of bacteria by endogenous periurethral flora, urinary oligosaccharides, and spontaneous exfoliation of uroepithelial cells, urinary immunoglobulins and mucopolysaccharide lining of the urinary bladder wall are the factors in prevention. Blood-group antigens, ABO, P, Lewis are also present on the uroepithelial cells. Presence of blood-group antigens on the uroepithelial cell surface obscure or inhibit the availability of the uroepithelial receptors for bacterial adhesions in secretors. From various documentations in the past, one can definitely state that it is probable that these components convey very slight changes in risk, but this is difficult to examine in any but well-designed genetic epidemiologic studies. In non-secretors the blood-group antigens are absent on the uroepithelial cells and hence exposes uroepithelium to adherence of bacteria. In many children in whom the urinary tract is normal, the increased susceptibility to UTI may be mediated by an increased capacity of the uroepithelium to bind the invading bacteria as they appear to be "stickier" than normal.

Escherichia coli is well studied for its virulence than any other organism. Serologic OKH types are found frequently associated with pathogenic virulence and APN. Adherence between bacteria and uroepithelial cells is essentially through receptors on uroepithelial cells and "adhesin" protein molecule on bacterial surface. In *E. coli* they are on the tips of pili or fimbriae, which are found radiating from the bacterial surface. Pili expressing characteristic receptor binding features are called P-fimbriae named after the P-blood group antigens, which also contains the same glycosphingolipid that is present in the uroepithelial receptors. P-fimbriae are detected in more than 90% of *E. coli* of urine of patients with APN. It is suggested that bacterial adhesion to uroepithelium may promote an inflammatory response by providing bacterial endotoxins and lipopolysaccharides more efficiently and directly to the renal tissues.

Virulence of *E. coli* cannot be modified at present. Occurrence of congenital urinary tract anomalies cannot be tackled straight away at present. The factor in between the two that is UTI can be tackled effectively if one is aware of the nature of UTI and the mind to correctly suspect it. Then treatment of UTI itself will reduce the parenchymal damage, the ultimate result of upper UTI.

CLINICAL FEATURES

Fever is of special importance as a clinical marker of renal parenchymal involvement (pyelonephritis). As also acknowledged by the American Academy of Pediatrics in its practice parameters, the presence of high fever ($\geq39°C$) with clinical diagnosis of UTI is an important indicator of pyelonephritis compared with no fever ($\leq38°C$) in those with cystitis.

Upper UTI presents during newborn period as septicemia or as fever with vomiting, lethargy, jaundice and seizures. In young children recurrent fever, diarrhea, vomiting, abdominal pain and poor-weight gain are the usual features. In older children, burning micturition, pollakiuria (frequent daytime urination), turbid or foul-smelling urine, secondary nocturnal enuresis and flank pain are other features. Urinary tract infection should be suspected in any infant or child with fever without focus beyond 3 days. Less common and unusual features include hematuria, diurnal or nocturnal incontinence resulting from uninhibited bladder contractions, acute hypertension and acute renal failure.

Cystitis is an inflammation of the lower urinary tract mucosa and usually is not invasive. The clinical features include dysuria, urgency and pollakiuria, suprapubic tenderness, voiding small volume urine and pyuria and absence of systemic manifestations such as fever. Hematuria may be commonly seen in cystitis and is termed as hemorrhagic cystitis. It manifests with large quantities of visible blood in the urine and is usually due to infection, bacterial or adenovirus types 1–47. When noninfectious in origin as in postchemotherapy situations, the signs and symptoms of infection may be absent. Adenovirus is a common cause and is self-limiting in nature. Hemorrhagic cystitis is often confused with glomerulonephritis, but hypertension and abnormal renal function are absent in hemorrhagic cystitis.

Clinical evaluation includes a search for structural abnormality like distended bladder, palpable and enlarged kidneys, tight phimosis in a boy, vulvar synechiae in a girl, palpable fecal mass in the colon, patulous anus, neurological deficit in lower limbs, and evidence of previous surgery of the urinary tract, anorectal malformation or meningomyelocele.

DIAGNOSTIC FEATURES

As it requires a minimum of about 24–48 hours before a urine culture result is known, rapid tests are often used to guide the initial management. Urine examined by dipstick and microscopy are two rapid tests. Rapid tests, like nitrite and leukocyte esterase, tests have problems of false positivity and negativity. Bacterial enzyme nitrate reductase can convert the urinary nitrate to nitrite, which can be detected. If sufficient time is not allowed for incubation of bacteria with urine, the tests become negative as in children with increased frequency. Even if UTI is caused by bacteria that do not contain nitrate reductase as in streptococcal species, false-negative results are seen. Similarly leukocyte esterase test detects leukocytes in urine, which can be present in UTI as well as in other conditions like interstitial nephritis or glomerulonephritis. More specificity is gained by combining a positive test for leukocyte esterase and nitrite in a child with clinicobiological features of UTI. Leukocyturia (> 5 WBC/HPF in centrifuged urine and >10 WBC/mm^3 in uncentrifuged urine) and bacteria on Gram stain can indicate UTI. In infants and children below 5 years pyuria may be absent in more than 50% of UTIs. We should note that pyuria need not indicate always UTI and can be seen in vaginitis, renal stone disease, interstitial nephritis, glomerulonephritis and rarely appendicitis. Enhanced urinalysis using uncentrifuged urine sample for leukocyturia in Neubauer counting chamber along with presence of any bacteria per 10 oil immersion field of Gram-stained smear is useful for supportive evidence of UTI. Urine Gram stained for bacteria has a better sensitivity (91%) and specificity (96%) than all other rapid tests used alone or in combination. A combination of positive enhanced urinalysis and rapid test will indicate UTI in 95% of the children. Ultimately the gold standard for the diagnosis of UTI, a positive urine culture is needed.

INITIAL EVALUATION

Clinical Evaluation

This evaluation becomes mandatory even at the stage of initial diagnosis of UTI, as this will give clues toward underlying anomalies and seriousness of the UTI. The following clinicobiological features should be noted. Degree of toxicity, dehydration and blood pressure recording should be noted. Bowel and bladder habits, straining during micturition, dribbling, double micturition, narrow stream of urine and prepuceal ballooning should be enquired. Voiding disorders, like nocturnal enuresis, should not be missed. Abdominal examination for renal and bladder masses and genital examination for prepuceal adhesions and phimosis in boys and vaginal synechiae in girls should be done. Central nervous system (CNS) examination of the lower limbs when voiding disorders are noted and rectal examination when history of constipation is present should not be overlooked.

Laboratory Evaluation

Elevated peripheral WBC count, polymorphonuclear leukocytosis, elevated C-reactive protein (CRP) levels and elevated ESR will aid in the diagnosis. Renal dysfunction is assessed by blood urea, serum creatinine and electrolytes estimation. Mild-to-moderate renal dysfunction can occur with severe APN more so if it involves both the kidneys or the single functioning kidney. Hyperkalemic metabolic acidosis may be a feature in APN especially when it occurs in a single functioning kidney. Ultrasound sonography (USG) examination is done to rule out underlying anatomical defects like obstruction and to assess the number, position, size and shape. Dilated collecting system, stone disease and pyelonephritis as suggested by unilateral nephromegaly, increased echotexture of the kidneys, pelvic wall thickening (pyelitis) and turbid urine in the collecting system can also be detected.

INITIAL MANAGEMENT

The need for hospitalization is decided on factors like the child's age, features suggesting toxicity and dehydration, ability to retain oral intake and the likelihood of compliance with medication, clinical urosepsis, laboratory evidence of bacteremia, immunocompromised state, lack of adequate outpatient follow-up and failure to respond to outpatient therapy. A sick, febrile child with inadequate oral intake or dehydration may require parenteral fluids. Paracetamol is used to relieve fever and it is always preferable to avoid the use of nonsteroidal anti-inflammatory agents. Prompt antibiotic treatment is needed to reduce the morbidity of infection, minimize renal damage and subsequent complications. Young infants less than 3 months of age and children with complicated UTI need hospitalization and are treated with parenteral antibiotics. Initial parenteral medications include ceftriaxone, cefotaxime, aminoglycoside and co-amoxiclav. Prelog et al. in retrospective study of children with febrile UTI showed that ampicillin and trimethoprim are insufficient as empirical monotherapy. Few advocate single daily dose of aminoglycoside in children with normal renal function. Subsequent treatment may be modified based on antimicrobial sensitivity. For the first 48–72 hours parenteral therapy is given and oral antibiotics are started with clinical improvement. Oral medications used in childhood UTI include cefixime, co-amoxiclav, ciprofloxacin and cefdinir. Children with only lower UTI and those above 3 months of age with upper UTI can be treated with oral antibiotics. With adequate therapy, there is resolution of fever and reduction of symptoms by 48–72 hours. Failure to respond to therapy may be due to presence of resistant pathogens, complicating factors or noncompliance and these children require re-evaluation. The duration of therapy is 10–14 days for infants and children with APN and 7–10 days for simple UTI. In children with severe pyelonephritis as in acute lobar nephronia (ALN) prolonged parenteral therapy may help to prevent progression to abscess. Following the treatment of the UTI, prophylactic antibiotic therapy is initiated in children below 1 year of age, until appropriate imaging of the urinary tract is completed. A repeat urine culture is not necessary, unless there is persistence of fever and toxicity despite 72 hours of adequate antibiotic therapy.

One should note the following important general guidelines in the management of childhood UTI. All febrile UTIs are treated only as upper tract infection in children. Short-course chemotherapy is better avoided in children for the fear of inadequate treatment. A 7–14 days of minimum therapy is ideal for every UTI but at least 5–7 days of parenteral therapy followed by 7 days of full oral therapy is useful in APN. Dose modification as per serum creatinine values are needed in UTI associated with renal failure for drugs, which are eliminated significantly by renal excretion like aminoglycosides. However, its nephrotoxic properties limit its use. When gentamicin or amikacin is used, kidney function should be monitored. Fluoroquinolones (ciprofloxacin) are effective for *E. coli*, but should not be used as first-line agents due to their questionable safety in children. Ciprofloxacin should be reserved for UTI caused by *Pseudomonas aeruginosa* or other multidrug-resistant organisms. Repeat urine culture and antibiogram are needed to decide treatment by 3rd day if the child continues to be symptomatic. After making the child asymptomatic with adequate parenteral followed by oral therapy, there is a role for antimicrobial prophylaxis in recurrent UTI, complicated UTI and UTI with VUR and/or dimercaptosuccinic acid (DMSA) showing cold areas.

Acute cystitis does not require any special medical care, other than appropriate antibiotic therapy and reassurance if urinary frequency and incontinence are a problem. On occasion, analgesics may be needed for dysuria or severe bladder spasms. The patient is usually treated with oral antibiotics, which is often initiated prior to receiving the report of bacterial antibiotic sensitivity. If clinical response is not good after 2–3 days, altering therapy may be necessary. If clinical response is satisfactory, therapy need not be altered, even if the laboratory data show that the bacteria were not susceptible to the antibiotic being used.

In general, 5–7 days of antibacterial therapy is adequate for treatment of children with cystitis. Sitz bath with warm water and salt twice a day for 3–5 days, often affords symptomatic relief for urethritis, prepuceal and vulval infections. At times, systemic analgesia with acetaminophen or bladder analgesia with phenazopyridine hydrochloride (may discolor urine) is very helpful. One should remember the risk of methemoglobinemia, hemolytic anemia, and other adverse reactions if phenazopyridine hydrochloride is used for more than 48 hours and hence use it for a shorter period. It is contraindicated in children with documented hypersensitivity and liver diseases. Do not use in children with renal failure when creatinine clearance is less than 50 mL/min/1.73 m². The dose is 12 mg/kg PO Q 8H. The other drug commonly used is flavoxate containing the active ingredient flavoxate hydrochloride as it has anticholinergic and antimuscarinic effects. Its muscle relaxant property is essentially due to a direct action on the smooth muscle, which relaxes the bladder wall muscle and reduces the unstable bladder contractions. This in turn, increases the bladder capacity and reduces the need to pass urine. It is not usually recommended for children under 10 years of age and always used with caution for a shorter period in 5–10 years age group. Side effects include headache, tachycardia, diarrhea, leukopenia, drowsiness, confusion, vertigo, palpitations, nausea and vomiting, nervousness, hyperpyrexia, blurred vision and dry mouth. It should not be used in children with gastrointestinal bleeding, intestinal obstruction, achalasia and obstruction of the urinary tract including urethra.

Extended-spectrum beta-lactamases (ESBL) producing organisms are plasmid-mediated enzymes capable of hydrolyzing broad-spectrum cephalosporins and monobactams but inactive against cephamycins and carbapenems. Widespread use of third-generation cephalosporins and aztreonam is believed to be the major cause of the mutations in these enzymes that has led to emergence of ESBLs. Infections due to ESBL producers range from uncomplicated UTI to life-threatening sepsis. The decision to treat ESBL producing organism should not be based on microbiology reports alone. An overall understanding of the patient's clinical condition and practical consideration such as cost, ease of antibiotic administration, patient compliance, adverse effects of antibiotics, antibiotic efficacy must form essential decision-making tools in deciding the most suitable clinical intervention. Decisions have to be taken whether the bacteria isolated from the patient represent infection or colonization, whether it could be treated with antibiotics alone or be treated without antibiotics. Lower colony counts from catheterized specimen of urine can be taken as significant when compared to lower colony counts from midstream urine specimen. These factors should be looked in combination rather than in isolation and generally temporal trends in diagnostic parameters are most significant than a single value. Nonantibiotic approach in the management of infections is a critical step in therapeutic decision-making. Removal of the source of infection is crucial in management of most infections and ESBL is no exception. When the source of infection is a catheter, removal of the device becomes all the more necessary because the devices are associated with biofilm formation. Beta-lactam-beta-lactamase inhibitor combinations (amoxicillin-clavulanate, piperacillin-tazobactam, etc.) are not the optimal therapy for serious infections due to ESBL producing organism. Although the inhibitors have significant activity against ESBL in vitro, their clinical effectiveness against serious infections due to ESBL producing organisms is controversial. The duration of the therapy depends on the source of infection. In an uncomplicated non-bacteremic UTI, 3 days of antibiotic therapy is considered sufficient. Whereas, complicated UTI would necessitate 2 weeks of treatment. One should note that ESBL producers are intrinsically resistant to cephalosporins and aztreonam. Quinolone antibiotics are usually avoided to treat ESBL infections.

IMAGING EVALUATION AFTER THE FIRST URINARY TRACT INFECTION

The aim of investigations is to identify patients at high risk of renal damage, chiefly those below 1 year of age, and those with VUR or urinary tract obstruction. Imaging studies are needed in all children with UTI. All infants should have an USG study, DMSA scintigraphy and a micturating cystourethrogram (MCUG) with first attack of febrile UTI (Flowchart 3.8.1). Ultrasound demonstrates renal size, number, location, renal anomalies, dilated or irregular pelvicalyceal system, renal parenchymal scars, urinary bladder anomalies and postvoid residual urine. Dimercaptosuccinic acid scintigraphy is done to identify APN during the acute phase of UTI and also to identify cortical scars on follow-up. Timing of DMSA scintigraphy is decided by the pediatrician treating the child. Many advocate that it should be done after 2–3 months of first

attack of acute febrile UTI to document the effect of infection in causing pyelonephritis and resultant scarring. But if it is done during the acute phase on first attack of febrile UTI it will help in identification of APN. This will help in adequate and complete treatment of UTI as APN. This can also aid the pediatrician to insist on full treatment for APN as there is evidence to show to the parents. We should remember with adequate antibiotics, fever subsides in 3–5 days and most of the parents take it as cure and discontinue the treatment even though the diagnosis of APN was made with clinicobiological features rather than with DMSA scintigraphy especially with first attack of febrile UTI more so in infants and children less than 5 years old, the period during which the renal cortex is susceptible to parenchymal damage. Micturating cystourethrogram detects VUR and provides anatomical and also functional status regarding the bladder and the urethra. Micturating cystourethrogram is done only after control of infection and the child is started on bacterial prophylaxis. A single dose of 1 mg/kg/dose of gentamicin given 60 minutes before doing MCUG is found to be useful in our experience. Follow-up studies in patients with VUR can be performed using direct radionuclide cystography. There is limited evidence that intensive imaging and subsequent management alters the long-term outcome of children with reflux nephropathy diagnosed following a UTI. With availability of antenatal screening, most important anomalies have already been detected and managed after birth. Therefore, there is considerable debate regarding the need and intensity of radiological evaluation in children with UTI.

The Expert Group of ISPN reviewed the current literature, keeping in view that in our country the diagnosis of UTI is often missed or delayed, and there are limitations of infrastructure and scarcity of resources for routine antenatal screening. Based on the above, it concluded that all children with the first UTI should undergo radiological evaluation. The detection of significant scarring, high-grade VUR or obstructive uropathy might enable interventions that prevent progressive kidney damage on the long-term. Since infants and young children are at the highest risk for renal scarring, it is necessary that this group undergo focused evaluation. It is recommended that all infants with UTI be screened by ultrasonography, followed by MCUG and DMSA scintigraphy. Since older patients (1–5 year old) with significant reflux and scars or urinary tract anomalies are likely to show abnormalities on ultrasonography or scintigraphy, an MCUG is advised in patients having abnormalities on either of the above investigations. Children older than 5 years are screened by ultrasonography and further evaluated only if this is abnormal. It is emphasized that patients with recurrent UTI at any age should undergo detailed imaging with ultrasonography, MCUG and DMSA scintigraphy. Ultrasonography should be done soon after the diagnosis of UTI. The MCUG is recommended 2–3 weeks later, while the DMSA scintigraphy is carried out 2–3 months after

FLOWCHART 3.8.1: Imaging evaluation following initial febrile urinary tract infection.#

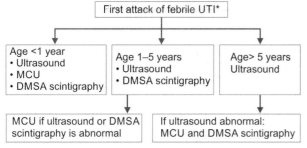

#Adapted from Guidelines of Indian Society of Pediatric Nephrology.

*All children with recurrent UTI need detailed evaluation with ultrasonography, DMSA scan and MCUG.

Abbreviations: MCUG, micturating cystourethrogram; DMSA, dimercaptosuccinic acid.

treatment. An early DMSA scintigraphy, performed soon after a UTI, is not recommended in routine practice as per ISPN guidelines. Patients showing hydronephrosis in the absence of VUR should be evaluated by diuretic renography using ^{99m}Tc-labeled diethylenetriaminepentaacetic acid (DTPA) or mercaptoacetyltriglycine. These techniques provide quantitative assessment of renal function and drainage of the dilated collecting system.

SUBSEQUENT EVALUATION

There is a consensus that children with recurrent UTI should have USG, DMSA scintigraphy and MCUG irrespective of age to detect underlying anatomical anomalies without ambiguity. In hydronephrosis, DTPA (diuretic renography using ^{99m}Tc-labeled DTPA) scan to assess the function of individual kidney and drainage of the dilated collecting system will be useful. Intravenous urogram (IVU) is being replaced by DTPA for this purpose.

Spinal dysraphism and radiopaque calculi are detected by X-ray of the kidney, ureter, and bladder region. Intravenous urogram is useful in double collecting system evaluation and for delineating the level of obstruction in obstructive uropathy associated with UTI. Areas of loss of renal parenchyma and clubbing and distortion of calyces as pointers for renal cortical scars can be identified by IVU. But in recent days for the evaluation of double system and ectopic insertion of ureter, MR urogram is found useful. Urine culture is always mandatory when child gets fever without focus. Children kept on long-term antimicrobial prophylaxis, need periodic follow-up.

PREVENTION OF RECURRENT URINARY TRACT INFECTION

General

Adequate hydration, frequent voiding, avoidance of constipation is recommended. Regular and volitional low-pressure voiding with complete bladder emptying should be encouraged in children with VUR who are toilet trained. To avoid postvoid residue, double voiding is stressed. Circumcision reduces the risk of recurrent UTI in infant boys, and might therefore have benefits in patients with high-grade reflux. Correction of vulvar synechiae in infant girls will prevent reinfection.

Bowel Bladder Dysfunction, Obstruction and Neurogenic Bladder

Recurrent UTI implicates complicating factors like VUR, obstruction of the urinary system, neurogenic bladder and voiding disorders. Since constipation is often associated with a functional voiding disorder, the condition is referred to as dyselimination syndrome or bowel bladder dysfunction. Features that suggest bowel bladder dysfunction include day time incontinence, recurrent febrile UTI, persistent high-grade VUR, constipation, impacted stools, maneuvers to postpone voiding (holding maneuvers, e.g. Vincent curtsy, squatting), voiding less than 3 or greater than 8 times a day, straining or poor urinary stream, thickened bladder wall greater than 2 mm, postvoid residue greater than 20 mL and spinning top configuration of bladder on MCUG. Approach to a voiding disorder needs initial recording of frequency and voided volume and fluid intake for 2–3 days. Personal study of the urinary stream and postvoid dribbling of urine is a valuable clinical urodynamic study. With limited availability of facility and experience, urodynamic studies are not done routinely. The management of voiding disorders should be carried out in collaboration with an expert in pediatric urology. Steps include essentially the exclusion of neurological causes, institution of structured voiding patterns and constipation management. In children with an overactive bladder, therapy with anticholinergic medications (e.g. oxybutynin) is effective. In children with bowel bladder dysfunction and large postvoid residues, timely voiding, bladder retraining and clean intermittent catheterization are needed.

Antimicrobial Prophylaxis

The use of antimicrobial prophylaxis has been a standard practice for many decades. The role of VUR in causing UTI and the use of antimicrobial prophylaxis to prevent UTI with or without VUR is a matter of controversial opinion. The need for higher-quality evidence to guide management is increasing. Until more evidence-based practices evolve, the pediatrician should be cautious when treating children with risk factors for recurrent UTI, including VUR. The pediatrician must decide whether the benefit of antibiotic use outweighs the risk and when surgical intervention might be a preferred option. Review of literature gives differing insight to the benefits of antimicrobial prophylaxis. A Cochrane review by Williams et al. in 2006 identified eight randomized studies (618 children) that compared antibiotics with placebo or no treatment to prevent recurrent UTI. Definitely antibiotics decreased the risk of positive urine culture compared with placebo. But, the authors concluded that more evidence in the form of properly randomized double-blinded trials is needed to support the routine use of antibiotic prophylaxis in preventing recurrent UTI. Garin et al. and Montini et al. in their studies reported no benefit with prophylaxis in children with or without VUR (Grades I–III). Study by Craig, et al. which was placebo-controlled, showed a reduction in the absolute risk of UTI (6 percentage points) that did not vary with any stratifying variable [age, sex, reflux status, history of more than one UTI, or susceptibility of the causative organism for Trimethoprim-sulfamethoxazole (TMP-SMX)]. Roussey et al. found no benefit to antibiotic prophylaxis in low-grade VUR except in boys with

Grade III reflux. Pennesi et al. documented no difference in UTI recurrence between prophylaxis and no prophylaxis in all patients less than 30 months. The Swedish Reflux Trial demonstrated that UTI recurrence rate in girls greater than 1 year with dilating VUR was higher than in boys and that this rate can be decreased with antibiotic prophylaxis and endoscopic treatment. There was no difference between the prophylaxis and endoscopic treatment groups. About 57% of patients in the surveillance group suffered a UTI recurrence during follow-up. The study also showed that girls had a significantly higher rate of new renal damage on DMSA than boys at 2 years. Renal damage was most common in the surveillance group and showed a strong association with recurrent febrile UTI. The results of these studies should be interpreted with caution because of some design-related limitations. In 2007, NICE published its recommendations that healthcare professionals in the United Kingdom do not use antibiotic prophylaxis routinely in infants and children following first-time UTI and only selectively in recurrent UTI.

With the advent of antibiotic prophylaxis, the morbidity of UTI has been greatly reduced. Low dose subpharmacological doses of antibiotics are used for this purpose. They are found to coat the receptors on the uroepithelial cells thereby modifying the pathogenic effect of bacterial invasions. They reduce the problem of recurrent febrile UTI with or without associated anomalies. Cotrimoxazole (2 mg/kg/night) in children above 6 months and cephalexin (10 mg/kg/night) in 0–6 month's age group are popular chemoprophylactic agents. Cefixime in a dose of 2 mg/kg/night is also found useful. The other drug commonly used is nitrofurantoin at a dose of 1–2 mg/kg/night, but is usually associated with gastrointestinal upset with vomiting. It is better given with food and avoided in less than 3 months of age and in children with G6PD deficiency and renal insufficiency. Duration of antimicrobial prophylaxis therapy is individualized ranging from 6 months to 2 years or till the child reaches the age of 5 years beyond which the chances of febrile UTI increasing the renal damage is relatively less. Children less than 5 years awaiting full radiological evaluation after first UTI, is started on antimicrobial prophylaxis. Children with VUR with or without DMSA abnormalities and children with DMSA showing renal scars even in the absence of VUR by MCUG will need antimicrobial prophylaxis. Antimicrobial prophylaxis is not advised in patients with urinary tract obstruction (e.g. posterior urethral valves), urolithiasis and neurogenic bladder, and in patients on clean intermittent catheterization. Breakthrough UTI results either from poor compliance or associated voiding dysfunction. The UTI should be treated with appropriate antibiotics. A change of the medication being used for prophylaxis is usually not necessary. There is no role for cyclic therapy, where the antibiotic used for prophylaxis is changed every 6–8 weeks

ASYMPTOMATIC BACTERIURIA

Asymptomatic bacteriuria is documentation of significant bacteriuria on screening in a child without symptoms. The incidence varies from 1% of girls to 0.05% of boys in their childhood period. Urinary tract infections without symptoms with normal CRP levels indicate ABU. A few studies have documented the chance of pyelonephritis in them and hence it is worthwhile to do an USG to rule out major anomalies especially in adolescent females. Low virulence E. coli is the usual organism, which prevents colonization of virulent strains. Aggressive treatment leads to colonization of virulent strains. About one-third of children with ABU have a past history of symptoms referable to the urinary tract. Pyuria is usually absent. Reflux was seen in 20–35% of these children and scarring was low in many studies. Asymptomatic bacteriuria is also observed in children with neurogenic bladder, particularly if the patient is on clean intermittent catheterization, but studies have not shown increased risk of renal scarring or the need for prophylactic antibiotics in this group. Patients with neurogenic bladder very often also have increased number of WBC in their urine, which makes UTI diagnosis difficult. Recent studies have suggested that renal function and renal growth of scarred and unscarred kidneys is equal in medically treated as well as untreated patients of ABU. The increased scarring would have been due to symptomatic UTI in the past, which was not diagnosed initially. The presence of ABU in a patient previously treated for UTI should not be considered as recurrent UTI.

VESICOURETERAL REFLUX

Vesicoureteral reflux (VUR) is diagnosed and graded by a conventional MCUG done with radio-contrast. The severity of VUR is graded in accordance with the International Study Classification from Grade I to Grade V. In addition to VUR documentation, the MCUG can show abnormalities of the bladder and urethra. Direct radionuclide cystogram using DTPA can also detect VUR, but its limitation are failure to grade the severity of VUR and identify terminal ureter and bladder anomalies like ureterocele, diverticulum and posterior urethral valve. Hence radionuclide cystogram is not useful as a screening procedure, as it will miss anatomical anomalies of the urethra and bladder. Radionuclide cystogram is found to detect VUR in some children where MCUG has failed. Radionuclide cystogram is more sensitive and specific compared to MCUG. Vesicoureteral reflux is seen in 40% of infants and 30–50% of children with recurrent febrile UTI with resultant renal cortical scars. Lower grades of VUR like Grades I–III are more likely to resolve over time. The presence of moderate to severe VUR, particularly if bilateral, is an important risk factor for pyelonephritis and renal scarring, with subsequent risk of hypertension, proteinuria and progressive kidney disease. The risk of scarring is highest among infants. Reflux nephropathy indicates renal parenchymal damage due to VUR. Clinical evidence of hypertension, laboratory documentation of proteinuria along with imaging evidence of renal scars will complete the diagnosis of reflux nephropathy on the background of VUR. Over the last decade it has been increasingly recognized that not all children with VUR benefit from diagnosis or treatment.

Antenatally diagnosed VUR, in some is associated with essential renal parenchymal damage developed during intrauterine period and presents as hypoplasia or dysplasia kidney at birth. Long-term outcome of these kidneys is subject of unconfirmed conclusions. The present view is for early diagnosis, adequate treatment of UTI and antimicrobial prophylaxis. Studies have shown that the ultimate outcome following surgical correction of VUR when compared to children managed with medical treatment in terms of breakthrough UTI and renal scars is the same.

Children with VUR and otherwise normal urinary tract are treated with long-term chemoprophylaxis with antimicrobial prophylaxis drugs like nitrofurantoin, cotrimoxazole, cephalexin or cefadroxil. Training the child for double or triple micturition to reduce the residual urine is also beneficial. Urine examination (microscopic and culture) is done if UTI is suspected on follow-up.

As per ISPN guidelines (2011), in Grades I and II VUR antibiotic prophylaxis is given up to 1 year of age and later they are followed up till 5–7 years of age. Antibiotic prophylaxis is restarted in them if there is breakthrough febrile UTI. In children with Grades III–V VUR, antibiotic prophylaxis is given up to 5 years of age. Beyond 5 years in this group, prophylaxis is continued for a sufficient period if there is bowel bladder dysfunction. Surgery for VUR is considered if breakthrough febrile UTI is a problem.

Recent American Urological Association's guidelines on primary VUR management (2010) should be noted at this point. In an infant, if VUR is diagnosed after febrile UTI, continuous antibiotic prophylaxis is recommended in all grades. If VUR is diagnosed through screening, prophylaxis is recommended in Grades III–V VUR and is only an option in Grades I and II VUR. In children above 1 year old, antibiotic prophylaxis is only an option if the child has VUR without recurrent febrile UTI, bowel bladder dysfunction or renal cortical anomalies. If there is recurrent febrile UTI, bowel bladder dysfunction or renal cortical anomalies in them, the continuous antibiotic prophylaxis is recommended.

Yearly radionuclide cystography can be done to assess VUR especially in Grades III–V. Grades I–III VUR resolve in good percentage of children and even higher grades may disappear in a small percentage. Surgical indications as per pediatric surgeons' experience will include nonresolution

of Grades III–V VUR by 5 years of age, VUR Grades III–V associated with bilateral renal scarring after 2 years of age, recurrent breakthrough UTI's in children with VUR on antimicrobial prophylaxis, in children of noncompliant parents, if parents prefer surgical intervention to prophylaxis or in children who show deterioration of renal function and VUR associated with paraureteric diverticulum or in duplex systems as resolution is uncommon in this subset. There are two surgical options for correction of VUR, subureteric injection of Deflux is a daycare technique, which is 70% effective in eliminating VUR in Grade III or IV. Cost of the implant is the only limiting factor. The other option is a daycare minimal access extravesical ureteric reimplant technique and is also suitable only for Grade III or IV VUR. The most effective method of reflux elimination is surgery by open ureteric reimplantation. The suprapubic scar can be placed in a transverse direction just above the pubic symphysis so that it becomes obscured by the pubic hair line. An evaluation for VD (based on history, voiding diary) should be done before surgery. Antibiotic prophylaxis is continued for 6 months after surgical repair.

Voiding dysfunction should be studied in recurrent UTI with or without VUR. Failure to recognize and manage VD may lead to recurrent UTI, failure of resolution of VUR, managed medically or surgically, renal parenchymal damage and chronic kidney disease. Elimination of constipation and correction of VD play a major role in the management of VUR in children. Reflux is inherited in an autosomal dominant manner with incomplete penetrance and 27% of siblings and 35% of offspring of children can have VUR. Ultrasonography is usually recommended to screen these children. Further imaging is required if ultrasonography is abnormal. Once this group develops febrile UTI the protocol for imaging evaluation of first febrile UTI should be followed.

LONG-TERM FOLLOW-UP

Children with renal scar (reflux nephropathy) are counseled regarding the need for early diagnosis and therapy of UTI and regular follow-up. Physical growth and blood pressure should be monitored every 6–12 months, through adolescence. Investigations include urinalysis for proteinuria and estimation of serum creatinine. Yearly ultrasound examinations are done to monitor renal growth. On follow-up, long-term therapy with angiotensin converting enzyme inhibitors and angiotensin-receptor blockers will be needed in them to stabilize the renal function. Children with complicated UTI need long-term follow-up into adulthood. Children with only DMSA abnormalities are kept on antimicrobial prophylaxis and followed-up as mentioned. Children with anatomical anomalies and VDs are treated accordingly and followed-up for a long period.

Usually UTI can be confidently treated by the primary pediatrician, but due to their potential for renal parenchymal damage, scarring and subsequent chronic kidney disease, children having essential risk factors that can predispose them to the complications should be managed by the pediatrician in consultation with pediatric nephrologist. The common indications for referral include recurrent UTI, UTI associated with bowel bladder dysfunction, VUR, underlying urologic or renal abnormalities and with renal scar, deranged renal functions and hypertension.

ACUTE LOBAR NEPHRONIA

Acute lobar nephronia, otherwise termed as acute focal pyelonephritis or acute focal bacterial pyelonephritis, is a nonliquefactive focal severe infection involving one or more of the renal lobules. It is a medical renal disease which presents as a febrile UTI. This falls in the spectrum of benign inflammatory lesions of the kidney with generalized pyelonephritis at one end, focal acute bacterial nephritis in the middle and renal abscess in the other end. All require intravenous higher antibiotics for a longer duration. As against the first and second in the spectrum, the last one the renal abscess requires a surgical drainage. About 25% of the children with ALN may progress into renal abscess if not treated with appropriate and adequate intravenous antibiotics. Even the duration of the therapy differs with APN needing 14 days of intensive antibiotic therapy whereas ALN definitely needs 3 weeks of the same.

The typical clinical presentations of ALN include fever, flank pain, leukocytosis, pyuria and bacteriuria, which are similar to those with renal abscess or APN. The blood parameters are similar to that of any deep-seated infections with neutrophilic leukocytosis and high CRP levels with the blood and urine cultures may or may not be sterile. The common organisms grown in a clean midstream sample or suprapubic aspirate are *E. coli, Klebsiella pneumoniae, P. aeruginosa, Staphylococcus aureus*, etc.

Imaging is vital in deciding on the further course of management of the disease. The basic ultrasonography is the gold standard in identifying the hypoechoic lesion in the kidney with or without areas of liquefaction. It has an observer variant but gives us adequate information by an expertise. It can mimic a spurious tumor. The nature of the lesion, consistency, liquefaction, perinephric extension, the inflamed thick renal capsule, perinephric space collection, involvement of hilum can be ascertained by USG of abdomen. Hence the use of ultrasound is of vital importance in the diagnosis and in follow-up of cases treated.

Enhanced CT scan with IV contrast has got better anatomical delineation with more information on the following aspects, which goes in favor of ALN. The lesion presents as focal or global enlargement of the kidney. It primarily appears to radiate from the papilla to the cortex similar to columns of Bertin. The corticomedullary differentiation is essentially blunted by edema with calyceal effacement. Due to edema, there is less vascularity of the lesion and hence gets poor enhancement by the IV contrast. The other features of inflammation include obliteration of renal sinus and perinephric fat planes as well as thickening of the pelvicalyceal wall and gerota's fascia.

Role of DMSA is important in follow-up of ALN as well as in identification of the lesion. Focal photopenic areas during the infective episode which may progress to form a renal scar with volume loss can be identified.

Once diagnosed to have ALN, child requires appropriate antibiotics by intravenous administration for a minimum period of 2 weeks followed by 1 week of oral antibiotics. This condition is a slow responder to antibiotics and usually the fever settles only by the end of 1 week of IV antibiotics and it is necessary to have an image follow-up in the 2nd week to ascertain that it does not have pus collection in the center of the lesion. A positive urine culture and *E. coli* growth is said to have poor response to the treatment.

Surgical intervention comes into play only in 25% of the cases where the lesion turns to renal abscess. This requires a surgical intervention to let out the pus. In case of a doubt of malignancy, then open biopsy of the lesion is warranted. The gold standard for diagnosis is to get a tissue diagnosis of the lesion. The other differential diagnosis for the ALN includes simple nephrogenic rests and xanthogranulomatous pyelonephritis (generalized disease).

Acute lobar nephronia is being recognized now more due to awareness of the condition and the excellent imaging services available. The availability of higher antibiotics, early identification, imaging support and appropriate treatment has started bringing down the incidence of scars in patients with ALN.

FUNGAL URINARY TRACT INFECTION

It is usually seen in infants and young children with immunosuppressives, broad-spectrum antibiotics and prolonged catheters. Infection reaches by ascending or hematogenous route. Organisms like *Candida, Aspergillus* or *Cryptococcus* are common. Children can present with urinary obstruction due to fungal balls. Ultrasound and other imaging studies are very much needed for the diagnosis. Management strategy includes removal or change of bladder catheter. Bladder irrigation with amphotericin B is advised for localized fungal infection with no systemic features and negative fungal cultures from other tissues and blood. Oral fluconazole is useful for candida cystitis. Intravenous amphotericin or fluconazole for 3–4 weeks is needed for upper tract involvement. Surgical measures are mandatory if obstruction is present and persistent.

CONCLUSION

Urinary tract infection is notorious for its vague symptomatology in infants and young children. Early diagnosis, adequate and aggressive management followed by appropriate evaluation reduces the morbidity and mortality of childhood UTI, but with vague symptoms and faulty culture techniques there is always a delay to the diagnosis and hence the treatment. Further with inappropriate usage of antibiotics and faulty laboratory facilities one may get a negative urine culture in spite of child suffering from acute febrile UTI. Hence, a negative culture on the background of clinicobiological features of UTI needs further evaluations to rule out APN. Infection is an important aspect we can tackle as the virulence of the organism and occurrence of congenital urinary tract anomalies cannot be tackled at present by us.

BIBLIOGRAPHY

1. Chaudhary U, Aggarwal R. Extended spectrum-lactamases (ESBL)—an emerging threat to clinical therapeutics. Indian J Med Microbiology. 2004;22(2):75-80.
2. Indian Society of Pediatric Nephrology, Vijayakumar M, Kanitkar M, et al. Revised statement on management of urinary tract infections. Indian Pediatr. 2011;48(9):709-17.
3. Nathisuwan S, Burgess DS, Lewis JS. Extended-spectrum beta-lactamases: epidemiology, detection, and treatment. Epidemiology, detection and treatment. Pharmacotherapy. 2001;21:920-8.
4. Pennesi M, Travan L, Peratoner L, et al. Is antibiotic prophylaxis in children with vesicoureteral reflux effective in preventing pyelonephritis and renal scars? A randomized controlled trial. Pediatrics. 2008;121(6):e1489-94.
5. Peters CA, Skoog SJ, Arant BS, et al. Summary of the AUA Guideline on Management of Primary Vesicoureteral Reflux in Children. J Urol. 2010;184(3):1134-44.
6. Roussey-Kesler G, Gadjos V, Idres N, et al. Antibiotic prophylaxis for the prevention of recurrent urinary tract infection in children with low grade vesicoureteral reflux: results from a prospective randomized study. J Urol. 2008;179(2):674-9.
7. Saadeh SA, Mattoo TK. Managing urinary tract infections. Pediatr Nephrol. 2011;26:1967-76.
8. Vijayakumar M, Bagga A. Reader's forum: definition of recurrent UTI. Indian Pediatr. 2006;43:148-9.
9. Vijayakumar M, Prahlad N, Sharma NL, et al. Urinatry tract infection. In: Recent Advances in Pediatrics-17: Hot Topics. New Delhi: Jaypee Brothers; 2007. pp. 240-60.
10. Vijayakumar M, Prahlad N. Urinary tract infection in children. In: Nammalwar BR, Vijayakumar M (Eds). Principles and Practice of Pediatric Nephrology, 1st edition. New Delhi: Jaypee Brothers; 2004. pp. 348-56.
11. Vijayakumar M, Srivastava RN. Urinary tract infection, vesicoureteric reflux and reflux nephropathy. In: Parthasarathy A (Ed). IAP Textbook of Pediatrics, 4th edition. New Delhi: Jaypee Brothers; 2009. pp. 750-3.
12. Williams GJ, Wei L, Lee A, et al. Long-term antibiotics for preventing recurrent urinary tract infection in children. Cochrane Database Syst Rev. 2006;(3):CD001534.

3.9   **INFECTIVE DIARRHEA**

Ketan Bharadva

INTRODUCTION

Derived from the Greek word "dia" meaning "through" and "rhien" meaning "to flow", "diarrhea" is increase in fluidity, volume or frequency of stools, more than three stools per day is the definition used epidemiologically. "Acute diarrhea" is of less than 14 days in duration. Acute childhood diarrhea is usually infective diarrhea, self-limited, but it can have a protracted course. "Persistent diarrhea" is of less than 14 days duration. Acute bloody diarrhea is known as dysentery.

Apart from acute losses, there is potentially large impact of long-term disability caused by repeated early childhood enteric infections. Despite being preventable to a great extent by better water supply, sanitation and vaccination, diarrhea leads the disease burden in developing countries thus assuming prime importance in public and personal health.

With improving technology better diagnostic utilities are available and newer organisms are being associated with infective diarrhea and increasing resistance patterns found. Globalization has changed eating habits, travel and transport, with spread of organisms beyond routine geographic territory.

EPIDEMIOLOGY

Diarrhea is a leading killer of children, accounting for 9% of all deaths among children under age 5 worldwide in 2015. Diarrheal disease affects far more individuals than any other illness, even in high-income countries. WHO estimated in 2004 that it accounts for 1,276.5 million episodes in Southeast Asia, a much higher incidence than lower respiratory tract, malaria and many other illnesses. For less than 5 years of age in developing countries, a median of 3.2 episodes of diarrhea per child-year and mortality of 4.9 per 1,000 per year occurs. Despite improving trends in mortality rate, diarrhea accounted for a median of 21% of all deaths of children less than 5 years, i.e. 2.5 million deaths per year. There has not been a concurrent decrease in morbidity rate.

In 0–14 years age, out of all causes of deaths of 2,123,600, diarrheal disease accounted for 303,200 deaths in India in April 2011. National Institute of Cholera and Enteric Diseases, Kolkata, estimated that in India, by 2016 disability-adjusted life-year will be 27,486,636.0 rising from 23,801,447.1 in 2006. The proportion of rural households with under-three children, experiencing an episode of diarrhea vary markedly across Indian states, the prosperity of the state has no influence. Incidence of diarrheal illness is influenced by more with maternal anemia, maternal illiteracy, low socioeconomic status, summer months, lack of sanitary latrines and waste disposal systems, unsafe water and poor domestic hygiene practices.[1] In India diarrhea remains in top 3 as killer in 1–5 years age in 11.1 per thousand live births with more deaths in girl child in a nationally representative mortality survey[2] or 14% under five child deaths.[3] According to NFHS-2 (< 3 years age) and NFHS-3 (< 5 years age) burden of diarrheal disease has reduced from 19.2% to 9% in 2 preceding weeks of survey.[3]

Poor sanitation, lack of potable water, poor personal hygiene causes about 88% of childhood diarrhea in India.[4] Ghosh S et al. identified diarrheagenic risk behaviors in rural setup in India as bottle feeding; nonuse of soap for cleaning feeding containers, storage of drinking water in wide-mouthed vessels and indiscriminate disposal of children's feces. Risk of diarrhea amongst children of mothers having risk practice without knowledge as compared to those who utilized their knowledge to avoid risk practice was found significantly higher except for bottle feeding. Well water contamination is often a lead to epidemic of diarrhea.

Dysentery accounts for 10% diarrheal diseases steadily over last 2 decades.[3]

ETIOPATHOGENESIS

Pathogens vary between developed and developing countries. Bacterial and viral infections cause most infective diarrhea in developing countries. Viruses account for up to 40% of cases. Concurrent infection with 2 or more pathogens is found in about 33.8% to 48% diarrheas, more in < 2 years age (65.9%) and 34% in 2–5 years age.[5,6]

The Organisms

Bacteria

- *Entamoeba coli:* It is the most common cause being identified as enteropathogenic (EPEC), enterotoxigenic (ETEC), enteroaggregative (EAEC), enteroinvasive, enterohemorrhagic (EHEC) or Shiga Toxin (STEC). Enterotoxigenic causes most traveler's diarrhea. Enterohemorrhagic causes hemorrhagic colitis and hemolytic uremic syndrome in outbreaks. Enterotoxigenic and rotavirus are the leading causes of dehydrating diarrheal disease among infants starting complementary feeding.
- *Shigella:* It accounts for highest incidence in age 1–4 and causes of 10–20% of all diarrheal episodes under the age of 5 worldwide. It is an important cause of diarrheal deaths in 3–5 million children aged less than 5 years in developing countries. The emergence of pandemic strains with multiple antimicrobial resistance and

severe illness is a matter of concern. It requires small inoculums, so direct person-to-person transmission is much more common than with any other bacterial enteric infection. It rarely causes bacteremia and is not more frequent in immunocompromised patients.

- *Salmonella species:* Acute nontyphoidal Salmonellosis usually results from ingestion of contaminated meat, dairy or poultry products. It requires a relatively large inoculums, so person-to-person transmission is rare. It is remarkably resistant to drying, often transmitted via commercially prepared dry or processed food and eggs. Spread from distant geographic areas by fruits and vegetables can occur. It is more common and severe in immunocompromised hosts.
- *Campylobacter jejuni:* It is hyperendemic in developing countries, most frequent in the 1st year of life and in young adult years. Its reservoirs include chickens and household dogs. Occasionally associated is mesenteric lymphadenitis, which causes profusely tender abdomen-mimicking appendicitis. Complications like toxic megacolon and colonic hemorrhage are common if antimotility agents are used for it.
- *Vibrio cholera:* It has major role in epidemics. Seafood poisoning is by *Vibrio parahemolyticus.*
- *Clostridium difficile:* It is the most common cause of pseudomembranous colitis, during or following a course of antibiotics. Almost all antibiotics have been implicated but Clindamycin is the most identified. Newborn infants may be colonized with toxigenic *Clostridium difficile* and yet remain well. It is spread easily from patient to patient within general ward.
- *Yersinia:* It occurs in colder countries. It affects lymphoid tissue in lamina propria mimicking appendicitis.
- *Other bacteria: Aeromonas* and *Plesiomonas shigelloides.*

Viruses

- *Rotavirus:* It is the single most important cause of dehydrating diarrhea in children younger than 2 years who require hospitalization worldwide, accounting for about 3.5 million cases per year and as many as 110,000 hospital admissions for diarrhea according to surveillance published in MMWR 2008. Ashokkumar and others found rotavirus to account for 4.6% to 89.8% variation in stool positivity rate from various parts of India, in hospitalized samples of under 5 children.[7] Indian National Rotavirus Surveillance Network found 39.6% under 5 years aged children hospitalized for acute gastroenteritis had rotavirus infection, more often in < 2 years age and in cooler months, and G1P8 strain accounted for 62.7% cases.[8] Bhan MK and associates found that in India 50% of all children hospitalized with rotavirus by age 5 were hospitalized by the age of 6 months, 75% by the age of 9 months and almost 100% by the age of 2 years. Rotavirus was most prevalent in 31% children between 7 and 12 months of age, 20% in

1 and 2 years of age, 13% in less than 7 months of age. It shows a distinct seasonal pattern being most in winter months in temperate climates. It is transmitted by fecal oral spread with secondary spread via respiratory route.
- *Norwalk virus:* It is responsible for outbreaks of short-lived gastroenteritis in older children and adults.
- *Enteric adenoviruses and astroviruses:* These are emerging as significant causes of diarrheal disease in developed countries. Enteric adenoviruses account for 5–20% of hospitalizations for acute diarrhea. They have a longer incubation period of 8–10 days and diarrhea lasts longer 5–12 days. Astroviruses and caliciviruses each account for 3–5% hospitalizations for acute diarrhea. Cytomegalovirus (CMGV) has emerged particularly in both acquired and iatrogenic immunodeficiency.
- *Severe measles:* This infection is often accompanied by severe diarrhea.
- *Other viruses:* This includes Torovirus, enteric Corona-viruses and Picobirnaviruses. Dengue and influenza viruses can have diarrhea in its symptomatology.

Parasites

- *Giardia lamblia:* It is most frequent amongst parasites with prevalence up to 30% in developing countries in young children. It may be carried asymptomatically. It multiplies in small bowel but rarely invades the mucosa. Its disease pattern is opposite to the usual acute diarrhea, with an insidious onset over 5–10 days. Staying frequently in duodenum it presents with increased gastrocolic reflex.
- *Cryptosporidium:* It is often an acute onset but tend to be more chronic.
- Other important diarrheal gut parasites include *Isospora belli, Strongyloides stercoralis, Trichuris trichiura, Entamoeba histolytica* and Cyclospora. They have a variable importance, depending on geographic location and immune status of the child.
- *Nonpathogenic isolates:* It includes *Escherichia coli, Endolimax nana, Iodamoeba butschlii* and *Blastocystis hominis.*
- *Shigella, Giardia* and *Cryptosporidium* species, EPEC, EAEC and *E. histolytica* may cause a protracted illness. Parasitic diarrhea may be a significant contributing factor to persistent enteric disease and malnutrition. Giardia can cause intermittent or persistent diarrhea with fat malabsorption.

Conditions Predisposing to Infective Diarrhea

- *Sickle cell disease*: It predisposes to *Salmonella* species diarrhea
- *AIDS:* It predisposes to *Mycobacterium avium*, in addition to the other bacteria, CMGV and rotavirus

viruses and protozoa *Cryptosporidium* species, *I. belli*, *G. lamblia*, *E. histolytica*, *Cyclospora* species and Microsporidia
- *Liver diseases or malignancy:* It predisposes to *Plesiomonas* species.
- *Close animal contact:* Like dogs and cats predispose to Campylobacter and turtles to Salmonella species
- *Traveler's diarrhea:* It is mostly caused by *E. coli* but may be caused by *Shigella, Salmonella, Campylobacter* and rotavirus
- Intestinal dysmotility, malnutrition, achlorhydria, hemolytic anemia (especially sickle cell disease), immunosuppression and malaria predispose to *Salmonella* spp.
- Agammaglobulinemia, chronic pancreatitis, achlorhydria, cystic fibrosis predisposes to Giardia spp. *Dysentery* is commonly associated by *Salmonella, Shigella, Campylobacter* spp and *Aeromonas.*

Spread

Oral ingestion is the primary route of infection, although rotavirus appears to be transmitted by respiratory or mucous membrane contact as well. Many host factors, particularly within the gastrointestinal tract are decisive of illness severity. Gastric acid, GIT flora and gastrointestinal motility are protective. Inoculum size and acid stability of pathogen also matters.

Pathogenesis

The suggested pathogenesis of various agents has been given in Table 3.9.1.

Diarrhea occurs when intestinal fluid output exceeds the absorptive capacity of the gastrointestinal tract. The primary mechanisms responsible for acute diarrhea are described in Table 3.9.2.

Staphylococcus or *Bacillus cereus* grows in high concentrations in the food rather than the intestine, and it often is impossible to culture the organism from the stool. Food poisoning due to them is caused by their enterotoxin ingested directly with food. These toxins are relatively heat stable. Enterotoxigenic or *V. cholerae* colonize the intestine but do not invade the small bowel or destroy enterocytes.

Table 3.9.1: Suggested pathogenesis.

Agent	Suggested pathogenesis
Viruses	• Enterocyte lysis • Interference with brush-border function leading to malabsorption of electrolytes and carbohydrate • Stimulation of cyclic adenosine monophosphate
Bacteria	• Production of toxin by enterotoxigenic bacteria • Invasion and inflammation of mucosa or combination of both
Parasitic	• Invasion of epithelial cells causing villus atrophy and eventual malabsorption

Table 3.9.2: Primary mechanisms responsible for acute diarrhea.

Mechanism	Characteristics
Osmotic diarrhea	• Blunting of the villous brush border causing malabsorption of intestinal contents leads to an osmotic diarrhea • Stool output proportional to intake of the unabsorbable substrate • Stools usually not massive • Illness promptly improves with discontinuation of the offending nutrient or fasting • Stool-ion gap is high and osmolarity > 100 mOsm/kg
Secretory diarrhea	• Toxins bind to specific-enterocyte receptors causing release of chloride ions into the intestinal lumen or they may be produced in the intestine by the infecting organism or ingested as pre-existing toxin • High purging rate • Lack of response to fasting • Normal stool-ion gap (i.e. 100 mOsm/kg or less), indicating that nutrient absorption is intact

Their infections are benign, without systemic symptoms except for the severe fluid loss. Such patients if kept hydrated have good appetite and do not feel sick.

Invasive infection leads to inflammation of mucosa. After colonization, enteric pathogens may adhere to or invade the epithelium; they may produce cytotoxins or enterotoxins (which elicit secretion by increasing an intracellular second messenger). They may also trigger release of cytokines attracting inflammatory cells, which contribute to the activated secretion by inducing the release of agents like prostaglandins or platelet-activating factor.

Bowel Involvement

The segment of the bowel involved in diarrhea has been presented in Table 3.9.3.

CLINICAL FEATURES

The infection can present as a spectrum of asymptomatic to life-threatening illness. The same organisms that typically cause an invasive or inflammatory pattern of illness also may cause a secretory or viral pattern. There are no pathognomonic features of any specific-diarrheal infection. Hence epidemiological history is more informative than clinical presentation.

History

It should include both clinical and epidemiological factors in all patients.
- *Clinical history:* Ask for type of onset, frequency, duration, and character of diarrhea; stool characteristics

Table 3.9.3: Bowel involvement.

Segment involved	Characteristics
Small bowel diarrhea	• Usually viruses, enterotoxigenic bacteria (*E. coli, Klebsiella, Clostridium perfringens, Cholera* species, *Vibrio* species) and parasites, like *Giardia* and *Cryptosporidium*, are involved • Stools are watery, large, without gross blood • pH < 5.5, reducing substances may be present • Stool leukocytes < 5 per high power field • Without leukocytosis.
Large bowel diarrhea	• Invasive bacteria (EHEC, *Shigella, Salmonella, Campylobacter, Yersinia, Aeromonas, Plesiomonas*), toxigenic bacteria like *C. difficile* and parasite like *Entamoeba* usually involve large bowel • Stools are in higher frequency and mucoid, with or without blood, smaller in size • pH > 5.5 • Greater than 10 leukocytes per high power field • Leukocytosis with bandemia may be there

Table 3.9.4: Assessment of diarrhea patients for dehydration.

Criteria	Column A	Column B	Column C
Look at condition[a]	Well, alert	Restless, irritable	Lethargic or unconscious
Look at eyes[b]	Normal	Sunken	Sunken
Look at thirst	Drinks normally, not thirsty	Thirsty, drinks eagerly	Drinks poorly or not able to drink
Feel skin pinch[c]	Goes back quickly	Goes back slowly	Goes back very slowly

Dehydration status is decided as follows:
"No dehydration": If signs are according to column A
"Some dehydration": If there are two or more signs from column B
"Severe dehydration": If there are two or more signs from column C

[a] Being lethargic and sleepy are not the same. A lethargic child is not simply asleep: the child's mental state is dull and the child cannot be fully awakened; the child may appear to be drifting into unconsciousness.
[b] In some infants and children the eyes normally appear somewhat sunken. It is helpful to ask the mother if the child's eyes are normal or more sunken than usual.
[c] The skin pinch is less useful in infants or children with marasmus or kwashiorkor, or obese children.
Source: Adapted from: "The treatment of diarrhea—A manual for physicians and other senior health workers-4th rev. WHO; 2005"

(watery, bloody, mucous, purulent, greasy), relative quantity of stool produced, presence of dysenteric symptoms (fever, tenesmus, blood and/or pus in the stool), symptoms of volume depletion (thirst, tachycardia, decreased urination, lethargy, decreased skin turgor), and associated symptoms and its frequency and intensity (nausea, vomiting, abdominal pain, cramps, headache, myalgias, altered sensorium).

- *Epidemiological history:* Inquire about travel history, consumption of unsafe foods (e.g. raw meat, eggs, or shellfish; unpasteurized milk or juices) or swimming in or drinking untreated fresh surface water from, e.g. a lake or stream, visiting a farm or petting zoo or having contact with reptiles or with pets with diarrhea. Contacts with sick individuals, seafood ingestion, possible ingestion of toxic substances, daycare center attendance or employment, recent or regular medications (antibiotics, antacids, antimotility agents); underlying medical conditions predisposing to infectious diarrhea (Sickle cell disease, AIDS, immunosuppressive medications, prematurity).
- For persons with AIDS, refer specific guidelines.

Clinical Findings

Dehydration

It is the principal cause of morbidity and mortality:
- *Early stage:* No signs or symptoms. Weight loss of less than 5% and fluid deficit less than 50 mL/kg
- *Some dehydration:* Thirst, restless or irritability, decreased skin turgor, sunken eyes, lack of tears and sunken fontanelle (in infants), weight loss 5–10% and fluid deficit 50–100 mL/kg
- *Severe dehydration:* Weight loss greater than 10%, fluid deficit greater than 100 mL/kg. Finding of some

dehydration become more pronounced and there are evidences of hypovolemic shock, including: delayed capillary refill, depressed consciousness, lack of urine output, cool moist extremities, rapid-feeble pulse, low-blood pressure, and peripheral cyanosis. Death follows soon.

The most accurate clinical indicator of the extent of dehydration is the percentage loss of body weight during the illness. Capillary refill time, skin turgor and abnormal respiratory pattern are next (Table 3.9.4).

Fever

- *Abdominal pain:* Nonspecific non-focal abdominal pain cramping not increasing with palpation is common. Focal pain worsened by palpation, rebound tenderness, or guarding suggest possible complications or noninfectious diagnosis.
- *Borborygmi, perianal erythema/excoriation:* It occurs particularly in young children due to carbohydrate malabsorption and acidic stools. Bile acid malabsorption can result in a severe lesion
- *Failure-to-thrive and malnutrition:* Assessment of nutritional status is a must. In malnourished child, signs of sunken eyes, skin turgor and irritability are less useful and have to be interpreted cautiously. Often it is impossible to distinguish reliably between some and severe dehydration. It is difficult to distinguish severe dehydration from septic shock
- *Non-intestinal infection:* Like pneumonia, sepsis-meningitis and malaria can present with diarrhea
- *Stools:* Mucus and blood.

Red-Flag Signs

- Teaching these signs to parents is critical in diarrhea-case management.
- Infancy
- Significant malnutrition
- Prematurity
- Chronic medical or concurrent illness
- Fever greater than or equal to 100.4°F for infants aged less than 3 months or greater than or equal to 102.2°F for children aged greater than 3 months
- Bloody stools
- High purging rate
- Persistent vomiting
- History and signs of significant dehydration
- Altered sensorium (irritability, apathy or lethargy)
- Suboptimal response to oral rehydration therapy (ORT) already administered
- Inability of the caregiver to administer ORT.

MODALITIES OF DIAGNOSIS

Microbiological investigations are generally not needed. Blood in the stool, fever or persistence of the diarrhea may call for laboratory tests of an etiologic agent but WHO recommendations limit laboratory exploration primarily to treatment failures.

Stool Test

Microscopy is required especially for polymorphs and guaiac test. Although a fresh-stool sample is preferable, several well-saturated rectal swabs can be utilized. Dysentery and fever have a high predictive value but low sensitivity for a bacterial pathogen. Stool polymorphonuclear cells have a high sensitivity (>80%) and lower predictive value (60%) for bacterial pathogens.

Stool Culture

It remains critical for testing antibiotic resistance and serotype-subtyping in bacterial outbreaks. Considering rapid emergence of resistance in Shigella culture should be mandatory when suspected so. Enteric viruses cannot be grown in routine laboratory.

Overall stool culture yields from 1.5% to 5.8% for enteric pathogens. So it is often considered having high cost per relative yield as most diarrheal illnesses are self-limited and provide little information directly relevant to clinical care. But this information may have great public health importance to detect and control outbreaks. The yield can be improved by proper selection of target organism and its growth media based on clinical and epidemiologic setting. Fresh stool on 1st day of illness before antimicrobials and specimens with evidence of an inflammatory process gives better yield. Samples submitted in hospitalized patient greater than

3 days usually give poor yield except in immunosuppressed conditions. Evidence of an inflammatory response is often not present in noninvasive toxin-mediated infections such as those due to STEC or enterotoxic *E. coli*.

Organism-specific diagnosis helps to prevent unnecessary procedures and treatment considering differential diagnosis of noninfectious conditions in protracted and atypical cases, contain spread by food handlers and healthcare workers, monitor complications like hemolytic uremic syndrome (HUS) (*E. coli* 0157:H7), emergence of resistant organism (e.g. Salmonella, Shigella) and establish area-specific sensitivity pattern and thus avoid overtreatment with wide-spectrum antimicrobials.

- *Cysts in the stool:* These are excreted episodically; at least three stool specimens must be tested if Giardiasis is suspected. Amebic cysts are found in many pediatric stools, the majority of infections do not cause symptoms.
- *Stools for pH or reducing substances:* There is no value in routinely testing it. They often come positive when lactose intolerance is clinically insignificant.
- *Clostridium difficile toxin assay:* Can be done from stool culture.
- *Immunoassays:* These are available for Group A rotaviruses, enteric adenoviruses, and astrovirus and neutrophil-marker lactoferrin.
- *New methods:* Enzyme immunoassay and DNA probe nonculture techniques are rapidly being developed and hold promise for improved sensitivity.
- *Additional diagnostic evaluations:* Like blood-cell counts, blood cultures, urinalysis, abdominal radio/sonography, anoscopy and endoscopy may be considered for selected cases in which disease severity or clinical and epidemiological features mandate such testing.
- *Serum electrolytes testing:* Rarely change the management except in severe cases in ICU and malnutrition. These values are often misinterpreted, leading to inappropriate treatment.

TREATMENT

Fluid Management in Diarrhea

Treatment Plan A (for "No Dehydration", Home Therapy to Prevent Dehydration and Malnutrition)

Give the child more fluids than usual, to prevent dehydration. Wherever possible, these should include at least one fluid that normally contains salt. Plain clean water should also be given. Fluids that mothers consider acceptable for children with diarrhea should be considered.

As a guide, after each loose stool, give children under 2 years of age 50–100 mL of fluid; children aged 2–10 years 100–200 mL and older children and adults as much fluid as they want.

A few fluids are potentially dangerous and should be avoided during diarrhea, especially drinks sweetened with sugar, which can cause osmotic diarrhea and hypernatremia, e.g. commercial carbonated beverages and fruit juices and sweetened tea. Avoid fluids with stimulant, diuretic or purgative effects, e.g. coffee, some medicinal teas or infusions.

Treatment Plan B (Oral Rehydration Therapy for Children with "Some Dehydration")

Children with "some dehydration" should be given ORT with ORS solution in a health facility. The approximate amount of 75 mL/kg body weight of ORS is required. If the patient wants more than that, give more. Encourage breastfeeding.

Vomiting often occurs during initial hours of treatment but rarely prevents successful oral rehydration since most of the fluid is absorbed. Wait 5–10 minutes after vomiting and then restart ORT more slowly.

While replacement of water and electrolyte deficit is in progress the child's normal daily fluid requirements must also be met by continuing breastfeeding and offering as much plain water to drink as they wish, in addition to ORS solution.

If overhydration occurs, stop giving ORS solution, but give breast milk or plain water and food. Do not give a diuretic.

The usual causes for "failures" are: continuing rapid stool loss (more than 15–20 mL/kg/hour), e.g. in cholera, insufficient intake of ORS solution owing to fatigue or lethargy and severe vomiting. Such children should be given ORS solution by nasogastric (NG) tube or Ringer's lactate solution intravenously (IV) (75 mL/kg in 4 hours). After confirming that the signs of dehydration have improved, it is usually possible to resume ORT successfully.

Oral rehydration therapy should not be given in cases of abdominal distension with paralytic ileus; in glucose malabsorption (when a marked increase in stool output occurs, failure of the signs of dehydration to improve and a large amount of glucose in the stool when ORS solution is given). In these situations, rehydration should be given IV until diarrhea subsides; NG therapy should not be used.

Treatment Plan C (for Patients with "Severe Dehydration")

Start IV fluids with Ringer's lactate or normal saline immediately. First 30 mL/kg should be given in 1st hour in infants below 12 months age and in 30 minutes in older children. Reassess, this dose can be repeated if radial pulse is still very weak or not detectable after the shot. Then 70 mL/kg should be given in next 5 hours in infants and 2 and half hours in older children.

Children, who can drink even poorly, should be given ORS solution by mouth until the IV drip is running.

In addition, all children should start to receive some ORS solution (about 5 mL/kg/hour) when they can drink without difficulty, which is usually within 3–4 hours (for infants) or 1–2 hours (for older patients). This provides additional base and potassium, which may not be adequately supplied by the IV fluid.

Patients should be reassessed every 15–30 minutes until a strong radial pulse is present. Thereafter, they should be reassessed at least every hour to confirm that hydration is improving. Then choose the appropriate treatment plan (A, B or C) to continue treatment at that juncture.

If IV therapy is not available nearby, trained health worker can give ORS solution by nasogastric (NG) tube, at a rate of 20 mL/kg body weight per hour for 6 hours (total of 120 mL/kg body weight). If the abdomen becomes swollen, ORS solution should be given more slowly until it becomes less distended.

Fluid Management in Malnourished Patients

It should take place in hospital. Rehydration should usually be by mouth; an NG tube may be used for children who drink poorly. Oral rehydration should be done slowly, giving 70–100 mL/kg over 12 hours. Intravenous infusion easily causes overhydration and heart failure; it should be used only for the treatment of shock.

Full-strength ORS solution should not be used for rehydration. It provides too much sodium and too little potassium. When using the new ORS solution containing 75 mEq/L of sodium, dissolve one ORS packet into 2 liters of clean water (to make 2 liters instead of 1 liter); add 45 mL of potassium chloride solution (from stock solution containing 100 gm KCl/L), and add and dissolve 50 gm sucrose. Such modified solutions provide less sodium (37.5 mmol/L), more potassium (40 mmol/L) and added sugar (25 gm/L), each of which is appropriate for severely malnourished children with diarrhea.

Rehydration

First priority is to treat shock and dehydration. Critical initial treatment is ORT with an oral glucose or starch-containing electrolyte solution in the vast majority of cases. Mild diarrhea cases can prevent dehydration by ingesting extra fluids; more severe diarrhea and reduced urination signify the need for more rehydration fluids.

Intravenous fluids are mandatory when oral therapy is impossible like in coma, significant glucose intolerance (sometimes seen in malnutrition or persistent diarrhea), severe dehydration, shock, paralytic ileus. It should be used cautiously in cases with malnutrition, cardiac and respiratory disorders. If there is no contraindication to oral intake, the child on IV therapy should also be offered ORT as soon drinking is possible as it provides additional base and potassium, which may not be adequately supplied by the IV fluid. If IV therapy is not available nearby, health workers who have been trained can give ORS solution by NG tube.

Addition of glucose to solution of sodium stimulates uptake of sodium and fluid by small bowel, even in impaired sodium absorption by bacterial toxins. This finding is the base of ORT. It is dramatically effective in diarrhea by ETEC bacteria.

Oral rehydration solution with the WHO recommended new improved hypo-osmolar (245 mOsm/L) electrolyte concentration (sodium and glucose each 75 mmol/L) is to be used universally. It is safe and efficacious in cholera and non-cholera diarrhea and diarrhea in severely malnourished too. It lowers need of IV fluid rescue, reduces vomiting and has similar rate of hyponatremia as compared to standard ORS. Diarrhea-associated electrolyte disturbances are all adequately treated by it. It also stimulates child's appetite due to improved water and potassium balance.

Oral rehydration therapy with hypo-osmolar and rice-based carbohydrate or amylase-resistant starch containing and food-based solutions have shown better clinical efficacy in treating cholera. Promising new approaches to oral rehydration and nutrition therapy, incorporating glutamine or its derivatives to further help mucosal-injury repair, are being developed.

Only 30–40% of children actually required ORS, and thus recently the emphasis has shifted to preventing dehydration using recommended home fluids containing salt after each loose stool. Plain clean water should also be given. Fluids that do not contain salt need to be supplemented with 3 g/L salt, e.g. water in which a cereal has been cooked (e.g. unsalted rice water), unsalted soup or yoghurt, green coconut water, unsweetened weak tea or fresh fruit juice. Avoid fluids sweetened with sugar as they are potentially dangerous by causing osmotic diarrhea and hypernatremia, e.g. commercial carbonated beverages and fruit juices, and sweetened tea. Avoid those with stimulant, diuretic or purgative effects, e.g. coffee, some medicinal teas or decoctions.

Major barrier to the adoption of ORT is little effect on symptoms. Vomiting diarrhea may continue despite rehydration and often mistaken as therapy failure. Another barrier is the big gap in knowledge (73%) and practice (43%) in ORT-ORS use as found in NFHS-3.[4] Researchers are trying smart phone decision support tools to help diarrhea management in remote and resource limited settings for a better rationale therapy.

Diet

Refeeding children immediately after rehydration is a major advance that is still to be appropriately and widely implemented. Optimal management of mild-to-moderate dehydration consists of ORT over 3–4 hours and rapid reintroduction of normal feeding of the previously consumed diet thereafter. Prolonged fasting periods have potentially deleterious effect on nutrition. Most children with watery diarrhea regain appetite after rehydration. Those with bloody diarrhea often eat poorly until the illness abates.

In breast-fed child encourage mother to breastfeed. It should be continued during initial 3–4 hours of ORT also.

There is no role of diluting or gradual reintroduction of feeds, special soy-based or lactose-free formulas. Fluids with high sugar content should not be used. Give as much nutrient-rich (energy dense with essential micronutrients) food as the child will accept. Potassium-rich foods are beneficial. Small feedings are tolerated better. To facilitate catch-up growth additional meal for a week after the illness should be planned until the child has regained normal weight-for-height.

In malnutrition or persistent diarrhea, when clinical milk intolerance often occurs, a low-lactose diet is recommended in the initial recovery phase. Milk intolerance is clinically important only when milk feeding causes a prompt increase in stool volume and a return or worsening of the signs of dehydration, often with loss of weight. In such case animal milk intake can be replaced with yoghurt or its amount be restricted but do not dilute it with water, rather mix with cereals. Low-lactose diet includes culturally-acceptable foods, including vegetables, potatoes, maize and beans, thus providing high-quality, relatively inexpensive protein.

Vitamin A

Diarrhea reduces absorption of and increases the need for vitamin A, precipitating complications in malnourished or in diarrhea with severe measles. Supplementation does not alter course of acute diarrhea but repletion should be considered in likely deficiency as it reduces overall mortality. It is seen to be more advantageous in children 6-59 months.[4]

Zinc

Zinc deficiency is common (30–50%) in developing countries and associated with impaired electrolyte and water absorption; decreased brush-border enzymes and decreased immunity. Intestinal zinc losses during diarrhea aggravate pre-existing deficiency. Supplementation either in prevention or in treatment of acute diarrhea in developing countries has shown a decrease in duration and severity of acute diarrhea, and reduces recurrence in next 2–3 months by 15 to 25%. WHO, UNICEF and IAP National Task Force recommend Zinc supplementation starting from beginning of the illness (14 days of 10 mg zinc in 2–6 month age and 20 mg in older ones).

Supplementary multivitamins and minerals should be given for 2 weeks in all children with persistent diarrhea.

Antimicrobials

Antimicrobials are not usually indicated on outdoor basis even in suspected bacterial cause because majority acute diarrheas are self-limited; their duration is not shortened by use of antimicrobials. Irrational overuse of antibiotics contributes to microbial resistance. Most often resistance is encountered against Ampicillin and co-trimoxazole. *E. coli* are often extended beta-lactamase producers.[9] Even multidrug resistance is also found.

Use of antimicrobials should be made on individual basis and selected according to local sensitivity pattern in following cases:

- Organisms needing antimicrobial the most are *Shigella* and *V. cholerae.*
- Organisms needing antimicrobials in selected circumstances are *E. coli* (EPEC if protracted, ETEC with continued severe diarrhea despite rehydration and supportive), *Campylobacter* in compromised hosts, *Yersinia* in sickle-cell disease, *Salmonella* in febrile very young or positive-blood cultures.
- Outbreaks of Shigellosis, Cryptosporidiosis or Giardiasis to eliminate carriage and control outbreak.
- All severely malnourished children should receive broad-spectrum antimicrobial treatment.
- Treatment for Amoebiasis should be given in dysentery if trophozoites of *E. histolytica* are seen in the stool or two different antimicrobials usually effective for *Shigella* in the area have been given without clinical improvement.
- Giardiasis should be treated only if cysts or trophozoites of *G. duodenalis* are seen in persistent diarrhea.
- Persistent diarrhea with diagnosed infections in intestines or outside it (pneumonia, sepsis, UTI and otitis media).
- Special needs of individual children (e.g. prematurity, immunocompromised or underlying disorders).
- Systemic sepsis, serious nonintestinal infections such as pneumonia.

Antibiotics may even prolong illness. Antimicrobials can increase susceptibility to other infections like resistant *Salmonella* spp. carrier status in *Salmonella* infection and risk of HUS in EHEC. Use of Metronidazole or vancomycin considering *C. difficile* diarrhea in hospitals increases colonization of vancomycin-resistant enterococci.

Antiemetics are generally not effective and can be avoided.

Probiotics

Lactobacillus GG and *Saccharomyces boulardii* are consistently effective as adjunctive therapy at dose of 10^{10} CFU/day, especially in young infants with viral diarrhea when started early in illness. Probiotics can assist treatment of *C. difficile* diarrhea, shorten the duration of Rotaviral and prevent antibiotic-associated diarrheal disease. The improvements have been modest but reproducible. But in developing countries it has not achieved a consensus acceptance due to high prevalence of bacterial diarrhea where it is less effective; cost factors and safety issues

related to immunosuppression. Lack of species specific RCTs in Indian children, having varied gut microbiodata and breastfeeding rates is the cause of insufficient evidence for recommendation. Before recommendation in India there is need of bulk evidences for strain specific kinetics on standardization, colonisation, dosage, duration of treatment and interactions especially with zinc.[10]

Intestinal Motility Reducers

Loperamide, diphenoxylate + atropine and opioid products alter intestinal motility but do not reduce fluid loss. They are banned due to risk of paralytic ileus, drowsiness, protraction of Shigellosis, toxic megacolon in Clostridia and HUS in *E. coli* infections.

Toxin Adsorption and Alteration of Secretions

Mineral or clay adsorbents (smectite) and dietary fiber (psyllium fiber) may alter the appearance of stool but not the net water balance. They may help acceptance of ORT, which makes many mothers and doctors more comfortable with early refeeding. There is no role of racecadotril, kaolin-pectin, attapulgite, activated charcoal or bismuth, cholestyramine. Bismuth subsalicylate gives modest reduction in the duration of diarrhea with concerns about toxicity but its treatment is rarely practicable.

Immunoglobulin

Enteral immunoglobulin is reserved for immunodeficient children with protracted diarrhea and is extremely expensive. Hyperimmune bovine antirotavirus colostrum may be a cheaper alternative but has failed to show a benefit in active diarrheal disease.

COMPLICATIONS

The several complications associated with diarrhea, which have been discussed in Table 3.9.5. In developing countries Shigella is a common cause of complicated illness with encephalopathy as high risk factor.

PREVENTION

Preventive strategies have been much less successful than expected. National Diarrheal Diseases Control Programme from 1978, has reduced child mortality from diarrhea to half from 1981 to 1990. Next since 1985 focus was on strengthening case management of diarrhea for children under age of 5 years and national ORT program was introduced, which later became part of child survival and safe motherhood program in 1992 and reproductive and child health (RCH) programme in 1997. Integrated Management of Neonatal and Childhood Illnesses (IMNCI)

Table 3.9.5: Complications associated with diarrhea.

Complication	Pathogen associated
Hemolytic uremic syndrome	STEC
Guillain-Barré syndrome	*C. jejuni*
Malnutrition	Enteroaggregative *E. coli*, *Cryptosporidium*, *Giardia* or other recurrent enteric infections
Toxic megacolon and colonic hemorrhage	*Campylobacter*
Autoimmune arthritis, terminal ileitis and mesenteric adenitis with appendicitis like picture	Yersiniosis
Seizures - Encephalopathy	*Shigella*, EHEC or an electrolyte imbalance
Systemic sepsis	
Other complications	**Characteristics**
Hypoglycemia	In severely malnourished due to inadequate gluconeogenesis
Hypernatremia	Occurs in cases with diets of mainly salt and other hypertonic solutions are and with loss of hypotonic fluids in profuse watery diarrhea Thirst or depressed sensorium out of proportion to apparently mild signs of dehydration Doughy-rubbery skin High-pitched cry Associated serious problem is convulsions, which usually occur when the serum-sodium concentration exceeds 165 mmol/L and especially when IV therapy is started
Hyponatremia	Occurs in diets with bland (salt-free) and dilute fluids (e.g. tea, rice water, dilute formula) Common in children with shigellosis and severe malnutrition with edema Causes lethargy but seizures are less frequent
Hypokalemia	Occurs especially in children with malnutrition Presents with lethargy and hypotonia (muscle weakness), paralytic ileus, impaired kidney function and cardiac arrhythmia Worsened when base (bicarbonate or lactate) is given to treat acidosis without simultaneously providing potassium

has been implemented under RCH phase II in many districts.[4]

Improving water safety in all its aspects including prevention of tube-well contamination, avoidance of pond water (contaminated heavily with animal and human excreta) and point-of-use water treatment, its easy access, sanitation and domestic hygiene are all equally important. The importance of soap as a "do-it-yourself" prophylactic against diarrheal diseases cannot be undermined. Proper hand washing after defecation and handling faeces and before handling food has potential to reduce diarrheal diseases up to 47%.[11] Use of ash or soil in hand cleaning did not have any beneficial effects.[3] Improving hemoglobin and literacy among women may add to it.

Breastfeeding has a protective effect against contracting gastroenteritis. It should not be stopped during diarrheal illness. It allows faster recovery, improved nutrition and protects against dehydration. Its most impact is seen at the time of introduction of complementary feeding when there is lack of availability of suitable complementary foods associated with obvious contamination and immaturity of the immune system in the infant.

Vaccines: Rotavirus vaccines have proven efficacy. It has been recommended to include rotavirus vaccine in Indian National Immunisation Programme in areas where under 5 mortality due to diarrheal disease is more than 10%.[12] Though measles vaccine is promoted as diarrhea prevention strategy there is no much evidence to support its role.[3] The currently available vaccines against cholera and *S. typhi* have varying efficacy. Vaccine trials underway include cholera, *Shigella*, *Campylobacter*, ETEC and EHEC.

It is postulated that prevention of unnecessary use of antibiotics before age of 6 months can prevent later diarrheal episodes.[13]

REFERENCES

1. Park K. Epidemiology of communicable disease. In: Textbook of Preventive and Social Medicine. 19th ed. Jabalpur: Banarsidas Bhanot; 2007. p. 142–7.

2. Million Death Study Collaborators F the MDS, Bassani DG, Kumar R, Awasthi S, Morris SK, Paul VK, et al. Causes of neonatal and child mortality in India: a nationally representative mortality survey. Lancet (London, England) [Internet]. 2010 Nov 27 [cited 2017 Sep 14];376(9755):1853–60. Available from: http://www.ncbi.nlm.nih.gov/pubmed/21075444

3. Shah D, Choudhury P, Gupta P, Mathew JL, Gera T, Gogia S, et al. Promoting Appropriate Management of Diarrhea: A Systematic Review of Literature for Advocacy and Action: UNICEF-PHFI Series on Newborn and Child Health, India. INDIAN Pediatr [Internet]. 2012 [cited 2017 Sep 14];627(16). Available from: http://www.indianpediatrics.net/aug2012/627.pdf

4. Lakshminarayanan S, Jayalakshmy R. Diarrheal diseases among children in India: Current scenario and future perspectives. J Nat Sci Biol Med [Internet]. 2015 [cited 2017 Sep 14];6(1):24–8. Available from: http://www.ncbi.nlm.nih.gov/pubmed/25810630

5. Shrivastava AK, Kumar S, Mohakud NK, Suar M, Sahu PS. Multiple etiologies of infectious diarrhea and concurrent infections in a pediatric outpatient-based screening study in Odisha, India. Gut Pathog [Internet]. 2017 [cited 2017 Sep 13];9:16. Available from: http://www.ncbi.nlm.nih.gov/pubmed/28400860

6. Nair GB, Ramamurthy T, Bhattacharya MK, Krishnan T, Ganguly S, Saha DR, et al. Emerging trends in the etiology of enteric pathogens as evidenced from an active surveillance of hospitalized diarrhoeal patients in Kolkata, India. Gut Pathog [Internet]. 2010 Jun 5 [cited 2017 Sep 15];2(1):4. Available from: http://www.ncbi.nlm.nih.gov/pubmed/20525383

7. Ashok Kumar, Sriparna Basu Vipin Vashishtha, Panna Choudhury. Burden of Rotavirus Diarrhea in Under-five Indian Children. Indian Pediatr [Internet]. 2016 [cited 2017 Sep 14];53:607-17. Available from: http://www.indianpediatrics.net/july2016/july-607-617.htm

8. Girish Kumar C, Venkatasubramanian S, Kang G, Arora R, Mehendale S. Profile and Trends of Rotavirus Gastroenteritis in Under-five Children in India (2012-2014): Preliminary Report of the Indian National Rotavirus Surveillance Network. INDIAN Pediatr [Internet]. 2016 [cited 2017 Sep 14];619(15). Available from: https://www.indianpediatrics.net/july2016/619.pdf

9. Chiyangi H, Muma JB, Malama S, Manyahi J, Abade A, Kwenda G, et al. Identification and antimicrobial resistance patterns of bacterial enteropathogens from children aged 0-59 months at the University Teaching Hospital, Lusaka, Zambia: a prospective cross sectional study. BMC Infect Dis [Internet]. 2017 Feb 2 [cited 2017 Sep 13];17(1):117. Available from: http://www.ncbi.nlm.nih.gov/pubmed/28152988

10. Bhatnagar S, Alam S, Gupta P. Management of Acute Diarrhea: From Evidence to Policy. INDIAN Pediatr [Internet]. 2010 [cited 2017 Sep 13];215(17). Available from: http://www.indianpediatrics.net/mar2010/215.pdf

11. Curtis V, Cairncross S. Effect of washing hands with soap on diarrhoea risk in the community: a systematic review. Lancet Infect Dis [Internet]. 2003 May [cited 2017 Sep 14];3(5):275–81. Available from: http://www.ncbi.nlm.nih.gov/pubmed/12726975

12. Ramesh Verma PK& SC. Rotavirus vaccine can save millions of children's lives in developing countries. Hum Vaccin Immunother [Internet]. 2012 [cited 2017 Sep 14];8(2):272–4. Available from: http://www.tandfonline.com/doi/pdf/10.4161/hv.18390?needAccess=true

13. Rogawski ET, Meshnick SR, Becker-Dreps S, Adair LS, Sandler RS, Sarkar R, et al. Reduction in diarrhoeal rates through interventions that prevent unnecessary antibiotic exposure early in life in an observational birth cohort. J Epidemiol Community Health [Internet]. 2016 May [cited 2017 Sep 13];70(5):500–5. Available from: http://www.ncbi.nlm.nih.gov/pubmed/26621194.

BIBLIOGRAPHY

1. Bhatnagar S, Lodha R, Choudhury P, et al. IAP Guidelines 2006 on management of acute diarrhea. Indian Pediatr. 2007;44(5):380-9.

2. Borooah VK. On the incidence of diarrhoea among young Indian children. Econ Hum Biol. 2004;2(1):119-38.

3. Davidson G, Barnes G, Bass D, et al. Infectious diarrhea in children: Working Group Report of the First World Congress of Pediatric Gastroenterology, Hepatology, and Nutrition. J Pediatr Gastroenterol Nutr. 2002;35(Suppl 2): S143-50.

4. Estimation of the burden of diarrheal diseases in India, 2005. National Institute of Cholera and Enteric Diseases, Kolkata.

5. Forsberg BC, Petzold MG, Tomson G, et al. Diarrhea case management in low- and middle-income countries-an unfinished agenda. Bull World Health Organ. 2007;85(1):42-8.

6. Ghosh S, Sengupta PG, Mandal SK, et al. Maternal behaviour and feeding practices as determinants of childhood diarrhea: some observations amongst rural Bengalee mothers. Indian J Public Health. 1994;38(2):77-80.

7. Global Burden Disease Death Estimates 2008. Department of measurement and health information April-2011 WHO.

8. Guandalini S, Cuffari C. Diarrhea Medscape Reference. April 8, 2010.

9. Guarino A, Albano F, Ashkenazi S, et al. European Society for Paediatric Gastroenterology, Hepatology, and Nutrition/European Society for Paediatric Infectious Diseases evidence-based guidelines for the management of acute gastroenteritis in children in Europe-based guidelines for the management of acute gastroenteritis in children in Europe. J Pediatr Gastroenterol Nutr. 2008:46(Suppl 2):S81-122.

10. Guerrant RL, Van Gilder T, Steiner TS, et al. Practice guidelines for the management of infectious diarrhea. Clin Infect Dis. 2001;32(3):331-51.

11. Guidelines for the control of shigellosis including epidemics due to Shigella dysenteriae type 1 WHO/FCH/CAH/05.3.

12. Jain V, Parashar UD, Glass RI, et al. Epidemiology of rotavirus in India. Indian J Pediatr. 2001;68(9):855-62.

13. Kosek M, Bern C, Guerrant RL. The global burden of diarrhoeal disease, as estimated from studies published between 1992 and 2000. Bull World Health Organ. 2003;81(3):197-204.

14. Northrup RS, Flanigan TP. Gastroenteritis. Pediatr Rev. 1994;15(12):461-72.

15. Ramakrishna BS, Venkataraman S, Srinivasan P, et al. Amylase-resistant starch plus oral rehydration solution for cholera. N Engl J Med. 2000;342(5):308-13.

16. Randy P Prescilla, Russell W Steele. Pediatric Gastroenteritis Treatment & Management. Medscape Reference 29 Nov, 2011.

17. Rotavirus surveillance—worldwide, 2001–2008. MMWR Morb Mortal Wkly Rep. 2008; 57(46):1255-7.

18. Sullivan PB. Nutritional management of acute diarrhea. Nutrition. 1998;14(10):758-62.

19. The Global Burden of Disease 2004 update, WHO.

20. The Management of Bloody Diarrhea in Young Children. WHO document WHO/CDD/94: 49.

21. The Rational Use of Drugs in the Management of Acute Diarrhea in Children. Geneva, World Health Organization; 1990.

22. The Selection of Fluids and Food for Home Therapy to Prevent Dehydration from Diarrhea: Guidelines for Developing a National Policy. WHO document WHO/CDD/93: 44.

23. The treatment of diarrhea. A Manual for Physicians and Other Senior Health Workers, 4th rev. WHO-2005.

24. Urvashi, Saxena S, Dutta R. Antimicrobial resistance pattern of Shigella species over five years at a tertiary-care teaching hospital in north India. J Health Popul Nutr. 2011;29(3): 292-5.

3.10 INTRA-ABDOMINAL INFECTIONS

Suhas V Prabhu

INTRODUCTION

The term intra-abdominal infection generally refers to infections within the abdomen but outside the solid organs and the retroperitoneal space, i.e. infection in the peritoneal cavity. When the infection is generalized within this peritoneal space it is called peritonitis. The peritoneal space extends from the floor of the pelvis to the undersurface of the diaphragm and is divided into two major compartments by the diagonally attached mesentery. In addition, it extends into several recesses like the lesser sac (behind the stomach), the right and the left subphrenic spaces (separated from each other by the falciform ligament), the left and the right paracolic gutters, the pouch of Douglas (in females), etc. and in each of these sites, the infection may be segregated to form localized intraperitoneal abscesses.

Chronic low-grade infections like tuberculous peritonitis also occur in the abdominal cavity but are not within the ambit of the term intra-abdominal infection, which usually refers to the acute infections and have not been discussed here.

PERITONITIS

The peritoneal cavity is normally a sterile space. When infection occurs without any demonstrable intra-abdominal source it is referred to as primary peritonitis or spontaneous bacterial peritonitis. In these instances, the organisms reach it by hematogenous or lymphatic route, transmigration from intestinal lumen or possibly ascending via the genital tract in females. More common however is secondary peritonitis which is due to spread of organisms from a perforated hollow viscus or directly from the exterior along the tract of a penetrating injury. It may also occur by extension from or rupture of an abscess in a solid intra-abdominal or retroperitoneal organ.

EPIDEMIOLOGY AND ETIOLOGY

Primary Peritonitis

Primary peritonitis is an uncommon condition accounting for less than 2% of all acute abdominal emergencies in children in Western literature. In one Indian study, however, the incidence of peritonitis as a reason for explorative laparotomy was higher at 5.68%. The vast majority of cases of primary peritonitis occur in children with a pre-existing ascites due to nephrotic syndrome or cirrhosis. In children with nephrotic syndrome, the incidence of peritonitis is estimated to be about 2% in Western literature but up to 9% in developing countries and is an important cause of mortality in this group. Conversely, peritonitis constitutes about 15% of all infections at different sites in children with nephrotic syndrome. Reduced complement and immunoglobulin levels result in increased chances of infection especially with capsulated organisms like the *Pneumococcus*. Primary peritonitis can also occur in children with chronic liver disease like cirrhosis. The presence of ascites along with reduced immunity secondary to liver dysfunction is the reason for this. Rarely, primary peritonitis may occur in otherwise previously healthy children.

The most common causative organism of spontaneous bacterial peritonitis in the past used to be *Streptococcus pneumoniae,* but its incidence is declining possibly due to increasing use of antibiotics and vaccination. Other causative gram-positive organisms are group A *streptococci, enterococci* and *staphylococci.* Gram-negative organisms, like *Escherichia coli, Enterobacter, Klebsiella* or *Acinetobacter,* account for about half the cases.

Acute Secondary Peritonitis

Acute secondary peritonitis commonly results from release of enteric flora by rupture, obstruction or infarction of the intestines or other hollow viscus. Common situations when this occurs are following appendicitis, gangrene of the bowel secondary to strangulation in a hernia, mesenteric vessel obstruction, etc. or spontaneous perforation after typhoid fever, inflammatory bowel disease or colitis. Disruption of a surgical anastomosis of the intestine is another common cause. In immunocompromised children, like those receiving chemotherapy for malignancy or with AIDS, peritonitis can occur following spontaneous perforation of the cecum. This condition, referred to as typhlitis, is difficult to recognize and often fatal. Contamination of the peritoneal cavity may also occur secondary to pancreatitis, suppurative cholangitis or a ruptured hepatic, splenic or tubo-ovarian abscess (in adolescent females). In the neonatal period, it may be a complication of necrotizing enterocolitis or meconium ileus.

Microbiologically, secondary bacterial peritonitis is a polymicrobial infection with a mix of aerobic and anaerobic bacteria. These would include primarily *E. coli* and other gram-negative organisms like *Klebsiella, Proteus* and *Enterobacter.* Other organisms often present are *Streptococcus viridans,* enterococci and anaerobic organisms like *Clostridium perfringens, Bacteroides fragilis* and *Bifidobacterium* spp. Ascending infection from the female genital tract in sexually active adolescent girls is often due to *Neisseria gonorrhoeae* or *Chlamydia trachomatis.* Infection after a penetrating injury or in the presence of a foreign body like a dialysis catheter can mean a predominance of skin organisms like *Staphylococcus epidermidis, Staphylococcus aureus* and *Candida albicans.*

CLINICAL FEATURES

Peritonitis is usually an acute febrile illness. Onset is rapid if after an injury or perforation but may be insidious in primary peritonitis or if patient is already on antibiotics as for example in the postoperative period. Usually, the patient is toxic with high fever (up to 104°F). Subnormal temperature, seen as the disease progresses, is an ominous sign. The child may be irritable and restless, or conversely, be lying entirely still in bed with knees flexed in order to decrease the abdominal pain caused by any movement. Tachycardia is almost always present and in advanced cases, the child may have hypotension or shock. The respiration is shallow and rapid due to the discomfort in the abdomen caused by breathing movements.

Local symptoms include a marked loss of appetite, nausea, vomiting, diarrhea and abdominal pain. Examination of the abdomen usually reveals a distended or tense abdomen with decreased respiratory excursions. Tenderness on palpation is a hallmark and is usually generalized but it may be more prominent in a certain region where the infection is localized and/or near the organ which is the source (in secondary peritonitis). Rebound tenderness indicates inflammation of the parietal peritoneum and the adjoining abdominal wall. Localized rigidity may be seen due to reflex spasm of the overlying abdominal wall muscles. Percussion may reveal dullness due to the pre-existing ascites (in primary peritonitis) or hyper-resonance with obliteration of liver dullness due to free air in the abdominal cavity released from a perforated viscus. The bowel sounds are usually subdued or totally absent due to paralytic ileus.

As remarked earlier, these signs and symptoms may be very subtle or absent in typhlitis, which hampers early diagnosis. Such may also be the case in patients with severe malnutrition, wasting diseases, those on corticosteroid therapies and in neonates. A digital rectal examination will reveal tenderness in case of a collection in the pouch of Douglas or a ruptured pelvic appendix.

INVESTIGATION

A high index of suspicion is required to be maintained in patients prone to primary peritonitis and aggressive attempts made at early diagnosis in this group. This includes patients with nephrotic syndrome, cirrhosis with ascites and immunocompromised children, especially those neutropenic due to chemotherapy.

A complete blood count (CBC) shows a poly-morphonuclear leukocytosis with a shift to the left, but this may be absent in advanced, moribund or immuno-compromised cases. An elevated acute phase reactant like C-reactive protein (CRP) is suggestive. Increase in serum creatinine and blood urea nitrogen may reflect dehydration and catabolic state or may be due to compromised renal perfusion. Metabolic acidosis may be present due to fasting, catabolism due to infection, compromised renal function or hypotension and shock. Hyperglycemia may be present if there is associated or preceding pancreatitis, in which case there are also very high levels of amylase and lipase in the serum.

Proteinuria along with pyuria and sometimes microscopic hematuria may be seen in pelvic peritonitis. Massive proteinuria will also of course be present if it is a case of nephrotic syndrome with primary peritonitis.

A plain X-ray of the abdomen shows dilated bowel loops and air under the diaphragm in case of intestinal perforation (if taken in the erect position). Sometimes a lateral decubitus or supine film may be required to show this free air in the peritoneal cavity. Presence of air-fluid level and obliteration of psoas shadow are other features that may be seen. Ultrasonography, usually resorted to as the next modality of imaging, generally does not yield much more information. Inability to properly press the ultrasound probe due to extreme tenderness as well as the air in the dilated bowel loops and the peritoneal cavity add to the poor quality of the sonographic images generated in these cases. However, sonography is useful to pick up localized collections in the subphrenic space, pelvis or around the appendix. It will also reveal pathology in the underlying solid organs (if any) or evidence of pancreatitis. A contrast enhanced computerized tomography (CT) of the abdomen is invaluable in evaluating intra-abdominal infection and has made the "exploratory laparotomy" obsolete. Therefore, although more expensive and time-consuming, if available, it should be preferred to ultrasonography except if the lesion is suspected to be in the right upper abdominal quadrant or pelvis where an ultrasonographic examination will usually be adequate. The CT can reveal not only the presence of peritonitis, but also its extent, localization and the possible underlying pathology leading to it.

Needle aspiration of the peritoneal cavity is helpful in confirming peritonitis as well as identifying the causative pathogen(s). Abdominal paracentesis is relatively easy in a child with primary peritonitis complicating a pre-existing ascites and must be done at the earliest suspicion to confirm the diagnosis. But, if the collection is small or localized as may happen with secondary peritonitis, it may be done under sonographic or CT guidance. A lavage may be attempted if the fluid yield is poor or absent. Often the aspirate appears obviously turbid or purulent to the naked eye and a cell count of greater than 250/mL with a majority of polymorphonuclear cells clinches the diagnosis. A pH of less than 7.35 or high lactate levels are other diagnostic indicators. A high amylase level in this aspirate suggests pancreatitis.

A Gram stain must always be done on the fluid thus aspirated, and the presence of the offending pathogen quickly confirmed. Cultures are important, especially in patients who have developed peritonitis after a long hospital stay or already receiving antibiotics (e.g. postoperative cases) as the organisms therein are likely to be resistant to the usual antibiotics used. Culture yields are much improved by inoculating the peritoneal fluid directly into blood culture bottles. In primary peritonitis, an aspirate that shows neutrophilic leukocytosis but is sterile on culture does not negate the diagnosis. This "neutrocytic culture-negative ascites" may be due to other causes like tubercular peritonitis or malignancy-related ascites but should be treated like a bacterial peritonitis if evidence for these alternative causes cannot be found. A positive blood culture which may be seen in about a third of these cases will provide corroborative evidence of bacterial etiology.

TREATMENT

All peritonitis cases should of course be treated as inpatients. Supportive care includes correction of hypoxia, dehydration, acidosis, electrolyte imbalance, hypotension and respiratory failure (if any). Initial aggressive fluid resuscitation and cardiovascular support in early stages can materially improve the outcome in severe cases. Careful monitoring of fluid and electrolyte balance and vital parameters might necessitate admission to intensive care units for the more sick cases.

A nasogastric (NG) tube should be inserted and suction done at frequent intervals to decompress the dilated gastrointestinal tract. The patient is kept nil by mouth till the clinical condition improves and bowel sounds return to normal. Feeding may then be cautiously started in small amounts and gradually increased as per the patient's tolerance. The prolonged inability to feed orally combined with the high nutritional drain of severe sepsis sometimes calls for parenteral nutrition support.

Parenteral antibiotics in full doses should be started as soon as the diagnosis is confirmed. There is data to suggest that speed of initiation of antibiotic therapy is important in ensuring a favorable outcome. The choice of antibiotics for use should be guided by the possible causative microorganism(s) as enumerated earlier in this chapter. Cefotaxime and an aminoglycoside are standard choices for primary peritonitis. Vancomycin may need to be added in cases of primary peritonitis in areas where there is high penicillin resistance in *S. pneumoniae*. In secondary peritonitis, anaerobic coverage needs to be added in the form of metronidazole or clindamycin. Higher antibiotics, like β lactam-β lactamase inhibitor combinations (cefoperazone-sulbactam or piperacillin-tazobactam), fluoroquinolones (moxifloxacin or ciprofloxacin), aztreonam or carbapenems (meropenem or imipenem), may be required in children who have already received the first-line antibiotics listed above before developing peritonitis or failed to respond to them. They may also be started based on the results of culture of the peritoneal fluid. Tigecycline or Colistin should be kept in reserve and used only for patients with very resistant extended-spectrum β-lactamase producing organisms. Vancomycin may be required to cover Enterococcus or MRSA if isolated. Use of antifungal agents in case *Candida*

spp. is detected in the peritoneal fluid is controversial. Most authorities agree that they may not be of much benefit unless the patient is either immunosuppressed, has inflammatory bowel disease or has postoperative or recurrent infection. An intra-abdominal foreign body like a dialysis catheter may however need to be replaced or removed in such cases. Therapy should be continued for 10–14 days with switch to oral therapy acceptable once the child is afebrile and clinically well.

Surgery is generally never required in primary peritonitis. In secondary peritonitis, it will be required but may be deferred till the patient is hemodynamically stable and antibiotic therapy has been started. Surgery is done with the following three aims:

1. To confirm the diagnosis (if in doubt), i.e. exploratory laparotomy
2. To repair the perforation of the hollow viscus (if present)
3. To lavage the peritoneal cavity and drain abscesses or collections (if any).

Intraoperative peritoneal lavage is a standard practice in such cases. The aim is to remove all the exudates, fecal matter, food particles and other foreign matter. The value of addition of antibiotics to intraperitoneal lavage intraoperatively or postoperatively through a drain is debatable as the therapeutic efficiency of this modality is unclear. Probably profuse irrigation with plain sterile saline intraoperatively is adequate. Irrigation with an antiseptic like povidone iodine is not recommended as this agent has been shown to be a potent inhibitor of neutrophil chemotaxis and phagocytosis and this may be detrimental to the host immune response. Postoperative drains are generally not placed because adhesions rapidly localize pockets of residual infection, which often cannot be adequately reached even with multiple drains in place.

COMPLICATIONS

Systemic complications are generally due to the spread of the peritoneal infection and include respiratory failure, septic shock and renal failure. Death may occur due to uncontrolled sepsis and refractory shock with disseminated intravascular coagulation triggered by endotoxins.

Local complications are generally seen only in secondary peritonitis and are related to the primary pathology leading to the peritonitis or the surgical modality employed. Failure of the primary repair of the intestinal rupture may occur if the edges of the anastomosis are avascular or nonviable. This will necessitate re-exploration and another attempt at repair, irrespective of the grave clinical situation that the child may be in. Postoperative intestinal adhesions leading to intestinal construction are also not uncommon. Conservative management with bowel rest and continuous NG drainage should be tried first as re-exploration implies a risk of further adhesions because of the insult from the second surgical intervention. Occasionally, peritonitis can be complicated by formation of an intraperitoneal abscess. The location of the abscess is usually at or around the site of the primary disease or extending in the direction of dependent peritoneal drainage.

Infection of the operative surgical wound can occur even in the best of centers but, with proper aseptic precautions and postoperative wound management, the incidence should be very low. Rarer postoperative complications are fistulas and these are more common in cases with intestinal perforation in tuberculous enteritis or Crohn's disease. Incisional hernias may be a late complication seen in patients with poor general health or nutritional status.

PROGNOSIS

In primary peritonitis, early intervention with correct antibiotic therapy usually leads to a cure. In patients with nephrotic syndrome and no underlying disease, survival rates are over 90%. Nevertheless, many cases are recognized late and this can lead to mortality. This is particularly true for immunocompromised patients with typhlitis. Other factors leading to poor outcome are hypothermia, shock, renal insufficiency, severe hypoalbuminemia and hyperbilirubinemia. This implies that the risk is highest in patients where the peritonitis complicates ascites due to chronic liver disease especially with associated hepatic encephalopathy. Bacterial peritonitis complicating ascites due to end-stage cirrhosis has a high mortality of 50% or more. Even those who survive one episode are likely to develop a second infection in the subsequent months and the 2-year survival rate is 20% or less. Hence even a single episode of spontaneous bacterial peritonitis in a patient with severe chronic liver disease is considered as an indication to consider a liver transplant.

Prognosis in secondary peritonitis is more variable and less predictable. It depends on the severity of the infection, the type on organism(s) causing the infection and its antimicrobial sensitivity as well as the underlying disease condition that lead to the peritonitis in the first place. Obviously, cases resulting from penetrating injuries or moribund patients who present late with drug-resistant organisms or severe systemic sepsis do poorly compared to the rest.

PREVENTION

In children with nephrotic syndrome, prevention should include completion of not only the regular immunization but also the pneumococcal conjugate vaccine in the number of doses appropriate for their age. If older than 2 years, this should be followed by the 23-valent unconjugated pneumococcal vaccine to broaden the scope of protection. Doses should be given preferably when the child is in remission and only when off immunosuppressive therapy. Regular antibiotic prophylaxis is not recommended for all nephrotics as it is not effective. There is some benefit however in giving penicillin prophylaxis to children under 2 years of age with frequently relapsing nephrotic syndrome who have already suffered from one pneumococcal infection. One study reports a reduction of infections (not peritonitis in particular) in children with nephrotic syndrome by repeated administration of intravenous immunoglobulin therapy, but this is too expensive to be considered routinely.

Patients with cirrhosis and ascites who have suffered one episode of primary peritonitis and recovered have a high risk of having a second episode within the next year. In such cases antibiotic prophylaxis may offer decrease in chances of a second infection. This must be weighed with the increased risk of developing infection with drug-resistant organisms. Randomized controlled trials with Norfloxacin or Co-trimoxazole have shown benefit is adults. One study in children of New Delhi showed no added advantage with addition of probiotics. There is however paucity of data in Indian children.

The incidence of secondary peritonitis following routine "clean" or "clean-contaminated" abdominal surgery varies from institution to institution and in fact from one surgeon to another. Reduced incidence can be attributed to cleaner operating rooms, better asepsis and skilled surgical technique to prevent contamination of the general peritoneal cavity by intestinal contents. The rate can be further reduced by appropriate perioperative antibiotic prophylaxis. Even for clean surgeries where the bowel, urinary or female genital tract is not opened, peritonitis can occur by contamination by skin flora. Antibiotic prophylaxis in these cases should be directed toward possible skin flora and a first generation cephalosporin like cefazolin is the standard recommendation. The basic principle here is to administer the antibiotic an hour before the procedure in order to have adequate levels of the same in the tissues at the time of surgery and to continue these levels for 24 hours after the surgery.

When there is a likelihood of spillage of intestinal contents at the time of surgery this is referred to as clean contaminated surgeries. Examples are appendectomy for appendicitis without rupture or resection and anastomosis of bowel for stricture or atresia. The chances of postoperative peritonitis are around 30% in these cases. In planned surgeries, the load of organisms in the intestine can be reduced by giving preoperatively a low residue diet, cathartics and enemas. This can be further reduced to as low as 4% by appropriate preoperative oral antibiotic prophylaxis to cover the intestinal flora such as neomycin for coliform organisms and erythromycin for anaerobic ones.

Peritonitis is a known hazard in patients with a semi-permanent catheter like the Tenckhoff catheter for continuous ambulatory peritoneal dialysis. Almost half the patients will suffer at least one infection in the 1st year if not the first 6 months. A 10-year retrospective analysis of 30 patients from Lucknow revealed that 15 of them had a total of 21 episodes of peritonitis. St. John's Hospital at Bengaluru in an analysis of peritonitis following in dialysis catheters (in both adults and children) found coagulase-negative *Staphylococcus spp.* to be the most common organism followed by Enterobacteriaceae (12.2%). Other organisms isolated were non fermenting gram-negative bacilli (4.4%), *Pseudomonas aeruginosa* (3.3%), α-hemolytic Streptococci (3.3%), *Candida spp.* (2.2%), *S. aureus* (1.1%), β-hemolytic Streptococci (1.1%) and Micrococci (1.1%). Recurrence rates after first infection are in the range of 20–30% and may require removal or replacement of catheter or even a switch to hemodialysis. Prevention is only by scrupulous hygiene while handling the catheter as use of oral or injectable antibiotics has not shown to be effective in prophylaxis. However, administration of perioperative antibiotics to cover skin flora (as described above) is recommended during surgical placement of the catheter.

ACUTE SECONDARY LOCALIZED PERITONITIS (PERITONEAL ABSCESS)

Etiology and Pathology

Intraperitoneal abscesses may develop in any recesses of the peritoneal cavity described in the paragraph on anatomy at the beginning of this chapter like subdiaphragmatic, pelvic, etc. In addition, localization of the infection by adhesions between the peritoneum and/or the omentum can cause localized abscesses to form at other sites (other abscesses within the abdomen like a retroperitoneal abscess, psoas abscess or an abdominal wall abscess are, strictly speaking, not peritoneal abscesses because, on anatomical grounds, they do not lie within the peritoneal cavity).

The most common peritoneal abscesses in children are those occurring as a complication of appendicitis with perforation. The site of this abscess will depend on the length and direction of the appendix. A short one in anterior position will lead to a periappendicular abscess, a long one directed downward may result in a pelvic abscess and a retrocolic one may be associated with a right paracolic abscess or, if long enough, even a right subphrenic abscess. Lesser sac abscesses usually follow pancreatitis or perforations of the duodenum or posterior wall of the stomach. A ruptured hepatic abscess will result in a right or left subdiaphragmatic or subhepatic abscess. A perisplenic abscess surrounds an infected (and often infarcted) portion of the spleen. Localized abscesses can also form along the track of a foreign body like a dialysis catheter or a blocked drain.

Because a peritoneal abscess is generally a complication of peritonitis, it is also polymicrobial in origin and the causative microbial agents are basically the same as those for peritonitis. However, a subdiaphragmatic abscess may also follow an amebic abscess of the liver due to *Entamoeba histolytica*.

Clinical Features

Unlike peritonitis, a peritoneal abscess may have a subacute presentation, sometimes with duration of symptoms of more than a month. If arising as a complication of obvious peritonitis, it will present acutely. It can be recognized by occurrence of some improvement in the general condition of the patient on treatment, followed by a failure of complete defervescence coupled with localized symptoms, like pain, tenderness and guarding, at the site of the abscess.

If arising de novo, the general symptoms are fever, anorexia, vomiting, local abdominal pain and lassitude. With an appendicular abscess, which can arise directly from a chronic appendicitis without intervening generalized peritonitis, the pain is localized to the right iliac fossa with possibly a palpable mildly tender "appendicular lump". Symptoms suggesting a pelvic location of the abscess are: frequency of bowel and bladder evacuation often with small mucoid stools and tenesmus. A digital per-rectal examination elicits tenderness anteriorly. The tenderness is on the lateral side of the palpating finger in case of a pelvic abscess complicating a tubo-ovarian infection.

Subphrenic abscesses may present with fever, anorexia and respiratory distress. On examination, they may have decreased respiratory movements and air entry on the affected side while palpation of the abdomen will be unremarkable and the diagnosis can only be confirmed by imaging. A localized peritoneal collection in a region of the peritoneal cavity not in contact with the anterior abdominal wall (such as a subphrenic abscess) may also lead to a lack of these signs except for the absent bowel sounds.

Investigation

A plain X-ray of the abdomen can suggest the position of the abscess in about half the cases by the showing a soft-tissue shadow of the abscess with displacement of the bowel loops to the other side. Rarely, when the infection is due to gas producing organisms, the abscess shadow shows an air-fluid level or a mottled appearance. Unlike in peritonitis complicating a perforation, there is no air under the diaphragm but air-fluid levels may be seen within the intestines due to presence of paralytic ileus. Sometimes the dilated fluid filled bowel loops may be localized to the region immediately surrounding the abscess.

In a subphrenic abscess, the X-ray of the chest may show a collapse of the adjacent lower bronchopulmonary segment with an elevated diaphragm and sometimes a pleural effusion. Fluoroscopy can be suggestive by showing decreased diaphragmatic movement but it is only other modalities of imaging like ultrasonography that can reveal the actual abscess collection nestled between the liver

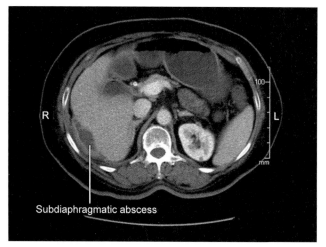

FIG. 3.10.1: Contrast-enhanced computed tomography abdomen showing subdiaphragmatic abscess.

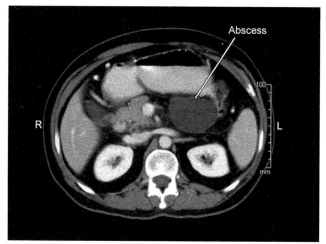

FIG. 3.10.2: Computed tomography abdomen showing collection in the lesser sac.

and the diaphragm. The ultrasonography is also generally adequate to show an appendicular or pelvic abscess. Smaller abscesses elsewhere can only be confirmed on a CT of the abdomen which will show the abscess as a low density mass surrounded by a well-defined enhancing capsule. Other imaging modalities, like MRI or Gallium scans, can also pinpoint the location of abscesses but are more expensive or not available everywhere. They are however hardly ever required as abdominal CT and sonography can pick up almost all the cases (Figs. 3.10.1 and 3.10.2).

General investigations, like CBC, show leukocytosis with polymorphonuclear predominance and elevation of acute phase reactants like CRP but imaging correlated with physical findings is primary in making a diagnosis.

Treatment

The axiom in any case of an abscess is to drain it and an intraperitoneal abscess is no exception to this rule. In the past, drainage involved surgery but small localized abscesses can now be drained percutaneously under ultrasonic or CT guidance provided the abscess is unilocular, well localized and a safe approach exists. It may also be necessitated by a poor general condition making the child unfit for exploration under anesthesia. The contents drained should be cultured to try to identify the pathogen(s) and their antibiotic sensitivity. Additionally, a drainage catheter may be left for a few days to ensure complete drainage. Drainage is usually by gravity but slow suction may be employed.

Antibiotic therapy is supplementary and is on the lines described for peritonitis and modified based on results of the antimicrobial tests. Initial therapy should be parenteral and continued till the abscess is completely drained and the child afebrile for several days.

BIBLIOGRAPHY

1. Alwadhi RK, Mathew JL, Rath B. Clinical profile of children with nephrotic syndrome not on glucocorticoid therapy, but presenting with infection. J Paediatr Child Health. 2004;40 (1-2):28-32.
2. Gulati S, Kher V, Gupta A, et al. Spectrum of infections in Indian children with nephrotic syndrome. Pediatr Nephrol. 1995;9(4):431-4.
3. Gupta S, Muralidharan S, Gokulnath, et al. Epidemiology of culture isolates from peritoneal dialysis peritonitis patients in Southern India using an automated blood culture system to culture peritoneal dialysate. Nephrology (Carlton). 2011;16(1):63-7.
4. Kioumis IP, Kuti JL, Nicolau DP. Intra-abdominal infections: considerations for the use of carbapenems. Expert Opin Pharmacother. 2007;8(2):167-82.
5. Levison ME, Bush LM. Peritonitis and intraperitoneal abscesses. In: Mandell BL, Bennett JE, Dolin R Mandell (Eds). Douglas & Bennett's Principles and Practice of Infectious Diseases, 7th edition. Churchill Livingstone; 2010. pp. 1011-32.
6. Prasad N, Gulati S, Gupta A, et al. Continuous peritoneal dialysis in children: a single-centre experience in a developing country. Pediatr Nephrol. 2006;21(3):403-7.
7. Runyon BA. The evolution of ascitic fluid analysis in the diagnosis of spontaneous bacterial peritonitis. Am J Gastroenterol. 2003;98(8):1675-7.

3.11 | SKIN AND SOFT TISSUE INFECTIONS

Sandipan Dhar

SCABIES

This extremely pruritic condition is caused by the mite *Sarcoptes scabiei*. The itching is worst at night when the patient is warm and the endogenous cortisol level is very low. The onset occurs 3–4 weeks after the infection is acquired and it coincides with a widespread eruption of inflammatory papules. The pathognomonic lesions of scabies are burrows which appear as slightly raised, brownish tortuous lesions. They occur commonly on the wrists, borders of the hands, the sides of the fingers and the finger-web spaces, the feet particularly the in-step and in the male, the genitalia. In babies the head and neck may be involved. With the development of hypersensitivity, itchy papules develop. Secondary changes may frequently confuse the clinical picture. Eczematous changes are common and may be widespread and severe. Secondary infection, manifests as folliculitis or impetigo, may also be severe and extensive (Figs. 3.11.1 to 3.11.3).

In infants, in addition to the more extensive burrows seen in older children and adults, vesicular and vesiculopustular lesions on the hands and feet are frequent. Extensive eczematization is often present. There may be multiple crusted nodules on the trunk and limbs. Many children with scabies develop persistent skin colored to reddish nodules over axillae, shoulders, groin, buttocks and scrotum. These lesions result from the hypersensitivity reaction to scabies mite and tend to persist for months together even after treatment of scabies.

Complications

Secondary infections of scabies lead to pustule formation and impetiginization. Nephritogenic strain of *Streptococcus* may rarely cause glomerulonephritis.

Eczema formation is mostly seen over the face. It can get confused with atopic dermatitis.

Treatment

Permethrin (5%) cream is the treatment of choice in infants and children. It is safe even in infants as young as 2 months of age. It is to be applied in adults and young children from neck to toes and in infants from head to toes including palms and soles. It is to be left on for 6–8 hours in infants and 12–14 hours in older children. If necessary, it may be repeated after 1 week.

Gamma benzene hexachloride (1%) is the most widely used antiscabetic because of its efficacy and it is being cheaper than permethrin. There are occasional reports of neurotoxicities, which are almost exclusively due to its inappropriate, prolonged or repetitive use or

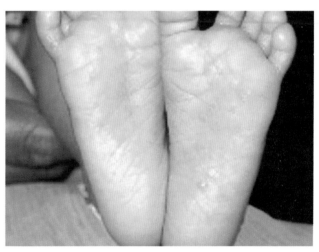

FIG. 3.11.2: Scabies lesions over soles.

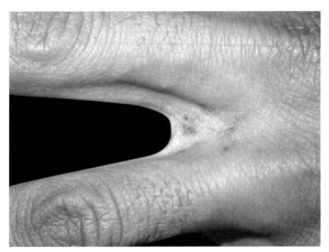

FIG. 3.11.1: Scabies lesions in web space.

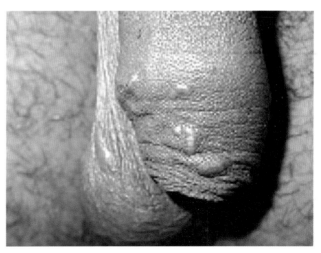

FIG. 3.11.3: Scabies burrows penis.

accidental ingestion by infants or young children. It is not recommended in infants and small children and cannot be applied over head and face. A second application after 1 week is a must. The current breakthrough in the treatment of scabies has been oral ivermectin. It is considered to be safe in children above 2 years of age. Two doses of 200 µg/kg of body weight at 1 week interval have been recommended. By and large its use is limited to cases of Norwegian scabies and scabies in HIV positive children.

PEDICULOSIS

Pediculosis or louse infestation is a worldwide problem but poor living conditions and poor personal hygiene contribute to epidemic proportions of the infestation in poor countries. The three types of lice-infest human beings are: (1) Pediculus humanus capitis (the head louse), (2) Pediculus humanus corporis (body louse), and (3) Phthirus pubis (crab louse).

Pediculosis Capitis (Head Louse Infestation)

It is caused by infestation of the scalp with Pediculus humanus capitis. Head louse is brown in color and lays about 50–150 ova (nits) during an average adult life of approximately 16 days and it measures 1–2 mm in length. They moult three times to develop into an adult over a period of an average of 2 weeks. Head louse infestation commonly affects females with long hair. The nits are firmly adhered to the hair and can slide along the hair but cannot be shed off like scales and the nits are greyish white, oval in shape and about 0.5 mm in length. The transmission is through close contact, sharing of headgear, combs and hairbrushes. In head louse, itching is the predominant symptom and secondary infection with enlargement of occipital lymph glands is the common presentation. Diagnosis is definitive when crawling lice can be seen on a naked eye but microscopic identification of the louse or the

stuck on nits on the hair shafts is confirmatory. Exudation, crusting, excoriations and red papules on the neck in females should arouse suspicion of pediculosis capitis (Fig. 3.11.4).

Treatment consists of treating the associated secondary infection if any. Treatment of pediculosis consists of application of gamma benzene hexachloride (1%) or malathion (0.5%) or permethrin (1%). Gamma benzene hexachloride and malathion both should be applied at night and should be left on for 10–12 hours and washed off in the morning. Permethrin should also be applied for 30–45 minutes and washed off. Repeated application after a week is usually given. To prevent reinfection, ensure that all family contacts and close friends are also treated simultaneously.

Pediculosis Corporis (Body Louse Infestation)

It is generally seen among the poor, homeless or mentally retarded subjects. Body lice generally thrive in conditions of poverty, war and natural disaster and in some neurological diseases (Figs. 3.11.5 and 3.11.6).

The body louse is about 4 mm in length and lives in the seams of cloths and lays about 270–300 ova during an average of 18 days of adult life. Nits incubate for 8–10 days and nymphs mature into adults over about 2 weeks.

Severe itching, excoriations, blood crusts and blood-stained cloths are the presentation of body louse infestation. In chronic cases hyperpigmentation and lichenification can also be seen. The diagnosis can be made by high degree of suspicion and demonstration or lice/nits from the seams of clothing.

Treatment consists of proper hygiene, laundering and ironing of clothes and application of insecticides to clothing. Application of permethrin or gamma benzene hexachloride to body hair may be helpful.

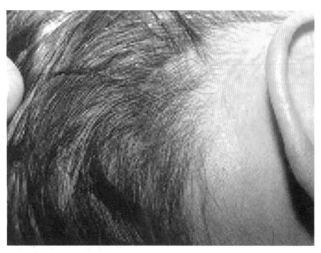

FIG. 3.11.4: Pediculosis capitis nits on scalp.

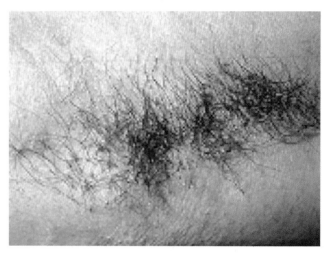

FIG. 3.11.5: Pediculosis corporis, nits on axillary hairs.

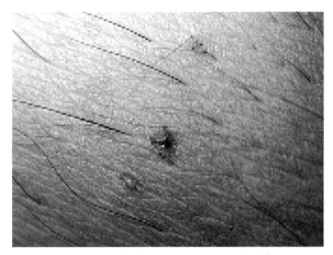

FIG. 3.11.6: Pediculosis corporis nits on body hair.

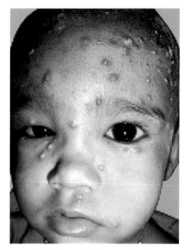

FIG. 3.11.8: Furunculosis.

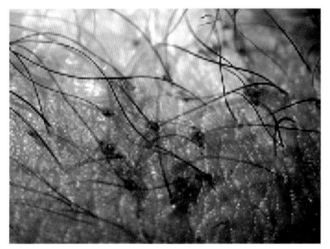

FIG. 3.11.7: Pediculosis pubis, nits on pubic hair.

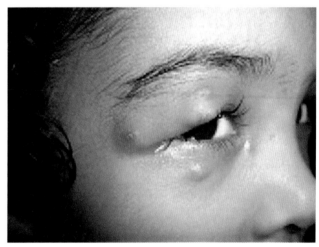

FIG. 3.11.9: Furuncle over eyelid.

Pediculosis Pubis

Pediculosis pubis is caused by crab louse. It is commonly spread by the sexual contact. However, it can be transmitted by clothing or towels. An adult female can lay about 25 eggs during their lifespan. It mainly attaches to the pubic hair but can be spread occasionally to axillary hair, eyebrows and eyelashes. The patient complains of itching and on examination bluish gray macules (maculae ceruleae) can be seen on the lower abdomen and thighs. The lice looks like brownish spots attached to the hair (Fig. 3.11.7).

Therapy consists of single gamma benzene hexachloride 1% or permethrin 1%. In case of eyelashes, application of petrolatum can be given 3–4 times a day for 7 days. Manual removal, shaving of hair and even oral ivermectin (1 mg/5 kg) can be employed as measures for eradication. Sexual partners should also be treated.

FURUNCULOSIS

This is an acute, usually necrotic infection of a hair follicle and perifollicular area with *Staphylococcus aureus*. A furuncle presents initially as a small, follicular papule, some inflammatory nodule, soon becoming pustular and then necrotic and healing after discharge of a necrotic core to leave a violaceous macule and ultimately a permanent scar. Tenderness is a constant feature. Lesions may be single or multiple and tend to appear in crops. The sites involved are the face and neck, the arms, wrists and fingers, the buttocks and the anogenital region. In some individuals, crops continue to develop for many months or even years (Figs. 3.11.8 and 3.11.9).

IMPETIGO

Impetigo is superficial pyogenic infection of the skin. Two main clinical forms are recognized, nonbullous and bullous impetigo. Bullous impetigo is caused by staphylococci, the nonbullous form may be caused by staphylococci or streptococci or both organisms together. The nonbullous form presents as a thin-walled vesicle on an erythematous base. However, the vesicle ruptures rapidly and so may be missed. The exuding serum dries to form yellowish-brown crusts. The lesions extend peripherally and often many

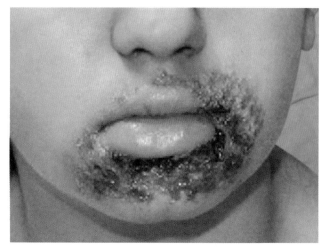

FIG. 3.11.10: Impetigo contagiosa.

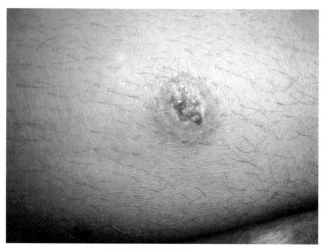

FIG. 3.11.12: Ecthyma.

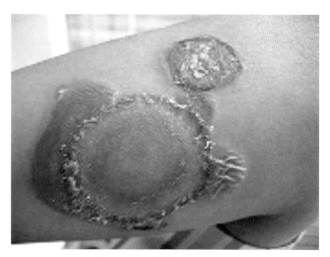

FIG. 3.11.11: Bullous impetigo.

lesions appear. The crusts eventually dry and separate out to leave erythematous skin which fades without scarring. The face and the limbs are commonly involved. Spontaneous recovery may occur in 2–3 weeks. In bullous impetigo, the bullae are less rapidly ruptured and become much large; a diameter of 1–2 cm is common but they may be of very considerable size and persist for 2 or 3 days. After rupture, thin, flat and brownish crusts are formed. The face is most commonly involved; however, the lesions may occur anywhere and may be widely and irregularly distributed (Figs. 3.11.10 and 3.11.11).

ECTHYMA

Ecthyma is a pyogenic infection of the skin that usually heals with scarring. It is characterized by the formation of adherent crusts beneath where ulceration occurs. It begins as small bullae or pustules on an erythematous base, which is soon surrounded by a hard crust of dried exudate. The base may become indurated and a red edematous areola

is often present. The crust is removed with difficulty, to reveal a purulent irregular ulcer. Healing occurs after a few weeks, with scarring. The buttocks, thighs and legs are most commonly affected. The lesions are usually few but new lesions may develop by autoinoculation over prolonged period of time (Fig. 3.11.12).

CELLULITIS AND ERYSIPELAS

Cellulitis results from inflammation of subcutaneous tissue. Erysipelas is a bacterial infection of the superficial and deep dermis. The two have similar bacteriology with streptococcal antigens being demonstrated in both lesions. Erythema, heat swelling and pain or tenderness are constant features. In erysipelas, the edge of the lesion is well-demarcated and raised, but in cellulitis it is diffuse blister formation, with hemorrhage into the blister is seen. Erysipelas and severe cellulitis can give rise to bullae formation and progression to dermal necrosis. Fasciitis and myositis are uncommon; however, lymphangitis and lymphadenopathy are frequent. The leg is most commonly involved followed by the face (Figs. 3.11.13 to 3.11.16)

Treatment

For furunculosis, impetigo, ecthyma either oral cloxacillin, amoxicillin and clavulanic acid combinations or erythromycin is to be given for 7–10 days. Topical mupirocin, fusidic acid or retapamulin cream/ointment can be applied over surrounding skin to prevent contamination.

For erysipelas and cellulitis either cefadroxil, cefixime, erythromycin may be chosen. In severe cases IV Benzyl penicillin at a dose of 600–1,200 mg 6 hourly is preferred and continued for 10 days to combat long-term carriage state of *S. aureus* (particularly in atopics) twice daily application of mupirocin cream inside nostril, external auditory meatus and perianal area for at least 6 months has been found to be very effective.

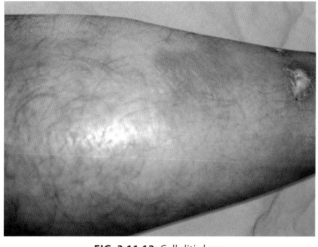

FIG. 3.11.13: Cellulitis legs.

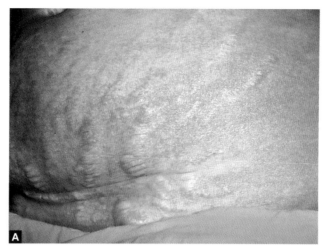

A

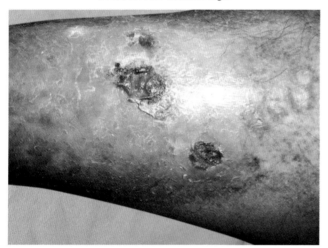

FIG. 3.11.14: Cellulitis (close-up).

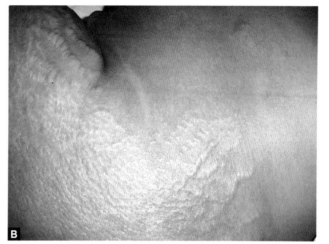

B

FIGS. 3.11.16A AND B: Erysipelas.

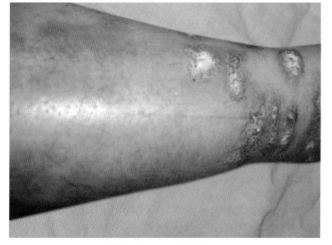

FIG. 3.11.15: Cellulitis.

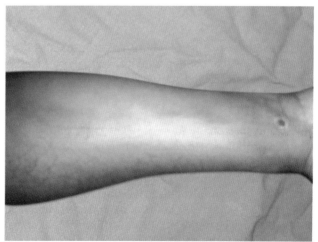

FIG. 3.11.17: Lymphangitis.

ACUTE LYMPHANGITIS

It is a streptococcal infection of lymphatic vessels of the subcutaneous tissue, seen as erythematous, linear streaks of varying width, extending from the local lesion toward the regional lymph nodes. The lymph nodes are tender and enlarged (Figs. 3.11.17 and 3.11.18).

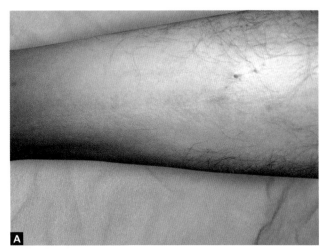

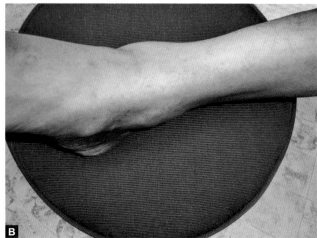

FIGS. 3.11.18A AND B: Lymphangitis over leg.

Differential Diagnosis

Lymphangitis needs to be differentiated from thrombophlebitis. In cases of thrombophlebitis, the red streak of inflamed vein corresponds to the course of a superficial vein and often a part of vein is visible as bluish line as continuation of the red line.

SYCOSIS BARBAE

Sycosis barbae is a subacute or chronic pyogenic infection involving the whole depth of hair follicle of the beard. It is most commonly seen in young adults and adolescent boys.

The essential lesion is an erythematous edematous papule and pustule with a hair at the center. The individual papule or pustule usually remains discrete. However, there is a tendency to coalesce at times and boggy plaques or noduloplaque lesions studded with pustules may be seen (Fig. 3.11.19).

Etiology

The causative organism is *S. aureus*. The bacteria are thought to be either coming from its nasal carriage sites or inoculated from shaving, mostly in a saloon or parlor.

Management

The diagnosis is made in most of the cases going by its typical morphology. However, one may carryout culture of pus for documentation.

The subacute forms can be controlled by topical antibiotics, e.g. mupirocin, fusidic acid, etc. However, in severe cases, several courses of antistaphylococcal antibiotics may be required. The newly introduced topical retapamulin ointment may serve as an alternative to systemic antibiotic therapy. Regular cleaning of the beard with soap and water is a must. During acute/subacute stage, it is better to avoid shaving for 7–10 days. Nasal carriage of *S. aureus* can be controlled by application of mupirocin cream twice daily for 3–6 months. Application of aftershave lotions is usually allowed.

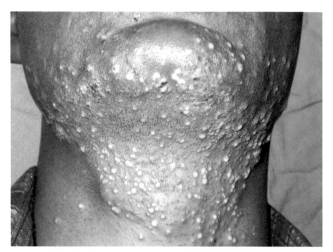

FIG. 3.11.19: Sycosis barbae.

LUPUS VULGARIS

This is a progressive form of cutaneous tuberculosis which occurs usually on the head or neck. The skin of and around the nose is frequently involved. The lesions consist of one or a few well-demarcated, reddish-brown patches containing deep-seated nodules, each about 1 mm in diameter. If blood is pressed out of the skin with a glass slide, these nodules stand out clearly as yellow-brown macules, referred to as apple-jelly nodules, because of their color. The disease is very chronic, with slow peripheral extension of the lesions. In the course of time the affected areas become atrophic, with contraction of the tissue. Characteristically, new lesions may appear in areas of atrophy. Superficial ulceration or verrucous thickening of the skin occurs occasionally (Figs. 3.11.20 and 3.11.21).

SCROFULODERMA

Scrofuloderma represents a direct intension to the skin of an underlying tuberculous infection, present most

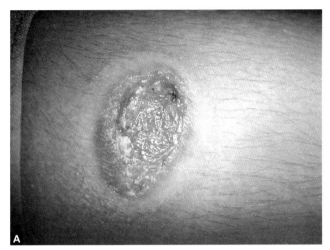 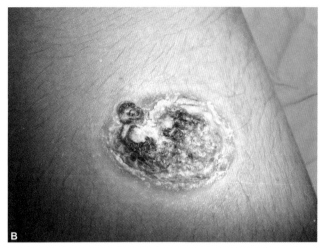

FIGS. 3.11.20A AND B: Lupus vulgaris.

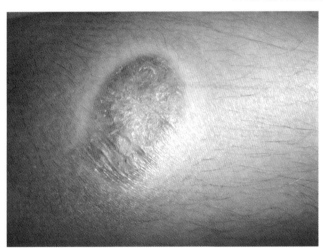 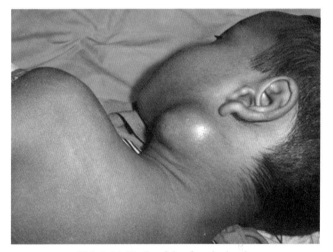

FIG. 3.11.21: Lupus vulgaris (healed).

FIG. 3.11.22: Scrofula of neck glands.

commonly in a lymph node or a bone. The lesion first manifests itself as a blue-red, painless swelling that breaks open and then forms an ulcer with irregular, undermined blue borders. Numerous fistulae may intercommunicate beneath ridges of a bluish skin. Progression and scarring produce irregular adherent masses, densely fibrous places and fluctuant or discharging in others. After healing, characteristic puckered scarring marks the site of the infection (Figs. 3.11.22 to 3.11.24).

TUBERCULOSIS VERRUCOSA CUTIS

This type of cutaneous tuberculosis results from inoculation in a person who has moderate or high degree of immunity. Laboratory workers, laborers and manual workers are often the victims and are secondary to trauma and commonly lower limbs are affected. It is an occupational hazard in veterinarians, pathologists, anatomists and butchers who handle the diseased tissue and hands are often affected (prosector's wart, butcher's wart) (Figs. 3.11.25A and B).

The clinical features are variable but large warty lesions of long duration affecting the hands or feet should arouse

suspicion. Initially, the lesions are dull red, deep-seated papule or nodule which slowly enlarge and become warty over the period. These lesions sometimes become warty over the period. These lesions sometimes become worse during summer season and may become crusted. On healing, there are atrophic scars left behind.

Treatment

Multidrug therapy has eased the treatment of cutaneous tuberculosis and the outcome is very good. The total duration of treatment is essentially 6 months, which is divided into initial 2 months intensive phase and continuation phase for 4–7 months. During intensive phase, various drugs used are isoniazid (5 mg/kg/day), rifampicin (10 mg/kg/day), pyrazinamide (30 mg/kg/day) and ethambutol (15 mg/kg/day). For cutaneous tuberculosis without any systemic involvement, 4 months' continuation phase is adequate. However, if there is underlying systemic involvement, the duration may need to be prolonged. During isoniazid therapy, pyridoxine supplementation is

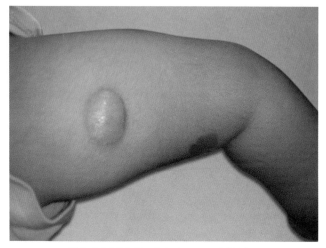

FIG. 3.11.23: Scrofuloderma at BCG site.

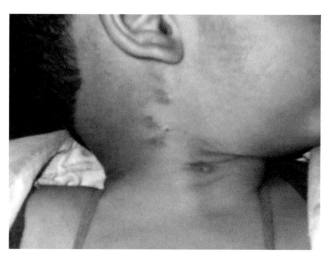

FIG. 3.11.24: Scrofuloderma scars.

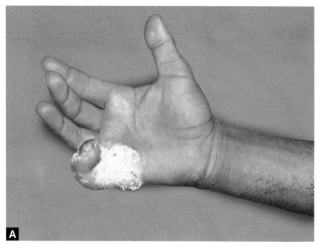

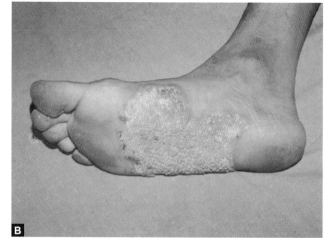

FIGS. 3.11.25A AND B: Tuberculosis verrucosa cutis.

routinely given. Associated malnutrition, if any, needs to be treated simultaneously.

MOLLUSCUM CONTAGIOSUM

This condition, caused by poxviridae, is characterized by the appearance of umbilicated skin nodules. The incubation period varies from 14 days to 6 months. The individual lesion is a shiny, pearly white, hemispherical, umbilicated papule which may show a central pore. It grows to a diameter of 5–10 mm in 6–12 weeks. The lesions spread frequently and are sometimes present in large number. After trauma or spontaneously after several months, inflammatory changes result in suppuration, crusting and virtual destruction of the base. The most common sites affected are the limbs. But it may also affect the scalp, face, oral mucous membrane or any other part of the body. Most cases are self-limiting in 6–9 months (Figs. 3.11.26A and B).

Treatment

Lesions are treated by chemical cautery by 50–60% trichloroacetic acid, phenol, cantharidin or silver nitrate. The

caustic is applied with either a needle or a tooth pick. Other options are electrodesiccation, cryotherapy or application of currently available imiquimod, an immunomodulator.

PITYRIASIS ROSEA

Pityriasis rosea is an acute and self-limiting disease characterized by a distinctive skin eruption and minimal constitutional symptoms. The etiology is considered to be infective with the appearance of the herald patch, which is larger and more conspicuous than the lesions of the later eruption, usually situated on the thigh, upper arm, the trunk or the neck. It is a sharply defined, bright-red, round or oval plaque soon covered by a fine scale, which reaches a size of 2–5 cm. After an interval of 5–15 days, the general eruption begins to appear in crops at 2–3 days interval over a week or 10 days. They appear in the form of discrete medallions, dull pink in color covered by fine dry, silvery-gray scales. The center tends to clear, assumes a wrinkled, atrophic appearance and a tawny color with a marginal collarette of scales attached peripherally, with the free

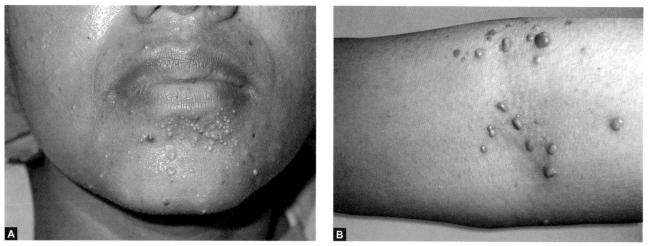

FIGS. 3.11.26A AND B: Molluscum contagiosum.

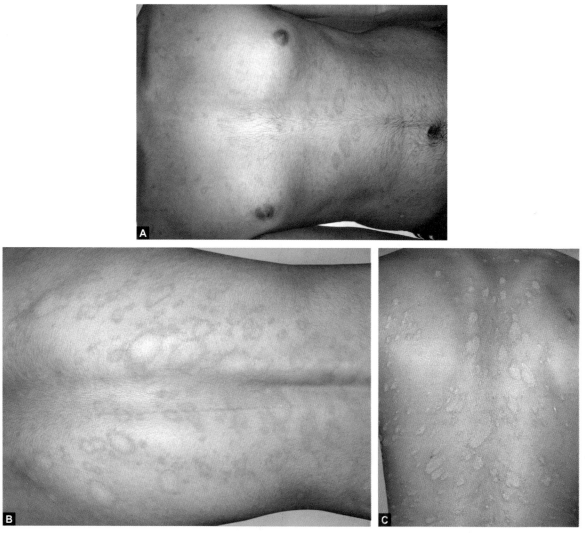

FIGS. 3.11.27A TO C: Pityriasis rosea.

edge of the scales internally. The medallions are commonly associated with pink macules of varying sizes. The lesions are usually confined to the trunk, the base of the neck and the upper third of the arms and legs. Involvement of the face and scalp are common in children. The skin lesions commonly fade after 3–6 weeks (3.11.27A to C).

Natural History

It is a self-limiting condition and resolves spontaneously in 2–4 weeks' time, although rarely it may persist up to 3 months or even longer.

Treatment

For mild itching, oral antihistamines are prescribed as well as local application of calamine. In severe cases, to cut down the severity of the disease and to improve the quality of life, oral corticosteroids at a dose of 10–30 mg is given for the duration of 7–21 days.

TINEA CORPORIS, TINEA CRURIS AND TINEA FACIEI

Tinea corporis is a dermatophyte infection of the glabrous skin typically occurring on exposed areas. Lesions are circular, sharply marginated with a raised edge. Single lesions occur or there may be multiple plaques. The degree of inflammation is variable. In inflammatory lesions, pustules or vesicles may dominate. Central resolution is common but not complete and the central skin may show

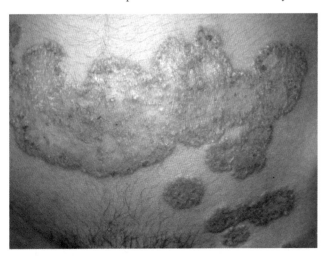

FIG. 3.11.28: Tinea corporis.

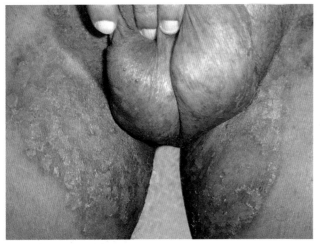

FIG. 3.11.29: Tinea cruris.

post-inflammatory pigmentation, a change of texture or residual erythematous dermal nodules.

Tinea faciei is an infection of the glabrous skin of the face with a dermatophyte fungus. Complaints of itching, burning and exacerbation after sun exposure are common. Lesions may be simple papular lesions or flat patches of erythema. Sometimes annular or circinate lesions, indurated lesions with raised margins may be seen (Figs. 3.11.28 to 3.11.30).

Management

For a single patch, topical antifungals are enough. Various topical antifungals used are clotrimazole (1%), miconazole (2%), oxiconazole (1%), ketoconazole (2%), terbinafine (1%), butenafine (1%) and ciclopirox olamine (1%). Once or twice a day application for 2–3 weeks is recommended.

Systemic antifungals are required for extensive and/or persistent infection, infection over scalp and nails. Griseofulvin is the drug of choice for tinea capitis and is also fairly effective for other types of dermatophytosis. Ultramicronized form of griseofulvin has enhanced bioavailability and lower dosage schedule. It is given in a dose of 5–10 mg/kg of body weight/day. For skin infections 4–6 weeks and for scalp infection 6–8 months courses are required.

In case of intolerance to griseofulvin other drugs which can be given are terbinafine 250 mg/day for older children and adolescents for 14 days. Ketoconazole 4–7 mg/kg/day for 2–4 weeks, fluconazole 50 mg weekly for 4–6 weeks, itraconazole 100 mg daily for 10–14 days are alternative drugs.

For kerion, along with antifungals oral antistaphylococcal antibiotics for 7–10 days and systemic corticosteroids for 7–14 days are to be given. Local application of clotrimazole or miconazole gel or lotion for 3–4 weeks prevents the spread of fungal spores to others.

TINEA PEDIS AND TINEA MANUUM

Tinea pedis is a fungal infection of the toe with predilection for web-space involvement. It is commonly seen in adolescents and sometimes in prepubertal children. While

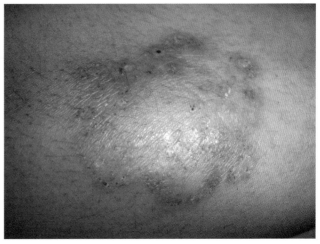

FIG. 3.11.30: Tinea faciei.

in some cases scaling and fissuring predominate (Figs. 3.11.31 and 3.11.32).

In others vesiculopustular lesions, erythema and maceration are found. The infection starts and may remain in between and along toes. However, the lesions can spread over the dorsal and plantar surfaces as well. Patients complain of intense itching and at times burning sensation. Similarly involvement of palm is known as tinea manuum.

Diagnosis

Diagnosis is confirmed by KOH preparation and culture of fungus.

Treatment

It is carried out by topical clotrimazole, miconazole, ketoconazole or recently available terbinafine creams in mild cases and in severe cases oral antifungals like griseofulvin, fluconazole or lately available terbinafine preparations.

TINEA CAPITIS

It is an infection of scalp hairs. There are three types of infection, black dot tinea, gray patch, kerion and favus. There is increased fragility and pluckability of hairs, itching at the patches and there is partial loss of hairs. Treatment consists of oral griseofulvin, terbinafine or itraconazole. Local application of clotrimazole, miconazole or oxiconazole, etc. will help (Figs. 3.11.33A and B).

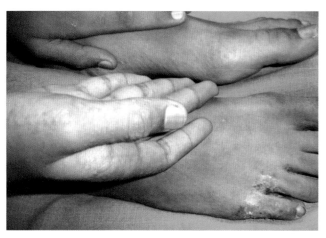

FIG. 3.11.31: Tinea pedis with id eruption.

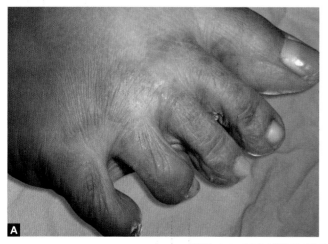

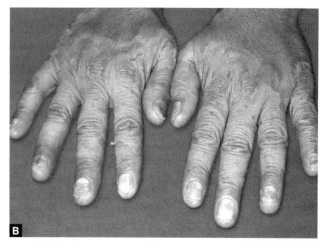

FIGS. 3.11.32A AND B: (A) Tinea pedis; (B) Tinea manuum.

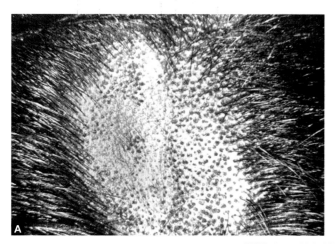

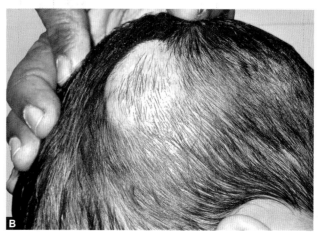

FIGS. 3.11.33A AND B: Tinea capitis.

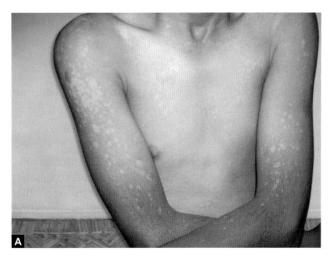
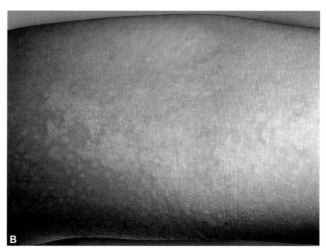

FIGS. 3.11.34A AND B: Pityriasis versicolor.

PITYRIASIS VERSICOLOR

This is a mild chronic infection of the skin caused by Malassezia yeasts and characterized by discrete or concrescent scaly discolored or depigmented areas mainly on the upper trunk. The primary lesion is a sharply demarcated macule characterized by a fine branny scaling. The eruption shows large confluent areas, scattered oval patches and outlying macules. The upper trunk is most commonly affected followed by the upper arms, the neck and the abdomen (Figs. 3.11.34 and 3.11.35).

Treatment

Topical application of 2.5% selenium sulfide solution once a week for 3–4 weeks, then once a month for 3–4 months is effective. Other agents are topical clotrimazole, ketoconazole, miconazole and terbinafine. For extensive and persistent lesions, various systemic antifungals which

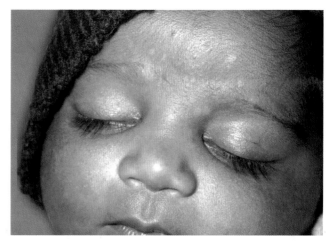

FIG. 3.11.35: Pityriasis versicolor in infant.

can be used are oral ketoconazole 20–200 mg/day for 5–7 days, fluconazole 50–100 mg single dose or itraconazole 100–200 mg/day for 5–7 days.

3.12 | BONE AND JOINT INFECTIONS

Nupur Ganguly

INTRODUCTION

Bone and joint infections are a significant cause of morbidity in infants and young children. Although with the advent of antibiotics incidence of osteomyelitis has decreased to some extent, yet it continues to be a major problem in our country. In the absence of early diagnosis and prompt treatment or failure of antibiotic therapy due to development of drug resistance, osteomyelitis can give rise to permanent sequelae. The increasing prevalence of methicillin-resistant *Staphylococcus aureus* (MRSA) in many hospitals, and infection caused by multidrug resistant and β-lactamase producing bacteria is posing a major challenge in the treatment. In children, bones of lower extremity are more often affected and of these, upper end of tibia and lower end of femur are more liable to infection as they have greater amount of growing bones in these areas. *S. aureus* is the most common organism throughout pediatric age group and the infection is mostly hematogenous. Infection caused by contiguous spread and vascular insufficiency is rare in children.

OSTEOMYELITIS

Classification

It can be classified by duration (acute or chronic), pathogenesis (trauma, contiguous spread, hematogenous, surgical), site, extent or type of patient. For all practical purposes it is classified as:
- Acute hematogenous osteomyelitis
- Osteomyelitis secondary to contiguous spread of infection after trauma, puncture wounds, surgery or joint replacement
- Osteomyelitis secondary to vascular insufficiency.

Epidemiology

The exact incidence of childhood osteomyelitis in India is unknown due to limited data. Other countries report a decrease in incidence in recent years. Approximately 50% of cases of osteomyelitis occur in the first 5 years of life. Boys are more likely to be affected than girls. The long bones of the lower extremities are most often involved, although any bone may be affected.

The most significant epidemiologic change regarding long-bone osteomyelitis, and all osteoarticular infections, is the ongoing rise of MRSA and other multidrug-resistant organisms.

Pathogenesis

Osteomyelitis may be caused by hematogenous spread, direct inoculation of microorganisms into bone, or from a contiguous focus of infection. A trivial skin infection may be the source of bacteremia or it may emerge as the result of a more serious infection such as acute or subacute bacterial endocarditis. Acute hematogenous osteomyelitis results from symptomatic or asymptomatic bacteremia. Hematogenous osteomyelitis usually involves the metaphysis of long bones because of its rich vascular supply. The infecting organism travels to metaphyseal capillary loops, where it replicates and causes local inflammation. As the bacteria replicate, they travel through vascular tunnels and adhere to cartilaginous matrix.

S. aureus increases bacterial adhesions to extracellular bone matrix and evade host defenses, attack host cells and colonize bone persistently. Further, bony metaphyses of children younger than 18 months are vascularized by the transphyseal vessels. These vessels enter the epiphysis and ultimately the joint space; hence they have a higher risk of joint space infection complicating osteomyelitis.

With hematogenous spread the joint space is usually spared in older children; however, it can get infected when the metaphysis is intracapsular, as is found at the proximal radius, humerus or femur.

The most common causes of direct inoculation osteomyelitis are penetrating injuries and surgical contamination. Contiguous osteomyelitis in children is seen in the setting of trauma, animal bites, puncture wounds, and direct extension of infection from an infected sinus, mastoid bone or dental abscess.

Pathology

Acute osteomyelitis presents as a suppurative infection accompanied by edema, vascular congestion and small vessel thrombosis. In early acute disease, the vascular supply to the bone is decreased by infection extending into the surrounding soft tissue. Large areas of dead bone (sequestra) may be formed when the medullary and periosteal blood supplies are compromised. Acute osteomyelitis can be arrested before dead bone develops, if treated promptly and aggressively with antibiotics and surgery (if necessary). In an established infection, fibrous tissue and chronic inflammatory cells form around the granulation tissue and dead bone. After the infection is contained, there is a decrease in the vascular supply to it, inhibiting an effective inflammatory response. Chronic osteomyelitis is the result of the coexistence of infected, nonviable tissues and an ineffective host response.

Microbiology

The type of infecting organism depends on the age of the child and underlying medical problem.

In infants, *S. aureus*, *Streptococcus agalactiae* and *Escherichia coli* are the most common pathogens isolated from blood or bone. However, in children more than 1 year of age, *S. aureus*, *Streptococcus pyogenes*, *Haemophilus influenzae* and *Kingella kingae* are commonly isolated. *S. pyogenes* causes approximately 10% of cases of acute hematogenous osteomyelitis with a peak incidence of disease in preschool-age and early school-age children. Children with *S. pyogenes* osteomyelitis often have a recent history of varicella infection and present with higher fever and white blood cell (WBC) counts compared with children infected with *S. aureus*.

Children with osteomyelitis caused by *S. pneumoniae* are more likely to have joint involvement.

Organisms causing bone infection in children with sickle cell disease include Salmonella and *S. aureus* and less commonly *E. coli*, Hib, Shigella and *S. pneumoniae*.

Kingella kingae is a fastidious gram-negative coccobacillary bacterium found in normal respiratory flora. Infection with this organism often is preceded by an upper respiratory tract infection or stomatitis; disrupted respiratory mucosa may facilitate invasion and hematogenous dissemination.

After 4 years of age, the incidence of *H. influenzae* infection decreases, and the overall incidence of *H. influenzae* as a cause of osteomyelitis is further decreasing with the use of *H. influenzae* vaccine.

Puncture wounds to the foot may result in osteomyelitis caused by mixed flora, including pseudomonas, *S. aureus*, enteric gram-negative bacteria and anaerobes. A series of cases describes osteomyelitis of the metatarsals occurring as a result of toothpick puncture injuries.

Anaerobes are a rare cause of pyogenic osteomyelitis in healthy children. Predominant organisms are *Bacteroides*, *Fusobacterium*, *Clostridium* and *Peptostreptococcus*.

Skeletal tuberculosis may occur as a result of hematogenous spread of *Mycobacterium tuberculosis* early in the course of a primary infection. On rare occasions, skeletal tuberculosis may be a contiguous infection from an adjacent caseating lymph node. Atypical mycobacteria, including *Mycobacterium marinum*, *Mycobacterium avium-intracellulare*, *Mycobacterium fortuitum* and *Mycobacterium gordonae,* all have been associated with osteoarticular infections. In addition, infections may also be caused by a variety of fungal organisms, including coccidioidomycosis, blastomycosis, cryptococcus and sporotrichosis.

Clinical Manifestations

The early signs of osteomyelitis are nonspecific and subtle, and high degree of suspicion is required for early diagnosis and management. Most children with acute hematogenous osteomyelitis are symptomatic for less than 2 weeks. Symptoms include acute, persistent and increasing pain over the affected bone.

In a neonate it is a serious infection. They may not have fever or appear ill hence the diagnosis is often delayed. There may be pain during movement of the extremity while changing the diaper. It often results from hematogenous spread of the organisms.

In infancy, the presenting signs and symptoms include fever, irritability, redness and swelling over the affected area and refusal to move the affected limb and diagnosis may be delayed because of nonspecific signs of illness. Infection involving multiple bones and contiguous joints and soft tissue is not uncommon.

Usually a single site of bone is involved and multiple site involvement is seen in less than 10% of cases; however, in neonates two or more bones are involved in half the cases.

Pelvic osteomyelitis is reported in 1–11% of all cases of acute hematogenous osteomyelitis and typically affects older children. Symptoms include hip, buttock, low back, or abdominal pain. Fever may be absent. Findings on physical examination include tenderness of the pelvic bones, pain with hip movement, decreased range of motion at the hip, and refusal or inability to bear weight. Any bone in the pelvis may be involved, but the ilium is more affected because of its rich blood supply. Many a time the symptoms and findings are nonspecific and poorly localized and are attributed to other diagnoses, such as pyogenic arthritis of the hip or appendicitis rather than osteomyelitis. This leads to delay in establishing the correct diagnosis.

Differential Diagnosis of Bone Pain

The differential diagnosis of bone pain in children includes trauma, malignancy and bone infarction in patients with sickle cell disease. Differentiation between bone infection and infarction in a child with sickle cell anemia is difficult because in both cases the acute onset of fever and bone pain is common. In addition, a patient may have infarction that predisposes to infection.

A Brodie abscess is a subacute osteomyelitis usually seen in the metaphyseal area of tibia. Classically, this may present after conversion as a draining abscess extending from the tibia out through the shin.

Chronic recurrent multifocal osteomyelitis is a poorly understood inflammatory illness characterized by recurrent bone pain and fever. Girls are predominantly affected and have radiologic evidence of multiple, often symmetric bone lesions involving primarily the long bones and clavicles. Associated findings include psoriasis vulgaris and palmoplantar pustulosis.

Diagnosis

The diagnosis of osteomyelitis depends primarily on clinical findings and corroborative laboratory and radiographic results. Every attempt should be made to establish a microbiologic diagnosis. In the case of hematogenous osteomyelitis, positive blood cultures often can eliminate the need for a bone biopsy, provided there is radiographic evidence of osteomyelitis. Otherwise, antibiotic treatment should be based on bone cultures taken at debridement or during bone biopsy. Whenever possible, cultures should be obtained before antimicrobial therapy has begun. Sinus tract cultures are reliable for confirming *S. aureus*, but they do not predict the presence or absence of gram-negative organisms that cause osteomyelitis.

A bacteriologic diagnosis can be made in 50–80% of cases if blood and bone cultures are obtained. In the case of culture-negative osteomyelitis that is not responding as expected to empirical therapy, a bone biopsy specimen should be obtained for histopathologic staining and for culture of bacteria, mycobacteria and fungi. Inoculation of bone or abscess material directly into an aerobic blood culture bottle facilitates isolation of *K. kingae*. Cultures for *K. kingae* and other fastidious organisms may need to be incubated longer than usual laboratory protocol.

The WBC count may be normal or increased. Erythrocyte sedimentation rate (ESR) is elevated in 80–90% of cases, and C-reactive protein (CRP) is elevated in 98% of cases. Erythrocyte sedimentation rate generally peaks 3–5 days after admission, and CRP peaks within 48 hours of admission. C-reactive protein typically returns to normal 7–10 days after appropriate therapy. Erythrocyte sedimentation rate may remain elevated for 3 or 4 weeks, even with appropriate therapy.

Patients who require surgical incision and drainage procedures may have prolonged time to normalization of ESR or CRP. Polymerase chain reaction is most sensitive in detecting *K. kingae*. It can detect *K. kingae* even after the use of antibiotic for 6 days.

Plain X-ray

They show soft-tissue swelling in the first few days of illness. Periosteal and lytic changes in the bone generally are not seen until substantial bone destruction has occurred, usually 10–21 days after onset of symptoms. In some cases of proven bacterial osteomyelitis, bone changes are never seen on plain film, presumably because prompt diagnosis and treatment prevented extensive bone destruction.

In cases of hematogenous osteomyelitis, radiographic changes usually lag at least 2 weeks behind the infection's evolution. The earliest changes seen are swelling of soft tissue, periosteal thickening and/or elevation, and focal osteopenia. Radiographs will usually not indicate lytic changes until at least 50–75% of the bone matrix is destroyed. Infected areas typically appear dark. The more diagnostic lytic changes are delayed and associated with subacute and chronic osteomyelitis. Similarly, radiographic evidence of improvements may lag behind clinical recovery. In contiguous focus osteomyelitis, radiographic changes are subtle and require careful clinical correlation to have diagnostic significance.

Bone Scan

Technetium 99m (^{99m}Tc) methylene diphosphonate is used for radionuclide bone imaging. It is very useful in early diagnosis, where the diagnosis of osteomyelitis is ambiguous or it is necessary to gauge the extent of bone and/or soft-tissue inflammation, and when there is multiple site involvement a three phase bone scan is done. Any increased area of blood flow or inflammation may cause increased uptake in the first and second phase but osteomyelitis causes increased uptake in the third phase (4–6 hours). Three phase imaging has the sensitivity of (84–100%) and specificity of (70–96%). However, the sensitivity in neonates is lower due to poor bone mineralization.

Radionuclide bone scans usually are positive within 48–72 hours of onset of symptoms. In some cases of osteomyelitis, vascular supply to the bone is compromised, with decreased uptake of technetium to the affected area, resulting in a "cold scan" whereas increased isotope accumulation is seen in areas of increased blood flow and new bone formation reactive to the infection. Some experts prefer bone scan as the initial study in the evaluation of suspected uncomplicated osteomyelitis of the long bones. It is less expensive than magnetic resonance imaging (MRI), sedation of the child is generally not necessary and it is particularly useful when multifocal osteomyelitis is suspected or the exact location of infection is not obvious on physical examination.

Radionuclide scans may be positive in other illnesses that result in increased osteoblastic activity, including malignancy, trauma, cellulitis, postsurgery and arthritis.

A negative ^{99m}Tc scan effectively rules out the diagnosis of osteomyelitis.

White Blood Cell Scans

It offers a marked improvement in specificity (80–90%) compared with bone scans, particularly when complicated conditions are superimposed. The white blood cell (WBC) scan was performed originally with indium-111 (^{111}In)-labeled WBCs and more recently with ^{99m}Tc hexamethyl propylene amine oxime-labeled WBCs. ^{111}Ic scans have sensitivity of more than 90% and specificity of 78%. Other promising diagnostic scans under evaluation are as below:

- The radiolabeled antibiotics scan is a fast-emerging diagnostic test for detection of infectious lesions because of their specific binding to bacterial components. These agents may prove to differentiate between infection and sterile inflammatory lesions.
- The fluorodeoxyglucose-positron emission tomography scan is a relatively novel technique that has demonstrated the highest diagnostic accuracy for confirming or excluding chronic osteomyelitis in comparison with bone scintigraphy, MRI or leukocyte scintigraphy. Positron emission tomography and single photon emission computed tomography are highly accurate

techniques for the evaluation of chronic osteomyelitis, particularly of the axial skeleton, allowing differentiation from soft tissue infection. Fluorodeoxyglucose-positron emission tomography should be avoided in the first 3–6 months after debridement surgery or trauma because of high false-positive results in postsurgical and traumatic bone healing. It has limited utility in differentiating infection with a failed prosthesis or a tumor.

- Recent studies show that use of superparamagnetic iron oxide MRI contrast agent for bone marrow imaging appears promising for differentiation between inflammatory lesions and neoplastic metastasis compared with the standard gadolinium complex MRI scans.

Magnetic Resonance Imaging

It gives excellent resolution of bone and soft tissue. It is particularly useful for visualizing soft tissue abscess associated with osteomyelitis, bone marrow edema and bone destruction and when the diagnosis of osteomyelitis is equivocal. Contrast enhancement with gadolinium is used to look for areas of abscess formation. If pelvic or vertebral body osteomyelitis is suspected, MRI is the imaging study of choice. It gives better spatial resolution than bone scan and is preferred if a surgical procedure to diagnose or drain an abscess is necessary. The typical appearance of acute osteomyelitis in an MRI scan is a localized area of abnormal marrow with decreased signal intensity on T1-weighted images and increased signal intensity on T2-weighted images. Limitations of MRI include the need for sedation in younger children, high cost and inability to assess easily whether other bones are affected.

Differentiating bone infarction versus infection can be difficult in a child with sickle cell disease. In both situations, children present with fever and bone pain and have elevated inflammatory markers. Biopsy and culture of affected bone is often necessary to establish the diagnosis. Some authors have used the pattern of MRI contrast enhancement to distinguish acute medullary bone infarction from osteomyelitis.

Differential Diagnosis

The differential diagnosis of osteomyelitis in children includes trauma, malignancy and bone infarction which causes bone pain and mimics osteomyelitis. Myositis and pyomyositis may also have the same clinical features like osteomyelitis like fever, local tenderness and limping. Malignancy and bone infarction in patients with sickle cell disease often simulate osteomyelitis. In such patients the differentiation between bone infection and infarction is also difficult as in both cases the acute onset of fever and bone pain is common. In addition, a patient may have infarction that predisposes to infection.

A brodie abscess is a subacute osteomyelitis usually seen in the metaphyseal area of tibia. Classically, this may present after conversion as a draining abscess extending from the tibia out through the shin.

Chronic recurrent multifocal osteomyelitis is a poorly understood inflammatory illness characterized by recurrent bone pain and fever. Girls are predominantly affected and have radiologic evidence of multiple, often symmetric bone lesions involving primarily the long bones and clavicles. Associated findings include psoriasis vulgaris and palmoplantar pustulosis.

Appendicitis, urinary tract infection and pelvic infection are considered in the differential diagnosis of pelvic osteomyelitis. Primary bone tumors are to be considered in the differential diagnosis of osteomyelitis.

Treatment

Successful treatment of osteomyelitis depends upon early diagnosis, appropriate selection and administration of antibiotics and surgical intervention when needed.

Empirical use of these antibiotics before organism identification and susceptibility testing depends on the age and the knowledge of likely bacterial pathogen for that age, severity of illness and incidence of MRSA in the community.

Common organism at different age group is shown in the Table 3.12.1.

Kingella kingae generally is susceptible to most beta-lactam antibiotics, including second-generation and third-generation cephalosporin. It is often resistant to clindamycin, and resistance to clotrimazole is reported.

When culture results are available, antibiotic therapy is modified depending on the organism and the susceptibility

Table 3.12.1: Common organism at different age group.

Age	Organism
Infants 0–2 months	Staphylococcus aureus
	Streptococcus agalactiae
	Gram-negative enteric bacteria
	Candida spp.
≤ 5 years	S. aureus
	Streptococcus pyogenes
	Streptococcus pneumoniae
	Kingella kingae
	Haemophilus influenzae type b (if child not completely immunized with conjugate Hib vaccine)
≥ 5 years	S. aureus; S. pyogenes
Adolescent	Neisseria gonorrhoeae

Note: S. aureus remains the most common cause of osteomyelitis till date in all age group.

pattern. If no organism is isolated, but the patient is improving, initial empirical coverage is continued. If the patient is not improving, further diagnostic testing should be considered, including bone biopsy for histopathology and culture if not previously obtained or imaging studies to rule out areas of infection that may require surgical drainage or debridement.

Infection caused by MRSA and CA-MRSA is increasing. Many isolates of CA-MRSA are susceptible to clindamycin. Isolates of *S. aureus* that are erythromycin resistant and clindamycin susceptible should be evaluated for the presence of inducible macrolide-lincosamide-streptogramin B (MLSB) resistance. This evaluation is done by means of a "D" test, performed by many hospital laboratories. Although some children treated with clindamycin for an infection with MRSA of the MLSB phenotype clear their infection, it is recommended that in the setting of serious infection, clindamycin should not be used if this phenotype is identified.

Alternative drugs to consider for treatment of osteomyelitis caused by MRSA include intravenous vancomycin and linezolid (Table 3.12.2).

For Gram-negative organisms amikacin, cefoperazone-sulbactam combination is also effective. Gentamicin once found to be most effective drug for the treatment of osteomyelitis has now become resistant. *P. aeruginosa* is developing resistance to gentamicin, ciprofloxacin and piperacillin. In various studies resistance of *P. aeruginosa* to ciprofloxacin has been reported. Multidrug resistance among pathogenic organisms poses a major challenge in the treatment of infections. A finding of greater concern is the progressively developing resistance to cefoperazone-sulbactam (beta-lactam + beta-lactamase inhibitor) combination among gram-negative isolates since antibiotics of choice in the treatment of infections due to β-lactamase-producing microorganisms are either limited to these combinations or to the carbapenems.

Duration of Therapy

It depends upon the extent of infection, clinical response and presence of underlying risk factors. In general, 3–6 weeks of antibiotic therapy is given depending on the clinical response. There is good evidence that treatment for less than 3 weeks results in an unacceptably high rate of relapse. Chronic infection is reported in 19% of children treated for less than 3 weeks compared with 2% in children treated longer than 3 weeks.

The decision to change from parenteral to oral therapy depends on the availability of an appropriate oral antibiotic, the child's ability to take the medication by mouth, reliable caregivers and the ability of the family to comply with frequent follow-up. Generally, oral therapy is begun when the child is afebrile, symptoms and signs of infection are resolving and CRP is returning to normal. Sequential intravenous to oral therapy is proven to be effective and safe, provided that close follow-up of the patient is ensured.

Oral Antibiotic

The dose of oral antibiotic is generally two to three times the usual dose for children when a beta-lactam antibiotic, such as dicloxacillin or cephalexin, is used. The usual recommended oral doses of clindamycin, trimethoprim-sulfamethoxazole, fluoroquinolone antibiotics and linezolid can be used because of the excellent bioavailability of these drugs. Vancomycin always must be given intravenously.

Doses of oral antibiotics used for bone and joint infections have been listed in Table 3.12.3.

Prognosis

Most children who receive appropriate therapy for osteomyelitis have no long-term sequelae. Recurrence of infection occurs in approximately 5% of cases. Risk factors for development of complications include delay in diagnosis, short duration of therapy and young age at the time of initial illness. The reported incidence of sequelae in neonates with osteomyelitis ranges from 6 to 50%.

Permanent abnormalities include disturbance in bone growth, limb-length discrepancies, arthritis, abnormal gait and pathologic fractures.

Table 3.12.2: Empirical parenteral antibiotic therapy for pediatric bone and joint infections.

Infants 0–2 months	Cloxacillin (150–200 mg/kg/24 hour q6 hourly IV) +
	Cefotaxime (150–200 mg/kg/24 hour q8 hourly)
	Amikacin may be used (but have reduced antibacterial activity in presence of low oxygen tension and low pH seen in tissue infection)
Children <5 years	Cloxacillin plus cefotaxime or ceftriaxone or cefuroxime
Children >5 years	Cloxacillin plus cefotaxime or ceftriaxone or cefuroxime
If MRSA is a concern (if local rates of MRSA are 5–10%),	
	Vancomycin (40 mg/kg/24 hour q6 hourly IV)
	or clindamycin (40 mg/kg/24 hour q6 hourly IV), as empirical therapy

Note: Alternative drugs, like teicoplanin and quinu pristine-dalfopristin, have also shown promising results.

Table 3.12.3: Doses of oral antibiotics used for bone and joint infections.

Antibiotic	*Dose (mg/kg/day)*	*Interval*
Cephalexin	100	q6–8h
Cloxacillin	100	q6h
Clindamycin	30	q6–8h
Linezolid	10	q–8h

Although it does not seem to be a significant difference in outcome for bone infections caused by MRSA compared with infections caused by methicillin-susceptible *S. aureus* children infected with MRSA tends to have longer duration of fever and prolonged hospitalization, complicated clinical course. Chronic osteomyelitis develops in less than 5% of children after acute hematogenous infection. It is observed more frequently after contiguous osteomyelitis.

Bone necrosis occurs as a result of chronic inflammation and vascular compromise. Extensive fibrosis eventually results. Signs and symptoms of chronic osteomyelitis vary from chronic vague symptoms of swelling, pain or intermittent drainage of the affected bone to acute exacerbations of fever, swelling, or redness over the bone. Effective management of chronic osteomyelitis usually requires surgical and medical management, with prolonged courses of antibiotics.

Conclusion

As *S. aureus* is the most common etiological agent of osteomyelitis, any first-line antibiotic should be primarily directed against this pathogen. For coverage of Gram-negative bacteria, beta-lactam + beta-lactamase inhibitor combination would be more useful. Use of monodrug therapy needs to be guided by sensitivity report. Finally continuous monitoring of susceptibility pattern needs to be carried out in individual setting so as to detect the true burden of antibiotic resistance among organisms and prevent their further emergence by judicious use of drugs.

PYOGENIC ARTHRITIS

Pyogenic arthritis or septic arthritis is a purulent invasion of a joint by an infectious agent which produces arthritis. It is a serious infection and can lead to devastating complications. It should be considered a medical emergency. If untreated, it may destroy the joint in a period of days and the infection may also spread to other parts of the body. The key to minimize irreversible damage is rapid initiation of treatment. The best results are obtained when treatment is instituted within 1 week of the onset of symptoms. Effective treatment involves antibiotics, joint drainage and decompression, and immobilization followed by rehabilitation of the affected joint.

Reactive arthritis is a sterile inflammatory process that usually results from an extra-articular infectious process.

Bacteria are the most significant pathogens because of their rapidly destructive nature. Viruses, fungal organisms and *M. tuberculosis* are uncommon causes of joint space infection. For this reason, the current discussion concentrates on the bacterial septic arthritis. Failure to recognize and appropriate treatment results in significant rates of morbidity and may even lead to death. Early diagnosis and treatment minimize further damage to synovium, adjacent cartilage and bone. An episode of septic

Table 3.12.4: Presentation of osteomyelitis and septic arthritis.

Osteomyelitis	Septic arthritis
• Subacute onset of limp/non-weight bearing/refusal to use limb	• Acute onset of limp/non-weight bearing/refusal to use limb
• Localized pain and pain on movement	• Pain on movement and at rest
• Tenderness	• Limited range/loss of movement
• Soft-tissue redness/swelling may not be present and may appear late	• Soft-tissue redness/swelling often present
• +/– Fever	• Fever

arthritis requires long-term follow-up to check for relapses and to assess the outcome of any residual joint damage.

There is considerable overlap in the presentation of osteomyelitis and septic arthritis (Table 3.12.4).

Pathogenesis

Pyogenic arthritis usually occurs as a result of infection of the vascular synovium by hematogenous spread of bacteria. An acute inflammatory response follows, resulting in migration of polymorphonuclear WBCs, production of proteolytic enzymes and cytokine secretion by chondrocytes. Degradation of articular cartilage begins 8 hours after onset of infection in children younger than 18 months of age; pyogenic arthritis can result from extension of a metaphyseal bone infection through transphyseal blood vessels. The growth plate, the epiphysis and eventually the joint space may be infected. Infection of the proximal femur and humerus often involves the hip and shoulder joints because the proximal metaphysis of each of these bones is intracapsular.

Epidemiology

Most cases of pyogenic arthritis occur in children 3 years old or younger. Cases are more frequent in boys. The joints of the lower extremities (hips, knees) are most often affected.

Microbiology

Staphylococcus aureus is the most common cause of pyogenic arthritis in all age groups, and infection with CA-MRSA is becoming more common. Infants younger than 2 months of age also may have infection caused by *S. agalactiae, Neisseria gonorrhoeae* and Gram-negative enteric bacteria. Arthritis caused by candida also is seen in the neonatal age group. *S. aureus, S. pyogenes, S. pneumoniae* and *K. kingae* are predominant organisms in the 2-month to 5-year age range. Children older than 5 years are most likely to have arthritis caused by *S. aureus* and *S. pyogenes. N. gonorrhoeae* arthritis occurs in sexually active adolescents. Arthritis caused by *K. kingae* has replaced Hib as the most common Gram-negative arthritis in the child 2 months to 5 years old with the better coverage of Hib vaccine. Primary viral infection of the joints are rare; however, arthritis accompanies many viral infection (mumps, rubella, many live vaccines, parvovirus) suggesting an immune-mediated pathogenesis. Candida arthritis may complicate systemic infection in neonates with or without indwelling catheters. *Borrelia burgdorferi* causes Lyme disease in endemic areas. Arthralgia is seen in early disseminated Lyme disease. Weeks to months after the initial infection, children may develop pauciarticular arthritis of the large joints, particularly the knees. *N. gonorrhoeae* infection should be considered in a sexually active adolescent with joint infection. Hematogenous spread of the organism can involve skin and joints (arthritis-dermatitis syndrome). Reactive arthritis is due to inflammation of a joint due to infection at some other site (gastrointestinal due to Shigella Salmonella, Campylobacter, *Yersinia enterocolitica*) or genitourinary tract infection. The arthritis associated with *N. gonorrhoeae* may also be reactive in nature.

Clinical Manifestations

Trauma or upper respiratory tract infection often precedes joint symptoms. Symptoms of pyogenic arthritis include acute onset of joint pain, fever, irritability and limp. Pain associated with pyogenic arthritis of the hip may be referred to the groin, thigh or knee. Findings on physical examination include redness, swelling and warmth over the affected joint. The child complains of pain with movement of the joint and restricted range of motion. Patients should be evaluated for signs of pharyngitis, rash, heart murmur, hepatosplenomegaly, and evidence of other joint or bone involvement.

Differential Diagnosis

The most common cause of hip pain in childhood is transient synovitis. Transient synovitis predominates in children 5–10 years old. The child generally has low-grade fever or is afebrile. Pain is usually unilateral, but may be bilateral in some cases. Pain ranges from mild to severe enough to wake the child up at night. Physical examination generally reveals a non ill-appearing child with decreased range of motion of the hip joint. Other causes of joint pain and swelling include reactive arthritis, juvenile rheumatoid arthritis, trauma and malignancy. Legg-Calvé-Perthes disease is an idiopathic avascular necrosis of the capital femoral epiphysis and may cause mild pain and limp in boys (mean age 7 years). Slipped capital femoral epiphysis is the most common hip disorder of adolescents; symptoms may include abnormal gait, pain and abnormal range of motion of the hip joint.

Diagnosis

Early diagnosis and treatment is most important to prevent damage to the articular cartilage. Every attempt should be made to grow the organism and establish microbiological diagnosis.

Blood and joint fluid should be obtained for aerobic and anaerobic cultures. Joint fluid should be inoculated directly into blood culture bottles to enhance identification of fastidious organisms such as *K. kingae*. Gram stain and cell count also should be performed on joint fluid. There is no specific laboratory test for septic arthritis. A WBC count of 50,000/mm³ or greater with a predominance of polymorphonuclear cells is suggestive of bacterial infection; however, it is also seen with rheumatologic disease. The peripheral WBC count, ESR and CRP are generally elevated, but are nonspecific to differentiate infection from other inflammatory process. C-reactive protein and ESR may be helpful to monitor the response to treatment or identifying complication. If *N. gonorrhoeae* is suspected, cultures of joint fluid, blood, pharynx, skin lesion, cervix, urethra, vagina and rectum should be obtained and inoculated onto special media. A throat culture for *S. pyogenes* should be sent if the patient has signs or symptoms of pharyngitis. Antibody titers to antistreptolysin O and anti-D Nase B also may be useful to diagnose infection with *S. pyogenes*. Serology for Lyme disease (Western blot) is used to diagnose Lyme arthritis in a patient with the appropriate exposure history. Plain radiographs of adjacent bone are useful in evaluating for other causes of joint pain and swelling, including trauma, malignancy and osteomyelitis. The prompt diagnosis of pyogenic arthritis of the hip is important to prevent serious permanent long-term sequelae. Untreated infection of the hip can result in vascular compromise and ischemic necrosis of the femoral head. Differentiation between pyogenic arthritis and transient synovitis of the hip is challenging. Most clinicians use fever and elevated inflammatory markers to diagnose and for the management of children with hip pain, but there is considerable overlap in the clinical and laboratory findings in children with pyogenic arthritis and transient synovitis. Close follow-up of the patients is needed.

Ultrasonographic Study

Ultrasound is highly sensitive in determining the fluid present in the hip joint where plain radiographs may be normal in more than 50% of cases. It is also used to guide joint aspiration. However, ultrasound cannot differentiate infected from noninfected fluid.

Radiographic Studies

Plain radiographs are obtained to rule out fracture, malignancy or osteomyelitis as the cause of pain. Plain films may show widening of the joint capsule, soft-tissue edema and obliteration of normal fat lines. Plain film of the hip may show medial displacement of the obturator muscle into the pelvis (obturator sign), lateral displacement of the gluteal fat lines and elevation of the Shenton line with the widened arc.

Computed Tomography and Magnetic Resonance Imaging

They are useful in confirming the presence of fluid in the joint space in case of suspected septic arthritis.

Management

The successful management of pyogenic arthritis depends on timely decompression of the joint space and institution of appropriate antibiotic therapy.

Aspiration of the affected joint usually is performed for diagnostic and therapeutic purposes. In the case of hip and shoulder joint infections, prompt surgical drainage of infected joint fluid usually is required.

The initial choice of empirical antibiotic therapy depends on the age of the child, clinical presentation and local patterns of antibiotic resistance.

In general, infants younger than 2 months are treated with cloxacillin and a third-generation cephalosporin to cover *S. aureus* and enteric Gram-negative bacteria.

Older children should receive antibiotic therapy active against *S. aureus, S. pyogenes* and *K. kingae*. If *N. gonorrhoeae* is suspected, ceftriaxone should be used.

Clindamycin is an appropriate antibiotic for most Gram-positive bacteria, including some strains of CA-MRSA. It is not active, however, against *K. kingae*.

Kingella kingae generally is susceptible to most beta-lactam antibiotics, including second-generation and third-generation cephalosporins. If MRSA is suspected, vancomycin should be used empirically until culture and susceptibility results are available as in osteomyelitis.

Intra-articular injection of antibiotics is not appropriate. Most antibiotics achieve high synovial fluid concentrations and the antibiotic may cause a chemical synovitis when directly injected into the joint.

As with osteomyelitis, a child should be treated with intravenous antibiotics until there is significant clinical improvement, inflammatory markers are returning to normal, and the child's oral intake is normal.

The doses of oral antibiotics used are the same as doses used to treat osteomyelitis. The duration of therapy for uncomplicated pyogenic arthritis depends on the response to therapy and the suspected organism. Generally, infections with *S. pneumoniae, K. kingae,* Hib and *N. gonorrhoeae* are treated for 2–3 weeks.

Infections caused by *S. aureus* or gram-negative enteric bacteria are treated for 3–4 weeks.

Dexamethasone in Septic Arthritis

A placebo controlled RCT examined the use of 4 days of IV dexamethasone (0.2 mg/kg/dose IV 8 hourly) in 123 children with acute septic arthritis. It significantly shortened the duration of acute phase and also reduced the dysfunction at the end of the therapy after 6 months and 12 months. Further studies are needed to confirm the benefits and risks of this treatment approach.

Prognosis

Complications of pyogenic arthritis include abnormal bone growth, limp, unstable articulation of the affected joint and decreased range of motion.

Complications are reported in approximately 10–25% of all cases. Risk factors for sequelae include delay in time to diagnosis of more than 4 or 5 days, onset of disease in infancy, infection with *S. aureus* or Gram-negative bacteria, and infection of adjacent bone.

Conclusion

The numbers of bone and joint infections resulting from vaccine-preventable infections, such as Hib and *S. pneumoniae*, have decreased in recent years.

S. aureus remains an important cause of pyogenic arthritis and osteomyelitis, and the prevalence of CA-MRSA is increasing. Transition from intravenous to oral antibiotic therapy remains the treatment of choice for uncomplicated pediatric bone and joint infections if the family is reliable and close follow-up can be ensured.

BIBLIOGRAPHY

1. Arnold SR, Elias D, Buckingham SC, et al. Changing patterns of acute hematogenous osteomyelitis and septic arthritis. Emergence of community-associated methicillin-resistant *Staphylococcus aureus*. J Pediatr Orthop. 2006;26(6):703-8.
2. Dubnov-Raz G, Ephros M, Garty BZ, et al. Invasive pediatric *Kingella kingae* infections. Pediatr Infect Dis J. 2010;29(7):639-42.
3. Gutierrez K. Bone and joint infections in children. Pediatr Clin North Am. 2005;52(3) 779-94.
4. Kaplan SL, Osteomyelitis, Septic arthritis. In: Kliegman RM, Stanton BF, St. Geme III JW, Schor NF, Behrman RF (Eds). Nelson Textbook of Pediatrics, 19th edition. Philadelphia: Saunders; 2011.pp.2394-400.

Common Bacterial Infections

Abhay K Shah

4.1 SALMONELLA INFECTIONS

Ajay Kalra

INTRODUCTION

Salmonella bacilli belong to the family Enterobacteriaceae. The organisms are motile, nonencapsulated, Gram-negative rods which remain viable at low temperatures for weeks and can survive for long periods in sewage, fecal matter and dried food. There are more than 2,500 serovars, all of which belong to a single species, designated *S. enterica*.

Salmonella serovars vary in their pathogenesis. *S. anatum*, *S. derby* and *S. newport* are usually limited to the intestine. *S. choleraesuis* rapidly enters the bloodstream and causes little damage in the intestine. *Salmonella typhi* bacteremia often leads to seedling of the liver and biliary tree.

Diseases caused by *Salmonella* organisms are divided into two categories:
1. *Enteric/Typhoidal*: *S. typhi* and *S. paratyphi* cause typhoidal disease.
2. *Nontyphoidal*: It results from other serovars that infect humans, the most common being *S. typhimurium* and *S. enteritidis*.

ENTERIC FEVER

The term "enteric fever" covers both typhoid and paratyphoid fevers. Nearly, 90% of the cases are typhoid while 10% are paratyphoid. Typhoid fever is an acute generalized infection of the intestinal lymphoid tissue, gallbladder and reticuloendothelial system. Typhoid organisms invade the reticuloendothelial system but have a remarkable predilection for gallbladder which gets invaded via retrograde spread from the gastrointestinal tract.

Etiological Agent

The organisms are gram-negative bacilli which are motile, nonacid fast, noncapsulated and having nonsporing flagellate, facultative anaerobe. The flagellate allows the organism to remain motile.

Salmonella typhi contains several antigens. Out of these, three are of importance. The first antigen, "O" antigen is heat stable polysaccharide which is a part of the liposaccharide of cell wall. The second antigen, "H" antigen is the flagellar antigen. It is heat and alcohol labile. Usually O antibodies appear on day 6–8 and H antibodies on day 10–12 after the onset of disease. Both these antigens are shared by *S. typhi, S. paratyphi A* and *S. paratyphi B*. They are important in the sense that antibodies formed against them are used in serodiagnosis of typhoid fever in Widal test. The third antigen, "Vi" antigen is called so because of its virulent nature. It is surface polysaccharide and heat stable, virtually present in all freshly isolated strains. Antibody formed against Vi antigen are shown to be protective in nature. Hence, Vi antigen is used for preparing vaccine.

Epidemiology

It is estimated that 33–60 million cases and 600,000 deaths occur annually due to typhoid fever worldwide. As the disease is primarily associated with poor hygienic and sanitary conditions, the major brunt of the disease occurs in developing countries. Around 5 million cases occur annually in India. Ten percent of cases occur in the infant age group when diagnosis may be difficult and mortality higher. A major problem in the last two decades of the twentieth century has been the emergence of plasmid encoded multidrug resistance ranging 17–90% as reported by various studies, especially to the quinolones. Children constitute 40–50% cases of multidrug resistant (MDR) typhoid fever with higher case fatality rates.

Humans are the only reservoir of *S. typhi* and they are the only known host at present that are susceptible to *S. typhi* infection. The peak incidence is in 5–15 years of age but cases are also reported frequently in infants and toddlers in developing countries. The frequent subclinical exposures make an individual partially immune as the age increases. There is no sex predilection. However, the disease is more common in males and chronic carrier state is more common in females. Fecal shedding for a year constitutes the chronic carrier state. The incidence of the disease is highest during summers and monsoon season, although they are frequently seen round the year.

Typhoid is essentially a food and water-borne disease. While water contamination can affect a sizeable group, yet, as the organism cannot multiply in water, the inoculums size may be too small to cause a disease because it would need a longer incubation period. On the other hand, food contamination introduces large inoculums which can cause disease within the short incubation period. Milk and milk products, vegetables grown in sewage irrigated farms, meat products and shell fish are common sources. House flies are well known for spreading the infection via food. Overcrowding, poor personal hygiene, poverty, illiteracy, poor sanitary and water supply situations, open defecation and parasitic infestations are important predisposing factors. *S. typhi* can survive for a long period in the environment. This may be 7 days in water, 30 days in ice and ice creams, 60 days in sewage irrigated soil and 20 days on the external surface of housefly.

PATHOGENESIS

Once ingested, the bacteria reach the small intestine. The inoculum size required to cause disease is 10^5–10^9 in order to survive in the normally lethal acidic pH of the stomach. In the small intestine, they adhere to the M cell of intestinal epithelium over the Peyer's patches. This results in invasion of the epithelium, multiplication in the submucosa and then drainage to the mesenteric lymph nodes. Hyperplasia of the Peyer's patches with necrosis and sloughing of the overlying epithelium leads to ulcer formation. Multiplication takes place in the mesenteric lymph nodes and also the organisms reach the thoracic duct. From there, the organisms enter the bloodstream and seed liver, spleen lymph nodes and Peyer's patches. Secondary multiplication occurs and bacteremia recurs leading to localized infection at various sites. The virulence of the organisms depends upon various factors which include genes (which regulate the invasion of Peyer's patches), inoculum size (the risk of getting typhoid is 25%, 50% and 75% after ingesting 10^5, 10^7, 10^9 organism respectively), gastric pH (acid ion in the stomach acts as a barrier to infection; gastric pH more than 1.5 promotes survival of bacilli in the gut lumen; this may occur when a person is on antacids), possession of Vi polysaccharide antigen by the bacilli which interferes with phagocytosis leading to more virulence, simultaneous harboring of *Helicobacter pylori* in the stomach which enhances the survival of the bacilli in the gut lumen, immunocompetence of the patients (cell mediated immunity is important) and presence of lipopolysaccharide endotoxin and enterotoxin.

In neonates, the infection is transmitted vertically. Antenatally, the mother has chorioamnionitis which can lead to abortion or premature delivery.

CLINICAL FEATURES

The incubation period for enteric fever is 3–60 days depending upon the inoculum size. Symptoms occur in 1–2 weeks. The clinical picture exhibits a wide range of clinical severity and varies according to the age of the patient. In neonates, the clinical manifestations begin within 72 hours presenting either with hypothermia or with hyperthermia, vomiting, diarrhea, abdominal distention, seizures, jaundice, hepatomegaly and failure to thrive. Infection is transmitted vertically.

In infants and children up to 5 years, the disease may be mild, presenting only as diarrhea or mimicking a viral illness. In older children and adolescents, the onset is insidious. There is a gradual rise in fever in stepwise manner and daily increments of 1°–2°F until after 5–7 days a sustained temperature of 102°–107°F is present. Without antimicrobial treatment, the temperature remains unremitting at this level for about 10–14 days. During convalescence, fever diminishes also in a stepwise fashion over several days. Anorexia, abdominal pain, malaise, myalgias, headache, cough and epistaxis may be associated features. Constipation is typical in older children while diarrhea may occur in younger children. In the second week, the symptoms become more severe with toxicity lethargy, delirium or coma supervening. A coated tongue, tender abdomen, anemia, bronchitis and hepatosplenomegaly are common. Spleen becomes palpable at the end of first week. Relative bradycardia is manifested in older children and adults. Rhonchi and rales may be present. Rose spots, which are blanching, erythematous papules may appear on 7–10 days in 10–20% of individuals. They are macular 2–4 mm size, 15–20 in number and appear in crops in periumbilical area and anterior chest, better appreciated in fair skinned persons. If the course remains uncomplicated, symptoms start abating by 2–4 weeks although lethargy and malaise may persist for 1–2 months. Complications occur in 10–15% patients and usually seen in second and third week of the infection. Relapse rates are 5–20% and occur 2–3 weeks after the fever subsides or stopping antibiotics. It mimics the original illness except that it is milder and has a shorter duration.

The morbidity and toxemia associated with MDR strain is higher in children due to greater virulence of the organisms.

DIFFERENTIAL DIAGNOSIS

It is to be differentially diagnosed from all fevers of about a week's onset and having a toxemic look.

COMPLICATIONS

Since it is a multisystem disease, complications have been reported in every system of the body. The most common complications are related to gastrointestinal (GI) tract with paralytic ileus and abdominal distension being the most frequent manifestations, others being intestinal perforation and severe hemorrhage. Occult blood in stools is detected in 10–20% of patients, 3% have melena and 0.5–3% patients may develop intestinal perforation followed by peritonitis (presenting as sudden tachycardia, hypotension, abdominal distension with guarding, rigidity and rebound tenderness). Perforation size may range from pinpoint to several centimeters. Gram-negative sepsis may ensue. Inadequate antimicrobial treatment, male sex and leukopenia have been found to be independent risk factors for enteric perforation. Intestinal bleeding usually occurs from multiple, variable sized punched out ulcers in the distal ileum and proximal colon.

Other complications include hepatitis, pancreatitis, cholecystitis, pneumonia (it may also occur by super infection with organism other than *S. typhi*), bronchitis (10%), toxic myocarditis, central nervous system manifestations (toxic encephalopathy, increased intracranial tension, cerebral thrombosis, acute cerebellar ataxia, chorea, aphasia, deafness, psychosis, transverse myelitis and peripheral and optic neuritis), fatal bone marrow necrosis, pyelonephritis, nephritic syndrome, meningitis, endocarditis, parotitis orchitis and suppurative lymphadenitis. Osteomyelitis and suppurative arthritis occur more commonly in children with hemoglobinopathies. The ocular complications include lid abscess, corneal ulcers, uveitis, vitreous hemorrhage and retinal hemorrhage, and are a result of direct microbial invasion. Other reported complications are disseminated intravascular coagulation (DIC), thrombocytopenia, hemolytic uremic syndrome (HUS). Overall mortality is less than 1% but higher in infants.

Laboratory Diagnosis

Hematological

None is specific. Total leukocyte count may be normal or decreased in 20–25% cases. There is relative lymphopenia and absence of eosinophils is quite characteristic. Transient thrombocytopenia may be seen in 10–15% cases after 1 week. Anemia because of the disease *per se* is rare but may be present some time as a late feature. Presence of significant anemia is a pointer of intestinal hemorrhage.

Biochemical

There is a mild elevation of serum glutamic-oxaloacetic transaminase (SGOT) and serum glutamic-pyruvic transaminase (SGPT) but seldom exceeds 2–3 times the normal levels. Serum bilirubin may be mildly elevated especially in infants and younger children. Prothrombin time and activated partial thromboplastin time (APTT) are also mildly prolonged.

Cultures

Definitive diagnosis is based on isolation of the organism on culture from blood, bone marrow, stool and urine. Culture of rose spots and aspirated duodenal fluid are also helpful although rarely used.

Blood culture: This is the gold standard and mainstay of diagnosis. Although more than 80% patients with acute typhoid fever have the causative organism in their blood, the sensitivity is about 50% and drops considerably with prior antibiotic treatment. The highest yield is in the first week of illness (90%). Thereafter, it is 75% in second week, 60% in third week and 25% in fourth week. The sample should be inoculated immediately at the time of withdrawing the blood. In case the sample has to be transported, it should be done at the room temperature. Since blood contains about 0.3 cfu/mL of bacteria, the optimum volume of blood for culture is 10 mL in adults and 5 mL in children to maintain a blood broth ratio of 1:5 to 1:10. Blood culture can be done easily in most laboratories in routine blood culture media (Hartey's blood agar, MacConkey agar). It does not need a special media. Automated blood culture system (Bactet) enhances recovery rate of bacteria.

Nalidixic acid resistance is a surrogate marker of quinolone resistance. If culture shows resistance to nalidixic acid, then irrespective of results of ciprofloxacin or ofloxacin sensitivity, quinolones should not be given.

Earlier, it was thought that clot cultures may be better as they obviate the inhibitory effect of serum, but it has now been found that there is no distinct advantage.

Bone marrow aspiration culture: Since *Salmonella* is predominantly an intracellular organism, bone marrow cultures have a very high yield with sensitivity between 80% and 95%. Further, it has the advantage that it also provides definitive diagnosis for patients who have already received antibiotics, have long history of illness and negative blood culture with recommended volume of blood. The concentration of bacteria in bone marrow is 5 times (9 cfu/mL) than that of peripheral blood in the first week and rising to 150 times in the third week. However, the invasive nature of this modality makes it more suitable for investigating pyrexia unknown origin (PUO) cases, where typhoid is a frequent diagnosis.

Stool culture: Stool culture is positive in 30% cases and that too only during the second and third week. Because of irregular shedding, several stool specimens are required. It needs to be processed within two hours after collection. In case of delay, the specimen should be stored at 4°C in refrigerator. Rectal swab culture has still poorer sensitivity.

Urine culture: It is also not recommended because of poor sensitivity.

Skin snip cultures from rose spots: This also has a high yield and has shown positivity in 63% cases. However, it is not very much in practice to use this modality.

Cultures of cerebrospinal fluid, peritoneal fluid, mesenteric lymph nodes, resected intestine, pharynx, tonsils, abscess and bone have also yielded the organisms in selected cases.

Serological Tests

Widal test: This is the most widely used serological test that measures agglutinating antibody levels against "O" and "H" antigens. O antibodies which are predominantly immunoglobulin M (IgM) appear usually on sixth to eighth day and "H" antibodies which are IgM and immunoglobulin G (IgG) appear on tenth to twelfth day after onset of disease. A high titer in first sample collected at the end of first week is highly suggested. A rising titer in a paired sample taken 2 weeks apart is also diagnostic but by that time the clinical tests become rather irrelevant to a clinician. Widal test is moderately sensitive and specific. In 30% of blood culture proved cases, it has been found to be negative. There are other serious limitations also of this test. In endemic areas like India, there exists a baseline antibody level in population following repeated exposures to *Salmonella* infection; hence interpretation of Widal titers becomes difficult unless these baseline values are known. Previous antimicrobial treatment may block antibodies response and Widal may be falsely negative. *S. typhi* shares "O" and "H" antigens with other *Salmonella* serotypes and has cross reacting epitopes with other enterobacteriaceae, so false positive test may occur. Widal test may also be false positive in malaria, typhus, sepsis with other organisms, cirrhosis, etc. Prior vaccination against typhoid by whole cell vaccines can also result in high baseline anti-O and anti-H levels.

There are two methods of doing Widal test: (1) the tube test and (2) the slide test. The tube test takes 6 hours while the slide test takes 2–5 minutes. However, the tube test is far better than the slide test and should be preferred over the slide test. The tube test can detect the antibody in the concentration of 1:1280 while the slide test can detect it only up to 1:320 concentration.

The antibody titer of *both (and not either)* "H" and "O" antibodies in the range of 1 in 160 dilution should be taken into account as cut off for diagnosis.

Typhidot/Enzyme immunoassay test (EIA): It is based on the detection of both IgM and IgG against a 50 KD outer membrane protein antigen of *S. typhi*. It is a simple, rapid, economic test with high specificity, sensitivity. However, in endemic areas because of a persistent high IgG levels following typhoid infection, this test cannot differentiate between acute and convalescent cases. It may also give false positive results because of previous infection with *S. typhi* or current reinfection in which secondary immune response significantly boosts IgG production and IgM becomes undetectable. To increase the diagnostic efficacy, a modified typhidot has been developed, called "*Typhidot M*" in which IgG is totally inactivated in the serum sample and only IgM is detected. However, this test is not available in India.

Typhidot test also has been mostly replaced by other serological tests which are described below:

IgM strip/dipstick test: This test is the most commonly used test today and has replaced the Widal and Typhidot tests. It

is based on binding of *S. typhi* specific IgM antibodies to *S. typhi* lipopolysaccharide antigen (LPS). It can be done on serum or whole blood and requires incubation for 3 hours at room temperature. Evaluation studies suggest that this method is 65–77% sensitive and 95–100% specific. It is a rapid and simple alternative for diagnosis of typhoid fever where culture facilities are not available. Moreover this test does not require trained persons or equipments.

IDL TUBEX test: Rapid and simple test which can detect IgM antibodies against 09 antigen specifically found in group D *Salmonella* within 2 minutes. It detects IgM and not IgG and is thus suggestive of recent infection. It is not positive with other serotypes including *S. paratyphi* and thus has a good specificity. A study showed that in a single blood sample collected on admission to hospital sensitivity of TUBEX test was 69.8% as compared with bone marrow culture and 86.5% as compared with blood culture.

Antigen detection tests: Using CIE, agglutination and immunoassay techniques to detect *Salmonella* somatic/flagellin/Vi antigen have been developed. The sensitivity and specificity is quite variable and as of now the tests are not of much utility.

Polymerase chain reaction (PCR): Since 1993, there have been some reports of PCR as a diagnostic modality with a very high sensitivity and specificity. There are, however, a few unanswered questions regarding effect of previous infections and vaccinations, false positivity and status in chronic carriers. At present, the last is best reserved for experimental purposes.

Management

Most of the cases can be safely treated on a domiciliary basis. Patients who have persistent vomiting, severe diarrhea, abdominal distension, toxemia and complicated typhoid would need hospitalization. The general supportive measures are in the form of fluids, nutrition and antipyretics. Contrary to popular belief, there is no need to restrict any type of diet in cases of typhoid.

Antibiotics

The mainstay of treatment of typhoid is specific antibiotic therapy. Today, the first and second generation antibiotics, like chloramphenicol, amoxicillin, ampicillin, cotrimoxazole, furazolidone, are no longer used ever since the emergence of multidrug resistant *Salmonella* (MDRS) since 1990.

Currently, the following are the antibiotics of choice:
- Third generation oral cephalosporins for domiciliary treatment:
  - Cefixime (20 mg/kg/day) given twice daily
  - Cefpodoxime (10 mg/kg/day) given twice daily has also been shown to be effective
- Third generation injectable cephalosporins for hospitalized and/or MDRS patients:

- Ceftriaxone (50–100 mg/kg/day) given once or twice daily
- *Fluoroquinolones (oral/IV)*:
  - Ciprofloxacin 15–20 mg/kg/day
  - Ofloxacin 10–20 mg/kg/day.

  In spite of the fact that the toxic effect on growing cartilage has been largely disproved even by the long-term usage of these drugs, it is not approved by Drug Controller General of India (DCGI) for use in pediatric patients and therefore has a limited utility. Moreover, there have been increasing reports of resistance to quinolones from various states in India and neighboring countries. When nalidixic acid resistance is reported, then a higher dose and prolonged duration of treatment has to be given while using ciprofloxacin and ofloxacin.
- *Macrolides*: Azithromycin 10–20 mg/kg/day orally—This has shown promising results in treating uncomplicated typhoid and quinolone resistant strains. Since *Salmonella* are intracellular organisms, azithromycin has good efficacy in cases of enteric fever especially during relapse.
- *Others*: Aztreonam 50–100 mg/kg/day in three divided doses in MDRS cases allergic to the cephalosporins. In complicated MDR typhoid, when there is no response to parenteral third generation cephalosporins, aztreonam is a good option.

Duration of antibiotic treatment: Typhoid fever takes time for defervescence. If this occurs within 24 or 48 hours of treatment, then one should review the diagnosis. Most of the children become afebrile within 7 days of treatment, but therapy should be continued for at least 14 days in uncomplicated fever or 7 days after defervescence.

Therapy of relapses: This varies with the type of drugs and is most common with beta lactams when used in shorter duration. They respond well and quickly to the same drug as used for primary therapy but in proper doses and right duration. Quinolones, if not used earlier, and azithromycin are also good alternatives.

Therapy of carriers: It is uncommon in children. When chronic carriage is demonstrated, treatment is with amoxicillin 100 mg/kg/day with probenecid 30 mg/kg/day or cotrimoxazole 10 mg/kg/day of TMP for 6–12 weeks. Alternatively quinolones can be given for 28 days.

Prognosis

The prognosis of a patient with typhoid fever depends upon the promptness of treatment, the age of the patient, the previous stage of health, the causative serotype and complications, if any. In developed countries, the mortality is less than 1%. In developing countries, the mortality rate is high (10%). This may be because of delay in diagnosis or hospitalization. Infants and children are with underlying debilitating disorders are at higher risk and this is all the more a problem in developing countries.

Prevention of Disease

A good system of sanitation and provision of clean treated bacteriologically monitored water supplies are the major requisites for prevention of typhoid in the community. This however still seems to be a far cry in our country. Till such a time, vaccination against the typhoid fever becomes a useful modality which can fill the gap.

Vaccines

The history of typhoid vaccines dates back to more than a century. The first whole cell typhoid vaccine was invented in 1896 by Wright, which was subsequently introduced in the British army. These vaccines were widely used in WHO sponsored large field trials in the 1950s to 1960s. However, because of the high incidence of severe side effects, these vaccines fell in to disrepute in spite of their efficacy. The need for a safe and effective vaccine was felt and a break through occurred in 1975 when Germainer and Fuer invented the Ty21a mutant typhoid strain. This leads to the availability of the first live oral typhoid vaccine. Another potential typhoid vaccine antigen the Vi capsular polysaccharide was identified way back in the 1930s; however, the process of extraction denatured it making ineffective for vaccine development. Dr Robbins group in the early 1980s isolated the undenatured Vi antigen and elucidated its protective role, which was subsequently validated in the field trials. The current stress in typhoid vaccines have been the development of conjugated polysaccharide vaccines and newer strains of oral typhoid vaccine.

- Parenteral whole cell typhoid vaccine (*not available now*): This was a killed (inactivated) vaccine. Initially, a combination of typhoid and paratyphoid A and paratyphoid B vaccines (therefore called TAB vaccine). Later paratyphi were omitted as these infections were uncommon and of low virulence but were resulting in lowering the immunogenicity of the vaccine. Thus, we had typhoid vaccine (T). The primary dose consisted of two doses given 4 weeks apart (0.25 mL in children 6 months to 10 years and 0.5 mL in children above 10 years and adults. Given subcutaneously, in upper arm over the deltoid region. Boosters were to be given every three years. This vaccine had better efficacy as compared to all other vaccines which have been tried so far in our country and it could be given to children even six months of age. Side effects ranging from fever, malaise, local reactions like swelling, pain, redness to severe rare reactions like shock and some deaths let to the withdrawal of this vaccine from the market.
- Oral Ty21A—a live vaccine (*not available now*): Using mutagenic techniques, a mutant strain of *S. typhi* was produced and used for making this vaccine. It is a live vaccine which has a good serum and secretory antibody response. Commercially, it was made available as enteric coated capsules to avoid being rendered ineffective by gastric acid juice to be given as three doses

on alternate days. Therefore, could be possible only in children above 6 years. No antityphoid antibiotics for a fortnight starting 5 days before start of first dose. Chloroquine and mefloquine to be avoided for 24 hours after vaccination. An interval of 4 weeks between any other oral vaccine dose and oral typhoid vaccine was needed. Therefore, the vaccine did not last long in the market. The side effects was very few (<1%) like nausea, diarrhea, vomiting, fever. The vaccine protection begins after a week of administration and lasts for 3–7 years. It had to be repeated every three years.

- Capsular Vi polysaccharide vaccine: New generation subunit vaccine containing highly purified antigenic fraction of Vi antigen of *S. typhi*. This is a polysaccharide antigen which stimulates B cells directly. As with other polysaccharide vaccine, it is not a good immunogen in children less than 2 years of age. It also fails to evoke booster effects as it is a T-cells independent vaccine. The efficacy of this vaccine ranges from 64 to 72%. Vaccine can be used only in children aged 2 years or above. Each dose contains 25 µg of purified polysaccharide in 0.5 mL of phenolic isotonic buffer. It has to be stored between 2–8°C. Can be given intramuscularly in anterolateral part of thigh or deltoid muscle or subcutaneously. The protection begins 2–4 weeks after immunization and lasts for 3–5 years. No protection against paratyphi A and B. The vaccine needs to be repeated every three years. Side effects are usually mild ranging from local reactions to systemic in less than 5% of the vaccines.
- Vi Conjugate vaccine first typhoid conjugate polysaccharide subunit vaccine, developed by Szu et al. by conjugation of Vi antigen with nontoxic recombinant *Pseudomonas aeruginosa* exotoxin A (Repa), has been evaluated in safety, immunogenicity and efficacy trials in Vietnam. It has been found immunogenic efficacious and safe. A conjugate vaccine with Vi capsular

polysaccharide being conjugated with tetanus toxoid has been licensed for use in the Indian market. The trials have been very limited, in a small sample size and there is incompatibility between sample and control groups in the study. The study has not been published in any peer reviewed journal. The manufacturer recommends two doses of 0.5 mL intramuscularly at an interval of 4–8 weeks followed by a booster dose every 10 years. In children, aged less than 2 years, an extra booster 2–2½ years after the first dose is recommended additionally. Since the immunogenicity trial assessed response to only a single dose, the dosing schedule requiring more than one doses recommended by the manufacturer seems arbitrary. The committee of immunization of IAP has not recommended the use of this vaccine in view of the discrepancies (Tables 4.1.1 and 4.1.2).

IAPCOI RECOMMENDATIONS

- For office practice, the IAPCOI recommends the administration of the currently available Vi polysaccharide vaccine 0.5 mL IM every three years beginning at the age of 2 years.
- A child with history of suspected/confirmed enteric fever may be vaccinated 4 weeks after recovery if he/she has not received the vaccine in the past 3 years.
- The committee does not recommend the use of the currently available conjugated typhoid vaccine. It also stresses the need for development of new vaccines against typhoid and paratyphoid fever.

NONTYPHOIDAL *SALMONELLA* INFECTIONS

These pathogens are responsible for bacterial diarrhea. More than 90% of nontyphoidal *Salmonella* infections are

Table 4.1.1: Comparison of the various typhoid vaccines.

Characteristics	Whole cell killed vaccines	Ty21a capsule vaccine	Vi polysaccharide vaccine	Vi polysaccharide conjugate vaccine
Type	Killed	Live	Subunit	Subunit
Route	IM/SC	Oral	IM/SC	IM/SC
Doses	2	3	1	2
Revaccination	3–5 years	3–5 years	3 years	?
Immunogenicity	++	+	+	+++
Efficacy	51–79%	35–67%	55–72%	91%
Duration of efficacy	65% at 7 years	62% at 7 years	55% at 3 years	91% at 2.3 years
Herd immunity	?	Yes	?	?
Side effects	++++	+	++	++
Age	>6 months	>6 years	>2 years	>6 weeks
Boosting	-	-	-	++
Mass vaccination	Unsuitable	Suitable	Suitable	Suitable
Availability	No	No	Yes	Yes (lacks data)

Note: All vaccines have long shelf life at 2–8°C, but should *never* be kept in the freezer.

Table 4.1.2: Summary of typhoid vaccines.

Vaccine	Content/dose	Nature	Storage	Dose, route, site	Schedule	Protective Efficacy	Major adverse effects	Contraindication
Vi typhoid	25–30 µg of Vi polysaccharide	Liquid vaccine	2–8°C	0.5 mL IM deltoid/thigh	Above 2 years single dose, revaccination of 3 years	60%	None	Serious hypersensitive
Vi Conjugate (not recommended by IAP COI due to lack of authentic data)	5 µg of Vi polysaccharide S. typhi conjugated to 5 µg of tetanus toxoid protein in isotonic saline	Liquid vaccine	2–8°C	0.5 mL IM deltoid/thigh	Between 3 months and 2 years two injections at interval of 4–8 weeks, followed by booster at 2–2½ years. Booster vaccination every 10 years	?	None?	Serious hypersensitivity?

food borne. The remainders 5% are nosocomial infections or acquired from pets like birds and reptiles. They may also occur from infected person or contaminated water, drugs or solutions. Outbreaks have been reported due to infection from eggs, cheese, fresh fruits and vegetables, juice, dry cereal and ice cream. *S. enteritidis* are reported to be transmitted transovarially from chicken to egg and under cooked eggs can lead to infection in a host. *Salmonella* organisms are commonly carried by farm animals, and antibiotic resistance particularly of *S. typhimurium* has been linked to use of antibiotics in animal feed.

Pathogenesis

The inoculum for *Salmonella* infection is approximately 10^5–10^9 organisms but is lower in infants, in persons with pernicious anemia and in persons taking antacids or H_2 receptor blockers. Additional risk facts are alteration of the endogenous bowel flora (e.g. by recent antimicrobial therapy), HIV infection, therapeutic immunosuppression, alteration of the reticuloendothelial system (e.g. malaria), sickle cell disease, splenectomy, diabetes, malignancy, rheumatologic disorders (including lupus). HIV-infected persons have 20–100 fold increased risk of *Salmonella* infection and a significantly increased risk of severe invasive disease. The development of disease depends upon the number of infecting organisms, their virulence and the host defense factors (stomach acidity and gastric transit time).

Salmonella organisms are ingested by specialized epithelial cells called intestinal M cells that overlie Peyer's patches and are present abundantly in the ileum. From here, the organisms are transported to the lymphoid tissue of the Peyer's patches from which they may enter the systemic circulation. *Salmonella* organisms have special mechanisms for survival inside macrophages. Induction of inflammatory cells in the Peyer's patches lead to their

enlargement and necroses after several weeks of infection. The organisms are also able to transit through some epithelial cells into deeper tissues, but ulcers are usually not found. Some organisms produced cholera like enterotoxins that increase cyclic adenosine monophosphate, leading to the efflux of water and electrolytes which is why nontyphoidal *Salmonella* organisms mainly cause acute gastroenteritis.

Clinical Features

Nontyphoidal *Salmonella* infections mainly cause gastroenteritis, but can also lead to bacteremia and extraintestinal focal infections like meningitis, pneumonia, endovascular infections, osteomyelitis and hepatic/splenic abscess.

Gastroenteritis

The incubation period for gastroenteritis caused by *Salmonella* organisms is 6–72 hours. Manifestations occur in the form of nausea, vomiting, fever, diarrhea and abdominal cramps. The stools are usually of moderate volume and do not contain blood. In rare cases, the manifestations may mimic appendicitis or inflammatory bowel disease. Diarrhea is generally self-limited, lasting for 3–7 days.

Fever of the range of 102°F (30°C) may occur for 1–2 days. A more prolonged or hectic fever pattern suggests bacteremia and/or metastatic foci. There is also mild abdominal tenderness and hyperactive bowel sounds may be present.

Laboratory tests: Microscopic examination of stool reveals leukocytes and rarely blood cells. *Salmonella* organisms can be cultured from stool or rectal swab. Since these sites contain a mixed bacterial flora, selective media which inhibit normal commensals (MacConkey's XLD, Bismuth sulfite or *Salmonella-Shigella* agar) should be used. The mean duration of fecal carriage after resolution of diarrhea for nontyphoidal *Salmonella* organisms is about 2 months in young children as compared to 1 month in adults.

Differential diagnosis: This includes infection caused by organisms like *Campylobacter, Shigella* and *Y. enterocolitica* and inflammatory bowel disease. A frank bloody diarrhea is more suggestive of *Shigella* or enterohemorrhagic *E. coli.*

Treatment: Since the condition is generally self-limited, antibiotics are not recommended for patients with uncomplicated gastroenteritis. As a matter of fact, antibiotic therapy may actually prolong intestinal carriage in these cases. In patients who are severally ill or at risk for extraintestinal spread of infection, including infants and patients with cardiac valvular or mural abnormalities or patients with prosthetic vascular grafts or patients who are receiving immunosuppressive therapy, effective antibiotics would include third generation cephalosporins and fluoroquinolones. Because of resistance to trimethoprim-sulfamethoxazole or ampicillin, they are not the preferred antibiotics these days. Duration of therapy should be only for 48–72 hours or until the patient becomes afebrile as longer therapy may increase the likelihood of long-term carriage.

Complications: Infants and children are at high-risk for central nervous system infection (meningitis) as *Salmonella* organisms invade the intestinal epithelium and enter the bloodstream, causing septicemia. Septicemia may also cause metastatic infection of other organs including lungs (pneumonia), endovascular sites (endocarditis/pericarditis), the hepatobiliary tract, the spleen (abscess) and bone (osteomyelitis).

Bacteremia and Vascular Infection

Nontyphoidal *Salmonella* organisms may colonize sites of vascular abnormality, such as prosthetic vascular grafts and aneurysms. The presence of high grade bacteremia (> 50% of three or more blood cultures positive) is suggestive of endovascular infection.

Patients with endovascular infection typically have high fevers that persist even after several days of therapy. Physical examination may reveal tenderness at the site of infection. Besides blood culture, echocardiography and other imaging studies may be helpful.

Treatment is by empirically giving *both* fluoroquinolone and a third generation cephalosporin antibiotic till sensitivity results are known. Therapy with Beta lactam antibiotics, like ampicillin or a cephalosporin, should be for 6 weeks, both in documented or suspected endovascular infection. For low-grade bacteremia, 7–14 days of IV therapy is recommended. Endovascular infection may require surgical intervention. However, in cases where surgical resection of infected grafts is not possible, lifelong oral suppressive therapy is recommended.

In patients with AIDS, a first episode of *Salmonella* bacteremia should be treated with 7–14 days of IV antibiotics followed by 4 weeks of oral fluoroquinolone. AIDS patients who experience relapses of *Salmonella* bacteremia should be treated within oral fluoroquinolone or trimethoprim-sulfamethoxazole for long-term suppression.

Carrier State

This is defined as carriage of *Salmonella* organisms in the stood for more than 1 year after initial infection and occurs in 0.2–0.6% of persons infected with nontyphoidal *Salmonella*. The site of chronic infection is the biliary tree. Long-term carriage may occur more rarely in urinary tract, as a secondary infection to an existing obstructive uropathy or tuberculosis or schistosomiasis.

The carrier state is generally asymptomatic and physical examination is unremarkable. It can be documented by culture of *Salmonella* organism.

Ampicillin or amoxicillin will eradicate the *Salmonella* organisms in 80% of carrier persons. Alternate therapy is trimethoprim-sulfamethoxazole or ciprofloxacin.

BIBLIOGRAPHY

1. Chitkara AJ, Adlakha N. Typhoid fever in children. In: Ghosh TK, Yewale V, Parthasarthy A, Shah NK (Eds). Pediatric Infectious Diseases. Mumbai: Indian Academy of Pediatrics; 2006. pp. 208-14.
2. Dubey AP, Mukherjee SB, Singh V, et al. Infectious diseases. In: Gupta S, Dubey AP, Kumar P (Eds). Pediatrics, 4th edition. New Delhi: Atlantic Publishers; 2009. pp. 252-6.
3. Goldberg MB. Salmonella infectious. In: Dale DC (Ed). Infectious Diseases. New York: Published WebMD Professional Publishing; 2003. pp. 336-40.

4.2   DIPHTHERIA

Yashwant Patil

INTRODUCTION

Diphtheria is an acute disease caused by *Corynebacterium diphtheriae*, less commonly by *Corynebacterium ulcerans*. Infection by toxigenic strains of *C. diphtheriae* causes diphtheria by production of an extracellular protein. Before invent of antitoxin diphtheria, throughout history, diphtheria has been one of the most feared infectious diseases globally causing devasting epidemics with high case-fatality rates, mainly affecting children and was a major cause of children mortality. It was called "strangling angel of children". Mention is made in works of Hippocrates.

Bretonneau coined the word diphtheria. He recognized in 1821 as a specific entity. Klebs stained the smear of membrane and identified the causative organism in 1983. Loffler grew organism on artificial media in 1884 and showed fatal illness in guinea pigs resembling human illness. Roux and Yersin in 1889 purified toxin and demonstrated that toxin alone could cause disease. *C. diphtheriae* and *C. ulcerans* appear grey on Loffler medium. On tellurite medium three diphtheria colony types can be identified. Mitis colonies are smooth, black, convex and hemolytic. Gravis colonies are grey, radially striate, semi rough and nonhemolytic. Intermedius colonies are small, smooth and have a black center and nonhemolytic. Intermedius strains were found to be more toxigenic than gravis and mitis. Diphtheria toxin is lethal in humans in an amount 130 microgram per kg body weight.

EPIDEMIOLOGY

Asymptomatic human carriers serve as reservoir for *C. diphtheriae* or a patient with active disease. Transmission occurs from person to person through droplets during coughing, sneezing and talking and through close physical contact. Rarely, it can spread by fomites or skin lesions. Infection leads to respiratory or cutaneous diphtheria. It is suggested that skin carriers are more infectious than either nose or throat carriers. Natural immunization is higher in areas with endemic skin lesions. Diphtheria has been documented by ingestion of infected unpasteurized milk from infected teats. *C. diphtheriae* has been isolated from horses, dogs and other domestic animals.

Diphtheria is endemic in India. Diphtheria is distributed worldwide and is endemic in developing world. The reported incidence of diphtheria in India during 1987 (before wide coverage of immunization) was about 12,952 cases, whereas during the year 2009 there were 3480 cases and 113 deaths showing a case fatality rate of about 3.25. The reported figure was 3,480 cases after vigorous

immunization with 113 deaths with a fatality rate of 3.25%. As per WHO-Review of the epidemiology of diphtheria 2000-2016, in the period 2011-2015, India had largest total number of reported cases each year, with a 5-year total of 18350 cases, followed by Indonesia and Madagascar with 3203 and 1633 reported cases respectively. The analysis further showed a significant under-reporting of cases to WHO, particularly from the African and Mediterranean regions. The true burden of disease is therefore likely to be greater than reported. Diphtheria however, remains endemic in countries in Africa, Latin America, Asia, the Middle East, and part of Europe, where childhood immunization with diphtheria toxoid-containing vaccines is suboptimal.

Incidence peaks during cooler months in autumn, winter and spring months. It occurs more in low socioeconomic population. Children between 1 year and 5 years are commonly infected. Preschool and school children are infected if inadequately or unimmunized. Infants of immunized mothers have antibodies for a few weeks in their system and therefore infection in infants younger than 6 months is rare. Subclinical infections give immunity in our population. Around 99% of Indian children are Schick positive by 5 years of age. A herd immunity of 70% is required to prevent epidemics. Some believe 90% herd immunity is needed to prevent epidemics. Contaminated objects like thermometers, cups, spoons, toys and pencils can spread the disease. Overcrowding, poor sanitation and hygiene, illiteracy, urban migration and close contact lead to outbreaks.

ETIOPATHOGENESIS

Pathogen *Corynebacterium* is a genus of gram-positive aerobic bacteria. Various species of the genus Corynebacterium exist. *Corynebacterium diphtheriae* is aerobic, club shaped, nonmotile, noncapsulated, non-sporing, irregularly staining gram-positive pleomorphic bacilli (Fig. 4.2.1). Corynebacterium diphtheriae enter into nose or mouth. Bacilli remain localized on mucus membrane of the respiratory tract. Ocular or genital mucus membrane may be infected occasionally. Intact skin is resistant to bacilli. It can infect pre-existing skin ulcers, cracks or wounds. After 2–6 days of incubation period, *C. diphtheriae* may elaborate toxin. Toxin is initially absorbed onto target cell membrane and later undergoes receptor-mediated endocytosis. Marked toxin-induced tissue necrosis occurs in the vicinity of *C. diphtheriae* colonies. There is marked inflammatory response. As infection progresses inflammation progress to patchy exudates

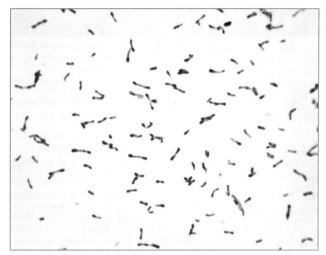

FIG. 4.2.1: *Corynebacterium diphtheriae.*
Source: Centers for disease control and prevention

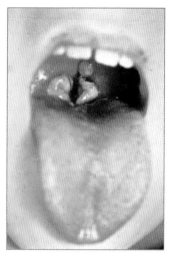

FIG. 4.2.2: Tonsillar diphtheria.
Source: Centers for disease control and prevention

which can be removed. As infection progresses, toxin causes centrifugal widening of the fibrinous exudate membrane, which bleeds on attempt to removal. Pseudomembrane consists of fibrin, inflammatory cells mainly neutrophils, red blood cells, organism and epithelial cells. Severe infections cause vascular congestion, edema, exudate and neutrophilic infiltration. The membrane may encroach and block airway. Respiratory embarrassment or suffocation can occur. Pneumonia may occur if exudates enter lung parenchyma.

Toxin produced from infected site is distributed via blood stream and lymphatics. Any tissue can be damaged by toxin but heart, nervous system and kidneys are markedly affected. Myocarditis manifests after 10–14 days. Nervous system takes 3–7 weeks to manifest.

Liver may undergo necrosis and hyaline degeneration leading to hypoglycemia. Adrenal hemorrhage and acute tubular necrosis of the kidney are known to occur in diphtheria. Renal manifestations include oliguria and proteinuria.

CLINICAL FEATURES

Signs and symptoms of diphtheria depend on the site of infection, immunization status of the patient and toxin circulation. The onset is usually relatively slow. Incubation period is 1–6 days (range 1–10 days). Classification can be done on the site of location. It can be nasal, pharyngeal, tonsillar, laryngeal or laryngotracheal, skin, eye and genitalia. There could be more than one anatomic site.

Nasal diphtheria may mimic common cold characterized by running of nose without systemic signs. Secretions from nose gradually become serosanguineous and later mucopurulent. Foul odor may follow. Nasal

mucosa may show a white membrane. Unilateral nasal discharge is quite pathognomonic of nasal diphtheria. Nasal diphtheria is a mild form as toxin absorption is low and slow. Accurate diagnosis of nasal diphtheria may be delayed due to paucity of systemic signs and symptoms.

Pharyngeal and tonsillar diphtheria begin with loss of appetite, malaise, low-grade fever and symptoms of pharyngitis. Membrane appears after 1 or 2 days (Fig. 4.2.2). In partially immune individual membrane may not develop. A white or grey membrane over tonsils, pharyngeal wall, uvula and soft palate may be seen. The membrane may extend into larynx and trachea. Bleeding takes place on removal of the membrane. Lymph nodes in cervical region enlarge. There may be edema of soft tissue of neck causing a "bull neck". Edema may be brawny, pitting, warm and tender on touch. Edema usually occurs with gravis or intermedius strain of *C. diphtheriae* (Figs. 4.2.3A and B).

The course of pharyngeal and tonsillar diphtheria depends on amount of toxin production. In severe cases, circulatory and respiratory collapse may occur. Disproportionate tachycardia compared to temperature is there. Fever is usually low grade. Palatal paralysis may occur associated with difficulty in swallowing, regurgitation or nasal twang of voice. Stupor, coma and death may occur in 7–10 days in severe cases. In less severe cases slow recovery with myocarditis or peripheral neuritis is there. In mild cases the membrane sloughs off in 7–10 days. Recovery is full and uneventful.

Laryngeal diphtheria is usually downward spread of the membrane from pharynx. Laryngeal diphtheria does not occur generally in primary disease. Noisy breathing, progressive stridor, hoarseness and dry barking cough may be there. Laryngeal obstruction may be associated with suprasternal, subcostal and supraclavicular retractions. These signs are directly proportional to laryngeal block.

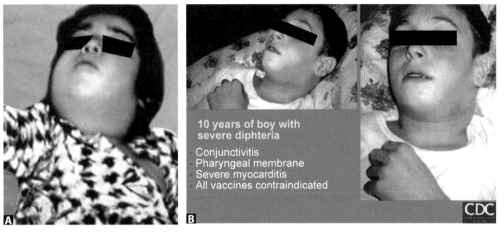

FIGS. 4.2.3A AND B: Diphtheria. Bull-neck appearance of diphtheritic cervical lymphadenopathy.
Sources: Centers for disease control and prevention

A detached membrane may block laryngeal opening and causing sudden signs and symptoms.

Cutaneous diphtheria is common in warm climates. Cutaneous diphtheria is more contagious than respiratory diphtheria. Skin lesions may begin as vesicles or pustules and turn into ulcers with a dark pseudomembrane. Lesions occur in legs, feet and hands. Pain is there for first 1–3 weeks. Healing takes place in 6–12 weeks (Fig. 4.2.4).

Conjunctival diphtheria is limited to palpebral conjunctiva. It is red and edematous. External ear and vulvovaginal diphtheria may occur. Ear infections are otitis externa, purulent and foul smelling.

Cases of septic arthritis are reported by *C. diphtheriae*. Myocarditis and nervous system involvement occurs in severe cases and delayed use of antitoxin.

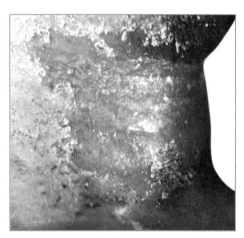

FIG. 4.2.4: Diphtheria. Skin lesion neck.
Sources: Centers for disease control and prevention

MODALITIES OF DIAGNOSIS

Diagnosis is based on clinical signs. Throat or skin swab should be sent for smear and culture. Isolation of *C. diphtheriae* confirms the diagnosis. Smear examination is a good supplement to clinical examination.

The Elek test can be used but takes 48 hours for results. Modified Elek test can be used for rapid diagnosis (16–24 hours).

A rapid enzyme immunoassay test is there for detection of diphtheria toxin. It takes about 3 hours. A rapid testing of diphtheria toxin by PCR specific for A or B portion of the toxic gene, "tox" is sensitive.

Schick test was used for immune status of the individual. It is not useful for early diagnosis as results are available after many days.

Complete blood counts are not helpful in diagnosis. Hypoglycemia, glycosuria, raised blood urea or abnormal electrocardiography (ECG) may help in detecting liver, kidney and heart involvement.

DIFFERENTIAL DIAGNOSIS

Mild diphtheria may mimic common cold. Congenital syphilis snuffle may resemble mild diphtheria. Sinusitis in older children should be differentiated from diphtheria. Adenoiditis and foreign body in nose are other conditions that mimic nasal diphtheria.

Streptococcal pharyngitis exudates need differentiation. There is high-grade fever while in diphtheria has low fever, angry red throat, more pain in swallowing in pharyngitis and no bleeding on dislodgement in pharyngitis.

Infectious mononucleosis has exudates in throat, lymphadenopathy, splenic enlargement and atypical lymphocytes in peripheral blood smear.

Thrush has membrane on tongue buccal mucosa and no systemic symptoms or signs.

TREATMENT

The treatment depends on clinical picture, throat swab smear and rapid diagnostic methods. Culture must be done. Sheet anchor of treatment is neutralization of toxin by antitoxin. Toxin circulating in system and absorbed onto the surface of a cell can be neutralized. Toxin embedded in a cell is not acted upon by antitoxin. Antibiotics should be used to reduce or eliminate toxin producing bacilli. Earlier the antitoxin used, less is the tissue damage. Intravenous administration of antitoxin should be done as early as possible. Antitoxin should be given in a single dose to minimize the chances of sensitization. Repeated doses are likely to sensitize the recipient.

A sensitivity test should be performed to know if patient is sensitive to antitoxin. About 0.02 mL of a 1:1,000 dilution of horse serum antitoxin should be introduced. Positive control histamine and negative control isotonic saline should also be used. A positive reaction should have a wheal of more than 3 mm in 15–20 minutes larger than the negative control reaction to isotonic saline. The erythema should be around the site of injection.

A sensitivity test could also be done with 1:100 dilution of antitoxin with superficial scratch, prick or puncture on the fore arm on the ventral aspect. If patient has an erythema more than 3 mm around the prick, the following desensitization should be done at an interval of 15 minutes (Box 4.2.1).

Intravenous route gives good control, though intradermal, subcutaneous and intramuscular routes are also used. If no reaction has occurred, the remaining calculated dose of antitoxin is given by slow intravenous infusion (Table 4.2.1). It starts neutralizing toxin in the throat from saliva. Intramuscular route is also equally effective. Reactions should be treated with aqueous epinephrine (1:1,000) provided intravenously.

This schedule applies to cases where diphtheria is diagnosed within 48 hours. A dose of 80,000–20,000 units is recommended where diphtheria is more than 48 hours duration and with brawny edema.

Diphtheria antitoxin if administered in time, is gold standard for diphtheria treatment, especially when there is medical emergency that often requires tracheostomy. However, global access to diphtheria antitoxin is limited as most manufacturers have ceased production.

Antibiotic treatment consists of a 14-day course of penicillin or erythromycin. Aqueous penicillin in dose of 100,000–150,000 units/kg/day in four divided doses intravenously, or procaine penicillin 25,000–50,000 units/kg/day in two divided doses (maximum 1.2 million units)

Box 4.2.1

Desensitization of erythema.
- 0.1 mL of a 1:1,000 dilution intravenously
- 0.3 mL of a 1:1,000 dilution intravenously
- 0.6 mL of a 1:1,000 dilution intravenously
- 0.1 mL of a 1:100 dilution intravenously
- 0.3 mL of a 1:100 dilution intravenously
- 0.6 mL of a 1:100 dilution intravenously
- 0.1 mL of a 1:10 dilution intravenously
- 0.3 mL of a 1:10 dilution intravenously
- 0.6 mL of a 1:10 dilution intravenously
- 0.1 mL of undiluted antitoxin intravenously
- 0.3 mL of undiluted antitoxin intravenously
- 0.6 mL of undiluted antitoxin intravenously
- 1 mL of undiluted antitoxin intravenously

Table 4.2.1: Doses of antitoxin.

Doses	Units
Pharyngeal or laryngeal diphtheria	20,000–40,000
Nasopharyngeal diphtheria	40,000–60,000
Severe laryngeal or pharyngeal diphtheria	80,000–120,000
Cutaneous diphtheria	20,000–40,000

intramuscularly. Procaine penicillin should be started after the clinical improvement to minimize injection number. As clinical improvement takes place and patient is able to tolerate oral medications penicillin V may be used in place of injections.

For patients, who are sensitive to penicillin, Erythromycin is recommended for diphtheria. Dose of erythromycin is 40–50 mg/kg/day in four divided doses for 14 days. Maximum dose is 2 gm/day. Antibiotic therapy is not enough, antitoxin must be given.

After 2 weeks of antibiotic therapy throat swab culture should be done. A positive throat swab will require erythromycin for 10 days in the same doses. Penicillin, amoxicillin, rifampin or clindamycin are other drugs used to eliminate *C. diphtheriae* from the throat.

A carrier state must be looked for. Throat swab cultures are done after 2 weeks of therapy. If positive, a single dose of benzathine penicillin is enough to eradicate *C. diphtheriae*. A dose of 600,000 units for children with a weight up to 30 kg, and 1,200,000 units for children with more than 30 kg, is given as a single intramuscular dose. Repeat cultures should be done after 2 weeks. There must be two to three cultures negative at the interval of 24 hours. If repeat culture is positive the individual should be again treated with antibiotics.

All contacts must be monitored for signs of diphtheria for 7–8 days. Either erythromycin or benzathine penicillin can be used for chemoprophylaxis.

Supportive Treatment

The child should have bed rest for 2–3 weeks. Hydration and nutrition of the patient should be maintained. Those unable to swallow may be given nasogastric or parental feeds. Monitoring of heart with echo and ECG is required for 6 weeks. Congestive cardiac failure needs age appropriate digitalis doses. Remember diphtheric myocardium is very sensitive to digoxin. Look for side effects of digitalis. Gavage feeding is recommended in patients of palatal paralysis with polyneuritis. Intubation, tracheostomy or mechanical ventilation may be required.

COMPLICATIONS

Respiratory tract obstruction by pseudomembrane may need urgent bronchoscopy, intubation or tracheostomy. Pneumonia by *C. diphtheriae* bacillus or other bacteria can occur. Myocarditis occurs in 10–25% cases of diphtheria accounting for 50–60% deaths.

Tachycardia, dyspnea, irregular or weak pulse or muffled heart sounds indicate myocardial involvement. Cardiac monitoring by Echo and ECG should be done at regular intervals. Signs of congestive cardiac failure should be monitored and treated timely. Palatal palsy may occur in 1–2 weeks after the onset. Nasal twang, difficulty in swallowing and regurgitation herald the paralysis of pharyngeal and laryngeal muscles. Facial nerve may also be involved. Ocular nerve palsy occurs after 3 weeks of onset. Generalized symmetrical paralysis occurs after 4–6 weeks of the disease. Careful monitoring for diaphragmatic muscle paralysis and keeping the ventilator ready are needed. Feeding by gavage is required to maintain nutrition and hydration. Neurological complications recover completely without a residue.

PROGNOSIS

It depends on how early the antitoxin therapy is started. Morbidity and mortality are mediated by the diphtheria toxin. Mortality is less than 1% if treatment started on day one. Mortality sharply rises to 20% if treatment delayed beyond 4–5 days. Gravis strains have maximum mortality. Laryngeal diphtheria increases risk of respiratory tract obstruction, increased absorption of toxin from the membrane site. Prognosis is guarded until complete recovery of myocardial complications, laryngeal obstruction, palatal, pharyngeal and peripheral neuritis may occur at various stages of the disease. Myocarditis, aspiration, regurgitation and obstruction of respiratory tract may prove fatal. The worldwide mortality is 5–10%.

PREVENTION

The control of diphtheria is based on primary prevention of disease by ensuring high population immunity through vaccination and secondary prevention of spread by the rapid investigation of close contacts to ensure prompt treatment of those infected. Immunization can prevent diphtheria. Therefore all children worldwide should be immunized against diphtheria.

There are single vaccines and mixed vaccines for diphtheria. To reduce number of injections and visits to health facility, it is better to combine various compatible vaccines without risking seroconversion. As diphtheria is almost exclusively available in fixed combinations with other antigens, immunization programs will need to harmonize immunization schedules between diphtheria, tetanus and pertussis. Diphtheria toxoid-containing vaccine can also be administered with other childhood and adolescence vaccines. The vaccine should be stored at 2-8°C. Vaccines should be used as early as possible after receiving at the sub-centre – ideally within a week. If vaccines have been frozen, they should not be used. Most diphtheria toxoid-containing vaccines are administered as a 0.5 ml dose, by intramuscular injection only. The anterolateral aspect of the thigh is the preferred site for immunization. Diphtheria toxoid is one of the safest vaccines available. Severe reactions are rare, and to date no anaphylaxis reactions attributable to the diphtheria component have been described. However, local reactions at the site of injection are common.

Diphtheria toxoid is available combined with tetanus toxoid and pertussis antigens as diphtheria, tetanus, and pertussis (DTP –First combination vaccine introduced in 1940s), *diphtheria-tetanus*-acellular pertussis (DTaP), diphtheria and tetanus toxoids (DT – Full dose/child dose diphtheria toxoid), diphtheria and tetanus toxoids adsorbed (Td – Low dose/adult dose diphtheria toxoid) and tetanus-diphtheria-pertussis (Tdap). The LF value of child diphtheria toxoid varies from 10 to 25 LF units. DTP or DTaP is also available combined with additional vaccine antigens such as hepatitis B surface antigen (HBsAg) and Hemophillus influenzea type B (HB) conjugate as Pentavalent vaccine and with inactivated polio vaccine (IPV) as Hexavalent vaccines. When IPV containing combination vaccine is not available, it is given along with oral polio vaccine.

The child dose diphtheria toxoid vaccine can be given up to 7 years of age. A complete primary immunization and booster doses shall prevent an epidemic and also reduce incidence of diphtheria. A primary series of 3 doses of diphtheria toxoid-containing vaccine is recommended, with first dose administered as early as 6 weeks of age. Subsequent doses should be given with an interval of at least 4 weeks between doses. The third dose of the primary series should be completed by 6 months of age if possible.

The interval between two doses should be 4–6 weeks. Shorter interval than 4 weeks may not have appropriate seroconversion. Longer than 8 weeks interval has no added advantage as per vaccinology. It may increase dropout rates.

Three booster doses of diphtheria toxoid-containing trivalent vaccine should be given in combination with tetanus toxoid and pertussis antigens using the schedule, i.e. at 15–18 months of age, 4–6 years of age, and 11–12 years of age, using age-appropriate vaccine formulations. The first booster i.e. fourth dose may be administered as early as age 12 months, provided at least 6 months have elapsed since the third dose of primary series. A booster dose, consisting of an adult preparation of Tdap is recommended at 11-12 years of age.

Because immunity wanes over time, subsequent additional boosters of reduced strength diphtheria toxoid – Td should be given every 10 years to maintain protective antibody levels. Levels of diphtheria antitoxin of 0.01 IU/ml or greater generally are accepted as protective.

DTaP/DT may be preferred to DTwP in children with history of severe adverse effects after previous dose/s of DTwP or children with neurologic disorders.

Schedule of Immunization:
- I dose at 6 weeks of age. (DPT/DTaP)
- II dose at 10 weeks of age. (DPT/DTaP)
- III dose at 14 weeks of age. (DPT/DTaP)
- I Booster dose at 15-18 months of age. (DPT/DTaP)
- II Booster at 4 - 6 years of age. (DPT/DTaP/DT)
- III Booster at 11-12 years of age (Tdap/Td)
- Followed by Td every 10 years.

Catch-up Vaccination

At any age opportunities should be taken to provide or complete the 3-dose diphtheria toxoid containing vaccine series for children aged ≥1year, adolescents and adults who were not vaccinated, or incompletely vaccinated, during infancy. Children who have missed I, II, III doses should receive age appropriate vaccination to update the immunization status.

For previously unimmunized children aged 1–7 years, the recommended primary schedule of 3 doses, with a minimum interval of 4 weeks between the first and second dose, and an interval of at least 6 months between the second and third dose, using DTP-containing vaccine and a first booster dose 6–12 months after the third dose of primary series. The second childhood booster is not required if the first booster was given after the age of 4 years; and if the first booster was given before 4 years the second booster is given between 4 and 6 years. Repeat boosters of Tdap/Td every 10 years.

After 7 years of age, the dose of diphtheria toxoid is 1/3–1/5 child dose (Td, Tdap). It works out to be 2–5 LF units per dose. After 7 years of age with child dose of toxoid there is risk of anaphylaxis. "D" denotes child toxoid and "d" refers to adult toxoid dose. The adult toxoid contains 2–2.5 LF units. Tdap or Td is approved for minimum 7 years and above, by Indian Academy of Pediatrics - Advisory Committee on Vaccines and Immunization Practices (IAP-ACVIP). For previously unimmunized older children >7 years, adolescents and adults use Td or Tdap combination vaccines; the recommended schedule for primary immunization is of 3 doses (Tdap, Td, Td), with a minimum interval of 4 weeks between the first (Tdap) and the second (Td) dose, and an interval of 6 months between the second and a third (Td) dose. Two subsequent booster doses using Td or Tdap combination vaccines are needed with an interval of at least 1 year between doses.

Adolescents 13–18 years of age who missed the Tdap or Td booster dose at 11–12 years or in whom it has been >5 years since the Td booster dose also, should receive a single dose of Tdap if they have completed the primary DTP/DTaP series.

To further promote immunity against diphtheria, the use of Tdap preferred over Td rather than TT is recommended during pregnancy after 20 weeks of gestation to protect against maternal and neonatal tetanus and pertussis in the context of prenatal care; and when tetanus prophylaxis is needed following injuries.

Special Populations

Diphtheria toxoid-containing vaccines can be used in immunocompromised persons including HIV-infected individuals. All health-care workers should up to date with immunization as recommended in their national immunization schedules. Travellers are generally not at special risk of diphtheria, unless they travel to an endemic country or outbreak setting. They should be immunized as recommended in their national immunization schedules.

Care of carriers is also important. Throat swab culture should be done. Those with positive culture should be treated with benzathine penicillin or erythromycin till at least two to three cultures at the interval of 24 hours are negative. Culture positive should be treated with antibiotics.

Chemoprophylaxis and immunization of the contacts is of paramount importance.

Children who contract disease and recover, should be followed-up for carrier state and treated as described above. These children do not develop immunity. They require age-specific immunization for diphtheria and vaccine preventable diseases. Combinations of vaccines for various vaccine preventable diseases are available although expensive.

Personal hygiene should be maintained. Washing of hands is important. There is a larger risk of contracting diphtheria with sharing of towels, cups, eating utensils, bed or bedroom and with overcrowding. Bath once a week or less is also associated with higher risk of contracting diphtheria from a reference case.

Complete immunization with primary and booster doses at regular recommended time should keep vaccine preventable diseases at bay.

BIBLIOGRAPHY

1. Buescher ES. Diphtheria. In: Kliegman RM, Stanton BF, St. Geme JW, Schor NF, Behrman RE (Eds). Nelson Textbook of Pediatrics, 19th edn. Philadelphia: Elsevier; 2012. pp. 929.
2. Centres for Disease Control and Prevention. Diphtheria, tetanus and pertussis: Recommendations for vaccine use and other preventive measures. MMWR. 1991;40:1-28.
3. Diphtheria vaccines: WHO Position Paper – August 2017. No 31: 2017, 92, 417-436.
4. Epidemiology and Prevention of Vaccine-Preventable Diseases, 10th edn. Department of Health and Human Services CDC; 2007.
5. Govt. of India (2010), National Health Profile. DGHS, Ministry of Health and Family Welfare, New Delhi; 2009.
6. Park K. Diphtheria. In: Park K (Ed). Park's Textbook of Preventive and Social Medicine, 21st edn. Jabalpur: M/s Banarsidas Bhanot Publishers; 2011. pp. 149-52.
7. Vashishtha VM, Chitkara AJ. Diphtheria, Tetanus and Pertussis Vaccines. In: Indian Academy of Pediatrics (IAP) Guidebook on Immunization 2013-14, 2014 edn. Advisory Committee on Vaccines and Immunization Practices (ACVIP) IAP. pp. 137.
8. WHO (2010), World Health Statistics, New Delhi, 2010.

V Poovazhagi

INTRODUCTION

Pertussis is a highly contagious acute bacterial infection caused by the bacilli *Bordetella pertussis*. Outbreaks of pertussis were first described in the 16th century. Sydenham first used this term "pertussis" meaning "intense cough". Pertussis is also known as "whooping cough" because of the "whooping" sound that is made when gasping for air after a fit of coughing. In some countries, this disease is called the 100 days' cough or cough of 100 days.

This was one of the major childhood illnesses before the advent of vaccine. Currently worldwide prevalence is diminished due to active immunization but pertussis remains a public health problem among older children and adults. Pertussis continues to be an important respiratory disease afflicting unvaccinated infants and previously vaccinated children as well as adults in whom immunity has waned.

EPIDEMIOLOGY

Pertussis occurs worldwide. Pertussis incidence has been increasing steadily in the last decade especially in industrialized countries despite the use of vaccination.[1-3] Adolescents and adults are the reservoir: no animal or insect reservoir exists. Transmission is through the respiratory route in the form of droplet infection. Pertussis is a highly communicable disease. Secondary attack rate is as high as 90% among household contacts. It is highly infectious in the catarrhal stage and 2 weeks after the onset of cough. Despite the revised guidelines for vaccination of adolescents and adults with tetanus-diphtheria-pertussis (Tdap) vaccine, the incidence of pertussis in this population has been on the rise.

ETIOLOGY

Bordetella pertussis is a small aerobic Gram-negative coccobacilli. The organism was first isolated in 1906. This is a fastidious organism which needs special media for isolation. The organism produces pertussis toxin, filamentous hemagglutinin, hemolysin, adenylate cyclase toxin, dermonecrotic toxin and tracheal cytotoxin, which are responsible for the clinical features and the immune response to one or more of these provide immunity to subsequent illness.

PATHOGENESIS

Pertussis is a toxin-mediated disease. The organism gets attached to the respiratory cilia and the toxin causes paralysis of the cilia. This also leads to inflammation and this interferes with the adequate clearance of pulmonary secretions. A mucopurulent-sanguineous exudate forms in the respiratory tract. This exudate compromises of the small airways (especially those of infants) and predisposes the affected individual to atelectasis, cough, cyanosis and pneumonia. The antigens also help the organism to evade the host defenses in that this causes lymphocytosis but impaired chemotaxis. There by the organism causes local tissue damage in the respiratory tract and systemic effects mediated through its toxin. Contrary to the previous thought that pertussis does not invade the tissues, it has been recently demonstrated to be present in the alveolar macrophages.

Clinical Features

Incubation period of pertussis is 7–10 days (range, 4–21 days). Infection usually lasts for 6 weeks but can present up to 10 weeks. Patients are infectious just prior to and for 21 days after the onset of cough if untreated. The clinical course is divided into three distinct stages:[4]

Stage 1 [Catarrhal stage (1–2 weeks)]: It is characterized by insidious onset of coryza, sneezing, low-grade fever, cough like common cold. Cough becomes more severe in the next 1–2 weeks (Catarrhal stage—cough and coryza).

Stage 2 [Paroxysmal cough stage (1–6 weeks)]: At this stage, pertussis is generally suspected. Cough occurs in bouts or paroxysms of numerous rapid coughs apparently due to the difficulty in expelling the thick mucous from the tracheobronchial tree. At the end of the paroxysm long inspiratory effort is followed by a whoop. In between episodes, child looks apparently well. During episodes of cough the child may become cyanosed, followed by vomiting, exhaustion and seizures. Apneic episodes may be life-threatening following cough. Apnea is more common in neonates and in infant less than 6 months. Infants less than 6 months of age may not be able to produce a whoop. Cough increases for 1–2 weeks, remains static for next 2–3 weeks and decreases over next 10 weeks. Absence of whoop and/or post-tussive vomiting does not rule out clinical diagnosis of pertussis.

Paroxysmal nature of cough of more than 2 weeks with or without whoop and/or post-tussive vomiting is the hallmark feature of pertussis.

Stage 3 [Convalescence stage]: Convalescence stage is a period of gradual recovery. The children may continue to have whoop with minor respiratory illness even up to 6 months. Disease occurring in vaccinated individuals, adults and adolescents vary from mild illness to severe cough like classic pertussis. They are unlikely to present with the characteristic whoop. Those with milder disease can also transmit the disease to susceptible population.

COMPLICATIONS

Young infants are at highest risk for the disease-related complications. Nearly 50% of infants with pertussis need hospitalization. Mortality is 1%. Common complications and the cause for mortality in infants with pertussis are due to secondary pneumonia (23%) and apneic spells (61%).[5] Neurological complications include seizures (1.1%) and encephalopathy (0.3%) due to hypoxia or due to the toxin itself or cerebral hemorrhage. Other complications include otitis media, anorexia and dehydration. Pneumothorax, epistaxis, subdural hematomas, hernia and rectal prolapse are the other complications that develop as a consequence of pressure effects of severe paroxysm. Complications are lesser in children and adults. Among the latter 5% need hospitalization. Pneumonia is encountered in 2%. They may present with weight loss (33%), loss of bladder control (28%) and rib fractures (4%).

DIFFERENTIAL DIAGNOSIS

Similar clinical picture can be encountered in infections with *B. parapertussis*, adenovirus, mycoplasma pneumonia and *Chlamydia trachomatis*. Other non-infectious causes for cough need to be included in differential diagnosis.

Foreign body aspiration, endobronchial tuberculosis and a mass pressing on an airway can present as pertussoid cough.

DIAGNOSIS

Diagnosis of pertussis is suspected on the basis of history and clinical examination and is confirmed by culture, genomics or serology. Laboratory confirmation is not necessary for diagnosis, but may be useful for infection control.

Elevated white blood cell (WBC) count with lymphocytosis is commonly encountered. The absolute lymphocyte counts of 20,000 or greater may give a clinical clue. It is one of the commonest causes of lymphocytic leukemoid reaction. This may not be always encountered in infants and children or in milder cases. Neonates present with higher counts in range of even more than 20,000 WBC/cmm. Normal WBC count does not rule out pertussis.

Culture is the gold standard for the diagnosis. *B. pertussis* isolated in the catarrhal stage is diagnostic. Nasopharyngeal swabs (NPS)/pernasal swabs (PNS) or nasopharyngeal aspirates (NPA) or throat swabs can be done. A saline nasal swab or swab from the posterior pharynx is preferred. The swab should be taken using dacron or calcium alginate and not cotton and has to be plated on to the selective medium. A cough plate can be used sometimes. Results may take as long as 2 weeks. Culture positivity depends on the stage of the disease and the yield is highest during the first 3–4 weeks of illness. Cultures are difficult to perform and are not recommended in clinical practice as the yield is poor because of previous vaccination, antibiotic use, diluted specimen and faulty collection and transportation of specimen.

Polymerase Chain Reaction

This is the most sensitive test to diagnose pertussis. Nasopharyngeal swab or aspirate can be used. It can be done even after antibiotic exposure and is more useful in infants where serology is difficult and culture yield is low. However, calcium alginate swabs cannot be used for polymerase chain reaction (PCR) testing. Polymerase chain reaction should always be used in addition with cultures and cannot replace the culture. Higher rates of false positivity and poor sensitivity are drawbacks with PCR for pertussis.

Direct Fluorescent Antibody Testing

It can be done with the nasopharyngeal specimen but has low sensitivity and variable specificity.

Serological Tests

Due to lack of association between the antibody levels and immunity in pertussis, these tests are difficult to interpret. This may be useful in adults or adolescents where the cultures may not be positive as they present late in the illness. Anti-pertussis toxin IgG becomes detectable 2 weeks after the onset of illness. A positive serology is confounded by maternal antibodies, primary or booster vaccination. The period of confounding may be up to 10 months post-primary vaccination and up to 3 years following preschool booster vaccination. Oral fluid testing for IgG antibodies is an alternate sample for children between 5 and 19 years of age.[6]

MANAGEMENT

Being a bacterial disease antibiotic has a role to play. Antibiotics are mainly used to reduce the period of communicability of the disease. Antibiotics started in catarrhal or early paroxysmal phase may reduce the severity and if started within two weeks of cough may reduce the spread to other children. The duration of cough is unaffected by antibiotic therapy. Macrolides are considered as the drug of choice. Erythromycin 40–50 mg/kg/day in 6 hourly divided doses for 2 weeks is the drug of choice. Alternatively azithromycin in dose of 10 mg/kg for 5 days in infants less than 6 months and for children older than 6 months 10 mg/kg on day 1, followed by 5 mg/kg from day 2 to 5 is recommended and tolerated better than erythromycin. Clarithromycin in dose of 15 mg/kg in two divided doses for 7 days can also be used and is preferred in infants below one month of age. Trimethoprim-sulfamethoxasole is the alternate drug used for older children. Respiratory co-infections may occur and may require modification of antibiotic. Avoidance of irritants, smoke, noise and other cough promoting factors form an important part of management.

Supplemental oxygen may be required in some children. Infants need to be watched for apneic spells during the episodes of cough. Hydration has to be taken care of in children if oral intake is inadequate due to spells of cough and vomiting. Humidified oxygen and ventilatory support may be required for seriously-ill patients. Cough mixtures and bronchodilators may be useful in individual cases. Respiratory isolation of cases is advised until greater than 5 days of erythromycin treatment.

Prophylaxis of Contacts

Postexposure antibiotic is indicated for all household contacts and those with high risk of developing pertussis if within 2 weeks of onset of cough in index case. High risk includes infants less than 12 months of age, people with certain pre-existing health conditions that may be worsened by a pertussis infection, such as immunocompromised patients and patients being treated for moderate to severe asthma and pregnant mothers in third trimester. Center for Disease Control and Prevention (CDC) recommends prophylaxis to anyone who will have close contact with the above groups too. Antibiotic dose is the same as for treatment. When continued transmission of pertussis is evident multiple rounds of antibiotics is not recommended. Mothers with pertussis or suspected to have pertussis deliver within 3 weeks of cough the neonates are treated with antibiotics. Children less than 7 years who have not completed the four primary doses of vaccination should complete the same at the earliest. Children less than 7 years, who have completed primary vaccination but not received the booster in the 3 years prior to exposure have to be given a single booster dose. Pregnant women exposed after 32 weeks need antibiotic and vaccine if not vaccinated in the past 5 years.

Vaccination

Every infant should receive three doses of pertussis vaccine and is to be followed by boosters at 15–18 months and at 5 years to make a total of five doses. Four doses of whole cell pertussis vaccine offer 70–90% protection and there is little or no protection at 5–10 years of last dose.

Acellular vaccine was developed in view of concerns over the safety issues. The immunogenicity of acellular vaccine is comparable to that of whole cell vaccine but reactogenicity in terms of fever, local pain, induration and systemic side effects are definitely low.

Diphtheria-tetanus-acellular pertussis (DTaP)and Tetanus-Diphtheria-Pertussis(DPT) are the two formulations available for primary vaccination. For vaccination, the same type of wP-containing or aP-containing vaccines should be given throughout the primary course and if unknown or unavailable interchange can be permitted.[7] Tetanus-*diphtheria*-acellular pertussis (Tdap) has been approved for use from 10 years or from 11 years to 64 years depending on the brand used for vaccination. Control of whooping cough rests mainly on adequate immunization of all infants, adolescents and adults. It is recommended that a single

Tdap dose be given for persons aged 11 through 18 years who have completed the childhood DPT/DT vaccination series[7] and for adults aged 19 through 64 years. Tdap in each pregnancy, preferably at 27 through 36 weeks gestation and if not received one dose postpartum is recommended to maximize passive transfer of antibody to infants.[8,9] The natural disease does not provide lifelong immunity as thought earlier, hence in view of waning immunity, vaccination is recommended following the natural disease. The strategies for prevention of infant pertussis by cocooning (immunization of all family members who could have a strict contact with a newborn aiming for reduction of infection) and neonatal immunization do not have evidence to be recommended as of now.[10,11]

REFERENCES

1. Vashishtha VM, Bansal CP, Gupta SG. Pertussis Vaccines: Position Paper of Indian Academy of Pediatrics. Indian Pediatr. 2013;50:1001-9.
2. Jackson DW, Rohani P. Perplexities of pertussis: recent global epidemiological trends and their potential causes. Epidemiol Infect. 2013;16:1-13.
3. Pertussis fact sheet for health care personnel. Public Health England pertusis reports .available from https://www.gov.uk/government/uploads/system/uploads/attachment_data/file/562472/HCW_Factsheet_Pertussis.pdf assessed on 25th august 2017.
4. Atkinson W, Wolfe S, Hamborsky J (Eds). Centers for Disease Control and Prevention. Epidemiology and Prevention of Vaccine-Preventable Diseases, 12th edition. Washington DC: Public Health Foundation; 2012.
5. Centers for Disease Control and Prevention. Complications of pertussis. https://www.cdc.gov/pertussis/about/complications.html accessed on 25.8.2017.
6. Guidelines for the Public HealthManagement of Pertussis in England- https://www.gov.uk/government/uploads/system/uploads/attachment_data/file/576061/Guidelines_for_the_Public_Health_Management_of_Pertussis_in_England.pdf accessed on 24.8.2017.
7. Centers for Disease Control and Prevention; American Academy of Pediatrics Committee on Infectious Diseases. Additional recommendations for use of tetanus toxoid, reduced-content diphtheria toxoid, and acellular pertussis vaccine (Tdap). Pediatrics. 2011;128(4):809-12.
8. Updated Recommendations for Use of Tetanus Toxoid, Reduced Diphtheria Toxoid, and Acellular Pertussis Vaccine (Tdap) in Pregnant Women—Advisory Committee on Immunization Practices (ACIP), 2012. MMWR. 2013 /62(07);131-5. https://www.cdc.gov/mmwr/preview/mmwrhtml/mm6207a4.html accessed on 25.8.2017.
9. Castagnini L, Healy MC, Rench MA, Wootton SH, Munoz FM, Baker CJ. Impact of maternal postpartum tetanus diptheria toxoids and acellular pertussis immunization of infant pertussis infection. Clin Inf Dis. 2012;54:78-84.
10. Libster R, Edwards KM. How can we best prevent pertussis in infants? Clin Infect Dis. 2012;54:85-7.
11. Wood N, McIntyre P, Marshall H, Roberton D. Acellular pertussis vaccine at birth and one month induces antibody responses by two months of age. Pediatr Infect Dis J. 2010;29:209-15.

4.4   TETANUS

Raju C Shah

INTRODUCTION

Tetanus historically called *'Lockjaw'* is an acute often fatal, severe exotoxin-mediated infection caused by *Clostridium tetani*. Rosenbach in 1886 demonstrated for the first time these slender bacilli. The disease first described by Carlie and Rattone is characterized by severe muscular spasms or acute spastic paralysis, is caused by the action of a potent neurotoxin produced during the growth of the bacteria in dead tissues.

EPIDEMIOLOGY

Tetanus occurs worldwide and is an important cause of neonatal death in developing world. The causative organism *C. tetani* is part of the normal flora in human and animal intestines and is disseminated through the excreta and found in soil and dust. In spore form, they are hard and long lasting in soil and dust. As the spores of *C. tetani* are ubiquitous, wound contamination is unavoidable. The contamination of wound, unhygienic and improper handling of the umbilical cord in newborns, lack of hygienic habits and aseptic care during and after delivery in women are the main risk factors for infection. Tetanus can occur in a child having chronic ear discharge.

It is the only vaccine preventable disease that is infectious but not contagious from person to person. Among the burden of vaccine preventable diseases world over, tetanus ranks fourth with 13% disease burden. The incidence is high in tropical countries with humid climate. According to WHO in 2009, global reported cases were 9,836 and estimated deaths in children <5 years were 61,000. The reported cases of tetanus in India in 2006 were 2587, of which 600 cases were neonatal tetanus. More cases are reported from rural than urban areas.

In 2010, there were 4797 reported Neonatal Tetanus cases globally with 373 cases from India. According to the Child Health Epidemiology Reference Group (CHERG) (2008), an estimated 60,000 newborns die of the disease each year. In April 2015, WHO included India in the list of countries which has eliminated neonatal tetanus. This means India has less than 1 case of neonatal tetanus per 1000 live births in every district.

2013 global figures
- 14,860 reported cases
- 72,600 estimated deaths in <5 years (in 2011)
- 84% estimated DTP3 coverage

ETIOLOGY

The causative organism *Clostridium tetani* is a Gram-positive, anaerobic, spore forming organism. It forms terminal spores resembling drumsticks. The spores are resistant to boiling, usual antiseptics and chemical agents like phenol. They can survive autoclaving at 121°C for 10–15 minutes.

Clostridium tetani usually enters the body through wound. The bacilli itself is noninvasive. The spores germinate in anaerobic conditions. They produce two types of toxins: tetanospasmin and tetanolysin. Of these, tetanospasmin is a neurotoxin and is responsible for the clinical signs and symptoms of the disease. Toxins act at several sites within the nervous system.

CLINICAL MANIFESTATIONS

The incubation period of tetanus is around 10 days (range 3–30 days). On the basis of clinical findings, three different forms of tetanus have been described:
- The most common type (80%) is "generalized tetanus".
- "Localized tetanus" produces pain and spasm of the muscles in proximity to the site of injury. Occasionally, this form of disease may precede generalized form.
- "Cephalic tetanus" is a rare form of the disease seen in children with otitis media.

Generalized Tetanus

It is usually present with a descending pattern. The first sign most of the time is trismus or lockjaw due to spasm of masseter muscle. Headache, restlessness and irritability may be early symptoms followed by stiffness of the neck, difficulty in swallowing and rigidity of abdominal muscles. The spasms can be precipitated by bright light, noise and even touch. The rigidity of facial muscles leads to the sardonic smile of tetanus or risus sardonicus, a typical grinning appearance. Rigidity and spasm of back and abdominal muscles causes arching (opisthotonus). Laryngeal and respiratory muscle spasm can lead to airway obstruction and asphyxia. Constipation and retention of urine may also occur. Hyperpyrexia, hypertension, excessive sweating, tachycardia and cardiac arrhythmia can occur due to sympathetic nerve involvement. Paralysis is evident in the first week, stabilizes in second week and ameliorates in the next 1–4 weeks.

Neonatal Tetanus

This typically occurs when the umbilical cord is cut with an unsterilized instrument and manifests within 3–12 days of birth. It is generalized tetanus, a serious condition and often fatal. Progressive difficulty in feeding (sucking and swallowing) with associated hunger and crying are generally seen. Paralysis and diminished movement, stiffness to touch, spasms with/without opisthotonus are the clinical features. Opisthotonus may be extreme or sometimes absent.

Localized Tetanus

This is painful spasms to the site of infection precede generalized tetanus. Cephalic tetanus with bulbar muscle involvement is seen with wounds of the head, face, nostrils or with chronic otitis media. Retracted eyelids, deviated gaze, trismus, risus sardonicus, spastic paralysis of the tongue and pharyngeal muscles are the presenting features.

DIAGNOSIS

Diagnosis is mainly clinical. The typical setting is an injured unimmunized patient or baby born to an unimmunized mother presenting within 2 weeks with trismus, rigid muscles and clear sensorium. The organism can be isolated from wound or ear discharge.

MANAGEMENT

It comprises of wound debridement, immunoglobulin administration, antibiotics and supportive care. The aim of therapy is to neutralize all toxins, eradication of *C. tetani* and wound environment conducive to anaerobic multiplication and supportive care.

Human tetanus immunoglobulin (TIG) 3,000–6,000 units IM is recommended to be given immediately. TIG has no effect on toxin which is already fixed to the neural tissue and does not penetrate the blood-CSF barrier. It can neutralize circulating tetanospasmin. If TIG is not available, human IVIG can be used. Antitetanus serum is recommended only when TIG is not available. It can be given in a single dose of 50,000–100,000 units, half the dose IM and the rest intravenously after skin test.

Penicillin is the antibiotic of choice for *C. tetani*. Penicillin G 200,000 units/kg body weight can be given intravenously in four divided doses for 10–14 days. Local wound, discharging ears, umbilical cord should be cleaned and debrided if needed.

All patients with generalized tetanus require muscle relaxant. Diazepam is preferred as it causes both muscle relaxation and seizure control. Initial dose is 0.1–0.2 mg/kg every 3–6 hours given intravenously. Midazolam, baclofen can also be used. The best survival rates with generalized tetanus are achieved with neuromuscular blocking agents like vecuronium and pancuronium. These drugs produce general flaccid paralysis which can be managed by mechanical ventilation.

Meticulous nursing care is imperative. The patient should be kept in a quiet, dark environment with minimum auditory or visual stimuli. Maintenance of nutrition, fluid and electrolyte balance, suctioning of secretions and cardiorespiratory monitoring should be done. Provision for tracheostomy should be kept ready.

Wound Management

All wounds should be cleaned, necrotic tissue and foreign material should be removed. As shown in Table 4.4.1, wounds which are not minor require human TIG except those in fully immunized patients. In patients with history of unknown or incomplete immunization, crush, puncture or bone projecting wounds, wounds contaminated with soil, saliva or feces, avulsion injuries, compound fractures, 250 units of TIG should be given IM. In cases where the wound could not be properly debrided or wound more than 24 hours old, 500 units of TIG should be given. Tetanus toxoid may be administered immediately depending on the immunization status of the child.

COMPLICATIONS

Aspiration of secretions leading to pneumonia is one of the major complications. Autonomic system irregularities in the form of cardiac arrhythmias, asystole, and labile blood pressure may be noted. Few children may get seizure related injuries, rhabdomyolysis, myoglobinuria, bone fractures and renal failure.

PROGNOSIS

The average mortality of tetanus is 45–55%. For neonatal tetanus, the mortality is 60–70%. The most important factor influencing outcome is supportive care. Recovery from tetanus does not confer immunity; therefore active immunization of the patients following recovery is imperative.

Table 4.4.1: Wound management.

History of tetanus toxoid doses	Clean minor wounds		All other wounds#	
	TT/Td/ Tdap	TIG	TT/Td/ Tdap	TIG*
Unknown, Less than three doses, Immunocompromised	Yes	No	Yes	Yes
More than three doses	No**	No	No***	No

Including, but not limited to, wounds contaminated with dirt, feces, soil, saliva; puncture wounds; avulsions; and wounds resulting from missiles, crushing, burns, and frostbite.
*TIG: Tetanus immunoglobulin (250–500 units IM).
**Yes, if more than 10 years since last dose.
***Yes, if more than 5 years since last dose.

PREVENTION

Tetanus is an entirely preventable disease. Active immunization is the best method to prevent tetanus. All children should be immunized with three doses of DPT at 6, 10 and 14 weeks followed by booster doses at 18 months and 5 years of age. Boosters should be given at 10 years and then every 10 years. Td or Tdap is the vaccine of choice above 7 years of age.

Neonatal tetanus could be prevented by immunizing the pregnant women with two doses of tetanus toxoid (preferably Td) between 16 weeks and 36 weeks of pregnancy, and with only one dose of Td in the subsequent pregnancies.

BIBLIOGRAPHY

1. Arnon SS. Tetanus. In: Kliegman RM, Jenson HB, Behrman RE, Stanton BF (Eds). Nelson Textbook of Pediatrics, 18th edition. Philadelphia: Elsevier; 2007. pp. 1228-30.
2. Centers for Disease Control and Prevention. Diphtheria, tetanus and pertussis: recommendations for vaccine use and other preventive measures. MMWR. 1991;40:1-28.
3. Epidemiology and Prevention of Vaccine-Preventable Diseases, 10th edition. Department of Health and Human Services CDC; 2007.
4. World Health Organization. The "high risk" approach: the WHO – recommended strategy to accelerate elimination of neonatal tetanus. Wkly epidemiol Rec. 1996;71:33-6.

4.5 CHOLERA

Alok Kumar Deb

INTRODUCTION

Cholera is the most feared of all diarrheal diseases, since it can cause severely dehydrating diarrhea and death within a few hours of onset even in the adults. Throughout history, populations all over the world have sporadically been affected by devastating outbreaks of cholera. Hippocrates (460–377 BC) and Galen (129–216 AD) described an illness that could possibly be cholera, and a cholera-like illness was also known in the Ganges delta region since antiquity.

Modern knowledge about cholera, however, dates only from the beginning of the 19th century when researchers began to probe different aspects of the disease. Despite the impressive advances in our understanding of the biology, ecology and epidemiology of the disease and the organism, cholera still poses a substantial health burden on the developing world. In addition, outbreaks of cholera also cause social and economic disruptions and impede the development of affected communities.

EPIDEMIOLOGY

The Indian subcontinent always played a crucial role in the global epidemiology of cholera. Since 1817, six out of seven cholera pandemics emerged from this region, killing millions of people across the globe. The ongoing seventh pandemic only originated in Indonesia in 1961. Hence, the state of West Bengal in India, together with neighboring Bangladesh, is often called the "homeland of cholera".

Cholera continues to be a public health challenge in the developing world due to lack of access to clean water and proper sanitation systems. Moreover, increasing travel across borders, rapid and unplanned urbanization, social and political unrest and natural disasters also result in spread and persistence of the disease. For example, devastating natural disasters perhaps caused a 30% increase in reported cholera cases in 2005 compared with 2004, while the 2010 outbreak of cholera in Haiti after a gap of 100 years illustrated the introduction of cholera through human activities from a distant geographic source. In 2010, 317,534 cholera cases were reported to WHO— an increase of 130% compared to 2000. However, 172,454 cases were notified to WHO in 2015, a 9% decrease from 190,549 cases reported in 2014. In contrast, Asia still witnessed a 14% increase in reported cholera cases during the same period (64,590 cases in 2015 vs. 56,787 cases in 2014). India contributed 889 cases and 4 deaths in 2015. Notably, only a small fraction of all cases are actually reported for various reasons, including inadequate surveillance and notification systems and fear of travel and trade-related sanctions. The actual global burden is estimated to be 1.3–4.0 million cases and 21,000–143,000 deaths per year.

Traditionally, cholera was thought to occur infrequently among young children. However, cholera has been found to be a significant contributor to morbidity in the pediatric population in India and many other developing countries where cholera is endemic. For example, in the urban slums of Kolkata in Eastern India, the incidence of cholera was highest among those less than 2 years of age at 9.3 cases per 1,000 child-years, while in all age groups the incidence was 2.2 cases per 1,000 person-years.

ETIOPATHOGENESIS

Cholera is caused by *Vibrio cholerae*, a Gram-negative, facultatively anaerobic rod in the family *Vibrionaceae*. In nature, vibrios most commonly reside in moderately saline tidal river and bay waters and proliferate in the summer months when water temperature exceeds 20°C. Consequently, the illnesses they cause, including cholera, also become more prevalent during these months. During inter-epidemic periods, the organism survives in a viable but nonculturable state.

Vibrio cholerae are subdivided into more than 200 serogroups based upon their somatic (O) surface antigens. Only O1 and O139 serogroups produce a potent enterotoxin, called "cholera toxin" that causes cholera. The O1 serogroup has three serotypes (Ogawa, Inaba and Hikojima) and two biotypes (classical and El Tor). El Tor biotype mostly causes mild or asymptomatic infections and predominates in most current infections. Recently, some new strains of El Tor (genetic hybrids having attributes of classical biotype) have been associated with more severe disease. In contrast, although *V. cholerae* O139 caused outbreaks in the past, it never spread outside Asia and currently detected only sporadically. The cholera toxin has two different types of subunits—the B subunit binds onto the intestinal epithelial cells while the A subunit enters into the epithelial cells and increases intracellular cyclic adenosine monophosphate (cAMP). This blocks absorption of sodium and chloride by microvilli and promotes secretion of water into intestinal lumen, causing watery diarrhea. The fluid loss mainly occurs in the duodenum and upper jejunum. The colon is less sensitive to the toxin and still can absorb some fluid; however, the large volume of secreted water overwhelms its absorptive capacity.

Cholera is usually transmitted through fecally contaminated water or food. Common sources of infection are contaminated drinking water, food, fruits and vegetables, and utensils washed with contaminated water. Owing to a very short incubation period (2 hours to 5 days), the number of cases can rise extremely quickly. To produce clinical disease, a relatively high infectious dose, 10^3–10^6 organisms in water or 10^2–10^4 organisms in food is required, as the bacteria is very susceptible to the acidity of the stomach. Thus, the risk of infection increases with drugs or conditions that decrease gastric acidity. Persons with blood group O also have an increased risk of infection.

Most people excrete *V. cholerae* in the feces and vomitus during diarrhea and for a few days after recovery. A few individuals carry the organism in the gallbladder for several months. Rare long-term carriers have also been reported. Organisms survive in feces for up to 50 days, in soil for up to 16 days and on fingertips for 1–2 hours. *V. cholerae* is susceptible to many common disinfectants such as 0.05% sodium hypochlorite, 70% ethanol, 2% glutaraldehyde, 8% formaldehyde, 10% hydrogen peroxide and iodine-based disinfectants.

CLINICAL FEATURES

About 75% of infected people remain asymptomatic. However, the pathogens stay in their feces for 7–14 days and their shedding may infect other individuals. Less than 20% of symptomatic cases develop typical cholera with signs of moderate or severe dehydration; others are of mild or moderate severity, indistinguishable clinically from other types of acute diarrhea. The symptoms mostly include a sudden onset of effortless high volume watery diarrhea, often followed by vomiting. Abdominal cramps and fever may also accompany in some children. The characteristic "rice water" stool may not be found in milder cases. The clinical signs correspond to the patient's degree of dehydration on presentation (Table 4.5.1).

Other signs may also help in assessing the dehydration status, for example dryness of tongue, decreased urine output, sunken anterior fontanelle in infants, weak or absent pulse, cold and moist extremities and fast breathing (in absence of cough or chest indrawing) due to acidosis. The assessment of dehydration is often difficult in children with severe undernutrition, which may alter many of the signs described above (e.g. general conditions, sunken eyes and diminished skin turgor).

DIAGNOSIS

Cholera can be diagnosed clinically (as suspected cases) or by laboratory methods (as confirmed cases). During outbreaks, a clinical diagnosis using WHO standard case definition is usually sufficient, along with sporadic testing. In endemic areas, although signs and symptoms of severe cholera may be unmistakable, the diagnosis is only confirmed by identifying the bacteria in stool sample. According to WHO, a case of cholera should be suspected in an area where (a) the disease is not known to be present and a patient aged 5 years or more develops severe dehydration or dies from acute watery diarrhea or (b) there is a cholera epidemic and a patient aged 5 years or more develops acute watery diarrhea, with or without vomiting. However, infants and young children bear the greatest burden of cholera in endemic areas.

Confirmation of cholera requires demonstration of presence of *V. cholerae* in stools/rectal swabs (a transport media such as Cary-Blair media may be used, if required) through various laboratory procedures such as (a) observing the organism's characteristic motility during direct, bright-field or dark-field microscopic examination of the feces; the addition of specific antibodies stops this motility, (b) isolation of the organism from distinctive yellow colonies grown on selective thiosulfate-citrate-bile salts-sucrose (TCBS) agar and serotyping using specific antisera and (c) identification through immunofluorescence, polymerase chain reaction (PCR) assay and other intensive methods. Whenever possible, microbiological confirmation of cholera should also accompany testing for antimicrobial sensitivity patterns.

A new rapid diagnostic test (dipstick), claimed to have sensitivity and specificity of more than 90% may allow quick bedside testing even in remote areas. Such rapid identification may also decrease death rates during cholera outbreaks. Till this test is fully validated, WHO suggests that all samples tested positive with this rapid test be retested using classic laboratory procedures for confirmation.

Table 4.5.1: Assessment of dehydration status in children with acute diarrheal diseases.

Dehydration status	Estimated fluid deficit	Clinical assessment criteria	Treatment plan
Severe	More than 10% of body weight	At least two of the following signs: • Lethargic/unconscious • Sunken eyes • Skin pinch goes back very slowly • Unable to drink/drinks poorly	WHO treatment plan C: • Intravenous (IV) fluid • Oral rehydration solution (ORS) • Antibiotics
Some	5–10% of body weight	At least two of the following signs: • Restless/irritable • Sunken eyes • Skin pinch goes back slowly • Drinks eagerly, thirsty	WHO treatment plan B: • ORS/home available fluids (HAF) • Antibiotics (selective cases)
No	Less than 5% of body weight	Not enough sign to classify as "some" or "severe" dehydration	WHO treatment plan A: • ORS/HAF

TREATMENT

The mainstay of cholera treatment is replacement and maintenance of fluid and electrolyte losses through timely, adequate and appropriate rehydration, using oral rehydration salts solution (ORS), various home available fluids (HAFs) and intravenous (IV) fluid replacement therapy according to the stage of dehydration (*see* Table 4.5.1). Antibiotics in severe cases and zinc supplements are also recommended.

Oral Rehydration Salts Solution

Based on the glucose-facilitated sodium, and hence, water absorption mechanism in the small intestine, which remains intact in secretory diarrhea such as cholera, ORS can adequately treat about 80% of cholera patients. Even when IV therapy is indicated, ORS should be used together whenever possible. The amount of ORS to be administered depends on the dehydration status. In "some" dehydration, the deficit of water is 50–100 mL/kg of body weight. If the child's weight is known, approximately 75 mL of ORS per kg should be given in the first four hours. If the weight is unknown, the amount can be determined using the child's age (Table 4.5.2), although this approach is less precise.

These estimates provide only a rough guide; the actual amount depends on the extent of thirst, stool losses and dehydration. In general, children should receive as much ORS as they want—with one teaspoonful every 1–2 minutes for children below 2 years of age, and frequent sips from a cup for older children. If the child vomits, stop ORS for 10 minutes and then resume more slowly. For breastfed children, continue breastfeeding along with ORS. For nonbreastfed infants below 6 months of age, also give 100–200 mL of clean water during the first 4 hours.

Home Available Fluids

In absence of ORS and when there is no dehydration, HAFs can also be used, although they are less efficient than ORS for treating dehydration. These may include soups, cereal gruels, cereal-salt solutions or home-made sugar-and-salt solutions. However, commercial soups and sweetened commercial fruit drinks or soft drinks as well as plain glucose solution should be avoided as their high concentrations of salt, sucrose or glucose may lead to hypernatremia, osmotic diarrhea or both. On the other hand, giving only plain water is less effective and may lead to hyponatremia.

Intravenous Therapy

Intravenous administration of fluids is indicated for children with severe dehydration and in situations when oral rehydration cannot be done, for example very rapid stool loss, severe repeated vomiting, paralytic ileus, glucose malabsorption and the child is unable to drink. Ringer's lactate is the preferred IV fluid; normal (0.9%) saline or half-normal saline with 5% glucose can be used in its absence. Oral potassium supplements may be required (e.g. in case of paralytic ileus), as these fluids have inadequate or no potassium. Early institution of ORS and feeding will also provide sufficient potassium and glucose.

Infants are given IV fluid as 30 mL/kg in the first hour, followed by 70 mL/kg in the next 5 hours (i.e. 100 mL/kg in 6 hours). The rate for older children and adults is 30 mL/kg within 30 minutes, followed by 70 mL/kg in the next 2.5 hours (i.e. 100 mL/kg in 3 hours). After administering the first 30 mL/kg, if the radial pulse is still very weak and rapid, a second infusion of 30 mL/kg should be given at the same rate. Small amounts of ORS solution should also be given by mouth (about 5 mL/kg/hour) as soon as the patient is able to drink.

When IV rehydration is not possible and the patient cannot drink, ORS can be given by nasogastric tube (size 6–8 French for a child, 12–18 for an adult). However, this is contraindicated in unconscious patients. The child's head should be kept slightly raised to prevent regurgitated fluid from entering the lungs. If severely dehydrated, administer about 120 mL of ORS per kg of body weight over 6 hours (i.e. 20 mL/kg/hour). This rate should be reduced if there is repeated vomiting or increasing abdominal distension.

The child needs careful monitoring during rehydration process. Increasing stool losses or repeated vomiting will require more fluid. If the child develops puffy eyelids, a sign of "overhydration", fluid should be stopped, although breastfeeding and provision of plain water should continue. The dehydration status should be reassessed at least every 4 hours of oral therapy or hourly for IV therapy. Treatment plans should change (or continue) accordingly.

Antibiotics

Antibiotics are indicated in severe cases of cholera and should be started even without bacteriologic confirmation. They reduce the stool volume, decrease shedding of organism and shorten the duration of diarrhea, but it cannot obviate the need for fluid replacement. Since antimicrobial resistance of *V. cholerae* is of great concern, especially in cholera-endemic areas, the choice of antibiotic should

Table 4.5.2: Oral fluid requirements during first four hours of rehydration.						
Age	*<4 months*	*4–11 months*	*1–2 years*	*>2–4 years*	*5–14 years*	*≥15 years*
Weight (kg)	<5	5–7.9	8–10.9	11–15.9	16–29.9	≥30
ORS (mL)	200–400	400–600	600–800	800–1,200	1,200–2,200	2,200–4,000

follow local susceptibility pattern. In Indian subcontinent, where 60–90% of clinical isolates show resistance to furazolidone, TMP-SMX and erythromycin, preferred antibiotics for childhood cholera may include single oral dose of doxycycline (2–4 mg/kg), azithromycin (20 mg/kg) or ciprofloxacin (20 mg/kg).

Others

Oral zinc supplementation as 20 mg of elemental zinc per day (10 mg/day if below 6 months of age) for 14 days reduces the severity and duration of diarrhea and prevents further occurrences in the next few months. Antidiarrheals including antimotility drugs (e.g. loperamide, diphenoxylate, codeine), adsorbents (e.g. kaolin), live bacterial cultures (e.g. lactobacillus, *Streptococcus faecium*) and charcoal do not offer any benefits, and may have dangerous side effects. Thus, no drug besides antibiotics and zinc for treatment of diarrhea or vomiting should be given.

COMPLICATIONS

Fluid and electrolyte imbalances, resulting from the disease process and/or inappropriate rehydration may lead to complications in cholera cases. For example, depletion of potassium due to large fecal losses, especially in infants and particularly dangerous among malnourished children, may cause general muscular weakness, cardiac arrhythmias and paralytic ileus. Occasionally, cases may develop convulsion due to hypernatremia or hyponatremia, hyperthermia or hypoglycemia. In addition, pulmonary edema may result from overhydration (usually through excessive IV fluid) and renal failure due to poor hydration. However, all these complications may also result from other causes and estimation of serum electrolytes, bicarbonate and pH should provide the necessary guidance.

PROGNOSIS

Cholera was a deadly disease in the 19th and early 20th century, when the case-fatality used to be as high as 40–50%. With better understanding of the disease, especially with the advent of oral rehydration therapy using ORS, the case-fatality has come down to less than 5% in most endemic areas. Complications are rare with appropriate rehydration and most cases will be cured within a week with/without antibiotics, as necessary. However, it still causes huge loss of lives in outbreak situations, particularly when introduced into a new community without pre-existing immunity, among the infants and young children, and among those with lower immunity, such as malnourished children or people living with HIV.

PREVENTION

Equally important to the treatment of cholera is the prevention of future infections. Since cholera spreads via the fecal-oral route, preventive measures mostly consist of providing clean water and proper sanitation. Boiling and chlorination of water can help to kill the bacteria. It is important to educate people about maintaining hygiene including hand washing with soap at appropriate times and food hygiene, and proper disposal and/or sterilization of infectious waste. Patient's bedding and clothing can be disinfected by stirring them for 5 minutes in boiling water. Bedding including mattresses can also be disinfected by thorough drying in the sun. Chemoprophylaxis using appropriate antibiotics can be offered selectively for close contacts of the patient, especially for those at higher risk. Mass chemoprophylaxis for a community, however, is not recommended since it has no effect on spread of cholera and may contribute to antimicrobial resistance.

There is a long history of development of vaccines against cholera. Currently, 3 WHO pre-qualified oral cholera vaccines are available—Dukoral, Shanchol and Euvichol—all are two-dose vaccines. Dukoral needs a buffer solution and 150 mL of clean water and provides 65% protection for 2 years. Shanchol and Euvichol are essentially same, produced by different manufacturers; they do not require buffer solution and offer 65% protection for 5 years. However, use of these vaccines in various settings require further assessment. For international travelers, vaccination is no longer required since the risk of contracting cholera is very small.

BIBLIOGRAPHY

1. Barua D. History of cholera. In: Barua D, Greenough III WB (Eds). Cholera. New York: Plenum Publishing Corporation; 1992. pp.1-36.
2. Centers for Disease Control and Prevention. Laboratory methods for the diagnosis of epidemic dysentery and cholera [WHO/CDS/CSR/EDC/99/8/EN]. CDC, Atlanta, USA; 1999.
3. Ghosh A, Ramamurthy T. Antimicrobials and cholera: are we stranded? Indian J Med Res. 2011;133:225-31.
4. Ramamurthy T, Bhattacharya SK (Eds). Epidemiological and Molecular Aspects on Cholera, 1st edition. New York: Humana Press, Springer Science+Business Media; 2010.
5. Sack DA, Sack RB, Nair GB, et al. Cholera. Lancet. 2004;363: 223-33.
6. World Health Organization. Oral cholera vaccines in mass immunization campaigns: guidance for planning and use. WHO: Geneva; 2010.
7. World Health Organization. Prevention and control of cholera outbreaks: WHO policy and recommendations. WHO, Regional Office for the Eastern Mediterranean [online]. Available from http://www.who.int/cholera/publications/en/[Accessed September, 2012].
8. World Health Organization. Cholera. Factsheet No. 107. Updated October 2016 [online]. Available from http://www.who.int/mediacentre/factsheets/fs107/en/[Accessed October, 2016].

4.6	*MYCOPLASMA* INFECTION

Somu Shivabalan

INTRODUCTION

The term "mycoplasma" is widely used to refer to any organism within the class Mollicutes, which is composed of five genera (*Mycoplasma, Ureaplasma, Acholeplasma, Anaeroplasma* and *Asteroloplasma*). It is a pleomorphic organism that, unlike bacteria, lacks a cell wall, and unlike viruses, does not need a host cell for replication. Only four species are well-established human pathogens:

*   *Mycoplasma pneumoniae*
*   *Mycoplasma hominis*
*   *Mycoplasma genitalium*
*   *Ureaplasma urealyticum*

Mycoplasma pneumoniae is one of three species of Mycoplasma that frequently produce infection in humans.

Mycoplasmas are ubiquitous and are the smallest bacteria that can survive alone in nature. It was first isolated in cattle with pleuropneumonia in 1898. In 1938, Reimann described the first cases of *Mycoplasma pneumoniae* in man and coined the term "primary atypical pneumoni". In 1944, Eaton discovered a specific agent as the cause of primary atypical pneumonia, thought it to be a virus and named it Eaton's agent. It was in 1961 that Eaton's agent was proved to be a *Mycoplasma* species.

PATHOGENESIS

The two properties that seem to cause direct injury in humans are: (a) its selective affinity for respiratory epithelial cell, and (b) its ability to produce hydrogen peroxide and superoxide causing cell disruption in the respiratory tract and damage to erythrocyte membranes. The prolonged paroxysmal cough seen in this disease is due to the toxic effect exerted on ciliated respiratory epithelium. Pathogenic features of infection with *M. pneumoniae* are believed to be immune-mediated rather than induced directly by the bacteria. Indirect immune-mediated mechanism is by antibodies produced against the glycolipid antigens of *M. pneumoniae that* may act as cross reacting autoantibodies against human red cells and brain cells.

Mycoplasma pneumoniae infection occurs around the year and is transmitted from person to person by infected respiratory droplets with an incubation period averaging about 3 weeks. It causes disease at all ages with a predilection for children above 5 years (school years). The attack rate amongst family members is about 9%, and immunity is not long lasting.

CLINICAL FEATURES

Mycoplasma has a mild presentation, and the severity is related to the patients underlying immune status and cardiopulmonary status. Mixed infections with both typical and atypical organism are about 10–20%. Multiple simultaneous infections might significantly interfere with pulmonary defense function and might cause pneumonia. *M. pneumoniae* exerts a toxic effect on ciliated human epithelium and invites other agents to invade and infect. Whether one of the pathogen serves as a co-pathogen that facilitates the penetration of the second pathogen which acts as pathogen or will both pathogen cause community-acquired pneumonia (CAP), by an additive, synergistic or perhaps even antagonistic clinical expression of both remains unclear.

Most infections are asymptomatic or nonspecific like headache, malaise, and low-grade fever. They can also cause significant respiratory (pulmonary) or extrapulmonary manifestation and none of these are unique or characteristic of *M. pneumoniae.*

Pulmonary Manifestations

Upper Respiratory Tract

Predominantly it causes more of upper respiratory symptoms with pneumonia only in a minority (3–10%). The upper respiratory manifestations can range from mild rhinorrhea, cough, pharyngitis and ear pain. A small percent (5%) can have severe ear pain resulting from hemorrhagic bullous myringitis. The cough can be intractable nonproductive or mildly productive in 75–100% cases.

Lower Respiratory Tract

It is known to cause "atypical pneumonia" in which the signs and symptoms are not characteristic of lobar consolidation. Atypical pneumonias accounts for approximately 15% of CAPs. The most common causes are by three zoonotic pathogens: (1) *Chlamydia psittaci* (psittacosis), (2) *Francisella tularensis* (tularemia) and (3) Coxiella burnetii (Q fever), and three nonzoonotic pathogens: (1) *Chlamydia pneumoniae*, (2) *M. pneumoniae* and (3) *Legionella*. These atypical agents, unlike the typical pathogens, often cause extrapulmonary manifestations. This description can also apply to disease caused by a variety of bacterial, viral and even protozoan organisms.

Box 4.6.1

Pulmonary complications of *Mycoplasma* infection.
- Lobar consolidation
- Abscess
- Necrotizing pneumonitis
- Bronchiolitis obliterans
- Acute respiratory distress syndrome
- Respiratory failure

However, clinically this etiological differentiation cannot be distinguished on the basis of clinical presentation. Wheezing and dyspnea may also occur, although dyspnea is not a common complaint. Despite having pneumonia, the chest may not have findings in early phase and might develop scattered rales, wheezes, or both later. With proper treatment, the pneumonia resolves without any serious complications. However, *M. pneumoniae* can cause severe pneumonia in children and has recently been associated with acute chest syndrome in sickle cell anemia. Rarely, it can cause severe complications which cannot be ignored (Box 4.6.1).

Mycobacterium pneumoniae and Chlamydophila (Chlamydia) pneumoniae infection may worsen asthma symptoms and can produce wheezing in children who do not have asthma. At follow-up, the patients infected with *M. pneumoniae* or *C. pneumoniae* were more likely to have recurrent asthma than those without these infections.

Extrapulmonary Manifestations

In mycoplasma infection, extrapulmonary abnormalities (Box 4.6.2) may suggest the diagnosis. The pathogenesis, as to whether it is caused by immune mechanisms or the direct action of the organisms is not clear.

These manifestations include hemolysis, skin rash, joint involvement, and symptoms and signs indicative of gastrointestinal tract, central nervous system (CNS), and heart disease. At times liver enzymes are also elevated.

Laboratory Investigations

The peripheral white blood cell (WBC) count is normal or slightly elevated with neutrophilia. Thrombocytosis can occur. Erythrocyte sedimentation rate (ESR) ranges from 20 to more than 100 mm/hour (higher value suggests more severe pulmonary disease). Routine laboratory tests are generally of limited benefit as they tend to be nonspecific or within the normal range.

Chest X-ray

In chest X-ray, there is no particular finding that is suggestive of *Mycoplasma*. It can be normal, hyperaerated or with features suggestive of bronchopneumonia, atelectasis, nodular infiltrates and hilar adenopathy. Small pleural effusions can be seen in 20% cases, and empyema is rare.

Box 4.6.2

Extrapulmonary manifestations of *Mycoplasma*.
Hematology:
- Hemolysis/Hemolytic anemia
- Immune thrombocytopenic purpura
- Coagulopathies

Skin disease:
- Mild erythematous maculopapular or vesicular rash
- Stevens-Johnson syndrome
- Urticaria
- Erythema nodosum

CNS involvement:
- Aseptic meningitis
- Encephalitis
- Meningoencephalitis
- Peripheral neuropathy
- Transverse myelitis
- Cranial nerve palsies
- Cerebellar ataxia
- Guillian-Barre syndrome

Gastrointestinal symptoms:
- Nonspecific pain abdomen
- Acute hepatitis
- Pancreatitis
- Loose stools

Rheumatologic symptoms:
- Arthralgia/Arthritis
- Myalgia
- Polyarthritis

Cardiac:
- Conduction abnormalities and rhythm disturbances
- Heart failure
- Chest pain
- Myocarditis
- Pericarditis

Renal:
- Membranoproliferative glomerulonephritis nephrotic syndrome
- Transient massive proteinuria
- Chronic renal failure due to cold agglutinin
- Acute interstitial nephritis
- Hemoglobinuria or hemolytic uremic syndrome
- Isolated hematuria, cystitis or urethritis

High-Resolution Computed Tomography

High-resolution CT (HRCT) scan is more sensitive for demonstrating abnormalities than is chest radiography but does not add to diagnose etiology.

In hemolytic anemia, *Coombs test* can be positive with elevated reticulocyte count.

Cold Agglutinins

Cold agglutinins are the presence of nonspecific high concentrations of circulating immunoglobulin M (IgM) antibodies against the erythrocyte I antigen. It is neither sensitive nor specific for *M. pneumoniae* infection in children. Cold agglutinin titers greater than 1:128 in patients with pneumonia may suggest mycoplasma in adults. Titer less than 1:64 can be due to many other respiratory pathogens (adenovirus, Epstein-Barr and measles viruses).

A quick bedside test can be performed by adding four drops of blood to a tube containing sodium citrate or other anticoagulant. The tube is placed in ice water (0°C to 4°C) in a freezer for about 30 seconds and immediately observed for coarse agglutination (grains of sand) by tilting the tube on one side. On rewarming the tube to 37°C, the agglutination should resolve, and it can be reproduced again by repeating the ice water cooling procedure. A positive bedside agglutinin test is equivalent to a laboratory titer of greater than 1:64. This test is practically possible when performed close to the place where sampling is done. This could be a side laboratory or bedside if freezing equipment such as cold box be taken to the ward.

In neurologic involvement, the cerebrospinal fluid (CSF) typically reveals a lymphocytic pleocytosis, elevated protein and normal glucose.

Gram Stains

Mycobacterium pneumoniae lacks a cell wall and cannot be stained.

Cultures

They are excreted from the respiratory tract for several weeks after the acute infection, isolation of the organism may not indicate acute infection and usually requires 7–21 days to grow (SP-4 medium), hence may not be of use to guide patient management so not done routinely. There is a considerable rate of healthy carriers in the community, hence even when isolated from the respiratory tract, it cannot be conclusively determined that it is the cause.

Serology

Serology is the mainstay of laboratory diagnosis, using complement fixation (CF), enzyme-linked immunoassay, and indirect hemagglutination of paired acute and convalescent sera. The most widely used approach for serodiagnosis is the CF test, which measures "early" IgM (predominantly) and immunoglobulin G (IgG) antibody (to a lesser extent) to *M. pneumoniae*. A positive result is defined as:

- A four-fold or greater increase in titer in paired sera (or)
- A single titer of greater than or equal to 1:32.

Antibody titers to rise 7–9 days after infection and peak at 3–4 weeks. A four-fold decline in titer is also diagnostic if late samples are obtained. In addition, although a single elevated IgM may be used to diagnose infection, this measurement cannot be used until almost 7 days into the illness.

Polymerase Chain Reaction

Polymerase chain reaction (PCR) can be done rapidly and has a high specificity in all phases of infection, including early periods when the serum may be negative for antibody. PCR had a sensitivity of 92% and a specificity of 98%. PCR can be performed on respiratory specimens such as throat swabs, sputum samples, bronchoalveolar lavage fluid and nasopharyngeal aspirates. PCR can also be done on CSF, but it has a low diagnostic yield.

Antigen Capture-Enzyme Immunoassay

Antigen detection by antigen capture-enzyme immunoassay (Ag-EIA), which may detect 10^4 cfu/mL (a level which should be present in the majority of infections), and the test is most often positive within 7 days of onset.

DIAGNOSIS

There is no clinical or radiologic manifestation that clearly distinguishes a *Mycoplasma* versus chlamydial, viral or other bacterial pneumonia. Compared to pyogenic pneumonia, *Mycoplasma pneumoniae* can have gradual onset of symptoms, less respiratory distress, and a normal WBC count. They are neither sensitive nor specific enough to exclude other etiologies. The gold standard cultures are difficult and time consuming rapid diagnostic tests have their limitations of variable sensitivity and specificity. High index of clinical suspicion is essential for early treatment of *M. pneumoniae* infection.

TREATMENT

Antimicrobials are effective in reducing the length of illness due to *Mycoplasma pneumoniae*. Beta lactams, like penicillins and cephalosporins, are ineffective, because the organism lacks a cell wall. The benefits of antimicrobial therapy for the treatment of upper respiratory tract symptoms caused by *M. pneumoniae* have not been adequately studied in children. However, limited data in children suggest that a macrolide (ML) antibiotic or tetracycline (>8 years of age) should be prescribed (Table 4.6.1) when a lower respiratory tract infection is likely to be caused by *M. pneumoniae*. The value of atypical coverage in antibiotic therapy for acute exacerbations

Table 4.6.1: Drugs and dosages for *Mycoplasma* infection.

Azithromycin	10 mg/kg OD on day 1 followed by 5 mg/kg OD for next 4 days
Clarithromycin	15 mg/kg/day BD for 10 days
Erythromycin	30–40 mg/kg/day QID for 10 days
Tetracycline	20–50 mg/kg/day QID for 10 days
Doxycycline	2–4 mg/kg/day OD or BD (maximum dose/day: 100–200 mg) for 10 days
Levofloxacin*	10 mg/kg/dose BD for 10 days (≥6 months to 5 years of age)
	10 mg/kg/day OD for 10 days (maximum daily dose: 500 mg) (≥5 years of age)
*Used greater than or equal to 18 years of age, used in younger age only if the benefits of therapy exceed the risks.	

of chronic bronchitis (chlamydia) and exacerbations of asthma (chlamydia and mycoplasma) is less clear. Suspect and initiate treatment against atypica organism when: (a) prolonged mild presentation with unexpected radiological finding on chest X-ray, (b) multisystem/extrapulmonary manifestation along with pulmonary involvement, (c) severe CAP or worsening of pneumonia despite appropriate therapy, instead of escalating antimicrobials also consider atypical either as sole etiology or coinfection as the conventional beta lactamase antimicrobials are not effective against them, (d) pneumonia worsening wheeze. Practically, treatment against *Mycoplasma* is claimed to decrease communicability and also decrease post-CAP asthma. Macrolide (ML) resistant mycoplasma was first isolated in 2000 from a 9-year-old girl with pneumonia. Since then the issue of ML-resistant mycoplasma is increasing in importance and has been reported in Asia, France, Italy, Israel, and the United States. Tetracyclines, doxycycline or fluoroquinolones (levofloxacin) are used for ML-resistant strains.

In hemolytic anemia or CNS involvement, antibiotics may not have a major therapeutic role as these disorders are thought to arise from immune-mediated mechanisms. However, anecdotal reports of various modalities in addition to antimicrobials are available.

- *Hemolytic anemia*: Warming the patient, steroid therapy, and plasmapheresis.
- *CNS disease*: Steroids, anti-inflammatory drugs, diuretics, and plasma exchange.

Duration of respiratory symptoms is reduced by treatment with MLs. It is still unclear whether treatment affects mortality because studies have showed spontaneous recovery of *M. pneumoniae* CAP without therapy. The role of therapy against atypical coinfection is not obvious. Coinfection may cause more severe manifestations and some studies report that they do not worsen disease leading to the belief that ML treatment is not necessary as there was no mortality even in cases of atypical coinfection treated with β-lactams alone. However, the role of coinfection in atypical pneumonia cannot be determined definitively until prospective trials are performed.

PROGNOSIS

Mortality rates for *M. pneumoniae* are relatively low. The same holds true even without treatment. The belief that antimicrobials reduce the duration of symptoms again is not certain at least in some, where the disease is self-limiting and the effect of therapy is doubtful. The clinical and radiologic manifestations of CAP caused by atypical pathogens are modulated by the immunologic and physiologic status of the host, and therefore are not pathogen-specific.

SUMMARY

- Atypical pathogens play a more important role in CAP than was recognized in the past, both as a single pathogen and as a copathogen.
- Their clinical and radiologic manifestations are modulated by the immunologic and physiologic status of the host.
- The effectiveness and importance of antimicrobial therapy in some patients with atypical pathogen CAP are unclear.
- Judicious use of MLs in recommended in view of global increase in emergence of ML-resistant mycoplasma.
- Microbiological confirmation of diagnosis is difficult. Due to lack of cell wall they are nonresponsiveness to beta-lactam therapy.
- In future, atypical pathogens (*M. pneumoniae*, *C. pneumoniae*, and *Legionella*) may no longer be called so as their presentation is similar to the *Pneumococcus* (clinically and radiographically) and they respond to a group of antibiotics (newer MLs and respiratory quinolones) that are effective against all the major causes of CAP. Their presence in the CAP spectrum is significant. The only difference between *S. pneumoniae* and these atypical organisms is that *S. pneumoniae* may be cultured from routine specimens.

BIBLIOGRAPHY

1. Blasi F. Atypical pathogens and respiratory tract infections. Eur Respir J. 2004;24(1):171-81.
2. Cunha BA. The atypical pneumonias: clinical diagnosis and importance. Clin Microbiol Infect. 2006;12(3):12-24.
3. Gupta SK. The role of atypical pathogens in community-acquired pneumonia. Med Clin North Am. 2001;85(6):1349-65.
4. Gupta SK, Sarosi GA. The role of atypical pathogens in community-acquired pneumonia. Med Clin North Am. 2001;85(6):1349-65.
5. Halm EA, Teirstein AS. Clinical practice: management of community-acquired pneumonia. N Engl J Med. 2002;347:2039-45.
6. Hindlyeh M, Carroll KC. Laboratory diagnosis of atypical pneumonia. Semin Respir Infect. 2000;15(2):101-13.
7. Kashyap S, Sarkar M. Mycoplasma pneumonia: clinical features and management. Lung India. 2010;27(2):75-85.
8. Lieberman D. Atypical pathogens in community acquired pneumonia. Clin Chest Med. 1999;20(3):489-97.
9. Restrepo MI. Antimicrobial treatment of community-acquired pneumonia. Clin Chest Med. 2005;26(1):65-73.
10. Salaria M, Singh M. Atypical pneumonia in children. Indian Pediatr. 2002;39:1061-2.

4.7   TUBERCULOSIS

Sangeeta Sharma

INTRODUCTION

Tuberculosis (TB) is an infection caused by *Mycobacterium tuberculosis* (MTB) complex comprising of *M. tuberculosis* in most cases, *Mycobacterium bovis* in few cases and *Atypical (Environmental) Mycobacterium* in immunodeficient children. TB was the only infectious disease to be declared a "global emergency" by the WHO in 1993.

EPIDEMIOLOGY

About 2 billion people worldwide are infected with MTB complex, with India contributing to about one-third of the global burden. There are 8.5 million TB patients prevalent at any point of time with addition of 1.8 million patients each year with half of them being sputum smear positive and contributing to transmission of disease. The global burden and the burden in endemic areas like Africa and Asia for childhood TB is still unclear due to lack of reliable epidemiological data on the incidence and prevalence of pediatric TB. It is estimated that with the annual risk of tubercular infection being 1–5% and an overall younger population globally, WHO has recently revised that 10–11% of the actual total caseload is estimated in children. Nearly 40 million children are likely to be exposed to the risk of TB globally with about 1.3 million new cases and 450,000 deaths occurring annually in children, majority being in developing countries. In a study from South India, a prevalence of 0.3% of radiological TB was observed in 1–14 year age group and 0.15% of bacteriological TB in 5–14 years age group out of a total 20,063 children. TB has also been found to be the most common infectious disease amongst admitted children in India.

ETIOPATHOGENESIS

Mycobacterium tuberculosis bacilli spread through the air droplets produced when a sputum positive patient coughs, sneezes or spits resulting in a large number of live bacilli being coughed into the air. They remain suspended for a variable period depending upon the size of the air droplet. When this droplet containing a few live, virulent tubercle bacilli is inhaled by a normal person, it results in a primary infection of the lungs, i.e. primary pulmonary tuberculosis (PTB). Thus, PTB is an air-borne infection. Other mode of infection, in a few cases, is ingestion of *M. bovis* infected unboiled or unpasteurized milk resulting in primary focus developing in the intestines. Generally, most infections in humans initially result in an asymptomatic latent TB infection (LTBI) or primary complex. Hematogenous dissemination from the primary focus, called primary bacteremia, occurs in all cases after the primary infection leading to the formation of microtubercles throughout the body. Further fate of these microtubercles depends upon the immunity of the individual with majority being cleared. But some may not be cleared and may remain dormant and localized only to be reactivated later. The presence of various high-risk host factors leads to a fall in the immunity, due to which about one-tenth of these LTBI eventually progress to an active disease. Active disease, if left untreated, kills more than 50% of its victims. If the fall in the immunity occurs at an early stage of primary infection, then the primary complex progresses either locally, leading to the development of progressive primary disease or hematogenously leading to dissemination and development of miliary TB, tubercular meningitis (TBM) or disseminated TB.

HIGH-RISK FACTORS FOR ACTIVE TUBERCULOSIS

- Infants and adolescents
- Poor immune status due to malnutrition, human immune deficiency virus (HIV) infection, any chronic debilitating disease, diabetes
- Drugs: steroids, chemotherapeutics or immunosuppressive medications
- Contact with an adult having active TB within last 2 years
- Overcrowding, poor unsanitary living conditions, immigration.

Primary complex, its further fate depending upon the host's immunity and the related clinical presentations of PTB and extrapulmonary TB (EPTB) disease, are discussed below in detail.

Primary Complex

Primary infection usually occurs in infants and young children with the commonest mode of infection being inhalation. Inhaled aerosol of mycobacteria lodges in the subpleural terminal alveolus usually in the mid zone to form the "primary complex" (Ghon focus and its draining lymph nodes) in the lungs, i.e. PTB, while when the mode of infection is ingestion of infected milk, then the ingested mycobacteria lodge in the submucosal Peyer's patches of the small intestine to form the primary complex along with the draining lymph nodes, i.e. primary EPTB. The child is usually asymptomatic with hardly any physical signs with the only evidence of infection being a positive skin tuberculin test.

Sometimes, the Ghon focus enlarges and reaches sufficient size or develops central caseous necrosis and liquefaction. Tubercle bacilli usually remain inhibited in the solid, caseous lesion due to the acidic pH, low oxygen tension and fatty acids. Thus, a solid lesion in all organs has a small bacillary load, i.e. 10^2–10^5 organisms. But in general,

Table 4.7.1: Forms of tuberculosis and time from infection to onset.

Forms of tuberculosis	Time from infection to onset
Immune conversion	4–8 weeks
Primary complex	4–12 weeks
Progressive primary TB	3–9 months
Pleural effusion (usually adolescents)	3–12 months
Miliary/Meningeal TB	Usually within 1 year
Bone-joint TB	12–36 months
Secondary breakdown (reactivation TB)	2–5 years onward
Skin TB	5 years onward
Renal TB	10 years onward

lung and kidney lesions have higher bacillary load than others. It then presents with meager nonspecific symptoms such as low-grade fever and general ill health. History of contact with an adult case of "open" sputum positive TB, hilar or mediastinal lymphadenopathy leading to pressure symptoms mainly cough, with/without opacity in unilateral lung may be present. These signs are difficult to diagnose clinically but are evident radiologically. Further, fate of the primary complex depends on interplay of cell mediated immunity and hypersensitivity and takes place according to an approximate time frame, as shown in Table 4.7.1.

Progressive Primary Disease

Sometimes, the Ghon focus or its draining lymph nodes enlarge and develop central caseous necrosis and liquefaction. Liquefaction is generally associated with the development of clinical disease. It then presents with meager nonspecific symptoms such as low-grade fever and general ill health. Expulsion of the liquefied caseous material through an airway leads to cavity formation or to an endobronchial spread with infiltrates scattered unevenly in one or both lung fields, being bigger than the size of millets. This needs to be differentiated from miliary TB where infiltrates are smaller, millets sized and distributed almost uniformly in both lung fields. There may be a local extension of the disease from the primary focus or from the ruptured lymph nodes to the lung parenchyma. Hilar or mediastinal lymphadenopathy may cause segmental or lobar collapse. These children may also present nonresolving pneumonia or persistent infiltrations (>4 weeks) despite a trial of 7–14 days of antibiotics. Majority of tubercles heal by fibrosis and calcification. The bacilli replicate poorly in fibrosed and calcified lesions but they can survive for years in the solid caseated lesions and may remain insensitive to chemotherapy.

Fibrocavitary Tuberculosis

Fibrocavitary disease is a common outcome of repeated reactivation or reinfection especially in older children and adolescents. Destruction of local tissue results in cavitary disease. Due to immunity, the disease usually remains localized to the lungs, often confined to a single lobe. However, in the walls of the cavity, as the oxygen tension is high, it promotes active growth and replication of the obligate aerobe TB bacilli, resulting in a population of 10^7–10^9 organisms. It heals by fibrosis, seen radiologically as fibrotic bands or destroyed lung causing in a mediastinal shift. Persistent fever, cough with expectoration, occasional hemoptysis, cachexia with deteriorating general health is the usual presentation. Physical signs are easily recognized, and patient is usually sputum smear positive.

Bronchiectasis

Bronchiectasis may develop due to active TB or a squeal of healed disease and may be caused by persistent atelectasis due to compression by an enlarged mediastinal lymph node. Cough with copious foul smelling sputum is the typical manifestation. Coarse crepitations over a localized area are often helpful sign.

Thus, the primary lesion in children usually has lower bacillary load than the progressive primary and reactivation type disease of the periadolescent age group. The lesions of PTB may vary from resolution, fibrosis and calcification, to liquefaction and cavity formation within same region of a lung or different regions of the same lung.

Extrapulmonary Tuberculosis

Hematogenous dissemination from the primary focus during primary bacteremia leads to the formation of microtubercles throughout the body. Majority of these microtubercles are cleared. But some may remain dormant and localized only to be reactivated later if there is a fall in the immunity leading to TB of that organ, i.e. EPTB. Almost any organ can be involved. In the decreasing order of involvement, lymph nodes, pleura, meninges, gastrointestinal tract, bones-joints, genitourinary tract, pericardium, etc. are the main sites involved, and the diagnosis is confirmed by relevant investigations depending upon the site. In our experience, lymph node TB (71.1%) was the commonest form for all ages followed by pleurisy 11.2%, bones-joint TB and abdominal TB in 6.4% cases each and 1.9% cases each of neuro TB and miliary or disseminated TB. Out of total 669 cases of lymph node TB, cervical tuberculous lymphadenitis (88.2%) was the commonest site for all ages followed by axillary lymphadenitis in 3.3%. TB lymphadenitis of other sites was seen in only 57 (8.5%) cases.

Pleural Disease

It can be caused by:
- Allergic reaction to a small subpleural focus results in an acute onset of large pleural effusion in a well-nourished child with good hypersensitivity. It presents

with high fever and transient chest pain followed by breathlessness depending upon the amount of fluid collected.

- Occasionally, tubercle bacilli may directly spill over in large amount into pleural cavity from adjacent lung due to bursting of a subpleural focus resulting in the formation of a bronchopleural fistula and tuberculous empyema.
- Rarely, pleural fluid may leak into the layers of the chest wall visible as a swelling on the chest known as *empyema necessitans.*
- Dry pleuritis without effusion is the result of poor hypersensitivity. Persistent chest pain and localized pleural rub with a normal chest X-ray helps in the diagnosis.

Miliary Tuberculosis

Miliary TB is an outcome of poor immunity without hypersensitivity. Fever may be the only symptom; other nonspecific symptoms include generalized weakness, anorexia and loss of weight or no weight gain. Night sweats may be complained of by older children. Hepatosplenomegaly, generalized lymphadenopathy along with miliary shadows on chest X-ray are good clues to the diagnosis. Miliary mottling may be demonstrated more clearly by CT scan of chest. Diagnosis may be confirmed by liver biopsy or abnormal cerebrospinal fluid (CSF) cytology.

Tubercular Meningitis

Tubercular meningitis is an outcome of poor immunity in very young children or infants. It usually develops within the first year of infection. Fever, convulsions, altered sensorium, neurological deficit with signs of meningeal irritation and raised intracranial tension confirmed by abnormal CSF cytology, biochemistry and Ziehl–Neelsen (ZN) staining and in some cases by CT scan of head.

CLINICAL FEATURES

Symptoms

The primary stage of TB usually does not cause symptoms. The presentations of childhood TB disease are protean and this varied clinical spectrum has been changing over the years, reflecting a trend toward an early age of reinfection or reactivation. In our experience, we have seen bilateral extensive fibrocavitary disease even in a 10-month old infant. This emerging trend along with the resurgence of TB has changed the clinical spectrum of childhood TB to an extent that every constellation of symptoms and signs is possible (Table 4.7.2).

MODALITIES OF DIAGNOSIS

The diagnosis of TB in children can sometimes be extremely challenging and time consuming due to

Table 4.7.2: Showing clinical features.

Symptoms

- Fever (usually moderate grade with an evening rise) and/or cough with expectoration for at least 2 weeks duration
- Hemoptysis
- Breathlessness, wheeze
- Chest pain
- Fatigue, lethargy
- Loss of weight or no weight gain
- Anorexia
- History of contact
- Enlargement of lymph nodes
- Oligohypomenorrhea in adolescent girls without genital involvement
- Symptoms related to the site of involvement for EPTB

Signs

On general physical examination (any of the following):
- Malnutrition
- Lymphadenopathy—single, multiple or generalized, 1–2 cm in size, firm, nontender, discrete, nonfluctuant/fluctuant but usually matted, not fixed to skin or underlying structures or develop overlying sinuses. Most common site is cervical followed by axillary, mediastinal, mesenteric and retroperitoneal
- Hepatomegaly and/or splenomegaly
- Meningeal signs: altered sensorium, neurological deficit, signs of meningeal irritation in a case of TBM

Chest signs
- Signs of pleural effusion or ascites in case of their involvement

difficulties in the demonstration of acid fast bacilli (AFB), which is the confirmatory diagnosis. A "golden triad" consisting of clinical features, an abnormal radiograph of chest and a positive tuberculin skin Mantoux test (1, 2 or 5 TU PPD RT23 with Tween 80 with an induration of >10 mm after 48–72 hours), with a history of contact or close exposure with an adult having active TB in the last 2 years, remains the most commonly employed method for diagnosing PTB, along with every effort to confirm this diagnosis by demonstration of AFB and isolation of MTB from the clinical specimens or histopathology [diagnostic algorithms in Flowcharts 4.7.1 and 4.7.2 for PTB and extrapulmonary (lymph node) TB].

Thus, based on these diagnostic algorithms, the commonly used methods for diagnosing TB in a child are as follows:

Mycobacterial Detection and Isolation

In order to establish a confirmatory diagnosis, detection of AFB or MTB by staining of appropriate clinical specimens is necessary. Since this is one of the confirmatory tests, attempts should always be made in each case to isolate and demonstrate the AFB despite its poor sensitivity.

Specimens to be Used

Depending on the location of the disease, examination of sputum, induced sputum, gastric lavage (GL), bronchial

FLOWCHART 4.7.1: Diagnostic algorithm for pediatric pulmonary TB.

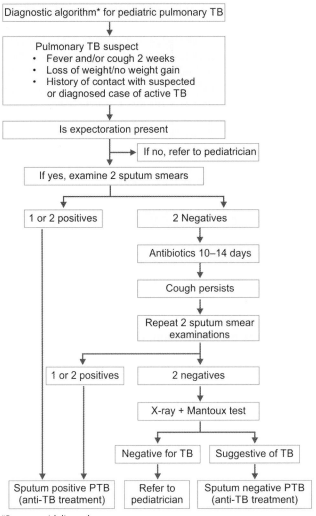

*Recent guidelines changes:
• Duration of fever and/or cough is for more than 2 weeks
• And only two sputum/GA examinations are to be done.

FLOWCHART 4.7.2: Diagnostic algorithm for TB lymphadenitis.

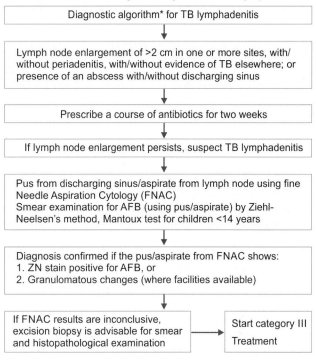

*Recent guidelines changes:
• Start category-I (New) and category-II (Retreatment) cases as category-III has been scrapped.

lavage, lung tissue, lymph node tissue, CSF, bone marrow, liver, blood, urine and stool may be undertaken.

Sputum, Induced Sputum, Gastric Lavage

Children less than 6 years of age are generally unable to expectorate unless and until endobronchial TB is present. However, where feasible, sputum analysis is best done in the morning. Recent recommendations of WHO and Revised National Tuberculosis Program (RNTCP) are to obtain a minimum of two samples (morning and spot) on same day. Saliva and nasopharyngeal secretions are not acceptable. In older children, adequate samples of deep bronchial secretions can be induced by stimulating cough with aerosolized isotonic saline (0.9%), although success is better with hypertonic saline (3–5%). Isotonic saline is better in cases of hyper-reactive airways, during exacerbation of asthma and severe asthma. Sputum may

be produced 30 minutes to even 24 hours after induction, so the patient may be sent home with sputum sample cups.

In younger children less than 6 years of age, GLs are used in lieu of sputum. The gastric aspirate (GA) or lavage should be obtained, after overnight fasting, first thing upon awakening for two consecutive days. The sensitivity of smears for identification of MTB is low (in the range of 25–30%) but specificity is very high (in the range of 90–99%). The yield of mycobacteria is high when the samples are repeated, in extensive pulmonary disease and in infants, where it is up to 60–70%.

Aspiration cytology: Fine needle aspiration (FNA) of cytological fluid from the lymph nodes, swellings and other involved areas can be used for either cytopathology or staining for AFB. In our study, out of total 622 (93%) cases of lymph node TB where fine needle aspiration and/or excision biopsy was done, it was positive (84.2%) and negative (15.6%) respectively for AFB or cytology, while it could not be done in 47 patients due to inaccessible sites.

Body fluid cytology: Lymphocytic exudative (protein >3.0 g/dL) fluid aspirates from the pleura, peritoneal or pericardial sacs is suggestive of TB. Occasionally, AFB staining of these aspirates may be positive for tuberculous bacilli. In our study on clinical profile and treatment outcome of tuberculous pleurisy in 106 children, diagnosis was made by X-ray chest in 92.5%, exudative pleural fluid

(100%) predominantly lymphocytic in 85.8%, positive AFB smear and culture in 4.7% and 5.7% cases respectively.

Histopathological Diagnosis

Pleural biopsy, lymph node, liver, bone marrow and transbronchial biopsy may reveal caseating granulomas, if these organs are involved.

Direct Smear

Smears made from sputum, induced sputum, body secretions or aspirates on a clean slide and stained with ZN stain for detecting AFB. Use of fluorescent dyes like Auramine O, etc. can improve the sensitivity of this test.

In our study, out of a total of 1,098 cases of PTB, sputum/induced sputum/GA was possible in only 818 patients. Out of these, 414 and 404 were smear positive and negative respectively while it could not be done in 280 patients. Sputum positivity increased with age. Smear positivity was highest (59%, 325/551) in 11–14 year age group followed by 6–10 years age group (34.7%; 68/196) and 0–5 years (29.6%; 21/71) for both new and retreatment cases combined. It increased significantly from age group of 6–10 years to 11–14 years (Or 3.42; 95% CI 2.0–5.86), whereas the increase was insignificant from 0–5 years to 6–10 years (Or = 1.26; 95% CI 0.70–2.28) stressing the fact that it was worth sending specimens like GA, induced sputum and "a deeply coughed up sputum after proper instructions" for microbiological examination for all PTB suspects. Also, simple measures like neutralization of GA within 1 hour of collection, liquefaction, decontamination and concentration of sputum, as was done in our study, increased bacterial yield appreciably. These procedures can be safely and effectively performed even for very small children.

Conventional Culture Techniques

Two types of solid media have traditionally been used: (1) an egg-based medium (Lowenstein Jensen) and (2) an agar-based medium (Middle brook 7H10 and 7H11). The growth of mycobacteria takes 6–8 weeks for colonies to appear and another 6–8 weeks for the drug sensitivity testing (DST). Sensitivity of culture methods in detecting mycobacteria is greater than direct smears.

Newer Rapid Growth Techniques

Several rapid techniques for detection of early growth (5–14 days as compared to 2–8 weeks with conventional methods) have been developed, which can help in obtaining the culture and sensitivity reports relatively early. Some commonly used rapid methods are based on principles of detection of radioactivity, immunofluorescence and colorimetry linked to bacillary growth and include the following:

- BACTEC system which is an automated radiometric culture method can detect the growth of mycobacteria more quickly than other conventional culture methods which use solid media. The system uses a liquid medium containing radio-labeled palmitic acid with radioactive carbon (^{14}C). Growth of mycobacteria within the system is measured as a daily growth index that detects the production of $^{14}CO_2$ by the living metabolizing organisms.
- Septicheck which is a biphasic broth-based system based on principle of growth detection by colorimetry
- Mycobacterial growth indicator tubes (MGIT) based on principles of growth detection by immunofluorescence.

Polymerase Chain Reaction

Polymerase chain reaction (PCR) is a promising tool for rapid diagnosis of TB but has the disadvantages of cost, technique, contamination and false positivity.

Rapid Identification of *Mycobacterium* Isolates

This can be done by lipid analysis, specific gene probes, PCR-RFLP methods or ribosomal RNA sequencing. Advances in knowledge about the complete genomic structure of tubercle bacillus has helped to develop gene probes and gene amplification methods for identification and detection of tubercle bacillus, either from culture specimen or directly from the clinical specimens. These rapid molecular techniques help in the fast detection of drug resistance also. While the gene probes can help in rapid identification of isolates, gene amplification methods (PCR as well as isothermal, real-time PCR) developed for diagnosis of TB is not only highly sensitive, especially in culture negative specimens, but also in children with paucibacillary forms of the disease. With these molecular methods and gene probes, drug resistant mutants to drugs like rifampicin can be detected with reasonable certainty within 90 minutes using the latest GeneXpert while combined rifampicin and isoniazid resistance and more recently probes to other first-line and reserve drugs can detect resistance within few hours using Line probe assays. These gene probes, gene amplification methods and *in situ* approaches offer unmatched sensitivity and specificity to enhance the diagnosis of TB in the future.

Radiological Examination

Chest roentgenograph is an important diagnostic tool in evaluating patients for PTB using posteroanterior and lateral views. Sometimes, apical (lordotic) and oblique films are helpful to assess the extent of lung involvement, apical lesions or extensive hilar adenopathy but are difficult to obtain in children. Lateral films can detect hilar adenitis not clearly appreciated in frontal films. Lateral decubitus views help to determine whether the effusion is freely moving or loculated.

Occasionally, lymphadenopathy may be detected on computed tomography (CT) as low attenuation lymph nodes with peripheral enhancement which may not be evident radiographically. In addition, CT findings, such as lymph node calcification, branching centrilobular nodules and miliary nodules, are helpful in making the diagnosis in cases where the radiograph is normal or equivocal. There is no radiological appearance specific to TB and chest X-ray can at best be just "suggestive of TB" with both interobserver and intraobserver discrepancies in radiographic reporting. In our study, out of a total of 1,098 cases of PTB, total of 427 (38.9%) patients had primary complex while 252, 163, 43, 24 and 189 patients had extensive parenchymal infiltrates, cavities, apical lesions, consolidation and combination of more than one type of radiological lesion respectively.

History of Close Contact

Close contact with an infectious case is of significance but it may not be clear-cut and may not be essentially in the household, e.g. a contact in the crowded day care center or classroom, in the close neighborhood of urban slums where a large number of people stay together in small poorly ventilated and poorly illuminated rooms.

Immunodiagnosis of Tuberculosis

- Mantoux test is a skin test based on hypersensitivity to TB antigen, that is 1, 2 or 5 TU PPD RT23 with Tween 80 is injected intradermally on the volar surface of left forearm and an induration of more than 10 mm after 48–72 hours is labeled as a positive test.
- Enzyme-linked immunosorbent assay (ELISA) using A60 or 38kDa antigen is one of the commonest tests used. Several recent studies have been conducted in children using ELISA to detect antibodies to various purified or complex antigens of MTB but none of these serodiagnostic tests has adequate sensitivity, specificity or reproducibility under various clinical conditions to be useful for routinely diagnosing TB in children.
- Interferon gamma radioimmunoassay (IGRA): These antigen-based tests are used to identify interferon producing peripheral mononuclear cells in patients of TB, namely IGRA, called QuantiFERON-Gold and enzyme-linked immunospot (ELISPOT) using CFP-10 and ESAT-6 antigen specific to MTB. These are used to measure the patient's immune reactivity to MTB. These are used for initial and serial testing of persons with risk of LTBI in developed countries, where the incidence-prevalence of TB is low. Sensitivity is comparable to the routinely used Mantoux test, being slightly more sensitive than the Mantoux test with results not influenced by the BCG vaccination, thus may be helpful in identifying true infections due to MTB but does not diagnose the disease.

Finally, the confirmation of diagnosis of childhood TB is difficult because of most primary disease being paucibacillary. The diagnosis is usually probable based on indirect evidences like prolonged symptomatology, history of contact, positive tuberculin test and roentgenographic abnormalities if many of these are present in conjunction. The clinical symptoms and signs of tubercular disease are so nonspecific and common that symptoms, like cough, fever, failure to gain weight, can lead to both over and under diagnosis. As these evidences are not very specific for the disease, confirmatory diagnosis should always be tried with all robustness. The search for a reliable test for diagnosing childhood TB continues to be one of the biggest challenges for our profession.

Differential Diagnosis

Nonresolving pneumonia can be due to atypical mycobacteria or *Mycobacterium* other than TB (MOTT), *legionella*, *Mycoplasma*, *Aspergillus* or *Pneumocystis jiroveci* pneumonia (PCP). These are diagnosed by bronchoalveolar lavage (BAL) culture and staining.

Atelectasis

History of any foreign body aspiration must be ruled out. High-resolution contrast-enhanced computed tomography (HRCECT) findings along with bronchoscopy is confirmative.

Immunological

Wegener's granulomatosis, allergic bronchopulmonary aspergillosis (ABPA), bronchiolitis obliterative organizing pneumonia (BOOP), idiopathic pulmonary fibrosis (IPF) all show usually bilateral disease with some family history with raised serum antibody titers.

Miscellaneous

Sarcoidosis diagnosed by positive Kveim test and sarcoid granuloma in transbronchial lung biopsy (TBLB); pulmonary alveolar proteinosis, a bilateral disease with onset since childhood.

TREATMENT

Basis of Combination Therapy

In general, combination chemotherapy is designed to kill the bacillary subpopulations, expected bacillary load based on the type of the disease and level of drug resistance. Four subpopulations of bacilli are present in a host, depending upon the metabolic activity:

- *Rapidly growing or multiplying bacilli:* Because the TB bacillus is an obligate aerobe, it is active and divides freely where oxygen tension is high and pH is neutral or alkaline. Such environmental conditions are prevalent in cavities, leading to a very large bacterial population.

- *Slow growing (intracellular)*: TB bacilli present within the macrophages, e.g. site of inflammation where pH is acidic.
- *Spurters*: Group of bacilli present in the caseous material are slowly dividing due to low oxygen tension and neutral pH.
- *Dormant*: Some bacilli remain dormant due to adverse environment and this dormancy period can be prolonged with most of the antitubercular drugs unable to act upon these dormant bacteria. Thus, these bacilli are the usual cause of subsequent relapse.

Children with primary PTB and EPTB are infected with a much less number of tubercle bacilli and expected bacillary load is paucibacillary. Another important bacteriologic consideration is the presence of naturally occurring drug-resistant mutants in bacterial subpopulation even before chemotherapy is started (primary resistance). Although most of the bacillary population is "drug susceptible", a subpopulation of drug resistant mutants occurs at a fairly predictable rate of about 10^{-6} bacterial divisions and varies slightly for various antitubercular drugs:

- Streptomycin 10^{-5}
- Isoniazid 10^{-8} to 10^{-9}
- Ethambutol 10^{-6}
- Rifampicin 10^{-8}

A closed caseous lesion containing 10^{2-5} tubercle bacilli has few or none drug-resistant bacilli while a cavity having 10^{7-9} bacilli has thousands of drug-resistant organisms respectively. Thus, three different subpopulations of drug-resistant organisms present in a host in varied proportions depending on history of prior antitubercular treatment (ATT) can be:

- Resistant to isoniazid alone
- Resistant to rifampicin alone
- Resistant to both isoniazid and rifampicin.

The occurrence of chance resistance to one drug is unrelated to that for other antitubercular drugs. For an organism to be 'naturally' resistant to two drugs (primary multidrug resistance) the population size would have to be 10^{11}–10^{17} which is comparatively rare in clinical practice. Thus, when three or more effective drugs are used in combination for treatment of TB, there are negligible chances of drug resistance and cross-resistance. In patients with multidrug resistant (MDR) TB, the proportion of the subpopulations of drug-resistant organisms resistant to both isoniazid and rifampicin, present in a host is much more than the other two subpopulations (resistant to isoniazid or rifampicin alone) and this is either due to sequential selection of drug resistant strains on repeated poor drug therapies or else due to transmission of infection from an infectious MDR case, as is more common in children.

Table 4.7.3: Pediatric dosages as mg/kg.

Drugs	RNTCP 2012 (Thrice a week)	WHO (2010) (Daily)	Major adverse effects
Isoniazid	12–18	10 (10–15)	Peripheral neuropathy, hepatotoxicity
Rifampicin	12–18	10 (10–20)	Hepatotoxicity, gastritis, flu like illness
Pyrazinamide	35–45	35 (30–40)	Arthralgia, hepatotoxicity
Ethambutol	30 (25–35)	30 (15–25)	Oculotoxicity
Streptomycin	15–25	15 (12–18)	Tinnitus

The combinations of various bacterial subpopulations, their size and the proportion of drug resistant mutations explain why a single antitubercular drug cannot be used to cure TB. In children with pulmonary cavities, extensive pulmonary infiltrates and disseminated TB, there are many bacilli resistant to at least one of the first line drugs necessitating the use of more than three antitubercular drugs. A single effective drug would allow the selection and final emergence of a dominantly resistant population. Children with progressive primary PTB and EPTB have moderate bacterial load where significant numbers of drug resistant mutants may/may not be present, and effective therapy requires at least two bactericidal drugs. But the recent WHO and RNTCP Guidelines recommend at least four drugs in the initial phase for all new patients irrespective of the extent of involvement. Table 4.7.3 lists the essential anti-TB drugs and their doses. Certain principles of anti-TB chemotherapy have emerged over the years (Box 4.7.1). These principles make the understanding of chemotherapy easier and more rationale.

Currently Prescribed Regimens

Different antitubercular drugs have different activities, i.e. some are bactericidal or bacteriostatic. Their action also differs in their sterilizing activity, bactericidal activity and prevention of emergence of resistance.

Rifampicin and isoniazid are active against all four subpopulations in intermittent short spans of only a few hours. Pyrazinamide has a very potent bactericidal activity against intracellular organisms, especially those inside macrophages in acidic environment. Clinical studies indicate that its maximum effect during the initial phase of therapy rather than throughout the full course of treatment and contributes to an early sterilization. Ethambutol is an oral drug and safe to use in children making it easier and cheaper to administer than injectable streptomycin and should be used for all age groups except in cases of optic neuritis and under ophthalmological supervision in cases of TBM.

Principles of antituberculosis treatment.
- Combination of various antitubercular drugs are used to kill different bacterial subpopulations and the drug resistant mutants, as single drug therapy is associated with a very high risk of developing resistance
- Number and inclusion of drugs in initial phase should take into account the prevalence of drug resistance in the infectious pool of the community
- Rifampicin, isoniazid, pyrazinamide form the backbone of all initial modern short-course chemotherapy regimens
- Continuing pyrazinamide beyond initial phase of 2–3 months is not usually recommended
- Ethambutol is relatively safe for all age groups and can be used in all types of the diseases including TB meningitis
- Most of the currently recommended short-course regimens include an initial intensive phase of 2 months of four drugs (rifampicin, isoniazid, pyrazinamide and ethambutol), followed by a 4-month continuation phase of two drugs (rifampicin and isoniazid) for all new patients (Refer Category I in the Treatment Table)
- Defaulter, failure or relapse requires retreatment should be treated with all the first line drugs of the armamentarium (refer Category II in the Treatment Table).
- Short course treatment for 6 months is efficacious for most situations and is as effective when used as daily or intermittent therapy
- Intermittent treatment should always be directly observed. Under directly observed treatment short-course (DOTS) strategy of WHO and Revised National Tuberculosis Control Program (RNTCP), thrice weekly regimens are given in patient-wise boxes (PWB) under direct observation
- Ensuring adherence and completion of treatment is a responsibility of the prescriber or provider
- A single drug should never be added to a failing regime

The intensive initial phase is designed to eradicate most of the tubercle bacilli in all four subpopulations quickly, whereas the continuation phase slowly eliminates the several logs that remain. Rifampicin, isoniazid, pyrazinamide form the backbone of all initial modern short-course chemotherapy regimens. Most of the currently recommended WHO and RNTCP regimens are of short duration and include an initial intensive phase of 2 months with four drugs (rifampicin, isoniazid, pyrazinamide and ethambutol), followed by a continuation phase containing two drugs (rifampicin and isoniazid) for all new patients. Isoniazid and rifampin are most commonly used drugs in the continuation phase because they kill bacilli in all four subpopulations. Continuation phase is prolonged to 10 months for patients with meningeal, disseminated or bone-joint TB with total treatment duration of 12 months.

Daily versus Intermittent Therapy

Prolonged treatment of minimum 6–8 months, number of adverse drug reactions associated with daily therapy and cost of therapy are important factors for noncompliance contributing toward treatment failure. To overcome this, studies on efficacy of intermittent therapy were attempted. The scientific basis of intermittent chemotherapy is the long

generation time (18–21 hours) of the tubercle bacilli after a culture of MTB is exposed to a particular anti-tubercular drug. The number of bacilli continues to fall for some time before re-multiplication begins again. This period when the drug is not available and before organisms begin to multiply again is called "Lag Phase". It is of variable duration depending on the type of drug used and the length of exposure to that drug. It is possible to suppress further replication of the bacilli if the next dose is given before the end of the lag period. This forms the basis of intermittent therapy. But intermittent therapy should always be given under direct observation and the patient actually swallows the drugs in front of a treatment supervisor, as even a single dose cannot be missed. The onus of treatment lies on the health worker to ensure adherence and compliance to treatment through proper interventions in all cases. Thus, self-administered intermittent therapy should be strongly discouraged.

Directly Observed Treatment Short-Course (DOTS) Strategy

Under directly observed treatment short-course (DOTS) strategy of WHO and RNTCP (Table 4.7.4) endorsed by the Government of India, thrice weekly regimens are given in patient-wise boxes (PWB) under direct observation. However, the same combination of drugs can also be given on a daily basis, if observation is not possible. It may not be out of place to emphasize that the healthcare providers (doctors and related staff) are fully responsible for ensuring free diagnosis and completing the full course of free treatment and the patient actually swallows the drugs in front of a treatment supervisor.

The recommended dosages given according to the child's weight as mg/kg are shown in (see Table 4.7.3) and the case definitions used for all cases diagnosed in (Table 4.7.4).

Patients with TBM are prescribed antitubercular drugs along with decongestive measures and steroids.

Indian Data on Directly Observed Treatment Short-Course (DOTS) Strategy

Directly-observed treatment short-course appears to be highly efficacious treatment strategy for pediatric PTB and EPTB as has been shown by our studies.

In our study on retrospective analysis of DOTS strategy for treatment of 1,098 patients of pediatric PTB, the cure rate was 92.4% (302/327) and 92% (80/87) for new and retreatment cases (χ_1^2=0.02, p=0.901), but the treatment completion rate was significantly higher for new cases (97%; 636/656) than retreatment cases (53.6%; 15/28) (χ_1^2=100.8, p <0.001). Overall success rate was 95.4% and 82.6% for new and retreatment cases respectively (χ_1^2=30.35, p <0.001). There was an overall 3% default rate, 1.9% failure rate and 1% death rate in the study.

Table 4.7.4: Revised National Tuberculosis Program treatment categories and regimens for children.

Category of treatment	Type of patient	Tuberculosis treatment regimens	
		Intensive phase	Continuation phase
Category I	New sputum smear-positive pulmonary tuberculosis (PTB) New sputum smear-negative PTB New extrapulmonary tuberculosis (EPTB)	$2 H_3R_3Z_3E_3$*	$4 H_3R_3$
Category II	Relapse Failure Treatment after default	$2 S_3H_3R_3Z_3E_3$** $+ 1H_3R_3Z_3E_3$	$5 H_3R_3E_3$

*In children, PTB includes all forms of PTB including primary complex. EPTB includes lymph node TB, skin TB, pleurisy, pleural effusion, TB meningitis (TBM), miliary TB, disseminated TB, TB pericarditis, TB peritonitis and intestinal TB, spinal TB with/without neurological complications, genitourinary TB and bone-joint TB.

**Prefix indicates month and subscript indicates thrice weekly.

For EPTB, retrospective analysis of 669 children of lymph node TB treated with DOTS strategy over 9 1/2 years showed an overall treatment completion rate was 94.9% and the default rate was 2.2% with a failure rate of 2.5%, death rate was 0.3%. While overall treatment completion rate was 94.3%, 4.7% default rate, 0.9% failure rate and no deaths for 106 children of tubercular pleurisy.

Adjunctive Treatment

Indications of Steroids

Given as 1 mg/kg body weight and tapered gradually over 6–8 weeks:

- Tuberculous meningitis—helpful in reducing vasculitis, inflammation and intracranial pressure to prevent long-term neurologic sequelae in patients with TBM
- Pericarditis and pericardial effusion
- Conditions causing severe respiratory distress or fall in oxygen saturation, e.g. miliary TB with alveolar-capillary block, endobronchial TB causing localized obstruction and emphysema, mediastinal lymph nodal compression
- Massive pleural effusions, peritonitis occasionally
- To suppress severe drug-related hypersensitivity reactions.

Indications of Pyridoxine
(in Dose of 40–100 mg/day)

Pyridoxine supplementation is not used routinely. However, pyridoxine is used to prevent and treat central and peripheral nervous system side effects of isoniazid which may develop in those having one or more of the following conditions: exclusively breastfed babies, severe malnutrition, HIV coinfection, chronic liver or renal disease, pre-existing peripheral neuropathy.

RECENT WHO (2010) AND RNTCP (2012) RECOMMENDATIONS

- Recommended dosages for children living in settings where the prevalence of HIV is high or where resistance to isoniazid is high or both, have recently been increased for isoniazid, rifampicin, pyrazinamide and ethambutol (preferably to be given daily in sick admitted patients or patients with confirmed HIV infection) (*see* Table 4.7.3). Previous experience suggests that these drugs are well tolerated with very low risk of toxicity when used in the revised dosages, at least in HIV-uninfected children.
- Weight gain in response to anti-TB therapy can be such that the child moves to another weight band during therapy requiring a higher dosage.
- Children with suspected or confirmed TBM, miliary TB and osteoarticular (OA) TB should be treated with a four-drug regimen (HRZE) for 2 months, followed by a two-drug regimen (HR) for 10 months; the total duration of treatment being 12 months.
- Tablets of fixed-dose drug combinations have several advantages over individual drugs including less likelihood of prescription errors and lesser pill burden.

Monitoring

Follow-up sputum examinations should be performed at 2, 4 and 6 months. Sputum examination is done as per Algorithm in Flowchart 4.7.3 and Table 4.7.5.

Table 4.7.5: Managing patients with interruptions in treatment.

Duration of therapy	Duration of interruption		Decision
Up to 4 weeks	<2 weeks		Resume original regime
	>2 weeks		Reassess and start treatment again
4–8 weeks	<2 weeks		Resume original regime
	2–8 weeks		Extend intensive phase by 1 month more
	>8 weeks		Consider Category II if diagnosis is still active TB
>8 weeks	<2 weeks		Resume original regime
	>2 weeks	Review activity	• No active disease: Continue same treatment • Active disease: Category II therapy

FLOWCHART 4.7.3: Algorithm for clinical monitoring.

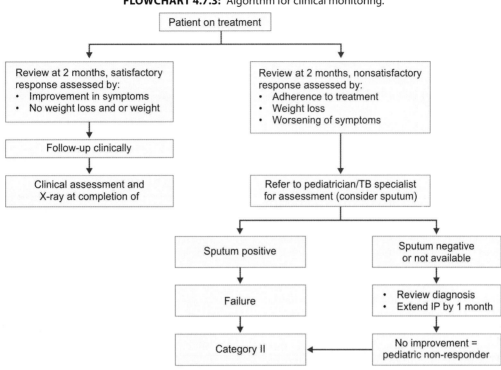

COMPLICATIONS

Drug Resistance

Drug resistance is an emerging problem in children. With the resurgence of TB, MDR (MTB bacilli strains resistant to rifampicin and isoniazid) and extreme-resistant (strains resistant to rifampicin, isoniazid plus injectable aminoglycoside and fluoroquinolone) strain is being increasingly found in children. Prolonged treatment, dependency on parents for finances and medicines, ignorance are important factors for nonadherence and poor compliance resulting in treatment failure and drug resistance. Various other factors, like poor drug prescription, use of substandard drugs, poor case management, HIV epidemic and, in addition population shift, are contributing to these problems.

Resistance can be primary, if the source of infection has resistant MDR-TB but can be secondary resistance in a child who has taken irregular ATT in the past, remains smear positive on category I or category II retreatment regimen with sputum AFB positive at 5 months or more (failure) or there is a fall and rise phenomenon, i.e. initially sputum smear becomes negative (or less positive) and later becomes persistently positive.

In all suspected cases, patients should be managed in a specialized unit. Bacteriological studies are mandatory on samples from sputum, induced sputum, GL, BAL, histopathology samples, fluid aspirates wherever available. Prompt diagnosis of drug resistance is made by specialized

Newer rapid investigations like MGIT/BACTEC culture and most recently GeneXpert or Line probe assay from a standardized WHO accredited laboratory. At present one intermediate reference laboratory (IRLs) has been set-up in every state while there are four national reference laboratories (NRLs) in the country with two laboratories blood sugar and HIV testing is also done.. These patients are prescribed reserve drugs in adequate doses which are very toxic, less effective and costly. Therefore, reserved drugs should be given as a daily regimen under direct observation until completion of full course of therapy, minimum of 2 years as DOTS-Plus. DOTS-Plus is being implemented in a phased manner with three types of PWB and have been made available for 16–25, 26–45 and more than 45 kg—three weight bands.

Dual infection with HIV, the lethal combination must be kept in mind when treating TB especially in cases of failure and suspected drug resistance. Thus, HIV testing should always be done. Antitubercular treatment and highly active antiretroviral therapy (HAART) should be started simultaneously in patients with dual infection. Other chronic debilitating diseases, diabetes, drug addiction, malignancy, use of steroids and chemotherapeutic agents should also be ruled out.

PROGNOSIS

Children with untreated latent infection act as a reservoir and may progress to disease. Among the infants (< 1 year), approximately 43% of those infected will develop the disease (usually primary), compared to 24% of children 1–5 years, 15% of adolescents and 10% of adults over a lifetime. Incidence is normally low between 5 and 10 years and then increases in adolescence (11–14 years) when PTB manifests like adult TB (postprimary disease). Our data suggests that the disease is more common in 11–14 years old and in females except for very small children where the sex ratio is reversed.

Moreover, the occurrence of MDR and extreme drug resistant (XDR-TB) MTB strains has been reported in children through isolated reports, both published and unpublished from our country, but it is yet not possible to estimate the exact magnitude and distribution from the available data in children. In India, there are almost 20,000 new MDR infections in 1 year. The prevalence of MDR-TB in adult and children combined, new smear positives (initial or primary resistance) is less than 3% while it is 12–17% amongst the previously treated smear positives (secondary or acquired resistance) respectively. Review of studies with representative samples does not indicate any increase in the prevalence of drug resistance over the years but this has definitely reduced the efficacy of ATT to the pre-treatment era. This is presenting an increasing threat to the global TB control and an added responsibility on the shoulders of all those involved in the management of these children. Nevertheless, documenting the level of drug-resistance in community is important in order to monitor the impact of national TB control programmed over time and also to ensure whether the treatment regimens being prescribed are appropriate.

PREVENTION

Chemoprophylaxis

Child contacts of smear-positive TB cases, especially those below 6 years of age, must be screened (Algorithm for chemoprophylaxis 4 in Flowchart 4.7.4. This is regardless of the bacillus of Calmette-Guérin (BCG) vaccination status.

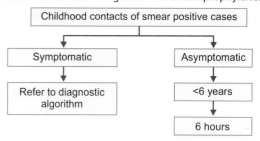

FLOWCHART 4.7.4: Algorithm for chemoprophylaxis.

BIBLIOGRAPHY

1. Chauhan LS, Arora VK, Central TB Division, et al. Management of pediatric tuberculosis under the Revised National Tuberculosis Control Program (RNTCP). Indian Pediatr. 2004;41(9):901-5.

2. Graham SM. Treatment of tuberculosis in children: revised WHO. Guidelines Paediatr Respir Rev. 2011;12:22-6.

3. Sharma S, Sarin R, Khalid UK, et al. Clinical profile and treatment outcome of tubercular pleurisy in pediatric age group using DOTS strategy. Indian J Tuberc. 2009;56: 191-200.

4. Sharma S, Sarin R, Khalid UK, et al. Clinical profile and treatment outcome of tuberculous lymphadenitis in children using DOTS strategy. Indian J Tuberc. 2010;57(1):4-11.

5. Sharma S, Sarin R, Khalid UK, et al. The DOTS strategy for treatment of pediatric pulmonary tuberculosis in South Delhi, India. Int J Tuberc Lung Dis. 2008;12(1):74-80.

6. Sharma S. Childhood tuberculosis. In: Arora VK, Arora R (Eds). Issues in Practical Approach to Tuberculosis Management, 1st edition. Delhi: Jaypee Brothers Medical Publishers Pvt Ltd; 2006. pp. 39-55.

7. Sharma S. Drug resistant tuberculosis in children. In: Ganguly N, Ghosh TK (Eds). Typhoid, Tuberculosis and Malaria, 1st edition. Kolkata: An IAP ID Chapter Publication; 2005.

8. World Health Organization. Treatment of tuberculosis in children WHO/HTM/TB/2010.13.

4.8 | LEPROSY

Rajeshwar Dayal

INTRODUCTION

Leprosy, also known as Hansen's disease, is a chronic granulomatous disease caused by *Mycobacterium leprae*. It can affect all the organs of the body but has predilection for the skin, peripheral nerves, mucosa of upper respiratory tract and eyes.

EPIDEMIOLOGY

World

The global registered prevalence of leprosy at the beginning of 2011 stood at 192,246 cases, and 228,474 new cases were detected during the year 2010. Previously highly endemic countries have now reached elimination (defined as reaching a prevalence of less than 1 leprosy case per 10,000 population) at the national level and are now intensifying their efforts at regional and district levels. However, pockets of high endemicity still remain in some areas of Angola, Brazil, Central African Republic, Democratic Republic of Congo, India, Madagascar, Mozambique, Nepal and the United Republic of Tanzania.

India

According to "WHO Global Leprosy Situation 2010", 87,190 cases of leprosy reside in India. All the countries of SEAR have now achieved the elimination target of less than 1/10,000 population. India achieved the leprosy elimination target at the end of 2005. Although the total number of registered cases of leprosy came down to 87,190 in 2010 in India, the new case detection rate did not reduce concomitantly. A total of 133,717 new cases of leprosy were detected in India in 2009.

Pediatric Leprosy

Pediatric leprosy constitutes about 10% of the total disease burden. The age group most commonly affected in the pediatric leprosy population is 5–14 years, although in very high endemic countries, prevalence in age groups 0–4 years is also significant. The prevalence is higher among males. Human immunodeficiency virus (HIV) infection has not been documented to alter the risk of leprosy in areas of high prevalence.

PATHOGENESIS

When *M. leprae* was discovered by GA Hansen in 1873, it was the first bacterium to be identified as causing disease in man. The etiological agent of leprosy, *M. leprae*, is a strongly acid-fast rod-shaped organism with parallel sides and rounded ends. In size and shape, it closely resembles the tubercle bacillus. It occurs in large numbers in the lesions of lepromatous leprosy, chiefly in masses within the lepra cells, often grouped together like bundles of cigars or arranged in a palisade. Chains are never seen. Most striking are the intracellular and extracellular masses, known as globi, which consist of clumps of bacilli in capsular material. It is believed that only leprosy bacilli which stain with carbol-fuchsin as solid acid-fast rods are viable and those bacilli which stain irregularly are probably dead and degenerating.

The bacteriological index (BI) is an expression of the extent of bacterial loads. It is calculated by counting six to eight stained smears under the 100 x oil immersion lens in a smear made by nicking the skin with a sharp scalpel and scraping it; the fluid and tissue obtained are spread fairly thickly on a slide and stained by the Ziehl-Neelsen method and decolorized (but not completely) which 1% acid alcohol. The results are expressed on a logarithmic scale (Box 4.8.1).

The bacteriological index is valuable because it is simple and is representative of many lesions but is affected by the depth of the skin incision, the thoroughness of the scrape and the thickness of the film.

The morphological index (MI) is calculated by counting the numbers of solid-staining acid-fast rods. Only the solid-staining bacilli are viable. It is important to recognize that measurement of MI is liable for observer variations and therefore not always reliable.

MODES OF TRANSMISSION

The only source of infection is the infected human being. The capacity of multibacillary leprosy patients to transmit the infection is 4–11 times that of patients with paucibacillary leprosy. For direct transmission, a prolonged and close contact is required. An "intrafamilial" contact with a patient is more risky than an "extrafamilial" one. It is transmitted via droplets from the nose and the mouth of untreated patients with severe disease, but is not highly infectious.

Box 4.8.1

Results expressed on a logarithmic scale.
- 1+ At least 1 bacillus in every 100 fields
- 2+ At least 1 bacillus in every 10 fields
- 3+ At least 1 bacillus in every field
- 4+ At least 10 bacilli in every field
- 5+ At least 100 bacilli in every field
- 6+ At least 1,000 bacilli in every field

Untreated lepromatous patients discharge as many as 100 million bacilli from their nasal secretions every day. These bacilli remain viable outside the human body in the nasal secretions for several days. Inhalation of these bacilli, via droplets, is now regarded as the most common mode of entry of leprosy bacilli into the contact person. After inhalation, these inhaled leprosy bacilli enter the respiratory system from where they are disseminated by blood to skin and peripheral nerves where depending on the host immune response, the disease may manifest either as tuberculoid leprosy (where there is good cell mediated immune response to *M. leprae*) or may manifest at lepromatous leprosy (where there is energy to *M. leprae*).

Other portals of entry include scratched, abraded or insect bitten skin which facilitates passage of organism via the droplets laden with leprosy bacilli through the epidermis into the dermis, and ingestion of infected breast milk. Occasionally, leprosy may spread by fomites being used by a patient suffering from multibacillary leprosy. Localized infections via infected syringes and tattooing needles have been reported.

CLINICAL FEATURES

Incubation Period

This varies from a few months to as long as 20 years with an average incubation time of 2–5 years.

Skin

A hypopigmented patch in the skin, present for a long duration, nonirritating with loss of sensation to touch, pain and temperature. There may be thickening of the skin, and it becomes more red and shiny in appearance than the surrounding parts; this is more prominent on face and hands. Loss of sensation, numbness, feeling of "pins and needles" or "crawling of ants", tingling sensation in any part of the body, especially in hands and feet are other common manifestations of leprosy in children. There may be paresis in hands and feet or difficulty in fine movements of fingers. Appearance of spontaneous blisters and ulcers, especially in the fingers, may occur.

Nerves

Thickened nerves, mainly peripheral nerve trunks constitute another feature of leprosy. A thickened nerve is often accompanied by other signs as a result of damage to the nerve. These may be loss of sensation in the skin and weakness of muscles supplied by the affected nerve. In the absence of these signs, nerve thickening by itself without sensory loss and/or muscle weakness is often not a reliable sign of leprosy. There may be involvement of one or more nerve roots or trunk. The nerve trunk becomes enlarged, hard, tender and later may form a nerve abscess. The affected nerves become thickened and tender,

producing sensory motor and trophic changes in their areas of distribution. This dysfunction leads to deformities, neuropathic ulcers and lagophthalmos, which may result in serious eye complications. The nerves most commonly involved in leprosy are ulnar, median, lateral popliteal, tibial, great auricular and rarely radial nerves. It also affects the V and VII cranial nerves.

CLINICAL VARIETIES OF LEPROSY

According to the classification laid down by Indian Association of Leprologists, the cases have been divided into five broad groups, viz. (1) indeterminate, (2) borderline, (3) tuberculoid, (4) lepromatous and (5) polyneuritic. The borderline group is further subdivided into mid borderline (BB), borderline lepromatous (BL) and borderline tuberculoid (BT) types.

Indeterminate Leprosy

This type of leprosy is seen in only 10–20% of infected individuals and is the earliest detectable form of leprosy and is characterized by the presence of a single hypopigmented macule measuring 2–4 cm in diameter, with a poorly defined border without any erythema or induration. Anesthesia may be minimal or even absent. Biopsy may show a granuloma but bacilli are rarely seen in the section. In 50–75% of patients, this lesion heals spontaneously, and in the remaining cases it gradually progresses to one of the classic forms.

Tuberculoid Leprosy

This type of leprosy occurs in persons with good cell mediated immunity. It is characterized by the presence of single or few asymmetrical, well defined, hypopigmented, erythematous or copper colored patches with sensory impairment. The entire patch or only its margins is raised above the level of the surrounding skin. At times, these patches may not be raised above the level of the surrounding skin. In this form of leprosy, the lepromin test is positive and skin smear fails to detect bacilli. On biopsy, foci of lymphocytes, epithelioid cells and Langhans giant cells are seen. This form of leprosy is the most common, especially in children, and is relatively benign and stable with a good prognosis.

Borderline Leprosy

Borderline leprosy is further classified into three subtypes on clinical and histological criteria.

Borderline Tuberculoid (BT) Leprosy

Here the lesions are greater in number but smaller in size than in tuberculoid leprosy. There may be small satellite lesions around older lesions and the margins of the borderline tuberculoid lesions are less distinct and the center is less atrophic and anesthetic. This form usually involves thickening of two or more superficial nerves.

Mid Borderline (BB) Leprosy

In this subtype, the lesions are more numerous and heterogeneous. The lesions may become confluent or even plaques may be present. The borders are poorly defined and the erythematous rim fades into the surrounding skin. Hyperesthesia is more common than anesthesia.

Borderline Lepromatous (BL) Leprosy

In borderline lepromatous leprosy, there are a large number of asymmetrically distributed lesions which are heterogeneous in appearance. Macules, papules, plaques and nodules may all coexist. Usually, the individual lesions are small unless confluent. Anesthesia is mild, and superficial nerve trunks are spared (Fig. 4.8.1).

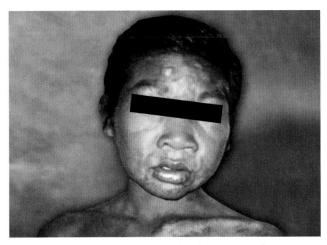

FIG. 4.8.1: A child with borderline lepromatous leprosy.

Lepromatous Leprosy

Most cases of lepromatous leprosy develop from borderline leprosy (BB or BL). This form of leprosy is relatively uncommon in the pediatric age group. There are two symptoms, which may precede the classical skin lesions by months or years, and serve to alert the physician to a possible early diagnosis. They are: (i) nasal symptoms and (ii) edema of legs. The nasal symptoms chiefly constitute, stuffiness, crust formation and blood stained discharge. Edema of legs and ankles is always bilateral, usually prominent late in the evening and disappears after overnight rest. Skin lesions may take the form of macules, papules, nodules and a combination of them. Numerous symmetrically distributed erythematous or coppery, shiny, macules with ill-defined margins are usually the first ones to appear. Patients may have a leonine facies due to loss of eyebrows and eyelashes. There is no sensory impairment in these lesions but as the disease progresses many peripheral nerves get symmetrically affected. Due to enormous bacillary infiltration, nerves are initially softer and larger than normal and are tender. In advanced cases, nerves become thin and hard due to fibrosis and result in extreme anesthesia. The skin smear is almost always positive and the lepromin test is negative. This form of lepromatous leprosy (LL) is the most infectious, prone to lepra reactions and, if left untreated, the prognosis is poor.

The features of these varieties of leprosy are summarized in Table 4.8.1. As age advances, the disease moves from tuberculoid end of the spectrum toward the lepromatous end.

Neuritic Leprosy

This may be of primary or secondary variety. In the former, the nerves are directly infected without any skin lesion while in the latter infection spreads up the nerves from leprous skin lesions. The affected nerves become thickened

Features	Types of leprosy				
	TT	BT	BB	BL	LL
Number of lesions	Single usually	Single or few	Several	Many	Very many
Size of lesions	Variable	Variable	Variable	Variable	Small
Surface of lesions	Very dry, sometimes scaly	Dry	Slightly shiny	Shiny	Shiny
Sensation in lesions	Absent	Markedly diminished	Moderately diminished	Slightly diminished	Not affected
Hair growth	Absent	Markedly diminished	Moderately diminished	Slightly diminished	Not affected
AFB in lesions	Nil	Nil or scanty	Moderate numbers	Many	Very many (plus globi)
AFB in nasal scrapings/in nose blows	Nil	Nil	Nil	Usually nil	Very many (plus globi)
Lepromin test	Strongly positive (+++)	Weakly positive (+ or ++)	Negative	Negative	Negative

Table 4.8.1: Differentiating points of various types of leprosy.

Abbreviations: AFB, acid-fast bacilli; TT, tuberculoid; BT, borderline tuberculoid; BB, mid borderline; BL, borderline lepromatous; LL, lepromatous leprosy.

and tender, producing sensory motor and trophic changes in their areas of distribution. This dysfunction leads to deformities, neuropathic ulcers and lagophthalmos, which may result in serious eye complications.

DIAGNOSIS

In an endemic country or area, a child should be regarded as having leprosy if he/she shows at least two of the first three cardinal signs given below or last sign independently:
• Characteristic skin lesions
• Partial or total loss of sensation in skin lesions
• Thickened nerves
• Acid fast bacilli in skin or nasal smear.

Smear Examination

In a small proportion of cases, rod-shaped, red-stained leprosy bacilli, which are diagnostic of the disease, may be seen in the smears taken from the affected skin when examined under a microscope after appropriate staining. Sites of bacteriological examination are usually the most affected parts of the lesion. If no definite patches or areas of thickened skin are visible, smear should be taken from ear lobules and buttock. Smears should be made by "slit and scrape" method and stained by Ziehl-Neelsen staining (Fig. 4.8.2). Smears are positive in LL, BL and some BB and BT cases. It is of limited help in TT and indeterminate lesions and patients with early atypical clinical presentation.

Bacillary Index

It is a semiquantitative estimation of the density of bacilli present in the skin smears and biopsies and is measured on two scales, namely the Dharmendra scale and the Ridley scale. It measures the total acid fast bacilli in microscopic field, which includes both live and dead bacilli.

Patients are labeled as having paucibacillary infection when there are less than five skin lesions and no bacilli on skin smears. They are labeled as having multibacillary

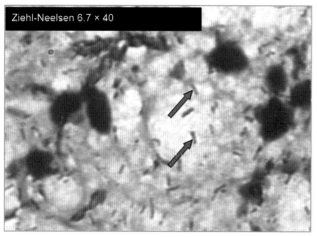

Ziehl-Neelsen 6.7 × 40

FIG. 4.8.2: Smear microscopy by Ziehl-Neelsen staining.

infection when there are greater than 6 skin lesions and bacilli are present on skin smears. The bacterial index can range from 0 (no bacilli in 100 oil immersion field) to 6 (> 1,000 bacilli per field).

Immunological Methods—Tests for Cell Mediated Immunity

Lepromin Test

Lepromin test is not a diagnostic test for leprosy but has been found to be useful for classifying the disease. This test is positive in cases of TT and BT, negative in LL, BL and weakly positive and variable in BB leprosy. The lepromin negative contacts have been found to be a much higher risk of developing disease, than the lepromin positive contacts. This test signifies immunity of person, i.e. cell mediated immunity against *M. leprae*, to its antigen. Two kinds of lepromin are commonly used: (a) crude antigen of Mitsuda and (b) the refined antigen of Dharmendra.

Serological Assays

Specific serological tests can detect subclinical infection. The major serological assays include the following:

Fluorescent Leprosy Antibody Absorption Test (FLA-ABS)

This technique is highly sensitive in detecting the antibodies against *M. leprae* antigen by immune-fluorescent technique and is useful in identifying healthy contacts of patients who are at risk of developing disease.

Radioimmunoassay (RIA)

It detects antibodies to the cell wall antigen of *M. leprae*.

Enzyme-Linked Immunosorbent Assay (ELISA)

PGL-ELISA was found highly positive in multibacillary cases, but positivity in paucibacillary and subclinical cases was quite low.

Further simplified dot ELISA and dipstick ELISA using a monoclonal antibody targeting PGL-1 have also been studied.

Serological testing is not useful for diagnosis as it does not detect most paucibacillary cases and it remains positive even after treatment of multibacillary patients.

MOLECULAR BIOLOGICAL APPROACHES

Identification of organisms can be done in a more rapid and specific way, both from culture and directly from clinical specimen, by recombinant DNA technology. Based on the gene sequences of *M. leprae*, several probes have been designed in recent years. Our institute has also studied the probes developed at Agra and found them to be of immense help for early diagnosis of the disease.

During the recent years, several gene amplification techniques (PCR) for amplifying *M. leprae* specific sequences from variety of specimens have been published. These have been reported to be highly sensitive and specific.

In Situ PCR

In situ PCR, also called slide PCR, is a method to run PCR directly on small tissue samples, tissue microarrays (TMA), or other small cell samples, rather than extracting DNA or RNA first, and then performing PCR, rtPCR, or qPCR from the extracted material. In our study, *in situ* PCR showed a positivity of 57.1% in early or localized form of leprosy (indeterminate or BT) and 61.5% in BB or BL group. When compared to histopathological examination, a significant enhancement of 15% in diagnosis was seen. Hence, we can conclude that *in situ* PCR, with added advantages of providing structural correlates and concomitant study of tissue pathology, improves diagnostic yield in early doubtful cases of leprosy and when histopathology in nonspecific.

In Situ Hybridization

In situ hybridization uses a labeled complementary DNA or RNA strand to localize specific DNA or RNA in a portion or section of tissue. Non-radioactive gene probes specific to 36 KD gene of *M. leprae* are used on histological specimens. If complementary nucleic acid strands of *M. leprae* are present in the specimen, the probe joins at the site (hybridization). This is indicated by a color change (brought about by immunoenzymatic reaction) and confirms the diagnosis. In our study on 22 patients, where histopathology confirmed the diagnosis in 27.2% cases only, *in situ* hybridization showed a positivity of 42.8% in early (I/BT) and 46.7% in BB/BL group, thus enhancing the diagnosis by 18.1%. This test allows concomitant study of histopathology. It augments the sensitivity of histopathological diagnosis.

In Situ PCR on Slit Skin Smears

Another latest in our series of molecular biological approaches is the utility of *in situ* PCR on the slit skin smears. It was found that with an average positivity of 72%. *In situ* PCR on slit skin smears was better than that on skin biopsies (60%). In addition, it has the added advantages of being minimally invasive and less cumbersome and can be performed even at sites from where skin biopsy is difficult.

TREATMENT

Leprosy patients should be treated with patience, perseverance and understanding. Besides the medical

Table 4.8.2: Dosage of antileprosy drugs for children with paucibacillary leprosy (indeterminate, TT, BT).

Age group (years)	Dapsone: daily dose unsupervised (mg)	Rifampicin: monthly dose supervised (mg)
3–5	25	150–300
6–14	50–100	300–450
15	100	600

Table 4.8.3: Dosage of antileprosy drugs for children with multibacillary leprosy (BB, BL, polyneuritic).

Age groups (years)	Dapsone: daily dose unsupervised (mg)	Rifampicin: monthly dose supervised (mg)	Clofazimine	
			Unsupervised dose (mg)	Monthly dose (mg)
3–5	25	150–300	100 once weekly	100
6–14	50–100	300–450	150 once weekly	150–200
15	100	600	50 daily	300

Table 4.8.4: Pharmacological effects of drugs applied for leprosy.

Rifampicin	Highly bactericidal
Dapsone	Bacteriostatic, weakly bactericidal
Clofazamine	Slow bactericidal
Ofloxacin	Bactericidal
Minocycline	Bacteriostatic

treatment, the patients and their parents need moral support and reassurance. Parents should be explained hygienic measures, proper diet and importance of taking treatment completely and regularly (Table 4.8.2).

It is now a well-known fact that simultaneous administration of several different antibacterial agents may prevent the emergence of drug resistant mutants.

Rifampicin is given once a month. No toxic effects have been reported in the case of monthly administration. The urine may be colored slightly reddish for a few hours after its intake; this should be explained to the patient while starting multi-drug therapy (MDT).

Clofazimine is most active when administered daily. The drug is well tolerated and virtually non-toxic in the dosage used for MDT. The drug causes brownish black discoloration and dryness of skin. However, this disappears within few months after stopping treatment. This should be explained to patients starting MDT regimen for MB leprosy (Tables 4.8.3 and 4.8.4).

DURATION OF THERAPY

The WHO study groups has recommended treatment of paucibacillary cases for only 6 months and of multibacillary cases for 12 months.

COMPLICATIONS

Reactions are acute exacerbations due to changes in the host-parasite immune relationship. They are common during initial years of treatment.

The following types are noted:

Type 1 (Reversal reaction): This is seen in borderline cases and consists of acute tenderness and swelling at the site of lesion. Irreversible nerve injury can occur if this reaction is not treated immediately.

Type 2 (Erythema nodosum leprosum reactions): This occurs in lepromatous and borderline lepromatous cases as a systemic inflammatory response. There is high fever, migrating polyarthralgia, orchitis, iridocyclitis and lymphadenitis. Tender red papules or nodules resembling erythema nodosum are seen characteristically.

Drugs commonly used in these conditions are antimalarials like chloroquine (given orally), antimonials, e.g. potassium antimony tartrate IV and fantosin IM, clofazimine, corticosteroids and thalidomide (all the three given orally). Symptoms, like iritis and neuritis occurring during reactions (or occurring independently), should be properly treated in order to avoid irreversible sequelae, i.e. deformities and neuropathic ulcers.

PREVENTION

Leprosy vaccine: There is no established vaccine against leprosy as yet.

The result of 5–9 years follow-up study conducted on 120,000 randomized individuals in South Africa, indicate that BCG booster vaccination (two dose BCG regimen given at 0 and 3 months) provides 50 to 75% protection against leprosy. The combined BCG *M. leprae* vaccine offered no additional benefit.

LEPROSY ELIMINATION STRATEGY

The main thrust of the leprosy elimination strategy is to:
- expand MDT services to all health facilities
- ensure that all existing and new cases are given appropriate MDT regimens
- encourage all patients to take treatment regularly and completely
- promote awareness in the community on leprosy so that individuals with suspicious lesions will report voluntarily for diagnosis and treatment
- set targets and time table for activities and make all efforts to achieve them
- keep good records of all activities in order to monitor the progress toward elimination.

BIBLIOGRAPHY

1. Dayal R, Agarwal M, Natrajan M, et al. PCR and in-situ hybridization for diagnosis of leprosy. Indian Journal of Paediatrics. 2007;74:645-8.
2. Dayal R, Singh SP, Mathur PP, et al. Diagnostic value of in situ polymerase chain reaction in leprosy. Indian Journal of Paediatrics. 2005;72:1043-6.
3. Park K (Ed). Leprosy. Textbook of Preventive and Social Medicine, 19th edition. Bhanot Publishers; 2007. pp. 264-76.
4. Powell DA. Hansen disease (*Mycobacterium leprae*). In: Kliegman, Behrman, Jenson, Stanton (Eds). Nelson Texbook of Pediatrics, 18th edition. Philadelphia: Elsevier Saunders; 2008. pp. 1255-8.
5. WHO Health Organisation: Leprosy. Global burden of leprosy at the end of 2010, Weekly Epidemiological Report, Sep. 2011.

Common Viral Infections

Digant D Shastri

5.1   MEASLES

Abhay K Shah

INTRODUCTION

Measles is an acute viral disease characterized by fever, cough, coryza, red eyes, a generalized maculopapular, erythematous rash called morbilliform rash, and pathognomonic enanthema (Koplik's spots).

A Scottish physician, Francis Home, demonstrated in 1757 that measles was caused by an infectious agent present in the blood of patients. Panum did classical studies on the epidemiology of measles in 1846. In 1954, the virus causing the disease was isolated by Ender and his colleagues from an 11-year-old boy from the United States. In 1958, measles vaccine was first used in a clinical trial, and in 1963 the live attenuated vaccine was licensed for use.

EPIDEMIOLOGY

Humans are the only natural hosts of the virus; no animal reservoirs are known to exist.

Measles is transmitted by direct contact with infectious droplets or, less commonly, by airborne spread. Measles is one of the most highly communicable of all infectious diseases. In temperate areas, the peak incidence of infection usually occurs during late winter and spring. In the prevaccine era, most cases of measles in the United States occurred in preschool—and young school aged children, and few people remained susceptible by 20 years of age. The childhood and adolescent immunization program in the United States has resulted in a greater than 99% decrease in the reported incidence of measles and interruption of endemic disease transmission since measles vaccine first was licensed in 1963.

Despite the safe and effective measles vaccine being available and despite efforts put in by various stakeholders over the past few decades, measles continues to kill 360 children every day worldwide. Measles is still common in many developing countries—particularly in parts of Africa and Asia, even though a safe and cost-effective vaccine is available.

More than 20 million people are affected by measles each year. The overwhelming majority (> 95%) of measles deaths occur in countries with low per capita incomes and weak health infrastructures. The primary reason for continuing high measles morbidity and mortality is the failure to deliver at least one dose of measles vaccine to all infants.

Indian Scenario

In India, measles is still considered an important contributor to child morbidity and mortality. Prior to immunization program, cyclical increase in the incidence of measles was recorded every third year. These cyclical peaks are decreased with improving immunization coverage. During 1987, about 2,47,000 cases were reported, whereas, after Universal Immunization Programme (UIP), the number of cases has gone down to 40,840 with 44 deaths in year 2009. A recent vaccination coverage survey in India showed overall 71% coverage for measles vaccination. Accepting 85% vaccine effectiveness, actual protection was offered to only 60% of birth cohort.

Measles cases in India have recorded a whooping drop by 43% between 2015 and 2016, number of measles cases being 17,250 in 2016 as against 47,418 in 2015. Still measles kills an estimated 49,000 children in India each year, which is about 37% of the global deaths due to this disease.

ETIOPATHOGENESIS

Etiological Agent

Measles, also known as rubeola or morbilli, is an infection of the respiratory system caused by a virus, specifically a paramyxovirus of the genus *Morbillivirus*. Morbilliviruses, like other paramyxoviruses, are enveloped, single-stranded; negative-sense RNA viruses. Only one serotype is known.

PATHOGENESIS

The essential lesions in measles are found in skin, mucosa of respiratory tract, conjunctiva and gastrointestinal tract. Serous exudates and proliferation of mononuclear cells and few polymorphs occur around the small capillaries. There is usually hyperplasia of lymphoid tissue, especially in the appendix, where multinucleated giant cells may be found. In the skin, reaction is notable around the sebaceous glands and hair follicles. Koplik's spots are due to proliferation of endothelial cells along with serous exudate. Interstitial pneumonia caused by measles virus takes the form of Hecht Giant cell pneumonia.

MODE OF TRANSMISSION

Measles is highly contagious and can be spread to others from 4 days before to 4 days after the rash appears (or from 1 to 2 days before the onset of symptoms and 4 days after the appearance of rash). This virus is so contagious that 90% of people without immunity sharing living space with an infected person will catch it.

The *incubation period* generally is 8–12 days from exposure to onset of symptoms. In family studies, the average interval between appearance of rash in the index case and subsequent cases is 14 days, with a range of 7–21 days.

INFECTIVITY PERIOD

An asymptomatic incubation period occurs 9–12 days from initial exposure and infectivity lasts from 2 to 4 days prior, until 2–5 days following the onset of the rash (i.e. 4–9 days infectivity in total). Patients with subacute sclerosing pan encephalitis (SSPE) are not contagious. The immunocompromized patients have prolonged excretion of virus in respiratory tract secretions.

RISK FACTORS

Risk factors for measles virus infection include the following:
- Children with immunodeficiency due to HIV, leukemia, alkylating agents, or corticosteroid therapy, regardless of immunization status
- Travel to areas where measles is endemic or contact with travelers to endemic areas
- Infants who lose passive antibody before the age of routine immunization.
- *Risk factors for severe measles and its complications include the following:*
  - Malnutrition
  - Underlying immunodeficiency

- Pregnancy
- Vitamin A deficiency.

SIGNS AND SYMPTOMS

Measles is an acute viral disease characterized by fever, cough, coryza, and conjunctivitis, followed by a maculopapular rash beginning on the face and spreading cephalocaudally and centrifugally. During the prodromal period, a pathognomonic enanthema (Koplik's spots) may be present.

The classical symptoms of measles include four-day fever and the three Cs—cough, coryza (cold) and conjunctivitis (red eyes) (Fig. 5.1.1).

Measles classically has three clinical stages:
1. Incubation period
2. Prodromal stage
3. Stage with rash and exanthema

The incubation period is usually 10–12 days from the day of exposure to onset of symptoms.

Prodromal stage lasts 3–5 days and consists of low to moderate fever with cough, coryza and conjunctivitis. Koplik's spots seen on day 2 or 3 of fever are pathognomonic for measles, but are not often seen, even in real cases of measles, because they are transient and may disappear within a day of arising. They are seen on the hard and soft palates as grayish-white dots with reddish areola and are often hemorrhagic. They tend to occur opposite lower morals but may spread irregularly over the rest of buccal mucosa. As they fade a spotty red discoloration of the mucosa may remain. Conjunctival congestion and photophobia are classical of measles and are seen before the appearance of Koplik's spot. Temperature rises abruptly as rash appears and may reach up to 40°C (104°F).

The characteristic measles rash is classically described as a generalized, maculopapular, erythematous rash that begins several days after the fever starts. The rash usually

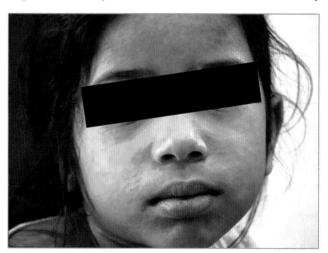

FIG. 5.1.1: Measles face.

begins as faint maculopapular rash on a person's face at the hairline and spreads downward to the neck, trunk, arms, legs and feet over next 24–48 hours. When the rash appears, a person's fever may spike to more than 40°C (104°F).

In uncomplicated measles, by the time rash appears on whole body and reaches to feet it starts disappearing from face and fades down in the same pattern. At this stage child begins to look essentially well. Measles rash are often itching. The rash is said to "stain", changing color from red to dark brown, before disappearing. The measles rash appears 2–4 days after initial symptoms, and lasts for up to 8 days. As the rash disappears it leaves behind the branny desquamation and brownish discoloration which disappears in 7–10 days.

The severity of the disease is directly related to the extent and confluence of rash. In severe cases the rash may be hemorrhagic. Sometimes the characteristic rash does not appear in immunocompromized children. In hemorrhagic measles (black measles) bleeding may occur from mouth, nose or bowels. Diarrhea and gastrointestinal symptoms are more common in malnourished and small children. Cervical lymphadenitis near the angle of jaw, mesenteric lymphadenitis and mild splenomegaly may be noted. Mesentic lymphadenitis and obliteration of appendicular lumen causes abdominal pain similar to acute appendicitis but they tend to subside with disappearance of Koplik's spots.

DIAGNOSIS

Diagnosis is mainly clinical. Clinical diagnosis of measles requires a history of fever of at least 3 days, with at least one of the three's (cough, coryza, conjunctivitis). Finding presence of Koplik's spots is also diagnostic of measles. Positive contact with other patients known to have measles adds strong epidemiological evidence to the diagnosis. The white cell count generally tends to be low, with a relative lymphocytosis.

Laboratory diagnosis of measles can be done with confirmation of positive measles immunoglobulin M (IgM) antibodies, a significant rise in measles immunoglobulin G (IgG) antibodies in paired acute and convalescent serum or isolation of measles virus RNA (by reverse transcriptase-polymerase chain reaction assay) from respiratory specimens.

The simplest method for establishing the diagnosis of measles is testing for IgM antibody on a single serum specimen obtained during the first encounter with a person suspected of having disease. The sensitivity of measles IgM assay varies and may be diminished during the first 72 hours after the onset of rash. If serum IgM is negative and patient has a generalized rash lasting for more than 72 hours, a second serum specimen should be obtained. Measles IgM is detectable for at least 1 month after the rash onset in unimmunized persons, but might be absent or present only transiently in people immunized with two doses of vaccine.

Isolation of measles virus is not recommended routinely, although viral isolates are important for molecular epidemiologic surveillance.

Genotyping of the virus isolates allows determination of patterns of importation and transmission, and genome sequencing can be used to differentiate between wild-type and vaccine virus infection. Monitoring of the genotypes isolated with a country or region can help to determine the status of measles circulation within that country or region.

Differential Diagnosis

The six classic rashes are measles, rubella, scarlet fever, exanthem subitum, erythema infectiosum and varicella. All, except varicella, are maculopapular and can thus be considered within the same differential diagnosis.

It includes the following:
- Rubella
- Roseolainfantum (exanthem subitum)
- Echovirus
- Coxsackie
- Adenovirus
- Infectious mononucleosis
- Scarlet fever
- Meningococcemia
- Kawasaki disease
- Drug fever

Measles is characterized by the four accepted clinical periods, with rising fever, profuse Coryza, disappearance of Köplik spots and morbilliform rash with onset in the retroauricular region which, within three days descends to the rest of the face, the trunk and the limbs.

Rubella is characterized by the triad of low-grade fever, swollen and tender glands and maculopapular rash, which is less intense than that of measles, with onset in the face and trunk and rapid progression to the limbs within 24 hours. The glands are painful in the retroauricular, posterior cervical and retro-occipital regions. Forchheimer's sign (petechiae in soft palate) may sometimes be observed. HHV-6 presents with sudden rash, although the profile may sometimes be similar to measles, with fever rash, cough, conjuntivitis and coryza. In Roseola infantum (exanthem subitum), the rash appears as the fever disappears.

The rashes of rubella and enteroviruses are less striking than that of measles, as do the degree of other symptoms and fever.

Parvovirus B19 and *Streptococcus pyogenes* are possibly the most-frequent causes of morbilliform rash. *Parvovirus B19* causes erythema infectiosum. However, it may also present different clinical profiles ranging from asymptomatic forms to aplastic crisis, morbilliform rash with fever or papular purpuric gloves- and-socks syndrome.

Streptococcus pyogenes causes scarlet fever, characterized by high fever, tonsillitis and a rough, erythematosus micropapular rash, predominantly in the skinfolds, with onset in the neck and progression to the limbs. The perioral region (triangle of Filatov) is respected. It may present with Forchheimer's sign and is accompanied by strawberry tongue and terminates with furfuraceous desquamation 7–10 days after onset of the rash. The diffuse fleshy papular rash with "goose flesh" texture is typical of scarlet fever.

In rickettsial infections cough and fever are less severe and rash usually spares the face.

The rash of meningococcemia may appear just like measles but conjunctivitis and cough are not there and patient is terribly serious.

Drug reactions may present with confluent, normally itchy maculopapular rash which may coexist with fever and other general symptoms such as arthralgia. Drug consumption suggests the possibility but there is no confirmatory test.

COMPLICATIONS

The most common compications include diarrhea and vomiting, often leading to dehydration, otitis media, infections of the respiratory system including bronchitis, laryngitis and pneumonia. Eye infetions including conjuctivitis, keratitis, corneal ulcerations and scarring are also reported. Rare complications include subacute sclerosing panencephalitis (SSPE), which can occur several years after measles, occurring in only 1 in every 25,000 cases. Noma of the cheeks may occur in rare instances. Gangrene elsewhere appears to be secondary to purpura fulminans or disseminated intravascular coagulation following measles. In underdeveloped nations with high rates of malnutrition and poor healthcare, fatality rates have been as high as 28%. In immunocompromized patients (e.g. people with AIDS) the fatality rate is approximately 30%. Measles virus itself can cause pneumonia, where the lesion is interstitial. Measles pneumonia in HIV patient is often fatal and not always accompanied by rash.

Post measles bronchopneumonia and pneumonia are quite common and are mostly associated with *Pneumococcus, Streptococcus,* and *Staphylococcus* and *Haemophilus influenzae* like infections. Exacerbation of existing tubercular lesion and temporary loss of hypersensitivity to tuberculin are quite frequent occurrence following measles episode. As many as 1 out of every 20 children with measles gets pneumonia, and about 1 child in every 1,000 who gets measles will develop encephalitis, that can lead to convulsions, and can leave the child deaf or mentally retarded. Neurological complications have been noted even in cases where measles is modified by immunoglobulin or by vaccine. Other neurological complications include Gullain-Barré syndrome, retro bulbar neuritis, hemiplegia and cerebral thrombophlebitis, but are rare. Myocarditis and transient ECG changes can occur following measles. Measles also can make a pregnant woman have a miscarriage, give birth prematurely, or have a low-birth-weight baby.

SUBACUTE SCLEROSING PANENCEPHALITIS

Subacute sclerosing panencephalitis (SSPE) is a very rare, but fatal degenerative disease of the central nervous system that results from a measles virus infection acquired earlier in life. It is characterized by behavioral and intellectual deterioration and seizures that occurs 7–10 years after wild type measles virus infection. A risk factor for developing this disease is measles infection at an early age. The first signs of SSPE may be changes in personality, a gradual onset of mental deterioration and myoclonia (muscle spasms or jerks). The diagnosis of SSPE is based on signs and symptoms and on test results, such as typical changes observed in electroencephalograms, an elevated antimeasles antibody (IgG) in the serum and cerebrospinal fluid, and typical histologic findings in brain biopsy tissue. All of the genetic analyses of viral material derived from brain tissue of SSPE patients have revealed sequences of wild-type measles virus, never vaccine virus. There is no evidence that measles vaccine can cause SSPE.

TREATMENT

There is no specific antiviral treatment for measles. Most patients with uncomplicated measles will recover with rest, adequate hydration and supportive treatment. Strong light may be avoided due to photophobia. Severe complications from measles can be avoided through supportive care that ensures good nutrition, adequate fluid intake and treatment of dehydration with WHO-recommended oral rehydration solution. Symptomatic treatment includes paracetamol to reduce fever and pain and, if required, a fast-acting bronchodilator for cough. Aspirin should not be used for the fear of Reye's syndrome. It is, however, important to seek medical advice if the patient becomes more unwell, as they may be developing complications.

Some patients will develop pneumonia, ear infections, bronchitis, and encephalitis as a sequel to the measles. While there is no specific treatment for measles encephalitis, antibiotics are required for bacterial pneumonia, sinusitis and bronchitis, and ear infection that can follow measles. *Staphylococci* and *Pneumococcus* are the two common organisms associated with post-measles LRTI. Humidification may be helpful for laryngitis with irritating cough.

Role of Vitamin A

The use of vitamin A in treatment of measles in the developing countries has been associated with decreased morbidity and mortality rates. This can help to prevent eye damage and blindness. Vitamin A supplements have been shown to reduce the number of deaths from measles by 50%. WHO recommends vitamin A for all children with acute measles, regardless of their country and residence. Vitamin A is administered once daily for 2 days, at the following doses:

- 2,00,000 IU for children 12 months of age or older
- 1,00,000 IU for infants 6–11 months of age
- 50,000 IU for younger than 6 months

An additional age specific third dose is given 2–4 weeks later to children with clinical signs and symptoms of vitamin A deficiency.

Isolation of the hospitalized patient:
In addition to standard precautions, airborne transmission precautions are indicated for 4 days after the onset of rash in otherwise healthy children and for the duration of illness in immunocompromised patients. Exposed susceptible patients should be placed on airborne precautions from day 5 after first exposure until day 21 after last exposure.

PROGNOSIS

While the vast majority of patients survive measles, complications occur fairly and may include bronchitis, pneumonia and pan encephalitis which is potentially fatal. About 30% of measles cases develop one or more complications, including the following:

- *Pneumonia*, which is the complication that is most often the cause of death in young children.
- *Ear infections* occur in about 1 in 10 measles cases and permanent loss of hearing can result.
- *Diarrhea* is reported in about 8% of cases.

Acute measles encephalitis is another serious risk of measles virus infection. It typically occurs 2 days to 1 week after the breakout of the measles exanthem, and begins with very high fever, severe headache, convulsions and altered sensorium.

PREVENTION OF MEASLES

Isolation

Isolation of patient is important from 7th day of exposure to 5 days after the appearance of rash.

Vaccine

Measles vaccines were first licensed in 1963. Currently, only live attenuated products are available in the market. Several live attenuated measles vaccines are available in combination with rubella, mumps, or varicella vaccines, or some combination of these. When using the combined measles–rubella (MR) vaccine, measles–mumps–rubella (MMR) vaccine, or measles–mumps–rubella–varicella (MMRV) vaccine, the protective immune response to each individual vaccine antigen is largely unchanged. Internationally available measles vaccines are safe, effective, and may be used interchangeably within immunization programs.

Measles vaccine contains live attenuated measles virus (Edmonston-Zagreb strain) propagated on human diploid cells (HDC). Each dose of 0.5 mL contains not less than 1,000 $CCID_{50}$ of measles virus. Vaccine is presented as lyophilized vaccine. The vaccine may be stored frozen or 2–8°C and protected from light at all times. Before use, the lyophilized vaccine is reconstituted with sterile diluent supplied by the manufacturers. Unconstituted vaccines remain viable for 2 years at 2–8°C but once reconstituted it should be used within 4 hours as vaccine does not contain any preservative or antibiotic.

Measles vaccines are licensed for use starting as early as 6 months of age. In countries where incidence and mortality from measles are high in the first year of life, manufacturers recommend that vaccination be initiated at 9 months or shortly thereafter. In countries where infection occurs later in life, vaccination can be delayed until 12–15 months of age. For primary immunization, 2 doses are recommended. The second dose of MCV is usually provided in the second year of life or at school entry, but it may be administered as early as 4 weeks after the first dose. The second dose is needed to protect children who did not develop protective immunity after the first dose. In general, countries with long-standing immunization programs reaching good coverage and low measles incidence offer both doses at older ages and rely on routine services for delivery. Countries with weaker health infrastructure use vaccination campaigns to increase coverage with 2 doses of MCVs. The diversity in measles vaccination schedules results from differences among countries in rates of endemic measles virus transmission, the health service infrastructure, as well as in the ability of programs to access children at different ages.

Immunogenicity, Efficacy and Effectiveness

Measles vaccine induces both humoral and cellular immune responses similar to those induced by wild-type measles virus infection, although antibody concentrations are usually lower. Vaccinating infants before or at the age of 6 months often fails to induce seroconversion due to the immaturity of the immune system as well as the presence of neutralizing maternal antibodies. Primary vaccination failures occur in up to 10–15% of infants vaccinated at age 9 months. Antibody avidity to measles virus is generally lower in children vaccinated at 6 or 9 months of age compared with the avidity obtained in children vaccinated at age 12 months. Therefore, the recommended age at vaccination must balance the risk of primary vaccine failure, which decreases with increasing age, with the risk of measles virus infection prior to vaccination which increases with age. Studies on revaccination in children who did not respond to their first dose of measles vaccine demonstrate that approximately 95% develop protective immunity after the second dose.

Vaccine Safety

Adverse reactions following measles vaccination are generally mild and transient. Within 24 hours of vaccination, vaccine recipients may experience slight pain and tenderness at the site of injection, which usually resolves in 2–3 days. Approximately 7–12 days after vaccination, systemic reactions occur in about 5–15% of recipients including fever of >39°C for 1–2 days. A transient rash occurs in about 2% of recipients. Adverse events, with the exception of anaphylactic reactions, are less likely to occur after MCV2 vaccination. Serious adverse events such as toxic shock syndrome, septicemia, and occasionally even fatal events, following measles vaccine administration (particularly when using multi-dose vials) can occur because of failure to adhere strictly to the manufacturer's recommendations when handling, reconstituting and administering measles vaccines. Allergic reactions to vaccine components including neomycin and the stabilizers have also been reported after measles vaccination. As with single-antigen measles vaccine, adverse events following administration of MMR and MMRV vaccines are mostly mild and transient, although the rate of febrile seizures occurring 7–10 days after the first dose in children vaccinated with MMRV is about double. (9/10 000) that in children who receive MMR and varicella vaccines separately at the same visit.

IAP ACVIP Recommendations

NTAGI's proposal of replacing the first and the second dose of measles containing vaccine (MCV) at 9 months and 16–24 months with measles-rubella (MR) vaccine in the universal immunization program (UIP) is already being implemented in few states of the country. However, MR is still not available in the private sector. Thus, Indian Academy of Pediatrics (IAP) Advisory Committee on Vaccines and Immunization Practices (ACVIP) after further considering the issue of morbidity following mumps infection, suggested that MMR be given instead of MR at both 9 months and 15 months and a third dose of the MMR vaccine at 4–6 years.

IAP ACVIP recommends that the varicella vaccine be given separately as MMR+V (varicella) at 15 months age and either the same (MMR+V) or MMRV be offered at 4–6

years of age. For catch up vaccination of children more than 48 months age, if both MMR and varicella vaccines not given earlier; two doses of MMRV or MMR + V separately be given 6 weeks to 3 months apart.

Immunization during an Outbreak

During outbreak immunization should be done to infants as young as 6 months of age. The seroconversion rates will be significantly lower if the vaccine is given at such a younger age. Therefore additional dose is needed at 12–15 months of age.

Use of Immunoglobulin

Immunoglobulins are used to prevent or to modify measles in a susceptible person within 6 days of exposure, in a dose of 0.25 mL/kg intramuscularly. The dose is 0.5 mL/kg in immunocompromized children. Immunoglobulin is particularly indicated in a household contact who are younger than 1 year, pregnant women and immunocompromised children for whom the risk of complications is highest. If Ig is used for such purposes, measles vaccine is given 6 months after the use of Ig, provided the child is more than 12 months of age. HIV infected children and adolescents and all children born to HIV infected mother should receive Ig prophylaxis in a dose of 0.5 mL/kg IM, irrespective of their measles immunization status.

Those who receive immune globulin intravenous (IGIV) regularly, the usual dose of 400 mg/kg is adequate for measles prophylaxis after exposure occurring within 3 weeks of IVIG administration.

Post-exposure Prophylaxis

- *Children less than 6 months:* No need for prophylaxis as the child is protected by maternal antibodies
- *6–12 months of age:* Vaccine has to be given within 72 hours in an unimmunized child
- *More than 12 months of age:* Vaccine has to be given as MMR within 72 hours, if not vaccinated previously
- *Immunocompromised child should receive Ig 0.5 mL/kg (maximum 15 mL) IM, irrespective of their immune status.*

Measles-Rubella Initiative Plan

Measles-Rubella Initiative Plan has a vision to achieve and maintain a world without measles, rubella and congenital rubella syndrome (CRS).

The Plan builds on the experience and successes of a decade of accelerated measles control efforts that resulted in a 74% reduction in measles deaths globally between 2000 and 2010. It integrates the newest 2011 World Health Organization (WHO) policy on rubella vaccination which recommends combining measles and rubella control strategies and planning efforts, given the shared surveillance and widespread use of combined measles-rubella vaccine formulations, i.e. measles-rubella (MR) and measles-mumps-rubella (MMR). The strategy focuses on the implementation of five core components.

1. Achieve and maintain high levels of population immunity by providing high vaccination coverage with two doses of measles- and rubella-containing vaccines.
2. Monitor disease using effective surveillance, and evaluate programmatic efforts to ensure progress.
3. Develop and maintain outbreak preparedness, respond rapidly to outbreaks and manage cases.
4. Communicate and engage to build public confidence and demand for immunization.
5. Perform the research and development needed to support cost-effective operations and improve vaccination and diagnostic tools.

BIBLIOGRAPHY

1. Available from http://www.who.int/mediacentre/factsheets/fs286/en/. WHO fact sheet no. 286. [Accessed October, 2012].
2. Barrero PR, Grippo J, Viegas M, et al. Wild-type measles virus in brain tissue of children with subacute sclerosing panencephalitis, Argentina. Emerg Infect Dis. 2003;9:1333-6.
3. Broy C, et al. A re-emerging infection. Southern Medical Journal. 2009:102(3):299-300.
4. CDC. Progress in global measles control and mortality reduction, 2000–2007. MMWR. 2008;57:1303-6.
5. Centre for Disease Control and Prevention. Notice to readers; lincesure of a combined live attenuated measles, mumps, rubella and varicella vaccine. MMRVMorb Mortal. Weekly Report. 2005;54(47):1212-4.
6. Dua HS, Ahmad MO, Singh AD. Cover illustration. Abu BakrRazi. British Journal of Ophthalmology. 2008;92(10):1324.
7. D'Souza RM, D'Souza R. Vitamin A for preventing secondary infections in children with measles—a systematic review. J Trop Pediatr. 2002;48(2):72-7.
8. Global Measles-Rubella Strategic Plan 2012–20. Available from https://www.unicef.org/videoaudio/PDFs/Measles_and_Rubella_StrategicPlan_2012–2020.pdf.
9. http://www.who.int/mediacenter/news/releases/2009/measles_mdq_20091203/en/
10. Huiming Y, Chaomin W, Meng M. Vitamin A for treating measles in children. Cochrane Database Syst. 2005:(4): CD001479.
11. Indian Academy of Pediatrics (IAP) Recommended Immunization Schedule for Children Aged 0 through 18 years—India, 2016 and Updates on Immunization, 2004. pp. 1026-32.
12. Karen S, Ray G, Dominguez Lee, et al. Reye's syndrome and salicylate use. Pediatrics. 1980;66(6):859-64.
13. Kukreja S, Aggarwal S. Measles, Mumps and Rubella. In: Ghosh TK, Yewale V, Parthsarthy A, Shah NK (Eds). IAP Speciality Series on Pediatric Infectious Diseases. 2006. pp. 235-8.
14. Live attenuated measles vaccine. EPI Newsl. 1980;2(1):6.
15. Maldonado Y. Measles. In: Behrman RE, Kliegman RM, Jenson HB (Eds). Nelson's Textbook of Pediatrics, 17th edition. Philadelphia: WB Saundes Company.
16. Measles in Red Book 2015. Report of the Committee on Infectious Diseases, 30th edition. pp. 543.
17. Perry RT, Halsey NA. The clinical significance of measles: a review. J Infect Dis. 2004;189(Suppl. 1):S4-16.
18. Rota JS, Heath JL, Rota PA, et al. Molecular epidemiology of measles virus: identification of pathways of transmission and implications for measles elimination. J Infect Dis. 1996;173:32-7.
19. Sension MG, Quinn TC, Markowitz LE, et al (1988). Measles in hospitalized African children with human immunodeficiency virus. American Journal of Diseases of Children. 1960;142(12): 1271-2.
20. The Millennium Development Report 2009. New York. Available at http://mdgs.un.org/unsd/mdg/resources/static/products/progress2009/mdg_report_2009_en.pdf.
21. WHO 2009, WEEKLY Epidemiological Record, No. 35,28 August, 2009.
22. World Health Organization, United Nations Children's Fund. Measles mortality reduction and regional elimination strategic plan 2001–2005. Geneva, Switzerland: World Health Organization. Available from http://www.who.int/vaccines-documents/docspdf01/www573.pdf [Accessed 2001].
23. World Health Organization. Global immunization vision and strategy 2006–2015. Geneva, Switzerland: World Health Organization. Available from http://www.who.int/vaccines-documents/docspdf05/givs_final_en.pdf [Accessed 2005].
24. Yewale V, Chaudhary P, Thacker N (Eds). Measles, mumps and rubella vaccine. In IAP Guide book on Immunization; 2009–2011. pp. 68-74.

5.2 | RUBELLA

P Ramachandran

INTRODUCTION

Rubella is generally a mild exanthematous infection in children with minimal morbidity and mortality. Infection in pregnancy may cause fetal infection resulting in congenital rubella syndrome (CRS) with considerable adversity for developing infants in the form of multisystem disease with sequelae.

Rubella was known as "German measles" due to the great interest shown by German physicians from 18th to 19th century. In 1866, a Scottish physician Veale gave the term "Rubella". In 1941, Gregg, an Australian ophthalmologist reported congenital defects (cataract, heart disease) in babies of mothers who had rubella in pregnancy. The viral agent was isolated in 1962. A worldwide pandemic of rubella occurred in 1962 to 1964. Live attenuated rubella vaccine was licensed in 1969.

VIRUS

Rubella virus is an RNA virus of genus Rubivirus under the family of Togaviridae. Human beings are the only hosts for rubella virus.

EPIDEMIOLOGY

Transmission of infection occurs through oral droplet or transplacental route. In community epidemics, attack rate in susceptible people is estimated to be 50–90%. During clinical illness virus is shed in nasopharyngeal secretions 7 days before exanthem and up to 7–8 days after its disappearance. Persons with subclinical disease are also infectious. The public health burden of rubella relates to the risk of infection of pregnant woman. Age stratified serological surveys reveal that average age at which infection occurs is 2–8 years in many developing countries. Rubella susceptibility among women of child bearing age in India is reported to vary from 4% to 43% in studies done 2–3 decades ago. The situation remains practically unchanged with some recent serological surveys reporting susceptibility (seronegativity) of adolescent girls to the tune of 17.8–23.4%. CRS remains a problem in many countries with WHO estimating that more than 110,000 children are born with CRS each year in developing countries.

ETIOPATHOGENESIS

Rubella infection manifests in two clinical syndromes: (1) Postnatal infection and (2) CRS. The risk of congenital rubella for the fetus and newborn depends on the month of pregnancy in which maternal infection occurs. Risk for congenital defects and disease is greatest when maternal infection occurs in the first trimester. Congenital infection occurs in about 90% of infants whose mothers acquire infection before 11th week of pregnancy decreasing to 10–20% by the end of first semester.

In pregnancies, complicated by rubella in 7–8 weeks, only 36% end in normal live births, 39% end in abortions or stillbirths, and 25% develop gross abnormalities. Infection with rubella virus confers lifelong immunity against clinical illness, but asymptomatic reinfection occurs. This asymptomatic reinfection in pregnant women is generally not considered a risk to the fetus, except in very rare instances. When maternal rubella infection occurs in first trimester it results in placental infection which persists throughout pregnancy affecting multiple organs. Fetal infection generally is subacute or chronic and may result in abortion, stillbirth, congenital malformations, manifestations at birth (thrombocytopenia, hepatitis, encephalitis) and rarely infected infants without defects. When maternal infection occurs after 16th week of pregnancy there is a low risk for congenital defects, but fetal infection may occur.

POSTNATAL INFECTION

Clinical Features

Incubation period of rubella infection is 14–21 days. Prodromal symptoms are more in adolescents and adults characterized by sore throat, eye pain, headache, fever, diarrhea and nausea. These symptoms precede the onset of rash by 1–5 days and may not be seen in many adults. Lymphadenopathy is a major clinical manifestation, characteristically involving suboccipital, retroauricular and posterior cervical lymph nodes, but generalized lymphadenopathy can also occur. Lymphadenopathy starts at least 24 hours before rash and remains for 1 week or more.

Exanthem

Discrete maculopapular rash starts over face and spreads over the whole body in about 24 hours. Rash may become confluent over face. Large areas of flushing over body are seen. Rash normally disappears by 3rd day. Rubella infection without rash is a common occurrence in up to 50%.

An enanthem in the form of discrete rose colored spots (Forchheimer spots) may be seen in the soft palate in 20% cases. They may coalesce and extend to over the fauces.

Incidence of polyarthritis or arthralgia varies considerably in rubella. It is seen more commonly in adults especially in women. Small joints of the hands are frequently involved, often knees and wrists are also involved, but practically any joint may be involved. The joint involvement lasts for several days to 2 weeks and rarely up to 3 months.

In some rubella infection is totally asymptomatic.

Diagnosis

Mild forms of measles, scarlet fever, roseola infantum, enteroviral infections and drug fever are to be considered in the differential diagnosis. A combination of exanthem and suboccipital lymphadenopathy can also occur in enteroviral or adenoviral infection, infectious mononucleosis and mycoplasma pneumonia infection in adolescents.

The diagnosis of rubella infection is confirmed by serology and viral culture. Rubella specific IgM (immunoglobulin M) antibodies identified in first few days of illness or fourfold rise in IgG (immunoglobulin G) antibodies in sequential sera are diagnostic. Rubella-specific IgM in saliva 7–42 days after onset of illness is also found to be sensitive and specific. IgG increase in paired sera can occur both in primary and reinfection. When high accuracy of diagnosis is required as in pregnancy, avidity of IgG is estimated. In primary infection the antibodies are of low avidity and in reinfection they are of high avidity. If facilities are available rubella virus can be cultured from nasopharynx and blood by tissue culture systems or identified by polymerase chain reaction (PCR).

To bring about uniform diagnostic criteria WHO has defined probable rubella infection as fever, maculopapular rash and cervical, suboccipital or posterior cervical lymphadenopathy or arthralgia/arthritis. Confirmed rubella is a probable case with IgM seropositivity within 28 days of onset of rash.

Complications

Encephalitis is a rare complication in postnatal rubella infection with a frequency of 1 in 5,000 cases with an overall mortality rate of 20%. Thrombocytopenic purpura can occur in 1 in 3,000 cases. Myocarditis and pericarditis are extremely rare.

CONGENITAL RUBELLA SYNDROME

Clinical Features

Congenital rubella syndrome (CRS) is the result of in utero fetal infection which usually occurs during first 12 weeks of pregnancy. Classical CRS comprises of triad of cataract, sensorineural hearing loss and congenital heart disease. It was later expanded to include many new anatomic findings. Many infants have only one or a few of those manifestations.

The following clinical features may be seen:
- *General:* Infant death and intrauterine growth retardation can occur in 50–85% of affected babies and they continue to suffer from growth retardation, postnatally also
- *Eye:* One-third of babies have bilateral or unilateral, cataract, mostly present at birth. Retinopathy with pigmentary changes of "salt and pepper" appearance can occur. Microphthalmia and congenital glaucoma are also seen.
- *Auditory defects:* Sensorineural deafness is the most common manifestation of CRS, seen in 80–90% of cases and it is generally bilateral. Frequently this is the only manifestation
- *Central nervous system (CNS):* 10–20% babies suffer from active meningoencephalitis at birth
- *Cardiovascular system (CVS):* Among structural cardio-vascular defects, patent ductus arteriosus (PDA) is the most common followed by pulmonary artery stenosis, VSD and ASD. In severe CRS with multisystem involvement, myocarditis may occur and often is the cause of death.

The clinical manifestations of CRS can be under three groups, which are described in Table 5.2.1. About 85% of infants born infected during first 8 weeks of pregnancy had congenital defects during first 4 years of life. The following rates of defects are noted at different periods of pregnancy when maternal infection occured: 9–12 weeks—52%; 13–20 weeks—16%; after 20 weeks—no defect.

Diagnosis of Congenital Rubella Syndrome

Viral isolation or identification by PCR from nasopharyngeal, urine or CSF specimen of infant is the best method, but difficult and not available in many places. Virus isolation may be possible for 6–12 months and occasionally for longer period.

Rubella-specific IgM is readily detected in first 6 months of life in infected infants and to a lesser extent up to 1 year

Table 5.2.1: Congenital rubella syndrome—clinical manifestations.	
Time of manifestation	*Features*
Manifestations of active infection seen at birth	• Hepatitis • Dermal erythropoiesis (blueberry muffin lesions) • Thrombocytopenic purpura • Anemia • Hepatosplenomegaly • Meningoencephalitis • Myocarditis
Permanent manifestations at birth through the 1st year	Deafness, cataract, structural cardiac lesions, microcephaly, mental and motor retardation
Delayed manifestations (not manifest in early life)	Deafness, endocrinopathies (thyroid deficiency, hyperthyroidism, insulin deficiency), vascular effects

of age. Its detection usually indicates prenatal rather than postnatal infection.

Persistence of rubella-specific IgG beyond 6 months can be seen in 95% of infants with CRS. It may also indicate a postnatal infection. Identification of low avidity IgG may indicate a prenatal infection.

Prenatal diagnosis of fetal rubella-infection can be confirmed by viral isolation or RT-PCR positivity from amniotic fluid or identification of rubella specific IgM in cord blood.

World Health Organization Case Definitions for Congenital Rubella Syndrome

Compatible CRS (when laboratory data are not sufficient for confirmation): Any two complications listed below in (a) or one from (a) and one from (b):
a. Cataract/congenital glaucoma, congenital heart disease, hearing loss, pigmentary retinopathy.
b. Purpura, splenomegaly, microcephaly, mental retardation, meningoencephalitis, radiolucent bone lesions, jaundice with onset within 24 hours of birth.

MANAGEMENT OF RUBELLA

The treatment of postnatally acquired rubella is symptomatic, for example, analgesics for arthritis.

Management of Exposed Pregnant Women

If a pregnant woman is exposed to a person with rubella infection, rubella antibody status is tested immediately in the woman. If rubella IgG antibodies are present, no further action is required. Susceptible women with no pre-existing antibodies are closely observed for 4 weeks for features of rubella infection: fever, rash, lymphadenopathy. If clinical illness occurs, nasopharyngeal specimen is sent for viral identification and serum for rubella IgM and a 2nd specimen after 1–2 weeks of illness for rising IgG antibodies. If seroconversion occurs (rise in IgG titers) or specific IgM is positive, fetal risk for intrauterine rubella is high. If IgM positive, repeat in another laboratory, and check for low avidity IgG antibodies to identify primary from reinfection. If positive, option for therapeutic abortion should be offered to mother.

Management in Congenital Rubella Syndrome

Isolation is required in nursery as these babies are actively infected at birth and contagious. Room isolation and urinary precautions are recommended. These babies should be cared only by persons who are seropositive for rubella.

Isolation at home may be required for up to 1 year. Exposure of pregnant women to these babies should be avoided.

Long-term Treatment

- *Deafness*: Early diagnosis of hearing loss and proper educational program are mandatory
- *Eye problems*: Glaucoma needs immediate attention. Cataract surgery is normally deferred until end of 1st year of life
- *Multiple handicaps*: Care of such infants requires a multidisciplinary team. Prognosis is poor, especially those with progressive neurologic symptoms.

Prevention

Principal goal of rubella vaccination is to prevent congenital rubella syndrome. RA 27/3 strain of rubella virus vaccine is widely used. Antibody response is seen in more than 99% vaccinees and protective efficacy is more than 90%. Indian Academy of Pediatrics (IAP) recommends a three dose regimen of MMR vaccine at 9 months, 15 months and 5 years of age.

BIBLIOGRAPHY

1. American Academy of Pediatrics. Rubella. In: Pickering LK, ED. Red book : 2012 Report of the Committee on Infectious Diseases. Elk Grove Village, Ill: American Academy of Pediatrics 2012. pp. 629-34.
2. Chaturvedi UC, Tripathi BN, Mathur A, et al. Role of rubella in congenital malformations in India. J Hyg (Lond). 1976;76:33-40.
3. Cherry JD, Adachi J. Rubella virus. In: Feigin RD, Cherry JD, Demmler-Harrison GJ, Kaplan SL, Hotez PJ, Steinbach WJ (Eds). Feigin and Cherry's Textbook of Pediatric Infectious Diseases, 7th edition. Philadelphia, USA: Saunders Elsevier; 2014. pp. 2195-225.
4. Panda SC, Panigrahi OP. Let us eliminate rubella. Ind J Pract Doc. 2006;3:203-6.
5. Plotkin SA, Reef SE, Cooper LZ, et al. Rubella. In: Remington JS, Klein JO, Wilson CB, Nizet V, Maldonado YA (Eds). Infectious Diseases of the Fetus and Newborn Infant, 7th edition. Philadelphia, USA: Saunders Elsevier; 2011. pp. 861-98.
6. Rachna R, Deepika D, Sarma S. Rubella serology in Indian adolescent girls and its relation to socio-economic status. J Obstet Gynecol India. 2005;55:167-9.
7. Reef SE, Strebel P, Dabbagh A, et al. Progress towards control of rubellla and prevention of congenital rubella syndrome: worldwide, 2009. J Infect Dis. 2011;204(S1):S24-7.
8. Seth P, Manjunath N, Balaya S. Rubella infection: the Indian scene. Rev Infect Dis. 1985;7:64-7.
9. Sharma HJ, Padbidri VS, Kapre SV, et al. Seroprevalence of rubella and immunogenicity following rubella vaccination in adolescent girls in India. J Infect Dev Ctries. 2011;5:874-81.

5.3 — MUMPS

Ashok Rai

INTRODUCTION

Mumps is an acute systemic viral infection characterized by swelling of one or more of the salivary glands, usually the parotid glands.

It is predominantly a disorder of childhood, almost 90% of cases presenting before adolescence. However, the infection is rare in infancy presumably because of persisting maternal antibodies.

It is not common in developed countries due to extensive vaccination programs but remains endemic in the developing countries, where extensive vaccination coverage is required.

ETIOLOGY

Mumps is caused by a single stranded RNA virus (Rubella virus) of Paramyxoviridae family. The virions are roughly spherical composed of an outer membrane enclosing an inner helical structure. The outer membrane is covered by projections extending 12–15 nm from the virion surface. It possesses both HN and F proteins. The mumps viruses are antigenically stable.

This virus exists as a single immunotype, and humans are the only natural hosts. Mumps virus are rapidly inactivated by chemical agents, ultraviolet light and heat.

PATHOGENESIS

Following infection, the virus replicates in the epithelium of upper respiratory tract and regional lymph nodes. After 12–25 days, a viremia occurs. During the viremia, the virus spreads to multiple tissues, including the meninges and glands, such as the salivary, pancreas, testes and ovaries. Mumps virus causes neurosis of infected cells and is associated with a lymphocytic inflammatory infiltrate.

EPIDEMIOLOGY

Mumps occurs worldwide and humans are the only natural hosts. Although, persons with asymptomatic or nonclassical infection can transmit the virus, but no carrier state is known to exist.

Virus spread from person to person by infected droplets or fomites; infectivity lasts from a week before salivary gland swelling starts to up to 9 days after; with a peak just before and at the onset of the parotitis. But the period of maximum infectiousness is 1–2 days before to 5 days after onset of parotid swelling. Incidence in India is still high due to poor vaccination coverage and strategy for mumps, measles and rubella (MMR). Exact incidence of mumps is not known for India due to lack of reporting and documentation in our country.

Mumps is seen round the year, with a slight increase during winters.

The US Centres for Disease Control and Prevention (CDC) and the American Academy of Pediatrics recommended an isolation period of 5 days after onset of parotitis for patients with mumps in both community and healthcare settings.

CLINICAL FEATURES

The incubation period of mumps is 12–25 days. The illness presents with a prodrome of fever, headache, malaise, neck pain and sore throat.

Parotitis is the most common manifestation and occurs in 30–40% of children. Parotitis usually starts unilaterally, but involves the other side in about 70–75% cases.

The swelling attains maximum size in 2–3 days, pushes the earlobe upward and outward, and the swelling subsided in 3–7 days.

Swollen gland is tender on palpation and painful. Ingestion of sour or acidic foods usually increases the pain in parotid area.

Approximately, one-third of infections does not cause clinically apparent salivary gland swelling and may manifest primarily as respiratory tract infections.

Other salivary glands namely submandibular and sublingual gland may also become inflamed, but in 10% of cases, these glands are involved in isolation. Edema over the manubrium and upper chest may also occur due to lymphatic obstruction in severe cases.

COMPLICATIONS

The most common complications of mumps are aseptic meningitis, encephalitis, orchitis or oophoritis.

Aseptic Meningitis

It is second to enterovirus as a common cause of viral meningitis and may be the presenting syndrome when only half have clinical evidence of parotitis.

Symptomatic involvement (headache, vomiting, neck rigidity) occurs in 10–30% of children suffering with meningitis and it resolves without sequelae in 3–10 days. This complication is more common in boys than girls (3:1 ratio), and adults are more at risk than children.

Meningoencephalitis

It usually develops 5 days after parotitis. It usually occurs due to primary infection of neurons by the viruses or may be postinfectious encephalitis with demyelination. Recovery is usually complete with rare fatalities. Occasionally meningitis or encephalitis may occur without parotitis.

Other less common neurological complications are transverse myelitis, facial palsy, aqueductal stenosis, ascending polyradiculitis and cerebellar ataxia.

Orchitis and Oophoritis

Orchitis with or without epididymitis is less common in prepubertal males. Orchitis was noted in 30–40% males after puberty. It is bilateral in approximately 30% of affected males.

It is usually associated with high grade fever, chills, malaise and rapid painful swelling of the testes and reddening of overlying scrotal skin. It may be associated with atrophy of testes but sterility is very rare even with bilateral involvement.

Oophoritis is rare in childhood and estimated to occur in 7% of female patients. It manifests with lower abdominal pain and tenderness.

Pancreatitis

Usually subclinical or mild infections are seen in cases of mumps; however, severe infections are rarely reported. It usually presents with fever, vomiting, epigastric pain and increase serum amylase level which are suggestive of the disease.

Deafness

It occurs in approximately 1 per 20,000 reported cases. It occurs due to neuritis of the auditory nerve and usually unilateral.

DIAGNOSIS

Diagnosis of mumps is clinical and suspected on the basis of clinical manifestations, particularly parotitis. A normal or low white blood cell count with relative lymphocytosis is the usual finding along with an elevated serum amylase during the first week of illness in these cases. A specific diagnosis of mumps should be made either by isolation of virus or serologic methods. The virus may be isolated from saliva, urine or cerebrospinal fluid (CSF); from the saliva within 4–5 days, urine up to 2 weeks, and CSF 8–9 days, after the onset of the illness.

Serology is the most convenient method of confirming mumps and enzyme immunoassay is more commonly used test. Demonstration of a fourfold rise or a single high titer antibody [immunoglobulin G (IgG)] to mumps is diagnostic. A negative serologic test, especially in a vaccinated person, should not be used to rule out a mumps diagnosis because the tests are not sensitive enough to detect infection in all persons with clinical illness.

DIFFERENTIAL DIAGNOSIS

Variety of illnesses may simulate mumps, but can be easily differentiated on the basis of clinical features. Parotitis may be caused by other viruses namely cytomegalovirus, parainfluenza virus types 1 and 3, influenza A virus, coxsackievirus and other enteroviruses, lymphocytic choriomeningitis virus, human immunodeficiency virus (HIV).

Purulent parotitis is usually caused by *Staphylococcus aureus* and other Gram-negative organisms, mainly occurs in debilitated patients, premature newborns and postoperative period. Recurrent parotitis is not rare in children and usually caused by salivary duct calculi. Collagen vascular disease, systemic lupus erythematosus (SLE) and certain drug reactions (e.g. phenylbutazone thiouracil) are the other causes of parotid swelling.

TREATMENT

Treatment of mumps is symptomatic and supportive. No specific antiviral drug is available for mumps. Antipyretics are used for reducing pain and fever. Adequate hydration should be maintained. Complications should be managed conservatively.

PROGNOSIS

Prognosis of mumps is usually excellent, although very rarely death has been reported in cases of meningoencephalitis. Permanent sterility or deafness is very rare sequelae.

PREVENTION

Prophylactic immunization is necessary to protect children against mumps and its complications. Complications are more commonly seen in adolescents and must be prevented by giving vaccine. Mumps vaccine is a live attenuated vaccine, available in India as MMR vaccine. Although mumps vaccine is also available as single antigen preparation, combined with rubella vaccine; combined with measles and rubella vaccine or combined with mumps, measles, rubella and varicella vaccine (MMRV).

Different strains of mumps virus are used for preparation of vaccine like Jeryl Lynn, Leningrad-Zagreb, Leningrad-3, Urabe, RIT 4385, etc. Leningrad-Zagreb (L-Z), Urabe and Jeryl Lynn strains containing vaccine are available for use in India by vaccine companies.

Seroconversion rate against mumps is more than 90%, but clinical efficacy and long-term protection is 60–90% with single dose, outbreaks have been reported in previously vaccinated population. Hence, two dosages are needed for double protection.

Mumps vaccine should be given as MMR vaccine routinely to children at 12–15 months of age, with a second dose of MMR at 4–6 years of age or any time 8 weeks after the first dose. The second dose of mumps vaccine provides an additional safeguard against primary and secondary vaccine failure. The recommended dose of MMR vaccine is 0.5 mL to be given subcutaneously.

Mumps vaccine is generally safe and, adverse reactions are very rare. Orchitis, parotitis and low-grade fever have been reported after immunization. This vaccine is contraindicated in pregnancy, severe immunodeficiency and patients with severe allergy to vaccine or its components.

BIBLIOGRAPHY

1. Agrawal KN. Mumps. Textbook of Pediatrics, 1st edition. Ana Book Pvt Ltd.; 2010. p. 124.
2. American Academy of Pediatrics. Mumps. In: Pickering LK (Ed). Red Book 2009: Report of the Committee on Infectious Diseases, 28th edition. American Academy of Pediatrics; 2009. pp. 468-71.
3. Ananthnarayan R, Paniker CKJ. Paramyxoviruses. In: Textbook of Microbiology, 7th edition. Orient Black Swan; 2006. pp. 512-3.
4. Ananthnarayan R, Paniker CKJ. Paramyxoviruses: In: Textbook of Microbiology, 4th edition. Pub Oriental Logman Ltd; Madras: 1990. pp. 496-8.
5. Atkinson W, Homborsky J, McIntyre L, et al. Mumps. In: Epidemiology and Prevention of Vaccine-Preventable Diseases, 10th edition. Centres for Disease Control and Prevention; 2007. pp. 149-54.
6. Committee on Immunization, Indian Academy of Pediatrics. In: Yewale V, Chaudhary P, Thacker N (Eds). IAP Guide Book on Immunization; 2011. pp. 73-4.
7. Ghosh TK, Yewale V, Parthasarathy A, et al. Mumps. IAP Speciality Series on Pediatric Infectious Diseases, 1st edition. Indian Academy of Pediatrics; 2006. pp. 237-8.
8. Kliegman RM. Mumps. In: Stanton BF, Schor NF, St. Geme JW, Behrman RE (Eds). Nelson Textbook of Pediatrics, 19th edition. Elsevier; 2012. pp. 1078-81.
9. Mandal BK, Wilkins EG, Dunbar EM, et al. Lecture Notes on Infectious Diseases, 5th edition. Blackwell Science Ltd; 1996. pp. 58-9.
10. Parthasarathy A. Mumps. IAP Textbook of Pediatrics, 3rd edition. New Delhi: Jaypee Brothers Medical Publishers (P) Ltd; 2006. pp. 242-3.
11. Robinson MJ, Roberton DM. Infectious diseases of childhood. In: Practical Pediatrics, 3rd edition. BI Churchill Livigstone Pvt. Ltd; 1995. pp. 277-8.
12. Thacker N, Shah NK. Mumps. Immunization in Clinical Practice, 1st edition (Reprint). New Delhi: Jaypee Brothers Medical Publishers (P) Ltd.; 2007. pp. 98-100.

AK Dutta

5.4 POLIOMYELITIS

INTRODUCTION

Poliomyelitis is one of the most crippling and potentially fatal, highly infectious disease caused by any of the three serotypes of poliovirus and is most often recognized by acute onset of flaccid paralysis. It is the most important cause of physical disabilities in children. The words polio (gray) and myelon (marrow, indicating the spinal cord) are derived from the Greek which describe the tissue most commonly affected in the spinal cord leading to the classic manifestation of paralysis. Once one of the most feared human infectious disease, poliomyelitis is now almost entirely preventable by proper immunization.

ETIOPATHOGENESIS

Poliovirus is a member of enterovirus subgroup, family Picornaviridae. There are three poliovirus serotypes (P1, P2 and P3) with minimal heterotypic immunity between them, i.e. immunity to one serotype does not protect against infection with other serotypes. However, immunity to each of the three serotypes is lifelong. Poliovirus type 1 has the highest ratio of paralytic infection to subclinical infection and is the most frequent cause of epidemics of paralytic disease. Poliovirus types 2 and 3 are less neurovirulent with type 2 being least paralytogenic. Clinical poliomyelitis can be caused by wild poliovirus and rarely by live attenuated vaccine virus strain. The virus is stable at acid pH and is ether insensitive but is rapidly inactivated by heat, formaldehyde, chlorine and UV light.

The virus enters human body through mouth and primary multiplication of the virus occurs at the site of implantation in the pharynx and intestine. The virus is usually present in the throat and stools before the onset of illness and continues to be excreted in stools for several weeks. From the site of implantation, virus invades the local lymphoid tissue, enters the blood stream causing viremia and then may infect the cells of the central nervous system (CNS). Replication of virus in anterior horn cells of spinal cord and brainstem results in cell destruction and typical manifestations of the disease. Paralytic cases represent only the tip of the epidemiological iceberg as most infections are subclinical and only about 1 in 200 (range 100:1–1000:1, depending on strain of poliovirus) primary poliovirus infection results in paralytic disease.

EPIDEMIOLOGY

Reservoir

Humans are the only known reservoir of poliovirus, which is transmitted most frequently by persons with inapparent infections. There is no asymptomatic carrier state except in immune deficient persons.

Transmission

Person-to-person spread of poliovirus via the fecal-oral route is the most important route of transmission but droplet spread can also occur.

Communicability

Poliovirus is highly infectious, with seroconversion rates among susceptible household contacts of children nearly 100%, and greater than 90% among susceptible household contacts of adults. Infected persons are most infectious from 7 to 10 days before and after the onset of symptoms but poliovirus may be present in the stool from 3 to 6 weeks.

Incubation Period

Typically 6–20 days (range: 3–35 days).

Temporal Pattern

Poliovirus infection typically peaks in the summer months in temperate climates. There is no seasonal pattern in tropical climates.

CLINICAL FEATURES

The response to poliovirus infection is highly variable and is categorized on the basis of severity and clinical presentation.

Inapparent/Asymptomatic Infection

This is the most frequent outcome after infection as up to 95% of all poliovirus infections are inapparent. However, infected persons without symptoms do shed the virus in stool and are able to transmit the infection.

Minor Illness/Abortive Poliomyelitis

This is the most frequent form of disease after infection. Approximately 4–8% of poliovirus infections result in minor nonspecific illness (indistinguishable from other viral illnesses) without clinical or laboratory evidence of CNS invasion. These mild symptoms are related to viremia and immune response against virus dissemination. Three syndromes observed with this form of poliovirus infection are: (1) upper respiratory infection (URI) (sore throat and fever), (2) gastrointestinal (GI) disturbances (nausea, vomiting, abdominal pain, constipation or rarely diarrhea) and (3) influenzae-like illness. There is complete recovery in less than a week.

Nonparalytic Poliomyelitis/Aseptic Meningitis

After a prodrome similar to that of minor illness, about 1–2% persons with infection have this outcome with symptoms of fever, headache, restlessness, irritability and stiffness of neck, back and/or legs and positive Kernig and Brudzinski sign. Typically these symptoms last 2–10 days followed by complete recovery.

Paralytic Poliomyelitis

Less than 1% of poliovirus infection results in flaccid paralysis. Paralytic symptoms generally begin 1–10 days after prodrome, progress for 2–3 days, reach a plateau which may last for days to weeks followed by some regain of function. Generally no further paralysis occurs after temperature returns to normal. The prodrome may be biphasic especially in children, with initial minor symptoms separated by 1–7 days from more major symptoms which include loss of superficial reflexes, increased deep tendon reflexes and severe muscle aches and spasm. Then the illness progresses to flaccid paralysis with diminished tendon reflexes. There is no sensory loss or change in cognition (Box 5.4.1).

Paralytic poliomyelitis is classified into three types depending on the level of involvement:

1. *Spinal polio*: It is the most common form and is characterized by asymmetrical flaccid paralysis, most often involving the legs.
2. *Bulbar polio*: Pure bulbar form of polio is uncommon and is characterized by weakness of muscles innervated by cranial nerves leading to dysphagia, dysphonia, vasomotor disturbances and respiratory muscle weakness.
3. *Bulbospinal polio*: Characterized by combination of spinal and bulbar manifestations.

Several factors have been shown to increase the risk of acquiring paralytic manifestations after infection including

Box 5.4.1

Distinguishing features of paralytic poliomyelitis.
- Fever at onset
- Rapid progression of paralysis within 2–3 days
- The legs are more commonly involved than the arms, and the large muscle groups are at greater risk than the small groups. The proximal muscles of the extremities tend to be more involved than the distal ones
- Asymmetrical distribution of paralysis with the most typical pattern being involvement of one leg only and less often one arm. It is less common for either both legs or both arms to be affected
- Quadriplegia is rare
- Preservation of sensory function with often severe myalgia
- Residual paralysis after 60 days·

intramuscular injection, stress, intercurrent infection, surgery (e.g. tonsillectomy), trauma and pregnancy.

Polio Encephalitis

It shows rare presentation with involvement of higher brain centers. The manifestations are similar to encephalitis due to any other cause and can be attributed to poliovirus only by specific viral diagnosis.

LABORATORY DIAGNOSIS

Virus Isolation

The laboratory diagnosis of polio is made by isolation of the poliovirus from stool, throat or cerebrospinal fluid (CSF). Stool cultures are most likely to yield the organism. The virus can be found in feces from 72 hours to 6 weeks after infection with the highest probability during the first 2 weeks after onset of paralysis. Isolation of virus from pharynx and CSF is less likely and is not recommended for routine use. If poliovirus is isolated from a person with acute flaccid paralysis (AFP), it must be further tested using oligonucleotide mapping (fingerprinting) or genomic sequencing to distinguish wild virus strains from vaccine strains.

Serology

Acute and convalescent serological tests can be done but are difficult to interpret as neutralizing antibodies appear early and may be at high level by the time patient develops paralysis. Therefore, a fourfold rise in antibody titer may not be demonstrated. Also, current serological tests cannot differentiate between wild virus and vaccine virus. These tests are, therefore, not recommended at present for diagnostic purpose.

Cerebrospinal Fluid Examination

In poliovirus infection, CSF usually contains an increased number of leukocytes (10-200 cells/mm³, primarily lymphocytes) and mildly elevated proteins (40–50 mg/dL) with normal glucose level.

TREATMENT

There is no specific antiviral treatment for polio. Treatment is supportive and aims to limit the disease progression and prevention of deformities during the acute phase and treatment of subsequent disabilities during rehabilitation.

Massage, intramuscular injections and surgical procedures should be avoided during acute phase of illness as they may result in progression of disease. Patient should be placed on complete bed rest.

Patient's vital functions should be carefully monitored with special focus on swallowing function, vital capacity, pulse and blood pressure. Some patients may develop respiratory failure due to depression of brainstem respiratory center (in bulbar polio) or paralysis of intercostal muscles and diaphragm, requiring ventilation. In bulbar poliomyelitis hypertension is not uncommon and may lead to hypertensive encephalopathy, if not recognized early.

Proper positioning with frequent change of posture— For comfort and prevention of skeletal deformities, suitable body alignment is necessary. Child should be made to lie on a firm bed in a neutral position with trunk and hip straight, knees in slight flexion (5-100) and feet at right angle at ankle joint. This position can be maintained with pillows, rolled towels or sand bags. Position should be changed in every 3-6 hours.

Warm moist fomentation with soft towels and analgesics are helpful to relieve muscle spasm and pain. Adequate diet and fluid intake should be maintained.

An orthopedist and physiatrist should see these patients early in the course of illness to assume responsibility of their care before fixed deformities develop.

Active and passive movements are indicated as soon as the pain has disappeared. All the joints of affected limb should be moved through their passive range of movement 2-3 times per day for about 10 times at each joint to prevent joint stiffness. This also helps in regaining muscle power.

Once acute phase is over, physiotherapy and other measures (orthotic devices) that facilitate recovery of movement and locomotion are helpful. Specific exercise programs for strengthening lower extremities are helpful to avoid contractures and muscle atrophy. In severe cases of contractures, patient may benefit from surgery to release the contracture and restore limb function.

PROGNOSIS

Some persons with paralytic poliomyelitis may recover completely and in most, muscle function returns to some degree, but large majority have permanent sequelae in the form of residual weakness and atrophy of affected limb. Weakness persisting beyond 12 weeks is usually permanent. Case fatality rate for paralytic poliomyelitis is about 2-5% among children and up to 15-30% for adults. It increases to 25-75% with bulbar involvement (Table 5.4.1).

PREVENTION

Prevention is the only cure available for poliomyelitis and vaccination is the only effective method for prevention. Although improvement in sanitation and personal hygiene may help to limit the spread of infection, immunization is necessary to break the chain of transmission.

There are two effective vaccines available against poliomyelitis: (1) the inactivated polio vaccine (IPV) and (2) live attenuated oral polio vaccine (OPV). IPV contains formaldehyde killed poliovirus, grown in monkey kidney/human diploid cells. It is highly immunogenic with seroconversion rates of 95-100% after two doses given after 6-8 weeks of age. The vaccine provides good mucosal as well as herd immunity and is very safe. OPV is a trivalent vaccine containing live attenuated poliovirus types 1, 2 and 3 grown in monkey kidney cells. It has excellent immunogenicity in developed countries. However, in developing countries

Table 5.4.1: Differential diagnosis of poliomyelitis.				
Signs and symptoms	*Poliomyelitis*	*Guillain-Barré syndrome (GBS)*	*Transverse myelitis*	*Traumatic neuritis*
Fever at onset	High, present	Not common	Rarely present	Present
Flaccidity	Asymmetrical and proximal	Symmetrical and distal	Symmetrical lower limbs (LL)	Asymmetrical limb
Deep tendon reflex (DTR)	Decreased or absent	Absent	Absent in LL early hyper-reflexia late	Decreased or absent
Sensation	Myalgia, no sensory loss	Cramps, tingling hypnoanesthesia of palms and soles	Loss of sensation with sensory level	Pain in gluteal region
Cranial nerves involvement	Only in bulbar and bulbospinal	Often present VII, IV, X, XI, XII	Absent	Absent
Cerebrospinal fluid (CSF), white blood cells (WBCs), protein	High WBCs normal or slight increase in protein	<10 WBCs, high protein	Normal WBC Normal or slight increase in protein	Normal WBC Normal protein
Bladder dysfunction	Absent	Transient	Present	Never
Nerve conduction velocity (NCV)—3rd week	Abnormal Anterior horn cell disease	Abnormal demyelination	No diagnostic value	Abnormal in sciatic nerve
Eelctromyogram (EMG)—3rd week	Abnormal	Normal	Normal	Normal

around the tropical and subtropical belt, immunogenicity is quite low with per dose efficacy as low as 9–13% in some regions of India. Thus, multiple doses of OPV are required before 90–95% children develop immune response to all the three serotypes. Because of low immunogenicity in developing countries including India, the herd effect seen in industrialized countries is not visible in India. Monovalent and bivalent OPVs are 2.5–3 times more efficacious than trivalent OPV and have been introduced for mass campaigns during National immunization days. Two risks associated with OPV use are vaccine associated paralytic poliomyelitis (VAPP) and outbreaks caused by circulating vaccine derived polioviruses (cVDPVs). OPV is contraindicated in immunodeficient patients and their household contacts.

Current IAP recommendation is to continue OPV use for birth dose, routine immunization at 6, 10 and 14 weeks, 18–24 months and at 5 years and on all NID's and SNID's as per recommendations of Government of India. If IPV is chosen then it should be given at 6, 10 and 14 weeks and 15–18 months. Also, under five children who have completed primary vaccination series with OPV can be given two doses of IPV at 2 months interval.

Vaccine-associated Paralytic Poliomyelitis and Vaccine-derived Polio Viruses

Vaccine-associated paralytic poliomyelitis is defined as those cases of AFP in whom residual weakness persists after 60 days of onset of paralysis, but from whose stool samples vaccine-related poliovirus (and not wild poliovirus) is isolated. It occurs due to loss of attenuating mutations and reversion to neurovirulence during replication of vaccine virus in the gut. These neurovirulent viruses may cause paralysis in vaccine recipients (recipient VAPP) or their contacts (contact VAPP). The risk of VAPP is higher with type 2 poliovirus, in patients with humoral immunodeficiency and with the first dose that takes (and not with the first dose). The incidence of VAPP has been estimated to be 1 per 4.1–4.6 million doses distributed and 1 per 2.8 million with first dose in India. Corresponding figure for developed countries, such as USA, is 1 per 2.4 million and 1 per 750,000 respectively. However, with eradication of type 2 polio virus from the world, the incidence of VAPP has dramatically reduced.

Vaccine derived polio viruses arise due to mutation and recombination in the human gut between vaccine virus and other neurovirulent enteric viruses and are 1–15% divergent from parent vaccine virus. These viruses are not only neurovirulent like those causing VAPP, but are also transmissible and thus capable of causing outbreaks of disease. In 2010, a total of five cases of type 2 VDPVs were reported in India. Recognition of VDPV is the primary reason for consideration of injectable polio vaccine in many parts of the world after the eradication.

POLIO ERADICATION

In 1988, WHO set out the goal for global eradication of poliomyelitis. This goal was defined as: (1) no cases of clinical poliomyelitis associated with wild poliovirus and (2) no wild poliovirus found worldwide despite intensive efforts to do so.

The strategies for achieving this goal are:
- Attaining high routine immunization (immunize every child aged under 1 year with at least three doses of OPV)
- National Immunization Days—to provide additional OPV doses to all under five children in a community within a short span of time so as to break the chain of transmission
- Acute flaccid paralysis surveillance—to identify all reservoirs of wild poliovirus transmission. This includes AFP case investigation and laboratory investigation of stool specimen from all AFP cases.

Acute Flaccid Paralysis Case Investigation

- Acute flaccid paralysis is defined as sudden onset of weakness and floppiness in any body part in a child aged less than 15 years or paralysis in a person of any age in whom poliomyelitis is suspected
- All AFP cases should be reported immediately to District Immunization Officer (DIO) and their stool samples collected within 14 days of onset of paralysis (up to 60 days)
- A 60 days follow-up examination is done between 60 and 90 days in certain cases to look for residual paralysis.

Laboratory Investigation

Two adequate stool specimens should be collected from every suspected case (adequate–collected 24–48 hours apart, within 14 days of onset of paralysis, of adequate volume ≈8–10 g, with proper documentation, in good condition, i.e. with no leakage or desiccation and with evidence that reverse cold chain has been maintained, i.e. with ice or temperature indicator).

An AFP case is "confirmed" as polio only if wild polio virus is isolated from any stool specimen. AFP case is classified as "Non Polio" if wild polio virus is not isolated from two "adequate" stool specimens or in case of inadequate stool samples, there is absence of residual paralysis on 60 day follow-up. A case is classified as "polio compatible" if stool samples are not adequate and there is residual paralysis on 60 day follow-up examination.

"Mopping-up" immunization—when poliovirus transmission has been reduced to well-defined and focal geographic areas, intensive house-to-house, child-to-child immunization campaigns are conducted over a period of days to break the final chains of virus transmission.

POST-POLIO SYNDROME

Post-polio syndrome (PPS) refers to the clinical deterioration experienced by many polio survivors several decades after their acute illness with symptoms of new muscle weakness, decreased muscle endurance, fatigue, muscle and joint pain. The pathogenesis of PPS is not fully understood, but a combination of distal degeneration of enlarged motor units caused by increased metabolic demands and the normal aging process, in addition to inflammatory mechanisms. It is not an infectious process and persons experiencing the syndrome do not shed poliovirus.

BIBLIOGRAPHY

1. Global Polio Eradication Initiative. [online] Available from http://polioeradication.org. [Accessed October, 2012].

2. Heymann D, Aylward B. Poliomyelitis. Available from www.orpha.net/data/patho/GB/uk_poliomyelitis.pdf [Not accessed].

3. Nathanson N, Kew OM. From emergence to eradication: the epidemiology of poliomyelitis deconstructed. Am J Epidemiol. 2010;172:1213-29.

4. National Polio Surveillance Project. [online] Available from http://www.npspindia.org. [Accessed October, 2012].

5. Poliomyelitis Eradication Field Guide. [online] Available from http://www.paho.org/english/ad/fch/im fieldguide_polio.pdf. [Not accessed].

6. Simoes Eric AF. Polio viruses. In: Kleigman R, Behrman R, Jenson HB, Stanton B (Eds). Nelson Textbook of Pediatrics, 18th edition. WB Saunders.

7. Sutter RW, Kew OM, Cochi SL. In: Plotkin SA, Orenstein WA, Offit PA (Eds). Vaccine, 5th edition. WB Saunders.

5.5 ACUTE VIRAL HEPATITIS

Malathi Sathiyasekaran

INTRODUCTION

Acute viral hepatitis (AVH) is a self-limiting disease with diffuse inflammation and/or necrosis of the hepatocytes caused by viruses and is characterized by an abrupt onset of symptoms with resolution of illness usually within 4 to 6 weeks. The necroinflammation may progress to acute liver failure or continue beyond 6 months resulting in chronic hepatitis. The term viral hepatitis is preferred when it is caused by hepatotropic viruses namely hepatitis A, B, C, D and E (HAV, HBV, HCV, HDV, HEV) are the recognized etiology for the illness.

Several other non-hepatotropic viruses, such as coxsackie, Epstein-Barr, HIV, cytomegalovirus (CMV) and dengue virus which cause systemic illness can also present with features of acute hepatitis. Non-viral agents, certain drugs and toxins are also well-known to cause acute hepatitis; however, in children viral etiology is more common than nonviral.

DEFINITION OF ACUTE VIRAL HEPATITIS

Acute viral hepatitis is an acute onset systemic viral infection marked by diffuse hepatic cell necrosis and inflammation, with a characteristic constellation of clinical (jaundice, nausea, vomiting, right hypochondrial pain), biochemical (elevated serum bilirubin and transaminases more than twice upper limit of normal) and pathological (hepatocellular inflammation and necrosis) features.

EPIDEMIOLOGY

The four common viruses presenting as AVH among this group of alphabetically named viruses are hepatitis A virus (HAV), hepatitis E virus (HEV), hepatitis B virus (HBV) and hepatitis C virus (HCV).

Hepatitis A virus: In India, sporadic AVH is caused by the two enterally transmitted viruses namely hepatitis A (60–70%) and hepatitis E (10–20%). About two decades ago it was not uncommon to identify children with natural protection against HAV following exposure to this virus. Improvement in socioeconomic status has resulted in a shift in epidemiology of HAV with children not acquiring protective antibodies in childhood and therefore being more susceptible to the infection later in life. The recent introduction of vaccines has also changed the etiological profile of viral hepatitis. The relative incidence of HAV is probably less than before, although it may still be high in some parts of the country.

Hepatitis E virus: It is more common in North India, especially in regions situated around the river Ganges. HEV has been isolated in all the major epidemics of hepatitis in India.

Hepatitis B and C viruses: The two parenterally transmitted viruses namely HBV (10–15%) and HCV (<1%) are less common causes of acute sporadic hepatitis.

The prevalence of hepatitis B surface antigen (HBsAg) positivity in India is approximately 2–7% whereas HCV is 1–2.5%. Infections due to HAV and HEV are self-limiting and do not progress to chronicity whereas HBV and HCV infections may resolve but can also progress to chronic hepatitis, cirrhosis and hepatocellular carcinoma (HCC).

ETIOPATHOGENESIS

Hepatotropic Viruses

All the major hepatotropic viruses are RNA viruses except HBV which is a DNA virus.

Hepatitis A is a 27 nm picornavirus spread by the orofecal route (Fig. 5.5.1). The necroinflammation is believed to be an immune response of the host to the hepatitis A virus.

Hepatitis E is a 30 nm RNA virus and is similar to HAV in the mode of transmission and incubation period. There are eight different genotypes identified till date. The mechanism of hepatocyte injury due to HEV is still unknown but is most probably due to an immune-mediated reaction.

Hepatitis B is a complex HEPA DNA virus which causes an immune-mediated injury. The intact HBV is the "Dane particle" or virion, which is double shelled and 42 nm in size (Fig. 5.5.2). Serologically, HBV is recognized by its three antigens namely surface (HBsAg), core antigen (HBcAg), and nucleocapsid/envelope (HBeAg) antigens and their corresponding antibodies namely anti-HBs, anti-HBc and anti-HBe. HBV DNA can be detected quantitatively and is a sensitive marker of active replication. HBV has been classified into A-H genotypes. A genotype is pandemic, B and C are prevalent in Asia, A and D are seen in India, E in Africa, F in USA, UK and France and H in Central America. The severity of the illness depends on the degree of immune response by the host. HBV is a very infectious virus and contact with 0.00002 mL of infected blood is sufficient to acquire the infection. The incubation period of HBV infection is 60–180 days, and HBV is transmitted by blood, blood products and body fluids including cervico-vaginal secretions, semen, breast milk, saliva, sweat, pharyngeal secretions and tears. Perinatal transmission of HBV is a unique problem seen in children and is more common in areas of high endemicity.

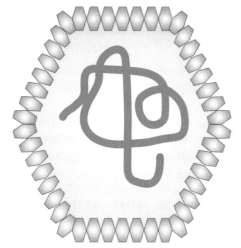

FIG. 5.5.1: Structure of hepatitis A virus.

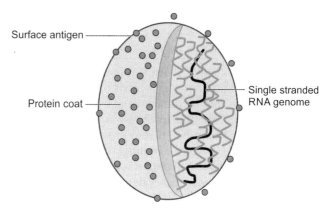

FIG. 5.5.3: Structure of hepatitis C virus.

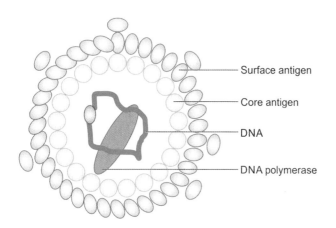

FIG. 5.5.2: Structure of hepatitis B virus.

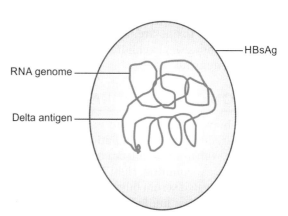

FIG. 5.5.4: Structure of hepatitis D virus.

Hepatitis B virus mutants: During the last decade numerous mutations have been described in the HBV genome. Mutation is defined as any change in the nucleic acid sequence of a genome. The various mutations that have been described are precore or core, vaccine escape and envelope mutants. The problems with these mutant strains are evasion of vaccine, drug resistance, change in tropism and change in pathogenesis.

Hepatitis C is a 30–80 nm RNA virus similar to a *flavivirus* and results in a complex immune response (Fig. 5.5.3). Recently non-immunologic genes have also been recognized to influence its clearance. HCV is less infective but more sinister than HBV and is spread by blood and blood products. Perinatal transmission occurs when mothers are anti-HCV positive with high viral load and if there is co-infection with HIV.

Hepatitis D (Fig. 5.5.4) is a defective virus with a small RNA molecule and an envelope constituted by HBsAg. This virus can infect only those who are HBsAg positive.

Hepatitis Viruses Non A-E

Several viral agents can cause non A-E hepatitis. They are either the less common hepatotropic viruses belonging to the *flaviviridae* hepatitis G virus/GB virus C [(HGV/GBV-C and yellow fever)] or Circoviridae family [Torque teno virus (TTV), SEN, etc].

Viruses such as Herpesviridae, severe acute respiratory syndrome (SARS), corona, parvovirus B19, dengue, measles, HIV, Lassa, Marburg and Ebola which cause systemic disease with transient liver involvement comprise a separate entity of non A-E hepatitis.

Flaviviridae

Yellow fever virus (YFV) is a RNA *flavivirus* which is spread by the mosquito vector *Aedes aegypti* and is endemic in South America and equatorial Africa. The hepatic injury has a characteristic mid-zonal pattern with sparing of hepatocytes around the central vein and the portal tracts.

The pathogenesis is still controversial and the hepatocyte injury may be due to tumor necrosis factor-α and cytokines produced in response to direct virus injury and the cytotoxic T cells involved in viral clearance.

CLINICAL FEATURES OF ACUTE VIRAL HEPATITIS

In the majority of children with AVH the illness is subclinical or anicteric whereas in the older age group the three classical stages of AVH namely the prodrome, icteric and convalescence may be more apparent.

The clinical presentation is common to all the etiological types of viral hepatitis with a prodrome which usually lasts for 2–7 days characterized by nausea, vomiting, high colored urine, fever and right hypochondrial pain followed by jaundice, pale stools and tender hepatomegaly.

The icteric stage lasts for 7–14 days, but may persist longer even for 12 weeks in older children. The child may present with pruritus which may be disturbing. The resolution of the illness is heralded by the disappearance of the constitutional symptoms, improvement in appetite and decrease in size of the liver. Certain features such as presence of ascites, firm liver may point to the existence of an underlying liver disease and a possibility of an acute on chronic liver disease should be considered. Prolonged fever, rash, arthralgia, arthritis, pallor, lymphadenopathy in a child with features of acute hepatitis may be clues to a diagnosis of non-viral hepatitis.

Some characteristic clinical features in the illness caused by the different hepatotropic viruses have been described and help in understanding the natural history.

Hepatitis A

Young children with icteric type of AVH have a benign illness and recover within 2 weeks. Older children with HAV infection may present with atypical manifestations, such as ascites, pleural effusion, firm hepatomegaly and disturbing pruritus. Cholestatic hepatitis is a distressing symptom of HAV infection more common in older children and may last for 12 weeks. Extrahepatic manifestations due to circulating immune complexes are uncommon and include evanescent skin rash, transient arthralgia, pancreatitis, vasculitis, thrombocytopenia, triggering of autoimmune hepatitis, red cell aplasia, myocarditis, nephritis, cryoglobulinemia and Guillain-Barré syndrome. Acute liver failure occurs in less than 1% of children. Relapsing hepatitis has been reported in children with HAV infection. Chronic hepatitis is not a feature of HAV infection.

Hepatitis E

Infection due to HEV is similar to HAV; however, it affects young adults more than children. The majority of clinical cases are icteric and extrahepatic manifestations are rarely reported. Chronicity is very rare but has been recently reported in immunosuppressed liver transplant individuals and in HIV infected patients. During HEV epidemics children usually have a milder or subclinical infection while pregnant women are more susceptible and present with acute liver failure which is associated with a high mortality of 1–20% and also increased still births. The reason for the severity during pregnancy is probably related to suppressed cellular immunity and hormonal factors. The immunological changes include down regulation of the p65 component of nuclear factor (NF-κB) with a predominant T-helper type 2 (Th2) bias in the T-cell response alongwith host susceptibility factors, mediated by human leukocyte antigen expression. Recent reports from Chennai, South India, have demonstrated a lower incidence of mortality in pregnancy probably due to difference in genotypes.

Hepatitis B

The majority of children with acute HBV infection are anicteric. Those with icteric hepatitis may be symptomatic for 1–2 months and present with nausea, jaundice and hepatomegaly. Immune-mediated extrahepatic manifestations, such as maculopapular or urticarial rash, migratory arthritis, nephritis and papular acrodermatitis of childhood or Gianotti-Crosti syndrome may be present. Most of the older children clear the virus by 6 months and seroconvert naturally. The risk of chronicity in HBV infection is inversely proportional to the age of acquisition of the illness. A neonate born to a mother who is HBsAg and HBeAg positive has a 90% chance of progressing to chronic infection. This incidence decreases to 30% if the age of acquisition is 1–5 years and 5–10% if acquired after the age of 5 years. When HBsAg is detected even after 6 months following an acute HBV infection it is considered as chronic HBV infection.

The stages of chronic HBV infection are immune tolerance, immune active HBeAg positive or negative, inactive HBsAg carrier and viral clearance.

They are categorized according to the level of transaminases and viral replication status.

In perinatal transmission the phase of immune tolerance where there is active viral replication, but minimal hepatic inflammation lasts for several years and is associated with a low annual HBeAg clearance.

HBV infection can therefore present as acute hepatitis, acute liver failure, chronic hepatitis which in turn can lead to cirrhosis and HCC. Progression of chronic hepatitis to cirrhosis is less common in children but there are few reports of HCC in adolescents.

Hepatitis C

Hepatitis C virus is an uncommon cause of acute hepatitis in children and has a benign and mild course with progression to acute liver failure in less than 1%. The symptoms of malaise, fatigue and jaundice are mild but the transaminases are elevated for a prolonged period. The incidence of chronicity is much more (40–50%) than seen in HBV infection. Chronic hepatitis can progress to cirrhosis and HCC. Sporadic hepatitis in children due to type C hepatitis is rare and is reported in children receiving multiple blood transfusions.

Hepatitis D

Hepatitis D virus infects only those children who are HBsAg positive. The clinical presentation depends on the status of the underlying HBV infection. Acute HDV infection can occur either as a co-infection with acute HBV infection or as a superinfection in an asymptomatic or symptomatic chronic HBsAg positive child.

Co-infection follows simultaneous exposure to both HBV and HDV. The incubation period is same as that for HBV infection. A biphasic illness occurs which is uncommon in other forms of hepatitis. The incidence of acute liver failure is as high as 10%.

Superinfection can occur in an asymptomatic HBsAg positive child or in those with symptomatic HBV related chronic liver disease. It results in deterioration of the pre-existing liver disease with the appearance or deepening of jaundice and worsening of ascites. Acute liver failure is as high as 20%.

ATYPICAL FEATURES AND COMPLICATIONS OF ACUTE VIRAL HEPATITIS, HAV AND G6PD DEFICIENCY

Acute viral hepatitis in children is usually a self-limiting illness. However, atypical manifestations can occur in all the types of viral hepatitis. The common presentation is the anicteric or classical hepatitis. In HAV infection some atypical manifestations are seen in older children. The jaundice may be prolonged and associated with cholestatic features. Relapsing hepatitis has also been described in 1–15% of individuals. The relapse may be mild presenting with elevation of transaminases. Other atypical features seen in children with AVH are prolonged fever, hyperbilirubinemia and triggering of autoimmune hepatitis in susceptible individuals. Ascites has been reported in 8.7% of children with HAV infection in a study done in Chennai. Ascitic form of sporadic AVH has been recognized as a separate entity in a report from Lucknow, India. The ascites resolved within 8 weeks in all these children.

A spectrum of extrahepatic manifestations have been reported in AVH such as aplastic anemia, glomerulonephritis, Guillain-Barré syndrome, myocarditis, pancreatitis, urticaria, polyarteritis nodosa, polyarteritis papular acrodermatitis, cryoglobulinemia. These are more common in HCV and HBV infection than in HAV infection.

The two major complications of AVH are acute liver failure and chronic hepatitis which increases the morbidity and mortality of the illness. Chronic hepatitis occurs only following HBV, HCV and HDV infection and is not a complication of AVH due to HAV or HEV. Co-infections with HAV and HEV have been reported with an increase in mortality however this finding has not been observed by others.

INVESTIGATIONS

Basic Blood Tests

The basic investigations in AVH include complete blood counts, urine for bile salts and pigments The characteristic biochemical feature of acute hepatitis is the detection of elevated transaminases more than twice the upper limit of normal with or without elevation of serum bilirubin In viral hepatitis alanine aminotransferase (ALT) is higher than aspartate aminotransferase (AST) indicating cytoplasmic rather than mitochondrial injury. The elevation is usually very marked more than 20 times upper of normal when the illness is due to the common hepatotropic viruses. Such high elevation is also seen in hypoxic or drug induced liver injury. The transaminases are elevated during the acute phase of the illness and decrease during recovery. The level of transaminases however does not correlate with severity of the illness. The total serum bilirubin is elevated when jaundice is present. Fractionation of bilirubin helps in diagnosing cholestasis (direct bilirubin elevated more than 20%) and hemolysis when it is predominantly unconjugated. In acute viral hepatitis the direct bilirubin is usually more than indirect.

Other liver tests such as total protein, serum albumin and alkaline phosphatase are not done routinely unless indicated. Prothrombin time is a useful test for assessing prognosis. Elevated prothrombin time and international normalized ratio (INR) more than two is not a good prognostic index and is a sign of acute liver failure even in the absence of encephalopathy. Blood glucose, urea, creatinine, electrolytes are included only if the child is hospitalized. Persistent hypoglycemia and hyponatremia and hypokalemia are also poor prognostic indices of acute hepatitis.

Serological Tests

Except screening for HBsAg, serological tests to confirm the etiological diagnosis of AVH are usually not done unless there are atypical features.

Acute HAV infection is confirmed by the presence of immunoglobulin M (IgM) antibodies to HAV which appears at the onset of illness and remains positive for 4–6 months. Anti-HAV immunoglobulin G (IgG) is detected in the sera within 8 weeks of onset of symptoms and remains positive indefinitely. Polymerase chain reaction (PCR) for detection of viral particles in stool or blood is not done routinely and reserved only for research purposes.

Acute HBV infection is diagnosed by the presence of the two markers: HBsAg and anti-HBcIgM. HBsAg is an early seromarker and is detected 6 weeks following infection and is normally positive only for 6 months whereas anti-HBcIgM is detected soon after the appearance of HBsAg and decreases in titre by 3 months and indicates recent infection. When HBsAg is positive for more than 6 months the infection is chronic. Anti-HBs, a protective antibody appears once HBsAg clears. HBeAg is detected in the sera soon after the appearance of HBsAg and is a marker of infectivity and active viral replication. It usually disappears by 6 weeks; persistence of this antigen for more than 6 weeks indicates progression to chronicity. It is detected in chronic hepatitis due to wild virus infection but not in precore mutant infection. HBV DNA is a marker of viremia and infectivity. It may appear 2–3 weeks before the appearance of HBsAg in those with acute HBV infection and remains detectable after HBsAg seroconversion. It is therefore of value only during the monitoring of a chronic HBV infection and not during the acute phase of hepatitis.

Acute HCV infection detection of antibodies to HCV and HCV RNA helps in the diagnosis of HCV infection. HCV RNA becomes positive within 2 weeks of exposure and anti-HCV within 8–10 weeks of exposure.

Acute HDV infection: Co-infection with HBV is diagnosed by the presence of HBsAg, anti-HBcIgM and low titres of anti-HDV IgM whereas in superinfection, HBsAg is present with high titres of anti-HDV IgM but in the absence of anti-HBcIgM.

Other Tests

When a child with features of acute hepatitis presents with atypical manifestations or has some unusual findings such as firm liver, early appearance of ascites, prominent abdominal veins or splenomegaly a diagnosis of acute on chronic liver disease (ACLD) should be considered. Prolonged fever, rash arthralgia, lymphadenopathy may be pointers of nonviral etiology such as bacterial hepatitis, Wilson's disease (WD), autoimmune hepatitis and hemophagocytic lymphohistiocytosis (HLH). Leptospira immunoglobulin M enzyme-linked immunosorbent assay (IgM ELISA), widal, blood culture, autoantibodies and work up for WD are included in the panel of investigations. Ultrasound examination is done to exclude liver abscess, gallstones and portal hypertension. Liver biopsy is not performed in children with acute hepatitis, but is essential in those with suspected acute on chronic liver disease or chronic hepatitis.

DIFFERENTIAL DIAGNOSIS

The differential diagnosis of AVH includes all conditions where the child presents with jaundice and elevated transaminases. There are two main differentials to be considered: (1) hepatitis caused by the non-hepatotropic viruses and (2) non viral hepatitis (both infective and non-infective causes). It is important that this group of non-viral hepatitis is recognized since specific therapy is available unlike in the viral marker positive hepatitis where only supportive therapy is recommended.

Nonhepatotropic Viruses

Several nonhepatotropic viruses can cause acute hepatitis and, although they are less common in older children, they form an important group in neonates and young infants. Children with this form of hepatitis usually present with features of the underlying illness such as the exanthem in measles or varicella in addition to hepatomegaly and elevated serum transaminases. Most of the times liver enzymes are moderately elevated and are not as high as AVH. The diagnosis is usually made clinically and if necessary confirmed serologically.

Epstein-Barr Virus

The Epstein-Barr virus (EBV) infects more than 90% of the world's population and thus is the most prevalent human viral infections. It belongs to the Gammaherpesvirinae family and causes infectious mononucleosis. The common clinical presentation is prolonged fever, sore throat, evanescent rash, lymphadenopathy, hepatosplenomegaly and transient self-limited elevation of transaminases. The liver damage is characterized by lack of expression of EBV antigens in hepatocytes instead the EBV latency proteins are seen in the lymphocytes. The cytotoxic T lymphocytes target EBV-infected B lymphocytes causing collateral liver damage. Chronic hepatitis and cirrhosis are not sequelae. The diagnosis is confirmed by the detection of IgM antibody to the viral capsid antigen.

Measles Virus

Measles presenting with anicteric hepatitis is an atypical manifestation of the illness and usually results in spontaneous recovery. Measles virus can trigger autoimmune hepatitis type I within 3 months of the infection in susceptible individuals.

Cytomegalovirus

Cytomegalovirus (CMV) is a ubiquitous herpes virus that infects majority of humans. CMV hepatitis in neonates presenting as prolonged cholestasis and later may progress to cirrhosis. In older children it may occur in recipients of renal or liver transplant. The disease resembles EBV related mononucleosis without pharyngitis or posterior cervical lymphadenopathy. CMV hepatitis is a major problem in liver transplant patients. The infection is usually primary although reactivation can also occur. The diagnosis is made by isolation of the virus from urine or saliva using PCR.

A fourfold rise in the antibody titre confirms diagnosis. Liver biopsy demonstrates the characteristic nuclear and cytoplasmic inclusion bodies. Quantification of CMV DNA by PCR is commonly used.

Parvovirus B19

Human parvovirus B19 can present with hepatic dysfunction, elevated transaminases and acute liver failure with or without aplastic anemia.

Herpes Simplex 1 and 2

Herpes simplex virus (HSV) hepatitis is usually rare beyond the neonatal period unless the child is immunocompromised. It may present as part of a generalized herpetic disease in infants. In older children it is rare and the mucocutaneous lesions may be absent. The diagnosis is made by the presence of IgM antibodies and the isolation of virus from the vesicles or other tissue. Liver biopsy shows the characteristic inclusion bodies.

Dengue Virus

Dengue fever presents with the characteristic features of fever, hepatomegaly, rash, pleural effusion and features of capillary leak. In addition, there is a moderate elevation of transaminases especially AST more than ALT. In the presence of dengue shock syndrome, the transaminases may be very high in several thousands due to ischemic or hypoxic hepatitis. This elevation of transaminases unlike in viral hepatitis is associated with a significant rise in LDH which drops sharply once the child is resuscitated. The diagnosis is confirmed by the high hematocrit, low platelet and the presence of IgM dengue antibodies.

Human Herpes Virus-6

Liver dysfunction in association with human herpes virus (HHV)-6 virus infection may present as infectious mononucleosis like syndrome, hepatitis or acute liver failure. HHV-6 could enhance allograft rejection and increase severity of other infections including CMV, HCV, ganciclovir and valganciclovir are active against HHV-6 infection.

Varicella Zoster

Varicella zoster virus causing liver disease is unusual except in immunosuppressed children with HIV infection or post-transplant recipients.

Human Immunodeficiency Virus

Infants with HIV hepatitis may manifest with cholestasis and later present with chronic hepatitis. Liver involvement in HIV infected individuals is indicative of a poor prognosis.

Echo, coxsackie and adeno virus may present in neonates and infants with acute liver failure.

Severe Acute Respiratory Syndrome—Coronavirus

Severe acute respiratory syndrome is a potentially lethal disease caused by SARS/coronavirus (CoV) which primarily affects the lung and intestine. Virus or viral products are also detected in the liver. Elevated ALT has been reported during the 1st week of illness and peaks by 2nd week. The liver disease due to SARS/CoV is of lesser significance compared the lung involvement.

Exotic Viruses

Marburg, Ebola and Lassa are dangerous viruses which primarily target the liver. Lassa fever is caused by an arena virus and transmitted from rodents to man or from man to man. It causes acute liver failure with high mortality. Ribavirin may be helpful. Marburg virus disease is caused by an RNA virus transmitted by monkeys. The illness is characterized by features of hemorrhage, encephalopathy and hepatitis. Ebola resembles Marburg illness.

Non-viral Hepatitis

Salmonella

Typhoid hepatitis can mimic AVH and is differentiated by the occurrence of toxemia, high fever and hepatosplenomegaly which is seen in typhoid fever. Some children may also have mild ascites and pleural effusion similar to primary liver disease. The transaminases are moderately elevated (3–20 times the upper limit of normal) with an ALT/LDH ratio less than four whereas in AVH it is more than four. The diagnosis is confirmed by a positive blood culture for *Salmonella typhi*. Specific therapy with cefatriaxone or quinolones offers excellent results.

Bacterial Sepsis

Bacterial sepsis should be considered in children presenting with fever, jaundice, hepatosplenomegaly and mild elevation of transaminases. Liver involvement is secondary to parenchymal or biliary invasion as a part of a systemic manifestation of sepsis. The prolonged prothrombin time and the mortality is due to disseminated intravascular coagulation (DIC) and sepsis rather than liver failure.

Tuberculosis

Tuberculosis hepatitis should be considered in those children presenting with fever of unknown origin, hepatomegaly, mild to moderate elevation of transaminases and high alkaline phosphatase. Liver biopsy shows the characteristic caseating granuloma.

Brucellosis

Brucellosis can occur in children who consume unpasteurized milk and presents with fever, lymphadenopathy and elevated transaminases. The diagnosis is confirmed by a high initial titer for Brucella antibody 1:160 or a rising titer done 2 weeks apart. Ultrasonography (USG) may show hepatic microabscess.

Leptospirosis

The clinical presentation may range from inapparent infection to features of acute hepatitis or fatal disease. Jaundice, hepatosplenomegaly, fever, myalgia, congested conjunctiva, bleeding manifestations, hematuria, anuria, minimal ascites and pleural effusion are the common clinical features. Apart from rise in serum bilirubin and transaminases the C-reactive protein (CRP) and creatinine phosphokinase (CPK) may be elevated which helps to differentiate it from viral hepatitis. A single high antibody titer by Microscopic Agglutination Test (MAT) or a rising titer 2 weeks apart helps in diagnosis.

Scrub Typhus

Scrub typhus or tsutsugamushi disease is a febrile illness caused by bacteria of the family Rickettsiaceae and named *Orientia tsutsugamushi*. It has also been reported in India and recently there have been several reports from South India. The clinical feature resembles dengue fever with thrombocytopenia and elevated transaminases. The eschar may be identified in less than 50% of patients. Diagnosis is confirmed by the presence of IgM antibody.

Malaria

Malarial hepatitis or malarial hepatopathy (term hepatopathy is preferable since inflammatory cells are not a characteristic feature on histology) is diagnosed when there is a threefold rise in ALT with or without rise in conjugated bilirubin, in the absence of clinical and serological evidence of viral and drug induced hepatitis and with a clinical response to antimalarials. It is usually seen with *Plasmodium falciparum* but may occur in *Plasmodium vivax* infection. The exact pathogenesis is unknown but could be due to impaired bilirubin transport caused by blockage of reticuloendithelial cells, microvilli damage or cytoadherence of parasites to the vascular endothelium leading to stagnant anoxemia.

Drug-induced Liver Injury

The common drugs causing hepatitis are anticonvulsants, antituberculous drugs, antimetabolites, nonsteroidal anti-inflammatory drugs (NSAIDs), paracetamol, herbals and indigeneous medications. It may be very difficult to differentiate drug induced liver injury (DILI) from viral hepatitis. The child presents with elevated transaminases with or without jaundice, rash and hepatomegaly. The absence of prodrome and the history of drug intake is a clue to diagnosis. The challenge is the onset of symptoms which occurs within 5–90 days of introducing the drug. On dechallenge, 50% drop in transaminases occurs within 8 days of stopping the drug.

Autoimmune Hepatitis

Autoimmune hepatitis (AIH) should be considered during the evaluation of acute hepatitis. It is a progressive inflammatory liver disease of unknown etiology presenting with elevated transaminases, hypergammaglobulinemia, interface hepatitis, non-organ and liver specific antibodies and good response to immunosuppressive treatment. Children may present with type I or type II hepatitis. In type I hepatitis, antinuclear antibody (ANA) and anti-smooth muscle antibody (ASMA) are present whereas in the latter liver/kidney microsomal type 1 (LKM1) is detected.

Obstructive Jaundice

Obstructive jaundice due to choledocholithiasis or biliary ascariasis can rarely mimic acute hepatitis. Abdominal pain and features of cholangitis are important clues to diagnosis. The direct bilirubin, alkaline phosphatase and ALT are elevated. Ultrasound helps in identifying the site and cause of obstruction.

Glycogen Storage Disease

In type I and III glycogen storage disease (GSD), the elevated transaminases may suggest anicteric hepatitis but the presence of massive hepatomegaly and other features such as short stature, doll-like faces, voracious appetite and early morning seizures will give a clue to a diagnosis of storage disorder. Jaundice is not a presentation. Fasting hypoglycemia, elevated lactate and uric acid levels are more suggestive of type I whereas elevated CPK and moderate elevation of transaminases especially AST are suggestive of type III. The liver biopsy shows swollen hepatocytes with glycogen [periodic-acid Schiff (PAS) positive and diastase sensitive] and steatosis in type I and PAS positive cells without steatosis in type III.

Wilson Disease

Wilson disease (WD) should be suspected in any child more than 3 years who presents with jaundice, elevated transaminases and a firm liver. Early appearance of free fluid, hemolysis, family history and a set back in school performance are pointers to suspect WD. The diagnosis is made by the presence of Kayser-Fleischer (KF) ring, decreased serum ceruloplasmin and elevated 24 hour copper and confirmed by liver biopsy, dry copper estimation and mutational studies.

MANAGEMENT OF ACUTE VIRAL HEPATITIS

Supportive Therapy

The majority of children with AVH will recover spontaneously and therefore require only supportive treatment. During the period of acute illness, the child should be provided adequate calories in the form of a nutritious diet. Undue physical exercise, hepatotoxic drugs and constipation should be avoided. It is of utmost importance to avoid unnecessary medications during the illness unless the drug is essential and its mechanism of action is well-understood. Water-soluble vitamins may be prescribed during acute hepatitis.

Hospitalization

Children with acute hepatitis do not require hospitalization unless there is persistent vomiting, fever, fluid retention, altered sensorium or gastrointestinal bleed. Ascites may be a presentation in some children with AVH and can be treated with a short course of spironolactone. Fever, if present, during AVH should be managed with tepid sponging and, if necessary, paracetamol is administered at half the dose. NSAIDs should be strictly avoided. If the child is on anticonvulsants, such as sodium valproate or phenytoin, it can be changed to phenobarbitone and if on antitubercular therapy with rifampicin, isoniazid and pyrazinamide, they should be withheld and ethambutol continued with streptomycin or fluoroquinolones. Older children and adolescents may present with significant and prolonged cholestasis or hyperbilirubinemia. Cholestasis can be treated with ursodeoxycholic acid 20 mg/kg/day.

Specific Therapy

Hepatitis A: Since the majority (> 95%) of children with acute hepatitis A recover spontaneously without any sequel no specific antiviral therapy is recommended.

Hepatitis E: Isolated hepatitis E infection in children is usually mild and does not require any specific treatment. Recently antiviral therapy with ribavirin has been reported with good results.

Hepatitis B: In acute hepatitis B no antiviral therapy is advised. These children should be followed up for 6 months to monitor spontaneous clearance of HBsAg.

Hepatitis C: Children and adolescents with acute hepatitis C acquired either by post transfusion or following IV drug abuse should be monitored closely for 12 weeks to establish spontaneous seroconversion. Those who have persistent viremia, i.e. HCV RNA positive for 12 weeks after the exposure are the candidates for treatment with interferon (IFN). Since, the genotype plays a major role in the prognosis and response to therapy it should be tested before therapy.

The current recommendation in adults is to initiate treatment with IFN-α or pegylated (PEG)-IFN as early as possible in asymptomatic patients infected with HCV genotype 1, while treatment may be delayed in icteric individuals with significant symptoms. Treatment can also be safely delayed in patients with genotypes 2 and 3 disease because these individuals clear acute hepatitis C more often than those with genotype 1 and treatment success in chronic HCV is much better. A shorter duration of therapy (12 weeks) compared to that required for the treatment of chronic hepatitis has been suggested.

Hepatitis D: Treatment is only supportive and liver transplant may be required.

TREATMENT OF ACUTE HEPATITIS DUE TO OTHER NONHEPATOTROPIC VIRUSES

The treatment of acute hepatitis due to other non-hepatotropic viruses is also usually supportive. Some specific antiviral agents such as acyclovir for herpes simplex, ganciclovir for CMV and highly active antiretroviral therapy (HAART) for HIV are available and may be used judiciously.

Prevention

The most important aspect of therapy in AVH is the prevention of the disease. The common viruses, such as HAV and HEV, can be prevented by improving personal, food and environmental hygiene since they are both spread by orofecal route. HBV, HCV, HDV can be prevented by avoiding unnecessary needle pricks; using disposable syringes and using only screened blood for transfusion. Active immunization is recommended against hepatitis A and hepatitis B.

BIBLIOGRAPHY

1. Craxi A, Stefano RD. Hepatitis due to non A-E viruses. In: Dooley JS, Lok Anna SF, Burroughs AK, Heathcote EJ (Eds). Sherlock's Diseases of the Liver and Biliary System, 12th edition.Wiley Blackwell Publication; 2011. pp. 427-37.
2. Kamath SR, Sathiyasekaran M, Raja TE. Profile of viral hepatitis A in Chennai. Indian Pediatr. 2009;46:642-3.
3. Mohan Prasad VG, Nathan V. Hepatitis A virus. In: Mahtab MA, Rahman S (Eds). Liver-A Complete Book on Hepato-Pancreatico Biliary Diseases. Elseiver India Pvt Ltd; 2009. pp. 201-5.
4. Schiff ER. Viral hepatitis section V. In: Schiff ER, Sorrell ME, Maddrey WC (Eds). Schiff's Diseases of the Liver, 10th edition. Philadelphia: Lippincot Williams & Wilkins; 2007. pp. 709-835.
5. Tagle M, Medina de Marioa, Schiff ER. Hepatitis A and E. In: Bacon BR, O'Grady JG, Di Bisceglie AM, Lake JR (Eds). Comprehensive Clinical Hepatology, 2nd edition. Mosby Elseiver; 2010. pp. 205-12.
6. Yachha SK, Goel A, Khanna V, et al. Ascitic form of sporadic acute viral hepatitis in children: a distinct entity for recognition. J Pediatr Gastroenterol Nutr. 2010;50(2):184-7.

Niranjan Mohanty

INTRODUCTION

Herpes simplex virus (HSV) infection is one out of nine human herpes viruses affecting children. HSV infection can cause morbidity and even mortality in neonates and children. The word "Herpes" means "to creep" in Greek. The earliest description of herpes as fever blisters was recorded by Hippocrates and Herodotous. In 1700s, Astrus described genital herpes lesion and in 1800s herpes was well described and in 1912 cultivation of HSV was done by Gruter on rabbit cornea.

Subsequently, the antigenic, biologic and epidemiologic characteristic of HSV-1 and 2 were delineated.

ETIOPATHOGENESIS

Herpes simplex virus has a double stranded DNA within an icosahedral capsid enveloped by a lipid bilayer with multiple glycoproteins. Manifestation of herpes simplex infection depends on the portal of entry, immunity status of host and whether the infection is primary or recurrent. Virus typically begins at a cutaneous portal of entry, e.g. oral cavity, ocular conjunctiva, genital mucosa or break in keratinized epithelia. HSV-1 has a greater propensity to cause recurrent oral infections, while HSV-2 has higher propensity to cause recurrent genital infection. HSV infection can manifest in three different ways:

1. *Primary infection*: It occurs in individuals who have not been previously infected with either HSV-1 or HSV-2. Due to lack of any seropositivity, these infections tend to be severe.
2. *Nonprimary infection*: It occurs in individuals who have been exposed previously to the either of the strains of HSV show some cross protection, making the infection less severe.
3. *Recurrent infection*: After primary or non-primary infection, HSV establishes a latent infection in regional sensory ganglion neurons. These can get reactivated periodically causing asymptomatic or a less severe symptomatic infection, depending on the immune status of the host.

Virus after entering the port replicates locally and enters the nerve endings and replicates in sensory nerve ganglions. Then moving through the neural arches causes the characteristic herpetic lesion. With reactivation, the viruses are transported to skin surfaces through the nerve fibers and produce the typical lesions. Immunocompromised hosts can manifest a very severe cutaneous form or hematogenous spread of the virus. Neonates are relatively immunocompromised. So, HSV infection transmitted during peripartum or postpartum can produce severe manifestation like pneumonia, encephalitis or severe viremia. Clinical manifestation depends on the virus type, portal of entry, gestational age of neonate and maternal immunity status.

CLINICAL FEATURES

Herpes simplex virus produces distinct clinical manifestations in immunocompetent and immunocompromised patients. The manifestations are dependent on whether the infection is primary, secondary or recurrent. In the later two (secondary and recurrent), the infection becomes less severe. Neonates manifest with a more severe form of disease due to their relative immune immaturity. Typical lesion in primary infection manifests as small to large vesicles surrounded by an erythematous base. The vesicles grow and eventually develop into ulcers. Reactivations are mainly asymptomatic and so unrecognized or manifest as small skin fissures or small erythematous non-vesicular lesions.

Orolabial Infections

Primary

The most common age of presentation is from 6 months to 5 years. Classic presentation of extensive orolabial HSV lesion with primary HSV infection in the young child is an extreme manifestation. When such symptomatic disease occurs, there are extremely painful lesions, high fever, irritability, drooling of saliva, refusal to feed, tender submandibular lymphadenopathy. Vesiculo-ulcerative lesions can develop on palate, gingiva, tongue, lips or facial area. Blisters along the vermilion border of the lips may develop, lesions known as herpes labialis. Herpes labials are associated with tingling, itching and pain prior to development of lesion and heal without scar formation in 6–10 days. Most common reason for hospitalization is the dehydration arising out of refusal to feeding and drinking. Symptomatic primary HSV infection is lengthy ranging 2–3 weeks. HSV pharyngitis occurs in older children and adults and is very difficult to distinguish from other viral or bacterial pharyngitis.

Reactivation

Reactivation of HSV from trigeminal ganglion is usually asymptomatic and usually follows manipulation of trigeminal nerve route or dental manipulation. Most common site is the vermilion border and ophthalmic division of trigeminal nerve.

Cutaneous Herpes

Cutaneous HSV infections result from muco-mucosal contact, exposure through open wounds or exposure to infections secretions. Commonly, it is seen in children who come in physical contact with children carrying the virus. The manifestations range from severe pain to burning and itching mainly before the eruption of lesion. Lesions start at the portal of entry as vesicles on erythematous base which progress to ulcers and heal without scaring. *Herpetic whitlow* refers to HSV infection of finger and toes. Whitlow results from digital contamination with oral secretions or genital secretions. Discrete vesicles erupt which coalesce over several days. These lesions are clinically confused with bacterial cellulitis. HSV infections of skin damaged by diaper dermatitis thermal burning or atopic dermatitis can be particularly severe.

Genital Herpes

Genital herpes is more common in older children who are sexually active. HSV-2 is more commonly associated but orogenital transmissions can be due to HSV-1.

Primary

Headache, fever, myalgia, backache develop within 7 days of incubation. Lesions evolve from vesicles and pustules to wet ulcers in about 10 days and then crust and heal in further 10 days. Lesions are distributed over the shaft of penis in males while the females can have lesions over labia, mons pubis, vaginal mucosa and cervix. Mucosal lesions heal faster. Tender inguinal lymphadenopathy appears in 2nd and 3rd week of infection.

Non-primary First Episode

Almost half of the patients with their first clinical outbreak of genital herpes have pre-existing heterologous antibodies. Lesions are less severe, associated with shorter duration of pain, more rapid healing and less severe complications.

Reactivation

Most recurrent forms of genital herpes are asymptomatic. Tender lymphadenopathy, dysuria, vaginal discharge and systemic complications occur less commonly. The carriers keep shedding the virus for long time.

Ocular Herpes

Herpes simplex virus ocular infections can occur through exposure to infected secretions or touching of a herpetic lesions from a different part of the body (like palm or hand after rubbing the genitals) or through peripartal route. Infection involves one or both eyes with a typical course of follicular conjunctivitis with pain, photophobia and tearing followed by chemosis, periorbital edema and preauricular tender lymphadenopathy. Pathognomonic dendritic corneal ulcers develop and are the most common ocular manifestation of recurrent herpes. Healing takes a prolonged period, usually greater than 1 month.

Central Nervous System Herpes

Herpes simplex virus is the most common cause of severe, sporadic, fatal encephalitis world over. It has a biphasic predilection, occurring in patients between 5 and 30 years and also those older than 50 years. Encephalitis can occur as a result of primary infection or more commonly post-reactivation. There occurs acute necrotizing inflammation of temporal and frontal lobe and limbic system with hemorrhagic discharge into the cerebrospinal fluid (CSF). Clinical manifestation may be nonspecific like fever, headache, vomiting with features of meningoencephalitis like nuchal rigidity, meningismus, seizures and altered sensorium. Other features due to temporal lobe or limbic system involvement like anosmia, loss of memory, aphasia and changes in speech, auditory hallucinations and focal seizures can occur. The disease has a very poor prognosis with coma and subsequent death occurring in 75% of cases. HSV is the leading cause of recurrent aseptic meningitis (Mollaret's meningitis).

In Immunocompromised Hosts

Children with compromised immune functions include neonates, the severely malnourished, those with primary and secondary immune deficiencies and those on immunosuppressive agents. Mucocutaneous infections, like mucositis and esophagitis, are most common. The skin and mucosal lesions slowly ulcerate, become necrotic, and extend to deeper tissues. Other common HSV infections are tracheobronchitis, pneumonia and anogenital infections. Viremia is quite common which leads to lodging of the virus is different body organs and presents with a disseminated sepsis like picture with liver, adrenal involvement. Shock and disseminated intravascular coagulation (DIC) can supervene. Retinal infections are also seen with disseminated herpetic infection. Skin lesions often become uncontrolled and spread over larger areas with lesions extending deep. In neonates (perinatal infections):

Herpes simplex virus infections in neonates can be acquired in utero, peripartum or postpartum.

Most cases of neonatal herpes are result of transmission to the baby during passage through a contaminated birth canal. Postpartum transmission can occur from a herpes labialis of mother or any person that the baby is exposed to. Risk of transmission is high if the gestational age is low and if the mother has primary genital herpes rather than recurrent herpes. Neonatal herpes is never thought to be asymptomatic. Infants who are exposed in utero present with skin vesicles, scars, chorioretinitis, or keratoconjunctivitis and microcephaly or hydranencephaly at the time of delivery. Neonates exposed peripartum may present with either 1 of the following patterns of the disease:
- Skin, eye, mouth (SEM) form
- Encephalitis with or without SEM
- Disseminated infection involving various organs.

Skin, eye, mouth form and disseminated form mainly presents within 5–11 days of life, while encephalitis form manifests at around 8–17 days of life. The disseminated from is difficult to distinguish from neonatal sepsis as manifestation are grossly similar. Why neonates present with such severe manifestation? The cause can be attributed to the relative neonatal immune system immaturity and the relative immunodeficiency. Around 50% of infants with encephalitic from succumb while 90% of infants with disseminated from die. The rest of the infants develop severe neurological sequelae.

COMPLICATIONS

Most of the complications of HSV infection are seen in immunocompromised hosts and neonates. Cutaneous HSV infections can be severe of life-threatening in patients who are immunocompromised or have disorders of the skin such as eczema herpeticum, pemphigus, burns and Darier's disease. If untreated, these lesions can lead to disseminated infection and death. Aseptic meningitis can be a complication of disseminated HSV infection. It can occur in 15% of cases of genital herpes. Encephalitis is one of the most grievous manifestations of HSV and leads to death in 75% of cases. Mollaret's meningitis or recurrent aseptic meningitis is one of the rare but under diagnosed complications of HSV-1 infection. Disseminated HSV infection can present as shock and disseminated intravascular coagulation (DIC). Ocular herpes can get complicated into a geographic corneal ulcer or progressive corneal scarring or may cause retinitis as well.

DIAGNOSIS

- *Culture:* It is the gold standard method for diagnosing herpes infection. HSV grows rapidly in cell culture. Cytopathological effect typical of HSV infection usually observed 1–3 days after inoculation. Methods of culture confirmation include—fluorescent antibody staining and enzyme immune assay. Those culture which remain negative by day 15, usually continue to be negative. Materials are collected by rupturing a vesicle and rubbing the base of lesion to collect fluids and cells usually gives better yield.
- Isolation of virus or viral DNA by polymerase chain reaction (PCR) is a diagnostic method of choice.
- Histologic examination and viral culture of a brain tissue specimen obtained by biopsy is the most definitive method of confirming the diagnosis of encephalitis.
- *Neonatal HSV infection*: Materials are collected through swaps from mouth, nasopharynx, conjunctiva for culture. Also specimens collected from skin vesicle, urine, stool, blood and CSF. If cultures become positive after 48 hours, it suggests infant infection.
- Direct detection of HSV antigen in clinical specimens has good specificity and rapidity also.

- Both time specific and nonspecific antibody to HSV has also been used for diagnosis. Immunoglobulin M (IgM) antibody estimation is unreliable, but immunoglobulin G (IgG) estimation in acute and convalescent serum which shows a fourfold rise bears significance. Presence of type-specific antibody to HSV-2 almost always indicates anogenital infection. But presence of HSV-1 antibody does not distinguish anogenital from orolabial infection.
- In routine blood count, there is usually a polymorphonuclear leukocytosis in mucocutaneous infection. In disseminated infections, thrombocytopenia, abnormal coagulation profile and raised liver enzymes are usually noted.
- In cerebrospinal fluid examination, increased numbers of mononuclear cells with raised protein, normal or decreased glucose with some RBC are usually found.

TREATMENT

Currently only three drugs are available in oral form:
1. Acyclovir
2. Valacyclovir
3. Famciclovir

Among them only acyclovir is available in syrup form and intravenous formulation:
- Acyclovir has poorest bioavailability, hence requires frequent dosing.
- Early initiation of therapy results in maximal therapeutic benefit.
- In acyclovir-resistant mutants—foscarnet and cidofovir are treatment of choice.
- Topical trifluorothymidine, vidarabine and idoxuridine are used in the treatment of hepres keratitis.

Acute Mucocutaneous Infection

For gingivostomatitis—oral acyclovir is given at a dose of 15 mg/kg/dose, five times a day for 7 days. The maximum amount of the dose must not exceed 1 g/day. If the treatment is started within 72 hours of onset, the severity and duration of the disease reduces significantly, also the duration of viral shedding.

Herpes Labialis

- Both oral and topical therapy has been evaluated in the treatment. But oral treatment is considered superior to topical therapy
- For treatment of recurrence in adolescent acyclovir is given 200–400 mg/dose, five times a day for 5 days. This treatment shortens the duration of episodes
- Long-term daily use of acyclovir (400 mg PO BID) or valacyclovir (500 mg PO OID) has been used to prevent recurrences in individual with frequent and severe recurrences

- Herpes gladiatorum in adolescent is treated with oral acyclovir (200 mg/dose, five times a day for 7–10 days or with valacyclovir (500 mg BID for 7–10 days) at the 1st sign of outbreak, which can shorten the course of recurrence
- Herpes simplex virus infection in patients can be severe/life threatening and should be treated with IV acyclovir (10–20 mg/kg IV 8 hourly).

Genital Herpes

Primary Infection

First episode should be treated antivirals. Treatment of initial infection decreases the severity and duration of illness, but has no effect on the frequency of subsequent recurrent infection. Oral therapy should be started within 6 days of onset of disease, shortens the duration of illness and viral shedding by 3–5 days. Oral therapy is almost equally efficacious for as IV acyclovir therapy.

Dosing Schedule

- In adolescents
  - Acyclovir (400 mg PO TID × 7–10 days)
  - Famciclovir (750 mg PO TID × 7–10 days)
  - Valacyclovir (100 mg PO BID × 7–10 days)
- *For small children*: Acyclovir (10–20 mg/kg/dose 4 times/day for 7–10 days is adequate. But the total dose should not exceed the adult dose
- The first episode is generally painful and use of analgesics along with antivirals is warranted.

Management of Recurrent Infections

In the management of recurrent infections, the choice of antiviral therapy depends up on many factors like:
- Frequently and seventy of recurrence
- Psychological impact of illness on patient
- Concern regarding the transmission of infection to sexual partners.

Therapeutic options being:
Episodic therapy: Treatment initiated at the first sign of outbreak in adolescents:
- Acyclovir (800 mg PO TID × 2 days)
- Valacyclovir (500 mg PO BID × 3 days)
- Famciclovir (100 mg PO BID × 1 day)

Long-term therapy: Long-term therapy is indicated in adults with frequent genital HSV, i.e. (six recurrences/year). It has advantage over the episodic therapy is that:
- It prevents outbreak
- Improves patients quality of life
- Also decreases the risk of sexual transmission after 1 year of daily treatment.

Therapeutic options being:
- *Acyclovir (400 mg PO BID)*: Generally given for 1 year. After 1 year of daily therapy, acyclovir is discontinued and recurrence is assessed. If recurrences occur again, additional therapy may be considered
- Famciclovir (250 mg PO BID)
- Valacyclovir (500–1000 mg PO QID).

Central Nervous System Infection

Older patient (other than neonates) who has herpes encephalitis treated with IV acyclovir 10 mg/kg/dose IV 8 hourly as 1 hour infusion for 14–21 days with supportive management of raised ICT and seizures and respiratory compromise. The presence of seizure at the time of onset of the therapy among young infants bears poor prognosis in the form of long-term neurologic morbidity.

Infection in Immunocompromised Persons

- Severe mucocutaneous infection and disseminated HSV infection should be treated with IV acyclovir 10 mg/kg IV 8 hourly until the resolution of infection is evident
- For less severe HSV infections oral therapy with acyclovir, famciclovir or valacyclovir can be used
- Drug resistant often occurs in these types of patients. In these cases foscarnet and cidofovir are the drugs which may be useful.

Perinatal Infection

Infants proven or suspected neonatal HSV infection should begin promptly on high dose, i.e. 20 mg/kg/dose IV 8 hourly. If laboratory shows no evidence of infection, it may be discontinued. Duration of treatment depends on the site of infection. So, infants with HSV infection limited to skin/eye/mouth, a 14 days therapy is adequate and if there is CNS or disseminated HSV infection, then 21 days of therapy is needed.

Ocular Infection

Several topical drugs 1% trifluridine, 0.1% iododeoxyuridine, 3% vidarabine have proved efficacy in superficial keratitis. For recurrent ocular lesions, additional treatment with oral acyclovir (80 mg/kg/day in three divided doses) may be of some benefit.

PREVENTION

In case of neonatal infection, the management of infants exposed to HSV during delivery differs according to the status of mother's infection, mode of delivery and expert's opinion.

In the newborns whose mothers have active genital herpes, the risk of infection is more than 50%. In these newborns avoidance of scalp monitors when possible and doing a cesarean section within 4–6 hours of membrane rupture significantly reduces the chance of infection. Many times anticipatory acyclovir started after birth, and cultures from nasopharynx and umbilicus are sent after delivery and at 48 hours of life. If cultures become negative, the acyclovir treatment is stopped. Some authors also recommend to start acyclovir after if the culture reports come positive.

In the newborns whose mothers have recurrent genital herpes, the risk of transmission is less (<5%). So, when doubt, cultures are sent and acyclovir is started if the culture at 48 hours comes positive.

In possibly exposed infants, the infant is observed for signs of vesicular lesions, respiratory distress, seizures and for other signs of sepsis. In the mean time, patient is also evaluating for HSV infection. Here, the testing of CSF by PCR is recommended. Acyclovir is started if anyone becomes positive.

The reduction in vertical transmission of HSV could be accomplished by reducing the maternal infection or the likelihood of transmission to neonate. The role of acyclovir in decreasing the HSV reactivation, and elimination of asymptomatic viral shedding is unclear. So, it is not recommended. To prevent transmission to others, the affected neonate with HSV infection should be hospitalized in a private room and managed with contact precautions for the duration of illness. Relapse can occur in neonates after the cessation of treatment, within first year.

PROGNOSIS

- Most infections are self-limiting—lasts from few days to 2–3 weeks and heals with scarring.
- Recurrent orofacial herpes can be severe and lead to scarring

Life-threatening events being:
- Neonatal herpes
- Herpes encephalitis
- Herpes simplex virus infections in immunocompromised patients
  - Severely malnourished infant and children
- Recurrent ocular herpes can lead to corneal scarring and blindness.

BIBLIOGRAPHY

1. Cook GC, Zumla AI. Cutaneous viral diseases. In: Cook GC, Zumla AI (Eds). Manson's Tropical Diseases, 22nd edition. Saunders Elseviers; 2009. pp. 845-6.
2. Fisher RG, Boyce TG. Acute encephalitis. In: Fisher RG, Boyce TG (Eds). Moffet's Pediatric Infectious Diseases, 4th edition. Philadelphia: Lippincott Williams and Wilkins; 2005. pp. 275-6.
3. Fisher RG, Boyce TG. Exposure during pregnancy. In: Fisher RG, Boyce TG (Eds). Moffet's Pediatric Infectious Diseases, 4th edition. Philadelphia: Lippincott Williams and Wilkins; 2005. pp. 644-5.
4. Fisher RG, Boyce TG. Neonatal sepsis and meningitis. In: Fisher RG, Boyce TG (Eds). Moffet's Pediatric Infectious Diseases, 4th edition. Philadelphia: Lippincott Williams and Wilkins; 2005. pp. 644-5.
5. Gutierrez KM, Arvin AM. Herpes simplex virus 1 and 2. In: Feigin R, Cherry J, Demmler-Harisson G, Kaplan S (Eds). Textbook of Paediatric Infectious Diseases, 6th edition. Philadelphia: Saunders Elsevier; 2009. pp. 1993-2021.
6. Pickering LK, Becker CJ, Long SS, et al. Herpes simplex. In: Pickering LK, Becker CJ, Long SS, McMillan JA (Eds). Red Book, 27th edition. New Delhi: CBS Publishers and Distributers; 2008. pp. 361-70.
7. Prober CG, Herpes simplex virus. In: Long S, Pickering L, Prober CG (Eds). Principles and Practices of Pediatric Infectious Diseases, 3rd edition. Churchill Livingstone Elsevier; 2008. pp. 1012-21.
8. Stanberry LR, Herpes simplex virus. In: Stanton B, Schor N, St Geme J, Berhman R (Eds). Nelson's Textbook of Paediatrics,19th edition. Philadelphia: Saunders Elsevier; 2012. pp. 1097-103.

5.7 PARVOVIRUS B19 INFECTION IN CHILDREN

Lalitha Kailas

INTRODUCTION

Parvoviruses are smallest DNA containing viruses that infect a variety of animal species. There are now four different types of parvoviruses known to infect humans: adeno-associated viruses (AAVs), parvovirus B19 (B19), human bocaviruses (HBoV). Parvovirus 4.B19 and HBoV are the only two parvoviruses known to be pathogenic in humans. B19 is the most well studied and clinically important of the human parvoviruses and the cause of erythema infectiosum or fifth disease. The more recently described human bocavirus is an emerging human pathogen.

Parvovirus B19 is a significant human pathogen that causes a wide spectrum of clinical manifestations ranging from mild, self-limting erythema infectiosum in immunocompetent children to lethal cytopenias in immunocompromised patients and intrauterine fetal death (IUFD) in primary infected pregnant women. The infection may also be persistent and can mimic or trigger autoimmune inflammatory disorders.

ETIOLOGY

Parvovirus B19: The virus was originally discovered in 1974, and the name B19 refers to the blood bank code by which the original positive sample was labeled human parvovirus B19 belongs to *Erythrovirus* genus within the parvovirus family named so because of a pronounced tropism for erythroid precursor cells. The virus replicates in the rapidly growing erythroid progenitor cells, which are found in human bone marrow, fetal liver, human umbilical cord and peripheral blood. The observed tropism of parvovirus is most likely due to its distribution of its cellular receptor P blood group antigen—globoside, which is found in high concentrations on red blood cells and their precursors. Rare individuals who lack P antigen are resistant to infection with parvovirus. The virus is very stable and often survives in blood products despite standard procedures for viral elimination.

EPIDEMIOLOGY

Parvovirus infections are most commonly recognized in school age children; approximately 70% of cases occurring between 5 years and 15 years of age. The seroprevalence increases with age, so that 15% of preschool children, 50% of younger adults and about 85% of the elderly show serologic evidence of past infection. Modes of transmission include contact with respiratory secretions, exposure to blood and blood products and vertical transmission from mother to fetus. *Respiratory transmission* is the most common form of transmission through close person-to-person contact, fomites, respiratory secretions and/or saliva. Young children are the main source of acquired B19, placing the pregnant women with young children at home at high risk of becoming infected. *Vertical transmission* can occur if a susceptible woman becomes infected during her pregnancy and the risk is greatest within first 20 weeks of gestation. *Transfusion transmitted* infections are more seen in those requiring multiple transfusions or blood products like IVIG. The virus is highly contagious and the transmission rate is 15–30% among susceptible household contacts. Nosocomial transmission also may occur and, although rare, is a potential risk in pediatric wards for immunocompromised children. Infection appears to confer lifelong immunity to immunocompetent hosts. Patients with erythema infectiosum are infectious before the onset of rash-not during the rash; whereas patients with aplastic crisis are likely to be most infectious at the time of acute presentation.

PATHOGENESIS

Incubation period ranges usually 4–14 days but can be as long as 21 days. Pathogenesis of erythroviral disease involves two quite separate components; first caused by the lytic infection of susceptible dividing cells and the second by interaction with the products of immune response. The virus, because of its unique tropism for human erythroid progenitor cells, leads to a progressive depletion of erythroid precursors and a transient arrest of erythropoiesis. Upon viral maturation, B19 causes cell lysis. The cytopathic effect induced during B19 infection can be seen in the form of giant pronormoblasts located in the patient's bone marrow. These cells, also called as lantern cells, are large and contain large eosinophilic nuclear inclusions, cytoplasmic vacuolization and immature chromatin. Some manifestations of B19 infection such as transient aplastic crisis (TAC) appear to be a direct result of viral infection whereas others, including exanthem and arthritis, appear to be post-infectious phenomena related to immune response.

IMMUNOLOGY

Viremia occurs 7–10 days after exposure and usually lasts approximately 5 days. Parvovirus B19 specific immunoglobulin M (IgM) antibodies are detected at day 10 through 12 and can persist up to 5 months; specific immunoglobulin G (IgG) antibodies are detectable about

15 days post-infection and persist long term. The close timing that exists between developing B19 specific IgM and IgG antibodies means that it is rare to find an IgM positive serum sample that is not also IgG positive. Development of the antibody response corresponds to virus clearance and subsequent protection from disease.

CLINICAL MANIFESTATIONS

The clinical presentations vary greatly, ranging from benign to life-threatening events, influenced by the age, hematological and immunological status of the individual. Many infections are clinically inapparent or exhibit mild nonspecific cold-like symptoms that are never linked to the virus. However, clinical conditions associated with infections include erythema infectiosum; arthropathy; transient aplastic crisis (TAC); chronic red cell aplasia and hydrops fetalis (Table 5.7.1). Papular purpuric eruptions on the hands and feet ("gloves and socks syndrome) is another not very common dermatologic manifestation of B19 infection.

Erythema Infectiosum (Fifth Disease)

The most common manifestation of parvovirus B19 is erythema infectiosum, which is a benign self-limited exanthematous illness of childhood. It is also referred to as "fifth disease" since it represents the fifth in a numeric classification of common childhood exanthems, each named in order of the dates they were described. The exanthems included: (1) measles, (2) scarlet fever, (3) rubella (4) Filatov-Dukes disease (a variant of scarlet fever—no longer recognized), (5) erythema infectiosum and (6) Roseola erythema infectiosum generally affects children between 4 years and 10 years of age and manifests as a biphasic illness. Approximately 1 week after the infection occurs, a nonspecific febrile illness with headache, malaise and myalgia develops; these symptoms last for 2–3 days, and coincide with the onset of viremia. This is followed by an asymptomatic period of approximately 7 days and then the exanthematous phase of the illness begins.

The exanthem usually occurs in three phases, which are not always readily distinguished. The initial stage

consists of an erythematous flushing of the face described as "slapped cheek" appearance with relative circumoral pallor. In the second stage the rash quickly or concurrently spreads to the trunk and proximal extremities as a diffuse macular erythema, followed by central clearing of the lesions giving a reticulated lacy appearance. Palms and soles are usually spared. This second stage rash lasts for 1–3 weeks. The third stage is characterized by periodic evanescence and recrudescence of the rash and lasts for 1–3 weeks. Mild pruritus may be present in older children and adults and rash may resolve spontaneously usually within 3 weeks without any desquamation; but may recur in response to a variety of nonspecific environmental stimuli such as sunlight, heat, exercise or emotional stress. By the time the rash develops, viremia has resolved, and the affected children are afebrile and do not appear ill. The rash is thought to be immunologically mediated. Lymphadenopathy is not a prominent or consistent feature.

Transient Aplastic Crisis

In a person with normal hematopoiesis, B19 infection produces a self-limited red cell aplasia that is clinically inapparent. In patients who have increased rates of red cell destruction or loss and who depend on compensatory mechanisms in red cell production to maintain stable red cell indices, B19 infection may lead to TAC. Patients at risk for TAC include those with hemolytic anemias (sickle cell disease, thalassemia, hereditary spherocytosis, etc.) and those with anemias associated with acute or chronic blood loss.

During this a transient arrest of erythropoiesis with a profound reticulocytopenia leads to a sudden fall in Hb requiring transfusions. This can be life-threatening, although most patients make a full recovery within 2 weeks. The precipitous drop in hemoglobin also may cause congestive failure, a cerebrovascular accident or acute splenic sequestration. White blood cell (WBC) and platelets also may fall. In contrast to children with erythema infectiosum, children with aplastic crisis are ill at presentation with fever and malaise, and signs and symptoms of profound anemia (pallor, tachycardia and so on). Rash is rarely present in these patients. The dramatic fall or absence of measurable reticulocytes is a hallmark laboratory finding in persons with B19 infection. Patients are highly contagious during aplastic crisis and should be isolated to prevent transmission of the virus. Humeral immunity is crucial in controlling infection. Specific IgM appears within 1–2 days of infection followed by IgG antibodies which leads to control of infection, restoration of reticulocytosis and a rise in hemoglobin.

A typical TAC may be the initial presentation of the underlying hemolytic condition in certain patients who are hemodynamically well compensated and under diagnosed, especially common to occur with hereditary spherocytosis.

Table 5.7.1: Clinical manifestations of parvovirus B19 infection.

Conditions	Usual hosts
• Erythema infectiosum (fifth disease) • Transient aplastic crisis • Polyarthropathy syndrome • Hydrops fetalis/congenital anemia • Chronic anemia/pure red cell aplasia • Persistent anemia • Myocarditis	• Normal children • Children with hemolytic anemias • Immunocompetent adults (more in women) • Fetus (first 20 weeks of pregnancy) • Immunocompromised hosts • Fetus/normal children/adults

Arthropathy

Arthropathy may be a complication of erythema infectiosum or a primary presentation of a parvovirus B19 infection. Approximately 8% of children infected with the virus have arthralgia. The arthropathy is particularly common in middle-aged women, and is characterized by a polyarthritis, typically involving the metacarpophalangeal joints, knees, wrists or ankles. In children, pattern can be symmetric or asymmetric and usually involves the knees (82%) and ankles. In some, arthritis may be prolonged, lasting for months and even mimics classical rheumatoid arthritis. The joint involvement however is not erosive and is probably immune mediated as it appears simultaneous with the circulating antibodies. Rheumatoid factor may also be transiently positive, leading to some diagnostic confusion.

Autoimmune Diseases

Apart from rheumatoid arthritis, B19 infection has also been associated with the onset of numerous autoimmune disorders including systemic lupus erythematosus (SLE), other connective tissue disorders and systemic vasculitis Henoch-Schönlein purpura, polyarteritis nodosa (HSP, PAN, etc.). The role of B19 in these disorders is not clear and in some cases, infection may be a pure coincidence and in some it may be a triggering factor or even a rare etiologic factor. B19 infection also can induce antibodies to double-stranded DNA, antinuclear soluble antigens, cardiolipin and rheumatoid factor. The autoantibody production most likely results from both polyclonal stimulation of immune responses and production. Although these responses are normally short duration, they can cause diagnostic difficulties.

B19 Infection in Immunocompromised Children

The clinical picture of acute and persistent B19 infection in the immunocompromised host differs significantly from immunocompetent subjects. They are at risk of developing chronic and recurrent infection with parvovirus B19. In the absence of an efficient humeral and/or cellular immune response, these persons do not have protective antibodies and the infection can cause persistent bone marrow suppression. Persistent anemia, sometimes profound reticulocytopenia is the most common manifestation of such infection which may also be accompanied by neutropenia, thrombocytopenia, or complete marrow suppression. But immune-mediated symptoms, such as rash and arthralgia, are not common. Susceptible children include children with congenital immunodeficiencies, HIV infection, leukemia, lymphoma, myelodysplastic syndrome and recipients of organ transplants. The severity of anemia is also more with B19 infection in patients with falciparum malaria.

Gloves and Socks Syndrome

A variety of atypical skin eruptions has been reported with B19 infection; most of these are petechial or purpuric in nature with evidence of vasculitis on biopsy. Among these rashes, papular-purpuric gloves and socks syndrome (PPGSS) especially occurs in young adults and presents as symmetric, painful erythema and edema of the feet and hands. The condition gradually progresses to petechiae and purpura and may develop into vesicles and bullae with skin sloughing. A hallmark of the syndrome is a sharp demarcation of the rash at the wrists and ankles, although other areas may be involved. Symptoms usually resolve within 1–3 weeks without scarring.

Fetal Infection

Vertical transmission of B19 from a primary infected mother may cause fetal infection and results in complications including miscarriage, intrauterine fetal death (IUFD) and/or non-immune hydrops fetalis. There is approximately 30% risk of vertical transmission to the fetus, mostly occurring in the first or second trimester as the placental P antigen, which may be necessary for the transmission becomes less frequent with increasing gestational age. Parvoviruses tend to infect rapidly dividing cells and can be transmitted across the placenta, posing a potential threat to the fetus. The fetus is at risk for serious disease because of both its hematologic status and immature status. The fetus is especially susceptible to the effects of B19 induced anemia due to its shortened red blood cell (RBC) half-life and expanding RBC volume. The relatively immature fetal immune system is also less able to effectively control virus infection. The presumed pathogenic sequence is as follows; maternal primary infection leads to transplacental transfer of B19 virus and infection of fetal hematopoietic cells. This causes arrest of red cell production, severe anemia (Hb <8 g/dL), high output cardiac failure and edema. Furthermore, B19 may cause fetal myocarditis, which can contribute to the development of hydrops. Parvovirus B19 has been implicated in approximately 10% of cases of fetal non-immune hydrops. Fetal B19 infection also can present with thrombocytopenia. Many fetuses are borne without symptoms, but there is a 2–6% risk of fetal loss. However, it is unlikely that parvovirus B19 is a cause for congenital anomalies. Hence therapeutic abortion should not be recommended in women infected with parvovirus during pregnancy. Rather, pregnancy should be followed with frequent examination and serial ultrasound scanning (USS) for signs of hydrops. B19 infection is a common cause of IUFD also in late gestation, but without fetal hydrops in a majority of cases. Congenital anemia, associated with intrauterine B19 infection has been reported in a few cases, mimicking other forms of congenital hypoplastic anemias.

Myocarditis

B19 infection has been associated with myocarditis in fetuses, infants, children and adults. This is because fetal myocardial cells contain P antigen; diagnosis is often based on serologic findings suggestive of a concurrent B19 infection mostly and demonstration of B19 DNA in a few cases. Also, dilated cardiomyopathy and isolated left ventricular diastolic dysfunction have been reported with parvovirus B19 infection.

Other B19 associated disorders include hepatitis, transient erythroblastopenia of childhood, meningitis, encephalitis glomerulonephritis, nephrotic syndrome, etc..

DIAGNOSIS

The diagnosis of erythema infectiosum is usually based on clinical presentation of the typical rash and rarely requires virologic confirmation. Similarly diagnosis of typical TAC in a child with hemolytic anemia is generally made on clinical grounds without virological testing.

Parvovirus B19 will not grow in standard tissue cultures because humans are the only hosts. Hence measurement of IgM and IgG antibodies in blood and B19 DNA in blood or tissue samples by polymerase chain reaction (PCR) are the most practical tests. Histological examination is also helpful in diagnosing B19 infection in certain situations. Examination of bone marrow aspirate in anemic patients reveals giant pronormoblasts or lantern cells against a background of general erythroid hypoplasia.

B19 specific IgM antibodies develop rapidly after infection and persist for 6–8 weeks and are the best markers for recent/acute infection. Anti B19 IgG antibodies become detectable a few days after IgM and persist for years and are the markers of past infection/immunity. Serology is unreliable in immunocompromised persons, and here methods to detect viral particles or viral DNA, such as PCR and nucleic acid amplification test (NAAT) are recommended to establish the diagnosis.

Prenatal diagnosis of B19 induced fetal hydrops can be accomplished by detection of viral DNA in fetal blood or amniotic fluid by these methods.

DIFFERENTIAL DIAGNOSIS

The rash of erythema infectiosum must be differentiated from rubella, measles, scarlet fever, enteroviral infections and drug reactions. Significant fever and typical coryzal prodrome of measles and the fever and pharyngitis of scarlet fever helps to differentiate.

TREATMENT

There is no specific antiviral drug against B19 infection; for most patients only supportive care is needed. Generally,

Table 5.7.2: Treatment options for parvovirus B19 infection.

Manifestation	Treatment options
Erythema infectiosum	None or symptomatic
Arthritis or arthralgia	Nonsteroidal anti-inflammatory drugs (NSAIDs)
Transient aplastic crisis	Transfusion if required
Fetal hydrops	Intrauterine transfusion (?)
Chronic infection with anemia	IVIG and transfusions

erythema infectiosum is self-limited and does not require treatment. Patients with arthralgia may require nonsteroidal anti-inflammatory drugs (NSAIDs). Patients in aplastic crisis may require hospitalization and anemia is often sufficiently severe (hemoglobin levels below 6 g/dL with few or no reticulocytes) to require transfusion until the patient's immune response eliminates the infection and red cell production returns. The usual course of parvovirus-associated anemia is spontaneous resolution within a few days to weeks. Beyond supportive red blood cell transfusion, more aggressive therapy with IVIG is generally limited to patients with chronic anemia related to a persistent parvovirus B19 infection. Doses recommended are either 400 mg/kg for 5 days or 1 g/kg for 3 days. There does not appear to be any role for immunoglobulin for patients with erythema infectiosum or aplastic crisis, as these are self-limited syndromes (Table 5.7.2).

There are no recommendations for the use of intravenous immunoglobulin (IVIG) in pregnancy with B19 infected fetuses. In the carefully followed pregnancy in which hydrops is worsening, intrauterine blood transfusions may be considered, especially if the fetal Hb is less than 8 g/dL. However, this procedure has significant attendant risks and B19 associated hydrops is known to resolve spontaneously and the fetus can be normal at delivery.

COMPLICATIONS

Arthralgia or arthritis associated with erythema infectiosum can be persistent after resolution of the rash especially in adolescents and adults. B19 infection may rarely cause thrombocytopenic purpura. Neurologic conditions including aseptic meningitis, encephalitis and peripheral neuropathy have been reported in association with B19 infection. B19 is also a cause of infection associated hemophagocytic syndrome, usually in immunocompromised persons.

PREVENTION

The only measures currently available to prevent B19 infection are those designed to interrupt virus transmission. However, because patients are viremic and infectious before the symptoms of erythema infectiosum, isolation of patients with fifth disease is not rational and the affected children can attend the school. But children are infectious during B19 induced TAC and demonstrate intense viremia and they should be isolated to prevent spread to susceptible patients and staff for 1 week until after resolution of fever.

The Centers for Disease Control and Prevention (CDC) recommends that patients with TAC be placed on droplet isolation precautions for seven days and that immunodeficient patients with chronic infection be placed on droplet precautions for the duration of their hospitalization.

The pregnant women are at high risk of developing fetal parvovirus disease when exposed to an infected household contact; school teachers and healthcare providers are more susceptible. Measurement of serum IgG and IgM levels and PCR may be useful to determine who is at risk or acutely infected after B19 exposure. For susceptible or acutely infected women, serial fetal ultrasonography is recommended to monitor fetal growth and the possible evolution of hydrops. Serial determinations of maternal serum alpha fetoprotein (a marker for fetal aplastic crisis in fetal parvovirus infection) are also helpful—AFP may rise up to 4 weeks before ultrasonography evidence of fetal hydrops, although this is often uncertain value.

No vaccine is currently available; however, prospects for vaccination are favorable with a B19 virus empty capsid vaccine is currently under development.

BIBLIOGRAPHY

1. Adler SP, Koch WC. Parvovirus infections. Krugman's Infectious Disease of Children, 11th edition; 2004. pp. 429-39.
2. Broliden K, Tolfvenstam T, Norbeck O. Clinical aspects of parvovirus infection. J Intern Med. 2006;260(4):285-304.
3. Brown KE. Human parvoviruses including parvovirus B19 and human bocavirus in Mandell, Douglas and Bennett's Principles and Practice of Infectious Diseases, 7th edition, 2010. pp. 2087-93.
4. Burchett SK. Viral infections. Manual of Neonatal Care, 7th edition; 2012. pp. 599-602.
5. Cherry JD, Schule DJ. Human Prvovirus B19 in Feign and Cherry 's Textbook of pediatric infectious diseases, 6th edition, 1902-1905;2:166.
6. Jordan JA. Clinical manifestations and diagnosis of human parvovirus B19 infection in Up2Date. In: Hirsch MS, Edwards MS (Eds), MD, updated: Dec 15, 2014.
7. Koch WC. Parvovirus B19 infections. Nelson's Textbook of Pediatrics, 20th edition; 251:1568-72.
8. Parvovirus B19 Infection (Erythema infectiosum) in Red book 2009—Report Committee on Infectious Diseases, 28th edition. Washington DC: AAP; 2009. pp. 491-3.
9. Servey JT, Reamy BV, Hodge J. Clinical presentations of parvovirus B19 infection. Am Fam Physician. 2007;75(3):373-6.

5.8 VARICELLA ZOSTER

Parang Mehta

INTRODUCTION

The varicella zoster virus is an alpha herpesvirus, and causes two types of disease in humans—chickenpox (varicella) and shingles (herpes zoster). The primary infection usually results in chickenpox, chickenpox but the virus remains dormant in dorsal root neurons in almost all patients. Reactivation of the virus (usually after many years) causes herpes zoster (shingles).

CHICKENPOX

This is a worldwide disease, and in the time before the vaccine became available, almost everyone would get it at some time in life. In western countries where universal vaccination against varicella is not practiced, the maximum incidence is between 1 years and 3 years of age, and almost all adults are immune through having the disease in childhood. In Asian countries, though, the incidence peak is shifted upwards, and adults are often non-immune.

Chickenpox is a highly infectious disease. With close exposure such as in the home, secondary attack rates can be as high as 100%. Lesser exposures such as in the classroom or playground have lower transmission rates.

The virus seems to be stable, and does not undergo changes in antigenic structure or virulence. Severe disease is caused by host factors rather than the agent. T-cells are more important than humoral immunity. Children with T-cell defects and AIDS are more likely to suffer disseminated and severe chickenpox.

Infection and Incubation

The infection is through the respiratory tract. The initial infection is followed by a primary viremia, during which the virus spreads to reticuloendothelial cells in the liver. Later, there is a secondary viremia, when the virus spreads to the skin. There is some evidence that skin infection occurs early, but replication of the virus is slow.

The incubation period for chickenpox is 10–21 days. Towards the end of this period, the virus is carried back to respiratory sites. This makes the person infective 24–48 hours before the first skin lesion.

Clinical Features

Chickenpox usually manifests 14–16 days after exposure, though it may be delayed as long as 3 weeks. It can be so mild as to escape diagnosis, but this is rare. Most children have symptoms for a day or two before the rash appears.

These consist of malaise, fever, headache, loss of appetite, and abdominal pain. The fever is rarely very high.

The rash begins on the face, scalp, or trunk, and the limbs are involved later. Lesions may appear in the mouth, conjunctivae, and vagina. Initial lesions are reddish macules that later form clear, fluid filled vesicles. Sometimes they have a surrounding margin of erythema, leading to the classical description of "pearl on a rose petal". The fluid becomes hazy after a day or two, and may show umblication. A characteristic feature of chickenpox lesions is itching, which can be severe enough to prevent sleep.

New lesions continue to appear as older ones evolve, and subside by drying and crusting. Crusts are shed as new skin is formed under them. New lesions may continue to appear for up to 7 days. Most children have less than 300 skin lesions, but having more than 500 lesions is common. This should not be taken as evidence of immunodeficiency.

Chickenpox is more severe in adolescents and adults. Young children usually have mild disease. Sunburn or skin trauma can cause severe rash in the affected areas. Usually the lesions heal without scarring, but the initial lesions sometimes involve deeper layers of th skin. These leave a shallow scar. Most lesions will leave areas of hypopigmentation, which fade to normal in a few weeks.

Differential Diagnosis

Smallpox was a major source of confusion, but that disease was eliminated in the 1970s. Other rashes that cause diagnostic problems are caused by enteroviruses, *Staphylococcus aureus*, drug reactions, insect bites, and contact dermatitis.

Complications

Infective Complications

The most common, and dangerous, complication is secondary bacterial infection. In otherwise healthy children with chickenpox, secondary infections are the most common cause of serious illness. Commonly involved are *Streptococcus pyogenes* and *Staphylococcus aureus*. The usual infections are impetigo and cellulitis. Subcutaneous abscesses, lymphadenitis, and necrotizing fasciitis are other, more destructive lesions. Cellulitis of the neck can sometimes cause respiratory obstruction.

Varicella gangrenosa is a rare but dangerous secondary infection, associated with *Streptococcus pyogenes*. Usually, one varicella lesion is involved, becoming red, warm, and painful. The surrounding skin becomes involved, often in only a few hours. Edema can be marked, and this progresses to necrotizing fasciitis, which needs emergency management.

Other infections are caused by entry of pathogens through the varicella lesions. Local infections like pneumonia, osteomyelitis and arthritis can occur following the transient bacteremia. Sometimes septicemia can occur, leading to high fever, shock, and disseminated intravascular coagulopathy (DIC).

Neurological Complications

Among noninfective complications, the most frequent are neurologic. CNS manifestations of chickenpox usually are seen 2–6 days after the rash appears, though they have been described (rarely) during the incubation period and after the resolution of the skin lesions. Varicella is a common cause of encephalitis, which is more common in children below 5 years of age. Cerebellar disease is also common, and ataxia, nystagmus and slurred speech can persist for several days.

The symptoms of encephalitis can overlap with meningitis and cerebellar disease. The child usually has abrupt onset of seizures, neck rigidity, altered consciousness, and extensor plantar reflexes. Some children may have only meningeal signs, with an intact sensorium and no seizures. Most children recover completely and rapidly; mortality or sequelae are uncommon. Some children may have long term seizures or neurologic deficits following varicella encephalitis.

Varicella was sometimes followed by Reye's syndrome, but this is rare, now that salicylates are not used for fever. Other rare complications are the Guillan-Barre syndrome and transverse myelitis.

Other Complications

Hematologic complications sometimes occur, with low platelet counts and bleeding into vesicles. Sometimes there is bleeding from the gums, gastrointestinal tract, nose, and hematuria. These manifestations are usually short lived, but thrombocytopenia may persist for weeks. Thrombocytopenia sometimes occurs after the chickenpox episode is over, and bleeding manifestations may persist for over a month. A rare but dangerous complication is purpura fulminans, caused by arterial thrombosis.

Hepatic complications are uncommon, and are often detected as disturbances of the enzymes without clinical manifestations. Nephritis, the nephrotic syndrome, and the hemolytic-uremic syndrome sometimes follow an episode of chickenpox. Other complications are arthritis, orchitis, pancreatitis, myocarditis, and pericarditis.

Chickenpox in Adolescents and Adults

Chickenpox is a mild disease in children, but can be serious in older age groups. Severe varicella is seen mainly in adults, among otherwise healthy population. One of the most dangerous manifestations is varicella pneumonia. It appears 1–6 days after the skin manifestations, and the first symptoms are usually cough and dyspnea. Some cases may have cyanosis, pleuritic chest pain, or hemoptysis. Radiology shows diffuse infiltrates on both sides with some nodular densities. Oxygen saturation can fall, sometimes more than is suggested by the clinical findings. Varicella pneumonia usually resolves in 2–3 days, but may sometimes progress to respiratory failure.

Chickenpox in Pregnancy

Chickenpox in pregnancy is very dangerous for both mother and unborn baby. The major risk to the mother is varicella pneumonia, which occurs in 10–20% of these patients. The mortality can be up to 40%.

Risks to the baby are intrauterine fetal death, spontaneous abortion, and premature delivery. The congenital varicella syndrome occurs in about 2% of babies who have been exposed to varicella in utero. The risk is highest if the exposure was in the first 20 weeks of gestation. The most common manifestations are skin scars, atrophy of a limb, hypopigmentation, encephalitis, cortical atrophy, mental retardation, joint abnormalities, and absent or malformed digits. The eyes may be involved, in the form of chorioretinitis, anisocoria, and microphthalmia. The later in gestation the exposure, the milder these manifestations.

If a woman has varicella at time of delivery, there is a 20% risk of transmission to the baby. If chickenpox onset was 5 days or more before delivery, the baby gets the infection, but also maternal IgG antibodies to varicella zoster virus, ensuring that severe disease will not occur. If the baby is born less than 4 days after onset of maternal varicella, or up to 2 days before the onset, there has not been time for formation and transfer of antibodies. These babies get only the virus, but no antibodies and are at high risk for severe varicella. Neonatal varicella is often associated with pneumonia and other serious complications. Mortality rates can be as high as 30%.

Maternal herpes zoster has very little risk of congenital varicella syndrome or neonatal complications. Possibly, because these women had the primary infection much earlier and have adequate circulating antibodies.

Diagnosis

Chickenpox is a clinical diagnosis, and laboratory studies are rarely required.

Most children with chickenpox have low white cell counts initially. Later, there may be a lymphocytosis. Hepatic enzymes are sometimes slightly raised.

Specific diagnosis of varicella zoster virus infection may be needed in immunocompromised children, to guide treatment. The virus is difficult to isolate by tissue culture, and rapid antigen methods are commonly used. Commonly used are in situ hybridization and polymerase chain reaction (PCR). Epithelial cells from the base of a vesicle show viral proteins when stained appropriately (Tzanck method).

Treatment

Treatment decisions are not straightforward in all cases. All children with chickenpox need some supportive therapy, but the need for specific antiviral treatment varies with age. Supportive therapy is usually needed for fever and itching. Paracetamol is the recommended antipyretic, and is effective and safe. Others like ibuprofen and mefenamic acid may be used. Salicylates should never be used in children with chickenpox because of the risk for Reye's syndrome.

Pruritus is so common as to be a part of chickenpox. It can lead to restlessness and lack of sleep, and scratching can cause secondary infection. Itching can be treated by daily bathing, cool compresses and antihistaminics. Older antihistamines are probably more effective; the newer (so-called non-sedating) drugs do not have as good an action on itching. Commonly used drugs are dimenhydramine and chlorpheniramine.

Among antiviral drugs for varicella, the nucleoside analog acyclovir has been most used in children. Other drugs like famciclovir and valacyclovir are structurally and functionally similar. They have better absorption after oral administration, but experience with their use in children is limited.

In normal children, acyclovir, if started within 24 hours of the appearance of the rash, will shorten the disease duration by one day. Since the benefit to normal children with varicella is so minor, acyclovir is not recommended for these children. The drug is recommended for adults especially pregnant women because the disease tends to be more severe. Oral acyclovir is recommended for most patients, but neonates, patients with varicella pneumonia, and immunocompromised patients should receive this drug parenterally. When given parenterally (IV) the dose is 30 mg/kg/day, in three divided doses. The oral dose is 80 mg/kg/day, divided into 4 doses.

Indications for acyclovir in children are:
- Neonatal age
- Malignancies
- Bone marrow transplantation
- Chemotherapy or high-dose steroid treatment
- HIV infection
- Severe varicella, like pneumonia or encephalitis
- Chronic skin disease
- Long term salicylate or steroid therapy
- Children over 12 years may be considered for antiviral therapy.

Acyclovir must be started in the first 24 hours after lesions appear, for the most benefit. It should be given for 7 days, or until no new lesions have appeared for 48 hours. It reduces the clinical symptoms of varicella, and diminishes the progression to severe varicella, the latter effect being its true value. The use of acyclovir does not reduce the host immune response in normal children, and immunity to varicella will develop.

Prevention

People with chickenpox are infectious for 1–2 days before skin lesions appear and diagnosis is made. Preventing children with chickenpox from attending school cannot, therefore, eliminate spread, though it will reduce it. Individual protection is required for prevention.

An episode of chickenpox gives lifelong immunity to the person. Second episodes of chickenpox are rare in immunocompetent people. A second episode of chickenpox should not lead to work up for immunodeficiency disorders. Parents reporting several episodes of chickenpox usually have not been diagnosed by a competent professional.

The varicella vaccine was developed in 1974, and has been in general use for over two decades now. It has been found to be safe and reasonably effective. The original recommendation was for a single dose for children 1–13 years of age. This was found to reduce the incidence of chickenpox to a large extent, and almost eliminate severe disease.

However, it was found that the protection wanes over time, and breakthrough varicella was a significant problem. Children with breakthrough varicella usually have mild disease, but are as infectious to others as unvaccinated children. Currently, two doses of this vaccine are recommended. This reduces the incidence of chickenpox to very low levels. Breakthrough varicella incidence rate in children vaccinated with one dose has been found to be 8.5 cases per 1,000 person years. Children who have received two doses have a much lower incidence of 2.2 cases per 1,000 person years.

The Indian Academy of Pediatrics Advisory Committee on Vaccines and Immunization Practices (ACVIP) recommends that the first dose should be given at the age of 15 months. The second dose should be given at the age of 4–6 years. For children not vaccinated at the recommended age, catch up vaccination can be started at any age. The second dose should be after 3 months in children under 13 years, and 4–8 weeks for children over the age of 13 years.

The vaccine is generally safe, and side effects are few and mild. The vaccine is contraindicated in:
- Immunodeficiency, congenital or acquired
- Symptomatic HIV infection
- High dose steroid therapy (2 mg/kg/day or higher)
- Blood dyscrasias
- Leukemia, lymphoma, and other malignancies
- Pregnancy
- Allergy to neomycin or other vaccine components.

The varicella vaccine is now available in combination with the measles, mumps, and rubella (MMR) vaccine.

This quadrivalent vaccine has the advantage of one less injection for the child. The IAP ACVIP and the Advisory Committee on Immunization Practices (USA) both recommend that this vaccine be given to children at the age of 4 years and above. For the 15 month doses, it is recommended that MMR and varicella vaccines be given separately to avoid the higher incidence of adverse effects with the quadrivalent vaccine.

Post-exposure Prophylaxis

Exposure to chickenpox is worrisome to parents, since it is known that the disease is highly infectious. Children who have suffered from chickenpox are immune, and no action need be taken. Children that are fully immunized are also immune. We need to take action for those children who have been exposed to chickenpox, and have no history of either the disease or the vaccine in the past.

If the child is over 1 year of age, the best option is the varicella vaccine, since it provides active immunity which is long lasting. When given as post-exposure prophylaxis, its effect is variable. The child may be fully protected, or may develop varicella. However, the disease will be attenuated. The vaccine must be given in a day or two after exposure.

The other options are varicella zoster immune globulin (VZIG) and acyclovir. Both of them are effective, and are especially useful when the vaccine cannot be used (infancy, immunodeficiency, pregnancy, etc). They provide protection for a short while only, and may prevent or attenuate the disease, depending on host factors and the time elapsed since exposure when intervention was begun. Some of the children given acyclovir will not develop immunity to chickenpox, and must be evaluated for the need for active immunization.

VARICELLA ZOSTER (SHINGLES)

This results from reactivation of dormant virus. Since this occurs several years after the initial infection, herpes zoster is rarely seen in children.

The disease manifests as a localized, one-sided vesicular rash, usually restricted to the skin distribution of a single sensory nerve. Vesicles resembling chickenpox appear in this delimited area, and progress and coalesce. The person may have pain, itching, and hyperesthesia. The acute skin lesions of herpes zoster subside by crusting in about 2 weeks. The most troublesome manifestation is post-herpetic neuralgia, which causes persistent pain and discomfort.

There does not appear to be any respiratory excretion during this time, so people with herpes zoster are not infectious through the airborne route. However, they remain a source of infection for unimmunized persons through direct contact.

Herpes zoster can be treated with acyclovir (IV, 30 mg/kg/day in 3 divided doses). This shortens the duration of the acute disease significantly, and reduces the incidence of post-herpetic neuralgia.

A live virus vaccine against herpes zoster is now available in some countries, and is recommended for people over sixty years of age.

BIBLIOGRAPHY

1. Indian Academy of Pediatrics, Advisory Committee on Vaccines and Immunization Practices (ACVIP). Vashishtha VM, Choudhary J, Jog P, et al. Indian Academy of Pediatrics (IAP) Recommended Immunization Schedule for Children Aged 0 through 18 years—India, 2016 and Updates on Immunization. Indian Pediatrics epub.
2. Lalwani S, Chatterjee S, Balasubramanian S, et al. Immunogenicity and safety of early vaccination with two doses of a combined measles-mumps-rubella-varicella vaccine in healthy Indian children from 9 months of age: a phase III, randomised, non-inferiority trial. BMJ Open 2015; 5:e007202.
3. Marin M, Broder KR, Temte JL, et al. Centers for Disease Control and Prevention (CDC). Use of combination measles, mumps, rubella, and varicella vaccine: recommendations of the Advisory Committee on Immunization Practices (ACIP). MMWR Recomm Rep. 2010;59(RR-3):1-12.
4. Seward JF, Zhang JX, Maupin TJ, et al. Contagiousness of Varicella in Vaccinated Cases: A Household Contact Study. JAMA. 2004;292:704-8.
5. Walker JL, Andrews NJ, Mathur R, et al. Trends in the burden of varicella in UK general practice. Epidemiol. Infect. 2017;145: 2678-82.
6. Zhu S, Zeng F, Xia L, et al. Incidence rate of breakthrough varicella observed in healthy children after 1 or 2 doses of varicella vaccine: Results from a meta-analysis. Am J Infect Control. 2017; pii: S0196-6553 (17);30945-8.

5.9   RESPIRATORY SYNCYTIAL VIRUS INFECTION

M Govindaraj

INTRODUCTION

Respiratory syncytial virus (RSV) is the major cause of respiratory tract infection in young children. All persons could have experienced RSV infection within the first few years of life. RSV infection is responsible for high mortality in under five children in developing countries.

The RSV is an extraordinarily successful respiratory virus that causes annual epidemics of respiratory disease. Although the virus is able to reinfect individuals throughout life, its greatest impact is on very young and elderly people. The major causes of acute viral bronchiolitis and pneumonia in admitted patients to the hospital are in this age group.

The RSV is an RNA virus belonging to the Pneumovirus family. It is closely related to the paramyxovirus. The virus was first isolated from a chimpanzee in 1956 and was originally called the "chimpanzee coryza virus". It was renamed because of its predilection for the respiratory system and its tendency to produce syncytial when inoculated into human cell lines.

The virus has been shown to cause respiratory disease in all parts of the world. The virus, without fail, produces yearly outbreaks of respiratory disease. In temperate climates, the disease commence in late autumn or early winter, rising rapidly to a peak and then falling away by late spring. Isolation of the virus in the summer is uncommon. In tropical and subtropical climates, epidemics tend to occur during the rainy season. It is still unclear why the epidemics follow such a regular pattern, the trigger for each epidemic remains to be defined. It has recently been demonstrated that the virus appears to be able to productively infect human dendritic cells during the RSV season, but out of the season it appears to lie dormant within these cells. Viral replication can be triggered by exogenous nitric oxide (NO), which may be relevant to the seasonality of the epidemics and the observation that the severity of illness is greatest in industrialized areas because of increased NO levels, in contrast to other pollutants, peak in the winter and are highest in industrialized areas, it is also of noted that exposure to cigarette smoke is associated with more severe disease.

The incubation period before the onset of symptoms appears to be in the range of 3–8 days. Spread of infection appears to be via large droplets of fomites. These droplets are transmitted to hands and fingers, and self inoculation that occur with transmission of virus into the eyes or nose, which acts as portals to the respiratory tract. Small droplet aerosol appears not to be an important form of transmissions. Survival of the virus on hands is variable but generally less than 1 hour. Shedding of virus by hospitalized infants continues even after significant clinical improvement, and the infants generally continue to shed virus for many days after discharge from hospital.

Almost all infants will have been infected by the virus by the end of their second winter, and half have experienced two infections during their first two winters. For most infants symptoms will be relatively mild with upper respiratory tract symptoms alone, however, up to 25% will develop lower respiratory tract symptoms. In most cases, these lower respiratory tract symptoms can be managed in the community, but between 0.5% and 1.5% of all infants are admitted to hospital during the winter epidemic following their birth with RSV lower respiratory tract symptoms. Those aged 1–4 months are at particular risk of severe disease include postnatal age, preterm birth, chronic lung disease of prematurity, cardiac disease with pulmonary hypertension, neurologic disease and immunodeficiency. Other factors increasing the likelihood of severe disease include attendance at day care exposure to tobacco smoke, overcrowding and having older siblings.

The poor herd immunity is probably attributable to the ability of the virus to inhibit the production of an effective long-term immune response or through hiding the important epitopes. Alternatively, antigenic variation may be more important than is currently appreciated. If so, this has important implications for the production of vaccines. Unfortunately, there is currently no immediate prospect of preventing these annual epidemics.

PHENOTYPES OF THE DISEASE

Over the past 30 years, researchers have been trying to identify possible specific immunopathologies that may explain the association of RSV with acute bronchiolitis and pneumonia.

As noted, the virus almost certainly influences the memory responses and as a consequence, certain aspects of the host viral interaction may differ from that observed with other respiratory viruses, and indeed any of the respiratory viruses, RSV may cause a simple coryzal illness, acute otitis media, bronchitis, laryngotracheobronchitis, bronchiolitis, pneumonia, virus-associated wheezing and viral exacerbations of asthma.

Acute Bronchiolitis

Surprisingly, despite the frequency and importance of this condition, there are still a number of controversies in the diagnosis and optimal management of infants with "acute bronchiolitis". This appears largely attributable to a failure to agree on the clinical features that characterize patients with acute bronchiolitis. In the United Kingdom, Australia and parts of Europe, the term acute bronchiolitis is limited to infants who present with the following clinical pattern. Upper respiratory tract symptoms with coryza and cough precede the relatively abrupt onset of lower respiratory symptoms after 2–3 days. Fever is common but frequently settles early in the course of the illness and may be absent when the patient presents to the hospital. The onset of lower respiratory symptoms is frequently acute, and, at presentation, the infant is dyspneic with a moist irritating cough. Difficulty feeding and agitation due to hypoxia are not uncommon. Wheeze may be present intermittently but is not characteristic. Tachypnea, hyperinflation of the chest with downward displacement of the liver and subcostal recession are typically present. However, the defining and characteristic clinical feature is that auscultation reveals widespread bilateral fine inspiratory crackles.

The diagnosis is essentially clinical, and most guidelines recommend that chest radiographs are not indicated unless there are atypical features because clinicians are frequently tempted to use antibiotics when there is evidence of apparent lobar consolidation or bronchopneumonia. These radiographic appearances may also encourage clinicians to inappropriately use the term pneumonia for such patients even though they have widespread crackles bilaterally. Most infants admitted to hospital with the typical phenotypic illness of acute bronchiolitis characterized by widespread crackles on auscultation will be less than 6 months old. Although older infants will also develop the same clinical picture, far fewer require admission to hospital as hypoxia and significantly impaired fluid intake are less common.

The acute inflammatory response in the airways of infants with this phenotype is dominated by an intense neutrophilia. Such a response also characterizes the response to other respiratory viruses such as rhinovirus. Inflammatory mediators such as human neutrophil elastase, myeloperoxidase and metalloproteases will induce mucus secretion, airways edema, coughing, and sneezing and hence are likely to play a major role in the induction of symptoms and dissemination of the virus. Indeed, there is some evidence that the peak of symptoms appears to correlate with the peak in neutrophil numbers, which lags behind the peak in viral titers. The support for the suggestion that neutrophils rather than virus-induced cytopathology are responsible for the generation of symptoms comes from experimental rhinovirus infection in adults in whom symptoms only occurred if there was significant neutrophilia within the airway and did not appear to correlate to evidence of viral replication. If symptoms are peaking as viral titers are falling, then it is perhaps not surprising that antiviral agents have not been shown to have a significant effect in this disease. It is probable that approaches that might reduce the intensity of the neutrophil response may prove to be more effective. There is evidence that neutrophils do have a role in reducing viral titers within the airways, although the mechanism remains to be elucidated.

There are overwhelming data indicating that there is no increase in atopy associated with this phenotype and that the pattern of subsequent respiratory morbidity does not appear to be asthmatic, in that it has yet to be shown that these symptoms respond to inhaled steroids or bronchodilators. The excess of respiratory symptoms experienced by hospitalized infants exhibiting this phenotype is most marked in the preschool years, is associated predominantly with subsequent intercurrent viral infections and is rarely severe enough to cause further hospitalization. The excess in respiratory morbidity declines rapidly through the early years of life with cohort studies suggesting that is excess has resolved by the beginning of the second decade of life.

Viral Pneumonia

Viral pneumonia in infancy is significantly less common than acute bronchiolitis, although viruses account for the majority of pneumonic illness in infancy. Infants with viral pneumonia, including those caused by RSV, typically exhibit a cough, are febrile, and develop significant respiratory distress. They are often more severely affected then those with acute bronchiolitis with a greater need for supportive and intensive care but, somewhat surprisingly, there are widespread nonlobar chest radiograph changes that often change and evolve over relatively short periods of time. There are no specific follow-up data in this group of patients.

Wheeze-associated Viral Infections and Exacerbations of Asthma (WALRI)

In many countries, including the United Kingdom and Australia, these patients would be described as having "Wheezing Bronchitis" or an "acute virus-associated wheezing episode". In contrast to those admitted with acute bronchiolitis as defined earlier, those patients admitted to hospital with this phenotype of illness characterized by wheezing without crepitation are generally older then 6 months.

This was based on the observation that the illness occurred at an age when passively acquired antibody levels are still generally high on the results of the trails using a formalin-inactivated vaccine in which infants receiving the vaccine had increased morbidity and mortality on subsequent natural exposure to the virus. The first hypothesis proposed that the condition results from an immune complex reaction between non-neutralizing antibody and virus. Subsequent theories have included the suggestion that there is a specific immunoglobulin E (IgE) response during the acute illness and the suggestions that the pathology is due to excessive cytotoxic T-cell activity, excessive Th2 activity or impaired macrophage activity due to infection of these cells.

COMPLICATIONS OF RESPIRATORY SYNCYTIAL VIRUS INFECTION

During RSV respiratory infections in very young infants, the two most serious complications are respiratory failure and apnea. Apnea is most common in the youngest patients, those born preterm, and those with chronic lung disease. Infants may present with apneas and progress to bronchiolitis, show signs of bronchiolitis and develop apneas or have apnea as the sole sign of RSV infection. Again RSV is not unique in its ability to induce apnea. RSV infection has been implicated in number of cases of "cot (or crib) death," and its ability to precipitate apnea may be relevant to this observation. A significant proportion of infants with RSV infection requiring assisted ventilation do so because of severe recurrent apneas rather than respiratory failure. The mechanisms leading to these apneas are unclear, but they tend to resolve within a few days. The use of apnea monitors is therefore important in young infants, those born preterm, and those with pre-existing lung disease.

It is well recognized that the clinical assessment of hypoxia is poor. Perhaps the most reliable clinical sign of respiratory failure is agitation, which, if not relieved by supplemental oxygen, can contribute to exhaustion and respiratory failure.

INVESTIGATIONS

Respiratory syncytial virus infection and other respiratory viruses can be identified using rapid diagnostic approaches such as immunofluorescent antibody method, enzyme-linked immunosorbent assay (ELISA) or polymerase chain reaction (PCR). Reliable commercial kits are now readily available and widely used, and indeed some are designed for use by the clinician at the bedside. Samples are generally obtained by means of nasopharyngeal aspirates, nasal lavage or nasal swabs. A positive result is valuable in supporting the diagnosis and in isolating infants with the virus. However, it should be remembered that all these methods require good-quality samples and a negative result does not exclude RSV infection, although ELISA technique appears more sensitive, serologic diagnosis are of little value because convalescent sera are required and hence results may take many weeks.

MANAGEMENT OF RESPIRATORY SYNCYTIAL VIRUS INFECTION

Although the morbidity associated with RSV infections in infancy is high, the mortality is fortunately low. While the virus is able to cause a variety of phenotypic illness, including acute bronchiolitis, pneumonia and wheeze-associated viral illness, management is essentially the same for each group of patients and has essentially remained unchanged for more than 40 years.

Good supportive care remains the cornerstone of therapy, with oxygen being vital in those with hypoxia. There is no convincing evidence that pharmacologic agents have any role in treatment of infants with RSV infection, but despite this, agents such as bronchodilators are still widely used. It is possible that patients less than 2 years of age with an RSV-induced viral exacerbation of asthma will benefit from traditional asthma therapies. However, it is difficult to differentiate those with their first significant exacerbation of asthma from those with wheeze-associated viral illness [bronchiolitis (wheezy bronchitis)] who represent the majority of patients in whom wheeze is a major feature. This difficulty probably underlies some of the apparent discrepancies in outcomes of trials assessing the role of bronchodilators in the treatment of bronchiolitis and is reflected in the American Academy of Pediatrics (AAP) bronchiolitis (diagnosis based on presence of wheeze) guidelines, which recommend that bronchodilators not be used routinely in the management of bronchiolitis. They suggest that a carefully monitored trail of adrenergic medication is an option, but the inhaled bronchodilators should be continued only if there is a documented positive clinical response to the trial, using an objective means of evaluation.

A small percentage requires more aggressive supportive care, which might include ventilation and even extracorporeal membrane oxygenation (ECMO), but most infants admitted with RSV infections have a brief, self-limiting illness. In North America, the United Kingdom and northern Europe, the mean duration of hospitalization is 3 days, compared with approximately 9 days in continental Europe. This may reflect differences in severity of patients admitted, differences in criteria for discharge or availability of hospital beds.

Oxygen

In the early 1960s, Reynolds and Cook noted that "oxygen is vitally important in bronchiolitis and there is little evidence that any other treatment is useful," and this is essentially true today with improved supportive care allowing correction. Oxygen at 30–40%, warmed and humidified and delivered via a headbox or nasal cannula, is sufficient to correct the hypoxia in most cases and rapidly relieves the distress and agitation observed in hypoxic infants. The AAP guidelines recommend the use of supplemental oxygen for those infants whose saturation falls below 90% although some centers would commence supplemental oxygen at higher levels.

Fluids

If uncorrected, the poor intake of fluid due to the respiratory distress and cough can lead to dehydration, and this tendency may be compounded by vomiting associated with the bouts of coughing. Hyponatremia due to inappropriate antidiuretic hormone secretion [syndrome of inappropriate diuretic syndrome (SIADH)] can occur, and hence it is sensible to restrict fluids to about two-thirds of maintenance.

Hypertonic Solution

This review was conducted to assess the effects of 3% saline solution administered via nebulizer, which can increase clearance of mucus, in these patients. We included seven randomized trials involving 581 infants with mild to moderate bronchiolitis. Meta-analysis suggests that nebulized 3% saline may significantly reduce the length of hospital stay among infants hospitalized for nonsevere acute bronchiolitis and improve the clinical severity score in both outpatient and inpatient populations. No significant short-term effects (30–120 minutes) of 1–2 doses of nebulized hypertonic saline were observed among emergency department patients; however, more trials are needed to address this question. There were no significant adverse effects noted with nebulized hypertonic saline when administered along with bronchodilators (*Source*: Cochrane Reviews).

Antiviral Agents

Ribavirin is a broad-spectrum virustatic drug first synthesized in 1972 whose exact mode of action is unclear. Since the initial enthusiasm that greeted its launch in 1986, concerns have been raised about its cost, safety and efficacy. A systematic review concluded that further large studies were required if a role for the drug were to be established. Most studies are now almost 20 years old, contained very few subject, and had remarkably high death rates compared with current practice. The drug is administered as an aerosol generated by a small-particle aerosol generator (SPAG). The aerosol is usually delivered into a headbox for 12–18 hours. No study to date has clearly demonstrated a significant impact on the course of the disease, and few units currently use the drug in previously healthy individuals or indeed those at risk of severe disease such as those with cardiac or pulmonary disease. Anecdotal reports suggest it is valuable in treating those with immunodeficiencies.

Antibiotics

Secondary bacterial infection appears uncommon in infants with RSV bronchiolitis, and hence antibiotics are rarely indicated even in those with patchy changes suggesting pneumonia. The clinical picture together with the rapid confirmation of RSV infection provides reassurance in most mild to moderately unwell infants. A large prospective study, covering a period of 9 years, found that secondary bacterial infection was more common in those given antibiotics than in those who did not receive them. However, dual infections with viruses and bacteria do occur, and it is not unreasonable to start antibiotics

in those who are particularly ill or in those with atypical features, and possible in some disadvantaged populations. Even in those ventilated, bacterial coinfection is relatively uncommon but is probably sufficiently frequent to justify the use of antibiotics in those requiring ventilator support while awaiting the results of bacterial cultures on samples obtained from the lower airway.

Although uncommon, it is also important to bear in mind that coincidental infections, such as urinary tract infections or meningitis, do occur in infants with RSV infections including bronchiolitis.

Bronchodilators

One of the greatest areas for contention in the management of acute bronchiolitis is in the role of bronchodilators. This probably stems in part form the desire of clinicians to have some form of therapy that they can offer beyond simple supportive therapy. Some of the differences may also be influenced by the types of clinical illness included in studies under the label of acute bronchiolitis. Published data suggest that bronchodilators, such as selective β-agonists and nonselective agents such as epinephrine and theophylline, are widely used particularly in North America, but to date there is no evidence that any of these interventions has a significant impact in those with acute bronchiolitis. These findings are perhaps not surprising in view of the marked mucus production and mucosal inflammation that are contributing to the airways obstruction. It should be borne in mind that one potential problem with studies in the age group is that it is extremely difficult to assess symptomatic improvement. For example, it would be inappropriate to assess the impact of bronchodilator on a child with moderately severe exacerbation of asthma by recording the time to discharge. The modest symptomatic relief obtained while awaiting the impact of systemic steroids clearly needs to be assessed using a different outcome measure. In infants, it is more difficult to objectively document symptomatic benefit as the patient cannot give his or her opinion.

More Intensive Supportive Care

Although the number of infants with acute bronchiolitis requiring ventilation can be minimized by good supportive care, a small proportion of infants admitted to the hospital may require ventilation for either recurrent apnea or respiratory failure. The majority of those admitted to intensive care are previously healthy individuals. Indications for intubation vary from unit to unit, but in general, infants are intubated for either recurrent apnea with significant oxygen desaturations or respiratory failure with persistent acidosis or hypoxia despite high oxygen requirements. Rising CO_2 levels of greater than 7–8 kPa would be viewed by some indication for intubation, but others would tolerate significantly higher levels in the absence of overt exhaustion, acidosis or uncorrected hypoxia. Patients should be weaned from the ventilator as rapidly as possible.

A number of units have reported a reduction in the need for assisted ventilation following the introduction of nasal continuous positive airway pressure (CPAP). Some infants who continued to deteriorate despite mechanical ventilation have been treated with ECMO and preliminary reports are encouraging. The role of NO, high-frequency ventilation, heliox and other agents, such as surfactant continue to be debated, and the role of these interventions, has still to be clearly determined.

Advances in supportive care have ensured that the prognosis for the vast majority to infants who develop acute bronchiolitis is very good, with an overall mortality rate significantly less than 1%. Mortality in previously well infants is extremely low, but the mortality rates in high-risk groups has historically been much higher with figures as high as 37% reported in infants with congenital heart disease. With improved supportive care, the mortality in infants from high-risk group who developed severe bronchiolitis is now generally below.

Specific Immunoglobulin

Studies have demonstrated that a humanized synthetic anti-E antibody preparation (palivizumab) administered intramuscularly at monthly intervals does reduce hospitalization in certain at-risk groups, including preterm infants, those with chronic lung disease, and those with hemodynamically important cardiac disease. The protection is incomplete, and, despite large numbers of subjects, the use of this preparation was not shown to have an impact on intensive care unit days or mortality, which is low even in these high-risk groups due to improved supportive care. As noted earlier, these high-risk groups represent a minority of those reaching the intensive care unit, and therefore this approach is unlikely to have a major impact on the workload of pediatric units during the winter. The cost-effectiveness of this approach is the subject of considerable debate in many countries.

VACCINES

For over two decades, much effort has been devoted for producing a vaccine able to prevent much of the respiratory morbidity associated with RSV bronchiolitis. The 1960s trails of a formalin-inactivated alum precipitated vaccine produced alarming results in that not only did the vaccine fail to protect infants but also there were excess morbidity and mortality in the immunized children when they subsequently were infected with the virus. Whether the enhanced disease severity noted on subsequent exposure to the virus was due to an abnormal response is unclear, although animal data suggest an aberrant response was induced.

Subsequent approaches have been to develop live attenuated strains, the generation of subunit vaccine, expression of viral glycoprotein genes on the surface of carrier viruses using recombinant gene technology, and the use of purified F protein obtained from tissue cultures. Debate continues as to whether injection, inoculation into the respiratory tract to produce local immunity or even administration to the mother would be most appropriate route, if an effective vaccine could be developed.

CONCLUSION

The prevention of acute RSV bronchiolitis in infancy remains a major challenge. The morbidity associated with this condition is considerable, and the financial constrain placed on health services is enormous. With improved supportive care, the mortality is now low even at-risk groups, but the condition still poses a major threat to the health of infants with underlying disease. A phenotypic approach to the management of infants infected with the virus appears to be important clinically while assessing the outcomes in clinical trails.

Despite an enormous amount of work aimed at preventing the annual influx of infants with acute bronchiolitis, it seems likely that the annual epidemics of RSV will continue to be the cause of season-affective disorder among pediatricians for the foreseeable future.

BIBLIOGRAPHY

1. American Academy of Pediatrics Subcommittee on Diagnosis and Management of Bronchiolitis. Diagnosis and management of bronchiolitis. Pediatrics. 2006;118: 1774-93.
2. Bont L, Steijn M, Van Aalderen WM, et al. Seasonality of long-term wheezing following respiratory syncytial virus lower respiratory tract infection. Thorax. 2004;59:512-6.
3. Bradley JP, Bacharier LB, Bonfiglio J, et al. Severity of respiratory syncytial virus bronchiolitis is affected by cigarette smoke exposure and atopy. Pediatrics. 2005;115:e7-14.
4. Elphick HE, Ritson S, Rigby AS, et al. Phenotype of acute respiratory syncytial virus induced lower respiratory tract illness in infancy and subsequent morbidity. Acta Paediatr. 2007;96:307-9.
5. Hall CB, Douglas RG Jr. Modes of transmission of respiratory syncytial virus. J Pediatr. 1981;99:100-3.
6. Published online: Published online March 16, 2011.
7. Reynolds EO, Cook CD. The treatment of bronchiolitis. J Pediatr. 1963;63:1205-7.

Anil K Prasad

INTRODUCTION

Influenza or flu is an acute, contagious viral respiratory illness, and is mostly ignored. Infection occurs in nose, throat, and at times descends to lungs. It can cause mild to severe illness, and when complicated with bacterial infection, particularly in risk population, can lead to serious consequences including death. It is estimated that all over the world, 3–5 million suffer with seasonal influenza and 300,000–500,000 die each year. Children and elderly people suffer more.

Infection spreads mainly by droplets, when people with flu, cough, sneeze or talk. Less often, a person also gets infected by using or by touching infected material or surface contaminated with flu virus and then touching their own mouth, eyes, and nose. Mostly very young children, acquire infection during fondling by others, who are already infected. School going children pick up infection at school and bring home or vice versa.

It is paradoxical as we all have suffered with influenza infection but yet we ignore this as common cold. Influenza is not just common cold, and if ignored specially in person with chronic conditions one could get into serious consequences and end fatally. The preventive vaccine is available from over 60 years but very much underused in developing countries.

Last century during the three influenza pandemics over 50–100 million people died all over the globe. The 1918-1919, the worst pandemic known as swine flu affected almost one fifth of the world population, killing almost 50 million people. India was worst affected and it is estimated over 20 million people died. There were two more flu pandemics in the last century (1957; 1967–1968). The best prevention of influenza is influenza vaccine, the single most cost effective.

This unpredictable virus kills approximately 500,000 people each year and goes un-noticed. USA uses preventive influenza vaccine in old/young and risk population and yet each year over 36,000 people die due to influenza and influenza complications. During 2014–2015 Ebola killed 11,000 worldwide and influenza kills between 250,000 to 500,000 in a year.

PEDIATRIC INFLUENZA

Protection is needed right from the time the embryo is growing in the mother's womb. This means influenza protection and prevention to the mother is very important for protecting the child in the mother's womb. This not only protects pre mature delivery, anatomical defects during embryo growth and other fatal complications.

Influenza virus is all the year round in circulation (1–5%) but increases during epidemic/pandemic 40–50% in elderly, children and in risk populations.

The alertness of influenza in pregnant women in recognizable degree was seen after the 2009 influenza pandemic. The pandemic virus (pH1N1) genetically reorganized and became a human pathogen with high invasive properties and assumed a pandemic role in 3 months time. Although the virus had low pathogenicity but due to high invasiveness, today this virus has replaced the old H1N1 virus, in the vaccine composition as well as influenza virus circulation. The old H1N1 also came from swine in 1918. Today the vaccine contains pH1N1 (from 2009 pandemic and H3N2 (from 1968 pandemic) and also in circulation.

HISTORY

The disease influenza is recognized for over 2,000 years. Hippocrates described this in 5th century. Since 1510 till 1930 some 30 widespread epidemic and pandemics have been described.

Influenza virus was first isolated in swine by Shope in 1930. The human influenza virus (type A) was first isolated by Smith et al. in 1933. The other two types: (1) influenza type B was isolated by Francis and Magill independently in 1940 and (2) influenza type C was isolated by Taylor in 1947. Epidemics due to influenza among man and animals are known from long time, and epidemiologists have been fascinated for the influenza outbreaks in the past.

VIRUS

Influenza is a single stranded RNA virus comprising of 3 types, A, B, and C which are determined by the nuclear material. Influenza A and B viruses are globally important human respiratory pathogens causing epidemics, usually during the winter season, and out of season sporadic cases and outbreaks. Influenza A viruses may also cause worldwide pandemics. Influenza type A has been the major pathogenic strain in human and animals including birds for all major outbreaks and pandemics. Whereas, type B and C are human pathogen, causing only localized outbreaks.

The virus is pleomorphic, spherical to filamentous in shape, 80–120 nm in size, single stranded, eight segmented RNA virus belonging to orthomyxoviruses. This virus has most of the time sprung surprise to most as a human pathogen of varied pathogenicity. Subtypes of influenza A viruses are determined by either hemagglutinin (HA) or neuraminidase (NA) activity types. There are sixteen serosubtypes of hemagglutinin and nine serosubtypes of neuraminidase. All these subtypes exist in birds. The human influenza virus subtypes contain H1 and H3, and N1 and N2. The H2—a human subtype pathogen, but it does not exist in circulation today.

Three types of HA (H1, H2 and H3) have a role in virus attachments to cells. Two types of NA (N1 and N2) have a role in viral penetration in cells. Minor point mutations causing small changes ("antigenic drift") in the HA gene enable the virus to evade immune recognition, resulting in seasonal influenza outbreaks during inter-pandemic years.. Antigenic shift is associated with major genetic changes , occurs in type A only and is responsible for pandemics.

The nomenclature to describe the virus is expressed in the following order:
• Virus type
• Geographic origin
• Strain number
• Year of isolation
• Virus subtype
  e.g. A/California/7/2009/H1N1.

Normally, when a new strain reappears, the older strain disappears from the circulation. But since 1977 when an old strain (H1N1) reappeared, this strain along with the H3N2 stain, both are in circulation. Influenza type A has been the major pathogenic strain in human and animals including birds for all major outbreaks and pandemics. Whereas, type B and C are human pathogen, causing only localized outbreaks.

Virus shows constant antigenic drift and shift, both in H and N surface antigens. This enables the virus to escape the existing host immunity. It, therefore, becomes essential that a close watch on the virus antigen for all the year around to incorporate the change in the viral vaccine. Most of the countries have established influenza multicentric surveillance watch for the prevailing virus. In India both, Indian Council of Medical Research (ICMR) and National Centre for Disease Control (NCDC), Government of India, are keeping watch on influenza through their over 20 such centers, spread all over the country.

GLOBAL INFLUENZA DISEASE BURDEN

Influenza occurs globally with an annual attack rate estimated at 5%–10% in adults and 20%–30% inchildren . Influenza spreads around the world in a yearly outbreak, resulting in about three to five million cases of severe illness and about 250,000 to 500,000 deaths. In the Northern and Southern parts of the world outbreaks occur mainly in winter while in areas around the equator outbreaks may occur at any time of the year. Children aged <5 years, and particularly those <2 years of age, have a high burden of influenza.

BURDEN OF INFLUENZA DISEASE IN INDIA

The incidence of influenza virus accounted to about 1.5% to 14.5% of all ARIs episodes and 33 to 44 per 1,000 children per year of the ALRI's in the past. A recent prospective study

carried out to determine the burden of influenza associated hospitalizations and seasonality of influenza activity during and three years following the 2009 pandemic showed that overall annual influenza associated hospitalization rate (all ages) was 35.8 per 10,000 population with the highest burden at younger ages (43.7 and 41.7 for 5–14 years and 15–29 years age groups respectively). The influenza associated annual hospitalization rate (all ages) was 46.8 per 10,000 during the pandemic year and 40.5, 29.3 and 43.2 per 10,000 in the 3 years post-pandemic. Influenza B accounted for a substantial 38% of the total influenza hospitalization burden.

SEASONAL INFLUENZA AND PANDEMICS

Seasonal human influenza outbreaks or epidemics are due to circulating influenza type A and B viruses undergoing drift in the virus. The seriousness of the disease and outbreak depends on the amount of the drift. In India, one observes two peaks in the influenza incidence. One, in and around rainy season and another during the winter months when there is sudden fall in the atmospheric temperature.

Minor drift in the surface antigen of influenza virus (H and N) is the reason for the yearly outbreak of the disease. Whenever there is a shift in the surface antigenicity, pandemic results. The notables in the past 100 years are pandemics of 1918–1919 (H1N1); 1957 (H2N2); 1968 (H3N2) and 2009 (p H1N1). Influenza pandemics has a singular disease that over 50-100 million people died; a fact unknown to have taken place due to any other human disease in a century. This figure is scary and makes one to think about influenza, which even today is ignored as common cold.

Influenza pandemic normally takes place in 10–30 years, when the virus has a shift in virus antigen either in H or N or both. World, including India, was anticipated influenza pandemic, for almost a decade, due to bird flu (H5N1) but to the surprise of all, in 2009 swine flu virus (H1N1), a triple re-assorted virus antigenically (material received from Swine, bird and human virus) appeared in Mexico and spread fast to assume the first influenza pandemic of the decade and century.

There have been 15,174 deaths reported from 209 countries till February 2010. In India, during this period the 1,135 deaths were reported. Already reports in 2012, about 13 deaths have occurred due to pH1N1 virus in Maharashtra, Rajasthan, Andhra Pradesh and Tamil Nadu.

INFLUENZA DISEASE SURVEILLANCE IN INDIA

The Indian Council of Medical Research conducts sentinel surveillance at twelve surveillance sites throughout India thereby generating crucial epidemiological and virological data. This surveillance improves the geographical representation, providing crucial insight into the geographical and seasonal variation of influenza transmission within India. The National Influenza Center (NIC) at Pune in addition has been sending timely isolates to CDC for antigenic analysis and has contributed cumulative weekly influenza surveillance data to the World Health Organization (WHO).

An extensive analysis of 4 years of seasonal influenza data has shown that seasonality varies according to geographical location of the site: Extreme North India demonstrates peak activity in winter and limited activity during rains. North (Delhi), Eastern and Western India demonstrate highest activity during rains and limited activity in winter. South India demonstrates a peak in the cooler season, during rains. Previously, India was only using Northern Hemisphere influenza vaccine, but these findings have led to importation of Southern Hemisphere vaccine.

Epidemiology

The Agent

Genetic sequencing shows a new sub type of influenza A (H1N1) virus with segments from four influenza viruses: North American Swine, North American Avian, Human Influenza and Eurasian Swine.

Host Factors

The majority of these cases have occurred in otherwise healthy young adults.

Transmission

The transmission is by droplet infection and fomites.

Incubation Period

About 1–7 days.

Communicability

From 1 day before to 7 days after the onset of symptoms. If illness persist for more than 7 days, chances of communicability may persist till resolution of illness. Children may spread the virus for a longer period.

There is substantial gap in the epidemiology of the novel virus which got re-assorted from swine influenza.

EPIDEMIOLOGY

The virus is prevalent all over the world. Overcrowdings, congested population, sudden cold and humid climate favor the virus circulation. Animal hosts, pigs and birds become the reservoir for the development of human influenza strains, in dual infection with human and animal influenza virus.

Today, among the emerging and re-emerging human viral diseases, influenza is a concern. The concern starts from the mother during pregnancy. Influenza infection during the second and third trimester can cause serious complications. The pregnancy can get aborted or the child may be deformed.

Although, influenza is a self-limiting infection but can cause a fatal complications in risk population. Infection starts suddenly and spreads fast over large areas. The disease disappears also as it starts.

CLINICAL FEATURES

High morbidity and low mortality is the characteristics of the disease. The disease has a short incubation period of 1–2 days and lasts for 3–5 days in uncomplicated case.

Symptoms include a combination of high fever, dry cough, sore throat, headache, muscle aches, fatigue, etc.
- Fever of 101 or higher
- Feeling feverish/chills
- Profound weakness/prostration
- Cough
- Sore throat
- Runny or stuffy nose, but not always (more common with a common cold)
- Muscle or body aches, and they can be quite debilitating;
- Headaches
- Fatigue (tiredness).

Some people experience vomiting and diarrhea, but this is more common with children.

Flu can present with croup, bronchiolitis, pneumonia, gastroenteritis, encephalitis or myocarditis, etc.

Complications from the flu include pneumonia, sinus and ear infections, and bronchitis.

SYMPTOM

The disease infection usually is seen with high fever, cough, sore throat, malaise, headache, vomiting in children and diarrhea.

Pregnant women are in high-risk group and show most of the above symptoms.

Sometimes, there is breathlessness with features suggesting acute lung conditions with hypoxia. In further deterioration there is acute respiratory distress syndrome (ARDS) and may lead to fatal results.

DIAGNOSIS

The diagnosis is based on history, clinical symptoms and physical examination, and confirmed by laboratory by virus isolation, serology, immunofluorescent microscopy, reverse transcriptase-polymerase chain reaction (RT-PCR), and chest radiograph.

Routine investigations required for evaluation and management of a patient with symptoms as described above will be required. These may include hematological, biochemical, radiological and microbiological tests as necessary.

Complete Blood Counts

Flu can present with leukopenia, neutropenia and lymphopenia but total WBC and neutrophil counts are significantly decreased four days after onset of illness compared with the counts over the first three days. The monocyte count and CRP levels also decreases 7 days after onset of illness compared with first 3 days after illness. In a patient presenting with two or more of influenza like symptoms (cough, sore throat, fever, rhinorrhea, malaise, headache, shortness of breath, chills) a decrease in WBC count and an neutrophil/lymphocyte ratio less than 2 indicate high possibility of swine flu (there are number quotes in literature). But the final diagnosis must be based on throat swab culture and virus isolation. N/L ratio less than two with typical features in a given epidemiological setting may serve a screening tool for isolation while awaiting throat swab culture reports.

Chest X-ray

X-ray can be normal as well. In patients with flu infection, the most common radiographic abnormality observed is consolidation in the lower zones more likely to have two or more lung zones involved. It can have changes of interstitial pneumonia with ground glass appearance, reticular pattern and at times even effusion but none of this is pathognomic.

Confirmation of influenza infection is through:
- Real time RT PCR or
- Isolation of the virus in culture or
- Four-fold rise in virus specific neutralizing antibodies.

For confirmation of diagnosis, clinical specimens such as nasopharyngeal swab, throat swab, nasal swab, wash or aspirate, and tracheal aspirate (for intubated patients) are to be obtained. The sample should be collected by a trained physician/microbiologist preferably before administration of the anti-viral drug. Keep specimens at 4°C in viral transport media until transported for testing. The samples should be transported to designated laboratories within 24 hours. If they cannot be transported then it needs to be stored at -70°C. Paired blood samples at an interval of 14 days for serological testing should also be collected.

COMPLICATIONS OF INFLUENZA

Complications of influenza can include bacterial pneumonia, ear infections, sinus infections, dehydration and worsening of chronic medical conditions, such as congestive heart failure, asthma or diabetes.

DISEASE BURDEN

There has been no systemic study report from India on the disease burden due to influenza. But, loss of school days, absence from work places, parents on leave due to sick children at home, industry losses of production hour, burden on the health budget and strain on attending hospital staff, etc. causes large economic losses. The general progress of the country gets slowed and at total derailment during pandemic.

TREATMENT

Treatment is symptomatic and palliative with bed rest. The patient is advised to increase fluid intake. In serious cases early use of antiviral and use antibiotics in case any bacterial infection is suspected.

Influenza is a self-limiting infection and in complication cases recovery takes place in 5–7 days with bed rest.

Antiviral treatment is advised in anticipation of serious influenza infection but needs to be used early, within 48 hours of the onset of the disease. Amantadine and rimantadine are M2 inhibitors and oseltamivir or zanamivir, which is neuraminidase inhibitor, are the choice of use.

Weight (kg)	Treating (dosing for 5 days)	Prophylaxis (dosing for 10 days)
Patients from 2 weeks to <1 year of age		
Any weight	3 mg/kg twice daily	Not applicable*
Patients from 1 to 12 years of age based on body weight		
15 kg or less	30 mg twice daily	30 mg once daily
15.1–23 kg	45 mg twice daily	45 mg once daily
23.1–40 kg	60 mg twice daily	60 mg once daily
40.1 kg or more	75 mg twice daily	75 mg once daily
It is also available as syrup (12 mg/mL) *Oseltamivir is not approved for prophylaxis of patients less than 1 year of age		

PREVENTION

It includes: General preventive measures and vaccination.

General Preventive Measures

- Wash hands frequently with soap and water or use alcohol-based hand cleaner* when soap and water are not available.
- Cover your mouth and nose with a tissue when coughing or sneezing
- Avoid touching your eyes, nose and mouth
- Avoid large gathering or crowd like malls, cinema halls, sport events and may be schools. School seems to be the place for children to pick up infection and for spread.
- Avoid close contact (i.e. being within about 6 feet) with persons with influenza-like illness (ILI).

VACCINATION

Influenza seasonal vaccination is the best prevention of the disease. At least the risk populations get covered by the seasonal influenza vaccine.

- Inactivated influenza vaccine (IIV)
  - Only trivalent vaccines (TIVs) are available
  - Qudrivalent
- Live attenuated influenza vaccines (LAIV).

The trivalent influenza vaccines are split products produced from detergent treated, highly purified influenza virus, or surface antigen vaccines containing purified hemagglutinin and neuraminidase. The development of quadrivalent influenza vaccine formulation for seasonal influenza vaccine is of interest in providing comprehensive protection against influenza B viruses.

Vaccine Schedule

Influenza vaccination is recommended every year, particularly for high-risk groups. TIV is administered intramuscularly. Children aged 6 through 35 months should receive a pediatric dose and previously unvaccinated children aged <9 years should receive 2 injections administered at least 4 weeks apart. A single dose of the vaccine is appropriate for children aged 9 years or more and healthy adults.

Any of the influenza vaccines can be administered at the same visit with all other recommended routine vaccines. All vaccines should be shipped and stored at 2°C to 8°C (35°F–46°F).

It is administered intramuscularly into the anterolateral thigh of infants and young children and into the deltoid muscle of older children and adults. The volume of vaccine is age dependent; infants and toddlers 6 months through 35 months of age should receive a dose of 0.25 mL/dose and all people 3 years (36 months) and older should receive 0.5 mL/dose.

LAIV is given as nasal spray, one dose only, but children aged 2–8 years should normally receive 2 doses, at least 4 weeks apart.

Recommendations

- Inactivated vaccines (containing killed virus): For use in 6 months of age and older, including healthy people, people with chronic medical conditions and pregnant women.
- The nasal spray flu vaccine: a vaccine made with live weakened flu virus that is given as a nasal spray (sometimes called live attenuated influenza vaccine (LAIV)]. The viruses in the nasal spray vaccine do not cause the flu. LAIV is approved for use in healthy people

2–49 years of age including those women who are not pregnant. LAIV is given as nasal spray, 1 dose only .
- Children aged 2–8 years who have not received seasonal influenza vaccine during the previous influenza season should receive 2 doses, at least 4 weeks apart
- LAIV cannot be prescribed to:
  - Children <2 years of age
  - High risk individuals
  - Pregnant women
- In about 2 weeks after vaccination, antibodies develop that protect against influenza virus infection. Influenza vaccines will not protect against flu-like illnesses caused by noninfluenza viruses. Protection against viruses that are similar antigenically to those contained in the vaccine extends for at least 6–8 months

The seasonal flu vaccine protects against the three influenza viruses that research suggests will be most common.

Vaccine Composition

For 2017–2018, three-component vaccines are recommended to contain:
- An A/Michigan/45/2015 (H1N1)pdm09-like virus (updated)
- An A/Hong Kong/4801/2014 (H3N2)-like virus
- A B/Brisbane/60/2008-like (B/Victoria lineage) virus
Quadrivalent (four-component) vaccines, which protect against a second lineage of B viruses, are recommended to be produced using the same viruses recommended for the trivalent vaccines, as well as a B/Phuket/3073/2013-like (B/Yamagata lineage) virus.

When to get Vaccinated against Seasonal Flu?

Yearly flu vaccination should begin in September or as soon as vaccine is available, and continue throughout the flu season which can last as late as May. This is because the timing and duration of flu seasons vary. While flu season can begin as early as October, most of the time seasonal flu activity peaks in January, February or later.

Ideal Time for Influenza Vaccination in India

- WHO classifies India under the 'South Asia' transmission zone of Influenza circulation
- Though India lies within the northern hemisphere, parts of the country have a distinct tropical environment being located close to the equator and behaves much like southern hemisphere seasonality with almost year round circulation and monsoon months peak, still northern India experiences another peak during winter just like northern hemisphere pattern.

Who is at High-risk for Developing Flu-related Complications?

- Children younger than 5 years, but especially children younger than 2 years old
- Adults 65 years of age and older
- Pregnant women
- People who have medical conditions including:
  - Asthma (even if it is controlled or mild)
  - Neurological and neurodevelopmental conditions [including disorders of the brain, spinal cord, peripheral nerve and muscle such as cerebral palsy, epilepsy (seizure disorders), stroke, intellectual disability (mental retardation), moderate to severe developmental delay, muscular dystrophy or spinal cord injury]
  - Chronic lung disease [such as chronic obstructive pulmonary disease (COPD) and cystic fibrosis]
  - Heart disease (such as congenital heart disease, congestive heart failure and coronary artery disease)
  - Blood disorders (such as sickle cell disease)
  - Endocrine disorders (such as diabetes mellitus)
  - Kidney disorders
  - Liver disorders
  - Metabolic disorders (such as inherited metabolic disorders and mitochondrial disorders)
  - Weakened immune system due to disease or medication (such as people with HIV, AIDS, cancer or those on chronic steroids)
  - People younger than 19 years of age who are receiving long-term aspirin therapy
  - People who are morbidly obese [Body Mass Index (BMI) of 40 or greater].

Who Else Should Get Vaccinated?

Other people for whom vaccination is especially important are:

- People who live in nursing homes and other long-term care facilities
- People who live with or care for those at high-risk for complications from flu, including:
  - Healthcare workers
  - Household contacts of persons at high-risk for complications from the flu
  - Household contacts and caregivers of children younger than 5 years of age with particular emphasis on vaccinating contacts of children younger than 6 months of age (children younger than 6 months are at highest risk of flu-related complications but are too young to get vaccinated).

IAP recommendations on 'target group prioritization' for seasonal influenza vaccination:

IAP believes that influenza vaccination should aim primarily at protecting vulnerable high-risk groups against severe influenza-associated disease and death contribution of risk group to the based on overall influenza disease burden in population, disease severity within individual risk group, and vaccine effectiveness in different age groups and categories.

Accordingly, following groups of individuals should be targeted for seasonal annual vaccination (1-Highest priority, 4-Lowest priority).

1. Elderly individuals (>65 years) and nursing-home residents (the elderly or disabled)
2. Individuals with chronic medical conditions including individuals with HIV/AIDS, and pregnant women (especially to protect infants 0–6 months)
3. Other groups: Healthcare workers including professionals, individuals with asthma, and children from ages 6 months to 2 years.
4. Children aged 2–5 years and 6–18 years, and healthy young adults.

Who Should not be Vaccinated Against Seasonal Flu?

Some people should not be vaccinated without first consulting a physician. They include:

- People who have a severe allergy to chicken eggs
- People who have had a severe reaction to an influenza vaccination in the past
- Children younger than 6 months of age (influenza vaccine is not approved for use in this age group)
- People who have a moderate or severe illness with a fever should wait to get vaccinated until their symptoms lessen.
- People with a history of Guillain-Barré Syndrome (a severe paralytic illness, also called GBS) that occurred after receiving influenza vaccine and who are not at risk for severe illness from influenza should generally not receive vaccine. Tell your doctor if you ever had GBS. Your doctor will help you to decide whether the vaccine is recommended for you.
- If you have questions about whether you should get a flu vaccine, consult your healthcare provider.

COUNTRIES WHICH PROTECTS FROM INFLUENZA

- Top ten countries in the world using preventive vaccine are Canada, Korea, USA, Japan, Australia, Spain, Germany, Italy, UK, Hong Kong SAR and yet people die due to this infection and complications.
- India after 2009 Influenza pandemic licensed four Indian vaccine manufacturing companies to manufacture

influenza vaccine but due to this disease not listed in the routine preventive vaccine.

BIBLIOGRAPHY

1. Baltimore D. Expression of animal virus genomes. Bacteriol Rev. 1971;35:235-41.
2. Compans RW, Meier-Ewert H, Palese P. Assembly of lipid-containing viruses. J SupramolStruct. 1974;2:496-511.
3. Gupte S, Gupte N. ECAB clinical update: seasonal influenza and pandemics. Complete Spectrum-1. Elsevier India; 2011. pp. 82-108.
4. Gupte S. Pediatric influenza revisited. Asian Pacific J Infect Dis. 2008;19:324-32.
5. Hoyle L. Morphology and physical structure. The Influenza Viruses. New York: Springer-Verlag; 1968. pp. 49-68.
6. Influenza (2nd Ed.: Wilschut, McElhaney & Palache (Mosby) (2006).
7. Khan; the Next Pandemic, Peruses Book Group (2016).
8. Lamb RA, King RM. Orthomyxoviridae. In: Fields BN, Knipe DM, Howley PM (Eds). Fields Virology, 4th edition. Philadelphia: Lippincott Williams and Wilkins; 2001. p. 1487.
9. Prevention and control of influenza with vaccines: recommendations of the Advisory Committee on Immunization Practices (ACIP) 2010. MMWR Recomm Rep. 2010;59:1-62.
10. Rao MI. ECAB clinical update: pediatrics. Influenza: Complete Spectrum-1. Elsevier India; 2011.p. 1.
11. Reena Wani: Fever in Pregnancy CBS Publishers & Distributors Pvt. Ltd (2016)
12. Webster RG. Influenza: an emerging disease. Emerg Infect Dis. 1998;4:436-41.

5.11 ROTAVIRUS

Monjori Mitra

EPIDEMIOLOGY

Rotavirus is the most common cause of severe, dehydrating gastroenteritis worldwide both in developed and developing countries. More than 500,000 deaths are attributed to rotavirus gastroenteritis annually worldwide, with the highest mortality in India, where 1 of 110 children is estimated to die due to rotavirus.

More than 85% of the deaths occur in low-income countries. Overall, rotavirus has been estimated to account for 20–31% of all childhood diarrheal deaths and 5% of all deaths among children less than 5 years of age.

The highest rates of rotavirus gastroenteritis occur among children 4 months to 3 years of age. Nearly 52% children below 6 months were infected with rotavirus as seen in Gladstone study in Vellore. Infants younger than 3 months of age have lower rates of infection, and are more likely to be asymptomatic when infected. Because natural infection confers protection against subsequent infection and disease, symptomatic illness is less common among children older than 5 years of age.

Although the virus is known to be democratic but the mortality is more in the developing countries than the developed countries because along with the rotavirus infection the underlying malnutrition, and coinfection with other virus or bacteria adds to the increase in the mortality and morbidity.

Overall in the United States, between 45,000 and 70,000 children less than 5 years of age are hospitalized for rotavirus annually. Similarly, studies in developing countries in Asia estimate that a median of 45% of gastroenteritis hospitalizations is attributable to rotavirus. Rotavirus infections account for a somewhat lower proportion of children presenting to clinics with mild disease, usually 5–15%, compared with the high rates found in severely ill children. Rotavirus is responsible for childhood diarrhea in 35% of hospitalized and 10–30% of community-based cases.

Rotavirus disease occurs in distinct winter seasonal peaks in temperate countries, and is uncommon in summer months. In tropical settings, rotavirus may circulate year-round, but often has seasonal peaks during the cool or dry months.

Rotaviruses are spread through fecal-oral contamination predominantly by close person-to-person spread. Spread through contaminated fomites is also common. Mostly the young child is affected with clinical illness and older children and young adults excrete the virus asymptomatically.

PATHOGENESIS

Rotaviruses are 70-nm icosahedral viruses that constitute a distinct genus of the family Reoviridae. The virus is composed of three layers (an outer and inner capsid and a core) that encase the genome of 11 segments of double-stranded RNA. Gene segments can be separated on the basis of their molecular weight by polyacrylamide gel electrophoresis (PAGE). When mixed infections with different rotavirus strains occur, the gene segments may reassort independently, producing various phenotypic and genotypic characteristics of the virus, which are used as vaccine candidate.

The virus comprises of six structural and six nonstructural proteins. Out of them the three major structural and one nonstructural protein of rotavirus are of interest in vaccine development. The outer layer of rotavirus contains two distinct proteins: (1) VP4 and (2) VP7, which elicits distinct serotype specific neutralizing antibodies and also cross reactive neutralizing antibodies. The most highly represented viral structural protein is VP6, which is found in the internal capsid and bears group-specific antigenic determinants.

The VP7 protein is glycosylated, and serotypes are termed G types; 14 rotavirus G serotypes have been identified. The VP4 protein is cleaved by the protease trypsin and serotypes are termed P types. The P protein presents in the form of 60-protein dimer spikes (the hemagglutinin), which extends beyond the VP7 surface while penetrating through the outer capsid to interact with VP6 on the inner capsid. Because of this extensive cross-reactivity among different P types, it was not possible to classify all P types and hence another additional system of P typing into genotypes identified by nucleic acid hybridization and nucleic acid sequencing studies. In this way 26 P genotypes have been identified leading to a complex binomial nomenclature. Table 5.11.1 shows the different serotypes of the rotavirus:

Rotavirus replication mainly occurs in the mature villous epithelial cells in the mucosal surface from the proximal to the distal of the small intestine. Rotaviruses do not appear to replicate in immature epithelial cells of the villous crypt or in M cells overlying Peyer's patches.

This replication causes several physiologic and morphologic changes. There is decreased capacity to absorb sodium, glucose and water, and have decreased levels of intestinal lactase, alkaline phosphatase and sucrase. These findings are consistent with an absorptive abnormality associated with an accelerated migration of immature epithelial cells toward the villous tip.

Table 5.11.1: Common human group A rotavirus serotypes.

P1A[8]	G1, G3, G4, G9, G8, G12
P1B[4]	G2
P2[6]	G9

The nonstructural proteins (NSP4) acts as a viral enterotoxin and its exposure to intestinal epithelial cells induces diarrhea, caused by excess chloride secretion by a calcium-dependent signaling pathway.

Rotavirus infections are more likely to be severe in children 3–24 months of age than in younger infants or older children and adults. Older children would be protected by a virus-specific immune response generated by repeated natural infections. In case of young infants it may be mediated by passively transferred, transplacental, maternal antibodies. Breastfeeding also clearly protects against rotavirus disease. Rotavirus entry into target cells is facilitated by cleavage of VP4, which occurs in the presence of trypsin, elastas, or pancreatin, which are decreased in intestinal fluid secretions of newborn infants compared with older infants and young children resulting in lesser incidence of rotavirus diarrhea in this age group.

Children in developing countries are more susceptible to severe rotavirus disease than those in developed countries because of malnutrition and concomitant infections with other viruses and enteropathogenic bacteria.

Although natural rotavirus infection protects against moderate to severe disease caused by reinfection, some children experience repeated episodes of diarrhea with the same serotype during the following rotavirus season, and a small number of children develop symptomatic rotavirus infection twice within the same season. These observations are consistent with the fact that the productions of virus-specific secretory immunoglobulin A (sIgA), are usually short-lived and that rotavirus-specific sIgA often is not detected at the intestinal mucosal surface within 1 year of symptomatic infection. Modification of the severity of rotavirus disease caused by reinfection is most likely mediated by production of virus-specific sIgA by memory rotavirus-specific B cells in the intestinal lamina propria.

CLINICAL FEATURES

Rotavirus has an incubation period of 1–3 days. It presents with fever and abrupt onset of vomiting and profuse watery diarrhea that can occur 8–20 times per day. It rarely has gross blood or visible mucus. Vomiting often precedes diarrhea and resolves in 1–3 days, while diarrhea can persist for 5–8 days (range in several studies of 2–23 days). Usually rotavirus diarrhea is associated with more severe gastroenteritis than other enteric pathogens resulting in more dehydration. Some children may have fever alone, without gastrointestinal tract symptoms, at first medical visit, presumably early in the illness. Symptoms and asymptomatic viral shedding can be prolonged substantially in immunocompromised patients.

Rare extraintestinal rotavirus manifestations have been reported like encephalitis, viremia and hepatitis, often without accompanying diarrheal illness, but these are extremely rare.

DIAGNOSIS

Rotavirus is diagnosed by enzyme immunoassay (EIA) or a latex agglutination (LA) format, and is 90% sensitive and greater than 90% specific compared with real-time polymerase chain reaction (RT-PCR) during the first few days of illness. RT-PCR is more sensitive than antigen detection for rotavirus infection especially late in the course or following resolution of symptoms when viral shedding has decreased. Electron microscopy and PAGE can both be used for detection, but are seldom used in favor of more convenient antigen test kits.

PREVENTION

The rotavirus vaccines currently available in the United States are both attenuated (weakened) live virus vaccines: RotaTeq is a pentavalent human-bovine reassortant rotavirus vaccine licensed in 2006 and Rotarix is a monovalent attenuated human rotavirus licensed in 2008.

Both vaccines are given by mouth in multiple doses, and are designed to replace a child's first exposure to wild-type rotavirus with strains that will not cause disease but will generate an adequate immune response to confer protection. Even so, distinct approaches to rotavirus immunization have been taken with respect to strain type (including the use of attenuated, human strains, nonhuman e.g, bovine, rhesus, and lamb strain and human-animal reassortants), number of strains in a vaccine (monovalent vs polyvalent), and the number of doses.

Observational data from the United States showed vaccine effectiveness against severe rotavirus gastroenteritis to be 85–95%. Sentinel laboratory surveillance demonstrated a decline in rotavirus activity in the United States during the first two seasons after the introduction of RotaTeq in 2006. During the 2007–2008 season, the onset of rotavirus activity was 11 weeks later than the median onset during 2000–2006, and the number of positive tests was 64% lower than in the pre-vaccination period. Although the number of positive tests was somewhat greater and the rotavirus season was longer during 2008–2009 compared with 2007–2008, rotavirus activity during both seasons was substantially lower than during 2000–2006. This decline was also noted in age groups other than those vaccinated, providing evidence of a potential herd protection effect.

Trials of rotavirus vaccines have been conducted in Asian and African countries that are classified within different child mortality strata; trials have also included countries where sanitation is poor and where there is high mortality from diarrheal diseases and a high maternal prevalence of HIV. Rotarix has been evaluated in Malawi and South Africa; RotaTeq has been studied in Ghana, Kenya and Mali in Africa, and in Bangladesh and Vietnam in Asia. The efficacies in the developing countries are less compared to the developed counties. Despite its lower efficacy in developing countries, the number of episodes of severe gastroenteritis prevented by vaccination was higher (3.9/100 vaccines) than in South Africa (2.5/100 vaccines) because of the higher incidence of severe rotavirus gastroenteritis in young infants in Malawi.

In the position paper on rotavirus vaccines published in 2007, WHO recommended the inclusion of rotavirus vaccination into national immunization programs in regions where efficacy data suggested that there would be a significant public health impact—that is, mainly in the America and Europe but not in the developing countries due to lack of evidence. However, taking into the account of a new evidence, WHO in 2009 recommends that infants worldwide be vaccinated against rotavirus.

There are 28 countries mostly in Africa which have been approved for each type of GAVI support as of 13 April, 2012 for rotavirus vaccination.

A previously released rotavirus vaccine, RotaShield was withdrawn from the market in 1999. RotaShield was a tetravalent reassortant rhesus-human rotavirus vaccine licensed by the Food and Drug Administration (FDA) in August 1998. However, in July 1999, after approximately 1 million children had been immunized with that vaccine, the CDC suspended its recommendation because they detected an increase in the number of children who developed a serious bowel disease called "intussusception". Investigators calculated that the risk of intussusception attributable to the vaccine was about 1/10,000 infants vaccinated which was about three times higher than unvaccinated children. That vaccine was voluntarily withdrawn from the market by the manufacturer in October 1999. Those who received the RotaShield vaccine in 1998 and 1999 do not have a continuing risk of developing intussusception.

DOSE AND SCHEDULE: IAPCOI RECOMMENDATION

Vaccination should be strictly as per schedule discussed below, as there is a potentially higher risk of intussusception if vaccines are given to older infants. Vaccination should be avoided if age of the infant is uncertain. There are no restrictions on the infant's consumption of food or liquid, including breast-milk, either before or after vaccination. Vaccines may be administered during minor illnesses. Although there is limited evidence on safety and efficacy of rotavirus vaccines in preterm infants, vaccination should be considered for these infants if they are clinically stable and at least 6 weeks of age as preterms are susceptible to severe rotavirus gastroenteritis. Vaccination should be avoided in those with history of hypersensitivity to any of the vaccine components or previous vaccine dose. Vaccination should be postponed in infants with acute gastroenteritis as it might compromise efficacy of the vaccine.

Immunocompromised infants are susceptible to severe and prolonged rotavirus gastroenteritis but safety and efficacy of either of the two vaccines in such patients is unknown. Risks versus benefits of vaccination should be considered while considering vaccination for infants with chronic gastrointestinal disease, gut malformations, previous intussusception and immunocompromised infants.

Human Monovalent Live Vaccine

Human monovalent live rotavirus vaccine contains one strain of live attenuated human strain 89-12 [(type G1P1A (8)] rotavirus. It is provided as a lyophilized power that is reconstituted before administration. Each 1 mL dose of reconstituted vaccine contains at least 106 median culture infective units of virus. The vaccine contains amino acids, dextran, Dulbecco's modified Eagle medium, sorbitol and sucrose. The diluents contans calcium carbonate, sterile water and xanthan. The vaccine contains no preservatives of thiomersal.

The vaccine and the diluents should be stored at 2–8°C and must not be frozen. The vaccine should be administered promptly after reconstitution as 1 mL orally. The first dose can already be administered at the age of 6 weeks and should be given no later than at the age of 12 weeks. The interval between the two doses should be at least 4 weeks.

Human Bovine Pentavalent Live Vaccine

Human bovine pentavalent live vaccine contains five reassortant rotaviruses developed from human and bovine parent rota viruses. Each 2 mL vial of vaccine contains approximately 2×10^6 infectious units of each of the five reassortant strains. The vaccine viruses are suspended in the buffer solution that contains sucrose, sodium citrate, sodium phosphate monobasic monohydrate, sodium hydroxide, polysorbate 80 and tissue culture media. Trace amounts of fetal bovine serum might be present. The vaccine contains no preservatives of thiomersal. The vaccine is available as a liquid virus mixed with buffer and no reconstitution is needed. It should be stored at 2–8°C. The recommended schedule is three oral doses at ages 2, 4 and 6 months. The first dose should be administered between ages 6–12 weeks and subsequent doses at intervals of 4–8 weeks. The manufacturer does not recommend re-administration of vaccine if a dose is spit out or regurgitated. Regardless of which vaccine is used, the first dose should be given between 6 weeks and 14 weeks 6 days of age. Immunization should not be initiated in infants 15 weeks or older because of insufficient safety data for vaccines use in older children. All the doses of either of the vaccines should be completed within 32 weeks of age. Both vaccines should not be frozen. Rotavirus vaccine must not be injected. Programmatic errors have been reported. Large vaccine volume requires full insertion of vial tip into infant's mouth. Contact with infant's mouth contaminates the vial and complicates development of multidose vials.

SPECIAL SITUATIONS

Regurgitation of Vaccine

Re-administration need not be done to an infant who regurgitates, spits out, or vomits during or after administration of vaccine although the manufacturers of human monovalent live vaccine recommend that the dose may be repeated at the same visit, if the infant spits out or regurgitates the entire vaccine dose. The infant should receive the remaining recommended doses of rotavirus vaccine following the routine schedule (with a 4-week minimum interval between doses).

Interchangeability of Rotavirus Vaccines

Ideally, the rotavirus vaccine series should be completed with the same product. However, vaccination should not be deferred because the product used for previous doses is unavailable. In such cases, the series should be continued with the product that is available. If any dose in the series was human bovine pentavalent vaccine, or if the product is unknown for any dose in the series, a total of three doses should be administered.

Missed Opportunity

It is not necessary to restart the series or add doses because of a prolonged interval between doses with either of the vaccines.

CONTRAINDICATIONS

Rotavirus vaccine should not be administered to infants who have a history of a severe allergic reaction (e.g. anaphylaxis) after a previous dose of rotavirus vaccine or to a vaccine component. Latex rubber is contained in the human monovalent vaccine oral applicator, so infants with a severe (anaphylactic) allergy to latex should not receive human monovalent vaccine. The human bovine pentavalent vaccine dosing tube is latex-free.

FUTURE OF ROTAVIRUS VACCINE DEVELOPMENT

Additional, vaccines are in the late stages of development and are expected to be available within the next few years. While most vaccines still in clinical development are live, orally administered vaccines, parenterally administered vaccines are also being investigated. Neither of the currently licensed vaccines, nor any vaccine in development, has yet been tested in countries where mortality because of rotavirus is high. Because past rotavirus vaccines have shown little efficacy in these settings, trials of rotavirus vaccines are underway; decisions about use of these vaccines in countries where mortality is high will await results of these trials.

BIBLIOGRAPHY

1. Clark HF, Offit PA, Parashar UD, et al. Rotavirus vaccines. In: Plotkin S, Orenstein W, Offit P (Eds). Vaccines, 5th edition. Saunders, 2008. pp. 715-34.
2. Cortese MM, Parashar UD. Centers for Disease control and prevention: prevention of rotavirus gastroenteritis among infants and children: recommendations of the Advisory Committee on Immunization Practices (ACIP). MMWR. 2009;58:1-25.
3. IAP Guidebook on Immunization—IAP Committee of Immunization 2009–2010. Available from www.iapcoi.com/hp/other_vaccination_resources.php [Accessed June, 2012].
4. Kapikian AZ, Chanock RM. Rotaviruses. In: Fields BN, Knipe DM, Howley PM, et al. (Eds). Fields Virology, 3rd edition. Philadelphia: Lippincott-Raven, 1996.pp.1657-708.
5. WHO. Weekly epidemiological record; No. 51-52, 2009, 84, 533–540. [online] Available from www.who.int/wer.
6. Zulfikar AB. Acute gastroenteritis in children. In: Kliegman R, Stanton B, Behrman R (Eds). Nelson: Textbook of Pediatrics, 19th edition. Saunders, 2011. pp.1323-38.

Swati Y Bhave

5.12   HUMAN PAPILLOMA INFECTION

EPIDEMIOLOGY

Human Papillomavirus

Human papillomavirus (HPV) is a double stranded DNA virus that infects the skin, upper respiratory and anogenital tracts. There are approximately 100 types of HPV of which about 40 infect the genital tract. The infection with HPV occurs all over the world. The only natural reservoirs of HPV are humans. Other species that can be affected are rabbits and cows. Most HPV types infect the cutaneous epithelium and cause common skin warts. Around 40 HPV types infect the mucosal epithelium. The classification is based on their propensity to cause malignant changes: (1) low-risk or non-oncogenic types (e.g. 6 and 11) that can cause benign or low-grade cervical cell abnormalities, genital warts and laryngeal papillomas and (2) high-risk or oncogenic type that act as carcinogens in the development of cervical cancer and other anogenital cancers (vulva, vagina, penis and anus). The various oncogenic types are 16, 18, 31, 33, 35, 39, 45, 51, 52, 56, 58, 59, 68, 69, 73, 82. The genital types of HPV may also cause some oral and pharyngeal cancers. In early 1980s, the DNA for HPV was demonstrated to be present in the cervical cancer cells. It took 10 years for the epidemiological studies to establish a significantly consistent association between HPV and cervical cancer. High-risk HPV types are detected in 99% of cervical cancers. Type 16 causes nearly 50% and together with type 18 about 70% of cervical cancers worldwide.

Indian Scenario

India has a population of 436.76 million women aged 15 years and older who are at risk of developing cervical cancer. Current estimates indicate that every year 1,22,844 women are diagnosed with cervical cancer and 67,477 die from the disease. Cervical cancer ranks as the first most frequent cancer among women in India, and the first most frequent cancer among women between 15 and 44 years of age. About 7.9% of women in the general population are estimated to harbor cervical HPV infection at a given time and 82.7% of invasive cervical cancers are attributed to HPVs 16 or 18. India has 27% of the global burden of cervical cancer. More than 185 women die every day.

Genital Warts

Approximately two-thirds of individuals who have sexual contact with an infected partner develop genital warts. The exact incubation time is unknown, but most investigators believe that the incubation period is approximately 3 months. In India, the incidence of genital warts has been reported to vary from 2% to 25.2% among STI clinic attendees.

ETIOPATHOGENESIS

Human papillomavirus infects the basal epithelium cells. As per the natural history of this infection, majority of HPV infections are transient and asymptomatic. Around 70% clear within 1 year, and approximately 90% clear within 2 years. Median duration of new infections is 8 months. The time between initial HPV infection and development of cervical cancer is usually decades. Nearly 80% appear to resolve spontaneously. In the other 20% again most resolve spontaneously, but a small proportion remains persistently infected, leading to cervical intraepithelial neoplasia (CIN). Low-grade CIN1 develops within a few years that again may spontaneously resolve. However, in some cases, persistent infection can directly progress to high-grade CIN2 or CIN3 which are cancer precursors. Again a small proportion of these may also regress, but majority of such cases, if undetected and untreated over years, can progress to cervical cancer. Infection with one type of HPV does not prevent infection with another type. It has been seen that 5–30% cases have infection with multiple types of the mucosal virus. Persistent infection with high-risk types of HPV is the most important risk factor for cervical cancer precursors and invasive cervical cancer. Since a persistent infection with a high-risk HPV type does not lead to cancer in a number of women, studies were done to detect other cofactors. These were found to be (a) young age at sexual initiation, i.e. less than 25 years; (b) number of sex partners; (c) lifetime history of sex partners; (d) inconsistent condom use; (e) number of pregnancies; (f) genetic factors; (g) smoking; (h) oral contraceptive use; (i) increased parity; (j) increased age; (k) other STIs and (l) immune suppression and other host factors. Circumcision of the male partner seems to act as a protective factor. Lack of circumcision of male partner and oral contraceptive use associated with smoking have a higher incidence. Risk of cervical cancer is also strongly related to the age at first intercourse. The relative risk for CIN and invasive cervical cancer increased with decreasing age at first intercourse. For example, the risk estimate for invasive cancer among women reporting their first intercourse before 18 years of age was 5-fold greater than that observed among women who reported their first intercourse after 22 years of age.

TRANSMISSION

Communicability can presumed to be high because of the large number of new infections estimated to occur each year. HPV is presumably communicable during the acute infection and during persistent infection. But this is difficult to confirm because of the inability to culture the virus. There is no known seasonal variation in HPV infection. Transmission occurs most frequently with sexual intercourse but can occur following non-penetrative sexual activity (finger to anus or genitalia, skin to genitals, anogenital, etc.) which are more common in adolescents. Hence consistent use of condom can reduce the incidence of HPV infection, although it cannot protect against the non-penetrative sexual intimacy.

Human papillomavirus infection is common among adolescents and young adults. In India, the current population of girls around 15 years of age is 336 million. Studies of newly acquired HPV infection demonstrate that infection occurs soon after onset of sexual activity. Cumulative risk of cervical HPV infection in female adolescents (UK 1988–1992), with only one sexual partner, is nearly 10% in the first month which rises to nearly 25% in the first year, 35% in the second year and is nearly 46% at 3 years. Cumulative incidence of HPV infection from time of first sexual intercourse, female college students (US, 1990–2000) is nearly 10% in the first month which rises to nearly 30% in the first year, 38% in second year and is over 40% at 3 years. Modeling estimates suggest that more than 80% of sexually active women will have been infected by age 50 years. We do not have any such robust study from India.

Nonsexual Routes

The uncommon nonsexual routes of genital HPV transmission include transmission from a woman to a newborn infant at the time of birth which can result in recurrent respiratory papillomatosis (RRP).

CLINICAL FEATURES

Most HPV infections are asymptomatic and result in no clinical disease. The various clinical manifestations of HPV infection are: anogenital warts, respiratory obstruction in infants due to RRP, cervical cancer precursors (cervical intraepithelial neoplasia) and cancers, including cervical, anal, vaginal, vulvar, penile, and some head and neck cancer.

MODALITIES OF DIAGNOSIS

So far, HPV has not been isolated from the culture. The infection is identified by detection of HPV DNA from clinical samples. Assays for HPV detection differ considerably in their sensitivity and type specificity. The detection rate can depend upon the anatomic region sampled and the method of specimen collection.

Digene Hybrid Capture 2 (HC2) high-risk HPV DNA test is approved by FDA. Results are reported as positive or negative and are not type-specific. The HC2 test is approved for triage of women with equivocal Papanicolaou (Pap) test results [atypical squamous cells of undetermined significance (ASC-US), atypical cells of undetermined significance] and in combination with the Pap test for cervical cancer screening in women over age 30 years. The test is not clinically indicated nor approved for use in men.

Serologic tests for HPV are VLP-based enzyme immunoassays. They are not very useful as the laboratory reagents used for these assays may not be standardized and there are no standards for setting a threshold for a positive result.

TREATMENT

There is no specific treatment. Management depends on treatment of the specific clinical manifestation of the infection (such as genital warts or abnormal cervical cell cytology). There are guidelines by many professional associations from various parts of the world for the management of the histopathological stages of the cervical mucosa. Anogenital warts may need excision for discomfort or cosmetic reasons. RRP can require emergency excision for obstruction. Recurrence of warts may need repeated excisions.

PREVENTION OF HUMAN PAPILLOMAVIRUS INFECTION

Primary Prevention

Abstaining from sexual activity (i.e. refraining from any genital contact with another individual) is the surest way to prevent genital HPV infection. For those who choose to be sexually active, a monogamous relationship with an uninfected partner is the strategy most likely to prevent future genital HPV infections.

Studies demonstrate a significant reduction in HPV infection among young women after initiation of sexual activity when their partners used condoms consistently and correctly; however, it cannot prevent transmission due to nonpenetrative sexual activity. Use of the HPV vaccine will considerably reduce the incidence of HPV infection thereby reducing the incidence of cervical cancer which is associated with high morbidity and mortality.

Primary Vaccination

According to the statement by WHO in 2006, HPV infection is sexually transmitted and is usually acquired within the first few years following sexual debut. Ideally, therefore, the vaccine should be administered before sexual debut, i.e. before any risk of exposure to HPV. Statement by SAGE (Strategic Advisory Committee of Experts) in 2009, WHO also supports that the most effective time to vaccinate is before exposure to HPV as the infection can be acquired soon after first sexual intercourse. There is minimal risk of exposure in 9–13 years old and hence this is the optimal time for vaccination.

The recommendations from various professional societies from various parts of the world have around the same recommendations. In India, Indian Academy of Paediatrics (IAP), Federation of Obstetrics and Gynaecological Societies of India (FOGSI) and Indian Medical Association (IMA) have supported primary and catch-up vaccination of adolescent girls.

There were two vaccines available the Bi-valent vaccine effective against Type 16 and 18 which are the oncogenic HPV viruses and the Quadrivalent vaccine which in addition has effectiveness against Type which are known to cause genital warts.

Primary vaccination consists of a three-dose schedule:
- 0 dose: 1 month and 6 months for the bivalent vaccine
- 0 dose: 2 months and 6 months for the quadrivalent vaccine.

Two Dose Schedule

With research studies, it has now been found that 2 doses also can be used for HPV vaccination for persons initiating vaccination before their 15th birthday.
- The recommended immunization schedule is 2 doses of HPV vaccine
- The second dose should be administered 6–12 months after the first dose (0, 6–12 months schedule).

For persons initiating vaccination on or after their 15th birthday, the recommended immunization schedule is 3 doses of HPV vaccine.
- The second dose should be administered 1–2 months after the first dose
- Third dose should be administered 6 months after the first dose (0, 1–2, 6 months schedule).

Newer HPV Vaccine

The Food and Drug Administration in December 10, 2014. Approved a 9-valent HPV vaccine (9vHPV). This vaccine targets HPV types 6, 11, 16, and 18, the types targeted by the quadrivalent HPV vaccine (4vHPV), as well as five additional types, HPV types 31, 33, 45, 52, and 58.

The Advisory Committee on Immunization Practices (ACIP) reviewed results of a randomized trial among approximately 14,000 females aged 16 through 26 years that showed noninferior immunogenicity for the types shared by 4vHPV and 9vHPV and high efficacy for the five additional types.

Other trials in the 9vHPV clinical development program included studies that compared antibody responses across age groups and females and males and concomitant vaccination studies. The evidence supporting 9vHPV vaccination was evaluated using the Grading of Recommendations, Assessment, Development, and Evaluation (GRADE) framework and determined to be type 2 (moderate level of evidence) among females and 3 (low level of evidence) among males; the recommendation was designated as a Category A recommendation (recommendation for all persons in an age- or risk-factor–based group).

Routine and Catch-up Age Groups

ACIP recommends routine HPV vaccination at age 11 or 12 years.

- Vaccination can be given starting at age 9 years. ACIP also recommends vaccination for females through age 26 years
- Fmales through age 21 years who were not adequately vaccinated previously
- Males aged 22 through 26 years may be vaccinated.

The new recommendations are:
- 9vHPV, 4vHPV or 2vHPV can be used for routine vaccination of females aged 11 or 12 years and females through age 26 years who have not been vaccinated previously or who have not completed the 3-dose series.
- 9vHPV or 4vHPV can be used for routine vaccination of males aged 11 or 12 years and males through age 21 years who have not been vaccinated previously or who have not completed the 3-dose series.
- ACIP recommends either 9vHPV or 4vHPV vaccination for men who have sex with men and immunocompromised persons (including those with HIV infection) through age 26 years if not vaccinated previously.

Adequately Vaccinated are those Persons

- Who initiated vaccination with 9vHPV, 4vHPV, or 2vHPV before their 15th birthday, and received 2 doses of any HPV vaccine at the recommended dosing schedule (0, 6–12 months), or 3 doses of any HPV vaccine at the recommended dosing schedule (0, 1–2, 6 months), are considered adequately vaccinated
- Who have initiated vaccination with 9vHPV, 4vHPV, or 2vHPV on or after their 15th birthday, and received 3 doses of any HPV vaccine at the recommended dosing schedule, are considered adequately vaccinated.

9vHPV may be used to continue or complete a vaccination series started with 4vHPV or 2vHPV.

For persons who have been adequately vaccinated with 2vHPV or 4vHPV, there is no ACIP recommendation regarding additional vaccination with 9vHPV.

Interrupted Schedules

- If the vaccination schedule is interrupted, the series does not need to be restarted
- The number of recommended doses is based on age at administration of the first dose.

Special Populations

- For children with a history of sexual abuse or assault, ACIP recommends routine HPV vaccination beginning at age 9 years
- For men who have sex with men, ACIP recommends routine HPV vaccination as for all males, and vaccination through age 26 years for those who were not adequately vaccinated previously

- For transgender persons, ACIP recommends routine HPV vaccination as for all adolescents, and vaccination through age 26 years for those who were not adequately vaccinated previously.

Medical Conditions

ACIP recommends vaccination with 3 doses of HPV vaccine (0, 1–2, 6 months) for females and males aged 9 through 26 years with primary or secondary immunocompromising conditions that might reduce cell-mediated or humoral immunity such as B lymphocyte antibody deficiencies, T lymphocyte complete or partial defects, HIV infection, malignant neoplasms, transplantation, autoimmune disease, or immunosuppressive therapy, because immune response to vaccination might be attenuated.

Papanicolaou testing and screening for HPV DNA or HPV antibody are not routinely recommended prior to vaccination at any age. Women who are given vaccination at a later age have to be given proper advice that this vaccine will not protect against the serotype with which they may have been already infected. Benefits may be limited to protection against HPV genotypes with which they have not been infected. Women infected with vaccine HPV-type and have cleared the cervical infection appears to have similar protective effects as in HPV naïve to the same vaccine HPV-type. Women with abnormal cytology can similarly be given the vaccine with proper counseling as above. Lactating women can receive the HPV vaccine and still continue breastfeeding because it is a vaccine without live viral DNA.

The use of the vaccine in pregnancy is not recommended, although no teratogenic effect by vaccine has been reported. No evidence to show that the HPV vaccine adversely affects fertility, pregnancy or infant outcome. Women planning to conceive are advised to defer vaccination until after delivery. Women, who become pregnant before completion of vaccination, postpone remaining dose until after pregnancy. Termination of pregnancy is not indicated for women who become inadvertently pregnant during course of vaccination.

Human papillomavirus vaccines can be given simultaneously with other vaccines such as hepatitis B and tetanus diphtheria and acellular pertussis.

Booster Doses

So far, clinical trials have shown both the vaccines to be effective for at least 5 years. Longer follow-up studies are being conducted and it would be clear. In the times to come about the need for a booster will become clearer.

Adverse Reactions Following Vaccination

The most common adverse reactions reported are local reactions like fever, nausea, dizziness, myalgia and malaise.

The most important side effect reported with quadrivalent vaccine is syncopal attack. This should be prevented by giving the injection in a lying down position and allowing her to continue in this position for at least 15 minutes before allowing her to go home.

Secondary Prevention

Routine Cervical Cancer Screening

Most cases and deaths from cervical cancer can be prevented through detection of precancerous changes within the cervix by cervical cytology using the Pap test.

The use of HPV vaccine does not eliminate the need for continued Pap test screening, since 30% of cervical cancers are caused by HPV types not included in the vaccine.

ACIP guidelines for cervical cancer screening recommendations have not changed for females who receive HPV vaccine. HPV types in the vaccine are responsible for approximately 70% of cervical cancers. Females who are vaccinated could subsequently be infected with an HPV type for which the vaccine does not provide protection. Furthermore, those who were sexually active before vaccination could have been infected with a vaccine type HPV before vaccination.

BIBLIOGRAPHY

1. ACOG Committee on Adolescent Health Care. Obstet Gynecol. 2004;104:891-8.
2. Bhatla N, Lal N, Bao YP, et al. A meta-analysis on human papillomavirus type-distribution in women from South-Asia: implications for vaccination. Vaccine. 2008;26:2811-7.
3. Bruni L, Barrionuevo-Rosas L, Albero G, et al. ICO Information Centre on HPV and Cancer (HPV Information Centre). Human Papillomavirus and Related Diseases in India. Summary Report 19 April 2017. [Accessed on 19th September 2017]
4. Collins S, Mazloomzadeh S, Winter H, et al. High incidence of cervical human papillomavirus infection in women during their first sexual relationship. BJOG. 2002;109:96-8.
5. Petrosky E, Bocchini JA, Jr Hariri S, et al. Use of 9-Valent Human Papillomavirus (HPV) Vaccine: Updated HPV Vaccination Recommendations of the Advisory Committee on Immunization Practices MMWR/Vol64/no 11/March 27 2015
6. https://www.nhp.gov.in/disease/reproductive-system/female-gynaecological-diseases-/cervical-cancer (Accessed on 19th Sep 2017)
7. https://www.cdc.gov/vaccines/vpd/hpv/hcp/recommendations.html (Accessed on 19th Sep 2017)
8. Kaarthigeyaaan K. Cervical cancer in India and HPV Vaccination .Indian J Med Pediatr Oncol. 2012;33(910):7-12.
9. La Vecchia C, Franceschi S, Decarli A, et al. Sexual factors, venereal diseases, and the risk of intraepithelial and invasive cervical neoplasia. Cancer. 1986;58:935-41.
10. Markowitz LE, Dunne EF, Saraiya M, et al. Quadrivalent human papillomavirus vaccine: recommendations of the advisory committee on immunization practices (ACIP). MMWR Recomm Rep. 2007;56(RR02):1-24.

11. Meeting of the Immunization Strategic Advisory Group of Experts, November 2008: conclusions and recommendations. Wkly Epidemiol Rec. 2009;84:1-16.
12. Meites E, Kempe A, Markowitz LE. Use of a 2-Dose Schedule for Human Papillomavirus Vaccination—Updated Recommendations of the Advisory Committee on Immunization Practices MMWR. 2016;65(49):14.
13. Patel MS, Kakkad KM, Patel SV. Human Papiloma Virus vaccination: Recent trends in prevalence and current trends in India JSAFOMS. J South Asian Feder Menopause Soc 2014;2(1):26-30.
14. Petrosky E, Bocchini JA, Hariri S, et al. Use of 9-Valent Human Papillomavirus (HPV) Vaccine: Updated HPV Vaccination Recommendations of the Advisory Committee on Immunization Practices MMWR. 2015;64(11):300-4.
15. Schiller JT, Frazer IH, et al. HPV Vaccines. In: Plotkin SA Orenstein WA, (Eds) Vaccines, 5th edn. Phiadelphia: Saunders 2008;243-77.
16. WHO/ICO Information Centre on HPV and Cervical Cancer (HPV Information Centre). Human Papillomavirus and Related Cancers in India. Summary Report 2010. Available from www.who.int/hpvcentre. (Accessed October 2012)
17. Winer RL, Lee SK, Hughes JP, et al. Genital human papillomavirus infection: incidence and risk-factors in cohort of female university students. Am J Epidemiol. 2003;157:218-26.
18. World Health Organization, United Nations Population Fund. Preparing for the Introduction of HPV Vaccines: Policy and Programme Guidance for Countries. World Health Organization; 2006.

5.13 — DENGUE ILLNESSES

Ashok Kapse

INTRODUCTION

Dengue-like illnesses with hemorrhagic manifestations were first found in the Chinese Encyclopedia of Symptoms during the Chin Dynasty (AD 265-420). It was known as "water poison" for its association with insects found near any water bodies. "Dengue" is a Spanish altered word evolved from the roots in the Swahili language as "Ki-dinga".

Dengue-like diseases were known to be present all over the world during the 18th and 19th century except in Antarctica. Till the mid 20s dengue was assumed to be an innocuous non-fatal disease but views on this changed in the 1950s as the disease went under some strange evolution. People started dying from dengue in the Southeast Asian countries and two major serious symptoms were found in these patients:
1. Bleeding diathesis
2. Shock.

Dengue was now named as "dengue hemorrhagic fever (DHF)-dengue shock syndrome (DSS)" and by 1975 because of this newly evolved disease many children were hospitalized and lost their lives.

In the 1980s, disease expanded and many Asian countries like India, Sri Lanka, Maldives, Bangladesh and Pakistan were hit by dengue. With invasion of every nook and corner India is one of the worst hit countries. Hyperendemicity that is circulation of multiple serotypes has become frequent. The recent epidemics in Sri Lanka and India were associated with multiple dengue virus (DENV) serotypes, although DEN-3 is clearly more prominent. By end of the last century, this disease moved on from Asia to the Pacific regions and the United States of America (Fig. 5.13.1). Currently, 50 million DENVs occur annually with the outcome of 500,000 hospitalization cases and deaths over 20,000.

TRANSMISSION

Virus

Four related yet antigenically distinct viruses cause dengue illnesses. These viruses belong to the *Flaviviridae* family which consists of nearly 70 viruses.

Vector

Dengue is arthropod borne viruses, they use mosquitoes as vector. *Aedes albopictus* although could be a suitable vector, the *Aedes aegypti* work as the most efficient carrier, vectors

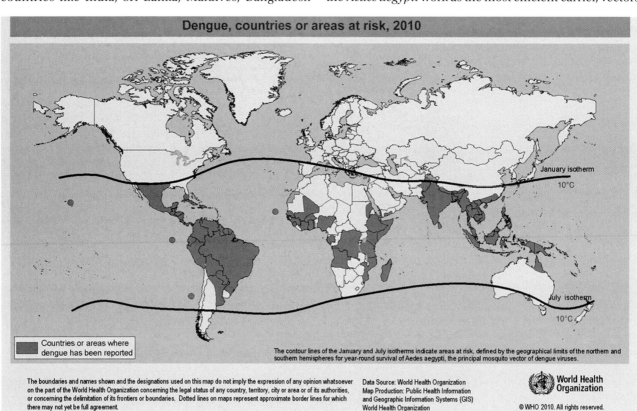

FIG. 5.13.1: Current global status (2010).

also serve to amplify viral replication. *Aedes aegypti*, the principal vector (Fig. 5.13.2) is a small, black-and-white, highly domesticated tropical mosquito that prefers to lay its (it's) eggs in artificial containers commonly found in and around homes, e.g. flower vases, old automobile tires, buckets that collect rainwater and trash in general. Containers used for water storage, such as large drums, cement cisterns and even septic tanks, are important in producing large numbers of adult mosquitoes in close proximity to human dwellings.

The adult mosquitoes remain indoors and feed on human blood at daytime. The two major periods when the feeding is at its highest is early in the morning 2–3 hours after daybreak and in the afternoon for many hours before dark. Female mosquitoes are anxious feeders and they are disrupted by just one movement when they switch to another person or the same person but probably at a different place. This particular behavior of *Aedes aegypti* makes it a very efficient epidemic vector. This female is a very effective mosquito and that is why there is no surprise in finding more than one person of the same household getting infected by dengue fever (DF) within 24–36 hours times.

After a person is bitten by this infected mosquito, the virus remains in him/her for 3–14 days and later the person may experience fever. This virus may circulate in the blood during this period of minimum 2 days or maximum 10 days. If any other *Aedes aegypti* mosquito bites this infected person in this period then they will carry the same virus and infect other people, with the incubation period of 8–12 days.

Climate also plays a major role for virus transmission. The rise and fall of the temperature and humidity, increases or decreases the virus transmission. As the temperatures go up, the mosquito larvae takes lesser time to mature and therefore is able to produce more eggs during this period. In warmer climates, mosquitoes feed frequently as the digestion of the blood is faster this time. World Health Organization (WHO) estimated that a temperature rise of 1–2°C could increase the vulnerable population by 700 million per annum.

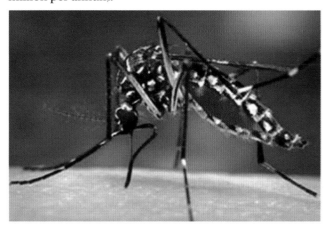

FIG. 5.13.2: *Aedes aegypti.*

Dengue Viruses

Dengue viruses are small spherical single stranded RNA viruses with a lipid envelope.

The viral genome encodes three structural proteins [Capsid protein (C), membrane protein (M), and envelope glycoprotein (E)] and seven nonstructural proteins (NS1, NS2a, NS2b, NS3, NS4a, NS4b and NS5).

The amino acid sequences of the E proteins determine the antibody neutralizing activity that classifies DENV into 4 serotypes: (1) DENV-1, (2) DENV-2, (3) DENV-3 and (4) DENV-4. The E protein also interacts with cellular receptor(s) which initiates viral entry.

Nonstructural proteins of DENV function in ribonucleic acid (RNA) replication and assembly and in viral protein processing. Along with working in viral replication, some nonstructural proteins can also modify the host immune system. Viral nonstructural proteins can influence type "I IFN" (type I interferon) signaling and induce cytokine production. NS1 is the only nonstructural protein with a soluble form that can be detected in circulation.

Infected by one dengue serotype provides lifelong immunity to that particular virus, but other serotypes have no cross protective immunity. Thus, persons living in an area of endemic dengue can be infected with three, and probably four, dengue serotypes during their lifetime.

Reasons for Recent Rise in Dengue and Dengue Hemorrhagic Fever

Sudden rise in density and geographic distribution of the *Aedes aegypti* and a large virus transmission geographically are the two principle factors responsible for the exponential increase in the emergence and re-emergence of DF and DHF.

The first factor is greatly influenced by changes in the demography which include the rise in population, and unplanned urbanization leading to bad housing and inadequate water supply and poor waste management systems.

Air travel gives the freedom to the virus to move about; different serotypes, strains, and even genotypes of virus from one place to another's outcome are hyperendemicity. Viremic individuals can then introduce virus in the new vulnerable population causing epidemics.

PATHOPHYSIOLOGY

Vascular Leak

The fundamental feature which differentiates DHF from DF is a transient increase in vascular permeability that results in the leakage of fluid from the plasma into the interstitium. The extravasated fluid is collected into serous cavities: peritoneum, pleura and pericardium; and the leakage results into hemoconcentration and hypovolemia. After some time, may be some hours to days, the increased vascular permeability spontaneously resolves, the extravasated fluid which gets reabsorbed and the recovery starts. A few patients suffer from a severe leak which leads to hypovolemia, hypotension and shock culminating into death.

Mechanism for Vascular Leak

The pathophysiological mechanisms underlying the capillary leak are ill understood. Although increase in microvascular permeability has been well documented using strain gauge plethysmography suggestive of endothelial dysfunction, however there is no evidence that the virus directly infects endothelial cells in vivo, and no structural endothelial abnormalities have ever been demonstrated. Strain gauge plethysmography well documents endothelial dysfunction yet there is no proof that the virus infects the endothelial cells in vivo directly, and no structural endothelial abnormalities have ever been demonstrated.

Luminal surface of the vascular endothelium has a layer of glycocalyx. Layer incorporates into it glycosaminoglycans (GAGs) which are complex, negatively charged polysaccharides. This layer creates a size selective physical barrier which allows the going of only some molecules between the fibers and an electrostatic barrier which works as a boundary for the access of negatively charged molecules underlying the cellular transport mechanisms. More than the endothelial cellular structures, it is the glycocalyx that shows the permselectivity. A recent research has pointed a change in the function of the endothelial glycocalyx at the time of dengue infection. The selective limitation on the negative charge is clearly impaired while on the other side the general size-dependent sieving mechanism is partially retained.

PATHOGENESIS

Dengue hemorrhagic fever usually occurs in two clinical settings: secondary dengue infection at any age and primary dengue infection in an infant. Lots of advances have worked toward the understanding of DENV biology in the past but still the pathogenesis explaining DHF in two different set of patients is still intriguing. Different factors like total viral virulence, virus burden, host immune response and genetic predisposition have been tagged as risk factors for DHF. But, still these factors are unable to explain the occurrence of DHF in both clinical settings.

The most noted risk factor for DHF is due to the pre-existence of non-neutralizing antibodies either from previous infection or transplacental mother-to-child transmission.

DENGUE VIRUS GENOTYPE AND PROTEINS

Dengue virus type-2 and DENV-3 are commonly associated with DHF, however, as no consistent correlation between a particular DENV serotype and genotype is ever established. In general, Asian genotypes appear to be more virulent than American and the South Pacific genotypes. Phylogenetic analysis showed that the Native American DENV-2 genotype was associated only with DF, whereas the Asian DENV-2 genotypes were more correlated with DHF cases. Subsequent studies demonstrated that an Asian genotype DENV-2 strain was capable of higher replication compared to the American genotype DENV-2 strains in human monocyte-derived macrophages (MDM) and dendritic cells (DCs). Nucleotide sequence variation is the most likely explanation for the genotype dependent divergent severity.

Higher Viral or Viral Protein Load

Not only the sequence variation but also other correlate of disease severity may also be the reason of virus and viral proteins in the bloodstreams of DF versus DHF patients. Many studies have given a positive correlation between peak levels of viremia and development of DHF for circulation serotypes.

The levels of "sNS1" in the bloodstreams of patients of DHF was to be found more than that of DF in some studies. Higher levels of "sNS1" were present in the plasma of patients who went ahead to develop DHF than in that of DF patients during the 3 days prior to onset of DHF, showing that "sNS1" may be useful as a prognostic marker of DHF as indicated by Avirutnan.

T-CELL IMMUNE PATHOLOGY

Coincident with defervescence, there is sudden surge of cytokines (Cytokine Tsunami) in symptomatic secondary dengue infections. This "Cytokine Tsunami" is believed to be responsible for pathognomonic DHF vasculopathy. Some of the noted changes are: high concentrations of soluble interleukin-2 receptor, soluble CD4, soluble CD8, interleukin 2 and interferon gamma, soluble tumor necrosis factor receptors, soluble CD8, soluble interleukin-2 receptors, interleukin 10, etc. Chemokine (CC motif) ligand 2 (CCL2), a protein that reduces tight junctions of vascular endothelium cells is found to be consistently high in DHF/DSS patients. Levels of these "cytokines" correlate with severity of dengue disease.

Massive activation of "T-lymphocytes" underlies this "cytokines" storm. "Dengue nonstructural protein NS3" is the predominant epitopes which react with antigen responsive "T-lymphocytes". Rothman and Ennis hypothesized that the number of cells presenting the dengue viral antigen to "T-lymphocytes" is markedly increased during a secondary infection; this in turn generates "T" cell immune pathology (abnormal T-lymphocyte activation).

NS1 Autoimmunity

Known immune activation along with immune cell dysfunction and altered platelet kinetics, has forced some researchers to suggest immune responses to certain components of DENVs which would contribute to autoimmune processes that result in DHF/DSS.

Antibodies directed against DENV NS1 cross-react with human platelets and endothelial cells. After binding to endothelial cells, anti-DENV NS1 antibodies induce nitric oxide mediated cellular apoptosis. These antibodies induce inflammatory endothelial cell activation of interleukins 6 and 8, and CCL2 also complement activation by the alternative pathway.

Durability of NS1 antibodies contradicts the autoimmune NS1 hypothesis. Vascular permeability and hemostatic dysfunctions are transitory whereas NS1 antibodies last for a longer period of time in DHF patients.

Role of Pre-existing Antibodies

Infection of a DENV in a dengue virgin body self-limits the febrile illness; recovery from this infection comes along with the generation of immunological responses. Epitopes present in E protein are capable of inducing homologous as well as heterologous neutralizing and non-neutralizing antibodies. These variations in the levels of antibodies have a central role for the dengue infection to change the infection to mild or serious disease.

Neutralizing antibodies to DENV are responsible for specific protection and infection with one such DENV serotype makes one immune to that infection serotype lifelong. Antibodies against E, prM proteins and to NS1 are capable of neutralizing DENV and providing protection against dengue infection.

The first infection also provides protection against other serotypes for the initial few months. However with a decline in neutralizing antibodies, heterotypic non-neutralizing antibodies result into antibody dependent enhancement (ADE). ADE is a phenomenon when the heterotypic antibodies form complexes with DNVs, which facilitate enhanced cellular infection. This occurs only during a secondary infection with a different serotype and when the heterotypic non-neutralizing antibodies are absent.

Antibody dependent enhancement theory proficiently elucidate observed occurrence of DHF in both clinical settings: primary infection in infants and during secondary infection at any age.

DISEASE CLASSIFICATION

Old Classification

Ranging from asymptomatic infection, to mild undifferentiated fever, to fatal shock, dengue illnesses have wide spectrum of clinical presentations. Till very recently WHO identified two types of dengue illnesses:
1. DF, a mild self-limiting febrile illness
2. DHF, a potentially fatal condition pathognomonic by leaky vasculopathy.

According to the disease severity DHF was further divided into four categories:

Grade I: Thrombocytopenia, hemoconcentration, positive Tourniquet Test (TT) and absence of spontaneous bleeding.

Grade II: Thrombocytopenia, hemoconcentration, positive TT and presence of spontaneous bleeding.

Grade III: Thrombocytopenia, hemoconcentration, positive TT and circulatory insufficiency (feeble pulse, drop of 20 mm Hg or greater in arterial blood pressure, cold extremities and apprehension).

Grade IV: Thrombocytopenia, positive TT, hemoconcentration, imperceptible pulse and blood pressure.

The Technical Advisory Committee at its meeting in 1974 at Manila, Philippines formulated the WHO case classification (DF/DHF/DSS). The classification to a large extent was based on the pioneering studies done at the Children's Hospital, Bangkok, Thailand in early sixties. The classification and guidelines for management were published by WHO; first published was in 1980 and with subsequent revision in 1986 and 1997.

Dengue Fever versus Dengue Hemorrhagic Fever: Central Theme in Previous Classification

Dengue fever is a nonspecific febrile illness and DHF is a potentially serious disorder caused by leaky vasculopathy, this major difference is the central theme in dengue disease classification. According to WHO guidelines, DHF cases must fulfill all four following criteria mentioned: (1) Fever or history of acute fever lasting 2–7 days, (2) hemorrhagic tendencies evidenced by at least one of the following: a positive TT, petechiae, purpura, ecchymoses; bleeding from mucosa, gastrointestinal tract, injection sites or other location hematemesis, and melena, (3) thrombocytopenia (platelets <100,000) and (4) evidences for plasma leakage in DHF: more than 20% rise in hematocrit, fluid in serous cavities documented by X-ray or ultrasonography (USG).

Difficulties with Previous Classification

Due to the spreading of dengue worldwide and to older age groups as well, clinicians and several investigators have felt and reported very many difficulties in the current system. Commonly reported difficulties are:
- The classification rigorously tries to distinguish between DF, DHF and DSS, although there is much overlap between the three for example bleeding or occult bleeding tendency (+ TT) and mild thrombocytopenia could occur in DF as well.
- Documentation of all four requirements for the WHO definition of DHF (fever, hemorrhage, thrombocytopenia and signs of plasma leakage) needs frequent assessment of packed cell volume and platelet counts which may not always be available or feasible, more over a properly fluid managed patient from early

stage of disease may fail to show 20% rise in hematocrit despite vascular leak.

- TT is an integral part of the existing scheme however test poorly differentiates between DF and DHF; moreover many children with "non-dengue" febrile illnesses may also have positive tests.
- The DF/DHF/DSS classification excludes severe dengue disease associated with organ involvement like hepatitis, encephalitis and myocarditis.
- Finally, the term DHF places undue emphasis on hemorrhage when the danger sign that should be watched for and managed is plasma leakage leading to shock.

New Classification

Realizing that the current classification of dengue into DF, DHF (Grades 1 and 2) and DSS (DHF Grades 3 and 4) would not be universally applicable for clinical management everywhere WHO convened a meet of global dengue experts in 2008 in Geneva. Committee recommended a new case classification for dengue illnesses and put forward revised guidelines in 2009 for the management of dengue illnesses. As per new guidelines this disease is now classified into three categories: (1) dengue, (2) dengue with warning signs and (3) severe dengue whereas the clinical course of the disease is divided in three phases: febrile, critical and recovery (Fig. 5.13.3).

CLINICAL PICTURE

Dengue

Febrile Phase

Following a short incubation period of 2–7 days, there is an abrupt onset of high grade fever. During fever whole body is invariably covered with bleachable erythematous flush (Fig. 5.13.4). With suffused and swollen face, injected eyes, reddened ears, crimson smaller area, swollen and purplish lips patients assume a measly look (Fig. 5.13.5). The flush deepens with advancing disease. In few of these patients, a classical maculopapular exanthema (Fig. 5.13.6) may erupt on the top of erythematous flush. Some patients may have sore throat, injected pharynx and conjunctival injection; however catarrh a typical characteristic of respiratory viruses is missing. Adolescents and older children often suffer from headache, retro-orbital pain, photophobia, backache, myalgia and arthralgia. Anorexia, nausea and vomiting are also not uncommon symptoms and these usually lead to dehydration. Mild hemorrhagic manifestations like petechiae (Figs. 5.13.7 to 5.13.9) and mucosal membrane bleeding (e.g. nose and gums, conjunctiva) may be seen (Fig. 5.13.10), however massive gastrointestinal bleeding commonly reported in adults during febrile phase is sporadic in children.

In the early febrile phase of the disease, it may not always be possible to distinguish dengue from non-dengue

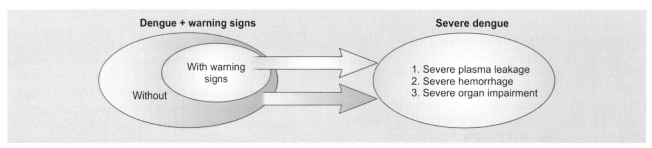

Criteria for dengue + warning signs		Criteria for severe dengue
Probable dengue	**Warning signs***	**Severe plasma leakage**
Live in/travel to dengue endemic area Fever and 2 of the following criteria: • Nausea, vomiting • Rash • Aches and pains • Tourniquet test positive • Leukopenia • Any warning sign	• Abdominal pain of tenderness • Persistent vomiting • Clinical fluid accumulation • Mucosal bleed • Lethargy, restlessness • Liver enlargement > 2 cm • Laboratory increase in HCT concurrent with rapid decease in platlet count	Leading to: • Shock (DSS) • Fluid accumulation with respiratory distress
		Severe bleeding As evaluated by clinician
		Severe organ involvement
Laboratory confirmed dengue (Important when no sign of plama leakage)	*Requiring strict observation and medical intervention	• *Liver:* AST or ALT >=1000 • *CNS:* Impaired consciousness • Heart and other organs

FIG. 5.13.3: Suggested dengue case classification and level of severity.

Abbreviations: DSS, dengue shock syndrome; HCT, hematocrit; AST, aspartate aminotransferase; ALT, alanine aminotransferase; CNS, central nervous system
Source: Guidelines for diagnosis, treatment, prevention and control, new edition. WHO TDR, 2009.

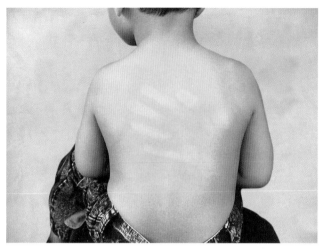

FIG. 5.13.4: Bleachable erythematous flush.

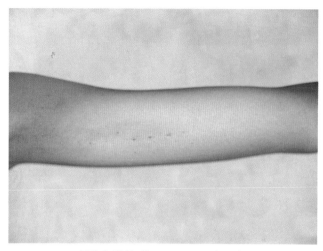

FIG. 5.13.7: Dengue purpuric rash.

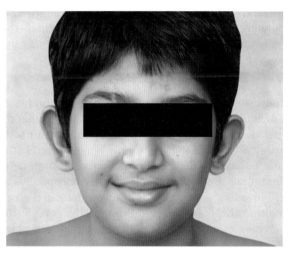

FIG. 5.13.5: Dengue facies.

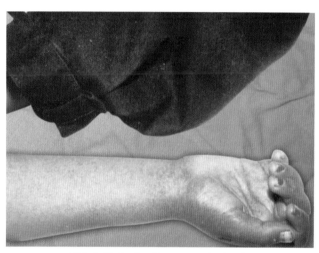

FIG. 5.13.8: Confluent petechial rash.

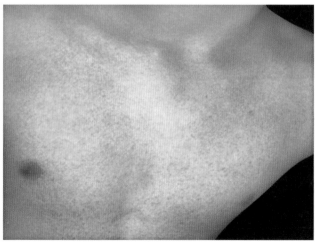

FIG. 5.13.6: Maculopapular rash.

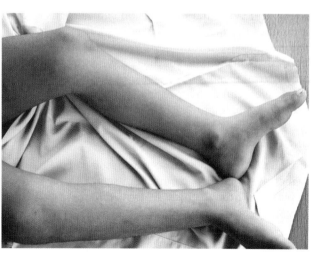

FIG. 5.13.9: Annular petechial rash.

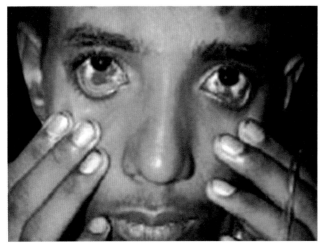

FIG. 5.13.10: Minor bleeds (conjunctival hemorrhage).

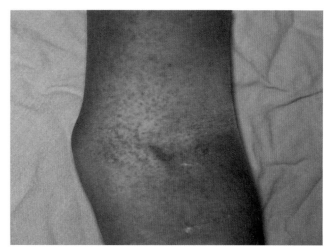

FIG. 5.13.11: Positive TT.

febrile diseases. A positive TT in this phase increases the probability of dengue diagnosis (Fig. 5.13.11).

Leukopenia, atypical lymphocytosis and mild thrombocytopenia are some of the commonly observed hematological changes during febrile phase of dengue illness.

After a period of 2–7 days majority patients make a smooth and complete recovery but some of the patients may deteriorate with defervescence, and they could pass into a critical phase. The initial clinical features are not clearly distinguishable between severe and non-severe dengue cases; therefore, it is imperative that the patient should be under strict monitoring for warning signs so that cases progressing to the critical phase could be timely identified.

Dengue with Warning Signs

Cases destined to pass into critical phase may display many of the following warning signs: persistent vomiting, abdominal pain, hepatic enlargement, lethargy restlessness, scanty urine, postural hypotension clinical signs of fluid accumulation (ascites, effusion, edema), rising hematocrit with progressive thrombocytopenia, mucosal bleeding (epistaxis, hematemesis, gum bleeding, metromenorrhagia, conjunctival bleeding). Presence of these warning signs should alert clinician for regular monitoring and prompt fluid therapy to improve patient's outcome.

Critical Phase

Around the time of defervescence, in some of the patients an increase in capillary permeability sets in. Extravasation of plasma, through these leaky capillaries result into progressive hemoconcentration. A parallel drop in platelets and progressive leukopenia usually precedes plasma leakage. Together these changes mark the beginning of the critical phase. Patients in this phase would display many of the above mentioned warning signs.

In majority of the cases, the leak is transient lasting for a few hours, once it stops patient quickly stabilizes and completely recovers. According to new classification these patients should be classified as dengue with warning signs.

Severe Dengue (Fig. 5.13.12)

With disease spreading to world over it was soon realized that dengue could have serious manifestations other than shock. Hepatitis, myocarditis, encephalitis and severe bleeding are few of the commonly encountered serious manifestations of a dengue illness. Some common serious presentations are hepatitis, myocarditis, encephalitis and severe bleeding. A new category: severe dengue is created to include these serious symptoms. This category has three types of patients: (1) patients with severe plasma

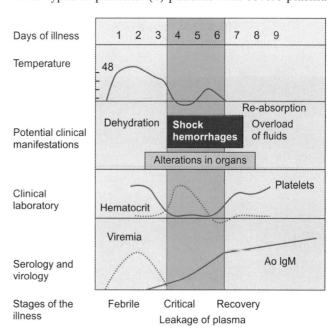

FIG. 5.13.12: Course of a dengue illness.

leakage: (a) shock (cold clammy peripheries, prolonged CRT, narrow pulse pressure, fall in systolic pressure), (b) fluid accumulation resulting into respiratory distress; (2) patients with profuse bleeding and (3) patients with significant organ involvement: (a) hepatic involvement (transaminases > 1,000), (b) patients with neurological involvement and (c) patients with cardiac involvement.

Dengue Shock

Patients with prolonged and prolific leak would deteriorate. These deteriorating patients will manifest signs of impending shock (cold and clammy extremities, feeble or imperceptible peripheral pulse, delayed capillary refill time, narrow pulse pressure, falling blood pressure).

In patients with massive leak, plasma may continue leaking for 2–3 days. Extravasated fluid collects primarily into serous cavities like peritoneum, pleura and pericardium (Fig. 5.13.13). Large ascites and pleural effusion are clinically detectable, however, small effusions would need X-ray chest and abdominal ultrasound for demonstration. Amount of vascular leak evidenced as degree of hemoconcentration is the primary determinant of prognosis.

Poorly monitored and inadequately managed patient may progressively pass into hypovolemia, hypotension and shock. Prolonged shock ensue organ hypoperfusion which may result in progressive organ impairment, metabolic acidosis and disseminated intravascular coagulation (DIVC). DIVC may incite severe uncontainable bleeding. A sudden fall in otherwise elevated hematocrit during critical phase should alert clinician for occult internal bleeding.

Recovery Phase

After a couple of days the leakage stops and the plasma which had extravasated during the leaky phase returns to circulation. Patient starts passing copious amount of dilute urine, develop bounding pulse, wide pulse pressure and rise in blood pressure. Appetite improves and patient feels better. Hemoconcentration resolves; due to dilutional effect hematocrit may go lower than normal. Around ninth day of the sickness, platelets start increasing and it becomes normal over next couple of days. Effusions are usually slow to resolve; patient may take few more days for complete recovery. In majority of cases disease recovers within 2 weeks.

Respiratory Distress

Patients with profound leak usually need massive resuscitative fluid therapy during critical phase. With the resolution of vascular leak, the extravasated fluid returns to the vascular compartment. This returning fluid may cause congestive heart failure (CHF) manifesting as tachycardia, tachypnea, muffling of heart sounds and basal rales; problem is particularly augmented with colloid uses. Massive pleural effusion and ascites (Fig. 5.13.14) may further add to respiratory distress. This phase most of the times last for 12–24 hours and intense monitoring is needed during this time. The respiratory distress might be so intense that the patient may need an oxygen support and decongestive (diuretics) therapy.

Author has serious reservations naming this stage of illness as recovery phase as during this stage of disease severe dengue patient is hemodynamically unstable and regularly needs close clinical observations and intensive therapy; which is against the tenet of recovery. In severe dengue, recovery would be considered only after uneventful passage of this stage of disease. It should better be named as congestive or regurgitation phase.

ORGANOPATHY

Hepatitis

Dengue viruses frequently inflict liver. Hepatomegaly and liver impairment in form of elevated transaminases is common occurrence in dengue illnesses. The intensity of these enzymes increase on the third day after the infection of

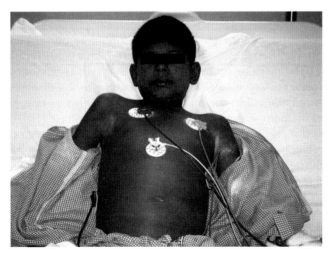

FIG. 5.13.13: Clinical ascites and puffy face (fluid overload).

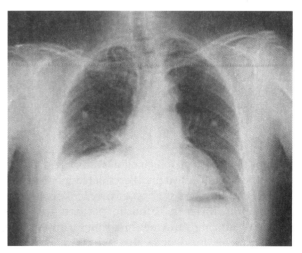

FIG. 5.13.14: Pleural effusion.

the disease; it reaches its highest point on the seventh or the eighth day and it decreases to normal values within 3–8 weeks approximately. In contrast to viral hepatitis the elevation in the level of serum glutamic oxaloacetic transaminase (SGOT) enzyme is normally greater than the elevation in the level of serum glutamic pyruvic transaminase (SGPT) in dengue patients.

This disease is self-limiting but severe hepatitis with elevated transaminases, hemorrhages and hepatic failure culminating into death is also seen in some patients. An elevated lactate dehydrogenase (LDH) enzyme is found to be a marker of life-threatening hepatitis in a recently concluded study at Surat. These types of cases always do not have pathognomonic dengue vascular leak but it could occur during the febrile phase and it is fortunate that severe hepatitis is not common in pediatric age group.

Neurological Complications

Dengue infections can cause variety of neurological manifestations; prominent among them are convulsion, unconsciousness, myositis, spasticity and paresis. Current research suggests that dengue especially DEN-2 and DEN-3 has strong neurotropism and can cause encephalitis due to direct viral invasion of the brain. Most neurological events are seen early in the febrile phase and are unrelated to the perfusion status.

Cardiac Complications

Heart can be affected with dengue viral infections. A global hypokinesia, low ejection fraction, electrocardiogram (ECG) changes and rhythm disturbances are noted in some of the recent studies. Majority changes are transient and reversible, however, a persistent cardiomyopathy is reported from Sri Lanka.

DENGUE CLINICAL MANAGEMENT

Proper dengue management has following principles:
- Suspicion of disease
- Assessments and management of early febrile phase
- Identifying patients with warning signs
- Recognizing early critical phase and initiating timely fluid therapy
- Recognizing and managing severe dengue shock, massive bleeding and severe organ impairment.

Suspicion of Disease

Clinicians need to keep a high clinical suspicion index as most of the patients have undifferentiated febrile illness. However, certain signs such as measly look, bloachable erythematous flush in a febrile patient presenting particularly during rainy season should immediately arouse suspicion for dengue illness. Respiratory viruses prevailing during rainy season could also present with similar erythematous flush however a significant catarrh differentiates them from dengue illnesses.

Assessments and Management of Febrile Phase

Clinical History

Suspected patient should be assessed for hydration status: history of voiding (frequency, amount and color), quantity of oral intake, excessive diaphoresis and history of diarrhea and vomiting. Vascular leak is a major dengue complication that occurs during peri-defervescence period hence date and timing of fever onset needs special noting. Frequent assessments for warning signs, dizziness and altered mental status are necessary to recognize complications at early stage.

Physical Examination

Vascular leak resulting progressively into dehydration, hypovolemia hypotension and shock is a major complication of dengue illnesses. Unraveling signs of dehydration and hypotension is therefore an important aim of clinical examination. Scanty urine, giddiness, inability to walk unsupported and narrow pulse pressure is some of the significant clinical findings of ongoing vascular leak. Signs of pleural and peritoneal effusion (dull percussion note, abdominal pain and distension) are other important clinical evidences for vascular leakage. Enlarged and tender liver with or without icterus may be suggestive of liver impairment. Abnormal mentation, impaired consciousness and convulsions may suggest early neurological dysfunction. Massive hemorrhages and mucosal bleed would be clinically apparent. However, diligent search is needed to find out petechiae, purpura and ecchymoses. A TT should always be performed; positive test suggests underlying bleeding tendency and augments probability of dengue diagnosis.

Investigations

A complete blood checkup (CBC) should be performed during first visit. A hematocrit test in the febrile phase forms a baseline value for the patient which serves as reference figure for any change during the course of the disease. A notable fall in the platelets with an analogous rise in hematocrit suggests progression to critical phase (DHF) of disease. These parameters exhibit a unique time-bound relationship with the disease. Changes start a little before the defervescence and peak around second or third febrile day. Degree of rise in hematocrit bears a distinct correlation with the severity of the disease. Serology may not become positive during febrile phase but NS1 a soluble antigen of dengue virus appears in patient's blood as early as second day of illness and may persist all through the disease period. Demonstrable by enzyme-linked immunosorbent assay

(ELISA); NS1 carries a high sensitivity and specificity for dengue diagnosis. Some important tests to be done are serum transaminases, creatinine and electrolytes. Clinical signs of fluid leakage may not be apparent in mild cases; a decubitus X-ray chest used to be employed by past clinicians for demonstrating mild pleural effusion however sonology has made the things convenient; as it can demonstrate the smallest amount of extravasated fluid in any of the serous cavity. Gallbladder edema is one of the unexplained yet a consistent sonological finding in dengue illnesses.

Management

Outpatient Management

Close clinical observations during the febrile period and 2–3 days beyond the defervescence is absolutely essential, however, majority of dengue patients could be treated as outpatients. Care takers should follow the given instructions:

- Give a set goal for child's fluid intake [100–150 mL/kg, body weight (BW)]. Fluids could be oral rehydration solution (ORS), water, milk, buttermilk, fruit juices, etc. The more the consumption of the fluid the less number of hospitalizations. Instruct parents to collect child's urine and compare the output against fluid intake; passing scanty urine with adequate oral fluid intake should alert clinician for vascular leak.
- Use only paracetamol for pain and fever, do not use aspirin, ibuprofen, mefenamic acid, nimesulide or other nonsteroidal anti-inflammatory drugs (NSAIDs) for fever or pain as these drugs interfere with platelet functioning.
- Warn parents for warning signs, viz scant urine, giddiness, restlessness, anxiety, severe abdominal pain and cold extremities.
- Carefully assess every patient exhibiting warning signs for impending shock, e.g. poor volume pulse, imperceptible pulses, narrowing of pulse pressure and fall in blood pressure. Patient with these symptoms need immediate hospitalization for intensive intravenous (IV) fluid therapy.
- In dengue illnesses, crucial pathophysiology starts with defervescence; hence any child deteriorating or failing to improve with subsidence of fever should be carefully assessed for progression to critical phase.
- Instruct the caregivers that the patient should be brought to hospital immediately if any of the following occur: no clinical improvement or deterioration around the time of defervescence, severe abdominal pain, persistent vomiting, cold and clammy extremities, lethargy or irritability/restlessness, bleeding (e.g. black stools or coffee-ground vomiting), not passing urine for more than 4–6 hours.

Majority patients without warning signs would tolerate oral fluids; however patients with anorexia, nausea and vomiting may need IV fluid therapy. Normal saline or Ringer's lactate with or without dextrose given at maintenance rate is sufficient in most of the cases. Switch over to oral fluids as soon as patients tolerate. Close medical supervision is mandatory for at least 3 days beyond defervescence.

Inpatient Management

A patient with severe dengue or warning signs should be admitted to the hospital; although not very common patients with profuse bleeding and with organ impairments need condition-specific management and also require hospitalization. In majority of the dengue illnesses IV fluid therapy of vascular leak is the most important aspect of management. In mild cases (dengue with warning signs, erstwhile DHF grades 1 and 2), plasma leakage is small and transient, and patients recover spontaneously or shortly after administration of IV fluid. In severe cases (severe dengue, former DHF grades III and IV), there are large plasma losses, hypovolemic shock ensues, and it can progress rapidly to profound shock. Volume replacement is the mainstay for the treatment of this type of severe dengue. The original guidelines for the IV fluid therapy in DHF were developed at the Children's Hospital, Bangkok, by Dr Suchitra Nimannitya. Guidelines were adopted by WHO and proposed as official recommendations in 1975 to 1999. High continuous fluid (7–10 mL/kg BW) replacement was the main theme of these recommendations. Over the last few years it was realized, that many complications and deaths were due to inappropriate fluid management leading to fluid overload, and it was felt that dengue vascular leak could be managed with lesser fluid therapy. In 2009 WHO came out with new set of guidelines with emphasis on resuscitation; accordingly shock is corrected with boluses of (10 mL/kg BW) isotonic fluid while replacement is done with much smaller doses.

Choice of Fluid

Two common types of IV fluids currently used in dengue shock are crystalloids and colloids. Colloid solutions tentatively are more advantageous than crystalloid solutions as they provide volume expansion over and above the actual fluid volume infused. The colloid molecules increase plasma oncotic pressure and reverse the net flux of fluid out of the intravascular compartment moreover pathophysiological studies indicate that there is preferential leakage of relatively small plasma proteins (e.g. albumin) as compared with larger molecules [e.g. immunoglobulin G (IgG)], which implies that resuscitation with colloid preparations of larger molecular weights may offer therapeutic advantages. However, these theoretical advantages have not been substantiated in clinical studies. A recent meta-analysis observed that colloids decrease the hematocrit and pulse rates of children with DSS after the first 2 hours of fluid resuscitation; however, these changes were transient and no significant advantage was found over crystalloids in reducing the recurrence of shock, the need for rescue colloids, the total amount of fluids, the need for diuretics and in reducing mortality. General consensus is crystalloids should be used for initial resuscitation while colloid boluses are reserved for patients presenting with hypotensive shock, recurrent shock and refractory hypotensive shock.

Management Plan

Dengue with Warning Signs

Patients displaying warning signs are likely to pass into critical phase; they need hospitalization for close clinical observations and IV fluid therapy. Platelet count and hematocrit should be checked before the fluid therapy. Initial values serve as reference for future changes.

Intravenous fluid therapy should be started with any of the isotonic solutions such as normal saline (0.9%) or Ringer's lactate. Patients may need 5–7 mL/kg/hour for 1–2 hours for initial hemodynamic stabilization. IV fluid is tapered off to 3–5 mL/kg/hour for 2–4 hours and then to 2–3 mL/kg/hour or less according to the clinical response. Use just enough IV fluid to maintain adequate perfusion. Frequent assessment should be done to keep a tab of hemodynamic status (pulse rate, pulse pressure, blood pressure, continuous real-time, urine output) and hematocrit. If the hematocrit remains the same or rises only minimally, continue with the same rate (2–3 mL/kg/hour) for another 2–4 hours.

Destabilization of hemodynamic status associated with increasing hematocrit during critical phase is the indication for stepping up the IV fluid rate. Bolus of to 5–10 mL/kg/hour may be given for 1–2 hours then modify fluid infusion rates as per the hematocrit.

After a variable period of few hours to few days (usually 24–48 hours) IV leak starts decreasing; increasing urine output along with decreasing hematocrit in a stable patient is the best indication of ending of critical phase. The critical phase comes to an end when the patient's IV leak starts decreasing, his/her urine increases and there is a decrease in hematocrit. This is seen only after a period of few hours to days (usually 24–48 hours).

All the patients should receive regular monitoring for vital signs, peripheral perfusion and detailed fluid balance till the risk period is over. The regularity of monitoring depends on the speed of the patient's recovery, however at least 1–4 hourly watch on vital signs and 4–6 hourly monitoring of urine output is obligatory. Hematocrit assessments every 6–12 hourly and additionally before and after every bolus fluid replacement is an essential recommendation from WHO; however it may not always be practicable as facility for microhematocrit is generally unavailable in field conditions. Regular check on urine output and hemodynamics can obviate the need for frequent hematocrit assessment.

Severe Dengue

(Dengue shock and/or fluid accumulation with respiratory distress, severe hemorrhages and severe organ impairment).

Patients with severe dengue need urgent hospitalization and emergency treatment. Hospital should have intensive care and blood transfusion facilities. In most of the cases astute resuscitation is the only intervention needed.

Dengue Shock

Over the last few years, IV fluid therapy has undergone a major conceptual shift. Currently, fluid therapy is separated as fluid resuscitation and fluid replacement. Fluid resuscitation is a strategy in which larger volumes of fluids (e.g. 10–20 mL boluses) are administered for a limited period of time under close monitoring. Goals of the resuscitation are to improve central and peripheral circulation and end organ perfusion. Plasma losses are constantly replaced with IV fluid over next 24–48 hours yet the recommendation for this fluid is much smaller; fluid just enough to maintain effective circulation and perfusion is advised. For resuscitation as well replacement only isotonic fluids must be used; hypotonic fluids have no place in dengue management.

From management view point compensated shock should be separated from hypotensive shock.

Compensated Shock

(Normal systolic pressure, rising diastolic pressure, narrowing pulse pressure < 30, postural hypotension).

Start IV fluid resuscitation with isotonic crystalloid solutions at 5–10 mL/kg/hour over 1 hour (Flowchart 5.13.1). Then reassess the patient's condition (vital signs, capillary refill time, hematocrit, urine output). The next steps depend on the situation. If the patient's condition improves, IV fluids should be gradually tapered to 5–7 mL/kg/hour for 1–2 hours, then to 3–5 mL/kg/hour for 2–4 hours, then to 2–3 mL/kg/hour. Patient with stable hemodynamic status may need only maintenance fluid therapy for next 24–48 hours.

Following the first bolus if vital signs are still unstable (i.e. shock persists), check the hematocrit. In patients with high or rising hematocrit, repeat a second bolus of crystalloid solution or colloid at 10–20 mL/kg/hour for 1 hour. After this second bolus, if there is improvement, reduce the rate to 7–10 mL/kg/hour for 1–2 hours, and then continue to taper as above. Patients may need further boluses during next 24–48 hours depending on their progress or regress of the situation.

FLOWCHART 5.13.1: Fluid management in compensated shock.

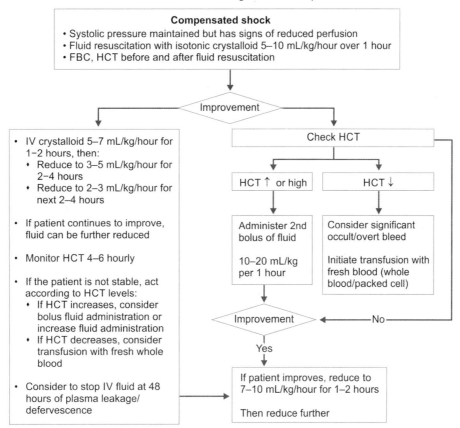

Abbreviations: IV, intravenous; FBC, full blood count; HCT, hematocrit

A falling hematocrit in a hemodynamically unstable patient indicates internal bleeding; timely blood transfusion could be life-saving in this type of clinical state.

Hypotensive Shock

A more aggressive approach is observed for hypotensive shock (Flowchart 5.13.2). An initial resuscitative bolus of 20 mL/kg BW of colloid is pushed over 15 minutes so as to rescue patient from shock. If patient improves a further bolus of IV fluid (crystalloid/colloid) 10 mL/kg/hour is infused over next 1 hour. In a hemodynamically stable, patient fluid is gradually tapered over following 6–8 hours. Further fluid replacement for subsequent 24–48 hours is undertaken with maintenance doses of isotonic crystalloid infusion.

In a hemodynamically unstable patient (i.e. shock persists), review the hematocrit before the first bolus. Low hematocrit indicates bleeding and needs blood transfusion. If the initial hematocrit was high compared to the baseline value; a second bolus of colloid solutions at 10–20 mL/kg is pushed over next 30 minutes to 1 hour. Review the hemodynamics after the second bolus if the condition stabilizes; reduce the rate to 7–10 mL/kg/hour for 1–2 hours, then change over to crystalloid solution and reduce the rate of infusion as mentioned above.

A patient with unstable hemodynamics, further management depends on the assessment of hematocrit. Decreasing hematocrit is an indication for blood transfusion while increasing hematocrit is signal for further colloid boluses. This practice is followed till the patient is stabilized. Once patient improves, reduce the rate to 7–10 mL/kg/hour for 1–2 hours, then change back to crystalloid solution and reduce the rate of infusion gradually over next 6–8 hours to maintenance doses. Multiple fluid boluses may need to be given during critical phase in a dengue shock patient. Extent and frequency of such boluses again depends on the patient's hemodynamic response. About 5% albumin boluses have found to be an effective treatment in unresponsive dengue shock patients.

Monitoring

Dengue shock has a highly dynamic clinical course; it is crucial that patient should be regularly monitored. Frequency of assessment generally is dictated by patient's condition; it should be at least hourly till patient is hemodynamically unstable. Regular monitoring (no less than 4 hourly) is mandatory even in a hemodynamically stable patient till fluid regurgitation is complete and patient is totally out of risk. Frequent assessment of vitals, pulse

FLOWCHART 5.13.2: Fluid management in decompensated shock.

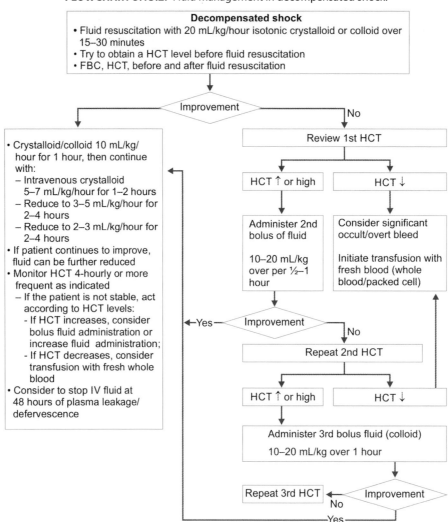

Abbreviations: FBC, full blood count; HCT, hematocrit; IV, intravenous

(peripheral pulses), blood pressure, pulse pressure, heart rate, abdominal girth, and urinary output are mandatory.

Peripheral Pulses

A nicely perceptible peripheral pulse is a sign of adequate perfusion. Imperceptible or feeble peripheral lower limb pulses (posterior tibialis and dorsalis pedis) particularly during replacement fluid therapy indicate higher fluid requirement.

Pulse Pressure

Dengue is unusual in that a slow leak occurs over several days, permitting compensatory mechanisms to operate. Before the development of overt cardiovascular collapse, the diastolic pressure rises to meet the systolic pressure, and the pulse pressure narrows; therefore narrowing of the pulse pressure is the most significant parameter for defining dengue shock. Maintaining pulse pressure of more than 20 mm Hg is the most important aspect of IV

fluid therapy. A narrow pulse pressure less than 20 mm Hg is an indication for stepping up IV fluid rate.

Urine Output

Maintaining fluid input-output chart is very important. Urine output gives vital information about end organ perfusion; it should be checked hourly till the patient is out of shock and there after 1–2 hourly until patient is out of risk. A continuous bladder catheter enables correct monitoring of urine output. An acceptable urine output would be about 0.5 mL/kg/hour.

Hematocrit

Hematocrit assessment is the central theme in dengue shock management; it should be monitored (before and after fluid boluses until stable, then 4–6 hourly). Changes in hematocrit are important therapeutic guide however these changes should always be interpreted along with the hemodynamic status. Following are the examples of correct hematocrit interpretation: (1) a rising or persistently high hematocrit together with stable hemodynamic status and adequate urine output does not require extra IV fluid. In this situation, it is likely that the hematocrit will start to fall within the next 24 hours as the plasma leakage stops; (2) a rising or persistently high hematocrit together with unstable vital signs (particularly narrowing of the pulse pressure) indicates active plasma leakage and the need for a further bolus of fluid replacement; (3) a falling hematocrit together with unstable vital signs (particularly narrowing of the pulse pressure, tachycardia, metabolic acidosis, poor urine output) indicates major hemorrhage and the need for urgent blood transfusion and (4) decrease in hematocrit together with stable hemodynamic status and adequate urine output indicates hemodilution and/or intravasation of fluids suggestive of stopping of further IV fluids.

Monitoring of arterial or venous blood gases, other organ functions such as: renal profile, liver profile, coagulation profile, should be performed as per individual case indication.

Severity Markers

Significant thrombocytopenia, clinical signs of vascular leak, and narrowed pulse pressure appearing early during febrile phase of sickness are indicators of serious course of disease.

Complications

Hemorrhagic Complications

Minor bleed: Little mucosal bleeding in the form of epistaxis, gum bleed, conjunctival hemorrhages might occur in dengue infected patients; these patients usually remain stable and need only fluid resuscitation/replacement; such bleeds rapidly improve during the recovery phase.

Major bleed: There are reports of unusual bleeding manifestations with some of the dengue outbreaks but generally major bleeding in pediatric age group is rare in dengue. Major bleed in the form of gastrointestinal and vaginal hemorrhages may occur in adult patients. Bleeding complications mostly take place in patients who have pre-existing acid peptic disease, are on anticoagulant therapy and/or are treated with NSAIDs agents. In pediatric patients major bleeding is almost always secondary to poorly managed shock culminating into multiorgan dysfunction and consequential DIVC.

Recognizing Major Bleed

As mentioned earlier gastrointestinal tract is the site where major internal bleeding takes place. It may destabilize hemodynamics in a critically placed dengue shock patient nevertheless hours may pass before it would manifest as "melena". Rapidly falling hematocrit together with unstable hemodynamic status is the early indicator of internal bleeding and should be taken as an urgent signal for blood transfusion irrespective of then absolute hematocrit level.

Plan for Treatment of Major Bleed

Ten milliliter/kg of fresh-packed red cells or 20 mL/kg of fresh whole blood should be transfused at an appropriate rate. Improvement in hematocrit, hemodynamic status and acid-base balance are some of indications for successful therapy. In case of inappropriate rise in hematocrit and inadequate clinical response, a repeat transfusion is indicated. Stored blood loses 2, 3 diphosphoglycerate (DPG), low levels of which impede the oxygen-releasing capacity of hemoglobin; resulting in functional tissue hypoxia therefore it is important that only fresh whole blood or fresh red cells are given.

Platelet Transfusion

Without significant bleeding platelets are not indicated even with a count as low as 10,000 per cu mm. Platelets transfusion are given only if significant bleeding occurs. Prophylactic transfusion with platelets and fresh frozen plasma do not produce sustained changes in coagulation status and platelet counts of DHF/DSS patients, on the contrary inappropriate transfusion of blood components increases the risk of pulmonary edema and respiratory.

Respiratory Distress

Causes

Acute pulmonary edema, severe metabolic acidosis from severe shock and acute respiratory distress syndrome (ARDS) are infrequent causes of respiratory distress however polyserositis (severe ascites and pleural effusions) due to fluid overload is the most common cause for this complication.

Fluid Overload

Causes for fluid overload are: (1) Excessive and/or too rapid IV fluids, (2) Erroneous use of hypotonic rather than isotonic crystalloid solutions, (3) Inadvertent continuation of IV fluids even after leakage has stopped, (4) Over use of colloids, (5) Inappropriate transfusion of blood products: fresh-frozen plasma, platelet concentrates and cryoprecipitates and (6) Comorbid conditions such as congenital heart disease, chronic lung and renal diseases.

Polyserositis in severe dengue may not always indicate fluid overload; in severe dengue vascular leak invariably is massive; infused fluid, however appropriate it may be, is bound to leak into serous cavities causing polyserositis.

Clinical Features

Tachypnea, dyspnea, wheezing, chest wall indrawing are some of the early signs of fluid overload. Tense ascites and pleural effusions may cause severe respiratory distress. Cough with frothy pink sputum herald the inception of pulmonary edema and CHF.

Management Plan

Intravasation of fluid starts as soon as the vascular leak is over and is indicated by the widening of pulse pressure, stable blood pressure, bounding peripheral pulses and increase in urinary output. Rapid gush of intravasating fluid would cause fluid overload and vascular congestion particularly if patient keeps receiving IV fluids.

Oxygen supplementation is a must for patients with respiratory distress, the management of fluid overload is dictated by hemodynamics, hematocrit and phase of the disease.

A falling hematocrit with wide pulse pressure and increased urinary output are indications to stop further IV fluid. Furosemide 0.1–0.5 mg/kg/dose intravenously once or twice daily helps in the reduction of respiratory distress in a fluid overloaded patient. Monitoring of serum potassium and correcting the ensuing hypokalemia is important for patients treated with furosemide. Avoid diuretic therapy if there is any doubt that critical phase (vascular leak) is still on.

Patient who is still in shock have low hematocrit levels and show signs of fluid overload might be suffering from occult hemorrhage. A fresh blood transfusion could vastly benefit such patients.

Repeated small boluses of a colloid solution would be of help if the patient remains in shock and has an elevated hematocrit.

Dyselectrolytemia, Blood Glucose Disturbances

Possibilities of electrolyte disturbances like hyponatremia, hypokalemia, hyperkalemia, serum calcium imbalances and metabolic acidosis should be kept in mind while treating dengue shock. Dyselectrolytemia is uncommon and occurs due either to incorrect uses of hypotonic solutions for resuscitation and replacement or diarrhea vomiting resulting into gastrointestinal electrolyte losses.

Regular blood sugar monitoring is necessary as both hypoglycemia and hyperglycemia could occur and destabilize a precariously positioned hemodynamics.

Adjuvant Therapy

Vasopressors and Inotropes

In a severe fluid unresponsive hypotensive dengue shock. Vasopressors and inotropes may be used as temporary measures, however vasopressors and inotropes should always be used as supportive measure and never as a substitute in a severe fluid unresponsive hypotensive dengue shock.

Avoidable Ancillary Treatment

Steroids, IV immunoglobulin, and of recombinant activated factor VII have been tried in some studies but none of them was found useful in dengue management.

Reasons for Mortality in Dengue Shock

Failing to appreciate that patient is passing in critical phase of disease.

In a febrile illness generally parents and treating physician tend to feel relieved when temperature subsides, unfortunately a dengue patient develops pathognomonic vascular leak with defervescence and worsens during this period; failure to appreciate this is the most common cause of death in dengue shock. Defervescence of fever is always considered as sign of clinical recovery both by care takers as well treating clinician, but unfortunately dengue patient develop the pathognomonic vascular leak with defervescence and the state worsens during this period. It is imperative for treating clinician to regularly assess every patient for warning signs during this stage of disease. Warning signs like anxiety, apprehension and giddiness at defervescence should alarm a physician for a possible development of shock and an impending death could be avoided by hospitalizing the patient for IV fluid therapy soon enough.

Failure to Appreciate Internal Bleeding

Although major clinical hemorrhages are uncommon in pediatric dengue; rarely however an occult massive bleed may prove life-threatening. Falling hematocrit and a destabilized hemodynamics should alert clinician for such an eventuality; a timely blood transfusion would save a patient.

Failure to Appreciate Vascular Congestion

Inadvertent continuation of IV fluid in the wake of intravasation of leaked out fluid would cause cardiac overload and consequential CHF and death. Falling hematocrit with increased urinary output is a pointer to intravasation of leaked out fluid and should be taken as signal to terminate IV fluid therapy.

Even though a complex disease DHF exhibits a set clinical pattern and observes a fixed time bound course of events. Awareness and familiarity with its course greatly facilitates diagnosis-making and proper therapy. With appropriate IV fluid management and frequent monitoring, mortality in dengue shock could be greatly minimized.

Organ Impairments

Organ specific standard management needs to be carried out in clinical situation of hepatitis, encephalopathy, encephalitis and cardiac abnormalities.

Dengue Antiviral Drugs

Recent clinical studies have noted that the viral load is much higher in blood of the patients who develop severe dengue (DHF, DSS) compared to with patients suffering from the milder DF. This observation suggests that any drug which could lower the viral load would be effective in curbing the disease progression and would halt the adverse morbidity. Search for molecules which could interfere with viral replication is going on. Several potential viral targets have been found out; currently the most advanced targets are the NS3/NS2B protease and NS5 RNA-dependent RNA polymerase.

Dengue Vaccine

Intense research is going on for dengue vaccine. The biggest challenge is to find out a tetravalent vaccine which can induce long-lasting protective immunity against all four viruses. Dengue vaccines in development are of four types: (1) live attenuated viruses, (2) chimeric live attenuated viruses, (3) inactivated or sub-unit vaccines and (4) nucleic acid-based vaccines. A DEN-DEN chimera is a dengue vaccine which is in advanced preclinical development stage. The tetravalent vaccine produced by combining the four chimeric dengue viruses is protective when administered to mice. Monkey challenge experiments have been conducted and preparations for clinical trials are underway.

Despite the stiff challenges posed by multiplicity of viral serotypes useful strides have been made in the fields of dengue antivirals as well in dengue vaccine.

BIBLIOGRAPHY

1. Bandyopadhyay S, Lum LC, Kroeger A. Classifying dengue: a review of the difficulties in using the WHO case classification for dengue haemorrhagic fever. Trop Med Int Health. 2006;11(8):1238-55.
2. Capeding RZ, Brion JD, Caponpon MM, et al. The incidence, characteristics and presentation of dengue virus infections during infancy. Am J Trop Med Hyg. 2010;82(2):330-6.
3. Chatarvedi UC, Nagar R. Dengue and dengue haemorrhagic fever: Indian perspective. J Biosci. 2008;33(4):429-41.
4. Clyde K, Kyle JL, Harris E. Recent advances in deciphering viral and host determinants of dengue virus replication and pathogenesis. J Virol. 2006;80(23):11418-31.
5. Deen JL, Harris E, Wills B, et al. The WHO dengue classification and case definitions: time for a reassessment. Lancet. 2006;368(9530):170-3.
6. Gubler DJ, Kuno G, Waterman SH. Neurologic disorders associated with dengue infection. proceedings of the international conference on dengue/dengue hemorrhagic fever. Kuala Lumpur: Malaysia; 1983. pp. 290-306.
7. Gubler DJ. Dengue and dengue hemorrhagic fever. Clinical Microbiol Rev. 1998;11(3):480-96.
8. Gubler DJ. Dengue and dengue hemorrhagic fever: Its history and resurgence as a global public health problem. In: Gubler DJ, Kuno G (Eds). Dengue and Dengue Hemorrhagic Fever. Wallingford, United Kingdom: AB International; 1997. pp. 1-22.
9. Guzmàn MG, Alvarez M, Rodriguez R, et al. Fatal dengue haemorrhagic fever in Cuba, 1997. Int J Infect Dis. 1999;3(3):130-5.
10. Guzmán MG, Kourí G. Dengue: An update. Lancet Infect Dis. 2002;2(1):33-42.
11. Halstead SB, Mahalingam S, Marovich MA, et al. Intrinsic antibody-dependent enhancement of microbial infection in macrophages: disease regulation by immune complexes. Lancet Infect Dis. 2010;10(10):712-22.
12. Halstead SB. Antibody, macrophages, dengue virus infection, shock, and hemorrhage: a pathogenic cascade. Rev Infect Dis. 1989;11(Suppl 4): S830-9.
13. Halstead SB. Dengue. Lancet. 2007;370(9599):1644-52.
14. Halstead SB. Is there an in apparent dengue explosion? Lancet. 1999;353(9158):1100-1.
15. Kalayanarooj S, Chansiriwongs V, Nimmannitya S. Dengue Patients at the Children's Hospital, Bangkok: 1995-1999 review. Dengue Bulletin. 2002;26:33-43.
16. Kalayanarooj S, Nimmannitya S. Clinical presentations of dengue hemorrhagic fever in infants compared to children. J Med Assoc Thai. 2003;86(Suppl 3):S673-80.
17. Kapse AS. A study of an epidemic of dengue at Surat, clinico-investigative analysis. In environment and health in developing countries. 1998. pp.339-50.
18. Kapse AS. Dengue illnesses. In: Parthasarthy A (Ed). IAP Text book of Pediatrics, 4th edition. New Delhi: Jaypee Brothers Medical Publishers (P) Ltd; 2009. pp. 396-403.
19. Kliks SC, Nimmanitya S, Nisalak A, et al. Evidence that maternal dengue antibodies are important in the development of dengue haemorrhagic fever in infants. Am J Trop Med Hyg. 1988;38(2):411-9.
20. Morens DM, Halstead SB. Disease severity-related antigenic differences in dengue 2 strains detected by dengue 4 monoclonal antibodies. J Med Virol. 1987;22(2):169-74.
21. Ngo NT, Cao XT, Kneen R. et al. Acute management of dengue shock syndrome: a randomized double-blind comparison of 4 intravenous fluid regimens in the first hour. Clin Infect Dis. 2001;32(2):204-13.
22. Nimmannitya S. clinical spectrum and management of dengue haemorrhagic fever. Southeast Asian j Trop Med Pub Health. 1987;18(3):392-7.
23. Premaratna R, Liyanaarachchi E, Weerasinghe M. Should colloid boluses be prioritized over crystalloid boluses for the management of dengue shock syndrome in the presence of ascites and pleural effusions?. BMC Infect Dis. 2011;11:52.
24. Rigau-Pérez JG. Severe dengue: the need for new case definitions. Lancet Infect Dis. 2006;6(5):297-302.
25. Srikiatkhachorn A. Plasma leakage in dengue haemorrhagic fever. Thromb Haemost. 2009;102(6):1042-9.
26. Sumarmo, Wulur H, Jahja E, et al. Clinical observations on virologically confirmed fatal Dengue infections in Jakarta, Indonesia. Bull World Health Organ. 1983;61(4):693-701.
27. Wahid SF, Sanusi S, Zawawi MM, et al. A comparison of the pattern of liver involvement in dengue hemorrhagic fever with classic dengue fever. Southeast Asian J Trop Med Public Health. 2000;31(2):259-63.
28. WHO. Dengue haemorrhagic fever: diagnosis, treatment, prevention and control. Geneva: WHO, 1975.
29. WHO and TDR. Dengue: Guidelines for diagnosis, treatment, prevention and control: 2009.
30. Wills BA, Nguyen MD, Ha TL, et al. Comparison of three fluid solutions for resuscitation in dengue shock syndrome. N Engl J Med. 2005;353(9):877-89.
31. Wills BA, Oragui EE, Dung NM, et al. Size and charge characteristics of the protein leak in dengue shock syndrome. J Infect Dis. 2004;190(4):810-8.

5.14 CHIKUNGUNYA FEVER

Rajniti Prasad

INTRODUCTION

Chikungunya is a viral fever caused by an Alphavirus and spread by bite of an infected *Aedes aegypti* mosquito. The disease was first discovered by Marion Robinson and WHR Lumsden in 1955 following an outbreak on the Makonde plateau. The name derives from a Kimakonde root verb, kungunyala, meaning 'to dry up or become contorted', specifically modified in early times to describe the bent posture of patients. Although primarily African and zoonotic, it is known chiefly for its non-African large urban outbreaks, which is transmitted by the same vectors as those of Dengue viruses. Since 1953, chikungunya virus (CHIKV) has caused numerous outbreaks and epidemics in both Africa and South-East Asia, involving hundreds and thousands of children.

EPIDEMIOLOGY

Chikungunya virus was probably an infection of primates in forests of Savannahs of Africa maintained by sylvatic Aedes mosquitoes. However, today, CHIKV is also responsible for extensive *A. aegypti* transmitted urban disease in the cities of Africa and major epidemics in Asia. In Africa, CHIKV is transmitted in the Savannahs and forests of tropical Africa by Aedes mosquito. The vertebrate portion of the cycle is provided by nonhuman primates, such as Cercopithecus, monkeys or baboons, which amplify and maintain virus circulation. It is thought that endemic circulation and epidemics in troops of primates are responsible for survival of the virus and local spillover into human population.

In India, after quiescence of about three decades, an outbreak of CHIKV is being reported from different parts of India. The current outbreak in India started in the end of 2005, when cases of suspected fever were reported from coastal parts of Andhra Pradesh and Karnataka. A number of suspected cases reported have varied from different sources ranging up to a million. The current outbreak has an attack rate of 4–45%. The confirmed cases of chikungunya fever have been reported from all over the country but more so from Andhra Pradesh, Karnataka, Maharashtra, Tamil Nadu, Madhya Pradesh and Gujarat states.

Chikungunya virus is commonly transmitted to humans through the bite of infected mosquitoes of the *Aedes* genus, which usually bite during daylight hours. Mother to child transmission, occupational exposure and occurrence in a health worker from careless handling a patient's blood has also been reported. In Africa, CHIKV appears to be maintained in sylvatic cycle involving wild primates and forest dwelling *Aedes* spp. Monkeys and possibly other wild animals may also serve as reservoirs of the virus.

Aedes aegypti, A. albopictus and *A. polynesiensis* are commonly involved in the transmission of virus, although Culex has also been reported for the transmission in some cases. *A. aegypti* is the principal vector of CHIKV in India. This vector species is anthropophilic, endophagic and bites during the day time. It mainly breeds in man-made containers such as rainwater barrels, cisterns, wells, water storage drums, pots, discarded bottles, tin cans, motor vehicle tyres, etc. A recent epidemic in the Indian Ocean islands suggested that Asian tiger mosquito, *A. albopictus* was responsible for spread. A mutation in the envelope protein gene (*E1-A226V*) was found in some strains of CHIKV causing epidemics on islands in the Indian Ocean. This mutation is directly responsible for CHIKV adaptation to the Asian tiger mosquito. Both *A. aegypti* and *A. albopictus* are present in the US and the Asian tiger mosquito in Europe. With the Global climate warming, CHIKV could expand to new geographic locations.

CHIKUNGUNYA VIRUS

Chikungunya virus, a positive strand, enveloped an RNA virus, is a member of the *Alphavirus* genus and belongs to the Togaviridae family. It is endemic in large parts of Africa, the Middle-East, India and South-East Asia, and is closely related to o'nyong-nyong viruses. Genetic analysis based on partial E1 envelope glycoprotein gene sequences showed the presence of three distinct phylogroups. The first contained all isolates from West Africa; the second comprised all Central, Southern and Eastern African strains (CSEA) and the third contained isolates from Asia. Phylogenetic studies have suggested that the West African CHIKV cluster was ancestral, the CSEA cluster diverged from West African ancestors, and the Asian and Indian Ocean clusters of genotypes had lately and independently evolved from CSEA variants.

Complete genomic sequence of CHIKV has been determined and found to have 11,805 nucleotides in length. Coding sequences consisting of two large open reading frames of 7,422 nucleotide and 3,744 nucleotide encoding the nonstructural polyprotein (2,474 amino acids) and the structural polyprotein (1,248 amino acids), respectively. The nonstructural polyprotein is the precursor of proteins nsP1 (535 amino acids), nsP2 (798 amino acids), nsP3 (530 amino acids) and nsP4 (611 amino acids) and the structural polyprotein is the precursor of protein C (261 amino acids), E3 (64 amino acids), E2 (423 amino acids), 6K (61 amino acids) and E1 (439 amino acids).

PATHOGENESIS

Chikungunya virus replicates in various human cells, including epithelial and endothelial cells, but primarily in fibroblasts and macrophages. T and B lymphocytes and monocyte-derived dendritic cells are not susceptible.

Viral entry occurs through a pH-dependent, endocytic pathway. CHIKV is highly cytopathic for mammalian cells, inducing apoptosis of infected cells. CHIKV replication is significantly inhibited by types I and II interferons (IFNs). In humans, CHIKV produces disease about 48 hours after mosquito bite. Patients have high viremia during the first 2 days of illness. Viremia declines around day 3 or 4 and usually disappears by day 5. Hemagglutination inhibition and neutralizing antibodies can usually be detected after day 5 with fading viremia. "Silent" CHIKV infections do occur, but how commonly this happens is not yet known. CHIKV infection (whether clinical or silent) is thought to confer lifelong immunity. A recent study has suggested CHIKV tropism for muscular satellite cells, which can act as small reservoirs for virus or virus-encoded components or both for longer than expected periods.

CLINICAL MANIFESTATIONS

Chikungunya is an acute infection characterized by abrupt onset fever and severe arthralgia, followed by other constitutional symptoms and rash lasting for a period of 1–7 days (triad: fever, rashes and arthralgia). The incubation period is usually 2–4 days, with a range of 1–12 days. All age groups are affected, including newborns.

Fever rises abruptly, often reaching 39–40°C accompanied by intermittent shaking chills, myalgias, headache and photophobia. This acute phase lasts 2–3 days. The temperature may remit for 1–2 days, after a gap of 4–10 days, resulting in a "saddle back" fever curve.

The arthralgias are polyarticular, migratory and predominantly affect the small joints of hands, wrists, ankles and feet with lesser involvement of larger joints. In acute stage, patients complain bitterly of pain when asked to move and assume an attitude of flexion. Pain on movement is worse in the morning, improved by mild exercise and exacerbated by strenuous exercise. Swelling may occur but fluid accumulation is uncommon. Patients with milder articular manifestation are usually symptom-free within a few weeks, but more severe cases require months to resolve entirely (Fig. 5.14.1).

Cutaneous manifestations include flushing of the face and trunk. This is usually followed by maculopapular rash. The trunks and limbs are commonly involved, but face, palms and soles may also show lesions. The rash may simply fade or desquamate. Petechiae may occur alone or in association with rash. They are observed during the acute stage of the illness, and others during convalescence or thereafter. Pigmentary changes have been reported to be the most common cutaneous finding

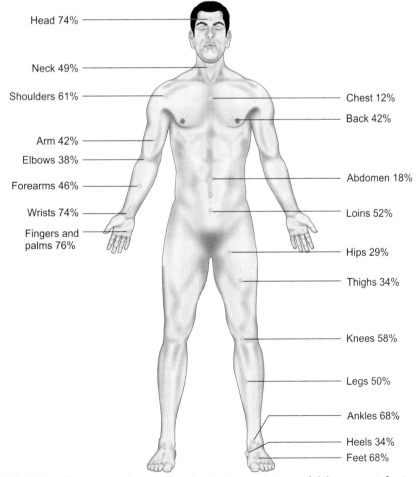

Head 74%
Neck 49%
Shoulders 61%
Arm 42%
Elbows 38%
Forearms 46%
Wrists 74%
Fingers and palms 76%

Chest 12%
Back 42%
Abdomen 18%
Loins 52%
Hips 29%
Thighs 34%
Knees 58%
Legs 50%
Ankles 68%
Heels 34%
Feet 68%

FIG. 5.14.1: Frequency of pain by location during acute stage of chikungunya infection.

(42%), followed by maculopapular eruption (33%) and intertriginous aphthous-like ulcers (21.37%). Exacerbation of existing dermatoses, such as psoriasis and unmasking of undiagnosed Hansen's disease, were also observed.

Iridocyclitis and retinitis are the most common ocular manifestations associated with chikungunya, with a typically benign clinical course. Less frequent ocular lesions include episcleritis. Diarrhea, vomiting and abdominal pain has been reported in about 50% of patients admitted in hospital. Neurological manifestations include encephalopathy, encephalitis (1%), febrile seizure, acute flaccid paralysis and Guillain-Barré syndrome. Other manifestations include congestive cardiac failure, pneumonia, fulminant hepatitis (2%), prerenal failure and respiratory failure. Hemorrhagic manifestations are rare, which is an important distinguishing feature from dengue fever.

Most symptomatic patients (93.7%) complained of a chronic stage of the disease, which is characterized by pains in joints and/or bones or both. This persisting pain was continuous (41.3%) or discontinuous with alternation of clinical remission and relapses (58.7%). Some infected individuals (11.7%) also mentioned fever at this stage.

The case fatality rate is about 1 in 1,000 during epidemics. The common causes of death are heart failure, multiple organ failure, hepatitis and encephalitis.

Diagnosis

Laboratory investigation is critical to establish diagnosis and initiate specific public health response. Three main laboratory tests are used for diagnosing chikungunya fevers: (1) virus isolation; (2) serological tests; and (3) molecular technique of polymerase chain reaction (PCR). Virus isolation is the most definitive tests. Between 2 and 5 mL of whole blood is collected during the first week of illness in heparinized tube and transported on ice to the laboratory. The CHIKV produces cytopathic effects in a variety of cell lines including BHK-21, HeLa and Vero cells. The cytopathic effects must be confirmed by CHIK specific antiserum and the results can take between 1 and 2 weeks. Virus isolation must only be carried in BSL-3 laboratories to reduce the risk of viral transmission.

Recently, a reverse transcriptase (RT)-PCR technique for diagnosis has been developed using nested primer pairs amplifying specific components of three structural gene regions: (1) capsid (C); (2) envelope E2; and (3) part of envelope E1. PCR results can be available within 1–2 days.

For serological diagnosis, an acute phase serum must be collected immediately after clinical onset and a convalescent phase, 10–14 days after the disease onset. The blood specimen is transported at 4°C and should not be frozen to the laboratory immediately. If testing cannot be done immediately, the blood specimen is separated into sera that should be stored and shipped frozen. Serologic diagnosis can be made by demonstration of four-fold increase in antibody in acute and convalescent sera or demonstrating immunoglobulin M (IgM) antibodies

Table 5.14.1: Diagnostic criteria of CHIK fever.

Criteria	Definition
Clinical criteria • Acute onset of fever >38.5°C and severe arthralgia or arthritis	Possible case when not explained by other medical condition: dengue or alpha virus infection, arthritic disease, endemic malaria
Epidemiological criteria • Residing in or visited epidemic area within 15 days before onset of symptoms	Probable case, if clinical and epidemiological criteria are met, other pathogens with similar clinical manifestations can cocirculate within the same geographical regions
Laboratory criteria After acute phase • Virus isolation • Presence of viral RNA • Specific IgM antibodies • Four-fold increase in IgG titers in paired samples	Confirmed case, if a patient tests positive for one of the laboratory, irrespective of clinical manifestations

specific for CHIKV. A commonly used test is the IgM antibody capture enzyme-linked immunosorbent assay (MAC-ELISA). Results of MAC-ELISA can be available within 2–3 days. Cross-reaction with other Flavivirus antibodies such as o'nyong-nyong and Semliki forest may occur in the MAC-ELISA; however, the latter viruses are relatively rare in South-East Asia but if further confirmation is required, it can be done by neutralization tests and hemagglutination inhibition assay (HIA). A positive virus culture supplemented with neutralization is taken as definitive proof for the presence of CHIKV. PCR results for E1 and C genome either singly or together constitute a positive result for CHIKV. The diagnostic criteria of CHIK fever is mentioned in Table 5.14.1.

Management

There is no specific treatment for CHIK fever. The illness is usually self-limiting and resolves with time. Supportive care with rest is indicated during the acute joint symptoms. Movement and mild exercise tend to improve stiffness and morning arthralgia, but heavy exercise may exacerbate rheumatic symptoms. Nonaspirin and nonsteroidal anti-inflammatory drugs (NSAIDs) are recommended. In unresolved arthritis refractory to NSAID, chloroquine (10 mg/kg/day) has proved to be useful. Chloroquine inhibits viral replication by blocking the pH-dependent endocytosis of CHIKV into host cells. Although chloroquine blocks CHIKV replication, the therapeutic (antiviral) index of chloroquine in cell cultures is rather narrow thus, one should be cautious when planning the use of chloroquine as an antiviral treatment in infected individuals.

Ribavirin has some antiviral activity against CHIKV and treatment with ribavirin showed moderate beneficial effect in alleviating arthralgia and swelling. Although ribavirin has some antiviral properties against CHIKV, IFN-α is more effective in inhibiting CHIKV replication.

Self-resolution occurs with cutaneous lesions. Patients with hyperpigmentation may be treated with sunscreens and topical steroids. All patients with only centrofacial involvement showed complete clearance during follow-up at 3 weeks. Patients with more diffuse involvement showed a slower resolution. Aphthous ulcers usually heal over 7–10 days with local cleaning and topical antimicrobials to prevent secondary infection. Iridocyclitis and retinitis have a typically benign clinical course. All the patients respond well to the treatment with preservation of good vision.

Infected persons should be protected from further mosquito exposure (staying indoors and/or under mosquito net during the first few days of illness) so that they cannot contribute to the transmission cycle.

Prevention and Control

Prevention is entirely dependent upon taking steps to avoid mosquito bites and elimination of mosquito breeding sites and include the following:

- Wear full sleeve clothes and long dresses to cover the limbs
- Use mosquito coils, repellents and electric vapor mats during the daytime
- Use mosquito nets to protect babies, old people and others who may rest during the day. The effectiveness of such nets can be improved by treating them with permethrin. Curtains can also be treated with insecticide and hung at windows or doorways, to repel or kill mosquitoes
- Drain water from coolers, tanks, barrels, drums and buckets, etc.
- Emptying coolers when not in use
- Remove from the house all objects, e.g. plant saucers, etc. which have water collected in them
- Cooperating with the public health authorities in anti-mosquito measures.

Vaccine

The widespread geographic distribution, recurrent epidemics and infection of military personnel, travelers and laboratory staff working with CHIKV have indicated the need for a safe and efficacious vaccine.

In Thailand, CHIK strain 15561 was used to develop a small lot of vaccine. The vaccine produced no untoward reactions and was highly immunogenic. The current live vaccine (Lot 1-85, TSI-GSD-218) was developed in the United States in United States Army Medical Research Institute for Infectious Diseases (USA MRIID) and was produced at the Salk Institute, from GMK strain 15561 by serial passage in MRC-5 cells. The results of phase I and phase II trials strongly suggest that the live vaccine is safe and well-tolerated and produces no severe or frequent symptoms than found in placebo recipients.

Surveillance

Epidemiological and entomological surveillance should be intensified. Reporting of fever cases should be monitored closely. Active surveillance by health workers using the case definitions for cases presenting with acute fever associated with arthralgia or arthritis (painful and stiff joints) to detect new cases early for treatment should be undertaken. This will help in identifying the affected areas, so that control measures may be initiated. Vector surveillance should also be done and will help in identifying the areas for initiating control measures and assess the impact of the measures taken. People need to be educated about the disease, mode of transmission, availability of treatment and adoption of control measures. The activities have to be identified particularly to effect changes in the practice of storage of water and personal protection.

BIBLIOGRAPHY

1. Briolant S, Garin D, Scaramizzino N, et al. In vitro inhibition of chikungunya and Semliki forest viruses replication by antiviral compounds: synergistic effect of interferon-alpha and ribavirin combination. Antiviral Res. 2004;61:111-7.
2. Burt FJ, Rolph MS, Rulli NE, et al. Chikungunya: a re-emerging virus. Lancet. 2012;379:662-71.
3. Chhabra M, Mittal V, Bhattacharya D, et al. Chikungunya fever: a re-emerging viral infection. Indian J Med Microbiol. 2008;26:5-12.
4. Chikungunya Fever Fact Sheet–CDC Division of Vector Borne Infectious Diseases. Available from *http://www.cdc.gov/ ncidod/chikungunya/chickfact.htm.2006*
5. Edelman R, Tacket CO, Wasserman SS, et al. Phase II safety and immunogenicity study of live chikungunya virus vaccine TSI-GSD-218. Am J Trop Med Hyg. 2000;62(6):681-5.
6. Inamadar AC, Palit A, Sampagavi VV, et al. Cutaneous manifestations of chikungunya fever: observations made during a recent outbreak in south India. Intern J Dermatol. 2008;47:154-9.
7. Khan AH, Morita K, Parquet MdMdel C, et al. Complete nucleotide sequence of chikungunya virus and evidence for an internal polyadenylation site. J Gen Virol. 2002;83:3075-84.
8. Lahariya C, Pradhan SK. Emergence of chikungunya virus in Indian subcontinent after 32 years: a review. J Vect Borne Dis. 2006;43:151-60.
9. Mahendradas P, Ranganna SK, Shetty R, et al. Ocular manifestations associated with chikungunya. Ophthalmology. 2008;115(2):287-91.
10. Mohan A. Chikungunya fever: clinical manifestations and management. Indian J Med Res. 2006;124:471-4.
11. Parola P, de Lamballerie X, Jourdan J, et al. Novel chikungunya virus variant in travelers returning from Indian ocean islands. Emerg Infect Dis. 2006;12:1493-9.
12. Pialoux G, Gaüzère BA, Strobel M. Chikungunya virus infection: review through an epidemic. Med Mal Infect. 2006;36:253-63.
13. Powers AM, Brault AC, Tesh RB, et al. Re-emergence of chikungunya and o'nyong-nyong viruses: evidence for distinct geographical lineages and distant evolutionary relationships. J Gen Virol. 2000;81:471-9.
14. Queyriaux B, Simon F, Grandadam M, et al. Clinical burden of chikungunya virus infection. Lancet Infect Dis. 2008;1:2-3.
15. Ravichandran R, Manian M. Ribavirin therapy for chikungunya arthritis. J Infect DevCtries. 2008;2:140-2.
16. WHO. Disease outbreak news. Chikungunya and dengue in the southwest Indian ocean, Geneva 17 March, 2006.

5.15 INFECTIOUS MONONUCLEOSIS

Narendra Rathi

INTRODUCTION

Infectious mononucleosis (IM) is an acute infection caused by Epstein-Barr virus (EBV), characterized by fever, lymphadenopathy, sore throat and atypical lymphocytes. Various names of IM are Pfeiffer's disease, Kissing disease, Druesenfieber, Glandular fever and "acute leukemia with spontaneous cure". Apart from IM, EBV is known to cause various lymphoproliferative diseases and epithelial malignancies like virus associated hemophagocytic syndrome, oral hairy leukoplakia, lymphoid interstitial pneumonitis, Burkitt lymphoma, Hodgkin disease, nasopharyngeal carcinoma and post-transplant lymphoproliferative disease.

EPIDEMIOLOGY

Seroprevalence

Infectious mononucleosis is frequently acquired during early childhood and is often asymptomatic. Various studies in India suggest that it has relatively high prevalence (70–80%) in normal adults. Age at primary infection and manifestations associated with primary infection varies markedly in different cultural and socioeconomic status. In developing countries and lower socioeconomic conditions, primary EBV infection occurs at an early age with most children becoming seropositive by 6 years of age and their primary infection is clinically silent or manifests as mild disease. In developed countries or higher socioeconomic status, primary EBV infection occurs later in life (adolescents and young adults) and is more likely to induce clinical symptoms in the form of IM syndrome.

Incidence

Various population based studies have reported incidence of IM as 50–100 cases per 100,000 population. One study from Chandigarh, India, has reported percentage of Paul-Bunnel antibody positivity of 11.1% among clinically suspected IM patients.

Viral Shedding

Virus is shed mainly in oropharyngeal secretions, although it is shedding in urine, uterine cervix, male reproductive tract and breast milk is also reported. After the acute attack, virus is shed regularly in oropharyngeal secretions for 6 months or longer and intermittently thereafter. Sixty percent of immunosuppressed patients continue to shed the virus.

Modes of Transmission

Intimate sharing of oral secretions is the major mode of transmission, although transmission via blood transfusion, intrauterine and perinatal transmission and sexual transmission are reported occasionally.

Incubation Period

Typical EBV—associated IM has incubation period of 30–50 days.

ETIOPATHOGENESIS

Epstein-Barr virus, the causative agent of IM, belongs to the family Herpesviridae and is a DNA virus. Its taxonomic name is human herpesvirus type 4, although it is popularly known by its historic name, i.e. EBV. Like any other herpesvirus, it has ability to remain in dormant or latent state after acute infection which allows for reactivation and recurrence of disease. Primary reservoir of EBV in body is latently infected B cells. Two genotypes of EBV, i.e. EBV-1 and EBV-2, were identified. Immunological effects of infected B cells are responsible for EBV associated disease manifestations. Detecting humoral antibodies against viral capsid [anti-viral capsid antigens (VCA)] and nuclear proteins [anti-Epstein-Barr nuclear antigens (EBNA)] establishes the diagnosis of acute infection while cellular immunity is important for effective control of EBV infection. During IM, there is generalized impairment in cell mediated and humoral immunity in spite of brisk immunological response to EBV. Sequential infection of oral epithelial cells, salivary gland, B lymphocytes and lymphoreticular system is seen after transmission of virus through saliva. The atypical lymphocytes are CD8+ T lymphocytes. The latent virus resides in oropharyngeal epithelial cells and memory B lymphocytes. Reactivation of EBV is asymptomatic.

More than 90% cases of IM are caused by EBV, while remaining 10% IM like illness are due to primary infection by cytomegalovirus, *Toxoplasma gondii*, HIV, adenovirus, rubella and hepatitis virus.

CLINICAL FEATURES

Clinical features of classic IM develops in mostly adolescents and adults after a primary EBV infection. Primary infection in younger children is silent or may result in mild clinical features, although classical IM is described rarely in young children. Clinical features of IM are described in three phases: (1) prodromal, (2) acute and (3) resolution.

Prodromal Phase

It lasts for around 1 week and like any other viral disease is accompanied by malaise, fatigue, fever, headache, myalgia and nausea.

Acute Phase

It consists of classical features of IM like fever, fatigue, sore throat, rashes, tonsillopharyngitis, hepatosplenomegaly and lymphadenopathy and lasts for 3–4 weeks. Fever begins abruptly, ranges between 38°C and 40°C, lasting usually for 2 weeks and rarely up to a month. Tonsillopharyngitis develops in 1st week of illness, resolves spontaneously in the second, usually symptomatic and consists of exudative inflammation similar to one seen in streptococcal infection. Although *Streptococcus pyogenes* is seen in 5% of cases of IM in pharynx, it represents carriage rather than concomitant streptococcal tonsillopharyngitis. Maculopapular rashes are seen in 3–15% of cases. Vasculitic, immune mediated, maculopapular, pruritic rashes are seen in 95–100% of adolescents treated with ampicillin or amoxicillin. These rashes develop 5–10 days after initiation of treatment and resolve spontaneously within few days once the offending drug is discontinued. Such "ampicillin rash" is less common in children with IM. Gianotti-Crosti syndrome (papular acrodermatitis of childhood) consisting of symmetric erythematous papules developing into plaques, involving cheeks, extremities and buttocks and lasting for 15–50 days is sometimes seen with primary EBV infection. Hepatosplenomegaly is seen in almost half of the patients, more common in younger children, develops in 2nd week and resolves by 4th week. Lymphadenopathy, commonly involving cervical lymph nodes (and sometimes generalized lymphadenopathy), is seen in almost 90% cases of IM and like hepatosplenomegaly most prominent from 2nd to 4th week of illness. Palatal enanthem and eyelid edema are sometimes seen in children with IM.

Resolution Phase

Gradual and uneventful resolution of all clinical features usually occurs although sometimes biphasic course is seen. Organomegaly and severe fatigue may take months to resolve.

DIAGNOSIS

Leukocytosis, absolute lymphocytosis and atypical lymphocytes (bigger lymphocytes with large, indented, folded and eccentrically placed nucleus) are common findings. Atypical lymphocytes are also seen with other infectious agents enumerated above leading to IM like illness. Thrombocytopenia and elevated hepatic enzymes are also commonly observed. For a typical uncomplicated case of IM, blood counts and heterophile antibody test are sufficient for presumptive diagnosis. Diagnosis can be confirmed further by specific EBV antibodies in cases which lack positive heterophile antibodies have atypical or severe manifestations of IM, develop chronic, lymphoproliferative or oncogenic features or in cases where one needs to confirm past-infection or determine susceptibility to future infection.

Heterophile Antibody Test

These antibodies agglutinate cells from different species. These IgM antibodies are known as Paul-Bunnell antibodies and are detected by Paul-Bunnell-Davidson test. These antibodies agglutinate sheep or horse RBCs but not guinea pig kidney cells. This test may be negative early in the course of disease and in children less than 4 years of age.

Specific EBV Antibodies

Antibodies to EBNA, Epstein-Barr virus early antigens (EBVEA) and VCA are specific EBV antibodies used for diagnosing EBV infections. Acute IM is characterized by immunoglobulin M (IgM) and immunoglobulin G (IgG) VCA and IgG EA. Anti-EBNA antibodies appear 3–4 months after the onset of infection, hence its presence indicates infection more than 3 months old and its absence (in presence of other antibodies) implies recent infection. IgM VCA is the most dependable antibody to confirm the diagnosis, although rheumatoid factor may give false- positive results.

Detection of EBV DNA by southern blot, in situ hybridization and PCR may be useful for diagnostic, epidemiological and pathogenetic purposes. Isolation of virus from body secretions and semiquantitative and quantitative viral load assay are available for research purposes.

DIFFERENTIAL DIAGNOSIS

- *Infectious mononucleosis like illnesses:* Heterophile negative IM is caused by various agents like CMV, toxoplasma, adenovirus, rubella virus and hepatitis virus.
- *Acute HIV syndrome:* This IM like syndrome is usually seen in adolescents at the time of initial burst of viremia, about 3–6 weeks after primary infection. It is of varying severity, most of the patients recovering spontaneously and followed by prolonged clinical latency.
- *Streptococcal pharyngitis:* Presence of hepatospleno-megaly and failure to respond in 3 days to appropriate antibiotics favors IM.
- *Leukemia:* Bone marrow examination may be necessary to differentiate from IM.
- *Scarlet fever:* Diffuse erythema, strawberry tongue, sandpaper feel and response to antistreptococcal antibodies favors the diagnosis of scarlet fever.
- *Rickettsial infections:* Evolving rash (from macular to popular to hemorrhagic), normal to low TLC, exposure to ticks and response to doxycycline are suggestive of Rickettsial infection.
- *Systemic onset juvenile idiopathic arthritis (SOJIA):* In absence of joint infection, SOJIA may be confused with IM. Evanescent rash at the height of fever, daily two spikes of fever, temperature dipping below baseline and thrombocytosis are in favor of SOJIA.

TREATMENT

Symptomatic treatment with rest, fluids and antipyretics is the mainstay of therapy as there is no specific treatment for IM. Although high doses of acyclovir reduced viral replication and oropharyngeal shedding, this therapy is of no use for resolution of signs and symptoms or reducing the rates of complications. Bed rest is important till there is debilitating fatigue. Avoiding contact sports and strenuous athletic activities in first 2–3 weeks of illness and till there is palpable spleen is of utmost importance in view of predisposition to splenic rupture. Imaging studies, like USG and CT abdomen, are neither accurate nor cost effective for predicting return to normal physical activities. A 2-week course of prednisone (1 mg/kg/day or equivalent for 1 week, followed by tapering doses over next 1 week) may be advocated with caution to some severely symptomatic patients (having high fever or severe pharyngitis). Corticosteroids are also used for complications of IM like stridor from massively enlarged tonsils or paratracheal lymphadenopathy, hematological complications like thrombocytopenia with bleeding or hemolytic anemia, neurologic complications like seizures or meningitis. Corticosteroids should not be used in uncomplicated cases of IM.

COMPLICATIONS

Most complications of IM are rare and transient. Significant hematologic, neurologic and pulmonary complications are seen in approximately 20% of IM cases.

- *Splenic subcapsular hemorrhage and rupture*: It occurs during 1st to 3rd week of illness and related to physical trauma to palpably enlarged spleen. Clinical features of splenic rupture are abdominal pain, orthostatic hypotension, syncope, tachycardia and left shoulder pain. Apart from a small subset of patients who are hemodynamically stable having low transfusion requirements and with normal sensorium which may be managed by medical therapy or endovascular intervention, most need emergency splenectomy.

- *Respiratory complications like airway obstruction, neck abscesses or pulmonary infiltrates*: Incidence of severe airway obstruction is 1–5% and can be due to enlargement of Waldeyer ring, edema of epiglottis or pharynx, pseudomembrane formation in airways or paratracheal lymphadenopathy. Drooling, stridor, dysphagia, odynophagia and dyspnea are the common manifestations. Various management options include head elevation, hydration, humidification, systemic corticosteroids, nasopharyngeal airway, tonsillectomy and tracheostomy.

- *Neurologic complications* are seen in 1–5% of patients with IM, mostly at the height of typical manifestations of IM. Various neurologic complications are aseptic meningitis, meningoencephalitis, cerebritis, cranial nerve palsies, Guillain-Barré syndrome and transverse myelitis. In view of nonspecific symptomatology and absence of typical IM symptoms, EBV should be considered a possible etiology for any child presenting with acute encephalitis.

- *Psychiatric complications* like Alice-in-Wonderland syndrome and chronic fatigue are described with IM. Alice-in-Wonderland syndrome or metamorphopsia is a visual illusion manifesting as a distortion in size, form, movement or color. This syndrome is also known to occur with migraine, epilepsy and hallucinogenic drugs apart from IM. It resolves in 4–6 weeks.

- *Hematologic complications* like thrombocytopenia, aplastic anemia, hemolytic anemia and neutropenia are described with IM. Immune-mediated thrombocytopenia is seen in 25–50% patients and resolves in 4–6 weeks. Corticosteroids and intravenous immunoglobulin (IVIg) are sometimes beneficial in severe, life-threatening cases.

- *Other complications* like hepatic failure, tubulointerstitial nephritis, nephritic syndrome, Reye syndrome and electrocardiographic abnormalities are occasionally seen.

PROGNOSIS

Complete recovery is almost a rule for healthy individuals with IM, although symptoms usually persist for 2–4 weeks before gradual recovery. Immunocompromised persons can have infection with different types of EBV but these episodes are always asymptomatic. Prolonged fatigue and malaise may last for few weeks to 6 months. Mortality in IM is extremely rare and usually attributed to splenic rupture, Guillain-Barré syndrome, secondary infection or massive bleeding.

PREVENTION

Standard infection control policies are recommended for hospitalized patients with IM. As EBV is spread in saliva and ubiquitous in occurrence, it is quite difficult to prevent the infection. Three doses of recombinant EBV subunit glycoprotein 350 candidate vaccine may be useful for prevention or reducing symptoms of IM.

BIBLIOGRAPHY

1. Jenson HB. Epstein-Barr virus. In: Kliegman RM, Stanton BF, Schor NF, Geme JWS, Behrman RE (Eds). Nelson Textbook of Pediatrics, 19th edition. Elsevier Saunders; 2011. pp. 1110-5.

2. Leach CL, Sumaya CV. Epstein-Barr virus. In: Feigin RD, Cherry JD, Demmler Harrison GJ, Kaplan SL (Eds). Textbook of Pediatric Infectious Diseases, 6th edition. Saunders Elsevier; 2009. pp. 2043-71.

3. Mishra B, Mohan B, Ratho RK. Heterophile antibody positive infectious mononucleosis. Ind Jour Ped. 2004;71:15-8.

5.16 | HIV/AIDS IN CHILDREN

Ira Shah

EPIDEMIOLOGY

In 2013 alone, the World Health Organization (WHO) estimated that 240,000 new HIV infections occurred among children less than 15 years old, and 190,000 children died of AIDS-related illnesses. Maximum cases of newly diagnosed HIV infection in children is reported from South East Asia and Africa while countries-like USA and western European countries report less than 1% of newly infected HIV positive children.

Antiretroviral therapy (ART) coverage among children in India is 29% whereby it is estimated that about 54100 children are on ART. However, ART coverage in children in both the American content is about 51% whereas in Europe it is estimated to be about 95%. Coverage in Africa stands at 22% though 630,300 children in Africa are on treatment.

TRANSMISSION AND PATHOGENESIS OF HIV

There are two main types of HIV: (1) type 1; and (2) type 2. There are geographic distributions of various subtypes of HIV-1 across the Globe. Within the predominantly gay male epidemic in North America and Europe, the virus is of subtype B. By contrast in sub-Saharan Africa predominant viruses are subtypes A, C, D, F and G. In India, the most common HIV-1 subtype circulating is subtype C. HIV-1 is more virulent, more infective. By contrast, HIV-2 has more limited variation and is less pathogenic than HIV-1 in humans and infection is limited to West Africa. Thus, our discussion in this chapter is limited to HIV-1 infection.

Human immunodeficiency virus transmission usually occurs through the mucosa of the lower genital tract or rectum in adults, and through the placenta or gastrointestinal tract in infants. Both free and cell-associated virions can enter mucosal tissue, where they encounter CD4+ T cells, which may be productively infected, or langerhans and dendritic cells, which can internalize HIV and transmit the virus to CD4+ T cells. Either way, reproduction of HIV in mucosal CD4+CCR5+ cells (memory T cells) occurs soon after infection, and rapidly spreads to local and distant mucosal sites.

Following entry of the HIV virus into the human cell, viral genome is released in the cellular cytoplasm, conversion of viral RNA to viral DNA occurs which is undertaken by the viral enzyme, reverse transcriptase (RT). RT is not very efficient, and errors in production of a true complementary gene base from parental viral RNA leading to mutations in the viral DNA. The single strand complementary cDNA is made into double stranded DNA by the viral polymerase and enters the cell nucleus for integration into the host cell genome. This is done by the integrase enzyme. Transcription of viral DNA to messenger RNA and genomic RNA is undertaken by host cell RNA polymerases. This is another source of potential variation in the resulting viral genome. A large polyprotein, comprising the gag and pol genes, is produced which is specifically cut by the viral protease enzyme. The protease enzyme recognizes specific cleavage sites and produces the correct proportion of the different resulting proteins, which include the capsid, matrix proteins and RT which is packaged within the virion for use when the virus enters the next infected cell. The virus then buds out of the cell.

Chronic immune activation is likely to account for much of the non-AIDS morbidity and mortality that occurs in HIV-infected individuals, because people live with a state of chronic inflammation, which has multiple effects on the body.

PERINATAL TRANSMISSION OF HIV

Human immunodeficiency virus can be transmitted vertically through the placenta (intrauterine transmission), exposure to vaginal fluids at the time of labor (intrapartum transmission) and through breast milk (breast-feeding—postpartum transmission). Pooled data from various cohort studies conducted prior to preventive interventions estimated the risk of *in utero* transmission to be approximately 10%, the risk of intrapartum transmission, i.e. during labor and delivery, to be approximately 15%, and the risk of postpartum transmission to be between 10% and 15%, depending on the duration of breast-feeding. Factors associated with rapid progression of HIV disease in vertically transmitted infants are:

- More advanced maternal disease is associated with more rapid infant progression
- *In utero* infected infants progress more rapidly than intrapartum-infected infants, which may relate to immaturity of the immune system
- High viral inoculum is related to rapid progression of the disease.

CLINICAL MANIFESTATIONS OF HIV

Infants

Among the early manifestations of HIV in children reported are HIV encephalopathy and opportunistic infections (OIs) especially with *Pneumocystis jiroveci* (PCP), cytomegalovirus (CMV), respiratory viruses and bacterial pneumonia. Recurrent gastrointestinal infections and oral thrush are commonly found. Lymphadenopathy, splenomegaly and hepatomegaly often are seen in the 1st year of life. The pathogenesis of these organ enlargements is not well understood, but relates to HIV activity and immune response. Effective treatment of the HIV leads to rapid reduction in organ size, usually to normal. Up to 10% of infants presenting with HIV have severe developmental delay and encephalopathy. Few infants (15–25% infected newborns in developed countries) may develop AIDS within the first few months of life and, if left untreated, they have a median survival time of 6–9 months. They are known as rapid progressors. Opportunistic infections (OIs) and neurological complications are features seen more commonly in this group. These are the children that are infected intrauterine with most of them showing positive HIV-1 culture and/or detectable viral load (VL) (median level 11,000 copies/mL) in blood in the first 48 hour of life. Between 5 and 15% of HIV-infected individuals do not experience clinical or immunological progression despite a long duration of infection in the absence of antiretroviral therapy (ART). They are known as long-term non-progressors. They maintain good CD4 counts and tend to have low VLs.

Children

Growth failure, fever, diarrhea and secondary infections are seen beyond infancy. Many children who present with HIV may have had mild symptoms for many years. They may present with recurrent ear infections with sinusitis, chronic parotitis, chronic otitis media, nail fungal infections and molluscum contagiosum. Hepatosplenomegaly and lymphadenopathy persist.

Older Children

Older children have growth failure, delayed puberty and subtle cognitive dysfunction. Systemic manifestations, such as HIV cardiomyopathy, idiopathic thrombocytopenic purpura (ITP), are seen in older children and adolescents.

End-stage HIV Disease

When the immune system has been exhausted by HIV replication, and the CD4 count is very low, then the individual becomes susceptible to all the severe and well-known OI. At this stage of disease, poor appetite, weight loss and wasting are common. Recurrent fevers, chronic diarrhea and bone marrow failure may be seen.

WORLD HEALTH ORGANIZATION STAGING SYSTEM FOR HIV IN CHILDREN

In 1986, World Health Organization (WHO) developed a provisional clinical AIDS case definition for adults and children to report AIDS cases in resource-constrained settings. In 2006, WHO revised the clinical staging in children less than 15 years of age. The clinical stage is useful for assessment at baseline (first diagnosis of HIV infection) or entry into long-term HIV care and in the follow-up of patients along with decision when to start cotrimoxazole prophylaxis and when to start ART. Table 5.16.1 and Box 5.16.1 depict the WHO staging system of HIV infection.

Table 5.16.1: WHO clinical staging of established HIV infection.

HIV-associated symptoms	WHO clinical stage
Asymptomatic	1
Mild symptoms	2
Advanced symptoms	3
Severe symptoms	4

Box 5.16.1

WHO clinical staging of HIV/AIDS for children with confirmed HIV infection.

Clinical Stage 1
- Asymptomatic
- Persistent generalized lymphadenopathy

Clinical Stage 2
- Unexplained persistent hepatosplenomegaly
- Papular pruritic eruptions
- Fungal nail infection
- Angular cheilitis
- Lineal gingival erythema
- Extensive wart virus infection
- Extensive molluscum contagiosum
- Recurrent oral ulcerations
- Unexplained persistent parotid enlargement
- Herpes zoster
- Recurrent or chronic upper respiratory tract infections (otitis media, otorrhea, sinusitis or tonsillitis)

Clinical Stage 3
- Unexplained moderate malnutrition or wasting not adequately responding to standard therapy
- Unexplained persistent diarrhea (14 days or more)
- Unexplained persistent fever (above 37.5°C intermittent or constant, for longer than 1 month)
- Persistent oral candidiasis (after first 6–8 weeks of life)
- Oral hairy leukoplakia
- Acute necrotizing ulcerative gingivitis or periodontitis
- Lymph node tuberculosis
- Pulmonary tuberculosis
- Severe recurrent bacterial pneumonia
- Symptomatic lymphoid interstitial pneumonitis
- Chronic HIV-associated lung disease including bronchiectasis
- Unexplained anemia (<8 g/dL), neutropenia (<0.5 × 10⁹ per liter) and or chronic thrombocytopenia (<50 × 10⁹ per liter)

Clinical Stage 4
- Unexplained severe wasting, stunting or severe malnutrition not responding to standard therapy
- Pneumocystis pneumonia
- Recurrent severe presumed bacterial infections (e.g. empyema, pyomyositis, bone or joint infection, meningitis, but excluding pneumonia)
- Chronic herpes simplex infection (orolabial or cutaneous of more than 1 month's duration or visceral at any site)
- Extrapulmonary tuberculosis
- Kaposi sarcoma

Contd...

Contd...

> *Esophageal candidiasis (or candida of trachea, bronchi or lungs)*
> - Central nervous system toxoplasmosis (outside the neonatal period)
> - HIV encephalopathy
> - Cytomegalovirus infection; retinitis or CMV infection affecting another organ, with onset at age over 1 month
> - Extrapulmonary cryptococcosis including meningitis
> - Disseminated endemic mycosis (extrapulmonary histoplasmosis, coccidioidomycosis, penicilliosis)
> - Chronic cryptosporidiosis
> - Chronic isosporiasis
> - Disseminated non-tuberculous mycobacteria infection
> - Acquired HIV-associated rectal fistula
> - Cerebral or B cell non-Hodgkin lymphoma
> - Progressive multifocal leukoencephalopathy
> - Symptomatic HIV-associated nephropathy or HIV-associated cardiomyopathy

DIAGNOSIS OF HIV

Diagnosis of HIV in Infants

All infants born to HIV-infected mothers carry maternal immunoglobulin G (IgG) antibodies which cross the placenta freely. These maternal antibodies may remain detectable in the infant's serum for up to 12–15 months after birth. As a result, serological diagnosis of HIV infection is only reliable after 15–18 months of age. Infants infected with HIV must be diagnosed as rapidly as possible to ensure the early institution of therapy to limit HIV-related morbidity and to prevent OI. Tests that can be done for diagnosis of HIV infection in children below 18 months of age are HIV culture, detection of HIV proviral DNA by polymerase chain reaction (PCR) or HIV antigen (p24). Detection of p24 antigen is cheaper, highly specific and easy to perform but it is less sensitive than other virologic tests. Also false negativity is high in younger children as most of the p24 antigen is bound to maternal antibodies. Polymerase chain reaction (PCR) is now the preferred tool for diagnosis of HIV in infants.

Human Immunodeficiency Virus Culture

Human immunodeficiency virus (HIV) culture is done from peripheral blood mononuclear cells (PBMCs) but is technically difficult and time consuming. It is expensive and done in research institutes. Positive results are available by 1–2 weeks but negative results are not reported till there is no evidence of HIV replication for 30 days. Sensitivity for detecting infection has been reported to be 50% at birth and 90% by 3 months of HIV. However, a single test is not conclusive of the diagnosis and should be confirmed by a repeat test or PCR test.

Polymerase Chain Reaction

Human immunodeficiency virus PCRs are of two types: (1) qualitative PCR and (2) quantitative. HIV DNA PCR has been found to be highly sensitive and specific for early diagnosis of pediatric HIV infection. Sensitivity of HIV PCR is less at birth and sensitivity increases rapidly to 95% at 4 weeks and to 99% at 6 months of age. Infants who have HIV DNA PCR positive during the first days of life are conventionally assumed to have been infected during pregnancy (in utero). Infants who test HIV negative in the first days of life but later are found to be positive are presumed to have been infected during labor and delivery (intrapartum) or through breastfeeding (postpartum). Thus, in nonbreastfed infants, HIV PCR can be done at 4–6 weeks after birth. In breastfeeding populations, HIV PCR should be done after 1 or 2 months after cessation of breastfeeding. HIV PCR can be done on dried blood sample transported to a laboratory on a filter paper or on whole blood. However, false positive and false negative results with HIV DNA PCR may occur. Repeating the PCR on independent samples may be required to reduce the test errors.

Diagnosis of HIV in Children above 18 Months of Age

Enzyme-linked immunosorbent assay (ELISA) is the time-tested reliable method for detection of anti-HIV antibodies with a sensitivity of more than 99.5% and specificity of 99%. However, a positive ELISA tests should be confirmed with a Western blot test or a repeat HIV ELISA test by a different kit. In Western Blot test, different viral antigens are separated using protein electrophoresis and antibodies are detected against individual antigens. It is considered positive if at least 2 out of 3 bands (p24, gp41, gp120/160) are positive. This reduces the chance of false positivity and false negativity. Western blot test is very expensive and in a resource limited setting like in our country, confirmation of positive HIV status can be done by 2 or 3 ELISA tests using different kits on the same sample.

MONITORING OF HIV DISEASE PROGRESSION IN CHILDREN

Immunological changes in HIV-1 infection include a decrease in CD4+ cells, a transient increase in CD8+ cells, total lymphocytes and inversion of the CD4/CD8 ratio. As HIV infection progresses, the CD4+ cells decline, while the CD8+ cells which may remain at high levels for long periods, eventually decrease but not to baseline levels. Plasma HIV-1 VL, CD4+ cell count and CD4 percentage are used to predict the clinical course and response to therapy in HIV infected adults and children. Guidelines issued by various organizations provide recommendations on the basis of CD4 count (or CD4 percentage which in children is found to be more accurate) and some also consider the criteria of VL.

CD4 Count Estimation

CD4 count is routinely measured in children with HIV-1 infection and used to evaluate the need of initiation of therapy and to monitor clinical progression. Assessment of the CD4 count in any child must be in relation to the appropriate count for age. For children above 5 years of age, absolute CD4+ counts are used in preference to percentages, and the levels are aligned with adult/adolescent cut-offs. The substantial intra-individual and inter-individual variation in absolute CD4 counts in young children led to the adoption of CD4 percentages as the preferred method of monitoring in pediatric practice. Box 5.16.1 depicts the WHO immunological classification for established HIV infection.

HIV and Viral Load

Perinatally infected infants acquire HIV before the immune system is fully matured and progress more rapidly to disease than older children or adults. Acute HIV infection in adults is characterized by high viremia, which rapidly declines as anti-HIV cytotoxic immunity emerge. In contrast, perinatally infected infants do not show the same dramatic fall in viremia, and HIV VLs only start to decline beyond infancy to reach an "adult" set point by approximately 5 years of age. The HIV plasma VL is predictive of mortality in older children. The relative risk of death is 2.1 times greater, if the presenting HIV RNA was more than 100,000 copies/mL.

Resistance testing: Development of drug resistance in HIV infected children with treatment failure is a major impediment to selection of appropriate therapy. Studies done on Indian population indicate that prevalence of HIV resistance mutations is around 9.6% in treatment naïve population and up to 81–96% in treatment experienced patients with virological failure. The pediatric population in particular is not only at a higher risk of developing resistance (due to greater viral loads and difficulty in adherence and accurate dosing), but resistance proves a greater challenge as they require longer term therapy than adults. There are two types of resistance testing available predominantly.

1. **Genotype tests:** They detect specific genetic mutations. They are based on amplification procedures and can detect mutations in plasma samples with more than 1000 copies/mL of HIV RNA. This involves the nucleotide sequencing of the relevant HIV genes, from which an amino acid sequence of the reverse transcriptase and protease enzymes is predicted. Genotypic testing is cheaper and more widely available compared to phenotypic testing.
2. **Phenotype tests:** Phenotypic assays measure the IC50 of the drug against the virus in vitro. Although, the sensitivity patterns of the virus tested can be determined, it may not detect minor species of resistant viruses.

In patients with HIV, genotypic resistance testing is preferred. Resistance testing should be performed by laboratories that have appropriate operator training, certification and proficiency assurance. Drugs for which

the virus requires only one mutation to develop high level resistance (such as Lamivudine and Nevirapine) will in fact generate very rapid resistance when used as monotherapy. For other drugs such as zidovudine (AZT), abacavir (ABC), tenofovir (TDF) and most PIs, high-grade resistance requires the serial accumulation of multiple mutations and is thus slower to emerge. Other drugs such as didanosine (ddI) and stavudine (d4T) are associated only with low level of resistance as measured in phenotypic assays predicting decreased efficacy.

Resistance testing is usually not required at the time of starting ART. It is recommended at the time of treatment failure when a switch in ART is planned. In virologically suppressed patients who are switching therapy because of toxicity or for convenience, viral amplification will not be possible and thus, resistance testing should not be done. Resistance testing is usually not recommended after 4–6 weeks after stopping the drug as drug resistant viruses usually constitute less than 10–20% of the circulating virus population and on stopping the drug, a wild type virus often re-emerges as the predominant population and resistance testing will not show the resistant mutations. Thus resistance testing is of greatest value when done before or within 4 weeks after drugs were discontinued.

ANTIRETROVIRAL THERAPY

Antiretroviral Drugs

Antiretrovirals are a group of drugs that are used in the treatment of HIV infected individuals to decrease the viral burden. They are potent inhibitors of viral replication. These drugs fall into 3 major classes—nucleoside reverse transcriptase inhibitors (NRTIs), non-nucleoside reverse transcriptase inhibitors (NNRTIs) and protease inhibitors (PIs). There are 3 new classes of drugs now approved for treatment of HIV in children. They are the entry inhibitors, integrase strand transfer inhibitors (INSTIs) and the CCR5 co-receptor antagonists.

Nucleoside Reverse Transcriptase Inhibitors (NRTIs)

The NRTIs were the first class of antiretroviral drugs that became available for treatment of HIV. They inhibit the reverse transcriptase enzyme (*See* the Chapter on Transmission and Pathogenesis). They have activity against both HIV-1 and HIV-2. The parent compounds need to undergo intracellular phosphorylation to become active against HIV. NRTIs act by competing with normal nucleoside triphosphates for incorporation into the growing proviral DNA chain. The abnormal nucleoside prevents the addition of further nucleosides to the chain, and viral replication ceases. Dual NRTI is the backbone of current combination of various antiretroviral therapies.

Drugs in this class include:
- Zidovudine (AZT/ZDV)
- Lamivudine (3TC)
- Stavudine (d4T)
- Didanosine (ddI)
- Abacavir (ABC)
- Emtricitabine (FTC)
- Tenofovir (TDF) – It is a nucleotide reverse transcriptase inhibitor (NtRTI). It affects the bone mineral density thus potentially limiting its use in pre-pubertal children. It also acts against Hepatitis B.

The drugs stavudine and didanosine are gradually being phased out from use in children due to their toxicity profile.

Non-nucleoside Reverse Transcriptase Inhibitors (NNRTIs)

NNRTIs were the second class of anti-HIV agents to be developed. The parent compounds are the active moieties, and are therefore immediately active on entering the cell. They inhibit HIV-1 reverse transcriptase by binding to a hydrophobic pocket on the enzyme close to the active site, thereby locking the enzyme in an inactive conformation. The NNRTI class of drugs rapidly reduce viral load; however drug resistance develops quickly after initiation of monotherapy and cross-resistance between drugs in this class is common. There are currently 3 NNRTIs used for treatment of HIV infection.
- Nevirapine (NVP)
- Efavirenz (EFV)
- Etravirine: Used in children >6 years of age and is considered a 'second generation' NNRTI, in part because it retains activity against HIV-1 isolates which are resistant to other NNRTIs.
- Rilpivirine (only approved for use in adults).

Protease Inhibitors (PIs)

The PIs inhibit the protease enzyme (See chapter on Transmission and Pathogenesis) by binding to the active site of the enzyme, thus preventing cleavage of precursor polyproteins at a late stage of viral replication. Virions are produced, but they are incomplete and non-infectious. PIs were the third class of ARVs to be developed. They are highly potent. They are active against both HIV-1 and HIV-2. PIs have a high genetic barrier to resistance, and PI resistance at regimen failure is uncommon.

The various PIs used for treatment of HIV infection are:
- Nelfinavir (NFV)
- Ritonavir (RTV)
- Lopinavir/Ritonavir (LPVr)
- Amprenavir
- Indinavir (IDV)
- Saquinavir (SQV)
- Atazanavir/Ritonavir (ATZr)
- Darunavir
- Tipranavir.

Boosted PIs: Low-dose ritonavir (RTV), itself a potent PI acts as a potent inhibitor of the cytochrome P450 3A4 (CYP3A4) isoenzyme, thereby inhibiting the metabolism of other PIs, and has been used in low doses combined with another PI as a "pharmacokinetic booster," increasing drug exposure by prolonging the second drug's half-life. Boosted PI-based regimens are commonly used in treatment of adults, but adequate pediatric data are only available for co-formulated lopinavir/ritonavir in children older than 6 weeks of age and for atazanavir, fosamprenavir, darunavir, and tipranavir with low-dose ritonavir in children age >6 years.

New Classes of Antiretroviral Drugs

Entry Inhibitors

These agents inhibit viral binding or fusion to host target cells. T-20 (Enfurvirtide) is the drug currently used and has to be given subcutaneously twice daily and is to be used only in children >6 years of age. It is a 36 amino acid peptide that binds to a region of the gp41 glycoprotein on the HIV cell surface and prevents virus-cell fusion. It is used as part of salvage regime in patients who have multi-antiretroviral therapy regime failures.

CCR5 Co-receptor Antagonist

Maraviroc blocks the chemokine CCR5 coreceptor on the CD4 cell surface (*See* Transmission and Pathogenesis Chapter) thereby preventing HIV from entering the cell. This was the first antiretroviral drug to be developed that does not actually target the virus itself. Maraviroc is effective as part of combination therapy in patients with multi-drug-resistant HIV-1. Before starting treatment with this drug, however, it is necessary to check for CCR5 or CXCR4 virus tropism. CCR5 antagonists will be inactive against CXCR4-tropic virus. Maraviroc is not yet routinely used in young children, but may be used in adolescents. There are considerable interactions with both PI and NNRTI classes, requiring alteration in maraviroc dosing depending on other drugs in the regimen.

Integrase Strand Transfer Inhibitors (INSTIs)

They block the integrase enzyme (*See* Chapter on Transmission and Pathogenesis) thereby preventing incorporation of viral DNA into human genome. Raltegravir, dolutegravir and elvitegravir are integrase strand-transfer inhibitors (INSTIs). These drugs have been found to be useful in the treatment of patients with multi-drug-resistant HIV-1. Raltegravir is FDA-approved for treatment of HIV-infected children aged ≥4 weeks and weighing ≥3 kg. Raltegravir has a favorable safety profile and lacks significant drug interactions. At this time, there are little data on raltegravir use as initial therapy in HIV-infected infants and children. Dolutegravir has recently been approved by the FDA for use in children aged ≥12 years and weighing ≥40 kg. The drug has a very favorable safety profile and can be dosed once daily in treatment of INSTI-naïve patients.

Cobicistat: It is in adolescents and adults used as a pharmacokinetic enhancer (boosting agent) of selected protease inhibitors (PIs) and the integrase inhibitor elvitegravir. Cobicistat is not interchangeable with ritonavir. It is not used in children less than 18 years of age.

Goals of Pediatric Antiretroviral

The aims of treatment with ARV drugs in HIV-infected children are to achieve and sustain full HIV RNA VL suppression and minimize short-term and long-term ARV drug toxicity. Sustained VL suppression should prevent the evolution of viral drug resistance and allow normal immune function, which in turn should prevent OIs, HIV encephalopathy, malignancy and progression of HIV disease, and allow normal growth and development.

Duration of Antiretroviral

Human immunodeficiency virus infection cannot be eradicated by the ARV drugs that are currently available. Proviral DNA persists in sanctuary sites such as the CNS and testis, while continued production of drug-sensitive virus has been demonstrated in children on highly active antiretroviral therapy (HAART) with plasma levels of HIV RNA below the limit of detection of current clinical assays (<50 copies/mL). Consequently, VL increases to pre-treatment levels within 1–2 weeks of stopping therapy, making lifelong treatment necessary. Also error-prone RT enzyme leads to mutations in the virus that prevents its eradication.

When to Start Antiretroviral Therapy

Decisions about when to start therapy, what drugs to choose in ARV-naïve children and how to treat ARV experienced children remain complex, and should be made in consultation with a specialist in pediatric and adolescent HIV infection. Treatment with ART depends on clinical condition, immune status of the child and HIV VL. Antiretroviral (ARV) drug-resistant virus can develop in both multidrug experienced children, and children who received initial regimens containing one or two drugs that incompletely suppressed viral replication. Additionally, drug resistance may be seen in ARV-naïve children who have become infected with HIV despite maternal/infant ARV prophylaxis. Thus, decisions about when to start therapy and what drugs to choose in ARV-naïve children

and on how to best treat ARV-experienced children remain complex.

Although implementing ART is complex, a number of guidelines are available to help practitioners to select effective regimens for particular patients. The decision to start ART depends on clinical, immunological and socioeconomic conditions. There are US guidelines, Penta guidelines, World Health Organization (WHO) guidelines and National AIDS Control Organization (NACO) guidelines that help in determining treatment protocols. There guidelines are regularly updated as and when newer research on treatment protocols and newer ARVs are available. The clinician treating HIV infected children should thus be aware of the latest treatment guideline. Table 5.16.2 depicts the WHO 2015 guidelines for starting ART. Before ART is started, it is essential that parents, caregivers and patients are counseled regarding the importance of adherence to the prescribed treatment regimen. The goal of therapy should ensure normal growth and development, avoiding OIs and organ dysfunctions due to HIV and maintaining as healthy and normal life style as possible. ART is never an emergency, and potential problems should be identified and resolved prior to starting therapy.

Prior to starting ART in HIV positive children, certain factors have to be considered:
- Children unlike adults usually acquire the infection through perinatal exposure
- HIV infection in children progresses rapidly and most affected children die by 4–6 years
- Children may have already been exposed to ARVs such as AZT and NVP as part of parent-to-child transmission prevention program

Table 5.16.2: WHO guidelines on when to start ART among people living with HIV (September 2015).

Adults	ART should be initiated in all adults living with HIV at any CD4 cell count
	As a priority, ART should be initiated in all adults with severe or advanced HIV clinical disease (WHO clinical stage 3 or 4) and individuals with CD4 count ≤350 cells/mm3
Adolescents (10–19 years old)	ART should be initiated in all adolescents living with HIV at any CD4 cell count
	As a priority, ART should be initiated in all adolescents with severe or advanced HIV clinical disease (WHO clinical stage 3 or 4) and individuals with CD4 count ≤350 cells/mm³
Children (1 to <10 years old)	ART should be initiated in all children 1 to <10 years old living with HIV at any CD4 cell count
	As a priority, ART should be initiated among all children <2 years old and those with severe or advanced HIV clinical disease (WHO clinical stage 3 or 4) and individuals with CD4% <25% (if <5 years old) or CD4 count ≤350 cells/mm³ (if ≥5 years old)
Children (<1 year old)	ART should be initiated in all children living with HIV younger than 1 year old at any CD4 cell count

- CD4 T cell count varies as per age in children and HIV VL is higher in the 1st year of life
- Pharmacokinetic parameters of the drugs change with the age. In adolescents with early puberty (Tanner Stages I and II), pediatric doses and schedules of ART are recommended whereas in those with late puberty, adult dosing schedule is recommended
- Availability of appropriate, palatable drug formulations and adherence to ARV treatment with their complexity of schedule and long-term and short-term side effects have to be considered
- Presence of co-morbidity may affect drug choice such as tuberculosis (TB), hepatitis B or C, chronic renal disease or liver disease, e.g. co-administration of rifampicin can significantly reduce drug levels of NVP and most PIs
- Minimum of triple drug therapy is recommended and drug interactions have to be kept in mind.

Which Antiretroviral Therapy Regimens

Triple combination therapy is recommended for treating all HIV-infected children. Combination therapy slows disease progression, improves survival, results in greater and more sustained virologic and immunologic response and delays development of virus mutations which may lead to resistance. *Monotherapy or dual therapy is no longer recommended to treat HIV infection.* Aggressive treatment with at least three drugs is recommended. Dual NRTI remains the backbone of any regimen in combination with either a protease inhibitor or an NNRTI. Although integrase strand transfer inhibitors (INSTIs) or CCR5 antagonists may be considered for first-line treatment of adults, there are insufficient data to recommend these agents as preferred agents for initial therapy in children and adolescents at this time. Some clinicians advocate using 2 NRTIs with an NNRTI to preserve the PI class for later. Others would start with a PI containing regimen due to concern about early resistance to NNRTI. Thus, regimen should be selected with individual patient in mind (Table 5.16.3).

Lamivudine and abacavir are the NRTI backbone of choice for most children less than 10 years of age, based on long-term follow-up. For children above 10 years of age, tenofovir and lamivudine (or emtricitabine) is the NRTI backbone. All PIs should be ritonavir boosted.

Prior to starting ART, a detailed history of any possible previous antiretroviral therapy (ART) given to the child and mother (or other likely source of infection) should be documented. Children should be examined clinically for opportunistic infections (OIs) and complications of HIV, including assessment of growth and development. All possible OIs should be treated first ideally prior to starting ART. Baseline pre-ART investigations should include HIV RNA viral load (if possible), CD4 count and percentage, testing for other blood-borne infections (especially hepatitis B and C), hematology and biochemistry profile, as

well as HIV resistance genotype (if prior exposure to ART) and HLA B*5701 genotype prior to abacavir (ABC) therapy. Tropism assay may be required if planning to give CCR5 receptor antagonist.

One special scenario is the choice of initial therapy for children <3 years of age. The only preferred regimens for children <3 years are co-formulated lopinavir/ritonavir-based therapy and nevirapine-based therapy. Infants exposed to nevirapine in the peripartum period as part of PPTCT strategy should not be treated with nevirapine-based combination therapy because of the established higher risk of treatment failure due to nevirapine resistance, and lopinavir/ritonavir-based combination therapy would be the only recommended, preferred initial regimen.

PI-based Therapy versus NNRTI-based Therapy

Advantages of PI-based regimens include excellent virologic potency, high barrier for development of drug resistance (requires multiple mutations), and sparing of the NNRTI drug class. However, the drugs have potential for multiple drug interactions due to metabolism via hepatic enzymes and may be associated with metabolic complications such as dyslipidemia, fat maldistribution, and insulin resistance. Factors to be considered in selecting a PI-based regimen for treatment-naïve children include virologic potency, dosing frequency, pill burden, food or fluid requirements, availability of palatable pediatric formulations, drug interaction profile, toxicity profile (particularly related to metabolic complications), and availability of data in children.

Use of NNRTIs as initial therapy preserves the PI class for future use, and less dyslipidemia and fat maldistribution have been reported with the NNRTI class than with the PI class. Additionally, there is generally a lower pill burden with these agents when compared with PI-based regimens for children taking solid formulations. The major disadvantages of the current NNRTI drugs approved for use in children are that a single viral mutation can confer drug resistance, and cross resistance develops between nevirapine and efavirenz and even other NNRTIs.

TREATMENT OF HIV IN SPECIAL SITUATIONS

Infants and Children Diagnosed with TB and HIV

Concomitant rifampicin substantially decreases concentration of both NVP and PI due to induction of P450 enzyme. Plasma levels of NNRTIs are decreased by 25–35% and plasma levels of PIs are decreased by more than 80%. Thus, PIs should be avoided when a child is on rifampicin and rifabutin should be used as it does not induce the

Table 5.16.3: Preferred and alternative first-line regimens for children according to the 2013 WHO consolidated guidelines.

Age group	Preferred first-line regimens	Alternative first-line regimens Children
Children < 3 years	ABC or AZT + 3TC + LPV/r	ABC or AZT + 3TC + NVP
Children 3–9 years and adolescents <35 kg	ABC + 3TC + EFV	ABC or AZT or TDF + 3TC (or FTC) + NVP or EFV
Adolescents (10–19 years) ≥35 kg	TDF + 3TC (or FTC) + EFV	ABC or AZT or TDF + 3TC (or FTC) + NVP or EFV

Abbreviations: ABC, abacavir; AZT, zidovudine; 3TC, lamivudine; LPV/r, lopinavir-ritonavir; NVP, nevirapine; EFV, efavirenz; FTC, emtricitabine; TDF, tenofovir

P450 enzymes and thus does not alter the levels of PIs. Dose of NVP should be increased by 20–30% when used concomitant with rifampicin to maintain the drug levels in the therapeutic range. However, a watch should be kept for hepatic toxicity.

Any child with active TB disease should begin TB treatment immediately, and start ART as soon as tolerated in the first 8 weeks of TB therapy, irrespective of CD4 count and clinical stage. The preferred first-line ARV regimen for infants and children less than 3 years of age, who are taking a rifampicin-containing regimen for TB, is 2 NRTIs + NVP. The preferred first-line ARV regimen for children more than 3 years of age, who are taking a rifampicin-containing regimen for TB, is 2 NRTIs + EFV. The preferred first-line ARV regimen for infants and children less than 2 years of age, who have been exposed to NVP and are taking a rifampicin-containing regimen for TB, is a triple NRTI regimen.

Children with Anemia

For a child or adolescent with severe anemia (<7.5 g/dL) or severe neutropenia (<500 cells/mm^3), AZT should be avoided.

RESPONSE OF ANTIRETROVIRAL THERAPY

Within 1 month of starting effective ART in children, plasma HIV RNA VL decreases substantially and the CD4 count starts to rise. Infants, who frequently start from a VL of between 10^5 and 10^7 copies/mL, can take many months to become undetectable.

MONITORING A PATIENT ON ANTIRETROVIRAL THERAPY

Antiretroviral drugs have their own side effects and while a child is on ART, screening for drug toxicity and adverse effect is essential. Child also has to be monitored for clinical, immunological and virological improvement.

Once children are established on treatment, clinical and laboratory monitoring should be undertaken on every 3–4 months in the same way as before starting treatment, with the important additions of monitoring adherence and for drug toxicities and interactions. The aim of ART is to achieve an undetectable VL (<50 copies/mL plasma) and CD4 reconstitution; VL and CD4 cell count should be monitored ideally every 3 months once established on ART. Blood biochemistry, complete blood count (CBC) and urine analysis should be done on every 3–4 monthly and lipid profile should be done once in 6 months.

ADVERSE EFFECTS OF ANTIRETROVIRAL THERAPY

Antiretrovirals are potentially toxic drugs and have adverse effects. Adverse effects to the tune of 30% may be seen in patients on ART and may be a major factor for poor adherence. The common adverse effects of ARVs are depicted in Table 5.16.4.

CHANGING ANTIRETROVIRAL THERAPY

Antiretroviral therapy regimen may be changed if there is failure of current regimen or there is toxicity or intolerance to current regimen.

Treatment Failure

Poor adherence, inadequate drug levels, prior existing drug resistance or inadequate potency of the drugs chosen can all contribute to ARV treatment failure. Treatment failure is considered as either clinical failure, immunological failure or virological failure.

Clinical Failure

It is defined as recurrent, persistent or new HIV-related illness after at least 3 months on ART. Also lack or decline of growth rate, development of encephalopathy or neuroregression is taken as clinical failure. Symptoms of OIs occurring in the first 3 months of ART concurrent with a rapid rise of CD4 values is termed as immune reconstitution inflammatory syndrome (IRIS) and is not failure of ART. Pulmonary tuberculosis alone is not indicative of treatment

Table 5.16.4: Adverse effects of antiretroviral drugs.

NRTI	Hepatitis, fatty liver, lactic acidosis, pancreatitis, myopathy, peripheral neuropathy, cardiomyopathy, bone marrow suppression
NNRTI	Rash, granulocytopenia, hepatotoxicity, psychosis
PI	Hyperglycemia, lipodystrophy, hyperlipidemia, osteoporosis, diabetes, increased bleeding tendencies

Abbreviations: NRTI, nucleoside reverse transcriptase inhibitors; NNRTI, non-nucleoside reverse transcriptase inhibitors; PI, protease inhibitors

failure and thus does not necessitate change is second-line therapy.

Immunological Failure

Immunological failure is considered if there is persistently declining CD4 cell count measured on at least two separate occasions or failure to increase age-related CD4 threshold despite an adequate trial of ART or developing or returning to the following age-related immunological thresholds after at least 24 weeks on ART, in a treatment-adherent child: CD4 count of less than or equal to 200 cells/mm^3 or percentage CD4+ ≤10% for a child more than 2 years to less than 5 years of age and CD4 count of less than and equal to 100 cells/mm^3 for a child 5 years of age or more.

Virologic Failure

Virological failure is suspected when there is inability of VL to below undetectable levels within 6 months of initiating therapy. In patients with alternative regimens, stabilization of VL below previous baseline may be an appropriate goal of therapy or there is repeated detection of virus in plasma after initial suppression to undetectable levels. Ensure that increase is not due to infection, vaccination or problems with test methodology. Increase should be at least threefold from lowest VL level.

When to Switch Antiretroviral Drugs for Treatment Failure

There are no data on when to switch ART in children with detectable viremia in order to minimize the evolution of drug-resistant virus. Available drug regimens, viral resistance profiles, adherence issues and readiness of the family and child to switch; all need to be considered. Adding or substituting single drugs in a failing ART regimen without resistance testing risks giving the new drug as effective monotherapy which may result in rapid development of further resistance. It is therefore recommended that all changes in therapy with detectable viremia be preceded by a resistance test unless it is unequivocal that there is no cross-resistance with previous drugs received. Ideally resistance testing should be performed while the patient is still on the old regimen or within a few weeks of stopping. Expert opinion should be sought in interpreting resistance genotypes. The general rule is to change all the drugs in the regimen after first-line ART failure with resistance. 3TC and ABC may be switched to ZDV and ddI or in adolescents, ZDV and tenofovir, which may be preferable as cross resistance, may occur between ABC and ddI. Failure of an NNRTI-based regimen is often as a result of viral drug resistance, and switching to a boosted PI is appropriate. Any change in regimen should be preceded by a thorough reassessment of adherence, and a plan for adherence monitoring of the new regimen.

PREVENTION OF PARENT-TO-CHILD TRANSMISSION OF HIV

With effective PPTCT programs risk of vertical transmission of HIV in children can be decreased to less than 2%. HIV transmission from infected mother to child is mainly prevented by ARV drug prophylaxis to mother and baby, replacement feeding and elective cesarean section (ECS). ARV prophylaxis acts by reducing VL in the mother and as post-exposure prophylaxis to the fetus and baby. Cesarean section before onset of labor or rupture of membranes has been used as an intervention for PPTCT to decrease risk of intrapartum transmission of HIV. The goal of effective PPTCT is to ensure minimum risk of transmission of HIV from mother to child and ensuring a healthy mother and child at the end of intervention. The year 2009 was the turning point for the prevention of postnatal transmission of HIV where three randomized controlled trials found that ARV prophylaxis in pregnant women and their infants coupled with breastfeeding could lead to a significant decrease in the vertical transmission of HIV.

World Health Organization Rapid Advise for Use of antiretroviral drugs for treating pregnant women and preventing HIV infection in infants. 2013: In pregnant women with confirmed HIV serostatus, initiation of antiretroviral therapy is recommended irrespective of gestational age and continued throughout pregnancy, delivery and thereafter. Infant born to these women should receive daily nevirapine (NVP) or zidovudine (AZT) from birth until 4 to 6 weeks of age. These women can then deliver their babies vaginally and also breastfeed their babies. A once-daily fixed-dose combination of TDF + 3TC (or FTC) + EFV is recommended as first-line ART in pregnant and breastfeeding women, including pregnant women in the first trimester of pregnancy and women of childbearing age.

CONCLUSION

With ART now freely available for children, HIV infected children are living longer and well into their adolescence. Thus newer issues in management of HIV now arise namely: toxicities of ARV drugs, resistance issues and psychosocial aspects of the adolescents which need specialized care and with complex treatment regimes. Promising results in the area of PPTCT of HIV leads one to think that the era of preventing the disease in children is not too far.

BIBLIOGRAPHY

1. Antiretroviral therapy for HIV infection in infants and children: towards universal access. Recommendations for a public health approach. 2010 revision. World Health Organization.

2. Centers for Disease Control and Prevention. 1994 revised classification system for human immunodeficiency virus infection in children less than 13 years of age. MMWR. 1994;43:1-10.

3. Lyall H. Diagnosis, staging and clinical presentation of HIV in children. Clinical and laboratory diagnosis. Available from www.eurocoord.net/contact_us/trinforpedhiv_2011.aspx [Accessed October 2012].

4. Parikh S, Shah I. Short term follow up of HIV-1 infected children without treatment: use of CD4/CD8 ratio as a marker of disease progression. J Trop Pediatr. 2011;57:235-6.

5. Pillay D. Overview of HIV in children. Biology and patho-physiology of HIV infection file. Available from www.eurocoord.net/contact_us/trinforpedhiv_2011.aspx [Accessed October 2012].

6. Read JS, Newell MK. Efficacy and safety of caesarean delivery for prevention of mother-to-child transmission of HIV-1. Cochrane Database Syst Rev. 2005;4:CD005479.

7. Shah I, Dhabe H, Lala M, et al. Assessment of adherence to antiretroviral therapy in HIV infected children—a preliminary Indian study. Pedicon 2007, Mumbai, January 2007.

8. Shah I, Dhabe H, Lala M. Prevention of maternal to child transmission of HIV: a profile in Indian children. 42nd National Conference of IAP (PEDICON—2005), Kolkata, January 2005; JF/08(P).

9. Shah I, Nadiger M. Long term non-progressors (LTNP) with vertically infected HIV children—a report from India. Ind J Med Res. Accepted for publication. 14th March 2012 (Research letter).

10. Shah I, Parikh S. HIV genotype resistance testing in antiretroviral (ART) exposed Indian children—a need of the hour. Indian J Pediatr. 2012.

11. Shah I, Parikh S. Reliability of absolute lymphocyte count as marker to assess need to initiate antiretroviral therapy in HIV infected children. J Postgrad Med. 2012;58:176-9.

12. Shah I, Swaminathan S, Ramachandran G, et al. Nevirapine and efavirenz blood concentrations and effect of concomitant use of rifampicin in HIV infected children on antiretroviral therapy. Indian Pediatr. 2011;48:943-7. Accepted for publication 26 November 2010 (Ref.No. IP/2010/276).

13. Shah I. Adverse effects of antiretroviral therapy in HIV-1 infected children. J Trop Pediatr. 2006;52(4):244-8.

14. Shah I. Age related clinical manifestations of HIV infection in Indian children. J Trop Pediatr. 2005;51:300-3.

15. Shah I. Correlation of CD4 count, CD4% and HIV viral load with clinical manifestations of HIV in infected Indian children. Ann Trop Paediatr. 2006;26(2):115-9.

16. Shah I. Diagnosis of perinatal transmission of HIV-1 infection by HIV DNA PCR. JK Science. 2004;6:187-9.

17. Shah I. Efficacy of HIV PCR techniques to diagnose HIV in infants born to HIV infected mothers—an Indian perspective. J Assoc Physicians India. 2006;54:197-9.

18. Shah I. HIV and pregnancy—is vaginal delivery a safe and viable option? Indian Pediatr. 2008;45:603-4.

19. Shah I. Is elective caesarian section really essential for prevention of mother to child transmission of HIV in the era of antiretroviral therapy and abstinence of breast feeding? J Trop Pediatr. 2006;52:163-5.

20. Singh HK, Gupta A, Siberry GK, et al. The Indian pediatric HIV epidemic: a systematic review. Curr HIV Res. 2008:6:419-32.

21. The mode of delivery and the risk of vertical transmission of human immunodeficiency virus type 1—a meta analysis of 15 prospective cohort studies. The International perinatal HIV Group. N Engl J Med. 1999;340:977-87.

22. World Health Organization (WHO). Guidelines on post-exposure prophylaxis for HIV and the use of co-trimoxazole prophylaxis for HIV-related infections among adults, adolescents and children: recommendations for a public health approach. 2014. Available at URL: http://apps.who.int/iris/bitstream/10665/145719/1/9789241508193_eng.pdf?ua=1.

23. World Health Organization (WHO). Rapid advice: use of antiretroviral drugs for treating pregnant women and preventing HIV infection in infants. 2010.

24. World Health Organization. Rapid advise for use of antiretroviral drugs for treating pregnant women and preventing HIV infection in infants. 2013.

Protozoal, Parasitic and Fungal Infections

Kheya Ghosh Uttam

6.1 | MALARIA IN CHILDREN

Santanu Bhakta

HISTORY

The name "malaaria" (meaning "bad air" in Italian) was first used in English in 1740 by H Walpole when describing the disease. The term was shortened to "malaria" in the 20th century. C Laveran in 1880 was the first to identify the parasites in human blood. In 1889, R Ross discovered that mosquitoes transmit malaria. Historical records suggest malaria has infected humans since the beginning of mankind. It has played a major role in human history, having arguably caused more harm to people than any other infectious disease. Malaria, despite being preventable and treatable, threatens the lives of 3.3 billion people around the world. Every year malaria accounts for 243 million cases and 863,000 deaths, 89% of which are in sub-Saharan Africa where a child dies every 45 seconds from malaria. High maternal mortality, low-birth-weight and maternal anemia are also consequences of this devastating disease. However, it is estimated that $5–6.2 billion is required each year if the global target of reducing 75% of malaria cases by 2015 is to be reached. Annual global financial commitments to malaria control currently total $1.7 billion (WHO World Malaria Report 2009).

ETIOLOGY

Malaria is an acute and chronic illness characterized by paroxysms of fever, chills, fatigue, anemia, sweating and splenomegaly. Malaria is caused by infection of red blood cells with protozoan parasites of the genus *Plasmodium* and transmitted to humans by female Anopheles mosquitoes. Of the four common species that cause malaria, the most serious type is *Plasmodium falciparum*. It can be life-threatening. The other three common species of malaria (*P. vivax, P. malariae* and *P. ovale*) are generally less serious and are usually not life-threatening. It is possible to be infected with more than one species of *Plasmodium* at the same time. In 2004, *P. knowlesi* (a primate malaria species) was also shown to cause human malaria, documented in Malaysia, Philippines, Singapore and Indonesia. Malaria can also be transmitted through blood transfusion, use of contaminated needles and from a pregnant woman to her fetus.

EPIDEMIOLOGY

It is a major worldwide problem, occurring in more than 100 countries. Principal areas of transmission are Africa, Asia and South America. *P. falciparum* and *P. malariae* are found in most areas. *P. vivax* is predominant in India, Bangladesh, Sri Lanka, Pakistan and Central America. *P. falciparum* is mainly found in Africa, Haiti and New Guinea. *P. ovale* is the least common species and is transmitted primarily in Africa. About 1.5 million malaria cases reported annually in our country, of which nearly 50% is due to *P. falciparum* and is on the rise in recent years. The magnitude of the problem is further enhanced by *P. falciparum* resistance to standard antimalarial drugs, particularly chloroquine.

PATHOGENESIS

Plasmodium species have a complex life cycle that enables them to survive in different cellular environments in the human host (asexual phase) and the mosquito (sexual phase).

Life Cycle of *Plasmodium* Species

There is a two-step process in humans, with the 1st phase in hepatic cells (exoerythrocytic phase) and the 2nd phase in the red cells (erythrocytic phase). The exoerythrocytic phase begins with inoculation of sporozoites into the bloodstream by a female Anopheles mosquito. Within minutes, the sporozoites enter the hepatocytes of the liver, where they develop and multiply asexually as a schizont. After 1–2 weeks, the liver cells rupture and release thousands of merozoites into the circulation. The tissue schizonts of *P. falciparum*, *P. malariae* and apparently *P. knowlesi* rupture once and do not persist in the liver. There are two types of tissue schizonts for *P. ovale* and *P. vivax*. The primary type ruptures in 6–9 days, and the secondary type remains dormant in the liver cell for weeks, months, or as long as 5 years before releasing merozoites and causing relapse of infection. The erythrocytic phase of *Plasmodium* asexual development begins when the merozoites from the liver enters the erythrocytes. Once inside the erythrocyte, the parasite transforms into the ring form, which then enlarges to become a trophozoite. These latter two forms can be identified with Giemsa stain on blood smear, the primary means of confirming the diagnosis of malaria (Figs. 6.1.1 and 6.1.2).

The trophozoite multiplies asexually to produce a number of small erythrocytic *merozoites* that are released into the bloodstream when the erythrocyte membrane ruptures, which is associated with fever. Over time, some of the merozoites develop into male and female gametocytes

that complete the *Plasmodium* life cycle when they are ingested during a blood meal by the female anopheline mosquito. The male and female gametocytes fuse to form a zygote in the stomach cavity of the mosquito. After a series of further transformations, sporozoites enter the salivary gland of the mosquito and are inoculated into a new host with the next blood meal.

Four important pathologic processes have been identified in patients with malaria:
1. Fever
2. Anemia
3. Immunopathologic events
4. Tissue anoxia

Fever occurs when erythrocytes rupture and release merozoites into the circulation. Anemia is caused by hemolysis, sequestration of erythrocytes in the spleen and other organs, and bone marrow suppression.

In contrast to malaria caused by *P. ovale*, *P. vivax*, and *P. malariae*, which usually results in parasitemias of less than 2%, malaria caused by *P. falciparum* can be associated

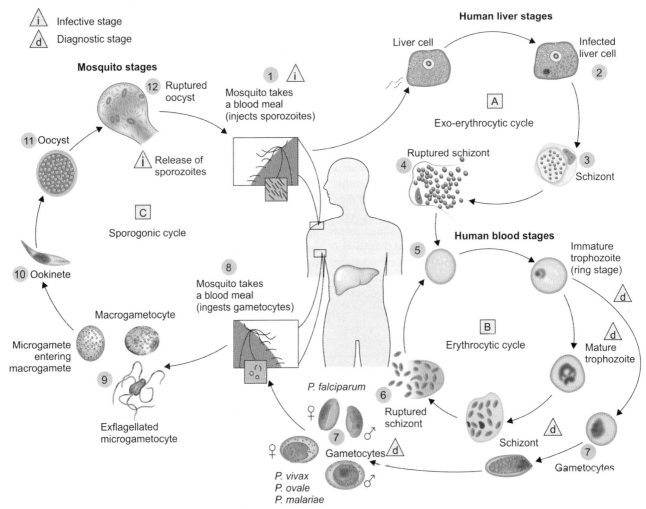

FIG. 6.1.1: Life cycle of *Plasmodium* species.

Source: Centers for Disease Control and Prevention: laboratory diagnosis of malaria

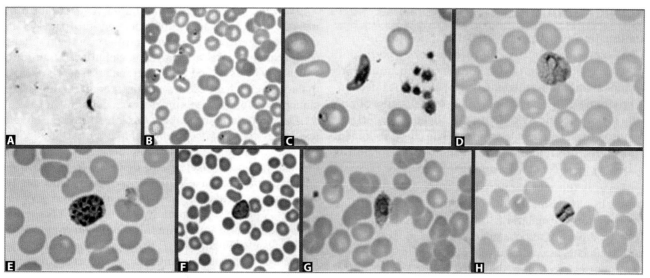

FIGS 6.1.2A TO H: Giemsa-stained thick (A) and thin (B to H) smears used for the diagnosis of malaria and the speciation of *Plasmodium* parasites; (A) Multiple signet-ring *P. falciparum* trophozoites, which are visualized outside erythrocytes; (B) A multiply infected erythrocyte containing signet-ring *P. falciparum* trophozoites, including an accolade form positioned up against the inner surface of the erythrocyte membrane; (C) Banana-shaped gametocyte unique to *P. falciparum*; (D) Ameboid trophozoite characteristic of *P. vivax*. Both *P. vivax* and *P. ovale* are infected erythrocytes which exhibit Schuffner's dots and tend to be enlarged compared with uninfected erythrocytes; (E) *P. vivax* schizont. Mature *P. falciparum* parasites, by contrast, are rarely seen on blood smears because they sequester in the systemic microvasculature; (F) *P. vivax* spherical gametocyte; (G) *P. ovale* trophozoite. *Note*: Schuffner's dots and ovoid shapes of the infected erythrocyte; (H) Characteristic band forms trophozoite of *P. malariae*, containing intracellular pigment hemozoin.

Source: A, B and F from Centers for Disease Control and Prevention: DPDx: laboratory identification of parasites of public health concern. www.dpd.cdc. gov/dpdx/C, D, E, G and H courtesy of David Wyler, Newton Center, MA, USA.

with parasitemia levels as high as 60%. The differences in parasitemia reflect the fact that *P. falciparum* infects both immature and mature erythrocytes, while *P. ovale* and *P. vivax* primarily infect immature erythrocytes, and *P. malariae* infects only mature erythrocytes.

Immunopathologic events include excessive production of proinflammatory cytokines such as tumor necrosis factor, that may be responsible for most of the pathology of the disease, including tissue anoxia; polyclonal activation resulting in both hypergammaglobulinemia and the formation of immune complexes; and immunosuppression.

Cytoadherence of infected erythrocytes to vascular endothelium occurs in *P. falciparum* malaria and may lead to obstruction of blood flow and capillary damage, with resultant vascular leakage of blood, protein, and fluid and tissue anoxia. In addition, hypoglycemia and lactic acidemia are caused by anaerobic metabolism of glucose. The cumulative effects of these pathologic processes may lead to cerebral, cardiac, pulmonary, intestinal, renal, and hepatic failure. Immunity after *Plasmodium* species infection is incomplete. Repeated episodes of infection occur because the parasite has developed a number of immune-evasive strategies, such as intracellular replication, vascular cytoadherence that prevent infected erythrocytes from circulating through the spleen, rapid antigenic variation, and alteration of the host immune

system resulting in partial immune suppression. Several alterations in erythrocyte physiology prevent or modify malarial infection. Erythrocytes containing hemoglobin S (sickle erythrocytes) resist malaria parasite growth, erythrocytes lacking Duffy blood group antigen are resistant to *P. vivax*, and erythrocytes containing hemoglobin F (fetal hemoglobin) and ovalocytes are resistant to *P. falciparum*. In hyperendemic areas, newborns rarely become ill with malaria, in part because of passive maternal antibody and high levels of fetal hemoglobin. Children from 3 months to 5 years of age have little specific immunity to malaria species and, therefore, suffer most. Immunity is subsequently acquired, and severe cases of malaria become less common. Severe disease may occur during pregnancy, particularly 1st pregnancy or after extended residence outside the endemic region. In general, extracellular *Plasmodium* organisms are targeted by antibody, whereas intracellular organisms are targeted by cellular defenses such as *T. lymphocytes*, macrophages, polymorphonuclear leukocyte, and the spleen.

Recrudescence may occur from the survival of erythrocyte forms in the bloodstream after a primary attack. Relapse is caused by release of merozoites from an exoerythrocytic source in the liver, which occurs with *P. vivax* and *P. ovale*, or from persistence within the erythrocyte, which occurs with *P. malariae* and rarely with *P. falciparum*.

CLINICAL MANIFESTATION

The usual incubation periods are 9–14 days for *P. falciparum*, 12–17 days for *P. vivax*, 16–18 days for *P. ovale* and 18–40 days for *P. malariae*. Children and adults are asymptomatic during this initial phase of malaria infection. A prodrome of 2–3 days is noted in some patients during which nonspecific symptoms, like headache, fatigue, anorexia, myalgia, slight fever and pain in chest, abdomen, and joints, are noted and high index of suspicion is necessary to detect malaria during this time.

Fever is the most important feature of malaria and comes in paroxysms alternating with periods of fatigue. Fever pattern in malaria is lassicly descibed as erratic. Febrile paroxysms are characterized by high fever, sweats and headache, as well as myalgia, back pain, abdominal pain, nausea, vomiting, diarrhea, pallor and jaundice. Paroxysms coincide with the rupture of schizonts that occurs on every 48 hours with *P. vivax* and *P. ovale*, resulting in fever spikes every other day. Rupture of schizonts occurs on every 72 hour with *P. malariae,* resulting in fever spikes on every 3rd or 4th day. Periodicity is less apparent with *P. falciparum* and mixed infections and may not be apparent early on in infection, when parasite broods have not yet synchronized. Children with malaria often lack typical paroxysms and have nonspecific symptoms, including fever (may be low-grade but is often >104°F), headache, drowsiness, anorexia, nausea, vomiting and diarrhea.

Distinctive physical signs may include splenomegaly (common), hepatomegaly, and pallor due to anemia. Typical laboratory findings include anemia, thrombocytopenia and a normal or low leukocyte count. The erythrocyte sedimentation rate (ESR) is often elevated.

Box 6.1.1

Clinical and laboratory criteria for severe malaria.

Clinical
- Impaired consciousness or unarousable coma
- Severe prostration
- Failure to feed
- Recurrent convulsion
- Respiratory distress from metabolic acidosis
- Circulatory collapse or shock
- Clinical jaundice plus evidence of other vital organ dysfunction
- Hemoglobinuria
- Abnormal spontaneous breathing

Laboratory
- Hypoglycemia (blood glucose <40 mg/dL)
- Metabolic acidosis (plasma bicarbonate < 15 mmol/L)
- Severe normocytic anemia (Hb <5 gm/dL)
- Hyperparasitemia (>2% or 100,000/mL)
- Renal impairment (serum creatinine >3 mg/dL)
- Pulmonary edema
- Hyperlactatemia (lactate >5 mmol/L)

Plasmodium falciparum is the most severe form of malaria and is associated with higher density of parasitemia and a number of complications. The most common serious complication is severe anemia (hemoglobin level <5 gm/dL), which also is associated with other malaria species. Severe malaria is characterized by one or more of the following clinical or laboratory features as shown in Box 6.1.1.

Plasmodium vivax malaria has long been considered less severe than *P. falciparum* malaria, but recent reports suggest that in some areas of Indonesia it is as frequent a cause of severe disease and death as *P. falciparum*. Severe disease and death from *P. vivax* are usually due to severe anemia and sometimes to splenic rupture. *P. ovale* malaria is the least common type of malaria. It is similar to *P. vivax* malaria and commonly is found in conjunction with *P. falciparum* malaria. *P. malariae* is the mildest and most chronic of all malaria infections. Nephrotic syndrome is a rare complication of *P. malariae* infection that is not observed with any other human malaria species.

Congenital malaria is acquired from the mother prenatally or perinatally and is a serious problem in tropical areas. In endemic areas, congenital malaria is an important cause of abortions, miscarriages, stillbirths, premature births, intrauterine growth retardation and neonatal deaths. Congenital malaria usually occurs in the offspring of a nonimmune mother with *P. vivax* or *P. malariae* infection, although it can be observed with any of the human malaria species. The 1st sign or symptom most commonly occurs between 10 and 30 days of age (range 14 hours to several months of age). Fever, restlessness, drowsiness, pallor, jaundice, poor feeding, vomiting, diarrhea, cyanosis and hepatosplenomegaly are primarily noted. Malaria is often severe during pregnancy and may have an adverse effect on the fetus or neonate, resulting in intrauterine growth retardation and low birth weight, even in the absence of transmission from mother to child.

DIAGNOSIS

Refer to Malaria Protocol in Chapter 8.

Differential Diagnosis

The differential diagnosis of malaria is broad and includes viral infections such as influenza and hepatitis, sepsis, pneumonia, meningitis, encephalitis, endocarditis, gastroenteritis, pyelonephritis, brucellosis, leptospirosis, tuberculosis, typhoid fever, amebic liver abscess, Hodgkin disease, and collagen vascular disease.

TREATMENT

For treatment of uncomplicated, complicated and severe malaria, refer to Malaria Protocol in Chapter 8.

BIBLIOGRAPHY

1. Brown AE, Kain KC, Pipithkul J, et al. Demonstration by polymerase chain reaction of mixed *Plasmodium falciparum* and *P. vivax* infections undetected by conventional microscopy. Trans R Soc Med Hyg. 1992;86:609-12.

2. Houwen B. Blood film preparation and staining procedure. Clin Lab Med. 2002;22:1-14.

3. IAP Textbook of Pediatrics.

4. Memorandum from a WHO meeting. Malaria diagnosis. Bull WHO. 1988;66:575-94.

5. Nelson's Textbook of Pediatrics, 19th edition.

6. Snounou G, Viriyakosol S, Jarra W, et al. Identification of the four human malaria parasite species in field samples by polymerase chain reaction and detection of high prevalence of mixed infection. Mol Biochem Parasitol. 1993;58:283-9.

7. WHO releases new malaria guidelines for treatment and procurement of medicines. March 9, 2010; Geneva.

8. World Health Organization. Approaches to the Diagnosis Malaria. New Perspectives Malaria Diagnosis. Report of a Joint WHO/USAID Informal Consultation; 2000. pp. 10-8.

9. World Health Organization. Diagnosis of Malaria in Management of Severe Malaria. A Practical Handbook, 2nd edition. Geneva: WHO; 2000. pp. 46-8.

10. World Health Organization. Severe and complicated malaria, 2nd edition. Trans R Soc Med Hyg. 1990:84(Suppl. 2);23-5.

6.2 KALA-AZAR

Nigam Prakash Narain, Rajesh Kumar

INTRODUCTION

Kala-azar (KA) or Visceral leishmaniasis (VL) remains a significant problem in the tropical and subtropical regions of the world being endemic in 97 countries and territories. In South East Asia Region (SEAR) an estimated 147 million people in 4 countries (India, Nepal, Bhutan and Bangladesh), are at risk with an estimated 1,00,000 new cases each year. In India, VL is endemic in 54 districts in 4 states viz. Bihar, West Bengal, Jharkhand and Eastern Uttar Pradesh with contributing for >70% cases. Sporadic cases are reported from Assam, Himachal Pradesh, Kerala, Madhya Pradesh, Sikkim and Uttarakhand. Approximately 50% of these new cases are children. Prolonged fever with anorexia and loss of appetite are the major presenting features. Marked enlargement of the spleen and liver (spleen larger than liver) with moderate to severe anemia are the other common features of this disease. Recent years have seen considerable advance in the diagnosis and treatment of Kala-azar. Because of a large pool of migrant population everywhere in India, it is customary for all the pediatricians of the country to know more about this disease.

EPIDEMIOLOGY

Natural Transmission

Natural transmission of *Leishmania donovani* takes place from man to man by bites of certain species of sandflies of genus Phlebotomus and Lutzomyia (Indian vector is *Phlebotomus argentipes*).

TRANSMISSION OF KALA-AZAR

Kala-azar is a vector borne disease. Sandfly of genus *Ps argentipes* are the only known vectors of kala-azar in India.

Indian kala-azar has a unique epidemiological feature of being anthroponotic; human is the only known reservoir of infection. Female sandflies pick up parasite [Amastigote or Leishman-Donovan (LD) bodies] while feeding on an infected human host. Parasite then undergo morphological change to become flagellate (Promastigote or Leptomonad), develops and multiplies in the gut of sandflies and move to mouth part. Healthy human hosts get infection when an infective sandfly vector bites them (Fig. 6.2.1).

KALA-AZAR VECTOR IN INDIA

There is only one sandfly vector of kala-azar in India called *Ps. argentipes*. Sandflies are small insects, about one-fourth of a mosquito. The length of a sandfly body ranges 1.5–3.5 mm.

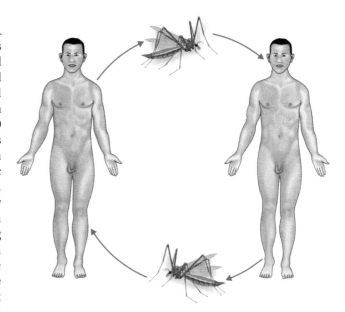

FIG. 6.2.1: Transmission of kala-azar.

Adult sandfly is a small fuzzy, delicately proportionate fly with erect large wings. The entire body including wings is heavily clothed with long hairs. Life cycle consists of egg, four instars of larvae, pupa and adult. The whole cycle takes more than a month; however, duration of cycle depends on temperature and other ecological conditions. They prefer high relative humidity, warm temperature, high subsoil water and abundance of vegetation. Sandflies breed in favorable microclimatic conditions in places with high organic matter that serve as food for larvae. These are ecologically sensitive insects, fragile and cannot withstand desiccation.

Agent: L. donovani is the causative agent of kala-azar [Visceral leishmaniasis (VL)]. The life cycle is completed in two hosts, one in vertebrate (man), i.e. Leishman-Donovan Bodies, and another in insect (sandfly), i.e. Flagellated Promastigote form.

Reservoir: Indian kala-azar is considered to be a non-zoonotic disease with man as the sole reservoir.

Host Factors

Age: All age groups including infants may be effected. Peak age group in India is 5–9 years.

Sex: Male female ratio is 2:1.

Population movements: Migrants, laborers, tourists, etc. moving from an endemic to a non-endemic area propagate the disease.

Socioeconomic status: Usual sufferers are the poorest of the poor.

Occupation: Those in farming, forestry and mining fishing are at increased risk.

Environmental Factors

Altitude: Kala-azar is mostly confined to plains and is unusual at altitude over 2,000 feet.

Season: In the past epidemics, two peaks, one in November and another in March-April were seen. In the 1977 Bihar epidemic, it was observed that most cases occurred between April and September. Generally, there is high prevalence during and after rains.

Vector: Sandflies (*Ps argentipes*) breed in cracks and crevices in soils and buildings, tree holes, caves, etc. Overcrowding, ill-ventilation and accumulation of the organic matter in the environment facilitate transmission. Their habits are primarily nocturnal. Only female sandflies bite.

INCUBATION PERIOD

Extrinsic incubation period in sandfly: Between 6–9 days. Intrinsic incubation period in man: Quite variable, generally 1–4 months with a range of 10 days to 2 years.

IMMUNITY

Dominant Th1 response is associated with healing, and Th2 response is associated with disease progression. Th1 cells produce interferon-gamma (IFN-γ), which is involved in cell mediated immunity. Th2 cells produce IL-4, IL-5 and IL-10; these are involved more in humoral immunity. Cytokine Il-12 promotes Th1 cell development. Phagocytic cells in response to infection with intracellular pathogens or I response to microbial products.

Th2 cytokines block intracellular killing of protozoa by macrophages and contribute to the pathological progression of kala-azar. Recent studies indicate that Il-12 may have an important curative role in human kala-azar. All these indicate that the induction of effective immunity in kala-azar depends on the induction of Th1 response. Immune response to kala-azar is protective and lasting.

CLINICAL FEATURES

Acute Onset

This is one of the rare presentations of kala-azar and is seen rarely in visitors or inhabitants of nonendemic areas. Fever is most common presentation and is either high intermittent or remittent in type and lasts for 2–6 weeks or longer. Spleen enlarges very rapidly being palpable even in few days.

Chronic Onset

Chronic onset is the most common way of presentation in endemic areas. The typical manifestation of kala-azar consists of high fever, abdominal discomfort, emaciation and pallor. Marked splenomegaly and moderate hepatomegaly generally appear approximately 6 months after the onset of illness.

Fever is generally high grade and intermittent with a double rise of temperature in a day (double quotidian), the characteristic finding not commonly seen nowaday. In spite of the high fever the children remain remarkably well and ambulant with reasonably preserved appetite.

Splenic enlargement is seen in nearly all cases. This becomes palpable by the first month of illness and thereafter enlarges at the rate of about one inch per month. It is huge, smooth, firm and non-tender unless there has been a recent infarct. Ultimately spleen is massively enlarged and firm.

Liver is usually enlarged but not to such an extent as the spleen. Hepatic functions remain unaltered. Jaundice with evidence of gross hepatocellular dysfunction is unusual and carries a grave prognosis.

Darkening of skin of face, hands, feet and abdomen that characteristically gave it the name of kala-azar was commonly seen earlier. But nowaday this feature is not commonly seen in children.

Features of Pancytopenia

Extreme degree of anemia can be found in a few cases, which is attributed to autoimmune hemolysis, hypersplenism, ineffective erythropoiesis, nutritional deficiencies and GIT blood loss.

Secondary infection is a common complication; most common association being tuberculosis. Other infections, which are commonly seen, are pneumonia, measles, otitis media, cancrum oris. Cough and diarrhea are also common.

Bleeding from mucous membrane in form of epistaxis and hematemesis, petechiae and purpura have been described with severe thrombocytopenia. But this is not a common presentation in endemic areas of Bihar.

DIAGNOSIS AND MANAGEMENT

Clinical description: An illness with prolonged irregular fever, splenomegaly and weight loss as its main symptoms. In endemic malarious areas, VL should be suspected when fever lasts > 2 weeks and no response has been achieved with antimalarial medicines (assuming drug resistant malaria has also been considered).

Laboratory Criteria for Diagnosis

1. Positive parasitology (stained smears from bone marrow, spleen, liver, lymph nodes, blood or culture of the organism from biopsy or aspirated material); and
2. Positive serology (IFAT, ELISA, rK39, direct agglutination test)
3. Positive PCR and related techniques.

Case Classification (by WHO Operational Definition)

A KA suspect case: History of fever of > 2 weeks and enlarged spleen and liver not responding to anti-malarial in patient from endemic area.

A case of KA: A person from endemic area with fever of > 2 weeks duration and with splenomegaly, who is confirmed by an RDT or a biopsy.

Lab Diagnosis

1. *CBC:* Leucopenia, anemia and thrombocytopenia. Leucopenia being very characteristic.
2. *Immunodiagnosis:*

Antigen detection—KAtex Test: It is latex agglutination test for detection of Leishmania antigen in urine and high sensitivity but poor specificity. It is especially useful in diagnosing case of VL- HIV co-infection and could help assess response to therapy. However it is still in field trial but a promising bed side test in future.

Antibody detection—IFA, ELISA, DAT: All these tests have high diagnostic values but are not user friendly in field conditions.

rK-39Rapid test for Kala-azar: It is rapid immunochromato-graphic dipstick test based on recombinant antigen 39 amino acid gene of L.Chagasi. It is highly specific, easy to perform, rapid and cheap. It is a bedside test for VL due to simplicity and easy availability, however, it cannot predict response to therapy. Diagnosis of Kala-azar case is done by using Rapid Diagnosis Test (RDT) Kits in the field and the results can be read in 10 minutes. These kits show > 90% specificity and sensitivity. These RD test kits are user friendly and interpretation of the test is also simple as two red lines indicate a positive result and only a single red strand indicate a negative result.

The rapid dipstick '**Rapid Diagnostic test**' has become the mainstay in the serological diagnosis and is the method of choice for diagnosis of Kala-azar. The test kit comprises of test strip (Usually 25 pouched test strips per kit box) and chase Buffer solution (Usually 2 vials per kit). Results are read in 10 minutes. Positive result is indicated by a red line appearing in the control line where the blood was placed and another red line appears where the blood has migrated through capillary action. There should be two red lines for the test to be positive. A faint red line also is considered positive. In negative result there is a red line where the drop of blood was placed but there is no red line where the blood has migrated by capillary action.

Storage and supply: The test strips and the buffer should be stored safely at room temperature between 20 and 30 degrees Celsius and should not be frozen since freezing deteriorates the quality of the reagent. Temperature in excess of 30 degrees can also reduce the quality of the test.

False positives results could be seen in hepatitis and TB cases. In situations where the clinical case definition is not followed, positive result should be interpreted with caution. Results could be falsely negatives in HIV patients where immune response is limited. The RDT can remain positive for months or years after treatment of VL. For this reason this test is not useful in the diagnosis of relapse cases. In PKDL it can be used only to rule out the disease if negative but not for confirmation. In these cases, parasitological diagnosis should be done, by bone aspirate or splenic aspirate.

PCR: It is a DNA detection method which recognizes parasite DNA and is highly sensitivity and specificity, capable of detecting a single parasite in specimen.

Parasite culture: L. donovani is cultured in NNN media. Although culture is expensive and time consuming, it can predict respond to treatment. It could differentiate between relapse and re-infection. However, its use is limited by it being very expensive and not user friendly.

Tissue smear examination: Demonstration of parasites (LD Bodies) in tissue smear of bone marrow or Spleen is gold standard for diagnosis of VL.

Diagnosis of PKDL: Cases of PKDL usually do not have any signs of Kala-azar like fever, splenomegaly, or anemia because 85–90% of them appear after the cure of Kala-azar. However, 5–6% of cases of PKDL cases occur without the preceding history of Kala-azar. They have only skin lesions that are varied. The lesions may be macular, papular nodular or mixed. Sometimes the lesions of PKDL are extensive. In PKDL cases, sensation over the lesions is preserved in contrast to leprosy where similar lesions have no sensations.

Case Definitions

Probable PKDL: A patient from a KA endemic area with multiple hypopigmented macules, papules, plaques or nodules, who are RDT positive.

Confirmed PKDL: A patient from a KA endemic area with multiple hypopigmented macules, papules, plaques or nodules, who is parasite positive in slit-skin smear (SSS) or biopsy.

Treatment Outcomes in PKDL

Initial cure: Clinical improvement at the end of treatment is defined as a considerable reduction in the number and size of skin lesions.

Final cure: Clinical cure 12 months after the end of treatment is defined as a complete resolution of macules, papules, plaques and nodules.

Co-infection with HIV: VL has emerged as an opportunistic infection in HIV patients. Atypical clinical presentations of these patients pose a diagnostic challenge. More than 1000 cases of co-infection with HIV and VL are reported from 25 countries. In these patients hepatosplenomegaly may be absent. Diagnosis is usually made by bone marrow examination as sensitivity of antibodies based immunodiagnostic test is low. Amastigotes may be demonstrated in buffy coat smear. PCR analysis of whole blood or its buffy coat may prove a useful screening test for these patients.

Treatment

Antimony compounds: Two compounds namely Sodium Stibogluconate (SSG) and Meglumine Antimonate have been in use for VL since 1930's. But since early eighties there was emergence of large scale SSG resistance in North Bihar and only 35–38% patients responded to SSG in Bihar and hence has gone out of favor. SSG may be used in dose of 20 mg/Kg body wt. IM or IV daily for 30 days in areas where they remain effective. Major adverse effects of these compounds are arthralgia, myalgia, metallic taste and cardiotoxicity.

Amphotericin-B: This antifungal drug has excellent anti-leishmanial activity and is 400 times more potent than SSG. Dose of conventional Amphotericin-B deoxycholate is 0.75–1 mg/kg slow IV infusion for 15–20 doses on alternate days. Total dose of 15 mg/kg achieves nearly 100% cure without any organ toxicity. Major side effects are infusion related, occasionally serious renal toxicity and electrolyte imbalance may occur.

Lipid formulations of amphotericin–B: They are the most important development in Chemotherapy of VL. Various lipid formulations available are: Liposomal amphotericin-B (Ambisome), Amphotericin-B lipid complex (Abelect), Amphotericin-B colloidal Suspension (Amphomul/Amphocil). **Conventional *Amphotericin-B requires prolonged hospitalization along with renal monitoring whereas Lipid formulations requires much shorter stay and relatively free from side effects with almost equal efficacy achieving cure rate of around 94% in VL.***

Liposomal Amphotericin B (Ambisome): It is recommended by WHO and included as the first line treatment by National Vector Borne Disease control programme (NVBDCP) in Accelerated Plan for Kala-azar Elimination-2017 due to it's ease of use, effectiveness and assured compliance. *It is much safer than conventional Amphotericin B, however, high cost is a limiting factor to its use. It is used in single dose of 10 mg/kg IV (for all age groups), dissolved in 5% dextrose and is administered over 2 hours.*

Miltefosine: It is one of the most important developments in the management of VL for adults, eliminating need for parenteral therapy and hospitalization. It is used in doses as followed; for children aged 2–11 years—2.5 mg/kg once daily after meals × 28 days, children >12 year weight < 25 kg—only one capsule of 50 mg daily × 28 days, children> 12 years and weight 25–50 kg—100 mg daily in two doses of 50 mg each after meals for 28 days and for >50 kg body wt—150 mg/day orally for 28 days in divided doses. Side effects of miltefosine include GIT symptoms (vomiting and diarrhea), asymptomatic transient elevation of hepatic enzymes and rarely nephrotoxic. It is a teratogenic drug, cannot be used during pregnancy and in females of child bearing age. It is presently being given as first line drug in North Bihar at PHC level on outdoor basis, however is not very successful in children due to GI intolerance.

Paromomycin: It is a aminoglycoside antibiotic marketed globally for >20 years. It is clinical efficacy in VL is established in clinical trials (Phase I/II) in Africa and India. It gas high overall cure rates (final cure: 94.6%) and is also effective in patients failing previous treatment. It is very affordable and safe to use.

Combination therapy: Various combination therapies are recommended for treatment of KA, viz., *Antimonial with Interferon-Gamma, Ambisome with Paromomycin, Ambisome with Miltefosine, Miltefosine with Paromomycin and SSG with Paromomycin.*

HIV/VL co-infected patients: LAmB is used in dose of 3–5 mg/kg daily or intermittently for 10 doses, days 1–5,10,17,24, 31 and 38, total cumulative dose of 40 mg/kg.

PKDL: First drug of choice is miltefosine orally for 12 weeks. Amphotericin 'B' deoxycholate injection could be used in dose of 1 mg/k/day by infusion for upto 60–80 doses over 4 months.

Therapeutic Options

- Use SSG only in responsive regions.
- Amphotericin B—Remains the most important drug and cure rate close to 100%

- *Lipid Ampho B*
  - Lipid formulations are most important development in chemotherapy of VL
  - Ambisome is wonder drug though cost is a limiting factor.
- *Miltefosine:*
  - Effective and Safe with great oral advantage
  - First line drug in Bihar on out-patient basis in adults and being distributed free by the public sector in North Bihar.
  - Limitations: Teratogenic, Expensive, Poor compliance in domiciliary care ?, GIT intolerance
- *Paromomycin:*
  - Safe effective and affordable
  - High cure rated reported only when used in combination with either Miltefosine or Amphotericin B

Treatment outcomes in Kala-azar: Treatment outcomes in Kala-azar have to be assessed twice: (1) At the last day of drug treatment (initial outcome) and (2) Six months after the last drug was taken(final outcome). *Four main outcomes are identified in Kala-azar elimination strategy:*

- *Cure*: A patient is considered clinically cured if he/she has completed full treatment and there are no signs and symptoms of KA.
- *Non-response*: Signs and symptoms persist or recur despite satisfactory treatment for more than two weeks.
- *Relapse*: any reappearance of KA signs and symptoms within a period of six months after the end of treatment.
- *Treatment failure*: non-response or relapse

Preventive strategies:
- Effective disease surveillance
- Early diagnosis and treatment of patients
- Vector control by effective IRS
- Effective environmental measures by IEC
- Kala-azar vaccine?

BIBLIOGRAPHY

1. Alvar J, et al. Leishmania and human immunodeficiency virus coinfection: the first 10 years. Clin Microbiol Rev. 1997;10:298-319.
2. A Publication of WHO/SEARO, WHO Regional Office for South-East Asia, 2008 (last updated: 15th May, 2012).
3. Attar ZJ, Chance ML, el-Safi S, et al. Latex agglutination test for the detection of urinary antigens in visceral leishmaniasis. Acta Trop. 2001;78:11-6.
4. Behrman RE, Kleigman RM, Arvin AM, et al. Leishmaniasis. Nelson's Textbook of Pediatrics, 15th edition.
5. Bhattacharya SK, Sinha PK, Sundar S, et al. Phase 4 trial of miltefosine for the treatment of Indian visceral leishmaniasis. J Infect Dis. 2007;196(4):591-8.
6. Bhattacharya SK, Sur D, Karbwang J. Childhood visceral leishmaniasis. Indian J Med Res. 2006;353-6.
7. Bora D. Epidemiology of leishmaniasis in India. National Medical Journal of India. 1999;12:62-8.
8. Braz RF, et al. The sensitivity and specificity of Leishmania chagasi recombinant K39 antigen in the diagnosis of American visceral leishmaniasis and in differentiating active from subclinical infection. Am J Trop Med Hyg. 2002;67:344-8.
9. Cabrera-Serra MG, Lorenzo-Morales J, Romero M, et al. In vitro activity of perifosine: a novel alkylphospholipid against the promastigote stage of Leishmania species. Parasitol Res. 2007;100:1155-7.
10. Cabrera-Serra MG, Valladares B, Piñero JE. In vivo activity of perifosine against Leishmania amazonensis. Acta Trop 2008;108:20-5.
11. Chatterjee KD. Parasitology, 12th edition. pp. 54-65.
12. Croft SL, Yardley V, Kendrick H. Drug sensitivity of Leishmania species: some unresolved problems. Trans R Soc Trop Med Hyg. 2002;96:127-9.
13. Davidson RN, et al. Liposomal amphotericin B (AmBisome) in Mediterranean visceral leishmaniasis:a multi-centre trial. Q. J. Med. 1994;87:75-81.
14. De Almeida Silva L, et al. Immunologic tests in patients after clinical cure of visceral leishmaniasis. Am J Trop Med Hyg. 2006;75:739-43.
15. de la Rosa R, et al. Influence of highly active antiretroviral therapy on the outcome of subclinical visceral leishmaniasis in human immunodeficiency virus-infected patients. Clin Infect Dis. 2001;32:633-5.
16. Deniau M, Canavate C, Faraut-Gambarelli F, et al. The biological diagnosis of leishmaniasis in HIV-infected patients. Ann Trop Med Parasitol. 2003;97(Suppl. 1):115-33.
17. Desjeux P. Leishmaniasis: current situation and new perspectives. Comp Immunol Microbiol Infect Dis. 2004;27:305-18.
18. Desjeux P. The increase in risk factors for leishmaniasis worldwide. Trans R Soc Trop Med Hyg. 2001;95:239-43.
19. El Tai NO, El Fari M, Mauricio I, et al. Leishmania donovani: intraspecific polymorphisms of Sudanese isolates revealed by PCR-based analyses and DNA sequencing. Exp Parasitol. 2001;97:35-44.
20. Fernandez Cotarelo MJ, et al. Effect of highly active antiretroviral therapy on the incidence and clinical manifestations of visceral leishmaniasis in human immunodeficiency virus-infected patients. Clin Infect Dis. 2003;37:973-7.
21. Gari-Toussaint M, Lelievre A, Marty P, et al. Contribution of serological tests to the diagnosis of visceral leishmaniasis in patients infected with the human immunodeficiency virus. Trans R Soc Trop Med Hyg. 1994;88:301.
22. Ghai OP. Essential Pediatrics, 8th edition
23. Hailu A, Berhe N. The performance of direct agglutination tests (DAT) in the diagnosis of visceral leishmaniasis among Ethiopian patients with HIV coinfection. Ann Trop Med Parasitol. 2002;96:25-30.
24. Hailu A. Pre- and post-treatment antibody levels in visceral leishmaniasis. Trans R Soc Trop Med Hyg. 1990;84:673-5.
25. Herwaldt BL. Leishmaniasis. Lancet. 1999;354:1191-9.

26. Jha TK, Olliaro P, Thakur CPN, et al. Randomised controlled trial of aminosidine (paromomycin) v sodium stibogluconate for treating visceral leishmaniasis in North Bihar, India. BMJ. 1998;316:1200-5.

27. Jha TK. Refractory Kala-azar—Diagnosis and Management: Medicine Update, 1998. pp. 137-44.

28. Krishna P, et al. Efficacy and safety of liposomal amphotericin B for Visceral leishmaniasis in children and adolescents at a tertiary care center in Bihar, India: Am J Trop Med Hyg. 2017;97(5):1498-1502.

29. Kuhlencord A, Maniera T, Eibl H, et al. Oral treatment of visceral leishmaniasis in mice. Antimicrob Agents Chemother. 1992;36:1630-4.

30. Kumar R, Pai K, Pathak K, et al. Enzyme linked immunosorbent assay for recombinant K39 antigen in diagnosis and prognosis of Indian visceral leishmaniasis. Clin Diagn Lab Immunol. 2001;8:1220-4.

31. Laguna F, et al. Treatment of visceral leishmaniasis in HIV-infected patients: a randomized trial comparing meglumine antimoniate with amphotericin B. Spanish HIV-*Leishmania* Study Group. AIDS. 1999;13:1063-9.

32. Lainson R, Shaw JJ. New World leishmaniasis–The Neotropical Leishmania species. In: Cox FEG, Kreier JP, Wakelin D (Eds). Topley & Wilson's Microbiology and Microbial Infections (volume 5), Parasitology. 9th edition New York: Oxford University Press; 1998 pp. 241-82.

33. Lodge R, Diallo TO, Descoteaux A. *Leishmania donovani* lipophosphoglycan blocks NADPH oxidase assembly at the phagosome membrane. Cell Microbiol. 2006;8:1922-31.

34. Lopez-Velez R, et al. Clinicoepidemiologic characteristics, prognostic factors, and survival analysis of patients coinfected with human immunodeficiency virus and Leishmania in an area of Madrid, Spain. Am J Trop Med Hyg. 1998;58:436-43.

35. Lopez-Velez R. The impact of highly active antiretroviral therapy (HAART) on visceral leishmaniasis in Spanish patients who are co-infected with HIV Ann Trop Med. Parasitol. 2003;97(Suppl. 1):143-7.

36. Manson-Bahr PEC. Diagnosis: The Leishmaniases in Biology and Medicine, vol 2, Clinical Aspects and Control. Peters W, Killick-Kendrick R (Eds). New York: Academic Press Inc; 1987. pp. 709-29.

37. Mira JA, et al. Frequency of visceral leishmaniasis relapses in human immunodeficiency virus-infected patients receiving highly active antiretroviral therapy. Am J Trop Med Hyg. 2004;70:298-301.

38. Moreno J, Canavate C, Chamizo C, et al. HIV–Leishmania infantum co-infection: humoral and cellular immune responses to the parasite after chemotherapy. Trans R Soc Trop Med Hyg. 2000;94:328-32.

39. Murray HW, Berman JD, Davies CR, et al. Advances in leishmaniasis. Lancet. 2005;366:1561-77.

40. Murray HW. Kala-azar as an AIDS-related opportunistic infection. AIDS Patient Care STDs. 1999;13:459-65.

41. Palma G, Gutierrez Y. Laboratory diagnosis of Leishmania. Clin Lab Med. 1991;11:909-22.

42. Park's Textbook of Preventive and Social Medicine, 18th edition. 2005.

43. Pasquau F, et al. Leishmaniasis as an opportunistic infection in HIV-infected patients: determinants of relapse and mortality in a collaborative study of 228 episodes in a Mediterreanean region. Eur J Clin Microbiol Infect Dis. 2005;24:411-8.

44. Pérez-Victoria FJ, Sánchez-Cañete MP, Seifert K, et al. Mechanisms of experimental resistance of Leishmania to miltefosine: implications for clinical use. Drug Resist Update. 2006;9:26-39.

45. Pizzuto M, Piazza M, Senese D, Scalamogna C, Calattini S, Corsico L, et al. Role of PCR in diagnosis and prognosis of visceral leishmaniasis in patients co-infected with human immunodeficiency virus type 1. J Clin Microbiol 2001;39:357-61.

46. Riera C, et al. Evaluation of a latex agglutination test (KAtex) for detection of Leishmania antigen in urine of patients with HIV–Leishmania coinfection: value in diagnosis and post-treatment follow-up. Eur J Clin Microbiol Infect Dis. 2004;23:899-904.

47. Ritmeijer K, et al. A comparison of miltefosine and sodium stibogluconate for treatment of visceral leishmaniasis in an Ethiopian population with high prevalence of HIV infection. Clin Infect Dis. 2006;43:357-64.

48. Rittig MG, Bogdan C. Leishmania–host-cell interaction: complexities and alternative views. Parasitol Today. 2000;16:292-7.

49. Rosenthal E, et al. Declining incidence of visceral leishmaniasis in HIV-infected individuals in the era of highly active antiretroviral therapy. AIDS. 2001;15:1184-5.

50. Rosenthal E, et al. HIV and *Leishmania* coinfection: a review of 91 cases with focus on atypical locations of Leishmania. Clin Infect Dis. 2000;31:1093-5.

51. Santa-Rita RM, Henriques-Pons A, Barbosa HS, et al. Effect of the lysophospholipid analogues edelfosine, ilmofosine and miltefosine against *Leishmania amazonensis*. J Antimicrob Chemother. 2004;54:704-10.

52. Santos-Gomes G, Gomes-Pereira S, Campino L, et al. Performance of immunoblotting in diagnosis of visceral Leishmaniasis in human immunodeficiency virus-Leishmania sp-coinfected patients. J Clin Microbiol. 2000;38:175-8.

53. Schallig HD, Schoone GJ, Kroon CC, et al. Development and application of 'simple' diagnostic tools for visceral leishmaniasis. Med Microbiol Immunol (Berl) 2001;190:69-71.

54. Schoone GJ, Hailu A, Kroon CC, et al. A fast agglutination-screening test (FAST) for the detection of anti-Leishmania antibodies. Trans R Soc Trop Med Hyg. 2001;95:400-1.

55. Sindermann H, Engel KR, Fischer C, et al. Oral miltefosine for leishmaniasis in immunocompromised patients: compassionate use in 42 patients with HIV infection. Clin Infect Dis. 2004;39:1520-3.

56. Singh S, Sivakumar R. Recent advances in the diagnosis of leishmaniasis. J Postgraduate Med. 2003;49:55-60.

57. Singh S. Diagnostic and Prognostic markers of anti-kala-azar therapy and vaccination. Proceeding of V Round Table Conference Series. No. 5. Gupta S and Sood OP (Eds). New Delhi: Ranbaxy Science Foundation; 1999. pp. 95-114.

58. Singh S. Newer developments in diagnosis of leishmaniasis. Indian J Med Research. 2006 .pp. 311-30.

59. Sinha PK, Pandey K, Bhattacharya SK. Diagnosis and management of leishmania/HIV co-infection. Indian J Med Res. 2005;121:407-14.

60. Sundar S, Chaterjee M. Visceral leishmaniasis—current therapeutic modalities. Indian J Med Res. 2006;123: 345-52.

61. Sundar S, Jha TK, Thakur CP, et al. Injectable paromomycin for visceral leishmaniasis in India. The New Eng J Med. 2007;356(25):71-81.

62. Sundar S, Murray HW. Availability of miltefosine for the treatment of kala-azar in India. Bull World Health Organ. 2005;83:394-5.

63. Vipolana C, Blanco S, Dominguiz J, et al. Noninvasive method for diagnosis of visceral leishmaniasis by a latex agglutination test for detection of antigens in urine samples. J Clin Microbiol. 2004;42:1853-4.

64. Weigle KA, de Davalos M, Heredia P, et al. Diagnosis of cutaneous and mucocutaneous leishmaniasis in Colombia: a comparison of seven methods. Am J Trop Med Hyg. 1987;36:489-96.

65. WHO. The World Health Situation of the Global Strategy for Health for All by the Year 2000, 8th Report, 2nd Evaluation, Vol. 1, Global Reviews, Geneva.

66. Williams, Leishmania JE, Trypanosoma. In medical parasitology. A practical approach. In: Gillespie SH, Hawkey PM, (Eds). London: Oxford University Press; 1995.

67. Wortman G, Sweeney C, Houng H-S, et al. Rapid diagnosis of Leishmaniasis by fluorogenic polymerase chain reaction. Am J Trop Med Hyg. 2001;65:583-7.

FUNGAL INFECTIONS

S Balasubramanian, Sumanth Amperayani

INTRODUCTION

Systemic fungal infection in normal hosts is commonly caused by three organisms: (1) Coccidioides, (2) Histoplasma, and (3) Blastomyces, and are restricted to certain geographic areas. Of these three, Histoplasma is notorious to relapse years later when the host is immunocompromised. Immunosuppression, foreign bodies (e.g. central catheters), ulceration of gastrointestinal and respiratory mucosa, broad-spectrum antimicrobial therapy, malnutrition, HIV infection and neutrophil defects are the major risk factors for opportunistic fungal infections.

HIGH INDEX OF SUSPICION IS YIELDING IN FUNGAL INFECTIONS

Fungal infections should be suspected when there is no or inadequate response to apt antibacterial therapy. Important predispositions include prolonged antibiotic therapy, intravascular catheters, parenteral nutrition, endotracheal intubation and mechanical ventilation. Candidiasis is the most common in pediatric age group followed by aspergillosis causing otomycosis or sinonasal infections. Aspergillosis may trigger hyper-reactive airway disease—allergic bronchopulmonary aspergillosis (ABPA). Cryptococcosis goes hand in hand with HIV and mucormycosis can cause pneumonia.

Fungal infections can be practically classified into superficial, subcutaneous, systemic infections—both in normal host and in immunocompromised patients. Table 6.3.1 gives a panoramic of mycoses.

FUNGAL INFECTIONS OF THE SKIN

Dermatophyte Infections

Dermatophytes become attached to the superficial layer of the epidermis, nails and hair, where they proliferate. They do not invade the lower epidermis or dermis and are limited to stratum corneum. Release of toxins from dermatophytes results in dermatitis. Fungal infection should be suspected with any red and scaly lesion.

Tinea capitis

Thickened, broken-off hair with erythema and scaling of underlying scalp are the pathognomonic features. In endemic ringworm, hair are broken off at the surface of the scalp, giving a "black dot" appearance. Pustule formation and a boggy, fluctuant mass on the scalp occurs in *Microsporum canis* and *Trichophyton tonsurans* infections. This is called kerion and represents an exaggerated host response to the organism. Diffuse scaling of the scalp may also be seen. Fungal culture is diagnostic.

Tinea corporis

Tinea corporis presents either as annular marginated plaques with a thin scale and clear center or as an annular confluent dermatitis. The most common organisms are *Trichophyton mentagrophytes* and *M. canis*. The diagnosis is made by scraping thin scales from the border of the lesion, dissolving them in 20% KOH, and examining for hyphae (KOH mount).

Table 6.3.1: Fungal infections.

Type	Fungus	Incidence	Diagnostic test	Treatment	Prognosis
Superficial	Candida Dermatophytes Malassezia	Very common	KOH preparation	Topical	Good
Subcutaneous	Sporothrix	Uncommon	Culture	Oral	Good
Systemic in normal host	Coccidioides Histoplasma Blastomyces	Common	CXR, serology, antigen detection, histology, culture of body fluids and tissue	Systemic	Good
Systemic in immunocompromised host	Candida Aspergillus Pneumocystis Mucorales Malassezia Pseudallescheria Cryptococcus	Uncommon	Tissue biopsy, culture, antigen detection	Systemic	Poor if treatment is delayed

Abbreviations: KOH, potassium hydroxide; CXR, chest X-ray

Tinea cruris

Symmetrical, sharply marginated lesions in inguinal areas occur with tinea cruris. The most common organisms are *Trichophyton rubrum*, *T. mentagrophytes* and *Epidermophyton floccosum*.

Tinea pedis

The diagnosis of tinea pedis is common in the prepubertal child. Presentation is with red scaly soles, blisters on the instep of the foot or fissuring between the toes. The lesions may be painful.

Tinea unguium (Onychomycosis)

Loosening of the nail plate from the nail bed (onycholysis), with yellow discoloration, may be the first give-away feature. Thickening of the distal nail plate then occurs, followed by scaling and a crumbly appearance of entire nail surface. *T. rubrum* and *T. mentagrophytes* are the most common culprits. The diagnosis is confirmed by KOH mount and fungal culture. Usually only one or two nails are involved. If all nails are involved, consider alternate diagnosis with systemic involvement like psoriasis, lichen planus.

Treatment: If hair is involved, systemic griseofulvin is the treatment of choice as topical antifungals do not enter hair or nails in sufficient concentration to eradicate the infection. The absorption of griseofulvin is enhanced by a fatty meal. The dosage of griseofulvin is 20 mg/kg/day. Fungal cultures should be repeated after 4 weeks once and treatment should be continued for another 4 weeks following a negative culture result. Itraconazole and terbinafine are second-line agents when griseofulvin fails. For nails, daily administration of topical ciclopirox 8% can be considered, as can pulsed-dose be itraconazole given in three 1-week pulses separated by 3 weeks.

Tinea corporis, tinea pedis, and tinea cruris can be treated effectively with topical medication after careful inspection to make certain that the hair and nails are not involved. Treatment with any of the imidazoles, allylamines, benzylamines or ciclopirox applied twice daily for 3–4 weeks is recommended.

Tinea Versicolor

Tinea versicolor is a superficial infection caused by *Pityrosporum orbiculare* (also called *Malassezia furfur*), a yeast-like fungus. Polycyclic hypopigmented macules and very fine scales in areas of sun-induced pigmentation are pathognomonic. In winter, the polycyclic macules turn reddish brown.

Treatment: Treatment consists of application of selenium sulfide, 2.5% suspension or topical antifungals. Selenium sulfide should be applied to the whole body and left on overnight. Treatment can be repeated again after 1 week and then monthly thereafter.

Candida albicans

Candida albicans is the most common pathogen in diaper dermatitis and also infects the oral mucosa, where it appears as thick white patches with an erythematous base (thrush); the angles of the mouth, where it causes fissures and white exudate (perlèche); and the cuticular region of the fingers, (candidal paronychia). Dermatitis is characterized by sharply defined erythematous patches, sometimes with eroded areas. Satellite lesions can occur and also in moist areas such as the axillae and neck folds. This is more common in children with prolonged antibiotic therapy.

Treatment: A topical imidazole cream is the drug of first choice for *C. albicans* infections and is best applied every 8–12 hours. In oral thrush, nystatin suspension is applied directly to the oral mucosa. It is not absorbed systemically and acts only topically. In candidal paronychia, the antifungal agent is applied over the area, covered with occlusive plastic wrapping, and left on overnight after the application is made airtight. Oral fluconazole may be contemplated for refractory candidiasis.

BLASTOMYCOSIS

The causative fungus, *Blastomyces dermatitidis*, is found in soil primarily in USA. Transmission is by inhalation of spores. Subclinical disease is common in children and does not have sex predilection. Severe disease is more common in adults.

Symptoms and Signs

Primary infection may be subclinical or may cause pneumonia. Acute symptoms, include cough, chest pain, headache, weight loss and fever occurring several weeks to months after inoculation, suggesting a long incubation period (30–45 days). Infection is usually self-limited in immunocompetent patients. Cutaneous lesions usually represent disseminated disease as local primary inoculation is rare. Skin lesions occur as progressive ulcerations with a sharp, heaped-up border or verrucous lesions. Bone disease is similar to any other form of chronic osteomyelitis. Lytic skull lesions in children are typical, but may involve long bones, vertebrae and the pelvis also. Extrapulmonary disease occurs in 25–40% of patients with progressive disease. A whole body radiographic examination is advisable when blastomycosis is diagnosed in the skin or another non-pulmonary site. The genitourinary tract involvement is rare in children. Lymph nodes, brain and kidneys may be involved.

Laboratory Findings

Diagnosis requires isolation or visualization of the fungus. Sputum, tracheal aspirates or lung biopsy may stain positive with conventional stains or fungal cell wall stains.

Primary response is suppurative followed by mononuclear cell infiltration, and then noncaseating granulomas. The budding yeasts are thick-walled, with refractile walls, and are large. Positivity of sputum specimens is 50–80% and that of skin specimens is 80–100%. The fungus is not fastidious and can be grown easily in 1–2 weeks. Serologic tests are not useful. An enzyme-linked immunosorbent assay (ELISA) antigen detection method, similar to that used for histoplasmosis, is useful for detecting blastomyces antigen in urine and other body fluids.

Imaging

Radiographic consolidation and fibronodular interstitial and alveolar infiltrates are common; effusions, hilar nodes and cavities are uncommon. Miliary pattern may also occur. Chronic pulmonary involvement may cause cavitation in upper lobes along with fibronodular infiltrations but unlike in tuberculosis or histoplasmosis, these rarely caseate or calcify. Thus, this can be differentiated from tuberculosis or histoplasmosis as the disease evolves.

Differential Diagnosis

Primary pulmonary infection mimics acute viral, bacterial or mycoplasmal infections. Subacute infection mimics tuberculosis, histoplasmosis and coccidioidomycosis. Chronic pulmonary or disseminated disease must be differentiated from cancer, tuberculosis or other fungal infections especially histoplasmosis.

Treatment

Mild pulmonary blastomycosis does not warrant treatment. Drug of choice for life-threatening (especially in the immunocompromised patient) or CNS infections is amphotericin-B (0.7–1.0 mg/kg intravenously for a total of 1.5–2.0 g). Itraconazole (6–8 mg/kg/day for 6 months) is preferred for other forms of blastomycosis. Bone disease may require 12 months of itraconazole. Surgical debridement is required for devitalized bone, drainage of large abscesses, and pulmonary lesions not responding to medical management.

CANDIDIASIS

Candidiasis is usually caused by *C. albicans*. Other *Candida* species causing systemic infection are *C. tropicalis*, *C. parapsilosis* and *C. glabrata*. Pathogenicity and response to azole therapy differ according to species. In tissue, pseudohyphae or budding yeast (or both) are seen. *Candida* grows on routine media more slowly than bacteria; growth is usually evident on agar after 2–3 days and in blood culture media in 2–7 days.

Candida albicans is ubiquitous and often presents in small numbers on skin, mucous membranes or in the intestinal tract. Normal bacterial flora, intact epithelial barriers, neutrophils and macrophages in conjunction with antibody and complement, and normal lymphocyte function by skin test reactivity are the host factors which prevent invasion. Disseminated infection is uncommon in immunocompetent individuals and almost always is preceded by prolonged broad-spectrum antibiotic therapy, instrumentation (including intravascular catheters) or immunosuppression. Patients with diabetes mellitus are especially prone to superficial infection most commonly thrush and vaginitis.

Symptoms and Signs

Oral Candidiasis (Thrush)

Adherent creamy white painful plaques on the buccal, gingival or lingual mucosa are seen. Lesions may be few or they may be extensive, extending into the esophagus. Thrush is very common in otherwise normal infants in the first week of life; it may last for weeks despite topical therapy. Spontaneous thrush in older children is unusual unless they have recently received antimicrobials or are immunosuppressed. Corticosteroid inhalation is the most common predisposing factor. Angular cheilitis is caused by *Candida* at the corners of the mouth, often in association with a vitamin or iron deficiency.

Vaginal Infection

Vulvovaginitis occurs in sexually active girls, diabetic patients and in those on prolonged antibiotic therapy. Patients present with thick, odorless, cheesy discharge with intense pruritus. The vagina and labia are erythematous and swollen. Catamenial response is common.

Diaper Dermatitis

Diaper dermatitis most commonly occurs due to *Candida*. Pronounced erythema with a sharply defined margin and satellite lesions are pathognomonic. Pustules, vesicles, papules or scales may be seen. Weeping, eroded lesions with a scalloped border are common. Moist areas such as axillae or neck folds, are frequently involved.

Congenital Skin Lesions

These lesions may be seen in infants born to women with *Candida* amnionitis or after prolonged rupture of membranes in an affected mother. A red maculopapular or pustular rash is characteristic.

Paronychia and Onychomycosis

These conditions may occur in immunocompetent children but are more commonly associated with immunosuppression, hypoparathyroidism or adrenal insufficiency (Candida endocrinopathy syndrome).

Chronic Draining Otitis Media

This is usually preceded by prolonged antibiotic therapy.

Enteric Infection

Esophageal involvement is most common in immuno-suppressed. It manifests as substernal pain, dysphagia, painful swallowing and anorexia. Nausea and vomiting are common in young children. Most patients do not have thrush. Stomach or intestinal ulcers also occur. A syndrome of mild diarrhea in normal individuals who have predominant *Candida* on stool culture, has also been described, although *Candida* is not considered a true enteric pathogen. Its presence more often reflects recent antimicrobial therapy.

Pulmonary Infection

Because the organism frequently colonizes the respiratory tract, it is commonly isolated from respiratory secretions. Thus demonstration of tissue invasion is needed to diagnose *Candida pneumoniae* or tracheitis. It is rare, being seen in immunosuppressed patients and patients intubated for long periods, usually while taking antibiotics. The infection may cause fever, cough, abscesses, nodular infiltrates and effusion.

Renal Infection

Candiduria may be the only manifestation of disseminated disease. More often, candiduria is associated with instrumentation, an indwelling catheter or anatomic abnormality of the urinary tract. Symptoms of cystitis may be present. Masses of *Candida* may obstruct ureters and cause obstructive nephropathy. *Candida* casts in the urine suggest renal tissue infection.

Other Infections

Endocarditis, myocarditis, meningitis, and osteomyelitis may occur in immunocompromised patients or neonates.

Disseminated Candidiasis

Skin and mucosal colonization precedes, but does not predict dissemination. This occurs in neonates—especially premature infants—in an intensive care unit setting, and is recognized when the infant fails to respond to antibiotics or when candidemia is documented. These infants have unexplained feeding intolerance, cardiovascular instability, apnea, new or worsening respiratory failure, glucose intolerance, thrombocytopenia or hyperbilirubinemia. Treatment for presumptive infection is often undertaken because candidemia is not identified in many such patients.

Hepatosplenic candidiasis occurs in immuno-suppressed, severely neutropenic patients with chronic fever, variable abdominal pain and abnormal liver function tests. Symptoms persist even when neutrophils return. Ultrasound or CT scan of the liver and spleen demonstrates multiple round lesions. Biopsy is confirmative.

Laboratory Findings

Budding yeast cells are easily seen in scrapings or other samples. A wet mount preparation of vaginal secretions is 40–50% sensitive; this is increased to 50–70% with the addition of 10% KOH. The use of a Gram-stained smear is 70–100% sensitive. The presence of pseudohyphae suggests tissue invasion. Culture is definitive. Ninety-five percent of positive blood cultures will be detected within 3 days; but in 10–40% cases, cultures may remain negative even with disseminated disease or endocarditis. *Candida* should never be considered a contaminant in cultures from normally sterile sites. Candida in any number in appropriately collected urine suggests true infection. Antigen tests are not sensitive or specific enough for clinical use. Antibody tests are not useful. The ability of yeast to form germ tubes when incubated in human serum gives a presumptive speciation for *C. albicans*.

Differential Diagnosis

Thrush may resemble formula (which can be easily wiped away with a tongue blade or swab, revealing normal mucosa without underlying erythema or erosion), other types of ulcers (including herpes), burns or oral changes induced by chemotherapy. Skin lesions may resemble contact, allergic, chemical or bacterial dermatitis, miliaria, folliculitis, or eczema. Candidemia and systemic infection should be considered in any seriously ill patient with the risk factors previously mentioned.

Complications

Failure to recognize disseminated disease early is the first and foremost complication. Arthritis and meningitis occur more often in neonates than in older children. Blindness from retinitis, massive emboli from large vegetations of endocarditis, and abscesses in any organ are other complications; the greater the length or degree of immunosuppression and the longer the delay before therapy, the more complications are seen.

Treatment

Oral candidiasis: In infants, oral nystatin suspension (100,000 units 4–6 times a day in the buccal fold after feeding until resolution) usually suffices. Clotrimazole troches (10 mg) 4 times a day are an alternative in older children. Painting the lesions with a cotton swab dipped in gentian violet (0.5–1%) is visually dramatic and messy, but may help refractory cases. Eradication of *Candida* from pacifiers, bottle nipples, toys or the mother's breasts (if the infant is breast-feeding) is essential to prevent reinfection.

Oral azoles, such as fluconazole (6 mg/kg/day), are effective in older children with candidal infection refractory to nystatin.

Skin Infection

Cutaneous infection usually responds to a cream or lotion containing nystatin, amphotericin-B or an azole. Diaper dermatitis may yield well with concurrent use of a topical mild corticosteroid cream, such as 1% hydrocortisone.

Vaginal Infections

Vulvovaginal candidiasis is treated with clotrimazole, miconazole, triazoles, or nystatin suppositories or creams, usually applied once nightly for 3–7 days. In general, nystatin is less effective and longer therapy is required. A high-dose clotrimazole formulation needs to be given for only a single night. Candida balanitis in sexual partners should be treated. A single 150 mg oral dose of fluconazole is effective for vaginitis.

Renal Infection

Candiduria is treated with a 7–14 days course of fluconazole, which is concentrated in the urine. Renal abscesses or ureteral fungus balls require intravenous antifungal therapy. Surgical debridement may be required. Removal of an indwelling catheter is imperative. Amphotericin-B may improve poor renal function caused by renal candidiasis, even though the drug is nephrotoxic.

Systemic Infection

Systemic infection is resistant to therapy. Surgical drainage of abscesses and removal of all infected tissue (e.g. a heart valve) are required for cure. Hepatosplenic candidiasis should be treated until all lesions have disappeared or are calcified on imaging studies. Treatment of systemic infection has traditionally utilized amphotericin B. Lipid formulations of amphotericin-B are indicated for patients who have a high likelihood of developing renal toxicity from such therapy. Fluconazole and the newer azole drugs, such as itraconazole (best absorbed from the liquid solution), voriconazole and a new class of drugs, echinocandins, are used interchangeably with amphotericin.

Flucytosine (50–75 mg/kg/day orally in four doses; keeps serum levels below 75 mcg/mL) may be synergistic to amphotericin-B. Unlike amphotericin-B, flucytosine has got better tissue penetration. Monotherapy with flucytosine is not indicated in serious infections as resistance develops rapidly.

Fluconazole, itraconazole and voriconazole are acceptable second line agents for non-neutropenic patients and are often effective as first-line therapy in immunocompromised patients. Infected central venous lines must be removed immediately; this alone is often curative. Persistent fever and candidemia suggest infected thrombus, endocarditis or tissue infection. If the infection is considered limited to the line and environs, a 14-day course (after the last positive culture) of a systemic antifungal agent following line removal is recommended for immunocompromised patients. Fluconazole dosage is 8–12 mg/kg/day in a single daily dose for initial therapy of severely ill children.

Prognosis

Superficial disease in normal hosts has a good prognosis; in abnormal hosts, it may be refractory to therapy. Early therapy of systemic disease is often curative if the underlying immune response is adequate.

COCCIDIOIDOMYCOSIS

Coccidioidomycosis is caused by the dimorphic fungus *Coccidioides immitis*. Infection results from inhalation or inoculation of highly contagious arthrospores. Human-to-human transmission does not occur. More than 50% of all infections are asymptomatic. Chronic pulmonary disease or dissemination occurs in less than 1% of cases.

Symptoms and Signs

Primary disease: The incubation period is 10–16 days (range, 7-28 days). Symptoms vary from mild fever and arthralgia to severe influenza-like illness, pleurisy, myalgias, arthralgias, headache, night sweats and anorexia. Upper respiratory tract signs are uncommon, but severe pleuritic chest pain may suggest this diagnosis.

Skin Disease

Up to 10% of children develop erythema nodosum or multiforme. Less specific maculopapular eruptions are more common. Skin lesions can occur following fungemia. Primary skin inoculation sites develop indurated ulcers with local adenopathy. Contiguous involvement of skin from deep infection in nodes or bone also occurs.

Chronic Pulmonary Disease

This is uncommon in children, but is characterized by chronic cough, hemoptysis, weight loss, consolidation, effusion, cavitation or pneumothorax.

Disseminated Disease

It is more common in infants, neonates and patients with immunosuppression. The most common sites involved are bone or nodes, meninges and kidney.

Laboratory Findings

Direct examination of respiratory secretions, pus, cerebrospinal fluid (CSF) or tissue may reveal large spherules (30–60 m) containing endospores. Phase-contrast microscopy is useful for demonstrating these refractile bodies; periodic acid-Schiff reagent, methenamine silver and calcofluor stains are helpful. Fluffy, gray-white colonies grow within 2–5 days on routine fungal and many other media. CSF cultures are usually sterile.

Peripheral blood eosinophilia is more common in coccidioidomycosis. Meningitis causes a mononuclear pleocytosis (70% with eosinophils) with elevated protein and mild hypoglycorrhachia.

Within 2–21 days, most patients develop a delayed hypersensitivity reaction to coccidioidin skin test antigen (Spherulin, 0.1 mL intradermally, should produce 5 mm induration at 48 hours). Erythema nodosum predicts strong reactivity; when this reaction is present, the antigen should be diluted 10–100 times before use. The skin test may be negative in immunocompromised patients or with disseminated disease. Positive reactions may remain for years and do not prove active infection. All this reads similar to Mantoux test for tuberculosis.

The extent of the complement-fixing antibody response reflects the severity of infection. Persistent high levels suggest dissemination. Serum precipitins usually indicate acute infection. Excellent ELISA assays are now available to detect immunoglobulin M (IgM) and immunoglobulin G (IgG) antibodies against the precipitin and complement-fixing antigens. The presence of antibody in CSF indicates central nervous system (CNS) infection.

Imaging

Approximately, 50% of symptomatic infections are associated with abnormal chest radiographs—usually infiltrates with hilar adenopathy. Pulmonary consolidation, effusion and thin-walled cavities may be seen. Bone infection causes osteolysis that enhances with technetium. Cerebral imaging may show hydrocephalus and meningitis.

Differential Diagnosis

Primary pulmonary infection resembles acute viral, bacterial or mycoplasmal infections; subacute presentation mimics tuberculosis, histoplasmosis and blastomycosis. Chronic pulmonary or disseminated disease must be differentiated from cancer, tuberculosis or other fungal infections.

Complications

Dissemination of primary pulmonary disease is associated with ethnic background, prolonged fever (>1 month), a negative skin test, high complement-fixation antibody titer and marked hilar adenopathy. Local pulmonary complications include effusion, empyema and pneumothorax. Cerebral infection can cause noncommunicating hydrocephalus due to basilar meningitis.

Treatment

Specific measures: Mild pulmonary infections in most normal hosts require no therapy. Antifungal therapy is used for prolonged fever, weight loss (>10%), prolonged duration of night sweats, severe pneumonitis, or any form of disseminated disease. Neonates, pregnant women and patients with high antibody titer also require treatment.

Amphotericin-B is used to treat severe disease (1 mg/kg/day until improvement, then reduce dose; total duration, 2–3 months). Posaconazole and voriconazole appear to be effective second line agent. For less severe disease and for meningeal disease, fluconazole or itraconazole are preferred (duration of therapy is >6 months, and is indefinite for meningeal disease). Measurement of serum levels is suggested to monitor therapy. Chronic fibrocavitary pneumonia is treated for at least 12 months. Lifelong suppressive therapy is recommended after treating coccidioidal meningitis. Itraconazole may be superior to fluconazole. Refractory meningitis may require prolonged intrathecal or intraventricular amphotericin-B therapy.

General Measures

Most pulmonary infections require only symptomatic therapy.

Surgical Measures

Excision of chronic pulmonary cavities or abscesses may be needed. Azole therapy should be given prior to surgery to prevent dissemination, and should be continued for 4 weeks arbitrarily or until other criteria for cure are met.

Prognosis

Most patients recover. Even with amphotericin-B, however, disseminated disease may be fatal. Reversion of the skin test to negative or a rising complement-fixing antibody titer is ominous.

CRYPTOCOCCOSIS

Cryptococcus neoformans is a ubiquitous soil yeast. It appears to survive better in soil contaminated with droppings from avian species, especially that of pigeons. Inhalation is the presumed route of inoculation. Children are rarely affected.

Symptoms and Signs

Pulmonary Disease

It is frequently asymptomatic. Pneumonia is the primary manifestation in one-third of patients and CNS disease in 50%. Symptoms are nonspecific.

Meningitis

The most common clinical disease is meningitis, which follows hematogenous spread from a pulmonary focus. Meningeal signs and papilledema are common. Cranial nerve involvement and seizures may occur.

Other Forms

Cutaneous forms are usually secondary to dissemination. Osteolytic areas are seen. Many other organs, especially the eye, can be involved with dissemination.

Laboratory Findings

The CSF usually has a lymphocytic pleocytosis. Direct microscopy may reveal organisms in sputum, CSF or other specimens. The capsular antigen can be detected by latex agglutination or ELISA, which are both sensitive (>90%) and specific. Serum, CSF and urine may be tested. The organism grows well after several days on many routine media; for optimal culture, collecting and concentrating a large amount of CSF (10 mL) is recommended, because the number of organisms may be low.

Imaging

Radiographic findings are usually lower lobe infiltrates or nodular densities. Single or multiple focal mass lesions (cryptococcoma) may be detected in the CNS on CT or magnetic resonance imaging scan.

Differential Diagnosis

Cryptococcal meningitis may mimic tuberculosis, viral meningoencephalitis, meningitis due to other fungi, or a space-occupying CNS lesion.

Complications

Hydrocephalus may be caused by chronic basilar meningitis. Significant pulmonary or osseous disease may ensure primary infection.

Treatment

Patients with symptomatic pulmonary disease should receive fluconazole for 3–6 months. Severely ill patients should receive amphotericin-B (0.7 mg/kg/day). Meningitis is treated with amphotericin-B and flucytosine (100 mg/kg/day). This combination is synergistic. Therapy is usually 6 weeks for CNS infections (or for 1 month after sterilization) and 8 weeks for osteomyelitis. CSF antigen levels should be checked after 2 weeks of therapy.

Prognosis

Treatment failure, including death, is common in immunosuppressed patients. Lifelong maintenance therapy may be required in these patients. Poor prognostic signs are the presence of extrameningeal disease; fewer than 20 cells/L of initial CSF; and initial CSF antigen titer greater than 1:32.

HISTOPLASMOSIS

The dimorphic fungus *Histoplasma capsulatum* is found in soil and contamination is enhanced by the presence of bat or bird feces. The small yeast form (2–4 m) is seen in tissue, especially within macrophages. Infection is acquired by inhaling spores that transform into the pathogenic yeast phase. Reactivation is very rare in children. The extent of symptoms with primary or reinfection is influenced by the size of the infecting inoculum. Human-to-human transmission and congenital infection does not occur.

Symptoms and Signs

Asymptomatic Infection (90% of Infections)

Asymptomatic histoplasmosis is usually diagnosed by the presence of scattered calcifications in lungs or spleen and a positive skin test, with its nearest differential being Ghon's focus.

Pneumonia

Approximately 5% of patients have mild to moderate disease. Acute pulmonary disease may resemble influenza, with fever, myalgia, arthralgia and cough occurring 1–3 weeks after exposure; the subacute form resembles infections such as tuberculosis, with cough, weight loss, night sweats and pleurisy. Chronic disease is unusual in children. The usual duration of the disease is less than 2 weeks, followed by complete resolution. Symptoms may last several months and still resolve without antifungal therapy.

Disseminated Infection (5% of Infections)

Fungemia during primary infection probably occurs in the first 2 weeks of all infections, including those with minimal symptoms. Resolution is the rule in immunocompetent individuals. Dissemination may occur in otherwise immunocompetent children; usually they are younger than age 2 years.

Other Forms

Ocular involvement consists of multifocal choroiditis and is common in adults. Brain, pericardium, intestine and skin (oral ulcers and nodules) are other involved sites. Adrenal gland involvement is common with systemic disease.

Laboratory Findings

Pancytopenia is present in many patients with disseminated disease. The diagnosis can be made by demonstrating the organism by histology or culture. Cultures may yield the organism after 1–6 weeks of incubation on fungal media. Detection of histoplasmal antigen in blood, urine, CSF and bronchoalveolar lavage fluid is the most sensitive diagnostic test (90% positive in the urine with disseminated disease; 75% positive with acute pneumonia). Antibodies may be detected by immunodiffusion and complement fixation. A single high titer or rising titer indicates a high likelihood of the disease.

Imaging

Scattered pulmonary calcifications in a well-child are typical of past infection. Bronchopneumonia (focal midlung infiltrates) occurs with acute disease, often with hilar and mediastinal adenopathy.

Differential Diagnosis

Pulmonary disease mimics viral infection, tuberculosis, coccidioidomycosis and blastomycosis. Systemic disease mimics disseminated fungal or mycobacterial infection, leukemia, histiocytosis, or cancer.

Treatment

Mild infections do not require therapy. Disseminated disease in infants may respond to as few as 10 days of amphotericin-B, although 4–6 weeks (or 30 mg/kg total dosage) is usually recommended. Amphotericin-B is the preferred therapy for moderately severe forms of the disease. Surgical excision of chronic pulmonary lesions is rarely required. Itraconazole (3–5 mg/kg/day for 6–12 weeks; achieve peak serum level of >1.0 μg/mL) appears to be equivalent to amphotericin-B therapy for mild disease and can be substituted for amphotericin-B in severe disease after a favorable initial response.

Prognosis

Patients with mild and moderately severe infections have a good prognosis. With early diagnosis and treatment, infants with disseminated disease usually recover.

SPOROTRICHOSIS

Sporotrichosis is caused by *Sporothrix schenckii*, a dimorphic fungus present as a mold in soil, plants and plant products. Spores of the fungus can cause infection when they breach the skin at areas of minor trauma. Sporotrichosis has been transmitted from cutaneous lesions of pets.

Symptoms and Signs

Cutaneous disease is by far the most common manifestation. Typically at the site of inapparent skin injury an initial papular lesion will slowly become nodular and ulcerate. Subsequent new lesions develop in a similar fashion proximally along lymphatics draining the primary lesion. This sequence of developing painless, chronic ulcers in a linear pattern is strongly suggestive of the diagnosis. Cavitatory pneumonia is an uncommon manifestation when patients inhale the spores.

Differential Diagnosis

The differential diagnosis of nodular lymphangitis (sporotrichoid infection) includes other endemic fungi, especially atypical mycobacteria.

Treatment and Prognosis

Treatment is with itraconazole (100 mg/day or 5 mg/kg/day) for 3–6 months. Prognosis is excellent with lymphocutaneous disease in immunocompetent children. Pulmonary or osteoarticular disease, especially in immunocompromised individuals, requires longer therapy, and surgical debridement may be required.

OPPORTUNISTIC FUNGAL INFECTIONS

These infections occur most commonly when patients are treated with corticosteroids, antineoplastic drugs, or radiation, thereby reducing the number or function of neutrophils and competent lymphocytes. Inborn errors in immune function (combined immune deficiency or chronic granulomatous disease) may also be complicated by these fungal infections.

Aspergillus species (usually fumigatus) and zygomycetes (usually mucorales) cause subacute pneumonia and sinusitis and should be considered when these conditions do not respond to antibiotics in immunocompromised patients. Aspergillus species are common invasive organisms in patients with chronic granulomatous disease. Mucormycosis is especially likely to produce severe sinusitis in patients with chronic acidosis, usually because of poorly controlled diabetes. This fungus may invade the orbit and cause brain infection. Mucormycosis also occurs in patients receiving iron chelation therapy. These fungal infections may disseminate widely. Imaging procedures may suggest the etiology, but they are best diagnosed by aspiration or biopsy of infected tissues. *Cryptococcus,* which can cause disease in the immunocompetent host, is more likely to be clinically apparent and severe in immunocompromised patients. This yeast causes pneumonia and is a prominent cause of fungal meningitis. *Candida* species in these patients cause fungemia and multiorgan disease, with lung, esophagus, liver and spleen frequently affected.

Malassezia furfur is a yeast that normally causes the superficial skin infection known as tinea versicolor. This organism is considered an opportunist when it is associated with prolonged intravenous therapy, especially central lines used for hyperalimentation. The yeast, which requires skin lipids for its growth, can infect lines when lipids are present in the infusate. Some species will grow in the absence of lipids. Unexplained fever and thrombocytopenia are common. Pulmonary infiltrates may be present. The diagnosis is facilitated by alerting the bacteriology laboratory to add olive oil to culture media. The infection will respond to removal of the line or the lipid supplement. Amphotericin-B may hasten resolution.

Opportunistic fungal infections are always included in the differential diagnosis for immunocompromised patients with unexplained fever or pulmonary infiltrates. These pathogens should be aggressively pursued with imaging studies and with tissue sampling when clues are available. These infections are difficult to treat. Amphotericin-B and appropriate triazole drugs are usually indicated. The echinocandins and voriconazole are now used to treat *Candida* and *Aspergillus* infections. Combinations of current antifungal drugs are being tested to improve the outcome. Many children who will have depressed phagocytic and T-cell, mediated immune function for long periods.

PNEUMOCYSTIS JIROVECI INFECTION

Although classified as a fungus on the basis of structural and nucleic acid characteristics, *Pneumocystis* responds readily to antiprotozoal drugs. It is a ubiquitous pathogen. Initial infection is presumed to occur asymptomatically via inhalation and tends to become a clinical problem upon reactivation during immune suppression. Severe signs and symptoms occur chiefly in patients with abnormal T-cell function such as occurs with HIV infection, hematologic malignancies and organ transplantation. It is one of the AIDS defining illnesses. Prophylaxis usually prevents this infection. Infection is generally limited to the lower respiratory tract. In advanced disease, spread to other organs occurs.

Symptoms and Signs

In most patients, a gradual onset of fever, tachypnea, dyspnea, and mild, non-productive cough occurs over 1–4 weeks. Hypoxemia out of proportion to the clinical and radiographic signs is an early finding. Respiratory failure and death occur without treatment. In children with AIDS or severe immunosuppression, the onset may be abrupt and progression more rapid. Acute dyspnea with pleuritic pain may indicate the related complication of pneumothorax.

Laboratory Findings

Laboratory findings are nonspecific. Serum lactate dehydrogenase levels may be elevated markedly as a result of pulmonary damage.

Imaging

Early chest radiographs are normal. The classic pattern in later films is that of bilateral, interstitial, lower lobe alveolar disease starting in the perihilar regions, without effusion, consolidation or hilar adenopathy. High-resolution CT scanning may reveal extensive ground-glass attenuation or cystic lesions.

Diagnostic Findings

Diagnosis requires finding characteristic round (6–8 mm) cysts in a lung biopsy specimen, bronchial brushings, alveolar washings, induced sputum, or tracheal aspirates. Because pneumonia in immunosuppressed patients may have many causes, negative results from tracheal secretions should prompt more aggressive diagnostic attempts. Bronchial washing using fiberoptic bronchoscopy is usually well tolerated and rapidly performed.

Several rapid stains—as well as the standard methenamine silver stain—are useful. The indirect fluorescent antibody method is most sensitive.

Differential Diagnosis

Chlamydia trachomatis pneumonia is the most common and nearest differential. In older immunocompromised children, the differential diagnosis includes influenza, respiratory syncytial virus, cytomegalovirus, adenovirus and other viral infections; bacterial and fungal pneumonia; pulmonary emboli or hemorrhage; congestive heart failure; and *Chlamydia pneumoniae and Mycoplasma pneumoniae* infections. *Pneumocystis pneumonia* is uncommon in children who are complying with prophylactic regimens.

Prevention

Children at high risk for developing *Pneumocystis* infection should receive prophylactic therapy. The prophylaxis of choice is trimethoprim-sulfamethoxazole (150 mg/m^2/day of trimethoprim and 750 mg/m^2/day of sulfamethoxazole) for three consecutive days of each week.

Treatment

General Measures

The patient should be in respiratory isolation.

Specific Measures

Trimethoprim-sulfamethoxazole (20 mg/kg/day of trimethoprim and 100 mg/kg/day of sulfamethoxazole in four divided doses intravenously or orally if well tolerated) is the treatment of choice. Methylprednisolone (2–4 mg/kg/day in four divided doses intravenously) should also be given to HIV-infected patients with moderate to severe infection (partial oxygen pressure < 70 mm Hg or alveolar-arterial gradient > 35 mm Hg) for the first 5 days of treatment. If trimethoprim-sulfamethoxazole is not tolerated or there is no clinical response in 5 days, pentamidine isethionate (4 mg/kg once daily by slow intravenous infusion) should be given.

Prognosis

The mortality rate is high in immunosuppressed patients who receive treatment late in the illness.

PEARLS IN INVESTIGATING A FUNGAL INFECTION

Diagnosis of a fungal infection is often made by clinical appearance alone. But laboratory examination of skin scrapings, hair or nail cuttings can help when the diagnosis is uncertain.

Fungal specimens are collected to confirm disease when the infection is chronic, severe or when considering systemic therapy. Laboratory fungal testing is also justifiable in the following circumstances:

- To confirm fungal infection before starting on oral treatment
- To determine the species of fungus to allow targeted oral treatment
- On epidemiological grounds.
- How to collect a suitable specimen?
- In most cases, collection of fungal specimens is performed at the laboratory.
- If this is not possible, ensure that the patient has not used antifungal medications for the previous three days.
- If collection of the specimen is proving difficult, then consider asking the patients to do it themselves, under supervision.
- Patients are often more aggressive at getting a good sample than a collector who is trying to be gentle.
- Laboratory analysis:
  ◆ At the laboratory, specimens are first examined under the microscope.
  ◆ Fungal elements are sometimes difficult to find, especially if the tissue is very inflamed.
  ◆ So a negative result does not rule out fungal infection.
  ◆ A sample is then cultured for about 3 weeks.
  ◆ Most positives are reported after 1–2 weeks. Testing has a reasonably low level of sensitivity.
  ◆ So a negative result still does not exclude the presence of a fungal infection.
- Specimen collection should be repeated after a negative result if fungal infection still appears likely, preferably prior to treatment.
- Consider a wide differential diagnosis as there are some other explanations for ring-shaped or scaly rashes, e.g. pityriasis rosea and discoid eczema.
- Negative results may be due to:
- Feature of methodology
- Incorrect initial clinical diagnosis

- Poor collection technique
  ◆ Inadequate specimen
  ◆ Nonviable hyphae elements in the distal region of a nail
  ◆ Uneven colonization
  ◆ Contaminant saprophytic fungi
  ◆ Antifungal treatment
  ◆ A delay in the specimen reaching the laboratory
  ◆ Incorrect laboratory procedures
  ◆ Slow growth of the organism.

Advances in Early Diagnosis

- Microscopy and culture of appropriate specimens remain the gold standard of mycological diagnosis.
- Modern imaging studies, detection of circulating fungal cell wall components and DNA in blood and other body fluids may enhance the laboratory diagnosis of invasive fungal infections (IFIs).
- CT findings characteristic in adults such as the halo and air crescent signs, are rather infrequent in pediatric patients with pulmonary aspergillosis.
- In immunocompromised children at risk, any radiological finding needs to be considered to represent invasive pulmonary mold infection and should prompt further evaluation.
- Hepatosplenic candidiasis can be detected early by ultrasound or MRI.
- MRI is useful to investigate other sites and to guide diagnostic and surgical interventions.
- Detection of cell wall markers—based on their performance in adults, two detection methods have been included in the MSG/EORTC diagnostic criteria developed for clinical research.
  ◆ The galactomannan antigen ELISA
  ◆ The beta-D glucan assay
- Detection of fungal DNA:
  ◆ Polymerase chain reaction (PCR) may be a powerful tool for early diagnosis of IFIs.
  ◆ Twice weekly screening in blood of high-risk children is yielding.
  ◆ Specific detection of fungal pathogens in tissue specimens has emerged as the most feasible clinical applications to date.

BIBLIOGRAPHY

1. Anstead GM, Graybill JR. Coccidioidomycosis. Infect Dis Clin North Am. 2006;20(3):621-43 [PMID: 16984872].
2. Blyth CC, Palasanthiran P, O'Brien TA. Antifungal therapy in children with invasive fungal infections: a systematic review. Pediatrics. 2007;119(4):772-84 [PMID: 17403849].
3. Bonifaz A, Saúl A, Paredes-Solís V, et al. Sporotrichosis in childhood: clinical and therapeutic experience in 25 patients. Pediatr Dermatol. 2007;24(4):369-72 [PMID: 17845157].

4. Burgos A, Zaoutis TE, Dvorak CC, et al. Pediatric invasive aspergillosis: a multicenter retrospective analysis. Pediatrics. 2008;121(5):e1286-94.

5. Catanzaro A, Cloud GA, Stevens DA, et al. Safety, tolerance, and efficacy of posaconazole therapy in patients with nonmeningeal disseminated or chronic pulmonary coccidioidomycosis. Clin Infect Dis. 2007;45(5):562-8 [PMID: 17682989].

6. Chayakulkeeree M, Perfect JR. Cryptococcosis. Infect Dis Clin North Am. 2006;20(3):507-44, v-vi [PMID: 16984867].

7. Denning D, Evans E, Kibbler C, et al. Fungal nail disease: a guide to good practice (report of a working group of the British Society for Medical Mycology). BMJ. 1995;311(7015):1277-81.

8. Gupta AK, Ryder JE, Chow M, et al. Dermatophytosis: the management of fungal infections. Skinmed. 2005;4(5):305-10 [PMID: 16282753].

9. Hidalgo A, Falcó V, Mauleón S, et al. Accuracy of high-resolution CT in distinguishing between *Pneumocystis carinii* pneumonia and non-*Pneumocystis carinii* pneumonia in AIDS patients. Eur Radiol. 2003;13(5):1179-84 [PMID: 12695843].

10. Hotez PJ, Molyneux DH, Fenwick A, et al. Control of neglected tropical diseases. N Engl J Med. 2007;357(10):1018-27 [PMID: 17804846].

11. Kalfa VC, Roberts RL, Stiehm ER. The syndrome of chronic mucocutaneous candidiasis with selective antibody deficiency. Ann Allergy Asthma Immunol. 2003;90(2):259-64 [PMID: 12602677].

12. Kauffmann CA, Bustamante B, Chapman SW, et al. Clinical practice guidelines for the management of sporotrichosis. Clin Infect Dis. 2007;45(10):1255-65 [PMID: 17968818].

13. Kaufman CA. Endemic mycoses: blastomycosis, histoplasmosis, and sporotrichosis. Infect Dis Clin North Am. 2006;20(3):645-62, vii [PMID: 16984873].

14. Kyle AA, Dahl MV. Topical therapy for fungal infections. Am J Clin Dermatol. 2004;5(6):443-51 [PMID: 15663341].

15. Kyle C (Ed). A Handbook for the Interpretation of Laboratory Tests, 4th edition. Auckland: Diagnostic Medlab; 2008.

16. LaRocque RC, Katz JT, Perruzzi P, et al. The utility of sputum induction for diagnosis of *Pneumocystis pneumonia* in immunocompromised patients without human immunodeficiency virus. Clin Infect Dis. 2003;37(10):1380-3 [PMID: 1453873].

17. Lindell RM, Hartman TE, Nadrous HF, et al. Pulmonary cryptococcosis. CT findings in immunocompetent patients. Radiology. 2005;236(1):326-31 [PMID: 15987984].

18. Mahindra AD, Grossman SA. *Pneumocystis carinii* pneumonia in HIV negative patients with primary brain tumors. J Neuro Oncol. 2003;63(3):263-70 [PMID: 12892232].

19. Maschmeyer G, Haas A, Cornely OA. Invasive aspergillosis: epidemiology, diagnosis and management in immuno-compromised patients. Drugs. 2007;67(11):1567-601 [PMID: 17661528].

20. Mennink-Kersten M, Verweij PE. Non-culture-based diagnostics. Infect Dis Clin N Am. 2006;20(3):711-27, viii.

21. Mongkolrattanothai K, Peev M, Wheat LJ, et al. Urine antigen detection of blastomycosis in pediatric patients. Pediatr Infect Dis J. 2006;25(11):1076-8 [PMID: 17072135].

22. Pappas PG. Managing cryptococcal meningitis is about handling the pressure. Clin Infect Dis. 2005;40(3):480-2 [PMID: 15668875].

23. Petrikkos G, Skiada A. Recent advances in antifungal therapy. Inter J Antimicrob Agents. 2007;30:108 [PMID: 17524625].

24. Reddy M, Gill SS, Kalkar SR, et al. Oral drug therapy for multiple neglected tropical diseases. JAMA. 2007;298(16):1911-24 [PMID: 17954542].

25. Ryan ET, Wilson ME, Kain KC. Illness after international travel. N Engl J Med. 2002;347(7):505-16 [PMID: 12181406].

26. Saubolle MA, McKellar PP, Sussland D. Epidemiologic, clinical, and diagnostic aspects of coccidioidomycosis. J Clin Microbiol. 2007;45(1):26-30 [PMID: 17108067].

27. Segal E. Candida, still number one—what do we know and where are we going from there? Mycoses. 2005;48(Suppl 1):3-11 [PMID: 15887329].

28. Shankar SM, Nania JJ. Management of *Pneumocystis jiroveci* pneumonia in children receiving chemotherapy. Paediatr Drugs. 2007;9(5):310-9 [PMID: 17927302].

29. Silveira F, Paterson DL. Pulmonary fungal infections. Curr Opin Pulm Med. 2005;11(3):242-6 [PMID: 15818187].

30. Silveira FP, Hussain S. Fungal infections in solid organ transplantation. Med Mycol. 2007;45(4):305-20 [PMID: 17510855].

31. Spellberg B, Edwards J, Ibrahim A. Novel perspectives on mucormycosis: pathophysiology, presentation, and management. Clin Microbiol Rev. 2005;18(3):556-69 [PMID: 16020690].

32. Spellberg BJ, Filler SG, Edwards JE. Current treatment strategies for disseminated candidiasis. Clin Infect Dis. 2006;42(2):244-51 [PMID: 16355336].

33. Subramanian S, Mathai D. Clinical manifestations and management of cryptococcal infection. J Postgrad Med. 2005;51(Suppl 1):S21-6 [PMID: 16519251].

34. Wheat LJ, Freifeld AG, Kleiman MB, et al. Clinical practice guidelines for the management of patients with histoplasmosis: 2007 update by the Infectious Diseases Society of America. Clin Infect Dis. 2007;45(7):807-25 [PMID: 17806045].

35. Wiley JM, Seibel NL, Walsh TJ. Efficacy and safety of amphotericin-B lipid complex in 548 children and adolescents with invasive fungal infections. Pediatr Infect Dis J. 2005;24(2):167-74 [PMID: 15702047].

36. Zaoutis T, Walsh TJ. Antifungal therapy for neonatal candidiasis. Curr Opin Infect Dis. 2007;20(6):592-7 [PMID: 17975409].

Sankaranarayanan VS

6.4   PARASITIC BOWEL DISEASES

INTRODUCTION

Protozoa and helminths constitute a significant cause of morbidity all over the country. Modern travel emigration and consumption of exotic cuisines allow intestinal helminths to appear in any locale. Many helminths survive for decades within a host, but surprisingly severe disease due to helminths is unusual. Nematodes (roundworms), cestodes (tapeworms) and trematodes (flukes or flat worms) are addressed in this chapter with special focus on epidemiology, life cycle, clinical manifestation, diagnosis and treatment.

Ascaris lumbricoides

Ascaris lumbricoides is the largest of the nematode parasites acquired by ingesting its eggs.

Epidemiology

It is distributed worldwide but more in developing countries with poor sanitation. Children acquire the parasite by playing in dirt contaminated with eggs whereas adults are infected by farming or eating raw vegetable, from plants fertilized with untreated sewage.

Life Cycle

Humans acquire the parasites by ingesting embryonated eggs containing third stage larvae. Fertilized eggs in the soil develop into embryo (molts twice) infective in 10–15 days. Eggs can survive in the soil for 7–10 years. Ingested eggs release larvae in the duodenum and penetrate infesting wall and enter mesenteric venules and lymphatics and enter lungs where they molt twice and ultimately reach small intestine (one more molting) and finally mature. Adult worms live for about 1 year (6–18 months). Worms mate in small intestine and females deposit about 200,000 eggs a day. *Ascaris* do not multiply in the host. Disease usually develops only in those with heavy worm burdens.

Clinical Features

Most infected persons are often asymptomatic or unexpectedly worms are seen in endoscopy or routine stool microscopic examination or in patients the parasite is passed per rectum or vomited rarely. Pulmonary ascariasis can manifest as consolidation or cough and wheeze (Loeffler's syndrome). Intestinal ascariasis can cause abdominal pain, distension, nausea and vomiting, partial or complete intestinal obstruction. Mature worms can enter the ampulla of vater and migrate into the bile or pancreatic ducts causing biliary colic, obstructive jaundice, ascending cholangitis, acalculous cholecystitis or acute pancreatitis. Pregnancy can promote biliary trespass.

Diagnosis

- Stool microscopy—direct smear
- Live adult worms in endoscopy or barium meal studies (long linear filling defects) or endoscopic retrograde cholangiopancreatography (ERCP).
- USG—hepatopancreatic biliary scan reveal long, linear echogenic strips without casting acoustic shadows.

Treatment

Albendazole 400 mg orally once, mebendazole 100 mg bid orally for 3 days or 500 mg once or pyrantel pamoate 11 mg/kg for 3 days (Table 6.4.1).

Table 6.4.1: Treatment of *Ascaris lumbricoides*.				
Indications	**Drug of choice**	**Mode of action**	**Dose**	**Side effects**
Intestinal worms	Albendazole	Paralyses the worms	400 mg orally once in 6 months	GI symptoms—common, elevated liver enzymes and leukopenia—rare
	Mebendazole	Same as albendazole	100 mg bid orally for 3 days	Not recommended below 2 years of age upper GI symptoms, raised SGOT, PT, rash and bone marrow toxicity
	Pyrantel pamoate	Depolarization of neuromuscular junction	11 mg/kg for 3 days	CI: hepatic dysfunction <1 year of age GI disturbances, dizziness
	Piperazine citrate	Paralyses and kills worms by hyperpolar-ization of neuromuscular junction. Useful in heavy worm load of ascaris with intestinal or biliary obstruction	75 mg/kg/day × 2 days	Upper GI symptoms
Pulmonary ascariasis	Albendazole 2 doses Glucocorticoids sometimes to reduce pneumonitis	First dose kills mature worms that finished migrating to the intestine and second dose kills worms that are in transit	400 mg orally 2 doses with 1 month apart	Nausea, vomiting, abdominal pain

STRONGYLOIDOSIS (*STRONGYLOIDES STERCORALIS*)

Introduction

Strongyloides stercoralis larvae infect by penetrating the skin of the feet, pass through the pulmonary phase and settle in the gut. There is no intermittent host to replicate. People at risk to develop strongyloidosis are children with immune suppression, glucocorticoid therapy, military veterans and prisoners of war. Autoinfection is possible. Dermatitis at the site of penetration, larva currens with moving edges in the perianal skin, Loeffler's syndrome, chronic diarrhea with protein-losing enteropathy, malabsorption and duodenitis are the likely manifestations. In immune suppressed hosts, hyperinfection and fatal disseminated strongyloidosis can result due to autoinfection.

Epidemiology

The parasite is endemic in tropical and subtropical soil. Poor sanitation, crowded living condition and warm moist soil contribute to its high level of transmission. Barefoot walkers get easily infected.

Life Cycle

Adult males and females live in soil and lay eggs. Eggs hatch to produce rhabditiform larvae which then mature to adults or develop to larger infective filariform larvae. The filariform larvae penetrate skin and migrate through dermis, enter venous circulation, go to lungs, break into the alveolar space and then enter bronchi. The worms are then swallowed; go to small intestine and remain embedded in jejunal mucosa. Only adult female worms inhabit the small intestine. Females lay fertile eggs and do not require males to reproduce. Rhabditiform larvae are passed in the stool. Autoinfection with filariform larvae is possible.

Clinical Features

Infected persons may present with larva currens migrating cuticare on buttock, thigh and lower abdomen due to external autoinfection. They may also present with wheezy cough, shortness of breath, eosinophilia, pulmonary infiltrates resembling Loeffler's syndrome. Adult worms can cause diarrhea, malabsorption, protein-losing encephalopathy, anorexia, pedal edema, bloody diarrhea in hyperinfection with superadded sepsis and peritonitis. Clinical picture may resemble ulcerative colitis but it is right-sided and eosinophilic colitis. Symptoms are minimal in balanced parasite burden. Massive auto-infection occurs in common variable immunodeficiency (CVID), HIV and AIDS, and may prove fatal due to disseminated fulminant strongyloidiasis and sepsis.

Diagnosis

- Peripheral blood eosinophils may be high.
- Enzyme-linked immunosorbent assay (ELISA) for immunoglobulin (18) G antibodies against *S. stercoralis* is 95% sensitive.
- Stool duct smears for rhabditiform larvae indicates active infestation though insensitive.
- Endoscopic duodenal mucosal biopsy for parasites, insensitive.

Treatment

The drug of choice is ivermectin 200 μg/kg/day for 1–2 days given orally followed by repeat dose after 2 weeks.

Mode of Action

Ivermectin paralyzes the intestinal adult worms, but not the larvae migrating through the tissues and, therefore, patients can develop recurrent infestation from migrating larvae. A repeat dose after two weeks helps to prevent this outcome.

TRICHURIASIS [WHIPWORM (*TRICHURIS TRICHIURA*)

Introduction

Trichuris trichiura, a nematode, inhabits the cecum and the ascending colon. They suck blood up to 0.005 mL/worm/day and cause chronic bloody diarrhea, prolapsed rectum and anemia. A mature female worm lays about 20,000 eggs a day and lives for 3 years.

Epidemiology

It is often seen in school-age children in temperate and tropical countries with poor sanitation. Embryonated parasite eggs are distributed worldwide. Infection develops after ingesting embryonated ova by direct contamination of hands, food or drinks. Transmission can also occur indirectly through flies or other insects.

Life Cycle

Ingestion of parasite egg is followed by escape of larvae in upper small intestine. Then they migrate to cecum, mature, mate and lay eggs in 3 months. Eggs are deposited with feces into the soil. Eggs are not infective till embryonated, so no multiplication in the host and no direct transmission to other persons occur.

Clinical Manifestations

Most infected persons are asymptomatic. Heavy infection produces symptoms like rectal prolapse, mucoid diarrhea, rectal bleed and anemia. Recurrence results in growth retardation.

Diagnosis

Stool examination for *T. trichiura* eggs (barrel shaped). Colonoscopy biopsy may show increase in mast cells. There is no significant eosinophilia.

Treatment

Mebendazole 100 mg bid for 3 days or alternatively albendazole 400 mg orally. Heavy infections may be treated with albendazole for 3 days.

ENTEROBIOSIS (*ENTROBIUS VERMICULARIS*)

Introduction

Enterobius vermicularis or pinworm infection is commonly seen in primary care providers due to ingestion of parasite eggs. Mostly the infected persons remain asymptomatic. Recurrence is common despite treatment for family members. *E. vermicularis* eggs that are ingested hatch out in the gut and inhabit at the cecum and appendix. The female worms migrate to perianal region, especially in the night to lay eggs. The eggs may remain viable for 3 weeks causing intense perianal itching, sleeplessness, vulvitis, nocturnal enuresis, colitis and salpingitis. Autoinfection and retroinfection are expected necessitating cyclical treatment.

Epidemiology

Enterobiasis spreads by contact with colonized persons. It is seen among all socioeconomic groups. School children suffer more, especially in overcrowded and if institutionalized. Eggs survive up to 3 weeks and they are chlorination resistant (e.g. swimming pools).

Life Cycle

"Hand-to-mouth" existence is common. Ingestion of parasite eggs from hands of the host followed by swallowing and hatching in duodenum. The larva mottled twice, migrates to cecum and ascending colon. The adult worm mates and migrates to rectum. Gravid females migrate at night and lay eggs in the perianal and perineal skin. Eggs from female parasite mature and are infective within 6 hours. Auto-infection from scratched hands with frequent reinfection and transmission to others is common.

Clinical Aspects

Mostly asymptomatic. Pruritus ani and restless sleeping is the most common manifestation. Rarely eosinophilic enteritis, vulvovaginitis in girls, granuloma of female genitalia and uterine adnexa due to dead worms and eggs may occur.

Diagnosis

Stool examination for parasite eggs is often negative. NIH cellophane tape test is diagnostic. Mostly 3–7 daily samplings may be required.

Treatment

Mebendazole 100 mg orally or albendazole 400 mg orally followed by same dose after 15 days. All members of family should be treated.

TRICHINELLA SPECIES (*T. SPIRALIS, T. BRITORIS, T. NELSONI, ETC.*)

Introduction

Seen in raw or undercooked meat often pork eaters which contain parasite larvae of *Trichinella*. Trichinosis is a systemic illness caused by any of the eight closely related *Trichinella* species. Trichinosis has both intestinal and systemic phases characterized sequentially by nausea and diarrhea, fever, myalgia and periorbital edema. Intense exposure can cause death due to severe myositis, neuritis and thrombosis. Treatment is albendazole and glucocorticoids.

Epidemiology

Carriers are pigs. Distribution is worldwide. All mammals including herbivores can transmit *Trichinella*.

Life Cycle

Infection occurs after ingestion of raw or undercooked meat like pork containing encapsulated parasite larvae. In the small intestinal mucosa, the mature worms mate within 30 hours. The females release larvae within a week and adults produce larvae in 4 weeks and then get expelled of the host. Larvae in circulation enter striated muscle but do not kill the myocyte. Larvae grow, become infective in 5 weeks and remain viable for many years.

Clinical Aspects

Adult worms can produce enteritis, abdominal pain, nausea, vomiting, low-grade fever and diarrhea. Symptoms develop 1–2 weeks after ingestion of contaminated meat often misdiagnosed as viral gastroenteritis or food poisoning. *T. spiralis* infests mice and rats also. The larval stage of parasite due to involvement of brain, spinal cord, heart may present as high fever, myalgia, periorbital edema, dysphagia, headache and paresthesia and lasts for 4–5 weeks. Myositis is usual with elevated eosinophilia and serum creatine phosphokinase (CPK).

Diagnosis

Not possible with routine stool examination or intestinal biopsy as *T. species* do not lay eggs. Diagnosis is often by muscle biopsy showing larvae within the nerve cells. Serology for parasites antibody is also useful.

Treatment

Albendazole 400 mg bid or mebendazole 5 mg/kg/day for 10–15 days. Symptomatic treatment with glucocorticoids in selective cases.

HOOKWORMS (ANCYLOSTOMA DUODENALE/NECATOR AMERICANUS)

Introduction

Hookworm infection is the infection caused by *Ancylostoma duodenale* or *Necator americanus* (nematodes) and may occur as single or mixed infection in the same person. *N. americanus* is predominant in South India, whereas *A. duodenale* in North India. Recently, another species, *A. ceylanicum* has been reported from a village near Kolkata. The heavily infected areas are found in Assam (tea gardens), West Bengal, Bihar, Odisha, Andhra Pradesh, Tamil Nadu, Kerala and Maharashtra. Morbidity and mortality from hookworm infection depends much on the worm load. Adult worms live mainly in jejunum attached to the villi and suck up to 0.2 mL of blood per worm per day. Eggs are passed in the feces in thousands. The rhabditiform larva molts in the soil and penetrates the skin usually feet within 5–10 days (ground itch), migrates via lymphatics and blood stream to lungs (Loeffler's syndrome) and reaches intestine by swallowing. Hookworm infestation causes chronic blood loss resulting in iron deficiency anemia, hypoalbuminemia and peptic ulcer like pain.

Life Cycle

Small adult worms (1 cm long) reside in the small intestine. Infection occurs by the larvae penetrating skin often between toes of barefooter and then enter capillaries, lungs, alveoli and ascend respiratory tract. It is then swallowed and enters intestine. Adult worms can live up to 14 years. Mild infestations cause no symptoms. Moderate-to-heavy hookworm infestation results in iron deficiency as the adult worms feed on intestinal epithelial cells and blood. Intestinal blood loss is estimated to be 0.01–0.04 mL/day per adult *N. americanus* and 0.05–0.3 mL/day per adult *A. duodenale*. Iron deficiency results when iron loss outstrips iron absorption. Local skin rash, itch and eosinophilia are found.

Diagnosis

Stool examination for typical eggs (three different days). Sometimes, the worms may be endoscopically visible and confirmed by direct smear for eggs. Stool concentration technique, sometimes, useful. Morphologic differentiation of *N. americanus* from *A. duodenale* is difficult.

Treatment

Albendazole 400 mg orally as a single dose or mebendazole 100 mg bid for 3 days.

CAPILLARIA (PARACAPILLARIA) PHILIPPINENSIS

Uncommon parasite in our set-up, acquired by eating raw fish that are infested with the parasite, replicates in the host producing intestinal worms. Birds not humans are natural hosts. Eggs are deposited in bird droppings into ponds and rivers, swallowed by fish, eating raw or undercooked, freshwater or brackish water fish containing parasite larva. Autoinfection is possible. Clinically manifests as sprue-like illness. Vague abdominal pain, borborygmi 2–3 weeks after infection, recurrent diarrhea, protein-losing enteropathy, edema, dehydration and hypokalemia. Sometimes untreated cases end fatally due to cardiac failure.

Diagnosis

Stool examination for typical eggs and larvae. No serologic tests available. Endoscopic mucosal biopsy may reveal the adult worm.

Treatment

Extended anthelminthic treatment with albendazole 200 mg daily orally bid for 10 days or mebendazole 200 mg orally bid for 20 days to prevent recurrence.

DIPHYLLOBOTHRIUM LATUM (SYN: FISH TAPEWORM)

Introduction

Diphyllobothrium latum is a cestode and is the largest human parasite (up to 12 meters). Infection results from eating raw or undercooked freshwater fish. *D. latum* absorbs dietary cobalamin and causes vitamin B_{12} deficiency over time. Habitat is small intestine. Clinically, megaloblastic anemia and neurologic symptoms are due to vitamin B_{12} deficiency. Diagnosis is by identifying *D. latum* eggs in stool which are abundant in stool.

Treatment

Praziquantel 10 mg/kg/oral single dose. Patient should be warned that he may pass a long worm 2–5 hours after taking the medication. Alternatively, albendazole 400 mg daily for 3 days also kills tapeworm.

HYMENOLEPIS NANA (DWARF TAPEWORM)

Introduction

Most common tapeworm of humans. Unlike other tapeworms, it can be transmitted from person to person.

In infected persons, anorexia, abdominal pain and diarrhea are the common symptoms. No intermediate host is required as the entire life cycle can be completed in humans. Ingested eggs—oncospheres—small intestinal mucosa, lymphatics of villi, cysticercoids larvae, proglottids of adult worms. Ineffective sanitation and lack of handwashing permits transmission to others.

Diagnosis

Repeated stool microscopic examination for eggs.

Treatment

Praziquantel 25 mg/kg single oral dose for adult worms and a repeat dose after 1 week for eggs. Treatment of family members after examination.

TAENIASIS

Introduction

Taenia saginata (beef tapeworm) and *Taenia solium* (pork tapeworm) are the two important cystode infections of zoonotic diseases. *T. saginata* is seen among beef eaters. The larval stage of *T. saginata* occurs almost all over the world. *T. solium* is endemic in India. Human cysticercosis caused by *T. solium* is a more important public health problem. Both *T. solium* and *T. saginata* pass their lifecycle in two hosts. In man, the adult parasites live in the small intestine. Man is the definitive, and cattle are the intermediate host for *T. saginata*. Man is the definitive host and pig is the intermediate host for *T. solium*. The larval stage of *T. saginata* and *T. solium* occurs in cattle and pig respectively. Man may also be infected causing muscular, ocular and cerebral cysticercosis. The encysted larvae may live up to 5 years and cause space-occupying lesions (such as neurocysticercosis in the brain). Persons who handle the pigs may also get the lesions.

TAENIA SAGINATA (BEEF TAPEWORM) AND TAENIA SOLIUM (PORK TAPEWORM)

Infection occurs following ingestion of eating raw or undercooked meat infested with cysticerci. Often asymptomatic but accidental endoscopic finding sometimes occurs. Ingestion of *T. solium* eggs causes cysticercosis. Ingested eggs—oncosphere—penetrates intestinal wall, blood vessels or lymphatics, subcutaneous tissue, muscle and organs, cysticerci live for several years in the intestine, scolex attaches to proximal jejunum, proglottids, strobila, stool in proglottids.

Clinically symptoms include mild abdominal discomfort, anorexia and change in stool pattern. Cysticercosis occurs when *T. solium* eggs are ingested; eggs release oncospheres—intestinal wall—disseminate through the body and form cysticerca. Cysticerci cause localized inflammation in the brain, spinal cord, eye and heart, and cause seizures.

Diagnosis

Diagnosis includes identification of eggs or proglottids in the stool, MRI brain and serology using a larval cyst antigen—specific immunoblot.

Treatment

Single oral dose of albendazole 10 mg/kg or albendazole 400 mg daily for 3 days. Patients with cysticercosis can be treated with albendazole 15 mg/kg daily for 8 days to kill the cysticerci.

ECHINOCOCCOSIS (HYDATID DISEASE)

Introduction

Hydatid disease is a zoonosis—a group of cystode infections of man caused by the infective larva of canine intestinal tapeworm, *Echinococcus*. Hydatidosis is prevalent in Andhra Pradesh and Tamil Nadu. Presently four species are seen namely *E. granulosis, E. multilocularis, E. oliganthus* and *E. vogeli*. Basically, it is a dog-sheep cycle with man as an accidental intermediate host. Man does not harbor the adult worm. Infection occurs when human eats vegetables contaminated by dog feces containing embryonated eggs. The eggs hatch in the small intestines and liberate oncospheres that penetrate the mucosa and migrate via vessels or lymphatics to the distal sites like liver, lungs, kidney, spleen, brain and bone in the order of frequency. In these organs, a hydatid cyst/cysts develop by vesticulation and produces thousands of protoscolices causing mass lesions rupture of the hydatid cyst may cause severe anaphylactic reactions.

CRYPTOSPORIDIUM INFESTATION

Introduction

Cryptosporidium parvum with two genotypes and *C. hominis* infect the gastrointestinal epithelium of wide range of vertebrates and cause most infections. These are spore-forming intestinal protozoa. Isospora, cyclospora and microsporidia are other spore-forming protozoa. But microsporidia has now been reclassified as fungi and it causes a broader spectrum of disease. Contaminated water or close contact with infected animals results in infection which occurs as a result of ingestion of oocysts. Multiplication occurs in lower ileum. Incubation period is 5–7 days. The protozoa attaches to enterocyte and in immune competent persons, it causes self-limiting diarrhea lasting for 1–4 weeks under 5 years of age. Upon ingestion of 1–10 oocysts, excystation and release of sporozoa in the presence of bile salts in small intestine occurs. The sporozoites attach to intestinal epithelium, enclosed inside the villi area and develop into merozoites which replicate asexually. Excystation and infection of neighboring cells follow. Both humoral and cellular immune responses are in control of *Cryptosporidium* infections and cause severe life-threatening diarrhea in children with immune deficiency, lymphocytic malignancies and low CD4-associated HIV.

Epidemiology

Infection is common under the age of 2 years. Autoinfection is common. Few cysts are adequate to cause infection. High-risk groups are HIV infection, severe combined immunodeficiency (SCID), agammaglobulinemia, leukemia or post-measles malnutrition. Infection lasts up to 2 weeks and discharges oocysts for several more weeks. Diarrheal symptoms may be associated with specific assemblages and assemblage B has been found to be more human restricted than assemblage A.

Clinical Aspects

Asymptomatic in healthy individuals or self-limiting watery diarrhea associated with nausea, vomiting and abdominal colic and, sometimes, dehydration, fever and lactose intolerance and persistent diarrhea.

Diagnosis

- Stool microscopic examination for oocysts using modified kinyoun acid—fast-stain technique
- Enzyme-linked immunosorbent assay for *Cryptosporidium* antigen in the stool
- Duodenal mucosal biopsy for parasites as well as villus atrophy.

Treatment

In normal children, it is supportive and in children with HIV, antiretroviral therapy in addition to nitazoxanide bovine immunoglobulin and azithromycin with paromomycin is recommended.

Prevention is important in immune compromised hosts. Handwashing is useful. Oocysts are susceptible to heat and drying.

Prevention of Parasitic Bowel Diseases in General

- Periodic en mass albendazole given at 6 monthly single dose especially in high endemic areas.
- Health education of parents regarding personal (such as handwashing after defecation, nail clipping) and environmental hygiene like proper disposal of human excreta, safe water supply, avoidance of barefoot walking and open air defecation and awareness to public through media are some of the prevention strategies. Maintenance of growth charts to detect malnutrition.
- Specific prevention strategies of organism.

BIBLIOGRAPHY

1. Gupta Y, Gupta M, Aneja S, et al. Current therapy of protozoal diseases. Indian J Pediatr. 2004:71(1):55-8.
2. IAP Textbook of Pediatrics, 4th edition. New Delhi: Jaypee Brothers; 2009. pp. 616-20.
3. Laishram S, Kang G, Ajjampur SS, et al. Giardiasis: a review on assemblage distribution and epidemiology in India. Indian J Gastroenterol. 2012;31(1):3-12.
4. Sleisenger, Fordtrans. Gastrointestinal and Liver Disease, 9th edition. 2010.pp.1905-39.
5. Sur D, Satha DR, Manna B, et al. Periodic de-worming with alabendazole and its impact on growth status and diarrheal incidence among children in an urban slum of India. Trans R Soc Trop Med Hyg. 2005;99(4):261-7.
6. Vohra P. Intestinal parasites in children. IAP Speciality Series on Pediatric Gastroenterology. New Delhi: Jaypee Brothers; 2008. pp.107-24.

Sutapa Ganguly

INTRODUCTION

Amebiasis is a parasitic infection caused by protozoon *Entameba histolytica*. Amebiasis is the third leading parasitic cause of death worldwide, surpassed by malaria and schistosomiasis. On a global basis, amebiasis affects approximately 50 million persons each year, resulting in nearly 100,000 deaths. This represents the tip of iceberg because only 10–20% of infected individuals become symptomatic.

The parasite has two forms: (1) a motile form called trophozoite, and (2) a cyst form, responsible for the person-to-person transmission of infection. The trophozoite of *E. histolytica* inhabits the large intestine to produce amebic colitis. Invasion of the colonic mucosa leads to dissemination of the organism to extracolonic sites, predominantly the liver. Faced with an adverse colonic environment, the trophozoite changes to the cystic form better adapted to survival.

PATHOPHYSIOLOGY

Amebiasis is acquired by the fecal oral route through consumption of fecally contaminated water or food. Direct oral anal contact can also be mode of acquisition of the infection. The ingestion of *E. histolytica* cysts is followed by excystation in the small bowel and invasion of the colon by the trophozoites. The incubation period varies from 2 days to 4 months. Invasive disease begins with the adherence of *E. histolytica* to colonic mucins, epithelial cells and leukocytes. Adherence of the trophozoites is mediated by a galactose and N-acetylgalactosamine-specific lectin.

The trophozoites of *E. histolytica* lyse the target cells by using lectin to bind to the target cells membranes and using the parasites ionophore like protein to induce a leak of ions (e.g. Na^+, K^+, Ca^+) from the target cell cytoplasm.

Spread of amebiasis to the liver occurs via the portal blood. The torphozoites ascend the portal veins to produce liver abscesses filled with a cellular proteinaceous debris. The material has the appearance of anchovy sauce. The trophozoites of *E. histolytica* lyse the hepatocytes and neutrophils which explain the paucity of inflammatory cells within the liver abscesses. The neutrophil toxins may contribute to hepatocyte necrosis. Triangular areas of hepatic necrosis may also occur due to ischemia caused by portal venous obstruction. The trophozoites of *E. histolytica* may be present along the periphery of these hepatic lesions.

Serum antibodies in patients with amebic liver abscess develop in 7 days and persist for as long as 10 years. *E. dispar* infections do not elicit antibody response, unlike asymptomatic *E. histolytica* infections. Mucosal immunoglobulin A (IgA) response to *E. histolytica* occurs during invasive amebiasis. However, no evidence suggests that invasive amebiasis is increased in incidence or severity in patients with IgA deficiency. Cell-mediated immunity is important in limiting the disease and preventing recurrences. Antigen-specific blastocemic responses occur, leading to production of lymphokines, including interferon-α (INF-α), which activates the killing of *E. histolytica* trophozoites by macrophages. During acute invasive amebiasis, T-lymphocyte response to *E. histolytica* antigen is depressed by a parasite-induced serum factor.

Reports suggest that amebic liver abscess is an emerging parasite infection in individuals with HIV infection in disease-endemic areas as well as nondisease-endemic areas.

CLINICAL FEATURES

The incubation period is commonly 2–4 weeks but ranges from a few days to years. Amebiasis is more severe in very young patients, in elderly patients and in patients receiving corticosteroids. The clinical spectrum of amebiasis ranges from asymptomatic infection to fulminant colitis and peritonitis to extraintestinal amebiasis, most commonly amebic liver abscess. The clinical expression of amebiasis may be related to geography. For instance, amebic colitis is the predominant presentation in Egypt, whereas amebic liver abscesses predominate in South Africa.

Asymptomatic infections are common following ingestion of the parasite. *E. dispar* does not cause invasive disease or antibody production. As many as 90% of *E. histolytica* infections are also asymptomatic. The infection is self-limited but may be recurrent. Only antigen detection tests can distinguish between *E. histolytica* and *E. dispar*.

Amebic colitis is gradual in onset, with symptoms presenting over 1–2 weeks, distinguishing it from bacterial dysentery. Diarrhea is the most common symptom. Patients with amebic colitis typically present with cramping abdominal pain, watery or bloody diarrhea, and weight loss. Fever is noted in 10% of patients.

Fulminant amebic colitis is a rare complication of amebic dysentery (< 0.5%). It presents with a rapid onset of severe bloody diarrhea, severe abdominal pain and high fever. Children younger than 2 years are at increased risk. Intestinal perforation is common. Patients may develop toxic megacolon, which is typically associated with the use of corticosteroids. Mortality rates with fulminant amebic colitis may exceed 40%.

Chronic amebic colitis is clinically similar to inflammatory bowel disease. Recurrent episodes of bloody diarrhea and vague abdominal discomfort develop in 90% of patients with chronic amebic colitis who have antibodies to *E. histolytica*. Amebic colitis should be ruled out prior to treatment of suspected inflammatory bowel disease because corticosteroid therapy worsens amebiasis.

A less common form of intestinal disease (e.g. ameboma) results from formation of annular colonic granulation in response to the infecting amebae, resulting in a large local lesion of the bowel. It presents as a right lower quadrant abdominal mass, which may be mistaken for carcinoma, tuberculosis, Crohn's disease, actinomycosis or lymphoma. Biopsy findings assist in establishing the correct diagnosis.

Amebic liver abscess is the most common form of extraintestinal amebiasis. It results from spread of the organisms from the intestinal submucosa to the liver via the portal system. However, approximately 40% of patients who have amebic liver abscess do not have a history of prior bowel symptoms. It occurs in as many as 5% of patients with symptomatic intestinal amebiasis and is ten times as frequent in men as in women. Approximately, 80% of patients with amebic liver abscess present within 2–4 weeks of infection and they present with fever and a constant, dull, upper right abdominal or epigastrium pain. Involvement of the diaphragmatic surface of the liver may lead to right-sided pleuritic pain or referred shoulder pain. Associated gastrointestinal (GI) symptoms occur in 10–35% of patients and include nausea, vomiting, abdominal distention, diarrhea and constipation. A small subset of patients with amebic liver abscess has a subacute presentation with vague abdominal discomfort, weight loss and anemia. Jaundice is unusual.

Pleuropulmonary amebiasis is most commonly the result of contiguous spread from a liver abscess rupturing through the right hemidiaphragm. However, a case of amebic lung abscess acquired through hematogenous spread has been reported. The typical age group is 20–40 years. The male-to-female ratio is 10:1. Approximately, 10% of patients with amebic liver abscess develop pleuropulmonary amebiasis, which presents with cough, pleuritic pain and dyspnea. A hepatobronchial fistula is an unusual problem characterized by the expectoration of sputum resembling anchovy paste. The trophozoites of *E. histolytica* may be found in the sputum sample.

Amebic peritonitis is generally secondary to a ruptured liver abscess. Left lobe liver abscesses are more likely to rupture. Patients present with fever and rigid distended abdomen. Roughly 2–7% of liver abscesses rupture into the peritoneum.

Amebic pericarditis is rare but is the most serious complication. It is usually caused by a rupture of the left liver lobe abscess and occurs in 3% of patients with hepatic amebiasis. It presents with chest pain and the features of congestive heart failure.

Amebic abscesses resulting from hematogenous spread have occasionally been described in the brain. Cerebral amebiasis has an abrupt onset and rapid progression to death in 12–72 hours. The patient presents with altered consciousness and focal neurologic signs. CT scanning reveals irregular lesions without a surrounding capsule or enhancement. A tissue biopsy sample reveals the trophozoites.

Genitourinary involvement may cause painful genital ulcers or may involve the fallopian tube.

LABORATORY STUDIES

Stool

- *Light microscopy:* Examination of a fresh stool smear for trophozoites that contain ingested RBCs is rather insensitive. Routine microscopy cannot distinguish the *E. dispar* and *E. moskovskii* (nonpathogenic amebae) from *E. histolytica*.
- An enzyme immunoassay kit to specifically detect *E. histolytica* in fresh stool specimens is commercially available.
- Polymerase chain reaction (PCR)-based diagnostic tests have been developed but are not widely available. Field studies that directly compared PCR with stool culture or antigen-detection tests for the diagnosis of *E. histolytica* infection suggest that these methods are equally comparable.
- Other stool tests:
  - The stool samples are always heme positive.
  - Fecal leukocytes may be absent.

Serum Tests

Antibody tests: Serum antibodies against amebae are present in 70–90% of individuals with symptomatic intestinal *E. histolytica* infection. Antiamebic antibodies are present in as many as 99% of individuals with liver abscess who have been symptomatic for longer than a week. Serologic examination should be repeated a week later in those with negative test on presentation. However, serologic tests do not distinguish new from past infection because the seropositivity persists for years after an acute infection. Several methods are commercially available for antibody detection.

Indirect hemagglutination antibody (IHA) test detects antibody specific for *E. histolytica*. The antigen used in IHA consists of a crude extract of axenically cultured organisms. Antibody titers of more than 1:256 to the 170-kd subunit of the galactose-inhibitable adherence lectin are noted in approximately 95% of patients with extraintestinal amebiasis, 70% of patients with active intestinal infection, and 10% of asymptomatic individuals. IHA is not useful in differentiating acute from previous infection because high titers may persist for years after successful treatment. False-positive reactions at titers higher than 1:256 are rare.

Enzyme immunoassay (EIA) is as sensitive and specific as the IHA test and has replaced IHA in most laboratories.

Immunodiffusion (ID) is simple to perform, making it ideal for the laboratory that has only an occasional request for amebic serology. However, it requires a minimum of 24 hours to complete, compared with 2 hours for the IHA or EIA test. ID is slightly less sensitive than IHA and EIA, but is equally specific.

Although detection of immunoglobulin M (IgM) antibodies specific for *E. histolytica* has been reported, sensitivity in patients with current invasive disease is only about 64%.

The galactose lectin antigen is present in the serum of 75% of subjects with amebic liver abscess and may be particularly useful in patients presenting acutely, before an immunoglobulin G (IgG) serum antiamebic antibody response occurs.

Imaging

Chest radiography may reveal an elevated right hemidiaphragm and a right-sided pleural effusion in patients with amebic liver abscess.

Ultrasonography is preferred for the evaluation of amebic liver abscess because of its low cost, rapidity, and lack of adverse effects. A single lesion is usually seen in the posterosuperior aspect of the right lobe of the liver. Multiple abscesses may occur in some patients. In an ultrasonographic evaluation of 212 patients, 34 (16%) had multiple abscesses, 75 (35%) had an abscess in the left lobe and the remaining 103 (49%) had a solitary abscess in the right lobe.

Computed tomography (CT) may be slightly more sensitive than ultrasonography. In cerebral amebiasis, CT shows irregular lesions without a surrounding capsule or enhancement.

Magnetic resonance imaging reveals high signal intensity on T2-weighted images. Perilesional edema and enhancement of rim are noted after injection of gadolinium (86%).

Complete resolution of liver abscess may take as long as 2 years. Repeat imaging is not indicated if the patient is otherwise doing well.

Other Tests

- Leukocytosis without eosinophilia is observed in 80% of cases.
- Mild anemia may be noted.
- Liver function tests reveal elevated alkaline phosphatase levels (in 80% of patients), elevated transaminase levels, mild elevation of serum bilirubin level, and reduced albumin levels.
- The erythrocyte sedimentation rate is elevated.

PROCEDURES

Endoscopy

Rectosigmoidoscopy and colonoscopy with biopsy or scraping at margin of colonic mucosal ulcer provides valuable materials for diagnostic information in intestinal amebiasis. Small mucosal ulcers covered with yellowish exudates are observed. The mucosal lining between ulcers appears normal (Fig. 6.5.1). Rectosigmoidoscopy and colonoscopy should be considered before using steroids in patients in whom inflammatory bowel disease is suspected. Biopsy results and a scraping of ulcer edge may reveal trophozoites.

Indications for endoscopy in suspected intestinal amebiasis include the following:
- Stool examination findings are negative, but the serum antibody test findings are positive.
- Stool examination findings are negative, but immediate diagnosis is required.
- Stool examination and antibody test results are negative, but amebiasis is strongly suspected.
- Evaluation of chronic intestinal syndromes or mass lesions is desired.

Aspiration

Aspiration of the liver abscess is occasionally required to rule out a pyogenic abscess. Aspiration amebic liver abscess yields an anchovy paste-like material that lacks WBCs due to lysis by the parasite. Amebae are visualized in the abscess fluid in a minority of patients with amebic liver abscess. Aspiration of liver is indicated only for large abscesses (>12 cm), imminent abscess rupture, failure of medical therapy or presence of left lobe.

TREATMENT

Antiamebic drugs are categorized into luminal and tissue amebicides. Tissue amebicides include 5-nitromidazoles, chloroquine and dehydroemetine, which are effective in

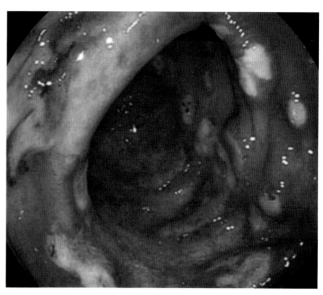

FIG. 6.5.1: Distinctive endoscopic findings of amebic colitis, multiple ulcerous lesions are present with exudate in the sigmoid colon.

the treatment of invasive amebiosis but are less effective in luminal conditions. Luminal amebicides include diloxanide furoate, diiodoquinol and paromomycin. Asymptomatic infections are not treated in endemic areas. However, in nonendemic areas, asymptomatic infection should be treated because of its potential to progress to invasive disease. Luminal agents that are minimally absorbed by the GI tract (e.g. paromomycin, iodoquinol, diloxanide furoate) are best suited for such therapy, but reinfection is quite common even after complete cure. It is recommended that persons when infected with *E. histolytica* should be specifically identified and treated; treatment with individuals with *E. dispar* is unnecessary.

Metronidazole is the mainstay of therapy for invasive amebiasis. Tinidazole has been recently approved by the US Food and Drug Administration (FDA) for intestinal or extraintestinal amebiasis. Other nitroimidazoles with longer half-lives (e.g. secnidazole, ornidazole) are currently available but experience in children is limited. Nitroimidazole therapy leads to clinical response in approximately 90% of patients with mild-to-moderate amebic colitis. Metronidazole is the most popular drug for management of both intestinal and extraintestinal forms of amebiasis. Till date, there is no evidence of resistance against this agent.

Amebic colitis is treated by metronidazole followed by a luminal agent to eradicate colonization. Fulminant amebic cholitis even with perforation may be managed conservatively with addition of antibiotics to deal with bowel flora. Radiographic monitoring of the abdomen by CT scan coupled with judicious use of percutaneous catheter drainage may aid in further management.

Most amebic liver abscesses, even of large size, can be cured without drainage. Most patients show a response to treatment (reduced abdominal pain and fever) within 72–96 hours. They should also receive a luminal agent to eliminate intestinal colonization. The role of ultrasound or CT-guided percutaneous therapeutic aspiration in the treatment of uncomplicated liver abscess is controversial. Large abscesses (> 300 mL) may benefit from aspiration with decrease duration of hospital stay and faster clinical recovery when compared to those manage medically alone. Abscess cavity resolves slowly over a period of several months.

Broad-spectrum antibiotics may be added to treat bacterial superinfection in a case of fulminant amebic colitis and suspected perforation. Bacterial coinfection of amebic liver abscess has occasionally been observed (both before and as a complication of drainage), and adding antibiotics to the treatment regimen is reasonable in the absence of a prompt response to nitroimidazole therapy.

Aspiration is usually reserve for individuals with following conditions:

Diagnosis is uncertain where pyogenic abscess or bacterial superinfection is a possibility.

Those who have not responded to metronidazole therapy characterized by persistent fever or abdominal pain after 4 days of treatment.

Individuals of large left lobe abscess, because of risk of rupture into pericardium.

Size more than 8–10 cm suggesting impending rupture and severely ill patients with an accelerated clinical course and large abscess suggesting of imminent rupture.

Aspiration, percutaneous catheter drainage or both improve outcomes in the treatment of amebic empyema after liver abscess rupture and percutaneous catheter drainage or surgical drainage could be life-saving in the treatment of amebic pericarditis.

PREVENTION

Improved sanitation is critical to preventing orofecal transmission of organisms such as *E. histolytica*. Travelers to developing countries should be advised to avoid consumption of unsafe food and water and practices that may lead to fecal-oral transmission. Eating only cooked food or self-peeled fruits in endemic areas minimizes the risk. Travelers should avoid eating raw fruits and salads, which are difficult to sterilize. The amount of chlorine normally used to purify water is inadequate in killing the cysts. Drinking water can be rendered safe by boiling, 0.22 µm filtration or iodination with tetraglycine hydroperiodide.

Disease transmission can be reduced by early treatment of carriers in nonendemic areas.

Development of a vaccine for invasive amebiasis is still in its infancy.

COMPLICATIONS

Complication of amebic colitis includes bowel perforation, GI bleeding, ameboma, toxic megacolon, stricture formation, fistula formation, intussusception, peritonitis.

Secondary bacterial infection of amebic liver abscess is an uncommon complication. Rupture of amebic abscess may lead to peritonitis, pericarditis, empyema, brain abscess.

PROGNOSIS

Intestinal infections due to amebiasis generally respond well to appropriate therapy. The severity of amebiasis is increased in the following individuals:
- Children, especially neonates
- Pregnant and postpartum women
- Those using corticosteroids
- Those with malignancies
- Malnourished individuals
- The mortality rate in patients with uncomplicated amebic liver abscess is less than 1%.
- Fulminant amebic colitis has a mortality rate of more than 50%.

- Pleuropulmonary amebiasis has a 15–20% mortality rate.
- Amebic pericarditis has a case fatality rate of 40%.
- Cerebral amebiasis is highly fatal with a 90% death rate.

GIARDIASIS IN CHILDREN

Introduction

Giardiasis is a major diarrheal disease found throughout the world. The flagellate protozoan *Giardia intestinalis* (previously known as *G. lamblia*), its causative agent is the most common protozoal intestinal parasite isolated worldwide.

Mode of Spread

The source of infection is unprotected contaminated water. Contaminated food is a less common etiology. Infection is more common in children than in adults. Because ingestion of as few as 10 *Giardia* cysts may be sufficient to cause infection, giardiasis is more common in daycare center, boarding schools and institutionalized patients. *G. intestinalis* is a particularly significant pathogen in people with malnutrition, immunodeficiencies or cystic fibrosis and travelers to highly endemic areas.

Giardia Life Cycle

Life cycle consists of two stages: (1) the trophozoite, which exists freely in human small intestine, and (2) the cyst, which is passed into the environment. No intermediate host is required. Upon ingestion of the cyst, contained in the contaminated water or food, excystation occurs in the stomach and the duodenum in the presence of acid and pancreatic enzymes. The trophozoites pass into the small bowel where they multiply rapidly with a doubling time of 9–12 hours. Trophozoites colonize the duodenum and proximal jejunum of the host, where they attach to the intestinal brush border causing damage to the microvilli of the small gut mucosa. As trophozoites pass into the large bowel, encystation occurs in the presence of neutral pH and secondary life starts. Cysts are passed into the environment, and the cycle is repeated. The organism is known to have multiple strains with varying abilities to cause disease, and several different strains may be found in one host during infections.

Clinical Features

Diarrhea is the most common symptom of acute *Giardia* infection, occurring in 90% of symptomatic subjects. A small number of patients develop abrupt onset of explosive watery diarrhea. These symptoms last for 3–4 days before

transition into the more common subacute syndrome. Most patients develop a more insidious onset of symptoms, which are recurrent or resistant.

Stools become malodorous, mushy and greasy. Stools do not contain blood or pus. Abdominal cramping, bloating and flatulence occur in 70–75% of symptomatic patients.

Symptoms of chronic infection include chronic diarrhea, malaise, nausea and anorexia. Marked weight loss is associated with chronic diarrhea which may continue for months. Post-infection lactose intolerance is a common finding, occurring in 2–40% of cases.

Extraintestinal manifestations are rare and include allergic manifestations such as urticaria, erythema multiforme, bronchospasm, reactive arthritis and biliary tract disease. The etiology of such extraintestinal symptoms is likely a result of host immune system activation and cross-reactivity.

Physical examination does not contribute to the diagnosis. Weight loss or failure to thrive may be evident, but no physical findings are attributable to giardiasis. In severe cases, evidence of dehydration or wasting may be present.

Complications of giardiasis may include:
- Development of chronic illness with weight loss
- Malabsorption syndrome
- Failure to thrive in children
- Disaccharidase deficiency
- Zinc deficiency in school children
- Growth retardation
- Persistent gastrointestinal symptoms.

Diagnosis

A diagnosis is made by microscopic examination of fresh stool specimen. At least three fresh specimens of stools collected on alternate days should be examined to achieve a sensitivity of 90%. There is no blood or pus cells in the stool. Enzyme-linked immunoabsorbent assay (ELISA) test and direct fluorescent antibody test for *Giardia* antigens have better sensitivity. Where diagnosis is strongly suspected but stool testing is negative duodenal aspiration or biopsy may yield high concentration of giardiasis when fresh mount is examined for trophozoites. Intestinal biopsy is rarely indicated when duodenal aspirate is negative for *Giardia* but there is suggestive setting like unexplained lactose malabsorption or absent secretory IgA or hypogammaglobulinemia.

Treatment

Treatment is given to all symptomatic cases of acute and persistent diarrhea, failure to thrive or malabsorption syndromes associated with giardiasis. Asymptomatic cyst carriers are not treated except in specific situations like outbreak control or prevention of ingestion from cases to immunocompromised family members.

Metronidazole and tinidazole are the most common treatment options. Metronidazole is given in a dose of 15 mg/kg/day q 8 hourly for 5–7 days. Its efficacy is 80–90% but has frequent adverse effects like nausea and vomiting. Tinidazole is used as a single dose of 50 mg/kg. It has an efficacy of greater than 90%. It has less adverse effects. Nitazoxanide is a newly introduced drug used in a dose of 100 mg/kg/q bid in children aged 1–4 years and 200 mg bid in children aged 4–12 years for a period of 3 days. Second-line alternatives include albendazole, furazolidine, paromomycin and quinacrine.

Prevention of Giardiasis in Children

Frequent washing of hands including under the fingernails should be practiced by the parents, caregivers. Children should not eat unwashed fruits unless peeled. Water should be boiled if there is any doubt about the source. Treatment of water with chlorine or iodine is somewhat less effective. Breastfeeding in infants is very helpful as breast milk contains glycoconjugates and secretory IgA that protects against giardiasis. Travelers to endemic area should avoid uncooked food.

BIBLIOGRAPHY

1. Abd-Alla MD, Jackson TF, Gathiram V, et al. Differentiation of pathogenic *Entamoeba histolytica* infections from nonpathogenic infections by detection of galactose-inhibitable adherence protein antigen in sera and feces. J Clin Microbiol. 1993;31(11):2845-50.
2. Chen Y, Zhang Y, Yang B, et al. Seroprevalence of *Entamoeba histolytica* infection in HIV-infected patients in China. Am J Trop Med Hyg. 2007;77(5):825-8.
3. Daly ER, Roy SJ, Blaney DD, et al. Outbreak of giardiasis associated with a community drinking water source. Epidemiol Infect. 2009;1-10.
4. Eisenstein L, Bodager D, Ginzl D. Outbreak of giardiasis and cryptosporidiosis associated with a neighborhood interactive water fountain—Florida, 2006. J Environ Health. 2008;71(3):18-22; quiz 49-50.
5. Escobeda AA, Cimerman S. Giardiasis: a pharmacotherapy review. Expert Opin Pharmacother. 2007;8:1885-902.
6. Freedman DO, Weld LH, Kozarsky PE, et al. Spectrum of disease and relation to place of exposure among ill returned travelers. N Engl J Med. 2006;354(2):119-30.
7. Gonzales ML, Dans LF, Martinez EG. Antiamoebic drugs for treating amoebic colitis. Cochrane Database Syst Rev. 2009; CD006085.
8. Grecu F, Bulgariu T, Blanaru O, et al. Invasive amebiasis. Chirurgia (Bucur). 2006;101(5):539-42.
9. Hardin RE, Ferzli GS, Zenilman ME, et al. Invasive amebiasis and ameboma formation presenting as a rectal mass: an uncommon case of malignant masquerade at a western medical center. World J Gastroenterol. 2007;13(42):5659-61.
10. Hill DR. *Giardia lamblia*. In: Mandell GL, Bennett JE, Dolin R (Eds). Principles and Practice of Infectious Diseases, 6th edition. Philadelphia, Pennsylvania: Churchill Livingstone—An Imprint of Elsevier Inc.; 2005. pp. 3198-203/277.
11. Hung CC, Chen PJ, Hsieh SM, et al. Invasive amoebiasis: an emerging parasitic disease in patients infected with HIV in an area endemic for amoebic infection. AIDS. 1999;13(17):2421-8.
12. Hung CC, Ji DD, Sun HY, et al. Increased risk for entamoeba histolytica infection and invasive amebiasis in HIV seropositive men who have sex with men in Taiwan. PLoS Negl Trop Dis. 2008;2(2):e175.
13. Huston CD. Intestinal protozoa. In: Feldman M, Friedman LS, Brandt LJ (Eds). Sleisenger & Fordtran's Gastrointestinal and Liver Disease, 8th edition. Philadelphia, PA: Saunders—An imprint of Elsevier Inc.; 2006. pp. 2420-3/106.
14. John CC. Giardiasis and Balantidiasis. In: Kliegman RM, Behrman BE, Jenson HB, Stanton BF (Eds). Nelson Textbook of Pediatrics, 18th edition. Philadelphia, PA: Saunders—An imprint of Elsevier Inc; 2007. pp. 1462-4/279.
15. Kiser JD, Paulson CP, Brown C. Clinical enquiries. What is the most effective treatment for Giardiasis? J Fam Pract. 2008; 57:270-2.
16. Loulergue P, Mir O. Pleural empyema secondary to amebic liver abscess. Int J Infect Dis. 2009;13(3):e135-6.
17. Nishi L, Baesso ML, Santana RG, et al. Investigation of *Cryptosporidium* spp. and *Giardia* spp. in a public water-treatment system. Zoonoses Public Health. 2009;56(5):221-8.
18. Pritt BS, Clark CG. Amebiasis. Mayo Clin Proc. 2008;83(10):1154-9; quiz 1159-60.
19. Rao S, Solaymani-Mohammadi S, Petri WA, et al. Hepatic amebiasis: a reminder of the complications. Curr Opin Pediatr. 2009;21(1):145-9.
20. Robertson L, Gjerde B, Hansen EF, et al. A water contamination incident in Oslo, Norway during October 2007; a basis for discussion of boil-water notices and the potential for post-treatment contamination of drinking water supplies. J Water Health. 2009;7(1):55-66.
21. Robertson LJ, Forberg T, Gjerde BK. *Giardia* cysts in sewage influent in Bergen, Norway 15–23 months after an extensive waterborne outbreak of giardiasis. J Appl Microbiol. 2008;104(4):1147-52.
22. Salles JM, Salles MJ, Moraes LA, et al. Invasive amebiasis: an update on diagnosis and management. Expert Rev Anti-infect Ther. 2007;5(5):893-901.
23. Snow MJ, Stanley SL. Recent progress in vaccines for amebiasis. Arch Med Res. 2006;37(2):280-7.
24. Stanley SL. Amoebiasis. Lancet. 2003;361(9362):1025-34.
25. Stanley SL. Vaccines for amoebiasis: barriers and opportunities. Parasitology. 2006;133(Suppl):S81-6.
26. Tanyuksel M, Petri WA. Laboratory diagnosis of amebiasis. Clin Microbiol Rev. 2003;16(4):713-29.

Emerging Infections

Vijay N Yewale

7.1 RICKETTSIAL INFECTIONS

Atul Kulkarni

INTRODUCTION

Rickettsiae comprise a group of microorganisms that phylogenetically occupy a position between bacteria and viruses. These are arthropod-borne bacteria belonging to the genus *Rickettsia* within the family *Rickettsiaceae* in the order Rickettsiales, α-proteobacteria.

Most of these bacteria are associated with ticks, which are their vectors and reservoirs, but some are vectorized by lice, fleas or mites.

Rickettsia species were classically divided into "spotted fever" and "typhus" groups based on serologic reactions. The outer membrane protein A (ompA) gene is present in spotted fever but not typhus group organisms. Complete genome sequences have further refined distinctions, and several species that possess ompA, but are genetically distinct from others in the spotted fever group (SFG), have been reassigned to a "transitional" group.

It is increasingly realized that rickettsial diseases are under-diagnosed and that they substantially contribute to the burden of preventable acute febrile illness, in many populations, all over the world. The greatest challenge to clinicians is the difficult diagnostic dilemma posed by these infections early in their clinical course, when antibiotic therapy is most effective. Early signs and symptoms of these illnesses are notoriously nonspecific or mimic benign viral illnesses, making diagnosis difficult. Rickettsial diseases continue to cause severe illness and death in otherwise healthy adults and children, despite the availability of low cost, effective antimicrobial therapy.

This article emphasizes those rickettsial diseases that are prevalent in Indian children.

HISTORY

The earliest records of Rocky Mountain spotted fever (RMSF), date to 1873. Early Western inhabitants and physicians grimly referred to this life-threatening illness as "spotted fever" or "black measles" for the dark and extensive petechial rash, and "blue disease" or "black fever" to describe the dusky appearance of moribund patients.

The genus *Rickettsia* is named after Howard Taylor Ricketts (1871–1910), who studied Rocky Mountain spotted fever (RMSF) in the Bitterroot Valley of Montana, and eventually died of typhus after studying that disease in Mexico City.

Napoleon's retreat from Moscow became inevitable when Typhus fever broke out among his troops during the period between 1917 and 1925. Twenty-five million cases of epidemic typhus with three million deaths were reported in Russia around the same period. Lenin said, "Either socialism will defeat the louse or louse will defeat socialism".

CLASSIFICATION

Classification of *Rickettsial* disease on the basis of clinical features and epidemiological aspects has been denoted in Table 7.1.1.

EPIDEMIOLOGY OF RICKETTSIAL INFECTIONS IN INDIA

Spotted fever disease was first observed in India by Megaw (1917) in the foothills of the Himalayas. Reports of Indian tick typhus (ITT) fever have come from all over the country including places like Jabalpur, Nagpur, Kanpur, Sagar, Pune, Lucknow, Bengaluru, Secunderabad, etc. Similarly, endemic typhus has been noted in many places in India like hills of Shimla, Mumbai, Jabalpur, Kashmir, Lucknow, Pune, etc.

Scrub typhus broke out in an epidemic form in Assam and West Bengal during Second World War. It was later found that scrub typhus was prevalent throughout India in humans, trombiculid mites and rodents. Recently, scrub

Table 7.1.1: Classification of Rickettsial disease on the basis of clinical features and epidemiological aspects.

Diseases	Rickettsial agent	Insect vectors	Mammalian reservoirs
Spotted fever group* a. Indian tick typhus b. Rocky Mountain spotted fever c. Tick-borne lymphadenopathy (TIBOLA)	R. conorii R. rickettsii R. slovaca	Tick Tick Tick	Rodents, dogs Rodents, dogs Wild boar
Typhus group a. Epidemic typhus b. Murine typhus	R. prowazekii R. typhi	Louse Flea	Humans Rodents
Scrub typhus group a. Scrub typhus	O. tsutsugamushi	Mite	Rodents
Transitional group a. Rickettsial pox b. Cat flea typhus	R. akari R. felis	Mite Fleabite	Mice Cats/dogs
Others a. Q fever b. Trench fever c. Ehrlichiosis d. Anaplasmosis	C. brunetti Rochalimaea quintana Ehrlichia Anaplasma Phagocytophilum	Nil Louse Tick Tick	Cattle, sheep, goats Humans Deer/dog Deer/dog

*More than 19 types of spotted fever varieties are described depending upon the geographical area where these are prevalent.

typhus has been reported from Delhi, Himachal Pradesh, Haryana, Karnataka, Kerala and Tamil Nadu.

Spotted fevers and typhus fever have been reported from Southern regions of India. Recent reports state that ITT is prevalent in many districts of Maharashtra (e.g. Solapur, Osmanabad, Latur, Ahmadnagar, Beed, Aurangabad, Nanded, Akola, Hingoli, Parbhani, Raigad, Pune, Mumbai), Karnataka (e.g. Vijayapura, Kalaburagi, Hubballi, Raichur), Tamil Nadu and Kerela. ITT is endemic in rural part of these areas. Serological surveys indicate that Q fever is present in animal as well as human populations in Haryana, Punjab, Delhi, Rajasthan and various other places in India.

ETIOLOGY AND MICROBIOLOGY

Rickettsia is a group of motile, gram-negative, non-spore forming highly pleomorphic bacteria that present as cocci (0.1 micron), rods (1–4 micron) or thread like (10 micron), obligate, intracellular parasites. To survive, these have to enter, grow and replicate in the cytoplasm or within the nucleus of the cell that they invade. They divide by binary fission and they metabolize host-derived glutamate via aerobic respiration and the citric acid (TCA) cycle. The cytoplasm of these bacteria contains ribosomes and strands of DNA and is limited by a typical gram-negative trilamellar structure made of a bilayer inner membrane, a peptidoglycan layer, and a bilayer outer membrane. The *Rickettsiae* have very small genomes of about 1.0–1.5 million bases.

Rickettsiae possess major antigens such as lipopoly-saccharide (LPS), lipoprotein, outer membrane proteins (OmpA, OmpB) of the surface cell antigen (SCA) family, and heat shock proteins. The Weil-Felix test, initially developed as a diagnostic test for rickettsioses, was based on the antigenic cross reactions among rickettsial antigens, mostly LPS, and *Proteus vulgaris* strains OX19 and OX2, and *Proteus mirabilis* OXK. *Rickettsia* cannot survive in artificial nutrient environments and hence are grown in either tissue or embryo cultures. Growth of *Rickettsia* is enhanced by the presence of sulfonamides.

METHOD OF TRANSMISSION

Tick, mite, flea and louse are the natural hosts, reservoirs and vectors of rickettsial organisms (except Q fever). These maintain the infection naturally by transovarial transmission (passage of the organism from infected ticks to their progeny) and transstadial passage. Ticks transmit the infectious agent to mammalian hosts (including humans) by regurgitation of infected saliva during feeding. Dogs and rodents serve as reservoir hosts for these vectors. These reservoir vectors can themselves develop the diseases and are important vehicles for bringing potentially infected vectors into the environment shared by humans.

PATHOPHYSIOLOGY

Adherence to the Host Cell

Rickettsiae are inoculated into the dermis of the skin by a tick bite or through damaged skin from the feces of lice or fleas. The bacteria spread through the bloodstream and infect the endothelium. Adherence to the host cell is the first step of rickettsial pathogenesis. The adhesions are presumed to be outer membrane proteins.

Invasion of Host Cells

Upon attaching to the host cell membrane, *Rickettsiae* are phagocytosed by the host cell. The *Rickettsiae* are believed to induce host cell phagocytosis because they can enter cells that normally do not phagocytose particles. Once phagocytosed by the host cell, *Rickettsiae* are observed to quickly escape from the phagosome membrane and enter the cytoplasm. The mechanism of escape from the phagosome membrane is not well understood, but it is thought to be mediated by a rickettsial enzyme, phospholipase A2.

Movement within and Release from the Host Cell

Observations in cell culture systems suggest that the mechanisms of intracellular movement and destruction of the host cells differ among the SFG and typhus group *Rickettsiae*.

Typhus group *Rickettsiae* are released from host cells by lysis of the cells. After infection with *Rickettsia prowazekii* or *Rickettsia typhi*, the *Rickettsiae* continue to multiply until the cell is packed with organisms and then bursts. Phospholipase A2 may be involved in cell lysis. Typhus group *Rickettsia*-infected host cells have a normal ultrastructural appearance.

Spotted fever group *Rickettsiae* seldom accumulate in large numbers and do not lyse the host cells. They escape from the cell by stimulating polymerization of host cell-derived actin tails, which propel them through the cytoplasm and into tips of membranous extrusions, from which they emerge. In scrub, typhus rickettsial organisms are released from the infected cell by budding. Infected cells exhibit signs of membrane damage associated with an influx of water, but the means by which rickettsiae damage host cell membranes is uncertain. There is evidence to suggest a role for free radicals of oxygen, phospholipase and a protease (Fig. 7.1.1).

Rickettsial microorganisms appear to exert their pathologic effects by adhering to and then invading the endothelial lining of the vasculature (microvasculitis) within the various affected organs.

Rickettsiae proliferate on the endothelium of small blood vessels, release cytokines which damage endothelial integrity, with consequent fluid leakage and platelet aggregation. Polymorphs and monocytes proliferate leading to focal occlusive endarteritis. This results in microinfarctions and typical "Typhus nodules of Wolhbach". This process especially affects the brain, cardiac and skeletal muscle, skin, liver, lungs and kidneys. This may also cause venous thrombosis and gangrene of the extremities.

The most important pathophysiologic effect is increased vascular permeability with consequent edema, loss of blood volume, hypoalbuminemia, decreased osmotic pressure and hypotension. On the other hand, disseminated intravascular coagulation (DIS) is rare and does not seem to contribute to the pathophysiology of *Rickettsiae*.

Vascular wall destruction consumes platelets, causing thrombocytopenia. Multiple factors lead to hypoalbuminemia (e.g. renal loss, decreased intake, hepatic involvement) and hyponatremia (e.g. renal loss, extracellular fluid shifts and cellular exchange of sodium for potassium).

IMMUNITY

Rickettsial infection stimulates an early innate immune response with activation of natural killer cells and production of gamma interferon (gamma IFN), which act in concert to dampen rickettsial growth. Acquired immunity develops with clonal expansion of CD4 and CD8 T-lymphocytes as well as antibody-producing B cells. Clearance of intraendothelial *Rickettsiae* is achieved by rickettsicidal effects due to cytokine activation of the infected endothelial cells themselves. Cell mediated immunity (CMI) plays an important role as expected in infection by an intracellular parasite, but antibodies (including those directed at epitopes of OmpA and OmpB) also play a role in protective immunity.

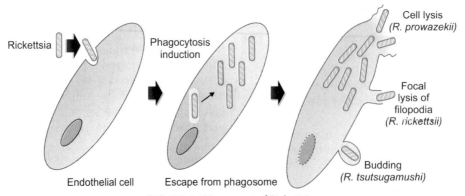

FIG. 7.1.1: Movement of *Rickettsia*.

CLINICAL MANIFESTATIONS

Incubation period in children varies from 2 to 14 days. It may extend up to 28 days with a median of 7 days. A history of exposure to tick or close contact with an infected pet animal may be forth coming. Often, history of travel from an endemic area or a similar illness in family members is available. Severity of manifestations varies from a mild, self-limiting illness to a life-threatening disaster.

Initially, the illness appears to be nonspecific and patients present with headache, fever, anorexia, myalgias and restlessness. Calf muscle pain and tenderness are common in children. Gastrointestinal symptoms include nausea, vomiting and diarrhea. Abdominal pain is a frequent complaint earlier in this disease. Skin rash is usually not present until after 2–4 days of illness. The typical triad of fever, headache and rash is observed in 44% of patients. Core body temperature may exceed 40°C and can be remain high or it can fluctuate dramatically.

Headache is severe, unremitting and usually unresponsive to analgesics.

Rash is initially discrete. Pale rose red blanching macules or maculopapules appear characteristically on the extremities including the ankles, wrist or lower limbs. Later, rash spreads rapidly to involve the entire body including palms and soles (Fig. 7.1.2). After several days, the rash becomes more petechial (Fig. 7.1.3) or hemorrhagic, sometimes with palpable purpura (Fig. 7.1.4). In severe form of the disease, petechiae may enlarge into ecchymosis, which can become necrotic (Fig. 7.1.5). Severe vaso-occlusive disease secondary to rickettsial vasculitis and thrombosis is infrequent but can result in gangrene of the digits (Fig. 7.1.6), toes, earlobes (Fig. 7.1.7), scrotum, nose or entire limbs. Painless eschar, the tache noire, may be seen at the initial site of tick attachment and regional lymphadenopathy.

Edema over the dorsum of hand or foot, periorbital edema and generalized edema are sometimes seen and so are hepatosplenomegaly and generalized lymphadenopathy.

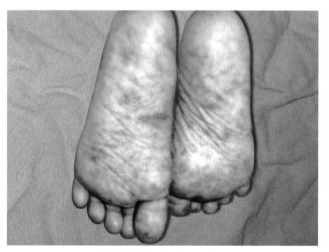

FIG. 7.1.2: Rash on sole.

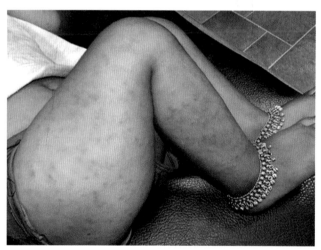

FIG. 7.1.4: Palpable purpura.

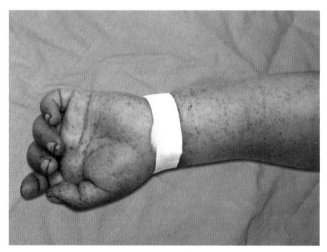

FIG. 7.1.3: Petechial rash.

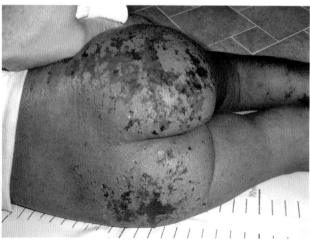

FIG. 7.1.5: Necrotic rash.

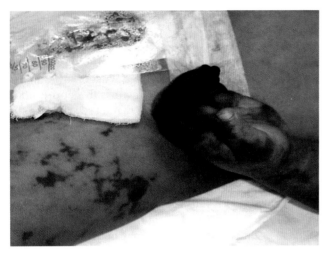

FIG. 7.1.6: Gangrene of digits.

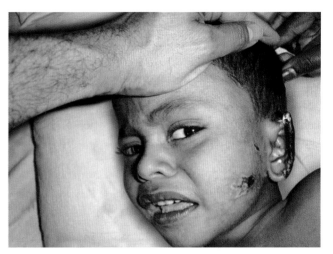

FIG. 7.1.7: Gangrene of earlobe (Kan kapya).

NEUROLOGIC INVOLVEMENT IN RICKETTSIAL DISEASES

The name typhus originated from the Greek word "typhos", which means smoky and refers to the cloudy sensorium of patients with typhus and other life-threatening rickettsioses. Rickettsial encephalitis manifests first as confusion or lethargy, as the disease progresses, stupor or delirium, ataxia, coma, deafness and seizures are observed. Involvement of blood vessels contiguous to the cerebrospinal fluid (CSF) leads to pleocytosis in 34–38% of patients, usually 10–100 cells/cumm with predominance of lymphocytes and macrophages. Occasionally, more than 100 cells/cumm with polymorphonuclear predominance are observed. The occurrence of coma or seizures is often associated with a fatal outcome.

PULMONARY INVOLVEMENT

The pulmonary microcirculation is heavily infected by *Rickettsiae* in severely, ill patients. This leads to non-cardiogenic pulmonary edema. Interstitial pneumonitis, alveolar edema and adult respiratory distress syndrome are the most severe manifestations.

OTHER INVOLVEMENT

More severe form of disease may include myocarditis, acute renal failure, DIC, hepatitis and vascular collapse.

Q FEVER

No vector is involved. Transmission is by inhalation of infected dust from soil previously contaminated by urine or feces of diseased animals. This fever is rarely reported in children. This presents in acute as well as chronic forms. Rash which is typical of variants of rickettsial fever is not seen in Q fever. Pneumonia, hepatitis and meningitis are some of the usual features of Q fever. Endocarditis is seen in chronic variety.

HOST RISK FACTORS FOR SEVERITY OF ILLNESS

Age is the host factor that most consistently influences the severity of illness. Mortality rate is significantly higher in older patients. Mortality is more common in male patients. Host factors related to underlying diseases and enhanced oxidative stress also appears to determine severity of rickettsioses. Patients with diabetes mellitus have an increased risk of a fatal outcome.

Anecdotal descriptions suggest that alcohol abuse and cardiovascular disease may be risk factors for severity of rickettsial illness. Sulfonamide treatment exacerbates the severity of illness caused by rickettsial infection. It is possible that sulfonamides increase oxidative stress, a pathogenic mechanism of cell injury in *R. rickettsii* infection in vitro.

Glucose-6-phosphate dehydrogenase deficiency is associated with the occurrence of fulminant spotted fever disease. Glucose-6-phosphate dehydrogenase is a component of the antioxidant protective mechanisms, and its deficiency could result in increased damage caused by oxidative stress.

COMPLICATIONS

Complications include non-cardiogenic pulmonary edema from pulmonary microvascular leakage, cerebral edema from meningoencephalitis, and multiorgan damage (hepatitis, pancreatitis, cholecystitis, epidermal necrosis and gangrene) mediated by rickettsial vasculitis and/or the accumulated effects of hypoperfusion and ischemia (acute renal failure). Hemophagocytics syndrome can rarely complicate the illness. Long-term neurologic sequelae are more likely to occur in patients who have been hospitalized for greater than or equal to 2 weeks and include paraparesis, motor dysfunction, hearing loss, peripheral neuropathy, and bladder and bowel incontinence. Language disorder and dysfunction of cerebellum and vestibule are also observed. Learning disabilities and behavioral problems are the most common neurologic sequelae among children who have survived severe disease.

DIFFERENTIATING FEATURES AMONG VARIOUS RICKETTSIAL DISEASES

Indian Tick Typhus

Until 1925, ITT was almost always diagnosed as RMSF because of the stark similarity in clinical presentation of these two entities. However, in 1925, Megaw put forth the view that tick typhus existed as a distinct entity in India—different from the tick typhus observed in the Rocky Mountains. Nevertheless, the etiological agent of Indian variety of tick typhus disease had never been isolated in patients. However, a SFG *Rickettsia* was isolated in 1950 from an *R. sanguineus* tick (Fig. 7.1.8) collected in India and it was assumed to be the agent for ITT. This bacterium, classified as *Rickettsia conorii*, was considered to be the cause of ITT. However, subsequent serological studies including cross adsorption and microimmunofluorescence serotyping demonstrated significant differences in antibody responses in patients suffering from ITT and Mediterranean spotted fever (MSF).

Using molecular methods, it was recently demonstrated that these *Rickettsiae* are closely related—even though they differ from each other as reflected in antigenic variation. Zhu et al. have recently proposed that the agent of ITT constitutes a subspecies of *R. conorii*, different from the agent of MSF, designated *R. conorii* subspecies Indica subspecies combination nova.

In a local Indian language, spoken in those parts of India where ITT is endemic, this disease bears graphically descriptive names—referring mainly to its devastating complications. For instance, *kan-kapya disease* (see Fig. 7.1.7), meaning the "disease that cuts one's ears"; refers to auto-amputation of ear-lobes due to microinfarcts. "*Bibtya*",

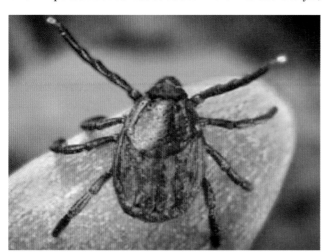

FIG. 7.1.8: An adult female *Rhipicephalus sanguineus* (brown dog tick).

meaning a spotted-leopard, refers to the papular rashes seen in ITT. "*MothaGovar*", meaning "*big measles*", refers to the rashes of ITT which are larger in comparison with measles rash. The name "*GhodyaGovar*" refers to the link between domesticated animals and spread of tick typhus.

Indian tick typhus is prevalent in many districts of Maharashtra, Karnataka and Tamil Nadu. The tick is the reservoir of infection. Various tick genera (e.g. *Rhipicephalus*, *Ixodes, Boophilus, Haemaphysalis*) have been incriminated as vectors. *Rickettsia* can be transmitted to dogs, various rodents and other animals, which constitute important links in the disease cycle and these animals bring this dangerous pathogen nearer to human beings.

Clinical presentation of ITT is similar to that of RMSF—although the manifestations are a less severe in ITT. Nevertheless, few recent Indian reports appear to suggest that ITT can present with clinical features as severe as RMSF. ITT differs from MSF in that the rash is frequently purpuric and an inoculation eschar at the bite site is seldom identified. However, recent Indian studies states in ITT rash is commonly popular, and eschar is uncommonly seen.

Rocky Mountain Spotted Fever

It is by far the most severe form of rickettsial fever. Here, the rash typically appears on the fourth day as blanching macules on the extremities and gradually becomes petechial as it spreads to the trunk, palms and soles over several days.

Epidemic Typhus

Here, the rash appears first in the axillary folds and on the trunk. It may later spread peripherally to the palms, soles and face. Severe clinical features, similar to RMSF, may be observed.

Murine Typhus

The rash is non-purpuric, non-confluent and less extensive. Renal and vascular complications are less common.

Scrub Typhus

Scrub typhus is an acute, febrile, infectious illness that is caused by *Orientia* (formerly *Rickettsia*) *tsutsugamushi*. It is also known as *tsutsugamushi disease*. Scrub typhus was first described from Japan in 1899. Humans are accidental hosts in this zoonotic disease.

Scrub typhus is endemic to a part of the world known as the "tsutsugamushi triangle", which extends from northern Japan and far-eastern Russia in the north, to northern Australia in the south, and to Pakistan in the west. Thus, India is an endemic zone for scrub typhus. The term scrub is used because of the type of vegetation (terrain between woods and clearings) that harbors the vector—however, this name is not entirely correct because certain endemic areas can also be sandy, semi-arid and mountain deserts.

Orientia sutsugamushi comes in five major serotypes: (1) Boryon, (2) Gilliam, (3) Karp, (4) Kato and (5) Kawazaki. Differentiation of serotypes is important for laboratory diagnosis. Scrub typhus is transmitted to humans and rodents by some species of trombiculid mites ("chiggers", *Leptotrombidium deliense and others*). The mite is very small (0.2–0.4 mm) and can only be seen through a microscope or magnifying glass. Humans acquire the disease from the bite of an infected chigger. The bite of the mite leaves a characteristic black eschar that is useful to the doctor in making the diagnosis.

Scrub typhus is difficult to recognize and diagnose because the symptoms and signs of this illness are often non-specific. The non-specific presentation and lack of the characteristic eschar in 40% of the patients often results in misdiagnosis and under-reporting of scrub typhus. Also, diagnostic facilities are not easily available in much of the areas endemic to scrub typhus. Therefore, the precise incidence of this disease is unknown. An estimated one billion people are at risk for scrub typhus and an estimated one million cases surface annually. Mortality rate in untreated patients ranges from 0% to 30%.

The chigger bite is painless and may become noticed as a transient localized itch. Bites are often found on the groin, axillae, genitalia or neck. An eschar is often seen in humans at the site of the chigger bite. The illness begins rather suddenly with shaking chills, fever, severe headache, infection of the mucous membrane lining the eyes (the conjunctiva) and swelling of the lymph nodes. A spotted rash on the trunk may be present. Symptoms may include muscle and gastrointestinal pains. Hearing loss concurrent with the onset of fever occurs in about one-third of cases and is a very useful diagnostic clue. However, true hearing loss must be distinguished from tinnitus, which sometimes coexists with hearing loss, and from transient hearing loss due to nasal congestion, also a common feature of scrub typhus. Sensorineural hearing loss was documented by audiometry in Thai patients during acute *O. tsutsugamushi* infection and resolved after treatment. Cough, sometimes accompanied by infiltrates on the chest radiograph, is one of the most common presentations of scrub typhus infection.

More virulent strains of *O. tsutsugamushi* can cause hemorrhaging and intravascular coagulation. Complications may include atypical pneumonia, overwhelming pneumonia with adult respiratory distress syndrome (ARDS)-like presentation, myocarditis and DIC. Patients with scrub typhus often exhibit leukopenia.

Acute scrub typhus appears to decrease viral loads in patients with HIV. This interaction is currently unexplained.

Prophylaxis

It has been shown that a single oral dose of chloramphenicol or tetracycline given every 5 days for a total of 35 days, with 5-day non-treatment intervals, actually produces active immunity to scrub typhus. This procedure is recommended under special circumstances in certain areas where the disease is endemic.

RICKETTSIALPOX

This disease is mild and the rash is in the form of vesicles. Surrounding erythema is sparse and the rash may resemble that of varicella.

Diagnosis

IAP Guidelines for Management

Case Definitions

Suspected case: A patient having compatible clinical scenario, suggestive epidemiological features and absence of definite alternative diagnosis should be termed as a suspected case of *Rickettsia*. Definition of 'compatible clinical scenario' and 'suggestive epidemiological features' and list of differential diagnosis is provided in Boxes 7.1.1 to 7.1.3, respectively. Alternative diagnosis can be searched from (but not limited to) the list of differential diagnoses (Box 7.1.4).

Box 7.1.1

Compatible clinical scenario for rickettsial infection.
One or more of the following:
- Undifferentiated fever of more than 5 days
- Sepsis of unclear etiology
- Fever with rash
- Fever with edema
- Dengue-like disease
- Fever with headache and myalgia
- Fever with hepatosplenomegaly and/or lymphadenopathy
- Aseptic meningitis/meningoencephalitis/acute encephalitic syndrome
- Fever with cough and pulmonary infiltrates or community acquired pneumonia
- Fever with acute kidney injury
- Fever with acute gastrointestinal or hepatic involvement

Box 7.1.2

Suggestive epidemiological features for rickettsial infections.
One or more of the following within 14 days of illness onset:
- Tick bite
- Ticks seen on clothes or in and around homes or in areas where children play
- Visit to areas which are common habitats of vectors like high uncut grass or weeds or bushes or rice fields or woodlands (where rodents share habitats with animals) or grassy lawns or river banks or poorly maintained kitchen gardens
- Animal sheds in proximity of homes
- Contact with pet or stray dog infested with ticks
- Living in or travel to areas endemic for rickettsial diseases
- Occurrence of similar clinical cases simultaneously or sequentially in family members, coworkers, neighborhood or pets
- Exposure to rodents

Differential diagnoses for rickettsial infections.
One or more of the following within 14 days of illness onset:
- *Viral diseases:* Enteroviral diseases, measles, dengue fever, chikungunya, infectious mononucleosis
- *Bacterial diseases:* Meningococcemia, leptospirosis, typhoid fever, scarlet fever, secondary syphilis, infective endocarditis
- *Protozoal diseases:* Malaria
- *Vasculitis:* Kawasaki disease, thrombotic thrombocytopenic purpura
- Adverse drug reactions
- Differential diagnoses pertaining to each systemic presentation

Suggestive laboratory features for rickettsial infections.
- Normal to low total leukocyte count with a shift to left in early stages and leukocytosis later on
- Thrombocytopenia
- Raised ESR and CRP
- Hyponatremia
- Hypoalbuminemia
- Elevated hepatic transaminases

Probable case: Suspected case having either eschar, or having rapid (<48 hours) defervescence with antirickettsial therapy, or having suggestive laboratory features (Box 7.1.4), or having Weil-Felix test positive with titer of 1:80 or more in OX2, OX19 or OXK or positive IgM ELISA for *Rickettsia* (optical density >0.5).

Confirmed case: Suspected case having rickettsial DNA detected in whole blood or tissue samples, or fourfold rise in antibody titers on acute and convalescent sera detected by immunofluorescence assay (IFA) or immunoperoxidase assay (IPA) [8]. In countries like India, where PCR and IFA are not commonly available, properly performed paired serological tests like ELISA have high positive predictive value.

ICMR Guidelines for Management

Case Definition

1. *Definition of suspected/clinical case:* Acute undifferentiated febrile illness of 5 days or more with/without eschar should be suspected as a case of Rickettsial infection. (If eschar is present, fever of less than 5 days duration should be considered as scrub typhus.) Other presenting features may be headache and rash (rash more often seen in fair persons), lymphadenopathy, multiorgan involvement like liver, lung and kidney involvement.
The differential diagnosis of dengue, malaria, pneumonia, leptospirosis and typhoid should be kept in mind.

2. *Definition of probable case:* A suspected clinical case showing titers of 1:80 or above in OX2, OX19 and OXK antigens by Weil Felix test and an optical density (OD) >0.5 for IgM by ELISA are considered positive for typhus and spotted fever groups of *Rickettsiae*. 3.1.3 Definition of confirmed case: A Confirmed case is the one in which: Rickettsial DNA is detected in eschar samples or whole blood by PCR • Or rising antibody titers on acute and convalescent sera detected by Indirect Immune • Fluorescence assay (IFA) or indirect immunoperoxidase assay (IPA).

Differential Diagnosis

Spotted fever can mimic a great number of febrile illnesses. Most important of these are meningococcemia, measles and enteroviral exanthemas. Other diseases included in differential diagnosis are typhoid fever, secondary syphilis, leptospirosis, toxic shock syndrome, scarlet fever, rubella, Kawasaki disease, parvo-viral infection, idiopathic thrombocytopenic purpura (ITP), thrombotic thrombocytopenic purpura (TTP), hemolytic uremic syndrome, Henoch-Schönlein purpura, acute abdomen, aseptic meningitis, hepatitis, dengue fever, infectious mononucleosis, drug reactions, malaria, tularemia, anthrax and other causes of pyrexia of unknown origin.

Laboratory Diagnosis of Rickettsioses

There is no widely available laboratory assay that provides rapid confirmation of early rickettsial fever. Treatment decisions must be based on epidemiologic and clinical clues, and should never be delayed while waiting for confirmation by laboratory results.

Laboratory findings are usually non-specific. Total leukocyte count may be initially normal or low but leukocytosis develops as the disease progresses. Blood smear microscopy might reveal presence of morulae in infected leukocytes, which is highly suggestive of HGA. Anemia, thrombocytopenia, hyponatremia, hypoproteinemia and elevated serum aminotransferases are some other features. CSF findings are usually normal but occasionally mononuclear pleocytosis (<10–300 cell/μL) may be found. Roughly, 20% of the patients may have elevated CSF proteins (200 mg/dL).

Specific Diagnosis

The diagnosis of a rickettsial illness has most often been confirmed by serological testing. Serological evidence of infection occurs not earlier than the second week of illness in any of the rickettsial diseases and hence a specific diagnosis may not be available until after the patient has fully recovered or worsened.

Isolation of *Rickettsia*

- Embryonated chicken egg yolk sacs
- Laboratory animals inoculation into guinea pigs, mouse, meadow voles, Sprague-Dawley rats has been used

- Cell cultures—Vero or L929 cells have been shown to allow better and faster isolation of *Rickettsiae*. Isolation of *Rickettsia* is reserved for reference lab which is not available in India
- Presumptive identification of a rickettsial isolate may be achieved by microscopic examination after staining. *Rickettsiae* appear as short rods which are not stained by staining with the Gram stain but are visible after Giemsa or Gimenez staining
- Serological diagnosis may be by Weil-Felix reaction or by specific tests using rickettsial antigens.

Weil-Felix Test

The basis of the test is the presence of antigenic cross-reactivity between *Rickettsia* species and certain serotypes of non-motile *Proteus* species, a phenomenon first published by Edmund Weil and Arthur Felix in 1916. The somatic (O) antigen that cross-reacted with anti-rickettsial antibodies, and furthermore, that different *Proteus* O antigens would cross-react with different species of *Rickettsia*.

- *Proteus vulgaris* antigen
- OX 2–Cross reacts with SFG
- OX 19–Cross reacts with typhus group, RMSF
- OX-K–Cross reacts with scrub typhus.

It is a slide agglutination test. The kit tests serum dilution from 1:20 to 1:320.

Significant titer is 1:80. Rising titers are more appropriate. Examination of paired serum samples obtained 2–3 weeks apart that demonstrate a rise in antibody titer is the most appropriate approach.

Weil-Felix test is a classic serological test, widely available but unacceptable for accurate diagnosis because of very low sensitivity and specificity. In conclusion, Weil-Felix test can be used in developing countries where other tests are not available for diagnosis of rickets infection. This test should be interpreted in conjunction with history and clinical presentation.

Immunofluorescence Assay

This is the gold standard test for serodiagnosis of rickettsial disease and allows for detection of immunoglobulin G (IgG) and immunoglobulin M (IgM). IgM titer, which is more than 1:640, suggests acute infection. IgM titer starts appearing at 5–10 days and peaks at 3–4 weeks after the onset of illness. IgG titer of more than 1:254 suggests acute infection. IgG >1:64 but ≤1:125 indicates previous infection. Serologic evidence of four fold change in serum antibody titer against *rickettsial* antigens between paired serum samples, as determined by IFA confirms diagnosis. Chief drawbacks of IFA are that it is expensive and not widely available.

Enzyme-linked immunosorbent assay (ELISA) was first introduced for detection of antibodies against *R. typhi* and *R. prowazekii*. The use of this technique is highly sensitive and reproducible, allowing the differentiation of IgG and IgM antibodies. This technique was later adapted to the diagnosis of RMSF and scrub typhus. ELISA has been demonstrated to be as sensitive and as specific as IFA for the diagnosis of rickettsial fever. It is now available in India and should be preferred for diagnosis.

The indirect *hemagglutination test* is rickettsial group specific test that detects both IgG and IgM antibodies. This test is not available in India.

The latex agglutination test is rapid (15 minutes) and does not require elaborate instrumentation. Latex agglutination is reactive with IgG and IgM antibodies. This test allows the demonstration of antibodies within 1 week after the onset of illness. Significant antibody titers disappear after 2 months. This test is also not available in India.

Immunoperoxidase assay: This is an alternative technique to VFA used in ploratorius lacking a UV microscope, in which peroxidase in used instead of fluorescein. It is both sensitive and specific. It is not available in India.

Immunohistochemistry for *R. conorii* and *R. typhi* of a biopsied skin lesion or autopsy tissues is useful for RMSF diagnosis. It is not available in India.

Western immunoblot assay with sodium dodecyl sulfate-gel electrophoresed and electroblotted antigens is a powerful serodiagnostic tool for seroepidemiology and confirmation of serologic diagnoses obtained by conventional tests. It is not available in India.

PCR-based detection: Detection of *Rickettsiae* from blood and tissues of infected patients. The technique of choice for early diagnosis (within first week) before seroconversion amplification of specific DNA by PCR provides a rapid method for detecting tick-borne rickettsial diseases (TBRD) infections. New techniques (e.g. real-time PCR) might offer the advantages of speed, reproducibility, quantitative capability, and low risk for contamination, compared with conventional PCR. It is not available in India.

TREATMENT AND SUPPORTIVE CARE

Delay in diagnosing and treating rickettsial disease may result in increased severity and at times may prove fatal. Since no reliable diagnostic test is available to confirm Rickettsial infection in the early stage, initial diagnosis and suitable treatment should be based on a high index of suspicion and appropriate clinical features. Epidemiological features (patient coming from an endemic area) and laboratory findings are important adjuvants.

Appropriate antibiotic treatment should be initiated immediately when there is a suspicion of rickettsial fever on the basis of clinical and epidemiologic findings. Treatment should not be delayed until laboratory confirmation is obtained.

Tetracycline and chloramphenicol are the two time-tested drugs to effectively treat rickettsial infections in patients of all ages including children with spotted fever. Doxycycline is the drug of choice for all age groups.

Chloramphenicol is reserved for patients with doxycycline allergy and for pregnant women. Tetracycline and doxycycline may cause discoloration of teeth in children who are less than eight years in age, whereas chloramphenicol can rarely cause aplastic anemia. Doxycycline can be used safely in young children because tooth discoloration is dose dependent and children are unlikely to require multiple courses. Furthermore the fact that increased mortality with chloramphenicol alone, compared with tetracycline alone, when other factors such as severity are considered have led to preference for doxycycline even in young children.

Recommended Treatment Regimens

- *Doxycycline:* 2.2 mg/kg/dose Bid PO or IV, maximum 200 mg/day
- *Tetracycline:* 25–50 mg/kg/dose 6 hourly PO, maximum 2 g/day
- *Chloramphenicol:* 50–100 mg/kg/day 6 hourly, maximum 3 g/day.
- *Azithromycin 10 mg/kg/day OD PO for 5 days.*

The therapy should be continued for a minimum of 5–7 days and for at least 3 days until the patient is afebrile in order to avoid relapse. Patients treated with one of these regimens usually become afebrile within 48 hours and thus the entire therapy lasts for less than 10 days.

Other Drugs

Mediterranean spotted fever has been effectively treated by azithromycin (10 mg/kg/day OD for 3 days), clarithromycin (15 mg/kg/day BID for 7 days) and fluoroquinolones besides doxycycline and chloramphenicol. However, doxycycline still remains the drug of choice. Specific fluoroquinolones regimens effective for children have not been established. Azithromycin or rifampicin may be used in doxycycline resistant scrub typhus.

Supportive Care

Most infections resolve rapidly with appropriate antimicrobial therapy and do not require hospitalization or other supportive care. On occasion, severe infections require intensive care. Particular attention to hemodynamic status is required in severely-ill children, because iatrogenic pulmonary or cerebral edema is easy to precipitate owing to diffuse microvascular injury of the lungs, meninges and brain. Judicious use of corticosteroids for meningoencephalitis has been advocated by some, but no controlled trials have been conducted.

Prevention

No vaccines are available. Known tick-infested areas should be avoided. Daily inspection of body for ticks is particularly important. Disinfection of dogs will minimize the tick population. Health education of people about mode of transmission by ticks and means of personal protection is equally important. Post exposure prophylactic antimicrobial therapy should not be administered because tetracycline and chloramphenicol are only rickettsiostatic.

FLOWCHART 7.1.1: Management algorithm for Rickettsial infections.

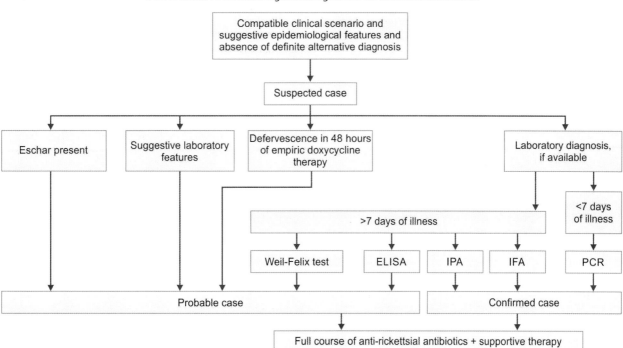

Abbreviations: ELISA, enzyme-linked immunosorbent assay; IPA, Immunoperoxidase assay; IFA, Immunofluorescence assay; PCF, Polymerase chain reaction.

Such therapy simply delays the onset of illness and confuses the clinical picture by prolonging the incubation period.

Prognosis

Delays in diagnosis and therapy are significant factors associated with death or severe illness. Before the advent of effective antimicrobial therapy for RMSF, the case fatality rate was 10% for children and 30% for adults. Diagnosis based on serology alone underestimates the true mortality of rickettsial fever, because patients often die before developing a serologic response. Deaths occur despite the availability of effective therapeutic agents, indicating the need for clinical vigilance and a low threshold for early empiric therapy. Even with administration of appropriate antimicrobials, delayed therapy can lead to irreversible vascular or end-organ damage and long-term sequelae or death. Early therapy in uncomplicated cases usually leads to rapid defervescence within 1–3 days and recovery within 7–10 days. A slower response may be seen if therapy is delayed. In those who survive despite no treatment, fever subsides in 2–3 weaks.

ACKNOWLEDGMENTS

I acknowledge Dr Sunil Vaidya, Dr PT Kulkarni, Dr Asawari Kulkarni, Dr LH Bidri, Dr VH Joshi, Dr Nandan Gadgil, Dr Chidgupkar Jyoti, and Dr SM Rudrakshi.

BIBLIOGRAPHY

1. Centre of Disease Control and Prevention (CDC). Rickettsial Diseases. [online] Available from http://www.cdc.gov/ncidod/diseases/sunmenus/sub_rickettsial.htm. [Accessed May, 2009].
2. DHR-ICMR Guidelines for Diagnosis and Management of Rickettsial Diseases in India 2015.
3. Kulkarni A, Vaidya S, Kulkarni P, et al. Rickettsial disease—an experience. Pediatr Infect Dis. 2009;1:118-24.
4. Kulkarni A. Childhood rickettsiosis. Indian J Pediatr. 2011; 78(1):81-7.
5. Mathai E, Lloyd G, Cherian T, et al. Serological evidence of continued presence of human rickettsiosis in Southern India. Ann Trop Med Parasitol. 2001;95:395-8.
6. Padbidri VS, Rodrigues JJ, Shetty PS. Tick-borne rickettsiosis in Pune district, Maharashtra, India. Int J Zoonoses. 1984;11:45-52.
7. Raoult D, Parola P. Rickettsial Diseases. New York: Informa Healthcare; 2007.
8. Rathi N, Kulkarni A, Yewale V, et al. IAP Guidelines on Rickettsial diseases. Indian Pediatrics. 2017;54:223-9.
9. Rathi N, Rathi A. Rickettsial infections: Indian perspective. Indian Pediatr. 2010;47:157-64.
10. Rathi NB, Rathi AN, Goodman MH. Rickettsial diseases in Central India: proposed clinical scoring system for early detection of spotted fever. Indian Pediatr. 2011;48:867-72.
11. Rathore MH, Steele RW. Rickettsial Infection. Available from http://emedicine.medscape.com/article/968385-overview.
12. Reller ME, Dumler JS. Rickettsial Infections. Nelson's Textbook of Paediatrics,19th edition. pp. 1038-53.
13. Scola B, Raoult D. Laboratory diagnosis of rickettsioses. J Clin Microbiol. 1997;33:2715-27.
14. Somashekar HR, Prabhakar DM, Sreeja P, et al. Magnitude and features of scrub typhus and spotted fever in children in India. J Trop Pediatr. 2006;52(3):228-9.
15. Sundhindra BK, Vijaykumar S, Kutti AK. Rickettsial spotted fevers in Kerala. Natl Med J India. 2004;17:51-2.
16. Todar K. Todar's Online Text Book of Bacteriology Rickettsial Diseases, including Typhus and Rocky Mountain Spotted Fever. Available from http://textbookofbacteriology.net/Rickettsia_2.html.
17. Walker DH. Rickettsiae and rickettsial infections: current state of knowledge. Clin Infect Dis. 2007;45(Suppl 1):S39-44.

Janani Sankar

7.2 LEPTOSPIROSIS IN CHILDREN

INTRODUCTION

Leptospirosis is a zoonosis of ubiquitous distribution, caused by infection with pathogenic *Leptospira* species. The spectrum of human disease caused by leptospires is extremely wide, ranging from subclinical infection to a severe syndrome of multiorgan infection with high mortality.

EPIDEMIOLOGY

Leptospirosis is presumed to be the most widespread zoonosis in the world. The source of infection in humans is usually either direct or indirect contact with the urine of an infected animal. The incidence is significantly higher in warm-climate countries than in temperate regions this is due mainly to longer survival of leptospires in the environment in warm, humid conditions. The disease is seasonal, with peak incidence occurring in summer or fall in temperate regions, where temperature is the limiting factor in survival of leptospires, and during rainy seasons in warm-climate regions, where rapid desiccation would otherwise prevent survival.

The usual portal of entry is through abrasions or cuts in the skin or via the conjunctiva; infection may take place via intact skin after prolonged immersion in water. Water-borne transmission has been documented; point contamination of water supplies has resulted in several outbreaks of leptospirosis. Inhalation of water or aerosols also may result in infection via the mucous membranes of the respiratory tract. Rarely, infection may follow animal bites. Direct transmission between humans has been demonstrated rarely. However, excretion of leptospires in human urine months after recovery has been recorded. It is thought that the low pH of human urine limits survival of leptospires after excretion.

The extent to which infection is transmitted depends on many factors, including climate, population density, and the degree of contact between maintenance and accidental hosts. Different rodent species may be reservoirs of distinct serovars, but rats are generally maintenance hosts for serovars of the serogroups lcterohemorrhagiae and ballum, and mice are the maintenance hosts for serogroup ballum. Domestic animals are also maintenance hosts; dairy cattle may harbor serovars hardjo, pomona and grippotyphosa; pigs may harbor pomona, tarassovi or bratislava; sheep may harbor hardjo and pomona; and dogs may harbor canicola. Distinct variations in maintenance hosts and the serovars they carry occur throughout the world. Knowledge of the prevalent serovars and their maintenance hosts is essential to understanding the epidemiology of the disease in any region.

CLINICAL FEATURES

Anicteric Form

The clinical presentation of leptospirosis varies widely. It can range from an acute febrile illness to a severe syndrome of multiorgan dysfunction. The more common, mild, anicteric form of the disease is characterized by nonspecific symptoms such as fever, headache, chills and severe myalgia restricting mobility. It may closely mimic acute infectious polyradiculomyelitis. Creatine phosphokinase (CPK) levels are usually very high. It may present with lymphadenopathy and generalized maculopapular rash mimicking mucocutaneous lymph node syndrome. Other manifestations include meningoencephalitis where children have severe headache and neck stiffness. Cerebrospinal fluid (CSF) shows mildly elevated protein and lymphocytosis. Neuroimaging may show leptomeningeal enhancement. CSF dark-field microscopy (DFM) for leptospires may be positive.

Similar to enteroviral infections, it can cause myocarditis which is more common in infants and toddlers. A short febrile illness with disproportionate tachycardia, muffled heart sounds and cardiomegaly with or without raised CPK MB is usually the clinical picture. Apart from parenteral crystalline penicillin these children need inotropes and hemodynamic monitoring. Polyserositis is usually seen in the form of pleural fluid, pericardial fluid, ascites and gallbladder wall edema. This is usually associated with reduced serum albumin and occasionally these fluids may test positive for DFM. Transient glomerular dysfunction which closely mimics nephrotic syndrome is seen in some children. Hepatorenal syndrome is a more serious condition which may require peritoneal or hemodialysis. It can involve the eyes and cause severe conjunctival congestion and uveitis.

Icteric Form (Weil's Syndrome)

This closely mimics acute viral hepatitis and the probable differentiating features may be the presence of polyserositis and cholecystitis. This is a severe form of the infection and occurs less commonly in children and can sometimes coexist with hepatitis A infection. When it coexists with hepatitis A infection the severity and the duration of illness is longer. Renal manifestations are common, with abnormal urine analysis (hematuria, proteinuria, and hyaline and granular casts) and azotemia, which is often associated with oliguria/anuria. Acute renal failure occurs in a few cases and is the most common cause of mortality. Both acute renal failure and jaundice are less common in children than in adults.

Institutional Experience

In a study done at Chennai in our hospital (Kanchi Kamakoti Childs Trust Hospital) over a period of 4 years (1999–2002), we had 139 children who were diagnosed as leptospirosis. Fifty-one percent of them were in the age group of 5–10 years with a male preponderance. Icteric type of leptospirosis was only in 25% of children. Nonspecific symptoms like fever and myalgia were seen in almost all children with anicteric form of leptospirosis. Fifty-three percent were DFM positive and microscopic agglutination test (MAT) was positive in 65% of children ranging from 1:200–1:600. Convalescent samples in 36 children revealed 2–4 fold rise in titer. The most common identified serovars were icterohemorrhagica in 39%, australis in 12%, grippotyphosa in 10%, hebdomadis in 9%, canicola in 17% and pomona in 6%. We also found that DFM 1+ and MAT 1:100 were positive in 29 healthy controls (13.3%) and this was attributed to endemicity of the infection.

DIAGNOSIS

Leptospirosis should be considered in all patients with acute febrile illness when there is a history of contact with animals or with soil/water contaminated with animal urine. A confirmed case of leptospirosis is one where the clinical specimens are culture positive for leptospira or the clinical symptoms are compatible with the disease and there is seroconversion or a fourfold rise in microscopic agglutination titer between acute and convalescent sera (taken at least 2 weeks apart and studied in same laboratory). A presumptive case is one where the clinical symptoms are compatible with the disease and microscopic agglutination titer is 1:100 or greater, there is a positive macroscopic agglutination slide test reaction on a single serum specimen obtained after onset of the symptoms, or there is a stable microscopic agglutination titer of 1:100 or more in two or more serum specimens obtained after onset of symptoms.

Although modified Faine's criteria are available for diagnosis of leptospirosis in adult, it has been found to be useful in older children. A high index of suspicion is required for the diagnosis when a patient presents with fever, headache and myalgia.

The Indian Leptospirosis Society's criteria for clinically suspecting leptospirosis is also very useful. According to these criteria, leptospirosis should be suspected in a child presenting with a history of abrupt onset of high fever (>39°C) and bodyache/headache, with any one or more of the following features: (i) jaundice, (ii) oliguria, (iii) cough and breathlessness, (iv) hemorrhagic tendency and (v) signs of meningeal irritation or altered sensorium or convulsions.

Modified Faine's Criteria (with Amendment) 2012

This criterion is found to be very useful in a presumptive case of leptospirosis while awaiting the lab reports. It applies clinical, epidemiological and laboratory criteria

Table 7.2.1: Modified Faine's criteria (2012).

Part A: Clinical data	
Question	Score
Headache	2
Fever	2
Temp >39°C	2
Conjunctival suffusion	4
Meningism	4
Muscle pain	4
Conjunctival suffusion	
+ Meningism	10
+ Muscle pain	
Jaundice	1
Albuminuria/Nitrogen retention	2
Hemoptysis /Dyspnea	2
Total score	
Part B: Epidemiological factors	
Question	Score
Rainfall	5
Contact with contaminated environment	4
Animal contact	1
Total score	10
Part C: Bacteriological and lab findings	
Isolation of leptospira in culture—diagnosis certain PCR	25
Positive serology	Score
ELISA IgM positive	15
SAT—Positive*	15
MAT—Single High titer+	15
Rising titer (paired sera)	15
Other rapid tests**	15

*Any one of the tests only should be scored   25
**Latex agglutination test/Lepto dipstick/Lepto tek lateral flow/Lepto Tek Dri-Dot Test
Presumptive diagnosis of leptospirosis is made of
Part A or Part A + B : 26 or more
Parts A, B, C (Total) : 25 or more
A score between 20 and 25 suggests leptospirosis as a possible diagnosis

with individual scores. It is more useful in older children (Table 7.2.1).

LABORATORY INVESTIGATIONS

The initial investigations to be done in an acutely febrile child suspected to have leptospirosis include, complete blood counts with differential leukocyte count and peripheral smear study. The total count is usually higher with polymorphonuclear predominance and careful examination of the peripheral smear shows toxic granulation in the neutrophils. The platelet count is usually reduced. C-reactive protein (CRP) may be positive and serum albumin levels may be low more so in children with polyserositis. Bilirubin and liver transaminases are raised in children with icteric form of leptospirosis. CPK may be raised in children presenting with myalgia and CPK MB may be raised in children with myocardial involvement.

For the specific diagnosis of leptospirosis the following tests are available.

Serological Tests

Serologic testing is mostly used for diagnosis. Enzyme-linked immunosorbent assay (ELISA) for detection of IgM antibodies (which is positive from the fifth day of illness onwards) and IgM-specific dot-ELISA tests are now recommended in clinical practice; these tests have sensitivity greater than 80–90% and are done at many regular pathological and microbiological laboratories. Between two and four fold rise in titer is suggestive of leptospirosis. Single high titer is usually seen during the 2nd or 3rd week of illness.

The slide agglutination method, Dri-Dot assay, LEPTO Dipstick, latex agglutination, complement fixation assay, indirect immunofluorescent test and indirect hemagglutination test are also available; these tests too have good sensitivity of up to 85%.

The microscopic agglutination test (serogroup-specific assay) using live antigen suspension of leptospiral serovars is the reference method. This test is available only in a few research institutes and is not helpful for diagnosing leptospirosis during the acute illness; however, it remains important for epidemiological research purposes. The test is read by dark-field microscopy for agglutination and the titers are determined; a fourfold or greater increase in titer in paired sera is confirmative. Agglutinins usually appear by the 12th day of illness and reach the maximum titer by the 3rd week. Due to lack of specific live serovars MAT is not regularly done. MAT titer of 1:400 in endemic areas and a titre of 1:100 in non endemic areas are considered diagnostic of infection. The limitations of MAT are:

1. Antibody titers rise and peak only in 2nd or 3rd week making it a less sensitive test.
2. High titers of past infection persist for long time and therefore interfere with diagnosis of current infection.
3. The cut-off titer for diagnosis of current infection depends on whether the area is endemic or nonendemic; the cut-off titers varies from 1/100–1/800. Therefore a second sample is usually required to diagnose current infection. Seroepidemiological studies are required for determining the cut-off values.
4. The test is complicated requiring dark field microscopy and cultures of live serovars.

Demonstration of Organism in Cultures

Although not commonly employed in routine practice, demonstration of the organisms in the patient's blood and culture of the organism can be used for diagnosis before the 10th day of the illness. Spirochetes can be demonstrated by phase-contrast or dark-field microscopy but these are not very sensitive tests. Leptospira are cultured on media containing rabbit serum or bovine serum albumin and long-chain fatty acids. Leptospira can be recovered from the blood or CSF during the first 10 days of illness and from the urine after 14 days.

Detection of DNA

Deoxyribonucleic acid hybridization techniques or nucleic acid amplification procedures, including polymerase chain reaction (PCR), can be used to detect the presence of leptospira in body fluids or culture supernatants within the first week of the disease.

TREATMENT

Leptospirosis usually responds to oral amoxicillin (50–100 mg/kg/day for 7 days), azithromycin (10 mg/kg/day for 3 days), cefixime (10 mg/kg/day for 7days) and doxycycline (5–10 mg/kg/day for 7 days).

Antibiotic administration especially before the 7th day of illness reduces the length of hospitalization and leptospiruria. Treatment with parenteral penicillin 50,000–100,000 U/kg/day or ceftriaxone 75–100 mg/kg/day is usually reserved for very sick children with meningoencephalitis, myocarditis and renal involvement.

Adequate attention to supportive care, including maintenance of the fluid-electrolyte balance, treatment of cardiovascular collapse and provision of dialysis for renal failure, is equally important. Frequent monitoring of vital parameters and hemodynamic assessment, careful charting of fluid input and output, and prompt use of ionotropes in patients with hypotension refractory to fluid therapy are important considerations in the management of the disease.

COMPLICATIONS

Complications are usually less common in children when compared to adults. However, severe forms can lead to renal failure, acute liver cell failure, acute respiratory distress syndrome (ARDS), myocarditis and meningoencephalitis.

PREVENTION

Important measures for prevention are rodent control and avoidance of contact with contaminated water and soil. Parents should instruct children not to wade through flood waters or play in puddles/stagnant water. Immunization of livestock (cattle, sheep, pigs and horses) and family pets (cats and dogs) has been recommended as a means of eliminating some of the animal reservoirs. Awareness of importance of environmental hygiene should be stressed and propagated.

BIBLIOGRAPHY

1. Azim P. Nelson Text Book of Pediatrics, 19th edition. Philadelphia: Saunders; 2011. pp. 984–5.
2. Stoddard R, Shadomy SV. CDC Health Information for International Travel 2012: The Yellow Book Chapter 3(71).
3. Terpstra WJ. Human Leptospirosis: Guidance for Diagnosis, Surveillance and Control. World Health Organization, International Leptospirosis Society; 2003.

INTRODUCTION

Brucellosis is one of the major bacterial zoonoses, and in humans is also known as undulant fever, Malta fever or Mediterranean fever. Expansion of animal industries, urbanization, lack of hygienic measures in animal husbandry and in food handling are the factors contributing to brucellosis. *Brucella* infection continues to be major public health problem worldwide. Humans are accidental hosts and acquire this zoonotic disease from direct contact with an infected animal or consumption of products of an infected animal. Brucellosis is widely recognized as an occupational risk among adults working with livestock. In children, *Brucella* infection is food-borne and is associated with consumption of unpasteurized milk products. Males are affected more commonly than females which may be due to risk of occupational exposure. However, in areas, where *Brucella melitensis* is endemic, pediatric cases are seen. Although brucellosis in human beings is rarely fatal, it can be severely debilitating and disabling. The disease has a tendency toward chronicity and persistence, becoming a granulomatous disease capable of affecting any organ system. The timely and accurate diagnosis of human brucellosis continues to challenge clinicians because of its nonspecific clinical features, slow growth rate in blood cultures and the complexity of its serodiagnosis. It is also a potential agent of bioterrorism.

EPIDEMIOLOGY

The epidemiology of brucellosis is complex and it changes from time to time. Wide host range and resistance of brucellae to environment and host immune system facilitate its survival in the population.

Worldwide, brucellosis remains a major source of disease in humans and domestic animals. It is more prevalent in Western parts of Asia, India, Middle Eastern, Southern European and Latin American countries. Human brucellosis is found to have significant presence in rural/nomadic communities where people live in close association with animals. Worldwide reported incidence of human brucellosis in endemic areas varies widely from less than 0.01 to greater than 200 per 100,000 populations. It has been estimated that the true incidence may be 25 times higher than the reported incidence, due to misdiagnosis and under-reporting.

In India, it is significant and increasing veterinary and public health problem. Eighty percent of the populations live in villages and small towns have close contact with domestic/wild animal population owing to their occupation. *B. melitensis* and *B. abortus* are two species which are of main concern in India. Bovine brucellosis is widespread in India due to increase in trade and rapid movement of livestock. Free grazing and movement with frequent mixing of flocks of sheep and goats also contribute to the wide distribution of brucellosis. As per various studies the prevalence of human brucellosis varies from 3% to 34%. In almost all states, brucellosis cases have been reported but the brucellosis situation varies widely between states.

Among children, however, geographic locations that are endemic for *B. melitensis* remain as areas of increased risk for the development of infection. In such locations, unpasteurized milk from goats or camels may be used to feed children, thus leading to the development of brucellosis. Consequently, a history of travel to endemic regions or consumption of exotic food or unpasteurized dairy or dairy products may be an important clue to the diagnosis of human brucellosis. But because of improved routine screening of domestic livestock and animal vaccination programs, brucellosis has become rare in industrialized countries.

ETIOLOGY

Agent

The agents are small, gram-negative rod-shaped, non-motile, nonsporing and intracellular coccobacilli of the genus brucella. Four species infect human: (1) *B. melitensis*, (2) *B. abortus*, (3) *B. suis* and (4) *B. canis*. *B. melitensis* is the most virulent and invasive species; it usually infects goats and occasionally sheep. *B. abortus* is less virulent and is primarily a disease of cattle. *B. suis* is of intermediate virulence and chiefly infects pigs. *B. canis* is a parasite of dogs (Table 7.3.1).

Reservoir of Infections

Main reservoirs of human infection are cattle, sheep, goats, swine, buffaloes, horse and dogs. In animals, the disease can cause abortion, premature expulsion of the

Table 7.3.1: Etiology of brucellosis.

Species	Natural host	Human pathogen
B. abortus	Cattle	Yes
B. melitensis	Goats, sheep	Yes
B. suis	Swine	Yes
	Hares	Yes
	Reindeer, caribou	Yes
	Rodents	Yes
B. canis	Dogs, other canids	Yes
B. ovis	Sheep	No
B. neotomae	Desert wood rat	No
B. maris (?)	Marine mammals	?

fetus or death. Cross infections can often occur between animal species. The infected animals excrete brucellae in the urine, milk, placenta, uterine and vaginal discharges particularly during a birth or abortion. The animals may remain infected throughout life.

Mode of Transmission

Transmission is usually from infected animals to human. There are some evidences of human to human transmission also.

The routes of spread are:
- *Food-borne infections*: Infection takes place indirectly by the ingestion of raw milk or dairy products (cheese) from infected animals. Fresh raw vegetables grown on soil and water contaminated with the excreta of infected animals may also serve as a source of infection.
- *Contact infection*: Most commonly, infection occurs by direct contact with infected tissues, abraded skin, mucosa, conjunctiva (mucocutaneous route), blood, urine, vaginal discharge, aborted fetuses, etc.
- *Air-borne infections*: The environment of a cowshed may be heavily infected. Few people living in such an environment can expose to inhalation of infected dust or aerosols. *Brucella* may be inhaled in aerosol form in slaughter houses and laboratories, so these infections are notified as occupational.
- *Transplacental infections*: Congenital and neonatal infections with these organisms have also been described. These have been transmitted transplacentaly, from breast milk, and through blood transfusions.
- *Person-to-person infection*: This is extremely rare. Occasional cases have been reported in which circumstantial evidence suggests close personal or sexual contact as the route of transmission. Of more potential significance is transmission through blood donation or tissue trans-plantation. Bone marrow transfer in particular carries a significant risk. It is advisable that blood and tissue donors be screened for evidence of brucellosis and positive reactors with a history of recent infection should be excluded. Transmission to attendants of brucellosis patients is most unlikely, but basic precautions should be taken.

Incubation Period

It is highly variable. Usually 1–3 weeks, but may be as long as 6 months or more. When brucellosis is suspected, the clinical laboratory should be alerted so the cultures can be maintained for greater than 21 days to ensure growth if the organism is present.

PATHOGENESIS

Brucella species are facultative intracellular bacteria that can multiply within phagocytic cells with human beings as end hosts. Brucella may enter the host via ingestion or inhalation or through conjunctiva or skin abrasions, contaminated meat or dairy products.

The risk for infection depends on the nutritional and immune status of the host, the route of inoculums, and the species of *Brucella*. For reasons that remain unclear, *B. melitensis* and *B. suis* tend to be more virulent than *B. abortus* or *B. canis*. The major virulence factor for *Brucella* appears to be its cell wall lipopolysaccharide. Strains containing smooth lipopolysaccharide have been demonstrated to have greater virulence and are more resistant to killing by polymorphonuclear leukocytes. These organisms are facultative intracellular pathogens that can survive and replicate within the mononuclear phagocytic cells (monocytes, macrophages) of the reticuloendothelial system. Even though *Brucella* is chemotactic for entry of leukocytes into the body, the leukocytes are less efficient in killing these organisms than other bacteria despite the assistance of serum factors such as complement.

Organisms that are not phagocytosed by leukocytes are ingested by the macrophages and become localized within the reticuloendothelial system. Specifically, they reside within the liver, spleen, lymph nodes and bone marrow, and result in granuloma formation (Fig. 7.3.1).

Antibodies are produced against the lipopolysaccharide and other cell wall antigens. This provides a means of diagnosis and probably has a role in long-term immunity. The major factor in recovery from infection appears to be the development of a cell-mediated response resulting in macrophage activation and enhanced intracellular killing. Specifically, sensitized T lymphocytes release cytokines (e.g. interferon-γ and tumor necrosis factor-α) which activate the macrophages and enhance their intracellular killing capacity.

Research suggests that the smooth, nonendotoxic lipopolysaccharides help to block the development of

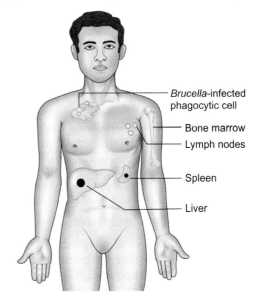

FIG. 7.3.1: Spread of *Brucella* in the body.

innate and specific immunity during the early stage of infection, and protect the pathogen from the microbicidal activities of the immune system. Rough (vaccine) strains (i.e. strains with lipopolysaccharide lacking the O-side chain) are less virulent because of their inability to overcome the host defense system.

CLINICAL MANIFESTATIONS

Brucellosis is a systemic illness that can be very difficult to diagnose in children without a history of animal or food exposure. Human brucellosis usually manifests as an acute or subacute febrile illness, which may persist, and progress to a chronically incapacitating disease with severe complications. Complaints may persist for weeks or months in absence of specific treatment. Symptoms can be acute or insidious in nature and are usually nonspecific, beginning 2–4 weeks after inoculation. The clinical features of brucellosis depend on the stage of the disease, and the organs and systems involved. Although the clinical manifestations do vary, the classic triad of fever, arthralgia/arthritis and hepatosplenomegaly can be demonstrated in most patients. Some patients present as a fever of unknown origin.

Brucella has been reported to compromise the central and peripheral nervous system, gastrointestinal, hepatobiliary, genitourinary, musculoskeletal, cardiovascular and integumentary systems. Despite major ongoing controversies in the taxonomy of *Brucella* species, the bulk of human disease is caused by two species: (1) *B. melitensis* and (2) *B. abortus*. On physical examination, the most common findings are hepatomegaly and splenomegaly, which occur in about one-third of patients. Lymphadenopathy is seen in about 10% of patients.

Gastrointestinal and Hepatobiliary Manifestations

Liver is a most commonly involved organ. Abdominal pain, constipation, hepatomegaly, jaundice, splenomegaly are also seen.

Osteoarticular Manifestations

Sacroiliitis, spondylitis, peripheral arthritis and osteomyelitis account for over half of the focal manifestations. The most common osteoarticular finding in children is monoarticular arthritis (usually of the knees and hips).

Cardiovascular Manifestations

Endocarditis with the aortic valve being the most commonly affected structure and multiple valve involvement being common within this subset of patients. It is the most serious problem, accounting for 5% total mortality rate of human brucella infections. Cardiac murmur is rare.

Genitourinary Manifestations

Glomerulonephritis, orchiepididymitis and renal abscesses can be found in 10% of cases.

Neurological Manifestations

This includes peripheral neuropathies, chorea, meningoencephalitis, transient ischemic attacks, psychiatric manifestations and cranial nerve compromise.

Skin Manifestations

Skin manifestations are erythematous papular lesions, purpura, dermal cysts and Stevens-Johnson syndrome, etc.

Pulmonary Manifestations

These include pleural effusion and pneumonias that can be found in up to 16% of complicated cases of brucellosis.

Congenital and Neonatal Manifestations

Congenital and neonatal infections with these organisms have also been described. The signs and symptoms associated with brucellosis are vague and not pathognomonic.

DIAGNOSIS

A history of exposure to animals or ingestion of unpasteurized dairy products is very helpful. A definitive diagnosis is made by recovering the organism from blood culture, bone marrow aspiration or other tissues. Routine laboratory examinations of the blood are not helpful; thrombocytopenia, neutropenia, anemia or pancytopenia may occur. Leukocytosis is observed in about 9% of patients, and, if found, focal complications should be excluded. Leukopenia (11% of patients) and thrombocytopenia (10% of patients) are seen in similar frequencies. Anemia is seen more frequently, affecting 26% of patients (Fig. 7.3.2).

CULTURE

Blood culture is the gold standard in the diagnosis of bacterial infections, including brucellosis. Although the biphasic Ruiz-Castañeda system is the traditional method for the isolation of *Brucella* spp from clinical samples, it has now largely been replaced by automated culture systems such as the lysis centrifugation method with increased sensitivity and reduced culture times. The sensitivity of blood culture depends on several factors, particularly the phase of the disease and previous use of antibiotics. For instance, in acute cases, the sensitivities of the Ruiz-Castañeda method and lysis centrifugation have been reported as high as 80% and 90% respectively, but as low as 30% and 70% respectively, in chronic cases.

Although automated culture systems and the use of the lysis centrifugation method have shortened the isolation

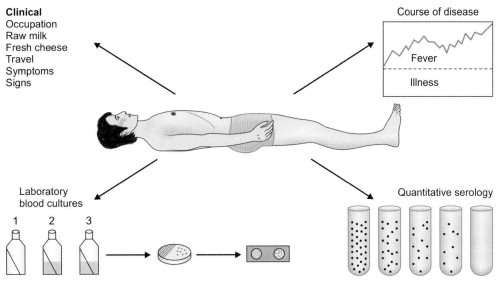

FIG. 7.3.2: History and physical examination.

time from weeks to days, it is prudent to alert the clinical microbiology laboratory that brucellosis is suspected. Isolation of the organism still may require as long as 4 weeks from a blood culture sample. Caution is also advised when using automated bacterial identification systems, because isolate have been misidentified as other gram-negative organisms (*Haemophilus influenzae type b*).

Bone marrow cultures may provide a higher sensitivity, yield faster culture times, and may be superior to blood cultures when evaluating patients with previous antibiotic use. *Brucella* can also be cultured from pus, tissue samples, and cerebrospinal, pleural, joint or ascitic fluid. Since brucellosis constitutes one of the most common laboratory-acquired infections, special care should be taken when using the lysis centrifugation method to avoid infection from contaminated aerosols.

SERODIAGNOSIS

Agglutination Tests

The serum agglutination test (SAT) detects antibodies against *B. melitensis, B. abortus, B. suis*. This method does not detect antibodies against *B. canis* because this organism lacks the smooth lipopolysaccharide. In the absence of culture facilities, the diagnosis of brucellosis traditionally relies on serological testing with a variety of agglutination tests such as the Rose Bengal test, the SAT and the antiglobulin or Coombs' test.

In general, the Rose Bengal test is used as a screening test, and positive results are confirmed by the SAT. These agglutination tests are based on the reactivity of antibodies against smooth lipopolysaccharide. These antibodies tend to persist in patients long after recovery; therefore, in endemic areas, high background values could occur that may affect the diagnostic value of the test (*Prozone effect*).

In addition the prozone effect can give false negative result in the presence of high titers of antibodies; to avoid this serum that is being tested should be diluted to greater than or equal to 1:320. Furthermore, the *Brucella* smooth lipopolysaccharide antigen tends to show cross reactivity with other gram-negative bacterias such as *Yersinia enterocolitica* 0:9, *Vibrio cholerae, Escherichia coli* 0:157, and *Francisella tularensis*, increasing the possibility of false-positive results.

No single titer is ever diagnostic, but most patients with acute infections have titers of greater than or equal to 1:160. Low titers may be found early in the course of the illness, requiring the use of acute and convalescent sera testing to confirm the diagnosis. Because patient with active infection have both an immunoglobulin M (IgM) and an immunoglobulin G (IgG) response, and the SAT measures the total quantity of agglutinating antibodies, the total quantity of IgG is measured by treatment of the serum with 2-mercaptoethanol. It is important to remember that all titers must be interpreted in light of a patient's history and physical examinations. Coombs' test may be more suitable for confirmation of brucellosis in relapsing patients or patients with persisting disease.

ELISA

Enzyme-linked immunosorbent assay (ELISA) has become increasingly popular as a well standardized assay for brucellosis. The sensitivity of ELISAs prepared in the laboratory may be high, especially when the detection of specific IgM antibodies is complemented with the detection of specific IgG antibodies. The specificity of ELISA, however, seems to be less than that of the agglutination tests. Since, ELISA for *Brucella* is based on the detection of antibodies against smooth lipopolysaccharide, the cut-off value may need adjustment to optimize specificity when used in endemic areas, and this may influence sensitivity.

Rapid Point-of-care Assays

Rapid tests such as the fluorescent polarization immunoassay (FPA) for brucellosis and the immunochromatographic *Brucella* IgM/IgG lateral flow assay (LFA), a simplified version of ELISA, have great potential as point-of-care tests. The FPA test is done by incubation of a serum sample with *Brucella* O-polysaccharide antigen linked to a fluorescent probe. The sensitivity of this test at the selected cut-off value is 96% for culture-confirmed brucellosis, and the specificity was determined to be 98% for samples from healthy blood donors.

The LFA uses a drop of blood obtained by fingerpick, does not require specific training. It is easy to interpret, and can be used at the bedside. The components are stabilized and do not require refrigeration for transportation or storage. The sensitivity and specificity of LFA are high (>95%), and the test can be used at all stages of disease. Another useful application for these tests is to screen the contacts of brucellosis patients.

Molecular Detection

Polymerase chain reaction (PCR) is a convenient tool for the diagnosis of human brucellosis that may improve sensitivity compared with culture. As per various studies PCR is found to be 100% sensitive and 98.3% specific to *Brucella* species, compared with 70% sensitivity for blood culture. PCR could be particularly useful in patients with specific complications such as neurobrucellosis, or other localized infections, since serological testing often fails in such patients. Relapsing brucellosis is another diagnostic challenge in which PCR could prove to be useful.

OTHER APPLICATIONS OF PCR

Polymerase chain reaction also appears to be useful in species differentiation and biotyping of isolates. PCR amplification of these variable repeats in more robust than classic typing methods for species and biovar identification. PCR was recently used to assess treatment efficacy.

Sonography of Abdomen

Microabscesses in spleen may be found in *Brucella* infection.

DIFFERENTIAL DIAGNOSIS

In Indian scenario, typhoid tuberculosis, cholecystitis, pyelitis, autoimmune disorders, etc. are more important differentials than tularemia, cat scratch disease, etc.

Brucellosis may be confused with other infections, such as tularemia, cat scratch disease, typhoid fever and fungal infections, due to histoplasmosis, blastomycosis or coccidioidomycosis. Infections caused by *Mycobacterium* *tuberculosis*, atypical mycobacteria, rickettsiae, and *Yersinia* can present in a similar fashion to brucellosis.

TREATMENT

Prolonged antimicrobial therapy is imperative for achieving a cure. Relapses generally are not associated with development of *Brucella* resistance but rather with premature discontinuation of therapy. Monotherapy is associated with a high rate of relapse; combination therapy is recommended. Many antimicrobial agents are active in vitro against the *Brucella* species, but the clinical effectiveness does not always correlate with these results. Doxycycline is the most useful antimicrobial agent and when combined with an aminoglycoside, is associated with the fewest relapses (Table 7.3.2).

Treatment failures with β-lactam antimicrobial agents, including the 3rd generation cephalosporins, may be due to the intracellular nature of the organism. Agents that provide intracellular killing are required for eradication of this infection. Similarly, it is apparent that prolonged treatment is the key to prevent disease relapse. Relapse is confirmed by isolation of *Brucella* within weeks to months after therapy has ended and is usually not associated with antimicrobial resistance.

The onset of initial antimicrobial therapy may precipitate a Jarisch-Herxheimer-like reaction, presumably due to a large antigen load. It is rarely severe enough to require corticosteroid therapy.

Evaluation of immunomodulation with levamisole plus conventional therapy in the management of chronic brucellosis has shown mixed results. Although initial reports of the addition of interferon α-2a to standard therapy in allergic patients seemed somewhat promising, this has not led to any practical application. Currently, extended treatment with standard drug combinations should be given to those patients with persisting signs and symptoms of recurrent disease.

Additionally, when treating focal infections, careful attention must be given to the penetration and activity of the drug in the particular tissue involved, and the choice and duration of therapy must be individualized with prolonged treatment in cases with specific complications such as endocarditis or central nervous system involvement. The more effective doxycycline-streptomycin combination is preferred in patients with more severe disease, such as spinal involvement, and the duration of therapy may be prolonged. Abscesses and specific localized forms of brucellosis including endocarditis, cerebral, epidural or splenic abscess might require surgical interventions since these forms are resistant to antibiotics.

COMPLICATIONS

Osteoarticular complications (sacroiliitis, spondylitis, peripheral arthritis and osteomyelitis) account for over half of the focal complications. Endocarditis with the aortic

Table 7.3.2: Recommended therapy for the treatment of brucellosis.

Age and condition	Antimicrobial agent	Dose	Route	Duration
> 8 years	Doxycycline	2–4 mg/kg/day; maximum 200 mg/day	PO	6 weeks
	+ Rifampin	15–20 mg/kg/day; maximum 600–900 mg/day	PO	6 weeks
	Alternative; Doxycycline	2–4 mg/kg/day; maximum 200 mg/day	PO	6 weeks
	+ Streptomycin	15–30 mg/kg/day; maximum 1 g/day	IM	2 weeks
	or Gentamicin	3–5 mg/kg/day	IM/IV	2 weeks
< 8 years	Trimethoprim-sulfamethoxazole (TMP-SMZ)	TMP (10 mg/kg/day; maximum 480 mg/day) and SMZ (50 mg/kg/day; maximum 2.4 g/day)	PO	4–8 weeks
	+ Rifampin	15–20 mg/kg/day	PO	6 weeks
Meningitis, osteomyelitis				
Endocarditis	Doxycycline	2–4 mg/kg/day; maximum 200 mg/day	PO	4–6 months
	+ Gentamicin	3–5 mg/kg/day	IV	2 weeks
	+ Rifampin	15–20 mg/kg/day; maximum 600–900 mg/day	PO	4–6 months

valve being the most commonly affected structure. Multiple valve involvement being common within this subset of patients is the most serious complication accounting for most of the 5% total mortality rate in human brucellosis.

Genitourinary complications (orchiepididymitis, glomerulonephritis and renal abscesses) can be found in around 10% of patients. Neurological complications include peripheral neuropathies, chorea, meningoencephalitis, transient ischemic attacks, psychiatric manifestations and cranial nerve compromise. Mucocutaneous complications include erythematous popular lesions, purpura, dermal cysts and Stevens-Johnson syndrome. Pulmonary complications including pleural effusions and pneumonias can be found in up to 16% of complicated cases of brucellosis.

PROGNOSIS

Before the use of antimicrobial agents, the course of brucellosis was often prolonged and may have led to death. Since the institution of specific therapy, most deaths are due to specific organ system involvement (e.g. endocarditis) in complicated cases. The prognosis after specific therapy is excellent if patients are compliant with the prolonged therapy.

PREVENTION

Isolation of the Hospitalized Patient

In addition to standard precautions, contact precautions are indicated for patients with draining wounds. since

human to human spread is extremely rare, isolation may give a wrong message for students.

Control Measures

In the Humans

Early diagnosis and treatment: In uncomplicated cases the antibiotic of choice is tetracycline.

In patients with skeletal or other complications, intramuscular streptomycin daily in addition to tetracycline usually achieves a cure.

Pasteurization of milk: Pasteurization of milk and dairy products for human consumption remain an important aspect of prevention.

Protective measures: The aim is to prevent direct contact with infected animals. Person at risk, such as farmers, shepherds, milkmen, abattoir workers, should observe high standards of personal hygiene.

Vaccination: No vaccine is currently available for use in children.

In the Animals

The most rational approach for preventing human brucellosis is the control and eradication of the infection from animal reservoirs which is based on the combination of the following measures:

Test and slaughter: Case finding is done by mass surveys. Skin tests are available. The complement fixation test is also recommended. Those animals infected with brucellosis are slaughtered with full compensation paid to farmers.

Vaccination: Vaccine of *B. abortus* strain 19 is commonly used for young animals. A compulsory vaccination program for all heifers in a given community on a yearly basis can considerably reduce the rate of infection. Control of the infection caused by *B. melitensis* in goats and sheep has to be based mainly on vaccination.

Hygienic measures: These comprise provision of a clean sanitary environment for animals, sanitary disposal of urine and feces, veterinary care of animal, and health education of all those who are occupationally involved.

BIBLIOGRAPHY

1. Abdoel TH, Smits HL. Rapid latex agglutination test for the serodiagnosis of human brucellosis. Diagn Microbiol Infect Dis. 2007;57:123–8.
2. Agasthya AS, Isloor S, Prabhudas K. Brucellosis in high risk group individuals (Journal Article). Indian J Med Microbiol. 2007;25(1):28-31.
3. Almuneef M, Memish ZA. Persistence of Brucella antibodies after successful treatment of acute brucellosis in an area of endemicity. J Clin Microbiol. 2002;40(6):2313
4. Almuneef MA, Memish ZA, Balkhy HH, et al. Importance of screening household members of acute brucellosis cases in endemic areas. Epidemiol Infect. 2004;132:533-40.
5. Araj GF. Enzyme-linked immunosorbent assay, not agglutination, is the test of choice for the diagnosis of neurobrucellosis. Clin Infect Dis. 1997;25:942
6. Bayindir Y, Sonmez E, Aladag A, et al. Comparison of five antimicrobial regimens for the treatment of brucellar spondylitis: a prospective, randomized study. J Chemother. 2003;15:466-71.
7. Chahota R, Sharma M, Katoch RC, et al. Brucellosis outbreak in an organized dairy farm involving cows and in contact human beings in Himachal Pradesh, India. Vet Arh. 2003;73:95-102.
8. Colmenero J, Queipo-Ortuno MI, Maria Reguera J, et al. Chronic, hepatosplenic abscesses in brucellosis. Clinico-therapeutic features and molecular diagnostic approach. Diagn Microbiol Infect Dis. 2002;42:159-67.
9. Ewals JA. Brucellosis as an imported disease in a young man with arthritis (Case Reports, English Abstract, Journal Article). Ned Tijdschr Geneeskd. 2005;149(50):2810-4.
10. Giannacopoulos I, Eliopoulou MI, Ziambaras T, et al. Transplacentally transmitted congenital brucellosis due to Brucella abortus. J Infect. 2002;45:209-10.
11. Gogia A, Dugga L, Dutta S. An unusual etiology of PUO (Case Reports, Journal Article). J Assoc Physicians India. 2011;59: 47-9.
12. Gokhale YA, Ambardekar AG, Bhasin A, et al. Brucella spondylitis and sacroiliitis in the general population in Mumbai (Journal Article, Research Support, Non-U.S. Govt). J Assoc Physicians India. 2003;51:659-66.
13. Greenfield RA, Drevets DA, Machado LJ, et al. Bacterial pathogens as biological weapons and agents of bioterrorism. Am J Med Sci. 2002;323:299-315.
14. Gur A, Geyik MF, Dikici B, et al. Complications of brucellosis in different age groups: a study of 283 cases in southeastern Anatolia of Turkey. Yonsei Med J. 2003;44:33-44.
15. Irmak H, Buzgan T, Evirgen O, et al. Use of the Brucella IgM and IgG flow assays in the serodiagnosis of human brucellosis in an area endemic for brucellosis. Am J Trop Med Hyg. 2004;70:688-94.
16. Irmak H, Buzgan T, Karahocagil MK, et al. The effect of levamisole, combined with the classical treatment in chronic brucellosis. Tohoku J Exp Med. 2003;201:221-8.
17. Kadri SM, Rukhsana A, Laharwal MA, et al. Seroprevalence of brucellosis in Kashmir (India) among patients with pyrexia of unknown origin (Journal Article). J Indian Med Assoc. 2000;98(4):170-1.
18. Kalla A, Chadda VS, Gauri LA, et al. Outbreak of polyarthritis with pyrexia in Western Rajasthan. J Assoc Physicians India. 2001;49:963-5.
19. Kochar DK, Gupta BK, Gupta A, et al. Hospital-based case series of 175 cases of serologically confirmed brucellosis in Bikaner. J Assoc Physicians India. 2007;55:271-5.
20. Kochar DK, Kumawat BL, Agarwal N, et al. Meningoencephalitis in brucellosis. Neurol India. 2000;48:170-3.
21. Kochar DK, Sharma BV, Gupta S, et al. Pulmonary manifestations in brucellosis: a report on seven cases from Bikaner (north-west India). J Assoc Physicians India. 2003;51:33-6.
22. Kumar S, Tuteja U, Sarika K, et al. Rapid multiplex PCR assay for the simultaneous detection of the Brucella Genus, *B. abortus, B. melitensis*, and *B. suis* (Evaluation Studies, Journal Article). J Microbiol Biotechnol. 2011;21(1):89-92.
23. Lapaque N, Moriyon I, Moreno E, et al. Brucella lipopolysaccharide acts as a virulence factor. Curr Opin Microbiol. 2005;8: 60-6.
24. Mangalgi S, Sajjan A, Mohite ST. Seroprevalence of brucellosis among Blood Donors of Satara District, Maharashtra (original article) Dept of Microbiology, Krishna Institute of Medical Sciences University, Karad (Maharashtra), India. JKIMSU. 2012;1(1):55-60 [ISSN 2231-4261].
25. Mantur B, Parande A, Amarnath S, et al. ELISA versus conventional methods of diagnosing endemic brucellosis (Comparative Study, Journal Article, Research Support, Non-U.S. Govt). Am J Trop Med Hyg. 2010;83(2):314-8.
26. Mantur BG, Akki AS, Mangalgi SS, et al. Childhood brucellosis—a microbiological, epidemiological and clinical study. J Trop Pediatr. 2004;50:153-7.
27. Mantur BG, Amarnath SK, Parande AM, et al. Comparison of a novel immunocapture assay with standard serological methods in the diagnosis of brucellosis (Comparative Study, Controlled Clinical Trial, Journal Article). Clin Lab. 2011;57(5-6):333-41.
28. Mantur BG, Mangalgi SS. Evaluation of conventional castaneda and lysis centrifugation blood culture techniques for diagnosis of human brucellosis (Comparative Study, Journal Article). J Clin Microbiol. 2004;42(9):4327-8.
29. Mirnejad R, Doust RH, Kachuei R, et al. Simultaneous detection and differentiates of *Brucella abortus* and *Brucella melitensis* by combinatorial PCR (Evaluation Studies, Journal Article, Research Support, Non-U.S. Govt). Asian Pac J Trop Med. 2012;5(1):24-8.

30. Palanduz A, Palanduz S, Guler K, et al. Brucellosis in a mother and her young infant: probable transmission by breast milk. Int J Infect Dis. 2000;4:55-6.

31. Purwar S, Metgud SC, Darshan A, et al. Infective endocarditis due to brucella (Case Reports, Journal Article). Indian J Med Microbiol. 2006;24(4):286-8.

32. Rahman AKMA, Dirk B, Fretin D, et al. Seroprevalence and Risk Factors for Brucellosis in a High-Risk Group of Individuals in Bangladesh. Food Borne Pathogens and Disease. 2012;9(3):190-7.

33. Renukaradhya GJ, Isloor S, Rajasekhar M. Epidemiology, zoonotic aspects, vaccination and control/eradication of brucellosis in India (Journal Article). Vet Microbiol. 2002;90(1-4):183-95.

34. Roth F, Zinsstag J, Orkhon D, et al. Human health benefits from livestock vaccination for brucellosis: case study. Bull World Health Organ. 2003;81:867-76.

35. Roushan MR, Gangi SM, Ahmadi SA. Comparison of the efficacy of two months of treatment with co-trimoxazole plus doxycycline vs. co-trimoxazole plus rifampin in brucellosis. Swiss Med Wkly. 2004;134:564-8.

36. Ruben B, Band JD, Wong P, et al. Person-to-person, transmission of Brucella melitensis. Lancet. 1991;337:14-5.

37. Ruiz-Mesa JD, Sanchez-Gonzalez J, Reguera JM, et al. Rose Bengal test: diagnostic yield and use for the rapid diagnosis of human brucellosis in emergency departments in endemic areas. Clin Microbiol Infect. 2005;11:221-5.

38. Sen MR, Shukla BN, Goyal RK. Seroprevalence of brucellosis in and around Varanasi. J Commun Dis. 2002;34:226-7.

39. Solera J, Geijo P, Largo J, et al. A randomized, double-blind study to assess the optimal duration of doxycycline treatment for human brucellosis. Clin Infect Dis. 2004;39:1776-82.

40. Tikare NV, Mantur BG, Bidari LH. Brucellar meningitis in an infant—evidence for human breast milk transmission (Case Reports, Journal Article). J Trop Pediatr. 2008;54(4):272-4.

Anju Aggarwal

INTRODUCTION

Anaerobic infections are caused by anaerobic bacteria. Anaerobic bacteria can be divided into strict anaerobes that cannot grow in the presence of more than 0.5% oxygen and moderate anaerobic bacteria that are able of growing between 2% and 8% oxygen.

Anerobic bacteria are:

- Gram-positive bacilli:
    - Spore-forming bacilli—*Clostridium* species
    - Nonspore-forming bacilli—*Actinomyces, Propionibacterium, Eubacterium, Lactobacillus* and *Bifidobac-terium* species
- Gram-negative bacilli—*Bacteroides, Prevotella, Porphyromonas, Fusobacterium, Bilophila, Sutterella*
- Gram-positive cocci—*Peptostreptococcus* species
- Gram-negative cocci—*Veillonella* species.

Infection with anaerobic bacteria occur alone or as mixed infections. We should suspect anaerobic bacteria if infection occurs near a mucosal surface as oropharynx, intestinal and genitourinary tract. Presence of putrid odor, tissue necrosis, abscesses, gangrene or fasciitis should make us suspect anaerobic infections. Another situation is when we fail to recover organisms by conventional methods, despite the presence of mixed pleomorphic organisms on smears.

Toxin mediated syndromes, such as botulism, tetanus, gas gangrene, food poisoning, pseudomembranous colitis, are due to anaerobic infections. At times thrombophlebitis and septicemic syndrome with jaundice or intravascular hemolysis can been seen. *Clostridium perfringens* causes bacteremia and wound infections. *Clostridium botulinum* can produce a paralytic toxin that causes a lethal illness in adults and a paralytic syndrome in infants. Many of the bacteroides species can produce the enzyme beta-lactamase. *Bacteroides fragilis* is most frequently involved in intra-abdominal infections, infections of the female genital tract, subcutaneous abscesses, and bacteremia. *Bacteroides melaninogenicus* and *Bacteroides oralis* are the predominant anaerobes in orofacial infections and aspiration pneumonia. Fusobacterium species are pathogens in aspiration pneumonia, brain abscesses and orofacial infections. Anaerobic gram-positive cocci can be recovered from all types of infections but predominate in respiratory tract and intra-abdominal infections.

Anaerobic infections affect all body systems. Various common infections caused by anaerobic bacteria are as follows.

NEONATAL INFECTIONS

Neonate is exposed to the cervical birth canal flora both aerobic and anaerobic and these have been seen in infant's gastric secretions, conjunctiva, which harbors aerobic and anaerobic bacteria. In high-risk infants, introduction of these organisms by exposure, aspiration or through fetal monitoring can lead to the development of infections. Most common organisms are *Bacteroides* species, *Clostridium* species and *Fusobacterium nucleatum*. Infant botulism will be discussed separately.

CENTRAL NERVOUS SYSTEM INFECTIONS

The seeding of anaerobic bacteria into the central nervous system is either through contiguous spread from chronic mastoiditis, sinusitis or otitis media, or through hematogenous seeding from a distant site (e.g. lung or abdomen). Anaerobes are frequently isolated from brain abscesses.

The most common organisms found in brain abscess are gram-positive anaerobic cocci, *Bacteroides* species (including *B. fragilis*), *Fusobacterium* and *Actinomyces*. There are few reported cases of anaerobic meningitis associated with shunts, surgical procedures or otitis media.

HEAD AND NECK INFECTIONS

Chronic, Recurrent Pharyngotonsillitis

Group A beta-hemolytic streptococci (GABHS), *Staphylococcus aureus*, and *Streptococcus pneumoniae* are traditionally associated with tonsillar and peritonsillar infections. However, anaerobes also have been isolated from the tonsils of children with chronic recurrent tonsillitis and peritonsillar abscesses. Beta-lactamase-producing strains of *B. fragilis*, *Fusobacterium* species, and *S. aureus* were isolated from the tonsils of about three-fourth of children with recurrent tonsillitis.

Suppurative infection of the lateral pharyngeal space beginning as pharyngitis is called Lemierre syndrome or postanginal sepsis. It may complicate Epstein Barr virus or other infections of the pharynx. It usually manifests as a unilateral septic thrombophlebitis of the jugular venous system with septic pulmonary embolization. Clinical signs include unilateral painful neck swelling, trismus and dysphagia culminating with signs of sepsis and respiratory distress. *Fusobacterium necrophorum* is the most commonly isolated organism, although polymicrobial infection may occur.

Suppurative Thyroiditis and Parotitis

Suppurative thyroiditis and parotitis were generally regarded to be due primarily to *S. aureus*; however, anaerobic bacteria, including Bacteroides species and *Peptostreptococcus* species, have recently been identified as causative organisms.

Chronic Sinusitis

When appropriate anaerobic microbiological techniques are applied, anaerobes are frequently recovered in this infection. The predominant anaerobes isolates are *Peptostreptococcus* species, *Bacteroides* species and *Veillonella* species. The isolation of anaerobes in brain abscess and meningitis occurs as a sequelae to sinusitis. Effective antibiotics should be introduced early for better management of such infections.

DENTAL INFECTIONS

Anaerobes are responsible, for periodontal infections in children. *Fusobacterium* species, *B. melaninogenicus*, anaerobic gram-positive cocci, and *Actinomyces* species are the significant pathogens associated with dental infections such as periodontitis and periodontal abscess. Acute necrotizing ulcerative gingivitis or trench mouth, also called Vincent's angina, is an acute, fulminating, mixed anaerobic bacterial-spirochetal infection of the gingival margin and floor of the mouth. It is characterized by gingival pain, foul breath and pseudomembrane formation. *Ludwig angina* is an acute, life-threatening cellulitis of sublingual and submandibular spaces, presumed to start from dental infections. This can lead to airway obstruction.

OTITIS MEDIA

Anaerobic infections are more likely as the chronicity of otitis or mastoiditis increases. Chronic ear infections are usually polymicrobial; the predominant aerobes are enteric gram-negative rods and *S. aureus*, whereas the predominant anaerobes are *Bacteroides* species, gram-positive anaerobic cocci, and *F. nucleatum*. Many of the organisms recovered from chronically infected ear produce the enzyme beta-lactamase. Antibiotics effective against polymicrobial pathogens can provide effective therapy in chronic otitis media.

INTRA-ABDOMINAL INFECTIONS

Anaerobes are commonly present in the intestines, most commonly in the colon. Contents of the gut may leak into the peritoneum following perforation leading to peritonitis, abscess formation. Secondary hepatic abscesses may then develop as complications of appendicitis, intestinal perforation, inflammatory bowel disease (IBD), or biliary tract disease. *Typhlitis* is a mixed infection of the gut wall usually beginning in the ileocecum and characterized by abdominal pain, diarrhea, fever and abdominal distention in neutropenic patients. Empirical antimicrobial therapy of fever and neutropenia may not be optimal against the anaerobes involved in typhlitis. Necrotizing enterocolitis, a mixed aerobic/anaerobic infection of the intestinal wall, and peritoneum is believed to be due to vascular insufficiency of the gut and hypoxia. Anaerobic bacteria have been more closely linked to intra-abdominal infections. *B. fragilis* is the most important pathogen in appendicitis-related infection.

PLEUROPULMONARY INFECTIONS

Anaerobes have commonly been identified as causative organisms in adult pleuropulmonary infections such as aspiration pneumonia, lung abscess, necrotizing pneumonia and empyema. Organisms isolated from these pleuropulmonary infections generally reflect the normal oral flora. Most common is *B. fragilis*, others being *B. ruminicola* subspecies brevis, *B. ureolyticus*, and *B. melaninogenicus*.

SKIN AND SOFT TISSUE INFECTIONS

Cutaneous abscesses are commonly encountered in children. *S. aureus* and GABHS are the organisms previously implicated in these infections. However, anaerobes, chiefly the *B. fragilis* group and *B. melaninogenicus* group, have been associated with cutaneous abscesses of the buttocks, perirectal, vulvovaginal, head and finger (paronychia) areas more frequently than other sites on the body. Although surgical drainage is the therapy of choice, the frequency with which the beta-lactamase producers *S. aureus* and *B. fragilis* are isolated from the abscesses supports the selection of an antibiotic that is resistant to beta-lactamase when treating these infections.

Decubitus ulcers are a complication of prolonged hospitalization in both adults and children. Anaerobic gram-positive cocci, *B. fragilis* and *F. nucleatum* were the most common anaerobes isolated whereas *S. aureus*, GABHS, *Haemophilus influenzae* and *Enterobacter* species were the most common aerobes. *Clostridial myonecrosis*, or *gas gangrene*, is a rapidly progressive infection of deep soft tissues, primarily muscles, associated with *C. perfringens*. *Necrotizing fasciitis* is a more superficial, polymicrobial infection of the subcutaneous space with acute onset and rapid progression that has significant morbidity and mortality. Group A streptococcus, known in the popular press as "the flesh-eating bacteria", and *S. aureus* are occasionally the causative pathogens. Commonly, necrotizing fasciitis is produced by combined infection of *S. aureus* or gram-negative bacilli and anaerobic streptococci, termed *synergistic gangrene*. This infection is often seen as a complication of varicella following secondary infection of cutaneous vesicles. Diabetic patients may have a particularly aggressive and destructive synergistic gangrene of the inguinal area and adjacent scrotum or vulva known as *Fournier gangrene*. Early recognition with aggressive surgical debridement and antimicrobial therapy is necessary to limit disfiguring morbidity and mortality.

BACTEREMIA

Anaerobes are rarely isolated from blood cultures of pediatric patients (<1%). It is a normal inhabitant of the skin. Many of these isolates reflect contamination of the blood cultures by skin flora. The cell walls of gram-negative anaerobes may contain endotoxin and can be associated with the development of hypotension and shock when present in the circulatory system. Clostridia produce hemolysins, and the presence of these organisms in the blood can herald massive hemolysis and cardiovascular collapse. Anaerobic organisms most commonly isolated from blood are *B. fragilis*, anaerobic gram-positive cocci and *Fusobacterium*. Infection usually occurs in patients with chronic debilitating disorders such as malignancy, immunodeficiency or chronic renal insufficiency, and usually carries a poor long-term prognosis. *Bacteroides* species were also frequently isolated following perforation of viscus and appendicitis.

Common complications of bacteremia are meningitis, peritonitis, subdural empyema and septic shock. Early recognition and treatment is important.

DIAGNOSIS

The diagnosis of anaerobic infection requires a high index of suspicion and proper collection and culture techniques. Swab samples from mucosal surfaces normally have anaerobes hence should not be swabbed for diagnosis. Aspirates of infected sites, abscess material, and biopsy specimens are appropriate. Specimens must be protected from oxygen. An anaerobic transport medium is used to increase the likelihood of recovery of obligate anaerobes. Gram staining of abscess fluid from suspected anaerobic infections is useful because even if the organisms do not grow in culture, they can be seen on the smear.

TREATMENT

Treatment of anaerobic infections requires adequate drainage of abscesses, debridement of necrotic tissue and appropriate antimicrobial therapy. Antibiotic therapy varies depending on the suspected or proven anaerobe involved. Aerobes are present with the anaerobes; hence broad-spectrum antibiotic combinations are required for empirical therapy. Specific therapy is based on culture results and clinical course.

Many oral anaerobic bacterial species are susceptible to penicillins, although some strains may produce a beta-lactamase. Drugs that are active against such strains include metronidazole, penicillins combined with beta-lactamase inhibitors (ampicillin-sulbactam, ticarcillin-clavulanate and piperacillin-tazobactam), carbapenems (imipenem and meropenem), clindamycin and cefoxitin. Penicillin and vancomycin are active against the gram-positive anaerobes.

For soft tissue infections, providing adequate perfusion to the area is critical. Drainage of infected areas is often necessary for cure. Bacteria may survive in abscesses because of high bacterial inoculum, lack of bactericidal activity and local conditions that facilitate bacterial proliferation. Aspiration is sometimes effective for small collections, whereas incision and drainage may be required for larger abscesses. Extensive debridement and resection of all devitalized tissue are needed to control fasciitis and myonecrosis. The therapeutic benefit of hyperbaric oxygen therapy remains uncertain.

Now, two common infections (tetanus and botulisms) have been discussed in detail.

TETANUS

Tetanus is characterized by increased muscle tone and spasms caused by the release of the neurotoxin tetanospasmin by *Clostridium tetani* following inoculation into a human host. *C. tetani*, a motile, gram-positive, spore-forming obligate anaerobe whose natural habitat worldwide is soil, dust and the alimentary tracts of various animals. *C. tetani* forms spores terminally, producing a drumstick or tennis racket appearance microscopically. Most cases of tetanus are caused by direct contamination of wounds with clostridial spores. Wounds, such as those with dead or devitalized tissue, a foreign body, or active infection, are ideal for germination of the spores and release of toxin.

Pathogenesis of tetanus is due to tetanospasmin, a zinc metalloprotease, is released in the wound and binds to the peripheral motor neuron terminal, enters the axon, and, via retrograde intraneuronal transport, reaches the nerve cell body in the brainstem and spinal cord. The toxin migrates across the synapse to presynaptic terminals where it blocks the release of the inhibitory neurotransmitters glycine and gamma-aminobutyric acid (GABA) by cleaving proteins crucial for the proper functioning of the synaptic vesicle release apparatus. One of these important proteins is synaptobrevin. This diminished inhibition results in an increase in the resting firing rate of the motor neuron, which is responsible for the observed muscle rigidity. The lessened activity of reflexes limits the polysynaptic spread of impulses (a glycinergic activity). Agonists and antagonists may be recruited rather than inhibited, with consequent production of spasms. Loss of inhibition may also affect preganglionic sympathetic neurons in the lateral gray matter of the spinal cord and produce sympathetic hyperactivity and high levels of circulating catecholamines. Finally, tetanospasmin can block neurotransmitter release at the neuromuscular junction, causing weakness and paralysis.

Tetanus occurs in several *clinical forms,* including generalized, cephalic, localized and neonatal disease. *Localized tetanus* develops when only the nerves supplying the affected muscle are involved. *Generalized tetanus* develops when the toxin released at the wound spreads through the lymphatics and blood to multiple nerve terminals. The blood-brain barrier prevents direct entry of toxin to the central nervous system (CNS).

Epidemiology of Tetanus

Tetanus occurs worldwide, most common form being, neonatal (or umbilical) tetanus. It causes approximately 500,000 infant deaths annually. This is due to lack of immunization of mothers and unhygiene delivery practices. Among children it occurs following wound infection or chronic otitis media. It is rare not to find history of trauma. Disease may also occur in association with animal bites, abscesses (including dental abscesses), ear and other body piercing, chronic skin ulceration, burns, compound fractures, frostbite, gangrene, intestinal surgery, ritual scarification, infected insect bites and female circumcision. There is no particular race or gender predilection. Age pattern depends on the soils exposure and immunization coverage.

Factors affecting severity and prognosis are:
- There is increased severity, if incubation period is less than 7 days
- Period of onset less than 48 hours
- Acquired from burns, surgical wounds, compound fractures, septic abortion, umbilical stump or intra-muscular injection
- Narcotic addiction
- Generalized tetanus
- Temperature greater than 104°F (40°C)
- Tachycardia greater than 120 beats/minute (>150 beats/minute in neonates) put period
- Neonatal tetanus and cephalic tetanus are always very severe.

Clinical Manifestations

Tetanus may be generalized or localized. Tetanus neonatorum has same features as generalized tetanus.

Generalized Tetanus

Generalized tetanus is the most common form of tetanus. The incubation period is 2–14 days, largely depending on the distance of the injury site from the CNS. Rarely, it may be longer. Trismus, that is inability to open the jaw

(masseter muscle spasm or lockjaw), is the most common presenting symptom. Other early features include irritability, restlessness, diaphoresis, and dysphagia with hydrophobia, drooling and spasm of the back muscles. These early manifestations reflect involvement of bulbar and paraspinal muscles, possibly because they are innervated by the shortest axons. The condition may progress for 2 weeks despite antitoxin. Sustained trismus may result in the characteristic sardonic smile (risus sardonicus) and persistent spasm of the back musculature may cause opisthotonus. Waves of opisthotonus are highly characteristic of the disease. With progression, the extremities become involved in episodes of painful flexion and adduction of the arms, clenched fists and extension of the legs. Laryngeal and respiratory muscle spasm can lead to airway obstruction and asphyxiation. Because tetanus toxin does not affect sensory nerves or cortical function, the patient unfortunately remains conscious, in extreme pain, and in fearful anticipation of the next tetanic seizure. Noise or tactile stimuli may precipitate spasms and generalized convulsions. Involvement of the autonomic nervous system may result in severe arrhythmias, oscillation of the blood pressure, profound diaphoresis, hyperthermia, rhabdomyolysis, laryngeal spasm and urinary retention. In most cases, the patient remains lucid.

Dysuria and urinary retention result from bladder sphincter spasm; forced defecation may occur. Fever, occasionally as high as 40°C, is common because of the substantial metabolic energy consumed by spastic muscles. Notable autonomic effects include tachycardia, dysrhythmias, labile hypertension, diaphoresis and cutaneous vasoconstriction. The tetanic paralysis usually becomes more severe in the 1st weak after onset, stabilizes in the 2nd weak and ameliorates gradually over the ensuing 1–4 weeks.

Localized Tetanus

Localized tetanus involves an extremity with a contaminated wound and widely varies in severity. This is an unusual form of tetanus and the prognosis for survival is excellent. In mild cases, patients may have weakness of the involved extremity, presumably due to partial immunity. In more severe cases, intense painful spasms occur and usually progress to generalized tetanus.

Cephalic Tetanus

Cephalic tetanus generally follows head injury or develops with infection of the middle ear. Symptoms consist of isolated or combined dysfunction of the cranial motor nerves (most frequently the seventh cranial nerve). It may remain localized or progress to generalized tetanus. This is an unusual form of tetanus with an incubation period of 1–2 days. The prognosis for survival is usually poor. Cranial nerve findings and rapid progression are typical. This form may remain localized or progress to generalized tetanus.

Tetanus Neonatorum

This is generalized tetanus that results from infection of a neonate. The usual cause is the use of contaminated materials to cut or dress the umbilical cord in newborns of unimmunized mothers. The usual incubation period after birth is 3–10 days, which is why it was referred to as the disease of the 7th day. Presenting symptom is progressive difficulty in feeding. The newborn usually exhibits irritability, poor feeding, rigidity, facial grimacing and severe spasms with touch. Physical examination findings are similar to generalized tetanus findings. The umbilical stump may have remnants of dirt, dung, clotted blood or serum.

Diagnosis

The diagnosis of tetanus is based entirely on clinical findings. Tetanus is unlikely if a reliable history indicates the completion of a primary vaccination series and the receipt of required booster doses. Wounds should be cultured in suspected cases. However, *C. tetani* can be cultured from wounds of patients without tetanus and frequently cannot be cultured from wounds of patients with tetanus. *C. tetani* is not always visible on Gram stain of wound material and is isolated in only about 30% of cases. The leukocyte count may be high. Cerebrospinal fluid examination is normal.

Differential diagnosis of trismus includes parapharyngeal, retropharyngeal, or dental abscesses or, rarely, from acute encephalitis involving the brainstem. Rabies may present as trismus with seizures but it can be differentiated from tetanus by hydrophobia, marked dysphagia, predominantly clonic seizures and pleocytosis. In strychnine poisoning presentation is of tonic muscle spasms and generalized seizure activity but there is relaxation in between spasms. Hypocalcemia may produce tetany that is characterized by laryngeal and carpopedal spasms. Trismus is absent in strychnine poisioning and hypocalcemic seizures.

Treatment

Management includes neutralization of all accessible tetanus toxins and removal of spores from the infected wound or wound hygiene. Surgical wound excision and debridement are required to remove the foreign body or devitalized tissue that created anaerobic growth conditions. Tetanus toxin be neutralized by tetanus immunoglobulin (TIG) before it has begun its axonal ascent to the spinal cord. TIG should be given as soon as possible. A single intramuscular injection of 500 U of TIG is sufficient to neutralize systemic tetanus toxin. In tetanus neonatorum practice of 250 IU intramuscularly and 250 IU intrathecally is recommended by some, although there is no specific indication for this. Another alternative is equine-derived or bovine-derived tetanus antitoxin (TAT). TAT is usually not available and a high incidence of serum sickness is seen with its use.

Penicillin G (100,000 U/kg/day divided every 4–6 hours IV for 10–14 days) remains the antibiotic of choice because of its effective clostridiocidal action and its diffusibility, which is an important consideration because blood flow to injured tissue may be compromised. Metronidazole (500 mg every 8 hour IV for adults) appears to be equally effective. Erythromycin and tetracycline (for persons >8 years of age) are alternatives for penicillin-allergic patients.

All patients with generalized tetanus need muscle relaxants. Diazepam provides both relaxation and seizure control. The initial dose of 0.1–0.2 mg/kg every 3–6 hour given intravenously is subsequently titrated to control the tetanic spasms, after which the effective dose is sustained for 2–6 weak before a tapered withdrawal. Magnesium sulfate, other benzodiazepines (midazolam), chlorpromazine, dantrolene and baclofen are also used.

Supportive Care

Quality of supportive care determines the prognosis. Supportive care in a quiet, dark, secluded setting is desirable. Because tetanic spasms may be triggered by minor stimuli, it may trigger spasms; therefore, the patient should be sedated and protected from all unnecessary sounds, sights and touch. Therapeutic and other manipulations must be carefully scheduled and coordinated. Endotracheal intubation should be done to prevent aspiration of secretions before laryngospasm develops. Cardiorespiratory monitoring, frequent suctioning and maintenance of the patient's substantial fluid, electrolyte and caloric needs are fundamental. Careful nursing attention to mouth, skin, bladder and bowel function is needed to avoid ulceration, infection and obstipation. Active immunization with tetanus toxoid is required at discharge with provision for completion of the primary series is mandatory.

Mortality is highest in the very young and the very old. A favorable prognosis is associated with a long incubation period, absence of fever and localized disease. Sequelae of hypoxic brain injury as cerebral palsy, diminished mental abilities and behavioral difficulties can be seen. Case fatality rates for generalized tetanus are 5–35%, and for neonatal tetanus they extend from less than 10% with intensive care treatment to greater than 75% without it. Cephalic tetanus has poor prognosis.

CLOSTRIDIUM DIFFICILE INFECTION

Clostridium difficile infection (CDI) or *Pseudomembranous colitis or antibiotic-associated diarrhea,* or *C. difficile-*associated diarrhea, refers to gastrointestinal colonization with *C. difficile* resulting in a diarrheal illness. *C. difficile* is a gram-positive, anaerobic bacillus capable of forming a spore that is resistant to killing by alcohol. Organisms causing symptomatic disease produce one or both of the following: toxin A and toxin B. These toxins affect intracellular signaling pathways, resulting in inflammation and cell death. Incidence is increasing with increasing use of antibiotics. Severity of the disease is also increasing.

Risk factors for CDI include use of broad-spectrum antibiotics, hospitalization, gastrointestinal surgery, IBD, chemotherapy, enteral feeding, proton pump-inhibiting agents and chronic illness. It can be nosocomial or community acquired. In children community acquired variety can be seen without antibiotic exposure.

Pathogenesis

Disease is caused by gastrointestinal infection with a toxin-producing strain. Toxins cause an inflammatory response and cell death leading to pseudomembrane formation and diarrhea. Intracellular signaling pathways and cytoskeletal organization are also affected.

Clinical findings vary from mild, self-limited diarrhea to explosive, watery diarrhea with occult blood or mucous, to pseudomembranous colitis, and even death. *Pseudomembranous colitis* describes a bloody diarrhea with accompanying fever, abdominal pain/cramps, nausea and vomiting. Rarely, small gut involvement, bacteremia, abscess formation, toxic megacolon and even death can occur. Symptoms of CDI generally begin less than a week after colonization and may develop during or weeks after antibiotic exposure. They are generally more severe in certain populations, including patients receiving chemotherapy, patients with chronic gastrointestinal disease (e.g. IBD), and some patients with cystic fibrosis.

Diagnosis

Clostridium difficile infection is diagnosed by the detection of a *C. difficile* toxin in the stool of a symptomatic patient. Most patients present with a history of recent antibiotic use. The standard for toxin detection is the tissue culture cytotoxicity assay. This assay detects only toxin B and requires 24–48 hour. Now enzyme immunoassay is the preferred technique, it gives results on the same day. Stool culture is a sensitive test, but it is not specific, as it does not differentiate between toxin-producing and nontoxin-producing strains. Pseudomembranous nodules and characteristic plaques may be seen on colonoscopy or sigmoidoscopy.

Treatment

There should be adequate fluid and electrolyte replacement. All unnecessary antibiotics should be discontinued. If symptoms persist antibiotics as oral metronidazole are required. Oral metronidazole (20–40 mg/kg/day) for 7–10 days should be given. Vancomycin should be reserved for severe disease. Vancomycin (25–40 mg/kg/day PO) for 7–10 days divided every 6 hours for 7–10 days) is widely approved for use against infection with *C. difficile*. Vancomycin is ideal as it is not absorbed in the gut. Nitazoxanide and fidaxomicin are other agents that are effective in treating CDI in adults.

Prognosis

Response to treatment is usually good but within 2–4 weeks 5–30% of cases recur. Recurrence may be due to incomplete eradication or reinfection with another strain. Initially, these should be treated with the original antibiotic. Multiple recurrences of CDI may be due to a suboptimal immune response, failure to kill organisms that have sporulated, or failure of delivery of antibiotic to the site of infection in the case of ileus or toxic megacolon. Tapered vancomycin may be used to decrease recurrences. Other antibiotics for this are (rifaximin or nitazoxanide), toxin-binding polymers (tolevamer), fecal transplantation and probiotics (*Saccharomyces boulardii or Lactobacillus* GG) have been used. Intravenous immune globulin (IVIG) may be required in some cases. At times postinfectious diarrhea may be due to other causes. CDI can be prevented by recognition of common sites of acquisition (hospitals, childcare settings, extended care facilities), effective environmental cleaning (i.e. use of chlorinated cleaning solutions), appropriate antibiotic prescription practices, cohorting of infected patients and proper handwashing with soap and water.

BOTULISM

Clostridium botulinum is a gram-positive, spore-forming anaerobe that naturally inhabits soil, dust, and fresh and cooked agricultural products. Three naturally occurring forms of human botulism are known: infant botulism, food-borne botulism and wound botulism. Two other forms, both human-made, also occur: inhalational botulism from inhaling accidentally aerosolized toxin and iatrogenic botulism from overdosage of therapeutic or cosmetic use of botulinum toxin. *C. baratii* and *C. butyricum* also produce botulinum toxin. Botulinum toxin is the most potent naturally occurring toxin known to humankind.

Pathogenesis

Food-borne botulism is not seen after eating fresh foods. Some methods of food preparation, such as home canning, produce an anaerobic, low-acid (i.e. pH >4.6), low-solute environment in which the toxin can be produced. A similar environment exists in wounds, thus providing an opportunity for wound botulism to develop.

In persons older than 1 year, the spores are unable to germinate in the gut; therefore, food-borne disease is the result of ingesting a preformed toxin. *C. botulinum* spores can germinate in the gut of infants younger than 1 year because of their relative lack of gastric acid, decreased levels of normal flora and immature immune systems (i.e. specifically lacking secretory immunoglobulin A). This environment is conducive to toxin production; therefore, infant botulism can arise from eating the spores present in unprepared foods.

All botulinum toxins are zinc metalloproteases that bind to different membrane proteins involved in fusion of the synaptic vesicle to the presynaptic membrane. This fusion allows release of acetylcholine into the synaptic junction. The toxins are classified as types A through G, although only types A, B, E and F cause human disease. Types A and E bind to synaptosomal-associated protein 25, type C binds to syntaxin and types B, D and F bind to vesicle-associated membrane protein. Inhibition of the proteins effectively blocks acetylcholine transmission across the synapse and functionally denervates the muscle. The magnitude of the clinical effect depends on the proportion of synapses blocked and the effects can range from weakness to flaccid paralysis and atrophy.

Clinical Features

In food borne botulism, gastrointestinal tract symptoms usually occur first, beginning 18–36 hours after ingestion (range, 2 hours to 8 days) and consist of nausea, vomiting and diarrhea followed by constipation. Involvement of cranial nerves and motor function follows. Patient may present with diplopia, blurred vision secondary to loss of accommodation, dry mouth. Later a rapidly progressive descending weakness or paralysis occurs. Autonomic dysfunction may lead to orthostatic hypotension, urinary retention or constipation. Because the toxin affects only motor and autonomic systems, sensation and mentation remain intact. Patients are usually afebrile.

Symptoms are same for wound botulism except history of injury. The incubation period is 4–14 days.

In infant, botulism incubation period is 2–4 weeks. The peak age of incidence is 2–4 months. Constipation is the usual presenting symptom, often preceding motor function symptoms by several days or weeks. Other signs of autonomic dysfunction usually present early as well, including those mentioned above. Gag reflexes are frequently impaired, which can lead to aspiration if the airway is unprotected. Infants with botulism are afebrile, suck poorly, and are lethargic and listless; they develop the same descending weakness and paralysis that occurs in those with food-borne disease. Breast-feeding may protect infants from lethal fulminant infant botulism, but exclusive breast-feeding is a risk factor for the disease, presumably because the relatively pristine bowel flora of the exclusively breastfed infant is more permissive for spore germination and toxin production.

Suspect botulism in patients with autonomic dysfunction (e.g. dry mouth, blurred vision, orthostatic hypotension), cranial nerve involvement (e.g. ptosis, mydriasis, decreased ocular motility, dysphagia, dysarthria) and muscle weakness or flaccid paralysis.

Differential Diagnosis

Due to a wide variety of symptoms botulism should be distinguished from dehydration, hypermagnesemia, hypothyroidism, poliomyelitis, organophosphate toxicity, Guillain-Barré syndrome, brainstem encephalitis.

Laboratory Studies

Although clinical suspicion should be sufficient to prompt supportive therapy for botulism, other differential diagnoses must be excluded. Obtain stool cultures in all patients, adding wound cultures if wound botulism is suspected. The bacterium, *C. botulinum*, produces a neurotoxin which causes the rare, but serious, paralytic illness, botulism. Approximately 60% of food-borne cases yield positive culture results; a positive finding in the presence of flaccid paralysis is diagnostic. Currently, specific assays for the toxin, including enzyme-linked immunoassays and polymerase chain reaction (PCR), are under investigation. Currently, the mouse inoculation test is the best test available and can be performed by the Centers for Disease Control and Prevention (CDC) in Atlanta, Georgia. In the assay, mice are injected with a serum sample from the patient and test results are considered positive for toxin if the mice die of respiratory arrest within 24 hours. The exact type of toxin is determined through pretreating each mouse in a set of mice with a different type-specific antitoxin, then injecting the serum. The mouse left alive the next day is the one pretreated with the antitoxin to the toxin affecting the patient. The sensitivity of this test in the diagnosis of wound botulism has been questioned; strong clinical suspicion should outweigh a negative mouse inoculation test. Multiplex PCR has been described. Lumber puncture findings can usually exclude Guillain-Barré syndrome, a condition that tends to elicit a higher protein level in cerebrospinal fluid (especially later in the course of the disease) than does botulism.

Perform CT scanning or MRI as clinically indicated to exclude stroke. Other tests are edrophonium chloride test to exclude myasthenia gravis, if indicated. Electromyelography (EMG) demonstrates nonspecific decreased amplitude of action potentials. Rapid repetitive EMG at frequencies of 20–50 Hz is more specific for botulism and useful in excluding Guillain-Barré syndrome, but this response does not distinguish botulism from Lambert-Eaton syndrome. Infant botulism is characterized by a pattern known as brief, small, abundant motor-unit action potential on EMG in clinically affected muscles.

Treatment

In patients with botulism, supportive care, especially ventilatory support, is essential. Patients need continued suctioning and may require intubation or tracheostomy. Antitoxin dramatically alters the course of the disease, especially if administered within the first 24 hours.

Antitoxins are agents that are used for food-borne and wound botulism. They are produced from horse serum stimulated with specific antibodies directed against *C. botulinum* and provide passive immunity. Botulism immune globulin, human (BabyBIG) is a solvent-detergent treated, and viral-screened immune globulin derived from pooled adult plasma from persons immunized with botulinum toxoid who developed high neutralizing antibody titers against botulinum neurotoxins types A and B. Indicated to treat infant botulism caused by types A or B *C. botulinum*. Botulinum antitoxin, heptavalent (HBAT) is an investigational antitoxin indicated for naturally occurring noninfant botulism. Equine-derived antitoxin that elicits passive antibody (i.e. immediate immunity) is against *C. botulinum* toxins A, B, C, D, E, F and G.

Each 20 mL vial contains equine-derived antibody to the seven known botulinum toxin types (A through G) with the following nominal potency values: 7,500 U anti-A, 5,500 U anti-B, 5,000 U anti-C, 1,000 U anti-D, 8,500 U anti-E, 5,000 U anti-F and 1,000 U anti-G.

Antibiotic therapy to clear clostridial gastrointestinal infection in infant botulism is contraindicated, because the treatment increases toxin release and worsens the condition. Antibiotics may be considered to treat secondary bacterial infections. Aminoglycosides, such as gentamicin or tobramycin, may potentiate the neuromuscular blockade; therefore, they are contraindicated. In patients with wound botulism, surgical debridement of the wound is indicated to remove the source of toxin production.

Prognosis

Timing of antitoxin administration greatly influences the prognosis. If antitoxin is used within 24 hours is associated with a 10% mortality rate, antitoxin administered more than 24 hours later is associated with a 15% mortality rate, and failure to administer antitoxin carries a 46% mortality rate. After recovery from acute illness, late symptoms may remain, primarily muscle weakness including diplopia and fatigue with exertion. Although some patients have reported feeling breathless, pulmonary function test results demonstrate that results in lung volumes, forced expiratory volume in 1 second (FEV$_1$)/forced vital capacity (FVC), maximum inspiratory and expiratory pressures, and ventilatory response to exercise fall within reference ranges.

BIBLIOGRAPHY

1. American Academy of Pediatrics. Botulism and infant botulism (Clostridium botulinum). Red Book: 2009 Report of the Committee on Infectious Diseases. 28th edition Elk Grove Village, IL: American Academy of Pediatrics; 2009. pp. 259-72.
2. Brook I. Anaerobic infections in children. Adv Exp Med Biol. 2011;697:117-52.
3. Clostridial infections. Nelson's Textbook of Pediatrics, 19th edition.
4. http://emedicine.medscape.com/article/961833-overview.

IAP Guidelines/Protocols

TU Sukumaran

8.1   IAP PROTOCOL ON KALA-AZAR

IAP ID Chapter

DISEASE BURDEN

The disease is endemic in three countries of WHO's Southeast Asian (SEA) region: Bangladesh, India and Nepal. Approximately 200 million people in the region are 'at risk' from the disease. Nearly 100,000 are estimated to occur in the region and 90% of these cases of kala-azar are found in Bihar itself. Worldwide, 9 out of 10 cases occur in Bangladesh, Brazil, India and Sudan. In the endemic countries kala-azar affects the poorest among the poor. The very poor have little knowledge about the disease and hence they are unlikely to seek early treatment, and most of those who start treatment cannot afford to complete it.

DIAGNOSIS

Clinical diagnosis of visceral leishmaniasis (VL) (kala-azar) is strongly suggested in a patient from endemic area with history of prolonged fever, weakness, cachexia, marked splenomegaly and hepatomegaly. The diagnosis becomes difficult and sequestration of parasite in reticuloendothelial system further complicates this issue.

Initial screening of patient with routine blood test (complete blood count), liver and kidney function tests and X-ray chest is done. Laboratories diagnosis of VL can be made by the following:

- Demonstration of parasite in tissue of relevance by light microscopic examination of stained specimen
- Immunodiagnosis by detection of parasitic antigen in tissues, blood or urine sample, by detection of nonspecific or specific antileishmanial antibodies (immunoglobulin) or by assay for leishmaniasis specific cell mediated immunity
- Detection of parasite DNA in tissue samples
- Indirect evidences supporting the diagnosis.

Direct Evidences

Demonstration and Isolation of Parasites

This is one of the most conclusive evidence and is gold standard for diagnosis of kala-azar. A parasitological diagnosis can be achieved by examination of following materials:
- Blood
- Biopsy material
  - Marrow obtained by sternal puncture
  - Splenic pulp tissue obtained by splenic puncture.

A stained peripheral blood film has often been successful in showing the presence of Leishman-Donovan (LD) bodies (amastigote forms) of the parasite.

The chances to find these can be adopting any of the following procedures:
- By making a thick film
- By producing a straight leukocyte edge
- By centrifuging a citrated blood. The sediment at the bottom is withdrawn by means of a capillary pipette, smears dried and stained.

Sternal puncture is a safer procedure but more painful. Aspirated material is stained with Giemsa or Leishman stain. Amastigotes appear as rod or oval body 2–3 μm in length and are found intracellularly in monocytes and microphages. After identification, parasite density can be scored microscopically by means of algorithmic scale ranging from 0 (no parasite/field) to +6 (>100 parasite/field). The sensitivity of the bone marrow smear is 60–85%.

Splenic puncture is one of the most valuable methods for diagnosis with sensitivity exceeding 95%. But it carries a risk of fatal hemorrhage in inexperienced hands. Splenic aspiration should not be done if the prothombin time is more than 5 seconds longer than that of the control or if the platelet count is below 40×10^9/L (40,000/mm³).

The two important factors for safety are that the needle remains within the spleen less than 1 second and the entry and exit axis of the aspirating needle are identical to avoid tearing of splenic capsule.

Liver biopsy is not usually done with the sensitivity of about 70%.

CULTURE

Immunodiagnosis

Antigen Detection

Latex test: A latex agglutination test detecting a heat stable, low molecular weight carbohydrate antigen in urine of VL patients has shown promising results. Its specificity and sensitivity are 100% and 48–87% respectively.

Advantages:
- Antigen can be detected quiet early during infection
- Decline rapidly following chemotherapy
- Useful diagnostic method in cases of immunodeficiency (AIDS).

Antibody Detection

Several tests detecting specific antileishmanial antibody have been developed but all have two major limitations:
- May remain detectable upto several years after cure (relapse cannot be diagnosed).
- A significant proportion of healthy individuals living in endemic areas are positive for antileishmanial antibody owing asymptomatic infection.

The available tests are:
- Indirect fluorescent antibody test (IFAT)
- Enzyme-linked immunosorbent assay (ELISA)
- Western blot.
  The above mentioned serological tests have shown high diagnostic accuracy in most studies but are poorly adapted to field settings.

Direct agglutination test (DAT): It is a semiquantitative test that uses microtiter plate in which increasing dilution of patient's serum or blood mixed with stained killed Leishmania donovani promastigotes. If specific antibodies are positive, agglutination is visible after 18 hours with naked eyes. It is 91–100% sensitive, and 72–100% specific.

Disadvantages
- Costly
- No prognostic value
- Not user friendly for field conditions.

rK39 ICT: It is a dipstick test based on cloned antigen of a 39 amino acid gene of *L. chopasi.* This recombinant antigen

rK39 which in the kinesin region is specific for antibodies in patient with VL. The sensitivity and specificity of this test are 93% and 95% respectively.

Advantages
- Easy to perform
- Rapid (10–20 minutes)
- Cheap and reproducible results
- Currently best available diagnostic tool for VL for use in remote areas.

Limitations

Cannot predict response to therapy or relapse.

Skin Testing
- Delayed type hypersensitivity test is a group specific response
- Montenegro skin test: It is specific to leishmaniasis but its role is limited as it is negative in acute cases of VL and positive after cure.

DNA Detection Method

Due to various limitations of other tests, new approaches such as DNA hybridization have been attempted. The development of polymerase chain reaction (PCR) has provided a powerful tool to the application of molecular biology techniques in diagnosis of VL.
- Ln PCR-Leishmania nested PCR

Kinetoplast DNA (kDNA): Seminested PCR (Sn PCR)
- Restriction fragment length polymorphism (RFLP).
- A positive PCR is related to the presence of living parasites, so result is negative after cure.

Advantage

Only test that can differentiate between relapse and reinfection.

Non-Leishmanial Tests
- Complete blood count usually shows the following features:
  – Anemia
  – Leukopenia
  – Thrombocytopenia
  – Relative lymphocytosis and monocytosis
  – Eosinopenia
- Elevated hepatic transaminase level
- Polyclonal hypergammaglobulinemia.
- *Leukocyte*: Erythrocyte ratio—1:2,000 to 1:1,000 (normal is 1:750)
- Raised ESR.

Diagnosis of HIV-Leishmania Coinfection

Atypical clinical presentation of VL in HIV infected patients poses a considerable diagnostic challenge:

- Diagnostic principles remain essentially same
- Amastigotes may be demonstrated in buffy coat preparation
- Amastigotes can be demonstrated in bone marrow
- Sensitivity of antibody based immunologic tests is low
- Leishmania amastigotes can be found at unexpected locations like the stomach, colon or lungs
- Polymerase chain reaction (PCR) analysis of the whole blood or its buffy coat preparation may prove a useful screening test for these patients.

TREATMENT

For more than half a century, the pentavalent antimony compounds meglumine antimonite and sodium stibogluconate (SSG) has remained the standard anti-leishmanial treatment worldwide except in India, where widespread resistance to these drugs is now being observed. The current alternative treatment of choice is amphotericin B, an antifungal agent that is highly effective in cases of kala-azar resistant to antimony compounds. Miltefosine, a new oral agent is a highly effective drug safe and affordable.

Amphotericin B

Amphotericin B, an antifungal agent, is a macrocyclic, polyene, antifungal antibiotic produced from a strain of *Streptomyces nodosus*. At present amphotericin B is extensively used in Bihar for all stibogluconate unresponsive cases and even as a first line drug. In Bihar, 100% resistance in cases of kala-azar in two villages of Darbhanga and Sitamarhi districts was observed; who failed to respond to SSG in WHO recommended doses. It intercalates with the episterol precursors of ergosterol in the parasite. The drug binds to ergosterol and damages the cell membrane. The drug is highly effective against kala-azar in India, and 90–95% long-term cure rate has been obtained in both antimonial unresponsive and previously untreated patients. The dose is 1 mg/kg intravenous (IV) on an alternate day schedule over a 30-day period (cumulative dose 7–20 mg/kg). The drug is administered as IV infusion in 5% dextrose solution at a concentration of 0.1 mg/mL over 6–8 hours, with a close vigil on febrile and allergic reactions. Adverse effects of this drug are mainly infusion related—fever, chill and bone pain. It is also associated with renal toxicity necessitating monitoring of renal function. The drawbacks of amphotericin B are its high cost and toxicity. Three new lipid-associated formulations of amphotericin B with improved therapeutic indices have been developed in the last decade and have been proven to increase the efficacy and to limit the toxicity of conventional amphotericin B. These formulations allow administration of considerably higher daily doses and simultaneously appear to target infected tissue macrophages via enhanced phagocytic uptake. Three lipid formulations are available:

- AmBisome®, (liposomal amphotericin B) which is a formulation using spherical, unilamellar liposomes that are less than 100 nm in size.
- Amphocil®, (amphotericin B cholesterol dispersion) which is dispersion with cholesterol sulfate in 1:1 molar ratio.
- Abelcet®, (amphotericin B lipid complex) which is a ribbon-like lipid structure using a phospholipid matrix.

In 1997, the USFDA approved AmBisome (in the dose of 3 mg/kg/day on days 1–5, 14 and 21) for the treatment of VL in immunocompetent children. Amphocil is given at dose of 2–4 mg/kg/day for 7–10 days in children with kala-azar. Abelcet is given at 5 mg/kg/day for 2 days.

By using the lipid formulations of amphotericin B, drug toxicity is minimized, and hospital stay can be reduced to 2–5 days from 30–40 days, which can offset the high cost of these drugs; however, these drugs still remain beyond reach for most of the Indian patients or those from other developing countries.

Pentavalent Antimony Drugs

Sodium stibogluconate remains the first line drug in treatment of kala-azar despite the availability of many newer drugs. In 1982, WHO recommended SSG in dose of 20 mg/kg/day IM/IV, once daily for 20–30 days in fresh cases and for double duration (40–60 days) in relapse cases; subsequently WHO (1990) recommended SSG in the dose of 20 mg/kg/day for 28 days. Total dose may be divided equally and given at an interval of 8–12 hours. Most children improve and become afebrile within less than a week, whereas hematological restoration and significant subsidence of splenomegaly usually occur within 2 weeks. While active elsewhere in India, SSG is no longer useful in northeastern state of India, where as many as 65% of the previously untreated patients fail to respond to or promptly relapse after therapy with SSG. Disadvantages of SSG include parenteral mode of administration, the long duration of therapy and the adverse reactions. Systemic toxicity normally relates to total dose administrated. Secondary effects (such as fatigue, body ache, abdominal discomfort, ECG abnormalities, raised aminotransferase levels and chemical pancreatitis) are frequent, albeit usually reversible. Severe adverse events remain rare. It has been proposed that instead of SSG, amphotericin B should be used in areas where high level (>50%) of resistance to SSG exists.

Refractory Kala-azar

- *Relapse*: Reappearance of signs and symptoms with positive parasite in bone marrow/splenic aspiration after initial cure with WHO recommended dosage of SSG, usually within 6 months

- *Primary unresponsiveness*: No clinical or parasitological improvement during or after the first course of treatment with SSG
- *Secondary unresponsiveness*: Occurs during relapse after one or more courses of apparently successful treatment.

Treatment of Relapse

- In case of relapse occurring after initial cure with WHO recommended dose of SSG, it seems unethical to use double duration of SSG in the same dose due to its poor response and high mortality. So, in these cases, second line drugs may be tried
- Relapse following incomplete, interrupted and substandard dose of SSG may be tackled by giving SSG at 20 mg/kg/day for 60 days.

Miltefosine

Miltefosine is hexadecylphosphocholine a phosphoryl-choline ester of hexadecanol, a membrane-active, alkyl phospholipid. It is the first effective oral agent for VL. Miltefosine was originally discovered and synthesized as an anti-cancer agent. Treatment with this agent has been almost 100% effective and well-tolerated in various studies conducted in India among newly diagnosed patients or patients unresponsive to pentavalent antimonial agents. Miltefosine has been shown to block the proliferation of Leishmania and to alter phospholipid and sterol composition. Leishmania have high levels of etherlipid and these are mainly found in the glycosylphosphophatidylinositol anchored glycoprotein and glycolipids present on the surface of the parasites. Miltefosine acts on key enzymes involved in the metabolism of ether lipids. Specifically miltefosine inhibits glycosomal alkyl-specific-acyl-CoA acyltransferase in a dose dependent manner. The anti-leishmanial activity of miltefosine is not only related to a direct cytotoxic effect on the parasite but is also related to the activation of cellular immunity which in turn takes care of the parasitic infection.

Dose

The recommended dose of miltefosine for the treatment of VL is 2.5 mg/kg/day for 28 days. The dose should be adjusted based on patient's weight so that a dose of 4 mg/kg/day is not exceeded. Miltefosine is well-tolerated with considerably fewer adverse effects as compared to antimonials and amphotericin B. The most commonly seen adverse effects are nausea and vomiting. There is an increase in aspartate aminotransferase (AST) and creatinine and/or blood urea and nitrogen (BUN) level which is mild. Grade III hepatotoxicity and renal damage

have also been reported in some cases. However, these changes are reversible in the face of continued treatment or after discontinuation of treatment. Diarrhea is common during first 2 weeks of treatment. Miltefosine although used as an antineoplastic agent is devoid of hematological toxicity. Miltefosine is now available under the name Impavido (10, 50 and 100 mg capsules). Based on the results available with this drug, it is hoped that this drug will eventually become the first line treatment for kala-azar in India. However, since the details in pregnant women are not fully known and it had not been tried on a large scale in such women, the use of miltefosine is not advocated in pregnancy.

Miltefosine is one of the few drugs which even though being an antineoplastic agent, stimulates the bone marrow rather than suppress it like other anticancer drugs. This in turn leads to correction of pancytopenia including hemoglobin which is a regular feature of VL. Miltefosine, being an oral agent can be easily given an outpatient basis. This drug has been recommended by the WHO in the kala-azar elimination program in India, Nepal and Bangladesh. The main limiting factor of this drug is its long half-life of about 5 days which can lead to development of early resistance besides its high cost.

Aminosidine (Paromomycin)

Aminosidine is an aminoglycoside antibiotic also known as paromomycin. An injectable formulation of 500 mg aminosidine sulphate (paromomycin) has been in the market in several countries for over 30 years for treating bacterial and parasitic infections. Aminosidine (paromomycin) was first shown to have antileishmanial activity in the 1960s and it has been shown to act synergistically with antimony drugs. Clinical trials with injectable aminosidine (paromomycin) for treating VL have been conducted in Africa (Kenya and Sudan), India (Bihar), and in complicated cases imported into the United Kingdom. Clinical trials on aminosidine (paromomycin) in comparison to SSG have been conducted in Bihar in India where the drug has been found to be highly effective. Aminosidine (paromomycin) given IM at 16 or 20 mg/kg/day for 21 days was significantly more effective in producing final cure than SSG 20 mg/kg/day for 30 days. Aminosidine (paromomycin) had a low incidence of adverse reactions including ototoxicity and renal toxicity, and was well tolerated. IM injection of aminosidine (paromomycin) 16 mg/kg/day for 21 days has been proposed as an alternative to SSG for VL in Bihar.

Sitamaquine (WR6026)

Sitamaquine, an 8-aminoquinoline (antimalarial), has been tried for VL (Sundar S et al. 2006). Sitamaquine was given in the dose of 2 mg/kg body weight for 21 days orally. The study revealed initial cure rate of 95% and the final cure rate of 85%. This drug has to be monitored for nephrotoxicity as it can cause acute glomerulonephritis. It is not to be given in patients with glucose-6-phosphate dehydrogenase deficiency as it can cause severe hemolysis. The drug can also cause cyanosis due to increase in the level of methemoglobinemia. Sitamaquine is still in a primitive trial stage and further trials are to be assessed before advocacy of this drug for the treatment of VL.

In view of minimizing the dose and duration of the existing anti-VL drug, the combination trial has just been started to compare the safety and efficacy of various combination like liposomal amphotericin B (AmBisome) with miltefosine, paromomycin with miltefosine and AmBisome with paromomycin. These are basically being tried for a shorter duration of treatment of VL, but can also prove to be a boon for treating patients with HIV-VL coinfection. These trials are still in a very early stage and the final outcome will be known after a few more years.

Other drugs which are being evaluated in the treatment of kala-azar include:
- Rifampicin and co-trimoxazole
- Dapsone
- Atovaquone
- Roxithromycin
- Gamma Interferon
- Allopurinol
- Pentamidine.

Thus the current status of diagnosis and treatment of kala-azar in endemic regions, including India, remains far from satisfactory. The development of rapid rK39 strip test is a good sign and its widespread use is expected to improve the diagnostic capabilities to a large extent. Therapy of kala-azar remains far from ideal. SSG is no more useful in India due to development of widespread resistance to this drug. The phenomenal cost of therapy with liposomal preparations of amphotericin B will keep it away from most patients in developing countries. Our hope for the future lies in miltefosine and the aminoglycoside aminosidine (paromomycin).

Response to Therapy

Evaluation of effectiveness of therapy of Kala-azar is very important. Response to therapy can be assessed clinically and repeat bone marrow/splenic examination. Acute phase reactants like C-reactive protein, serum amyloid A protein and Alpha-1 acid glycoprotein are less invasive tests for monitoring of therapy. The role of rK39 test in predicting response to therapy is also being evaluated.

Splenectomy

It should be reserved for cases that are unresponsive to both first and second line drugs to kill the residual parasites.

Splenectomy should be followed by SSG in recommended dose schedule.

Leishmania/HIV Coinfection

Kala-azar has been increasingly recognized as an opportunistic infection associated with HIV infection and has been reported from several countries including India. Leishmaniasis may also result from reactivation of a long standing subclinical infection. HIV infection and kala-azar are locked in a vicious circle of mutual reinforcement. Kala-azar accelerated the onset of full blown AIDS and shortens the life expectancy of HIV infected people, while HIV spurs in the spread of kala-azar. Opportunistic infections like TB, toxoplasmosis and candidiasis are more frequent in these patients. Frequently there is an atypical clinical presentation of kala-azar in HIV infected individuals, with prominent involvement of the gastrointestinal tract and absence of the typical hepatosplenomegaly. Bone marrow examination remains the safest and the most sensitive technique.

Due to destroyed immune response system, drug resistance, drug toxicity and overabundance of Leishmania in almost every tissue of the body, relapses are frequent. The use of triple therapy (by reducing the virus, increasing the number of cells responsible for immune response and preventing opportunistic infections), may improve the prognosis in these patients.

Option for combination therapies in VL with HIV/AIDS includes the following:
- SSG 20 mg/kg/day × 28 days + parmomycin 15 mg/day × 28 days
- SSG 20 mg/kg/day × 28 days + amphotericin B 1 mg/kg/day × 28 days
- SSG 20 mg/kg/day × 28 days + allopurinol 20 mg/kg/day × 28 days
- SSG 20 mg/kg/day × 28 days + interferon gamma for 28 days
- Pentamidine 4 mg/kg/day + parmomycin 15 mg/kg/day × 28 days
- Miltefosine 2.5 mg/kg/day × 28 days + SSG 20 mg/kg/day × 28 days.

Presently amphotericin B, paromomycin and miltefosine appear to be good drugs for VL with a very high cure rate and few side effects. The first two are injectable drugs whereas the other one is an oral preparation. Amphotericin B requires hospitalization and electrolyte monitoring, which is not the case with miltefosine as it can be given on an outpatient basis. The future of the other drug sitamaquine is still not very clear and paromomycin is in the Phase IV stage. The future of combination treatment is still not very clear. Further keeping in view the rising trend of unresponsiveness to sodium antimony gluconate (SAG) and the increasing incidence of HIV-VL coinfection, which is very prone to relapses as well as lack of an effective vaccine for VL, warrants future drug trials.

Leishmania: The Scope of Vaccine

The immune response to Leishmania is protective and is relatively easy to induce and maintain. Leishmania do not undergo significant antigenic variation and they have a single host cell (macrophage). A single morphological form (Amastigote) is associated with the pathology. Most species of Leishmania share many important antigens which may be advantageous for the development of the vaccine. All these facts signify that leishmaniasis is an excellent candidate for the development of safe and effective vaccine. Some antigens (a 44-46 kDa antigen of *L. amazonensis*, GP63 antigen and LACK antigens) have been extensively studied to look for expansion of leishmanial antigen-specific Th1 cells producing interferon (IFN)-gamma and promoting parasite destruction within macrophages and to down regulate Th2 response. First generation vaccines consist of killed whole Leishmania parasites, as have been tested in clinical trials in Iran, Sudan and Latin America. Second generation vaccines are comprised of recombinant antigens. Several recombinant antigens offer promise as candidate leishmaniasis vaccines, but there is need for further development. A vaccine composed of autoclaved Leishmania major promastigotes mixed with a low-dose of Bacillus Calmette-Guerin (BCG) (as adjuvant) has been tested in Sudan, Iran and Brazil has given encouraging results. More recently, a DNA vaccine containing the cDNA for a 15kD protein isolated from the saliva of sandfly (named SP15) has been found to confer significant immunity against leishmaniasis. Trials are underway to develop further vaccines based on salivary gland proteins or their cDNA as viable vaccine targets.

PREVENTION AND CONTROL OF KALA-AZAR

Government of India has formulated a kala-azar elimination program between years 2001–2012 with these targets:
- No death due to kala-azar by 2004
- Zero incidence of kala-azar by 2007
- Zero prevalence of post kala-azar dermal leishmaniasis (PKDL) by 2010
- Extended surveillance till 2012.

Strategies

The elimination program should ensure access to health care and prevention of kala-azar for people at risk with particular attention to the poorest and marginalized groups. The strategies will be implemented in four phases—preparatory phase, attack phase, consolidated phase and maintenance phase.

Major strategies are:
- Effective disease surveillance
- Early diagnosis by dipstick and complete treatment
- Effective vector control through Integrated Vector Management with a focus on indoor residual spray, insecticide treated nets and environmental management
- Social mobilization of the population at risk
- Clinical and operational research to support the elimination program.

Early Diagnosis and Complete Case Management

Effective case management of kala-azar requires improved home care management (improved healthcare practices) and increased healthcare seeking from trained healthcare personnel (including doctors and nurses), reliable laboratory facilities and adequate supply of medicines. Early diagnosis and complete treatment strategy would help to reduce case fatality rates and increase the credibility of the health system in order to increase the utilization of health services by people suspected to be suffering from the disease. It is proposed to use an agreed case definition of the disease as a starting point. The case definition for suspecting kala-azar agreed at the informal country consultation (2003) and endorsed by the Regional Technical Advisory Group (2004) is: history of fever for more than 2 weeks in a patient with no response to antibiotics and antimalarials. This case definition is likely to be sensitive but not specific. Additional signs that are useful include weight loss and enlarged liver and spleen. However, these are not likely to be recognized by health workers and health volunteers. Patients with the above mentioned symptoms should be screened by 'rK39' or DAT and, if positive, treated with an effective drug. Confirmation of kala-azar can be done by examination of bone marrow aspiration but this is difficult and invasive. Therefore, it can be done only in some hospitals (District hospitals in Bangladesh and India and zonal hospitals in Nepal). The effective and safe oral drug recommended is miltefosine. This drug has been registered in India. It cannot be used in early pregnancy and in women of reproductive age who are not using contraceptives regularly. If possible, miltefosine should be administered as directly observed treatment in order to retain its efficacy and delay in the appearance of drug resistance. Use of treatment cards is likely to contribute to better compliance. Paromomycin, an injectable drug, is promising and is undergoing phase III trials. Amphotericin B and liposomes are rescue drugs in the treatment of kala-azar.

Integrated Vector Management and Vector Surveillance

The mainstay of vector control is indoor residual spraying. While dichlorodiphenyltrichloroethane (DDT) can be used for the control of kala-azar in India, suitable alternatives have to be selected for Bangladesh and Nepal since DDT is not available or is not recommended as a national policy. Pyrethroids can be considered although these are very expensive and rapid development of resistance is a constraint. Adoption of a uniform insecticide strategy is advisable through inter-country cooperation. Through geographical information system (GIS) and remote sensing (RS), water bodies should be identified in the district selected and spraying operations carried out within a radius of 1 km of these water bodies. Mapping of the district for water bodies would be useful in limiting spraying operations to those areas where maximum impact is likely to occur. This will help to economize on insecticide consumption and help to control environmental degradation. Community mobilization is required to get maximum cooperation from households. Surveillance of *P. argentipes* vector is important to determine the distribution, population density, major habitats and spatial, and temporal risk factors related to kala-azar transmission. It would be important to monitor the levels of insecticide resistance. The information on vector surveillance would be crucial for planning and programming integrated vector management (IVM) strategy, integrated disease and vector surveillance is recommended for kala-azar elimination.

Effective Disease Surveillance through Passive and Active Case Detection and Vector Surveillance

Cases of kala-azar for surveillance should be classified into three parts: (1) suspect; (2) clinical and (3) confirmed cases. Adoption of this approach will help in the use of uniform criteria. Surveillance includes reporting of cases of PKDL since these are responsible for continued transmission of the disease.

Currently, surveillance through passive case detection (PCD) is done in government institutions. This does not give a true picture since (a) a majority of cases of kala-azar go to private doctors including quacks and there is no reporting from these healthcare providers; (b) treatment is often started without a definitive diagnosis of kala-azar and (c) many cases do not seek health care at all because of poverty and sociocultural constraints. Despite the above constraints, PCD and reporting is used to monitor the trends of the disease. The strategy will be to strengthen reporting through improved diagnosis and treatment and to establish partnership with private healthcare providers including private doctors and to ensure that community is empowered with knowledge of risks of seeking services of quacks for diagnosis and treatment, as an effort to make appropriate treatment available to the community through qualified professionals. For improved surveillance, kala-azar should be made a notifiable disease in the affected areas. Disease surveillance for kala-azar should comprise monthly reporting and feedback at district level, and evolving a system of regular reporting mechanism with state and national authorities. Reporting to WHO should be done on an annual basis (if possible twice a year) and endemic countries should send reports on an agreed reporting format.

As the program improves and capacity is increased, PCD should be supplemented with active case detection (ACD) that is supported by laboratory diagnosis. While ACD is recommended at least once a year in the beginning (if possible two times per year), ACD will become more important as the number of cases reported by PCD declines. ACD should also be supplemented by laboratory confirmation of suspected cases.

Social Mobilization and Building Partnerships

Behavioral change interventions are important in the elimination of kala-azar and for the success of early diagnosis and treatment adherence. Effective behavioral change can also help in promoting early care seeking. Participation of community and families in indoor residual spraying and in reducing human vector contact is necessary. Social mobilization should be an integral part of the elimination program right from inception. National programs should plan adequate resources for effective behavioral change.

Partnerships will be necessary at all levels, i.e. at district and state levels, at national level and with international stakeholders. Some of the elimination and eradication program (polio, leprosy, lymphatic filariasis) owe their success to multi-partner leadership.

Partnerships networking and collaboration will be required with other programs like vector-borne disease programs (malaria, dengue, filaria) and others, e.g. HIV/AIDS, TB and leprosy. Anemia control, improvement in nutritional status and poverty alleviation programs should be made partners of kala-azar elimination program.

Clinical and Operational Research

Diagnostic and therapeutic tools are available for elimination of kala-azar. More clinical research is required to enable the addition of new drugs and diagnostics. The available diagnostic tests should be validated under field conditions. Additional research is needed to identify and evaluate techniques for rapid assessment and mapping of the disease, to develop a mechanism for monitoring the effectiveness of intervention strategies. Operational research is recommended to establish monitoring of drug resistance, drug efficacy and quality of drugs used in the program. Research is also needed to optimize the effectiveness of drugs including the use of combination drugs in the treatment of kala-azar. Research is also needed in searching for cases of PKDL and for satisfactory treatment of cases of PKDL. This is at present a serious constraint in the elimination of kala-azar. Implementation research is required in pilot districts where the program should be monitored closely to identify constraints and lessons learnt.

BIBLIOGRAPHY

1. A Publication of WHO/SEARO, WHO Regional Office for South-East Asia 2008 (Last updated: 26 May 2006).
2. Bhattacharya SK, Sinha PK, Sundar S, et al. Phase 4 trial of miltefosine for the treatment of Indian visceral leishmaniasis. J Infect Dis. 2007;196(4):591-8.
3. Bhattacharya SK, Sur D, Karbwang J. Childhood visceral leishmaniasis. Indian J Med Res. 2006;123(3):353-6.
4. Das VN, Ranjan A, Singh VP, et al. Magnitude of unresponsiveness to sodium stibogluconate in the treatment of visceral leishmaniasis in Bihar'. Natl Med J India. 2005;18 (3):131-3.
5. Harith AE, Kolk AH, Kager PA, et al. A simple and economical direct agglutination test for serodiagnosis and sero-epidemiological studies of visceral leishmaniasis. Trans R Soc Trop Med Hyg. 1986;80:583-7.
6. Jha TK, Olliaro P, Thakur CPN, et al. Randomised controlled trial of aminosidine (paromomycin) v sodium stibogluconate for treating visceral leishmaniasis in North Bihar, India. BMJ. 1998;316:1200-5.
7. Jha TK. Refractory kala-azar—diagnosis and management. Medicine Update. 1998;137:44.
8. Kuhlencord A, Maniera T, Eibl H, et al. Oral treatment of visceral leishmaniasis in mice. Antimicrob Agents Chemother. 1992;36:1630-4.
9. Osman OF, Oskam L, Zijtsra EE, et al. Use of polymerase chain reaction to assess the success of visceral leishmaniasis treatment. Trans R SocTrop Med Hyg. 1998;92:397-400.
10. Park's Textbook of Preventive and Social Medicine, 18th edition 2005.
11. Piarroux RF, Gambarelli F, Dumon H, et al. Comparision of PCR with direct examination of bone marrow aspiration, myeloculture and serology for diagnosis of visceral leishmaniasis in immunodeficiency type 1. J Clin Microbiol. 1994;32:746-9.
12. Shyam Sundar, Jha TK, Thakur CP, et al. Injectable paromomycin for visceral leishmaniasis in India. The NEJM. 2007;356(25);2571-81.
13. Singh S, Sivakumar R. Recent advances in the diagnosis of leishmaniasis. J Postgrad Med. 2003;49:55-60.
14. Sinha PK, Pandey K, Bhattacharya SK. Diagnosis and management of leishmania/HIV co-infection. Indian J Med Res. 2005;121:407-14.
15. Sundar S, Chatterjee M. Visceral leishmaniasis-current therapeutic modalities. Indian J Med Res. 2006;123:345-52.
16. Sundar S. Diagnosis of kala-azar. An important stride. J Assoc Physicians India. 2003;51:753-5.
17. The leishmaniasis. Report of WHO expert committee. World Health Organ Tech Rep Ser. 1984;701:1-40.
18. Vilaplana C, Blanco S, Domínguez J, et al. Noninvasive method for diagnosis of visceral leishmaniasis by a latex agglutination test for detection of antigens in urine samples. J Clin Minobiol. 2004;42:1853-4.
19. WHO. The world health situation of the global strategy for health for all by the year 2000. 8th report, 2nd evaluation. Vol. 1, Global Reviews, Geneva.
20. Zijlstra EE, Daifalla NS, Khalil EPG, et al. rK39 enzyme-linked immunosorbent assay for diagnosis of leishmania donovani infection. Clin Diag Lab Immunol. 1998;5:717-20.

DIAGNOSIS OF ENTERIC FEVER

The correct and rapid diagnosis of enteric fever is of paramount importance for instituting appropriate therapy and also for avoiding unnecessary therapy.

Complete Blood Count

For practical purposes, the complete blood count (CBC) in enteric fever is unremarkable. The hemoglobin is normal in the initial stages but drops with progressing illness. Severe anemia is unusual and should make one suspect intestinal hemorrhage or hemolysis or an alternative diagnosis like malaria. The white blood cell (WBC) count is normal in most cases and leukocytosis makes the diagnosis less probable. Leukopenia perceived to be an important feature of typhoid fever and has been reported only in 20–25% cases. The differential count is usually unremarkable except for eosinopenia. Eosinopenia often absolute may be present in 70–80% cases. Presence of absolute eosinopenia offers a clue to diagnosis but does not differentiate enteric fever from other acute bacterial or viral infections. Conversely, a normal eosinophil count does make typhoid fever a less likely possibility. Platelet counts are normal to begin with and fall in some cases by the second week of illness.

Cultures

Blood Culture

Blood cultures are the gold standard diagnostic method for diagnosis of enteric fever. The sensitivity of blood culture is highest in the first week of the illness and reduces with advancing illness. Overall sensitivity is around 50% but drops considerably with prior antibiotic therapy. Failure to isolate the organism may be caused by several factors which includes inadequate laboratory media, the volume of blood taken for culture, the presence of antibiotics and the time of collection. For blood culture it is essential to inoculate media at the time of drawing blood.

Salmonella can be easily cultured in most microbiologic laboratories with the use of routine culture media (Hartley's media, Blood agar and MacConkey agar). Automated blood culture systems such as BACTEC, certainly enhance the recovery rate. Sufficient amount of blood should be collected for culture as the median bacterial count in the peripheral blood is only 0.3 CFU/mL (interquartile range 0.1–10; range 0.1–399). At least 10 mL of blood in adults and 5 mL in children should be collected. Dilution should be appropriate in order to adequately neutralize the bactericidal effect of serum and a ratio of 1:5–1:10 of blood to broth is recommended. Clot cultures, wherein the inhibitory effect of serum is obviated have not been found to be of superior sensitivity as compared to blood cultures in several clinical studies. In the laboratory, blood culture bottles should be incubated at 37°C and checked for turbidity, gas formation and other evidence of growth after 1, 2, 3 and 7 days. For days 1, 2 and 3 only bottles showing signs of positive growth are cultured on agar plates. On day 7 all bottles should be subcultured before being discarded as negative.

Bone Marrow Culture

Salmonella typhi is an intracellular pathogen in the reticuloendothelial cells of the body including the bone marrow. Studies have revealed that the median bacteremia in the bone marrow is 9 CFU/mL (IQR, 1–85; range, 0.1–15,805) compared to 0.3 CFU/mL (IQR, 0.1–10; range, 0.1–399) in blood. This bone marrow, peripheral blood ratio which is around 4.8 (IQR, 1–27.5) in the first week of the illness increases to 158 (IQR, 60–397) during the third week owing to disappearance of bacteria from the peripheral blood. The overall sensitivity of bone marrow cultures ranges from 80% to 95% and is good even in late disease and despite prior antibiotic therapy.

Stool, Urine and Other Cultures

Stool specimen should be collected in a sterile wide mouthed container. Specimens should preferably be processed within 2 hours after collection. If there is a delay the specimen should be stored in a refrigerator at 4°C or in a cool box with freezer packs. The sensitivity of stool culture depends on the amount of feces cultured and the positivity rate increases with the duration of the illness. Rectal swabs should be avoided as these are less successful. Stool cultures are positive in 30% of patients with acute enteric fever.

Antimicrobial Sensitivity Testing

The crucial issue here pertains to fluoroquinolone susceptibility testing. Fluoroquinolones were introduced in 1989 and during the past decade there has been a progressive increase in the minimum inhibitory concentrations (MICs) of ciprofloxacin in *S. typhi* and *S. paratyphi*. Since the current MICs are still below the National Committee for Clinical Laboratory Standards (NCCLS) susceptibility breakpoint, laboratory reports will continue to report *S. typhi/paratyphi* as ciprofloxacin/ofloxacin sensitive. However, use of fluoroquinolones in this scenario is associated with a high incidence of clinical failure. It has also been demonstrated that resistance to nalidixic acid is a surrogate marker for high ciprofloxacin MICs, predicts fluoroquinolone failure and hence can be used to guide antibiotic therapy (i.e. if culture results show resistance to nalidixic acid irrespective of the results of ciprofloxacin/ofloxacin sensitivity, quinolones should not be used or if used high doses should be given). Since MIC testing is not within the scope of most laboratories, nalidixic acid susceptibility testing is mandatory to help guide the choice of antibiotics.

Serologic Tests

WIDAL Test

This test first described by F Widal in 1896, detects agglutinating antibodies against the O and H antigens of *S. typhi* and H antigens of *S. paratyphi A* and *S. paratyphi B*. The 'O' antigen is the somatic antigen of *S. typhi* and is shared by *S. paratyphi A, S. paratyphi B*, other Salmonella species and other members of the Enterobacteriaceae family. Antibodies against the O antigen are predominantly immunoglobulin M (IgM), rise early in the illness and disappear early. The H antigens are flagellar antigens of *S. typhi, S. paratyphi A* and *S. paratyphi B*. Antibodies to H antigens are both IgM and immunoglobulin G (IgG) rise late in the illness and persist for a longer time. Usually, O antibodies appear on day 6–8 and H antibodies on days 10–12 after the onset of disease. The test is usually performed on an acute serum (at first contact with the patient). A convalescent serum should preferably also be collected so that paired titrations can be performed.

Conventionally, a positive WIDAL test result implies demonstration of rising titers in paired blood samples 10–14 days apart. Unfortunately this criterion is purely of academic interest. Decisions about antibiotic therapy cannot wait for results from two samples. Moreover antibiotics may dampen the immune response and prevent a rise in titers even in truly infected individuals. Establishing appropriate cut-offs for distinguishing acute from past infections is thus important for the population where the test is applied. In one study from Central India, anti O and anti H titer of more than 1:80 was seen in 14% and 8% respectively of a study sample of 1,200 healthy blood donors.

While interpreting the results of the WIDAL test, both H and O antibodies have to be taken into account. There is controversy about the predictive value of O and H antibodies for diagnosis of enteric fever. Certain authorities claim that O antibodies have superior specificity and positive predictive value (PPV) because these antibodies decline early after an acute infection. Other studies report a poorer PPV of O antibodies probably due to rise of these antibodies in other Salmonella species, Gram-negative infections, in unrelated infection and following typhoid-paratyphoid A and B (TAB) vaccination. For practical purpose and for optimal result this test should be done after 5–7 days of fever by tube method and level of both H and O antibodies of 1 in 160 dilution (fourfold rise) should be taken as cut-off value for diagnosis. H antibodies once positive can remain positive for a long-time.

The WIDAL test as a diagnostic modality has suboptimal sensitivity and specificity. It can be negative in up to 30% of culture-proven cases of typhoid fever.

Not withstanding these problems, the WIDAL test may be the only test available in certain resource poor set ups for diagnosis of enteric. In Vietnam, using a cut-off of more than 1/200 for the O agglutinin or more than 1/100 for H agglutinin test performed on acute-phase serum, the WIDAL test could correctly diagnose 74% of blood culture for positive typhoid fever; however, 14% results would be false positive and 10% false negative. Hence, it is important to realize the limitations of the WIDAL test and interpret the results carefully in light of endemic titers so that both over diagnosis and under diagnosis of typhoid fever and the resulting consequences are avoided.

Other Serologic Tests

In view of the limitations of the WIDAL test and need for a cheap and rapid diagnostic method, several attempts to develop alternative serologic tests have been made. These include rapid dipstick assays, dot enzyme immunoassays and agglutination inhibition tests.

Enzyme Immunoassay Test or Typhidot® Test

A dot-enzyme immunoassay (EIA) that detects IgG and IgM antibodies against a 50 KD outer membrane protein distinct from the somatic (O), flagellar (H) or capsular (Vi) antigen of *S. typhi* is commercially available as Typhidot. The sensitivity and specificity of this test has been reported to vary from 70% to 100% and 43% to 90% respectively. This dot EIA test offers simplicity, speed, early diagnosis and high negative and PPVs. The detection of IgM reveals acute typhoid in the early phase of infection, while the detection of both IgG and IgM suggests acute typhoid in the middle phase of infection. In areas of high endemicity where the rate of typhoid transmission is high the detection of specific IgG increases. Since IgG can persist for more than 2 years after typhoid infection, the detection of specific IgG cannot differentiate between acute and convalescent cases. Further more, false positive results attributable to previous infection may occur. On the other hand, IgG positivity may also occur in the event of current reinfection. In cases of reinfection there is a secondary immune response with a significant boosting of IgG over IgM, such that the later cannot be detected and its effect masked. A possible strategy for solving this problem is to enable the detection of IgM by ensuring that it is unmasked. The original Typhidot® test was modified by inactivating the total IgG in the serum samples. Studies with modified test, Typhidot® M, have shown that inactivation of IgG removes competitive binding and allows the access of the antigen to the specific IgM when it is present.

The Typhidot M that detects only IgM antibodies of *S. typhi* has been reported to be slightly more specific in a couple of studies.

IDL Tubex® Test

The Tubex® test is easy to perform and takes approximately 2 minutes time. The test is based on detecting antibodies to a single antigen in *S. typhi* only. The 09 antigen used in this test is very specific found in only serogroup D *Salmonella*. A positive result always suggests a *Salmonella* infection but not which group D *Salmonella* is responsible. Infection by other serotypes like *S. paratyphi A* gives negative result. This test detects IgM antibodies but not IgG which is further helpful in the diagnosis of current infections.

IgM Dipstick Test

The test is based on the binding of *S. typhi* specific IgM antibodies to *S. typhi* lipopolysaccharide (LPS) antigen and the staining of the bound antibodies by an antihuman IgM antibody conjugated to colloidal dye particles. This test will be useful in places where culture facilities are not available as it can be performed without formal training and in the absence of specialized equipment. One should keep in mind that specific antibodies appear a week after the onset of symptoms so the sensitivity of this test increases with time.

Antigen Detection Tests

Enzyme immunoassay's, counter-immune electrophoresis and coagglutination tests to detect serum or urinary somatic/flagellar/Vi antigens of *S. typhi* have been evaluated. Sensitivity of Vi antigen has been found to be superior to somatic and flagellar antigen and has been reported as ranging from 50% to 100% in different studies. Similarly specificity estimates have been reported to vary from 25% to 90%. The suboptimal and variable sensitivity and specificity estimates, inability to detect *S. paratyphi* infection and Vi antigen negative strains of *S. typhi* are serious limitations of the Vi antigen detection tests.

Molecular Methods

The limitations of cultures and serologic tests advocate for development of alternative diagnostic strategies. Polymerase chain reaction (PCR) as a diagnostic modality for typhoid fever was first evaluated in 1993 when Song et al. successfully amplified the flagellin gene of *S. typhi* in all cases of culture proven typhoid fever and from none of the healthy controls. Moreover, some patients with culture negative typhoid fever were PCR positive suggesting that PCR diagnosis of typhoid may have superior sensitivity than

cultures. Over the next 10 years a handful of studies have reported PCR methods targeting the flagellin gene, somatic gene, Vi antigen gene, 5S-23S spacer region of the ribosomal RNA gene, invA gene and hilA gene of *S. typhi* for diagnosis of typhoid fever. These studies have reported excellent sensitivity and specificity when compared to positive (blood culture proven) and healthy controls. The turnaround time for diagnosis has been less than 24 hours. These reports should be viewed within the context of certain limitations.

Conclusion

The CBC is the logical first investigation. Presence of a normal or low leukocyte count with eosinopenia points to possible enteric. It also helps in evaluation of alternative diagnoses such as malaria, dengue and other bacteremias. Blood cultures remain the most effective investigations for diagnosis of enteric till date. They should be sent early in the course of the illness and prior to starting antibiotic therapy. Susceptibility testing for nalidixic acid should be routinely done for all isolates to aid choice of antibiotics. Bone marrow culture is a highly sensitive diagnostic test even in late stages of the illness and with prior antibiotic therapy. It should be performed in all patients with prolonged pyrexia if routine investigations have failed to establish a diagnosis. The WIDAL test has several limitations and should be requested for the second week of the illness and its results interpreted with caution. Data on baseline titers in the local population should be generated by appropriate studies to help in determining appropriate cut-offs for the WIDAL. The modified WIDAL test, Typhidot, Tubex and Vi antigen tests need to be evaluated further before their routine use can be recommended. Molecular methods are still experimental.

TREATMENT OF ENTERIC FEVER

Antimicrobial Therapy

Since 1990s *S. typhi* has developed resistance simultaneously to all the drugs used in first line treatment (chloramphenicol, cotrimoxazole and ampicillin) and are known as multidrug resistant typhoid fever (MDRTF). There are some reports of re-emergence of fully susceptible strain to first line drugs. But these reports are few and unless antibiotic sensitivity testing shows the organisms to be fully susceptible to first line drugs they are not advocated for empirical therapy in typhoid.

Fluoroquinolones are widely regarded as the most effective drug for the treatment of typhoid fever. But unfortunately some strains of *S. typhi* have shown reduced susceptibility to fluoroquinolones. On routine disc testing with the recommended breakpoints, organisms showing susceptibility to fluoroquinolones shows poor clinical response to actual treatment. These organisms when tested by disc testing with nalidixic acid shows resistance to it. So in other words resistance to nalidixic acid is a surrogate marker which predicts fluoroquinolones failure and can be used to guide antibiotic therapy. The resistance to fluoroquinolones may be total or partial. The nalidixic acid resistant *S. typhi* (NARST) is a marker of reduced susceptibility to fluoroquinolones.

With the development of fluoroquinolones resistance third generation cephalosporins were used in treatment but sporadic reports of resistance to these antibiotics also followed.

Recently azithromycin are being used as an alternative agent for treatment of uncomplicated typhoid fever.

Aztreonam and imipenem are also potential third line drugs which are used recently.

There is now considerable amount of evidence from the long-term use of fluroquinolones in children that neither they cause bone or joint toxicity nor impairment of growth.

Ciprofloxacin, ofloxacin, perfloxacin and fleroxacin are common fluoroquinolones proved to be affective and used in adults. In children, the first two are only used in our country and there is no evidence of superiority of any particular fluroquinolones. Norfloxacin and nalidixic acid do not achieve adequate blood concentration after oral administration and should not be used. Fluoroquinolones have the advantage of lower rates of stool carriage than the first line drugs. However, fluoroquinolones are not approved by Drug Controller General of India to be used under 18 years of age unless the child is resistant to all other recommended antibiotics and is suffering from life-threatening infection.

Of the third generation cephalosporins oral cefixime has been widely used in children. Amongst the third generation cephalosporins in injectable form ceftriaxone, cefotaxime and cefoperazone are used of which ceftriaxone is most convenient.

Fluoroquinolones like ofloxacin or ciprofloxacin, are used in a dose of 15 mg/kg of body weight per day to a maximum of 20 mg/kg per day.

Of the oral third generation cephalosporins, oral cefixime is used in a dose of 15–20 mg/kg per day in 2 divided doses. Parenteral third generation cephalosporins include ceftriaxone 50–75 mg/kg per day in 1 or 2 doses; cefotaxime 40–80 mg/kg per day in 2 or 3 doses and cefoperazone 50–100 mg/kg per day in 2 doses.

Azithromycin is used in a dose of 10–20 mg/kg given once daily.

Fluoroquinolones are the most effective drug for treatment of typhoid fever. For nalidixic acid sensitive *S. typhi* (NASST) 7 days course are highly effective. Although shorter courses are advocated but they should be reserved for containment of epidemics. For nalidixic acid resistant *S. typhi* (NARST) 10–14 days course with maximal permitted dosage is recommended. Courses shorter than 7 days are not satisfactory.

In case of uncomplicated typhoid oral third generation cephalosporins, e.g. cefixime should be the drug of choice as empiric therapy. Fever defervescence in enteric fever can take at least 5 days. There is currently an outbreak of XDR typhoid in Sindh, Pakistan where more than 300 XDR typhoid cases have been reported since November, 2016. XDR typhoid means resistance to three first-line drugs (chloramphenicol, ampicillin, and trimethoprim-sulfamethoxazole) as well as fluoroquinolones and third-generation cephalosporins. Hence, it is extremely important to judiciously use Azithromycin as this is the only currently available oral antibiotic alternative in such a situation.

For complicated typhoid the choice of drug is parenteral third generation cephalosporin, e.g. ceftriaxone. In severe life- threatening infection fluoroquinolones may be used as a last resort. Aztreonam and imipenem may also be used.

Combination therapy though practiced all over needs substantiation with adequate data from studies.

In Tables 8.2.1 and 8.2.2, various antibiotics are given which are used in the management of both complicated and uncomplicated typhoid with different sensitivity patterns.

Management of Relapse

Relapses involving acute illness occur in 5–10% of typhoid fever cases that have been apparently treated successfully. Cultures should be obtained and standard treatment should be administered. They are sensitive to same antibiotics which were given for the first episode and should be given for a period of 5–7 days.

Prognosis

The prognosis depends on the patient population and geographic area. In an epidemic in developed countries patients will be generally seen and treated promptly, have case fatality rate is less than 1%. The majority of patients in the endemic area will be treated as out-patients and have case fatality and complication rates comparable to those expected in epidemic in developed countries.

The factors associated with poor prognosis are late diagnosis and late initiation of treatment, extremes of age (children of < 2 years and elderly), multidrug resistant (MDR) organism, severe enteric at the time of presentation, associated conditions like HIV infection, sickle cell disease, and if complications are identified late and with its delayed management.

Four baseline variables such as abdominal pain, low systolic blood pressure, hypoalbuminemia and laboratory evidence of disseminated intravascular coagulation are independently associated with severe complication and can be used as prognostic indicators.

In developing countries like India, severe typhoid is common among hospitalized patients. These patients have mortality rate as high as 50%, if not treated with high doses of dexamethasone.

A delay in appearance of agglutinins may indicate severe illness. Toxemic circulatory failure is the most common cause of death which can be relieved by the

Table 8.2.1: Treatment of uncomplicated typhoid.

Susceptibility	First line oral drug			Second line oral drug		
	Antibiotic	Daily dose (mg/kg)	Days	Antibiotic	Daily dose (mg/kg)	Days
Fully sensitive	3rd generation cephalosporine, e.g. cefixime	15–20	14	Chloramphenicol Amoxicillin TMP-SMX	50–75 75–100 8 TMP 40 SMX	14–21 14 14
Multidrug resistant	3rd generation cephalosporine, e.g. cefixime	15–20	14	Azithromycin	10–20	14

Table 8.2.2: Treatment of severe typhoid.

Susceptibility	First line parenteral drug			Second line parenteral drug		
	Antibiotic	Daily dose (mg/kg)	Days	Antibiotic	Daily dose (mg/kg)	Days
Fully sensitive	Ceftriaxone or Cefotaxime	50–75	14	Chloramphenicol Ampicillin TMP-SMX	100 100 8 TMP 40 SMX	14–21 14 14
Multidrug resistant	Ceftriaxone or Cefotaxime	50–75	14	Aztreonam	50–100	14

Note: Imipenem are potential second line drug and fluoroquinolones can be used in life-threatening infection resistant to other recommended antibiotics.

steroids. Second most common and serious cause of death is intestinal perforation.

The prognosis for the neurological deficit is usually good. In most of the cases the recovery is slow and complete, but in some cases deficit may persists for long.

Periostitis may cause symptoms for months but recovery usually ensues. Postenteric mania has good ultimate prognosis. Immunity following enteric fever is partial.

BIBLIOGRAPHY

1. Ananthanarayan R, Panikar CKJ. Textbook of Microbiology. Chennai: Orient Longman. 1999. pp.244-9.
2. Background document: the diagnosis, treatment and prevention of typhoid fever. Communicable Disease Surveillance and Response, Vaccines and Biologicals. World Health Organisation. May 2003. WHO/V & B/03.07.
3. Bhutta ZA, Mansurali N. Rapid serologic diagnosis of pediatric typhoid fever in an endemic area: a prospective comparative evaluation of two dot-enzyme immunoassays and the WIDAL test. Am J Trop Med Hyg. 1999;61(4):654-7.
4. Bhutta ZA. Impact of age and drug resistance on mortality in typhoid fever. Arch Dis Child. 1996;75:214-7.
5. Cardona-Castro N, Agudelo-Florez P. Immunoenzymatic dot-blot test for the diagnosis of enteric fever caused by Salmonella typhi in an endemic area. Clin Microbiol Infect. 1998;4:64-9.
6. Chiu CH, Tsai JR, Ou JT, et al. Typhoid fever in children: a fourteen-year experience. Acta Pediatr Taiwan. 2000;41:28-32.
7. Choo KE, Davis TM, Ismail A, et al. Rapid and reliable serological diagnosis of enteric fever: comparative sensitivity and specificity of Typhidot and Typhidot-M tests in febrile Malaysian children. Acta Tropica. 1999;72:175-83.
8. Crump JA, Barrett TJ, Nelson JT, et al. Reevaluating fluoroquinolone breakpoints for Salmonella enterica serotype typhi and for non-typhi salmonellae. Clin Infect Dis. 2003;37:75-81.
9. Deshmukh CT, Nadkarni UB, Karande SC. An analysis of children with typhoid fever admitted in 1991. J Postgrad Med. 1994;40:204-7.
10. Duthie R, French GL. Comparison of methods for the diagnosis of typhoid fever. J Clin Pathol. 1990;43:863-5.
11. Dutta P, Mitra U, Dutta S, et al. Ceftriaxone therapy is ciprofloxacin treatment failure typhoid fever in children. In J Med Res. 2001;113:210-3.
12. Eustache JM, Hreis DJ. Typhoid perforation of the intestine. Arch Surg. 1983;118:1269-71.
13. Farooqui BJ, Khurshid M, Ashfaq MK, et al. Comparative yield of Salmonella typhi from blood and bone marrow cultures in patients with fever of unknown origin. J Clin Pathol. 1991;44:258-9.
14. Gasem MH, Smits HL, Goris MG, et al. Evaluation of a simple and rapid dipstick assay for the diagnosis of typhoid fever in Indonesia. J Med Microbiol. 2002;51:173-7.
15. Gupta A, Swarnkar NK, Choudhary SP. Changing antibiotic sensitivity in enteric fever. J Trop Ped. 2001;47:369-71.
16. Handojo I, Dewi R. The diagnostic value of the ELISA-Ty test for the detection of typhoid fever in children. Southeast Asian J Trop Med Pub Health. 2000;31:702-7.
17. Haque A, Ahmed N, Peerzada A, et al. Utility of PCR in diagnosis of problematic cases of typhoid. Jpn J Infect Dis. 2001;54:237-9.
18. Hatta M, Goris MG, Heerkens E, et al. Simple dipstick assay for the detection of Salmonella typhi-specific IgM antibodies and the evolution of the immune response in patients with typhoid fever. Am J Trop Med Hyg. 2002;66:416-21.

19. Hirose K, Itoh K, Nakajima H, et al. Selective amplification of tyv (rfbE), prt (rfbS), viaB, and fliC genes by multiplex PCR for identification of Salmonella enterica serovars typhi and paratyphi A. J Clin Microbiol. 2002;40:633-6.

20. Hoffman SL, Punjabi NH, Kumala S. Reduction in chloramphenicol treated severe typhoid by high dose of dexamethasone. N Engl J Med. 1984;310:82-8.

21. Jackson AA, Ismail A, Ibrahim TA, et al. Retrospective review of dot enzyme immunoassay test for typhoid fever in an endemic area. Southeast Asian J Trop Med Pub Health. 1995;26:625-30.

22. Jesudason M, Esther E, Mathai E. Typhidot test to detect IgG and IgM antibodies in typhoid fever. Indian J Med Res. 2002;116:70-2.

23. Kapil A, Renuka, Das B. Nalidixic acid susceptibility test to screen ciprofloxacin resistance in Salmonella typhi. Indian J Med Res. 2002;115:49-54.

24. Khan M, Coovadia Y, Connolly C, et al. Risk factors predicting complications in blood culture-proven typhoid fever in adults. Scand J Infect Dis. 2000;32:201-5.

25. Khosla SN. Changing patterns of typhoid fever. Asian Med J. 1982;25:185-98.

26. Kim JP, Oh SK, Jarrett F. Management of ileal perforation due to typhoid fever. Ann Surg. 1975;181:88-91.

27. Lakohotia M, Gehlot RS, Jain P, et al. Neurological manifestation of enteric fever. J Indian Acad Clin Med. 2003;4:196-9.

28. Lim PL, Tam FC, Cheong YM, et al. One-step 2-minute test to detect typhoid-specific antibodies based on particle separation in tubes. J Clin Microbiol. 1998;36:2271-8.

29. Massi MN, Shirakawa T, Gotoh A, et al. Quantitative detection of Salmonella enterica serovar typhi from blood of suspected typhoid fever patients by real-time PCR. Int J Med Microbiol. 2005;295:117-20.

30. McKendrick GDW. Salmonella infections. In: Scott RB (Ed). Price's Textbook of the Practice of Medicine, 12th edition. Norfolk: ELBS; 1978. pp.39-44.

31. Meier DE, Imediegw OO, Tarpley JL. Perforated typhoid enteritis: operative experience with 108 cases. Am J Surg. 1989;157:423-7.

32. Nsutebu EF, Ndumbe PM, Koulla S. The increase in occurrence of typhoid fever in Cameroon: overdiagnosis due to misuse of the Widal test? Trans R Soc Trop Med Hyg. 2002;96:64-7.

33. Olopoenia LA, King AL. Widal agglutination test–100 years later: stIll plagued by controversy. Postgrad Med J. 2000;76:80-4.

34. Osuntokum BO, Bademosi O, Ogunremi K, et al. Neuro-psychiatric manifestations of typhoid fever in 959 patients. Arch Neurol. 1972;27:7-13.

35. Pandey KK, Srinivasan S, Mahadevan S, et al. Typhoid fever below five years. Indian Pediatr. 1990;27:153-6.

36. Pandya M, Pillai P, Deb M. Rapid diagnosis of typhoid fever by detection of Barber protein and Vi antigen of Salmonella serotype typhi. J Med Microbiol. 1995;43:185-8.

37. Parry CM, Hien TT, Dougan G, et al. Typhoid fever. N Engl J Med. 2002;347:1770-82.

38. Parry CM, Hoa NT, Diep TS, et al. Value of a single-tube WIDAL test in diagnosis of typhoid fever in Vietnam. J Clin Microbiol. 1999;37:2882-6.

39. Prakash P, Mishra OP, Singh AK, et al. Evaluation of nested PCR in diagnosis of typhoid fever. J Clin Microbiol. 2005;43:431-2.

40. Punjabi NH, Hoffman SL, Edmand DC, et al. Treatment of severe typhoid fever in children with high dose of dexamethasone. Pediatr Infect Dis J. 1988;7:598-600.

41. Punjabi NH. Typhoid fever. In: Rakel RE (Ed). Conn's Current Therapy, 52nd edition. Philadelphia: WB Saunders; 2000. pp.161-5.

42. Rao PS, Prasad SV, Arunkumar G, et al. Salmonella typhi Vi antigen co-agglutination test for the rapid diagnosis of typhoid fever. Indian J Med Sci. 1999;53:7-9.

43. Richens J. Typhoid fever. In: Weatherall DJ, Ledingham JGG, Warrell DA (Eds). Oxford Textbook of Medicine, 3rd edition. New York: Oxford University Press; 1996. pp.560-8.

44. Rodrigues C. The Widal test more than 100 years old: abused but still used. J Assoc Physicians India. 2003;51:7-8.

45. Rogerson SJ, Spooner VJ, Smith TA, et al. Hydrocortisone in chloramphenicol-treated severe typhoid fever in Papua New Guinea. Trans Roy Soc Trop Medi Hyg. 1991;85:113-6.

46. Rowland HAK. The treatment of typhoid fever. J Trop Med Hyg. 1961;64:101-11.

47. Saha SK, Talukdar SY, Islam M, et al. A highly ceftriaxone resistant Salmonella typhi in Bangladesh. The Ped Infect Dis. 1999;18:297-303.

48. Sanchez-Jimenez MM, Cardona-Castro N. Validation of a PCR for diagnosis of typhoid fever and salmonellosis by amplification of the hilA gene in clinical samples from Colombian patients. J Med Microbiol. 2004;53:875-8.

49. Sharma M, Datta U, Roy P, et al. Low sensitivity of counter-current immuno-electrophoresis for serodiagnosis of typhoid fever. J Med Microbiol. 1997;46:1039-42.

50. Shukla S, Patel B, Chitnis DS. 100 years of WIDAL test and its reappraisal in an endemic area. Indian J Med Res. 1997;105: 53-7.

51. Sood S, Kapil A, Das B, et al. Re-emergence of chloramphenicol sensitive Salmonella typhi. Lancet. 1999;353:1241-2.

52. Thong P Le, Hoffman SL. Typhoid fever. In: Guerrant RL, Walker DH, Weller PF, (Eds). Tropical Infectious Diseases. Philadelphia: Churchill Livingstone; 1999. pp.277-95.

53. Van Basten JP, Stockenbrugger R. Typhoid perforation. A review of the literature since 1960. Trop Geo Med. 1994;46:336-9.

54. Vidyasagar S, Nalloor S, Shashikiran U, et al. Unusual neurological complication of typhoid fever. Calicut Med J. 2004;2:3.

55. Wain J, Pham VB, Ha V, et al. Quantitation of bacteria in bone marrow from patients with typhoid fever: relationship between counts and clinical features. J Clin Microbiol. 2001;39:1571-6.

56. Woodward TE, Hall HE, Dias-Rivera R, et al. Treatment of typhoid fever. II. Control of clinical manifestations with cortisone. Ann Intern Med. 1951;34:10-9.

57. Woodward TE, Smadel JE. Management of typhoid fever and its complications. Ann Intern Med. 1964;60:144-57.

8.3 GUIDELINES FOR RABIES PROPHYLAXIS IN CHILDREN

MK Sudarshan

INTRODUCTION

Rabies is fatal encephalitis caused by a single-stranded negative sense RNA virus belonging to the genus Lyssavirus of the family Rhabdoviridae. This is a zoonotic disease and transmission to humans occurs by bite of an infected animal. In India, the transmitting animal is dog in more than 96% cases. As per a national multicentric rabies survey (2003), about 20,000 human rabies deaths occur in this country, of which it is 65% in adults and 35% in children. This survey also revealed that the incidence of animal bites is 1.7% annually, i.e. about 17 million bites occur annually. Over 96% of these bites are due to dogs both by pet and stray dogs. The same survey provided an estimate of 28 million pet or household dogs in the country and yet there is no official statistics of dog population in India.

Although rabies is fatal once symptoms of the disease develop, it is almost 100% preventable, if the state-of-the-art modern prophylactic measures are instituted soon after the exposure. Potent and safe modern rabies vaccines and immunoglobulins are available in India for the past three decades but rabies deaths continue to occur. There are several reasons for this paradoxical situation. The public awareness about the disease is still poor, at least half the bite victims resort to indigenous treatment consisting of application of chili powder or paste, herbal extracts, etc. and even those who approach qualified medical practitioners, do not receive rabies immunoglobulin (RIG) which is life-saving in Category III exposures. Most bite victims are administered with only vaccines and the use of immunoglobulins is limited to about 2% of bite victims.

The Association for Prevention and Control of Rabies in India (APCRI) and Rabies in Asia Foundation, India, chapter are now actively working for increasing public awareness and professional education about this disease, and trying to get more attention of the government on the continued rabies deaths. The use of highly reactogenic semple (sheep brain) vaccine was discontinued in December, 2004 and potent and safe cell culture vaccines (CCVs) were made available in government run antirabic treatment centers. However, following vaccine shortages, Government of India in 2006 approved intradermal (ID) administration of these vaccines, which used about one-fifth or one-tenth volume of vaccine and there by reduced the cost of rabies prophylaxis by almost 60%.

Problem of Rabies in Children

In India and other developing countries, children suffer almost a two times more attacks or bites by dogs than adults. There are several reasons as to why children are more susceptible: (1) Children play in the streets and are more prone for dog bites. Because of their playful nature they also tend to tease dogs and in consequence, dogs attack them. (2) Due to their short stature, bites on heads and neck and upper part of the body are more common and bites tend to be severe. This results in greater risk for rabies infection with relatively shorter incubation period. Because of their short stature, even bites on lower parts of the body including genitals may result in shorter incubation period. (3) Many times, because of fear of painful injections that are given, children tend to hide the fact that they were bitten. (4) As children have soft skin even minor scratches and trivial bites may result in severe exposures.

Keeping in view all these factors it becomes very essential that children bitten by dogs and other animals get immediate state-of-the-art prophylactic treatment which includes wound treatment, rabies vaccines and immunoglobulins. A high level expert committee meeting took place at National Institute of Communicable Diseases [now National Centre for Disease Control (NCDC)], Delhi, in 2007 to update the existing national guidelines for rabies prophylaxis. Although it addressed all these issues in a general way, management of animal bites particularly in children was not addressed separately. The infectious disease chapter of Indian Academy of Pediatrics (IAP) came forward to update the treatment guidelines especially for children. A committee was constituted with national rabies experts from APCRI, Rabies in Asia Foundation (RIA) and IAP. It is sincerely hoped that pediatricians both in private practice and in service will find this manual useful in treating children exposed to rabies following bites from dogs and other animals. Children constituted 35% of human rabies. The animal bite incidence in children is more (2.5%) when compared to adults (1.3%).

POSTEXPOSURE PROPHYLAXIS

In rabies endemic country like India, where every animal bite is suspected as a potentially rabid bite, the treatment should be started immediately. Because of long and variable incubation period, which is typical of most cases of human rabies, it is possible to institute rabies prophylaxis following a rabies exposure. This must be started at the earliest to ensure that the individual will be effectively immunized or protected before the rabies virus reaches the nervous system. The risk of infection occurring in children depends on severity of bite; the amount of virus inoculated at the site of wound, virulence of the virus and some as yet unknown host factors. The post-exposure prophylaxis (PEP) depends on the severity of exposure and for many years during the era of semple (sheep brain) vaccine the classification of exposures advocated by Central Research Institute, Kasuali and Pasteur Institute,

Table 8.3.1: Type of contact, exposure and recommended PEP.

Category	Type of contact	Type of exposure	Recommended PEP
I	Touching or feeding of animals Licks on intact skin	None	None, if reliable case history is available
II	Nibbling of uncovered skin Minor scratches or abrasions without bleeding	Minor	Wound management Antirabies vaccine
III	Single or multiple transdermal bites or scratches, licks on broken skin Contamination of mucous membrane with saliva (i.e. licks)	Severe	• Wound management • Rabies immunoglobulin • Anti-rabies vaccine

Note: After carefully assessing the category of exposure, the treating doctor should evaluate the course of action to be taken, based on the following general considerations. He should also keep in the mind that in doubtful situations the presently available CCVs or purified duck embryo vaccine (PDEV) are safe to offer treatment rather than withhold.

Coonoor was followed to start appropriate PEP. With the advent of modern CCVs, the WHO has come out with new recommendations for categorization of rabies exposures or wounds and for administration of vaccines and immunoglobulins. To ensure standardization and uniformity globally, the classification of animal bites or rabies exposures for PEP has been based on these WHO recommendations (Table 8.3.1).

Vaccination Status of the Biting Animal

Although unvaccinated animals are more likely to transmit rabies, vaccinated animals can also do so, if the vaccination of the biting animal was ineffective for any reason. A history of rabies vaccination in an animal is not always a guarantee that the biting animal is not rabid. Animal vaccine failures may occur because of improper administration or poor quality of the vaccine, poor health status of the animal, and the fact that one dose of vaccine does not provide long-lasting protection against rabies infection in dogs.

Provoked versus Unprovoked Bites

Whether a dog bite was provoked or unprovoked should not be considered a guarantee that the animal is not rabid as it can be difficult to understand what a dog considers provocation for an attack.

Observation of Biting Animal

The treatment should be started immediately after the bite. The postexposure vaccination may be modified if the biting animal (dog and cat only) remains healthy throughout an observation period of 10 days as by then three doses of vaccine due on days 0, 3 and 7 would have been given. Subsequently, PEP may be modified and made beneficial and effective for future by giving the fourth dose of vaccine as the truncated and last dose on day 14 as per new CDC schedule. To reiterate again the observation period of 10 days is valid for dogs and cats only. The natural history of rabies in mammals other than dogs and cats is not fully understood and therefore the 10-day observation period is not applicable to other animals.

Bite by Wild Animals

Bites by all wild animals including foxes, wild dogs, jackals and mongooses and others should be treated as Category III exposure.

Bites by Other Domestic and Peridomestic Animals

Bites by monkeys should be given PEP depending on the category of exposure. Bites by other mammals, such as horses, pigs, cattle, donkeys and camels, should be evaluated based on circumstances of bite. Bites by house rats, squirrels and rabbits ordinarily do not require PEP, but when exposures occur in strange/peculiar situations and when in doubt the physician may consider providing rabies PEP. The bites by snakes, lizards, birds and insects do not require rabies PEP.

Bat Rabies

Bat rabies has not been conclusively proven in India and hence exposure to bats does not ordinarily warrant treatment.

Human-to-human Transmission

The risk of rabies transmission from a human rabies case to other person is very minimal and there has never been a well-documented case of human-to-human transmission, other than the few cases resulting from organ transplant. However, children who have been exposed closely to the secretions of a patient with rabies may be offered PEP one dose of rabies vaccine given on days 0, 3, 7 and 14 (and no RIG) as a precautionary measure.

It is re-emphasized that treatment should be started as early as possible after exposure. However, it should not be denied to person reporting late for treatment as explained previously.

Approach to Postexposure Prophylaxis

The PEP consists of three components. All three carry equal importance and should be done simultaneously as per the category of the bites or exposure:

- Management of animal bite wound(s)
- Passive immunization: RIGs
- Active immunization: Antirabies vaccines (ARV).

Management of Animal Bite Wounds

Wound toilet: Since the rabies virus present in the saliva of the rabid animal, enters the human body through a bite or scratch, it is imperative to remove as much saliva as possible, and thereby the virus from the wound by an efficient and gentle wound toilet without causing additional trauma. Since the rabies virus can persist and even multiply at the site of bite for a long time, wound toilet must be performed even if the patient reports late (Table 8.3.2).

Prompt and gentle thorough washing with soap or detergent and flushing the wound with running water for up to 15 minutes would suffice. If soap and detergent are not immediately available, wash with running water for up to 15 minutes. Avoid direct touching of wounds with bare hands. Considering the importance of this step the anti-rabies clinics should have wound washing facilities.

The application of irritants (like chili powder or paste, oil, turmeric, lime, salt, herbal extracts, etc.) is unnecessary and damaging. In case, irritants have been applied on the wound, enough gentle washing with soap or detergent should be done to remove the extraneous material especially oil followed by flushing with copious amount of water for up to 15 minutes immediately.

It should be noted that the immediate washing of the wound is a priority. However, the victim should not be deprived of the benefit of wound toilet as long as there is an unhealed wound, which can be washed even if the patient reports late. The maximum benefit of the wound washing is obtained when fresh wound is cleaned immediately. In children, having multiple bites or wounds it is very important to identify and wash all wounds.

Application of antiseptic: After thorough washing and drying of the wound(s), any one of the following available chemical agents in appropriate recommended dilution should be applied, viz. povidone iodine (betadine/

wokadine), alcohol, chloroxylenol (Dettol), chlorhexidine gluconate and cetrimide solution (Savlon).

Local infiltration of rabies immunoglobulins: In Category III bites, RIG should be infiltrated as anatomically feasible in the depth and around the wound(s) to inactivate the locally present virus as described below. All care should be taken in this process to avoid injuring nerves and blood vessels.

Suturing of wound should be avoided as far as possible. If surgically unavoidable, minimum loose sutures should be applied after adequate local treatment along with proper infiltration of RIGs.

Cauterization of wound is no longer recommended as it leaves very bad scar, and does not offer any additional advantage over washing the wound with water and soap.

Tetanus toxoid injection should be given to those children who have not received a booster dose. To prevent sepsis in the wound, a suitable course of an antibiotic must be prescribed.

Rabies Immunoglobulin

The antirabies serum or RIG provides passive immunity in the form of ready-made antibody to tide over initial phase of infection. Antirabies serum or RIG has the property of binding to rabies virus, thereby resulting in neutralization of the virus.

Two types of RIGs are available.

Equine Rabies Immunoglobulin

Equine rabies immunoglobulin is of heterologous origin raised by hyperimmunization of horses. However, currently manufactured ERIGs are highly purified and enzyme refined so that only antigen binding portion (Fab) of the immunoglobulin molecules are present. With these preparations, the occurrence of adverse events has been significantly reduced. The currently available ERIGs are indigenously produced in India.

Human Rabies Immunoglobulin

Human rabies immunoglobulins (HRIG) are prepared from the serum of healthy people hyperimmunized with modern rabies vaccines. As it is homologous HRIG is free from the side effects encountered in a serum of heterologous origin, and because of their longer half-life, are given in half the dose of equine anti-rabies serum. The HRIGs are imported from abroad.

The antirabies sera which are stored in the refrigerator between 2°C and 8°C should always be brought to room temperature (20–25°C) before injection.

Dose of Rabies Immunoglobulin

The dose of ERIG is 40 IU/kg body weight of patient and is given after testing for sensitivity. Its dosage is up to a maximum of 3,000 IU. The ERIG produced in India

Table 8.3.2: Wound management.		
Do's		
Physical	Wash with running tap water for up to 15 minutes	Mechanical removal of virus from the wound
Chemical	Washing the wound with soap and water, dry and apply antiseptic	Inactivation of the virus
Biological	Infiltration of rabies immune-globulins in the depth and around the wound in category III exposures	Neutralization of the virus
Don'ts		
• Touch the wound with bare hand		
• Apply irritants like soil, chilies, turmeric, oil, herbs, chalk, betel leaves, etc.		

contains 300 IU/mL. The dose of the HRIG is 20 IU/kg body weight (maximum 1,500 IU). HRIG does not require any prior sensitivity testing. HRIG preparation is available in concentration of 150 IU/mL.

Administration of Rabies Immunoglobulin

As much of the calculated dose of RIG as is anatomically feasible should be infiltrated into and around the wounds (Fig. 8.3.1).

Multiple needle injections into the wound should be avoided. Any RIG remaining after all wounds have been infiltrated, should be administered by deep intramuscular (IM) injection at an injection site distant from the site of vaccine injection. Animal bite wounds inflicted can be severe and multiple, especially in small children. In such cases, the calculated dose of the RIG may not be sufficient to infiltrate all wounds. In such situations, it is advisable to dilute the RIG in sterile normal saline to a volume sufficient for infiltration of all wounds. The total recommended dose of RIG must not be exceeded as it may interfere or suppress the antibody production following antirabies vaccination in the child.

If RIG was not administered when antirabies vaccination was begun, it can be administered up to 7th day after the administration of the first dose of vaccine. Beyond the 7th day, RIG is not indicated since an antibody response to antirabies vaccine is presumed to have occurred. RIG should never be administered in the same syringe or at the same anatomical site as rabies vaccine.

Skin Sensitivity Test before Administration of ERIG

With antisera of equine origin, rarely adverse events or reactions may occur and hence skin sensitivity test (SST) is recommended before giving ERIG. Skin test may be

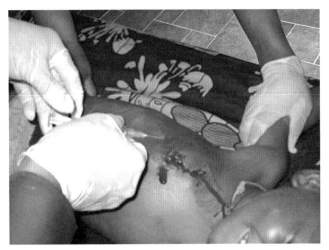

FIG. 8.3.1: Infiltration of rabies immunoglobulin (RIG) into/around the wound in a child.
Courtesy: Dr DH Ashwath Narayana

performed as per the manufacturer's instructions given in the product insert. However, general guidelines may be used which have been discussed in Box 8.3.1.

A negative skin test must never reassure the physician that no anaphylactic reaction will occur. Those administering ERIG should always be ready to treat early anaphylactic reactions with adrenalin. The dose is 0.5 mL of 0.1% solution (1 in 1,000 1 mg/mL) for adults and 0.01 mL/kg body weight for children, injected subcutaneously or IM. If patient is sensitive to ERIG, HRIG should be used.

However, WHO has recently recommended abolishing the SST as it is considered not predictive of adverse events or reactions to occur. However, in India it is obligatory on the part of physician to do it as mentioned in the product insert due to prevailing drug laws and until it is withdrawn.

Approach to a Patient Requiring Rabies Immunoglobulin When None is Available

In circumstances where RIG is not available greater emphasis should be given to proper wound management followed by Essen schedule of modern rabies vaccine with double dose of vaccine on day 0 at two different sites intramuscularly (one dose each on left and right deltoid) followed by one dose each by IM on days 3, 7, 14 and 28. It is emphasized that doubling the first dose of CCV is not a replacement to RIG. However, all efforts should be made to refer the patient to the nearest facility providing RIG to receive the same within 7 days of starting rabies vaccine.

Tolerance and Side Effects

With RIG, there may be transient tenderness at the injection site and a brief rise in body temperature, which do not require any treatment. The incidence of anaphylactic reaction is 1:45,000 cases and till date none has died of anaphylaxis following ERIGs. The hypersensitivity reaction to the skin test is 1–11%. Consequently, ERIGs are lifesaving in all Category III cases and their benefits clearly outweigh the remote risk of anaphylaxis. Serum sickness occurs in 1–6% of patients usually 7–10 days after injection of ERIG, but it has not been reported after treatment with HRIG.

Box 8.3.1

General guidelines.
- Inject 0.1 mL ERIG diluted 1:10 in sterile physiological saline intradermally into the flexor surface of the forearm to raise a bleb of about 3–4 mm diameter
- Inject an equal amount of sterile normal saline as a negative control on the flexor surface of the other forearm
- After 15 minutes an increase in diameter to >10 mm of induration surrounded by flare, swelling, pseudopodia, etc. is taken as positive skin test, provided the reaction on the saline test is negative
- An increase or abrupt fall in blood pressure, syncope, hurried breathing, palpitations and any other systemic manifestations should be taken as positive test

Rabies Monoclonal Antibody (R-Mab)

In November, 2017, the Serum Institute of India, Pune, launched the world's first rabies monoclonal antibody (R-Mab). It is a novel human rabies single monoclonal antibody against rabies G protein (glycoprotein) manufactured by recombinant DNA technology on Chinese hamster ovary (CHO) cells. This R-Mab is known to neutralize a wide variety of terrestrial and bat isolates of rabies virus worldwide including all rabies strains in India. The clinical studies conducted have shown that it induced rabies virus neutralizing activity which was non-inferior to HRIG regimen when used in Essen PEP schedule. Consequently, it is considered as an effective alternative to blood derived RIGs.

Each of vial of 2.5 mL contains 100 IU of R-Mab, having a potency of 40 IU per mL and the dosage is 3.33 IU per kg body weight. One vial would suffice for a person weighing approximately 30 kg. There is no need for skin sensitivity test and it is administered on the same lines of HRIG.

Antirabies Vaccines

Active immunization is achieved by administration of safe and potent CCVs or PDEV. The dosage schedule is same irrespective of the body weight or age of the children.

Storage and Transportation

Although most CCVs or PDEV are marketed in freeze dried (lyophilized) form, which is more tolerant of vagaries of temperature, yet it is recommended that these vaccines should be kept and transported at a temperature range of 2–8°C. Freezing does not damage the lyophilized vaccine but there are chances of breakage of ampoule containing the diluent. Liquid suspension or adsorbed vaccines should never be frozen.

Reconstitution and Storage

The lyophilized vaccine should be reconstituted just prior to use with the diluent provided with the vaccine. After reconstitution if there is delay it should be used within 6–8 hours.

Adverse Effects with Cell Culture Vaccines/ Purified Duck Embryo Vaccine

The CCVs or PDEV presently in the market are safe and generally do not produce any side effects. Occasional local or systemic side effects may be seen. Commonly seen local side effects are pain and tenderness at the injection site. Systemic side effect may include fever, malaise, urticaria and rarely lymphadenopathy. Generally these side effects are self-limiting and occasionally require medication.

Switch over from One Brand/Type of Vaccine to the Other

Shifting from one brand or type of CCV or PDEV to other brand or type should not be encouraged as literature supports that good immunity is best achieved with same brand. However, under unavoidable circumstances, available brand or type of rabies vaccine may be used to complete PEP.

Protective Level of Antirabies Antibody

Humoral antibodies play an important role in protection against rabies and a titer of 0.5 IU/mL or more in serum as tested by Rapid Fluorescent Focus Inhibition Test (RFFIT) is considered as adequate or protective. The facility for this test is available at the Department of Neurovirology, National Institute of Mental Health and Neurosciences, Bengaluru-560029 (Phone: 080-26995128/29).

Currently available CCVs and PDEV are administered by Essen IM regimen. Some CCVs which are also approved for ID use can be administered by cost-effective ID regimens.

Intramuscular Regimen

The currently available vaccines and regimens in India for IM administration are described below.

Vaccines

1. *Cell culture vaccines:*
   – *Human diploid cell vaccine (HDCV)*: Produced locally in private sector. It is an adsorbed (liquid) vaccine
   – *Purified chick embryo cell vaccine (PCECV)*: Produced locally in private sector
   – *Purified vero-cell rabies vaccine (PVRV)*: Imported and produced locally in public and private sectors.
2. *Purified duck embryo vaccine* (PDEV): Produced locally in private sector.

Note: All CCVs and PDEV used for PEP should have potency (antigen content) greater than 2.5 IU/IM dose irrespective of whether it is 0.5 mL or 1.0 mL vaccine by volume.

Regimen

Essen schedule: Five dose IM regimen—the course for PEP consists of IM administration of five injections on days 0, 3, 7, 14 and 28. Day 0 indicates the date of first injection and may not be the day/date of bite/exposure.

Site of inoculation: The anterolateral thigh region is ideal for the inoculation of these vaccines. Gluteal region is not recommended because the fat present in this region retards the absorption of antigen and hence impairs the generation of optimal immune response.

Intradermal Regimen

Intradermal regimens consist of administration of a fraction of IM dose of CCVs at multiple sites in the layers of dermis of skin. The use of ID route leads to considerable savings in terms of total amount of vaccine needed for full pre-exposure or postexposure vaccination, thereby reducing the cost of active immunization. Single dose (0.5 mL/1 mL) of rabies vaccine or antigen when given by IM route gets deposited in the muscles. Thereafter the antigen is absorbed by the blood vessels and is presented to antigen presenting cells which triggers immune response. Whereas, in ID route, small amount (0.1 mL) of rabies vaccine or antigen is deposited in the layers of the skin at two or more sites. The antigen is directly taken up by the antigen presenting cells (Langerhan's cells) within the layers of the skin, which then migrate to regional lymph nodes generating a stronger and quicker antibody response.

Immunity is believed to depend mainly upon the CD 4+ T-cell dependent neutralizing antibody response to the G protein. In addition, cell-mediated immunity has long been reported as an important part of the defense against rabies. Cells presenting the fragments of G protein are the targets of cytotoxic T-cells and the N protein induced T helper cells. The immune response induced by intradermal rabies vaccination (IDRV) is adequate and protective against rabies.

General Guidelines for Use of Intradermal Rabies Vaccination

- Vaccines to be applied by ID route of administration should be approved by Drugs Controller General of India (DCGI)
- The vaccine package leaflet should include a statement indicating that the potency as well as immunogenicity and safety allow safe use of vaccine by ID pre-exposure and postexposure
- Postmarketing surveillance (PMS) data should be maintained for a minimum of two years by vaccine manufacturers on a predesigned and approved protocol
- Intradermal injections must be administered by staff trained in this technique
- Vaccine vials must be stored at 2–8°C after reconstitution
- The total content of reconstituted vial should be used as soon as possible, but at least within 8 hours
- Any leftover of reconstituted vaccine should be discarded after 8 hours of reconstitution or at the end of the day
- Rabies vaccines formulated with an adjuvant or PDEV should not be administered intradermally
- Vaccine when given intradermally should raise a visible and palpable bleb in the skin

- In the event that the dose is inadvertently given subcutaneously or intramuscularly or in the event of spillage, a new dose should be given intradermally in nearby site
- Animal bite victims on chloroquine therapy (antimalarial therapy) should be given ARV by IM route.

Vaccines and Regimen Approved for ID Use in the Country

Considering the recommendations on ID application of rabies by WHO and results of safety, efficacy and feasibility trials conducted in India, Drug Controller General of India (DCGI) approved the use of reduced dosage ID vaccination regimen for rabies PEP. The use of this route leads to considerable savings in terms of the total amount of vaccine needed for a full postexposure vaccination, thereby reducing the cost of active immunization.

Currently, the following vaccines have been approved by DCGI for IDRV.

Vaccines

- *Purified vero cell rabies vaccine*: Verorab, Aventis Pasteur (Sanofi Pasteur), Lyon, France
- *Purified chick embryo cell vaccine*: Rabipur, Chiron Behring Vaccines Pvt. Ltd., Mumbai
- *Purified vero cell rabies vaccine*: Pasteur Institute of India, Coonoor
- *Purified vero cell rabies vaccine*: Abhayrab, Human Biologicals Institute; Indirab, Bharath Biotech, Hyderabad

Note: Since PDEV (Vaxirab, Zydus Fortiza, Ahmedabad) is a suspension; HDCV (Rabivax, Serum Institute of India, Pune) is an adsorbed (with an adjuvant) vaccine these are not recommended for ID administration.

Potency of Approved Vaccines

The vaccines should have stated potency of more than 2.5 IU/IM dose, irrespective of reconstituted volume. The same vaccine is used for ID administration as per stated schedule. 0.1 mL of vaccine, irrespective of reconstituted volume, is administered per ID site as per schedule below.

Regimen

Updated Thai Red Cross Schedule (2-2-2-0-2)

This involves injection of 0.1 mL of reconstituted vaccine per ID site and on two such ID sites per visit (one on each deltoid area, an inch above the insertion of deltoid muscle) on days 0, 3, 7 and 28. The day 0 is the day of first dose administration of IDRV and may not be the day of rabies exposure or animal bite.

Maintenance of vaccine vial in use:

- Use aseptic technique to withdraw the vaccine
- Store in a refrigerator at 2–8°C
- Reconstituted vaccines should be used as soon as possible or within 6–8 hours, if kept at 2–8°C. The unused (reconstituted) vaccine at the end of 6–8 hours must be discarded.

Materials required:

- A vial of rabies vaccine approved for IDRV and its diluent
- Disposable 2 mL syringe with 24 G needle for reconstitution of vaccine
- Disposable 1 mL (insulin) syringe (with graduations up to 100 or 40 units) with a fixed (28 G) needle (Fig. 8.3.2)
- Disinfectant swabs (e.g. 70% ethanol, isopropyl alcohol) for cleaning the top of the vial and the patients' skin.

Intradermal Injection Technique

Using aseptic technique, reconstitute the vial of freeze-dried vaccine with the diluent supplied by the manufacturer. With

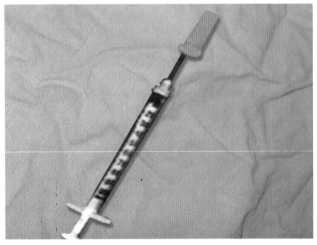

FIG. 8.3.2: 1 mL syringe with hypodermic needle (insulin syringe).

1 mL syringe draw 0.2 mL (up to 20 units if a 100 units syringe is used or up to 8 units if a 40 units syringe is used) of vaccine needed for one patient (i.e. 0.1 mL per ID site × 2 sites, 0.2 mL) and expel the air bubbles carefully from the syringe thereby removing any dead space in the syringe.

Using the technique of bacillus Calmette-Guérin (BCG) inoculation, stretch the surface of the skin and insert the tip of the needle with bevel upward, almost parallel to the skin surface (Fig. 8.3.3) and slowly inject half the volume of vaccine in the syringe (i.e. 0.1 mL; either 10 or 4 units) into the uppermost dermal layer of skin, over the deltoid area, preferably inch above the insertion of deltoid muscle. If the needle is correctly placed inside the dermis, considerable resistance is felt while injecting the vaccine. A raised papule should begin to appear immediately causing a peau d'orange (orange peel) appearance (Fig. 8.3.4). Inject the remaining half the volume of vaccine (i.e. 0.1 mL; either 10 or 4 units) on the opposite deltoid area.

If the vaccine is injected too deeply into the skin (subcutaneous), papule is not seen. Then the needle should be withdrawn and reinserted at an adjacent site and the ID vaccine given once more. If it fails for the second time then the vaccine has to be administered by the IM route.

Antirabies treatment centers which meet the following criteria may use ID administration:

- Have adequately trained staff to give ID inoculation of antirabies vaccine
- Can maintain cold chain for vaccine storage
- Ensure adequate supply of suitable syringes and needles for ID administration
- Are well-versed in management of open vial and safe storage practices.

Postexposure Prophylaxis for Previously Vaccinated Children

Children who have received previously full rabies PEP or preexposure vaccination (either by IM or ID route) with a

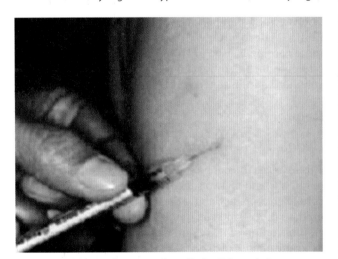

FIG. 8.3.3: Insertion of needle for ID inoculation.

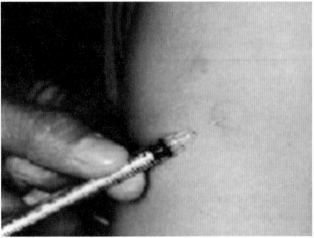

FIG. 8.3.4: Bleb raised on ID inoculation.

potent cell-culture vaccine/PDEV should now be given only two booster doses, either intramuscularly (0.5 mL/1 mL) or intradermally (0.1 mL at one site only, using ID compliant vaccine) on days 0 and 3 irrespective of the duration of previous vaccination. Proper wound toilet should be done. Treatment with RIG is not necessary. In case of travellers who cannot come for the second visit, a single day/visit four site (0.1 mL × 4 ID sites, viz. two deltoids and two suprascapular or thighs) ID booster may be given as per the recent recommendation of WHO.

Managing Re-exposure Following Post-exposure Treatment with Nerve Tissue Vaccine

Children who have previously received full postexposure treatment with nerve tissue vaccine (NTV) should be treated as fresh case and given treatment as per merits of the case.

Postexposure Prophylaxis of Immunocompromised Children

Children with immunodeficiency disorders and HIV infection may also be exposed to rabies. It has been shown that children in whom CD4 cell count is less than 200, antibody response may be impaired after vaccination. In such situations, proper and thorough wound management and antisepsis accompanied by local infiltration of RIG followed by antirabies vaccination are of utmost importance. In fact, administration of RIG is life saving in such situations. Even immunocompromised children with Category II exposures should receive RIG in addition to a full postexposure vaccination. Preferably, if the facilities are available, antirabies antibody estimation should be done 10 days after the completion of course of vaccination.

PRE-EXPOSURE VACCINATION/ PROPHYLAXIS OF CHILDREN

As rabies is virtually cent percent fatal disease and children are at special risk, it may be advisable to vaccinate children after they attain the age of 3 years as they start playing in the streets and come in contact with street or pet dogs. It has been shown by several studies that a course of pre-exposure vaccination will elicit a good immune response and the memory cells generated will last for many years. In fact some studies have also shown that protective levels of antibodies may persist for up to a decade. If such children are exposed to rabies following animal bites, two booster doses given on days 0 and 3 (or single visit four site ID) will elicit a rapid and stronger secondary immune response which will neutralize the virus and prevents its ascent to the CNS. There is no need for local or systemic administration of RIG. Advocating a course of pre-exposure vaccination to children becomes especially important as RIG is expensive, may produce some side effects and is also in short supply. Additionally, as bites in children may be

severe, multiple and incubation period tends to be short, a course of pre-exposure rabies vaccination will sensitize the child's immune system for rabies antigen and two booster doses administered following rabies exposure will elicit a strong humoral and cell mediated immune response. By this practice, treatment failures can be completely avoided and mortality in children can be prevented. As the presently available CCVs and PDEV are very safe and effective, pre-exposure vaccination should be advocated to children in endemic countries like India. It may not be possible presently to incorporate this in the national immunization program but should be advised as an optional vaccination to those children whose parents can afford three doses of any modern CCV or PDEV. The cost of vaccination can be further reduced if it is given by the ID route. As many parents are ready to immunize their children with expensive vaccines for diseases that are not fatal, offering a course of pre-exposure vaccination to a fatal disease like rabies will go a long way in reducing its mortality and save the lives of thousands of children every year.

SCHEDULE OF VACCINATION

Intramuscular

Three doses of any CCV or PDEV (1 mL or 0.5 mL depending on the brand) administered on the anterolateral thigh on days 0, 7 and 28.

Intradermal

The dose is same for all (ID compliant) vaccine brands and 0.1 mL is administered intradermally over the deltoid on days 0, 7 and 28.

Recent Advances

WHO position paper, April 2018, Rabies vaccines: Recently the World Health Organization issued new guidelines to replace the previous 2010 guidelines. A list of it as relevant to rabies prophylaxis is given vide below:
1. *New PEP regimens:*
   - *Intramuscular:* (i) Two-week IM PEP regimen/4-dose Essen regimen/1-1-1-1-0; Duration of entire PEP course: between 14 and 28 days. (ii) Three-week IM PEP regimen/Zagreb regimen/2-0-1-0-1; Duration of entire PEP course: 21 days.
   - *Intradermal:* One-week, 2-site ID regimen/Institut Pasteur du Cambodge (IPC) regimen/2-2-2-0-0; Duration of entire PEP course: 7 days.
2. *New PrEP regimens:* (i) 2-site ID vaccine administered on days 0 and 7. (ii) 1-site IM vaccine administration on days 0 and 7.
3. *Use of RIGs in category III (severe) exposures:* WHO no longer recommends injecting the remainder of the calculated RIG dose IM at a distance from the wound. Instead, the calculated RIG dose can be fractionated

in smaller, individual syringes to be used for several patients. This requires handling and storage in aseptic conditions. Unused fractionated doses and open vials of RIG should be discarded by the end of the day.

However, for introducing these new guidelines in India, revised national guidelines are to be issued by Government of India and this is under active consideration.

SOME TIPS ABOUT HOW TO AVOID DOG BITES

- Typical warning signs of unfriendly dogs are snarling or a stiff stance, ears laid back and fur or hair on back standing up
- Train your dog not to bite. Train your dog to obey simple commands (sit, stay, come and no)
- Do not play aggressive games like wrestling or tug-of-war with your dog
- Do not stare at dogs or provoke any animal
- Do not leave children unattended with dogs. More bites involve children under 12
- Talk to your children about avoiding strange dogs and growling dogs
- Teach children not to take food and toys away from dogs
- Do not run past a dog. They naturally love to chase and catch things. Hence more attacks are seen in children.

BIBLIOGRAPHY

1. Association for Prevention and Control of Rabies in India. Assessing Burden of Rabies in India, WHO sponsored national multi-centric rabies survey, May 2004, KIMS, Bangalore, India. [online] Available from www.apcri.org [Accessed October, 2012].
2. Association for Prevention and Control of Rabies in India. Manual on RIG administration. 2009, Bangalore, India. [online] Available from www.apcri.org [Accessed October, 2012].
3. Centers for Disease Control and Prevention (CDC), Use of a Reduced (4-Dose) Vaccine Schedule for Post-exposure Prophylaxis to Prevent Human Rabies: Recommendations of the Advisory Committee on Immunization Practices. 59, RR-2, 2010, Atlanta, USA.
4. Serum Institute of India Pvt. Ltd . Rabishield . Product Monograph, Pune-28, India, 2017.
5. Sudarshan MK. Rabies Prevention. Rapid Consult. Delhi, India: MacMillan Publishers, 2010.
6. World Health Organization (WHO). Rabies vaccines, WHO position paper. Weekly Epidemiological Record. 2010;32(85): 309-20, Geneva, Switzerland.
7. World Health Organization (WHO). Rabies vaccines, WHO position paper. Weekly Epidemiological Record. 2018;16(93): 201-20, Geneva, Switzerland.
8. World Health Organization. WHO expert consultation on rabies, first report, Technical Report Series, 931, 2005, Geneva, Switzerland.

Vaccines and Immunization

Rohit Agrawal

Vipin M Vashishtha

9.1 PRINCIPLES AND PRACTICE OF IMMUNIZATION

9.1.1. PRINCIPLES OF VACCINATION

INTRODUCTION

Although immunology is a complicated subject but understanding of the basic function of the immune system is useful in order to understand both how vaccines work and the basis of recommendations for their use.

Immunity is the ability of the human body to tolerate the presence of material indigenous to the body (self), and to eliminate foreign (nonself) material. This discriminatory ability provides protection from infectious disease, since most microbes are identified as foreign by the immune system. Immunity to a microbe is usually indicated by the presence of antibody to that organism. Immunity is generally specific to a single organism or group of closely related organisms.

ACTIVE AND PASSIVE IMMUNITY

There are two basic mechanisms for acquiring immunity: (1) active and (2) passive. 'Active immunity' is protection that is produced by the person's own immune system. This type of immunity is usually permanent. 'Passive immunity' is protection by products produced by an animal or human and transferred to another human, usually by injection. Passive immunity often provides effective protection, but this protection wanes (disappears) with time, usually within a few weeks or months.

Active Immunity

Active immunity is stimulation of the immune system to produce antigen-specific humoral (antibody) and cellular immunity. Unlike passive immunity, which is temporary, active immunity usually lasts for many years, often for a lifetime. One way to acquire active immunity is to survive infection with the disease-causing. In general, once people recover from infectious diseases, they will have lifelong immunity to that disease.

Another way to produce active immunity is by vaccination. Vaccines interact with the immune system and often produce an immune response similar to that produced by the natural infection, but they do not subject the recipient to the disease and its potential complications.

The immune system is a complex system of interacting cells whose primary purpose is to identify foreign (nonself) substances referred to as antigens. Antigens can be either live (such as viruses and bacteria) or inactivated.

The most effective immune responses are generally produced in response to a live antigen. However, an antigen does not necessarily have to be alive, as occurs with infection with a virus or bacterium, to produce an immune response. Some proteins, such as hepatitis B surface antigen, are easily recognized by the immune system. Other materials, such as polysaccharide (PS), are less effective antigens, and the immune response may not provide as good protection.

Many factors may influence the immune response to vaccination. These include the presence of maternal antibody, nature and dose of antigen, route of administration and the presence of an adjuvant (e.g. aluminum-containing material added to improve the immunogenicity of the vaccine). Host factors, such as age, nutritional factors, genetics and coexisting disease, may also affect the response.

Passive Immunity

Passive immunity is the transfer of antibody produced by one human or animal to another. Passive immunity provides protection against some infections, but this protection is temporary. The antibodies will degrade during a period of weeks to months, and the recipient will no longer be protected.

The most common form of passive immunity is that which an infant receives from its mother. Antibodies are transported across the placenta during the last 1–2 months of pregnancy. As a result, a full-term infant will have the same antibodies as its mother. These antibodies will protect the infant from certain diseases for up to a year. Protection is better against some diseases (e.g. measles, rubella and tetanus) than others (e.g. polio, and pertussis).

Many types of blood products contain antibody. Some products (e.g. washed or reconstituted red blood cells) contain a relatively small amount of antibody, and some (e.g. intravenous immune globulin and plasma products) contain a large amount.

In addition to blood products used for transfusion (e.g. whole blood, red cells and platelets) there are three major sources of antibody used in human medicine. These are homologous pooled human antibody, homologous human hyperimmune globulin and heterologous hyperimmune serum.

Homologous pooled human antibody is also known as immune globulin. It is produced by combining (pooling) the immunoglobulin G (IgG) antibody fraction from thousands of adult donors. Because it comes from many different donors, it contains antibody to many different antigens. It is used primarily for postexposure prophylaxis for hepatitis A, measles and treatment of certain congenital immunoglobulin (Ig) deficiencies.

Homologous human hyperimmune globulins are antibody products that contain high titers of specific antibody. These products are made from the donated plasma of humans with high levels of the antibody of interest. However, since hyperimmune globulins are from humans, they also contain other antibodies in lesser quantities. Hyperimmune globulins are used for postexposure prophylaxis for several diseases, including hepatitis B, rabies, tetanus, and varicella.

Heterologous hyperimmune serum is also known as antitoxin. This product is produced in animals, usually horses (equine), and contains antibodies against only one antigen such as antitoxin for treatment of diphtheria. A problem with this product is serum sickness, an immune reaction to the horse protein.

Immune globulin from human sources is polyclonal; it contains many different kinds of antibodies. 'Monoclonal antibody' is produced from a single clone of B-cells, so these products contain antibody to only one antigen or closely-related group of antigens. Monoclonal antibody products have many applications, including the diagnosis of certain types of cancer, treatment of cancer, prevention of transplant rejection, and treatment of autoimmune diseases and infectious diseases. A monoclonal antibody product is available for the prevention of respiratory syncytial virus (RSV) infection. It is called palivizumab. It is a humanized monoclonal antibody specific for RSV. It does not contain any other antibody except RSV antibody, and so will not interfere with the response to a live virus vaccine.

Humoral and Cell-mediated Immunity

Vaccines confer protection against diseases by inducing both antibodies and T-cells. The former is called 'humoral' response and the latter, 'cellular' response or 'cell-mediated immunity'. Antibodies are of several different types (IgG, IgM, IgA, IgD and IgE) and they differ in their structure, half-life, site of action and mechanism of action. Humoral immunity is the principal defense mechanism against extracellular microbes and their toxins. B lymphocytes secrete antibodies that act by neutralization, complement activation or by promoting opsonophagocytosis.

Cell-mediated immunity (CMI) is the principal defense mechanism against intracellular microbes. The effectors of CMI, the T-cells are of two types. The helper T-cells secrete proteins called cytokines that stimulate the proliferation and differentiation of T-cells as well as other cells including B lymphocytes, macrophages and natural killer (NK) cells. The cytotoxic T-cells act by lysing infected cells.

VACCINATION VERSUS IMMUNIZATION

Broadly speaking both terms appear to be same and frequently used interchangeably. However, there is minor technical difference. 'Vaccination' is a process of inoculating the vaccine/antigen into the body. The vaccine may or may not seroconvert to vaccine whereas the process of inducing immune response, which can be 'humoral' or 'cell-mediated' in the vaccine is called 'immunization'.

Vaccines can be administered through different routes, e.g. nasal mucosa, gut mucosa or by injection which may be given intradermal, subcutaneous or intramuscular (IM). This process is called 'vaccination' or 'active immunization'. In case immunoglobulins or antisera are administered, it is called 'passive immunization'. Thus, administration of immunoglobulins or antisera is not vaccination, although it provides immunity or protection for a short period.

BIOLOGY OF VACCINES

There are two basic types of vaccines: (1) live attenuated and (2) inactivated. The characteristics of live and inactivated vaccines are different, and these characteristics determine how the vaccine is used.

Live attenuated vaccines are produced by modifying a disease-producing (wild) virus or bacterium in a laboratory. The resulting vaccine organism retains the ability to replicate (grow) and produce immunity, but usually does not cause illness.

Inactivated vaccines can be composed of either whole viruses or bacteria, or fractions of either. Fractional vaccines are either protein-based or PS-based. Protein-based vaccines include toxoids (inactivated bacterial toxin) and subunit or subvirion products. Most PS-based vaccines are composed of pure cell wall PS from bacteria. Conjugate PS vaccines contain PS that is chemically linked to a protein. This linkage makes the PS a more potent vaccine.

Live Attenuated Vaccines

Live vaccines are derived from "wild", or disease-causing, viruses or bacteria. These wild viruses or bacteria are attenuated, or weakened, in a laboratory, usually by repeated culturing. To produce an immune response, live attenuated vaccines must replicate (grow) in the vaccinated person. A relatively small dose of virus or bacteria is administered, which replicates in the body and creates enough of the organism to stimulate an immune response. Anything that either damages the live organism in the vial (e.g. heat, light) or interferes with replication of the organism in the body (circulating antibody) can cause the vaccine to be ineffective.

Although live attenuated vaccines replicate, they usually do not cause disease such as may occur with the "wild" form of the organism. When a live attenuated vaccine does cause "disease", it is usually much milder than the natural disease and is referred to as an adverse reaction.

The immune response to a live attenuated vaccine is virtually identical to that produced by a natural infection. The immune system does not differentiate between an infection with a weakened vaccine virus and an infection with a wild virus. Live attenuated vaccines produce immunity in most recipients with 1 dose, except those administered orally. However, a small percentage of recipients may not respond to the 1st dose of an injected live vaccine [such as mumps, measles, and rubella (MMR) or varicella] and a 2nd dose is recommended to provide a very high level of immunity in the population.

Live attenuated vaccines may cause severe or fatal reactions as a result of uncontrolled replication (growth) of the vaccine virus. This only occurs in persons with immunodeficiency [e.g. from leukemia, treatment with certain drugs or human immunodeficiency virus (HIV) infection].

A live attenuated vaccine virus could theoretically revert to its original pathogenic (disease-causing) form. This is known to happen only with live (oral) polio vaccine.

Active immunity from a live attenuated vaccine may not develop because of interference from circulating antibody to the vaccine virus. Antibody from any source (e.g. transplacental, transfusion) can interfere with replication of the vaccine organism and lead to poor response or no response to the vaccine (also known as vaccine failure). Measles vaccine virus seems to be most sensitive to circulating antibody. Polio and rotavirus vaccine viruses are least affected.

Currently available live attenuated viral vaccines are measles, mumps, rubella, vaccinia, varicella, zoster (which contains the same virus as varicella vaccine but in much higher amount), yellow fever, rotavirus, oral polio vaccine (OPV) and influenza (intranasal). Live attenuated bacterial vaccines are bacille Calmette–Guérin (BCG) and oral typhoid vaccine.

Inactivated Vaccines

Inactivated vaccines are produced by growing the bacterium or virus in culture media, then inactivating it with heat and/or chemicals (usually formalin). In the case of fractional vaccines, the organism is further treated to purify only those components to be included in the vaccine (e.g. the PS capsule of pneumococcus).

Inactivated vaccines are not alive and cannot replicate. The entire dose of antigen is administered in the injection. These vaccines cannot cause disease from infection, even in an immunodeficient person. Inactivated antigens are less affected by circulating antibody than are live agents, so they may be given when antibody is present in the blood (e.g. in infancy or following receipt of antibody-containing blood products).

Inactivated vaccines always require multiple doses. In general, the 1st dose does not produce protective immunity, but "primes" the immune system. A protective immune response develops after the second or 3rd dose. In contrast to live vaccines, in which the immune response closely resembles natural infection, the immune response to an inactivated vaccine is mostly humoral. There are little or no cellular immunity results. Antibody titers against inactivated antigens diminish with time. As a result, some inactivated vaccines may require periodic supplemental doses to increase, or "boost", antibody titers.

Currently available whole-cell inactivated vaccines are limited to inactivated whole viral vaccines (polio, hepatitis A and rabies) and whole inactivated bacterial vaccines (pertussis). Inactivated whole virus influenza vaccine and some whole inactivated bacterial vaccines, like typhoid, cholera and plague, are no longer available. Fractional vaccines include subunits [hepatitis B, influenza, acellular pertussis, human papillomavirus (HPV), anthrax] and toxoids (diphtheria, tetanus).

Polysaccharide Vaccines

Polysaccharide (PS) vaccines are a unique type of inactivated subunit vaccine composed of long chains of sugar molecules that make up the surface capsule of certain bacteria. Pure PS vaccines are available for three diseases: (1) pneumococcal disease, (2) meningococcal disease, and (3) *Salmonella typhi*.

The immune response to a pure PS vaccine is typically T-cell independent, which means that these vaccines are able to stimulate B-cells without the assistance of T-helper cells. T-cell independent antigens, including PS vaccines, are not consistently immunogenic in children younger than 2 years of age. Young children do not respond consistently to PS antigens, probably because of immaturity of the immune system.

Repeated doses of most inactivated protein vaccines cause the antibody titer to go progressively higher or "boost". This does not occur with PS antigens; repeat doses of PS vaccines usually do not cause a booster response. Antibody induced with PS vaccines has less functional activity than that induced by protein antigens. This is because the predominant antibody produced in response to most PS vaccines is IgM, and little IgG is produced.

In the late 1980s, it was discovered that the problems noted above could be overcome through a process called conjugation, in which the PS is chemically combined with a protein molecule. Conjugation changes the immune response from T-cell independent to T-cell dependent, leading to increased immunogenicity in infants and antibody booster response to multiple doses of vaccine.

The first conjugated PS vaccine was for Hib A conjugate vaccine for pneumococcal disease was licensed in 2000. A meningococcal conjugate vaccine was licensed in 2005.

Recombinant Vaccines

Vaccine antigens may also be produced by genetic engineering technology. These products are sometimes referred to as recombinant vaccines. Four genetically engineered vaccines are currently available. Hepatitis B and HPV vaccines are produced by insertion of a segment of the respective viral gene into the gene of a yeast cell. The modified yeast cell produces pure hepatitis B surface antigen or HPV capsid protein when it grows. Live typhoid vaccine (Ty21a) is *S. typhi* bacteria that have been genetically modified to not cause illness. Live attenuated influenza vaccine (LAIV) has been engineered to replicate effectively in the mucosa of the nasopharynx but not in the lungs.

Adjuvants

Adjuvants are agents which increase the stimulation of the immune system by enhancing antigen presentation (depot formulation, delivery systems) and/or by providing costimulation signals (immunomodulators). Aluminum salts are most often used in today's vaccines. Hence, the adjuvants improve the immunogenicity of vaccines. Many new generations of adjuvants are in fact analoges of toll-like receptors (TLRs), for example CpG-ODN used in new generation of Japanese encephalitis vaccines.

Most non-live vaccines require their formulation with specific adjuvants to induce danger signals and trigger a sufficient activation of the innate system. These adjuvants may be divided into two categories: (1) delivery systems that prolong the antigen deposit at site of injection, recruiting more dendritic cells (DCs) into the reaction and (2) immune modulators that provide additional differentiation and activation signals to monocytes and DCs. Although progress is being made, none of the adjuvants currently in use trigger the degree of innate immune activation that is elicited by live vaccines, whose immune potency far exceed that of nonlive vaccines.

IMMUNOLOGY OF VACCINES

Innate and Adaptive Immunity

Innate immunity comprises of the skin and mucosal barriers, phagocytes (neutrophils, monocytes and macrophages) and the NK cells. It comes into play immediately on entry of the pathogen and is nonspecific. Adaptive immunity is provided by the B lymphocytes (humoral/antibody-mediated immunity) and T lymphocytes (cellular/CMI).

The innate immune system triggers the development of adaptive immunity by presenting antigens to the B lymphocytes and T lymphocytes. Adaptive immunity takes time to evolve and is pathogen specific (Table 9.1.1 and Fig. 9.1.1).

B-cells and T-cells

Immune system almost does not exist at birth; maternal antibodies transferred transplacentally provide some protection during early childhood. After birth, baby comes in contact with microbes which gradually activate immune system. B-cells form the most important component of immune system in the body. These are produced in liver in fetal life and mature in bone marrow in humans. In other species these cells mature in an organ called "bursa of Fabricius", thus these lymphocytes are called B-cells. On activation by an antigen contained in microorganisms and vaccines, the B-cells proliferate and get converted to plasma cells, which in turn produce antibodies. For effective production of antibodies, B-cells need help from T helper cells.

T lymphocytes are the cells that originate in the thymus, mature in the periphery, become activated in the spleen/ nodes if: (1) their T-cell receptor bind to an antigen presented by a major histocompatibility complex (MHC) molecule and (2) they receive additional costimulation signals driving them to acquire killing (mainly CD8+ T-cells) or supporting (mainly CD4+ T-cells) functions.

B-cells have Ig surface receptor, which binds with the appropriate antigen present on the infective pathogen. The processed antigen stimulates the B-cell to mature into antibody secreting plasma cell and generate IgM. T helper

Table 9.1.1: Comparison of innate and adaptive immunity.

Nonspecific immunity (innate)	*Specific immunity (adaptive)*
Its response is antigen-independent	Its response is antigen-dependent
There is immediate response	There is a lag time between exposure and maximal response
It is not antigen-specific	It is antigen-specific
Exposure does not result in induction of memory cells	Exposure results in induction of memory cells
Some of its cellular components or their products may aid specific immunity	Some of its products may aid non-specific immunity

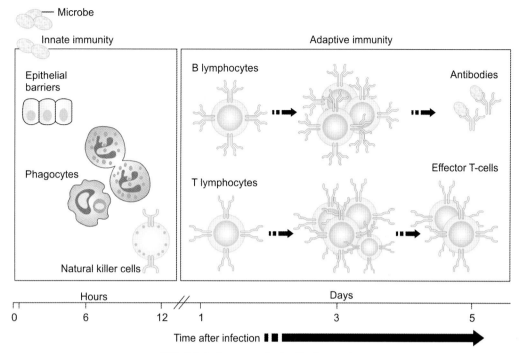

FIG. 9.1.1: Innate and adaptive immunity.

2 (Th2) cell leads to switch in the production from IgM to IgG, IgA or IgD. The B-cells can directly respond to the antigen and process the antigen, but the T-cells do not react with the antigen directly unless processed and presented by special cells called antigen presenting cells (APCs).

Antigen Presenting Cells and Dendritic Cells

Antigen presenting cells are the cells that capture antigens, process them into small peptides, display them at their surface through MHC molecules and provide costimulation signals that act synergistically to activate antigen-specific T-cells. APCs include B-cells, macrophages and DCs, although only DCs are capable of activating naïve T-cells (Fig. 9.1.2).

Dendritic cells are major APC in the body in addition to the B-cells and the macrophages. The major role of these cells is to identify dangers, which is done by the special receptors on the APC named TLRs. Vaccine antigens are taken up by immature DCs activated by the local inflammation, which provides the signals required for their migration to draining lymph nodes. During this migration, DCs mature and their surface expression of molecules changes. DCs sense "danger signals" through their TLRs and respond by a modulation of their surface or secreted molecules. Simultaneously, antigens are processed into small fragments and displayed at the cell surface in the grooves of MHC (HLA in humans) molecules. As a rule, MHC class I molecules present peptides from antigens that are produced within infected cells, whereas phagocytosed antigens are displayed on MHC class II

molecules. Thus, mature DCs reaching the T-cell zone of lymph nodes display MHC-peptide complexes and high levels of costimulation molecules at their surface. CD4+ T-cells recognize antigenic peptides displayed by class II MHC molecules, whereas CD8+ T-cells bind to class I MHC peptide complexes.

Antigen-specific T-cell receptors may only bind to specific MHC molecules (e.g. HLA A2), which differ among individuals and populations. Consequently, T-cell responses are highly variable within a population.

Immune Responses Elicited by Live Attenuated and Nonlive Vaccines

Live viral vaccines do efficiently trigger the activation of the innate immune system, presumably through pathogen-associated signals (such as viral RNA) allowing their recognition by pattern recognition receptors (PRR)-TLRs. Following injection, viral particles rapidly disseminate throughout the vascular network and reach their target tissues. This pattern is very similar to that occurring after a natural infection, including the initial mucosal replication stage for vaccines administered through the nasal/oral routes. Following the administration of a live viral vaccine and its dissemination, DCs are activated at multiple sites, migrate toward the corresponding draining lymph nodes and launch multiple foci of T-cell and B-cell activation. This provides a first explanation to the generally higher immunogenicity of live versus nonlive vaccines.

The strongest antibody responses are generally elicited by live vaccines that better activate innate reactions and thus better support the induction of adaptive immune

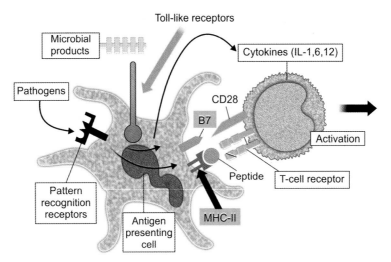

FIG. 9.1.2: Schematic presentations of a dendritic cell and its activation by pathogens.
Source: Siegrist CA. Vaccine immunology. In: Plotkin SA, Orenstein W, Offit P (Eds). Vaccines, 5th edition. Saunders Elsevier; 2008.pp.17-36.

effectors. Nonlive vaccines frequently require formulation in adjuvants of which aluminum salts are particularly potent enhancers of antibody responses, and thus included in a majority of currently available vaccines. This is likely to reflect their formation of a deposit from which antigen is slowly deabsorbed and released, extending the duration of B-cell and T-cell activation, as well as the preferential induction of IL-4 by aluminum-exposed macrophages.

Very few non-live vaccines induce high and sustained antibody responses after a single vaccine dose, even in healthy young adults. Primary immunization schedules therefore, usually include at least two vaccine doses, optimally repeated at a minimal interval of 3–4 weeks to generate successive waves of B-cell and germinal center (GC) responses. These priming doses may occasionally be combined into a single "double" dose, such as for hepatitis A or B immunization. In any case, however, vaccine antibodies elicited by primary immunization with non-live vaccines eventually wane (Table 9.1.2).

Germinal Centers and Marginal Zone

Germinal centers (GCs) are dynamic structures that develop in spleen/nodes in response to an antigenic stimulation and dissolves after a few weeks. GCs contain a monoclonal population of antigen-specific B-cells that proliferate and differentiate through the support provided by follicular DCs and helper T-cells. Ig class switch recombination, affinity maturation, B-cell selection and differentiation into plasma cells or memory B-cells essentially occur in GCs.

Marginal zone is the area between the red pulp and the white pulp of the spleen. Its major role is to trap particulate antigens from the circulation and present it to lymphocytes.

An "epitope", also known as antigenic determinant, is the part of an antigen that is recognized by the immune system, specifically by antibodies, B-cells or T-cells. The part of an antibody that recognizes the epitope is called a "paratope".

The antibody "affinity" refers to the tendency of an antibody to bind to a specific epitope at the surface of an antigen, i.e. to the strength of the interaction. The "avidity" is the sum of the epitope-specific affinities for a given antigen. It directly relates its function.

Toll-like Receptors and their Role in Vaccine Immunogenicity

Toll-like receptors are a class of proteins that play a key role in the innate immune system. They are single membrane-spanning noncatalytic receptors that recognize structurally conserved molecules derived from microbes. Once these microbes have breached physical barriers, such as the skin or intestinal tract mucosa, they are recognized by TLRs which activates immune cell responses. TLRs are a family of ten receptors (TLR1 to TLR10) that present at the surface of many immune cells, which recognize pathogens through conserved microbial patterns and activate innate immunity when detecting danger. TLRs are a type of PRR and recognize molecules that are broadly shared by pathogens but distinguishable from host molecules, collectively referred to as pathogen-associated molecular patterns (PAMPs). TLRs together with the interleukin-1 receptors form a receptor super-family, which are known as the "interleukin-1 receptor/toll-like receptor super-family"; all members of this family have in common a so-called TIR (Toll-IL-1 receptor) domain. The TLRs appear to be one of the most ancient, conserved components of the immune system.

T-cell Dependent and T-cell Independent Immune Responses

Certain antigens, primarily proteins, induce both B-cell and T-cell stimulation leading to what is called T-cell-dependent immune response. Infants of 6 weeks of age

Table 9.1.2: Correlates of vaccine-induced immunity.

Vaccines	Vaccine type	Serum IgG	Mucosal IgG	Mucosal IgA
Extended Program on Immunization Vaccines				
Diphtheria toxoid	Toxoid	++	(+)	
Pertussis, whole cell	Killed	++		
Pertussis, acellular	Protein	++		
Tetanus toxoid	Toxoid	++		
Measles	Live attenuated	++		
Polio Sabin	Live attenuated	++	++	++
Polio salk	Killed	++	+	
Tuberculosis (BCG)	Live mycob			
Nonextended Program on Immunization Vaccines				
Hepatitis A	Killed	++	(+)	
Hepatitis B (HbsAg)	Protein	++		
Hib polysaccharide (PS)	PS	++	(+)	
Hib glycoconjugates	PS-protein	++	++	
Influenza	Killed, subunit	++	(+)	
Influenza intranasal	Live attenuated	++	+	+
Meningococcal PS	PS	++	(+)	
Meningococcal conjugate	PS-protein	++	++	
Mumps	Live attenuated	++		
Pneumococcal PS	PS	++	(+)	
Pneumococcal conjugate	PS-protein	++	++	
Rabies	Killed	++		
Rotavirus	VLPS	(+)	(+)	++
Rubella	Live attenuated	++		
Typhoid PS	PS	+	(+)	
Varicella	Live attenuated	++		
Yellow fever	Live attenuated	++		

onward are capable of T-cell dependent response. This type of response usually results in higher titers of IgG type and long lasting. It also shows booster effects with repeated exposures.

On the other hand T-cell independent response being only B-cell mediated is not possible below 2 years of age. It is predominantly IgM type with low titers. The response is short lasting, repeated doses of vaccine does not lead to boosting effect. IgA is not produced and hence there is no local mucosal protection with this type of antigens, while in case of T-cell dependent response IgA antibodies are also produced which helps in providing mucosal protection and eradication of the carrier state. Few examples of T-cell independent vaccines include bacterial PS vaccines such as *Streptococcus pneumoniae*, *Neisseria meningitidis*, *Haemophilus influenzae* and *S. typhi*.

T-cell-independent response being B-cell mediated younger children do not respond to such vaccines. A T-cell independent antigen like PS can be made into T-cell dependent by the technique of conjugation.

Such conjugated vaccines can also be administered to children less than 2 years of age. This technique is used to produce conjugated Vi typhoid, Hib, pneumococcal and meningococcal vaccines.

THE MAIN EFFECTORS OF VACCINE RESPONSES

The nature of the vaccine exerts a direct influence on the type of immune effectors that are predominantly elicited and mediate protective efficacy (Table 9.1.3). Capsular PS elicit B-cell responses in what is classically reported as a T-independent manner, although increasing evidence supports a role for CD4+ T-cells in such responses. The conjugation of bacterial PS to a protein carrier (e.g. glycoconjugate vaccines) provides foreign peptide antigens that are presented to the immune system and thus recruits antigen-specific CD4+ Th cells in what is referred to as T-dependent antibody responses. A hallmark of T-dependent responses, which are also elicited by toxoid,

Table 9.1.3: Comparison of immune responses between live and nonlive vaccines.

Nonlive vaccines	Live vaccines
Phagocytes (monocytes, macrophages and dendritic cells) take up vaccine Ag in local tissues	Dendritic cells take up vaccine Ag in multiple tissues
Transport Ag primarily to local draining lymph node, no replication	Generalized dissemination, replication
Transport Ag to spleen and lymph nodes in many regions	Site and route of administration is unimportant
Poor activation of innate immune responses	Efficiently trigger the activation of the innate immune system and better support the induction of adaptive immune effectors
Repeated boosters are needed to maintain adequate antibody level	Immunity is robust and lifelong or at least for several decades
Frequently require formulation in adjuvants to elicit potent immune response and also to extend the duration of B-cell and T-cell activation	Adjuvants are not needed
Primary vaccination include usually at least two doses for induction	Usually a single dose is sufficient
No toll-like receptors (TLR) recognition; hence no T cell activation, no memory cell formation and no class switch	Permits TLR recognition, T-cell activation, memory cell formation and high affinity antibody formation after class switch

protein, inactivated or live attenuated viral vaccines is to induce both higher-affinity antibodies and immune memory. In addition, live attenuated vaccines usually generate CD8+ cytotoxic T-cells. The use of live vaccines/vectors or of specific novel delivery systems (e.g. DNA vaccines) appears necessary for the induction of strong CD8+ T-cell responses.

Most current vaccines mediate their protective efficacy through the induction of vaccine antibodies, whereas BCG-induced T-cells produce cytokines that contribute to macrophage activation and control of *Mycobacterium tuberculosis*. The induction of antigen-specific immune effectors (and/or of immune memory cells) by an immunization process does imply that these antibodies, cells or cytokines represent surrogates or even correlates of vaccine efficacy. This requires the formal demonstration that vaccine-mediated protection is dependent in a vaccinated individual upon the presence of a given marker such as an antibody titer or a number of antigen-specific cells above a given threshold. Antigen-specific antibodies have been formally demonstrated as conferring vaccine-induced protection against many diseases.

The neutralization of pathogens at mucosal surfaces is mainly achieved by the transudation of vaccine-induced serum IgG antibodies. It requires serum IgG antibody concentrations to be of sufficient affinity and abundance to

result into "protective" antibody titers in saliva or mucosal secretions. As a rule, such responses are not elicited by PS bacterial vaccines but achieved by glycoconjugate vaccines, which therefore prevent nasopharyngeal colonization in addition to invasive diseases.

Under most circumstances, immunization does not elicit sufficiently high and sustained antibody titers on mucosal surfaces to prevent local infection. It is only after having infected mucosal surfaces that pathogens encounter vaccine-induced IgG serum antibodies that neutralize viruses, opsonize bacteria, activate the complement cascade and limit their multiplication and spread, preventing tissue damage and thus clinical disease. That vaccines fail to induce sterilizing immunity is thus not an obstacle to successful disease control, although it represents a significant challenge for the development of specific vaccines such as against HIV-1. Current vaccines mostly mediate protection through the induction of highly specific IgG serum antibodies. Under certain circumstances, however, passive antibody-mediated immunity is inefficient (tuberculosis).

Prevention of infection may only be achieved by vaccine-induced antibodies, whereas disease attenuation and protection against complications may be supported by T-cells even in the absence of specific antibodies. The understanding of vaccine immunology thus requires appraising how B-cell and T-cell responses are elicited, supported, maintained and/or reactivated by vaccine antigens.

IMMUNE RESPONSES AT CELLULAR LEVEL

The First Steps after Immunization

Following injection, the vaccine antigens attract local and systemic DCs, monocytes and neutrophils. These activated cells change their surface receptors and migrate along lymphatic vessels, to the draining lymph nodes where the activation of T and B lymphocytes takes place. In case of killed vaccines there is only local and unilateral lymph node activation. Conversely for live vaccines there is multifocal lymph node vaccination due to microbial replication and dissemination. Consequently, the immunogenicity of killed vaccines is lower than the live vaccines; killed vaccines require adjuvants which improve the immune response by producing local inflammation and recruiting DCs/monocytes to the injection site. Secondly, the site of administration of killed vaccines is of importance; the IM route which is well-vascularized and has a large number of patrolling DCs is preferred over the subcutaneous route. The site of administration is usually of little significance for live vaccines. Finally, due to focal lymph node activation, multiple killed vaccines may be administered at different sites with little immunologic interference. Immunologic interference may occur with multiple live vaccines unless they are given on the same day at different sites or at least 4 weeks apart.

Immune Responses of T-cell Independent Antigens at the Cellular Level

On being released from the injection site these antigens are usually nonprotein, PSs in nature, reach the marginal zone of the spleen/nodes and bind to the specific Ig surface receptors of B-cells. In the absence of antigen-specific T-cell help, B-cells are activated, proliferate and differentiate in plasma cells without undergoing affinity maturation in GC.

The antibody response sets in 2–4 weeks following immunization, is predominantly IgM with low titers of low affinity IgG. The half-life of the plasma cells is short and antibody titers decline rapidly. Additionally, the PS antigens are unable to evoke an immune response in those aged less than 2 years due to immaturity of the marginal zones. As PS antigens do not induce GCs, bona fide memory B-cells are not elicited. Consequently, subsequent re-exposure to the same PS results in a repeat primary response that follows the same kinetics in previously vaccinated as in naïve individuals. Revaccination with certain bacterial PS of which group C meningococcus is a prototype—may even induce lower antibody responses than the first immunization, a phenomenon referred to as hyporesponsiveness whose molecular and cellular bases are not yet fully understood.

Immune Responses of T-cell Dependent Antigens at the Cellular Level

T-cell dependent antigens include protein antigens which may consist of either pure proteins (hepatitis B, hepatitis A, HPV, toxoids) or conjugated protein carrier with PS antigens (Hib, meningo, pneumo). The initial response to these antigens is similar to PS antigens. However, the antigen-specific helper T-cells that have been activated by antigen-bearing DCs trigger some antigen-specific B-cells to migrate toward follicular dendritic cells (FDCs), initiating the GC reaction. In GCs, B-cells receive additional signals from follicular T-cells and undergo massive clonal proliferation, switch from IgM toward IgG/IgA, undergo affinity maturation and differentiate into plasma cells secreting large amounts of antigen-specific antibodies.

Most of the plasma cells die at the end of GC reaction and thus decline in antibody levels is noted 4–8 weeks after vaccination. However, a few plasma cells exit nodes/spleen and migrate to survival niches mostly located in the bone marrow, where they survive through signals provided by supporting stromal cells and these results in prolonged persistence of antibodies in the serum.

Hence, following possible immune reactions can occur at cellular level following immunization with a T-cell dependent antigen:

- *Extrafollicular reaction:* Similar to PS antigen in the marginal zones of spleen/lymph nodes
- *GC reactions:*
  - Clonal proliferation of B-cells followed by affinity maturation and differentiate into plasma cells secreting large amounts of antigen-specific high affinity antibodies
  - Formation of long-lasting plasma cells in the bone marrow
  - Generation of memory B-cells in response to T dependent antigens.

Memory B-cell Response

Memory B-cells are those B lymphocytes that generate in response to T dependent antigens, during the GC reaction, in parallel to plasma cells. They persist there as resting cells until re-exposed to their specific antigens, when they readily proliferate and differentiate into plasma cells secreting large amounts of high-affinity antibodies that may be detected in the serum within a few days after boosting. These cells also undergo affinity maturation in GC.

These cells are only generated during T-dependent responses inducing GC responses. These cells are resting cells that do not produce antibodies. Memory B-cells undergo affinity maturation during several (4–6) months. A minimal interval of 4–6 months is required for optimal affinity maturation of memory B-cells. Memory B-cells rapidly (days) differentiate into antibody-secreting plasma cells upon re-exposure to antigen. Memory B-cells differentiate into PCs that produce high(er) affinity antibodies than primary plasma cells. As plasma cells and memory responses are generated in parallel in GCs, higher post-primary Ab titers reflect stronger GC reactions and generally predict higher secondary responses. During induction, a lower antigen dose at priming results in inducing B-cells differentiation away from PCs, toward memory B-cells. Box 9.1.1 summarizes the implications of immune memory on immunization programs.

Immune Response to Live Vaccines

The live vaccines induce an immune response similar to that seen with protein vaccines. However, the take of live vaccines is not 100% with the 1st dose. Hence, more than one dose is recommended with most live vaccines. Once the vaccine has been taken up, immunity is robust and lifelong or at least for several decades. This is because of continuous replication of the organism that is a constant

---

Box 9.1.1

Impact of immune memory on immunization programs.

Immune memory—implications for immunization programs:

- Immunization schedule should never be started "all over again" regardless of duration of interruption
- Regular boosters are not required to maintain immune memory during low risk periods (travelers)
- Certain immunization schedules may not need boosters if exposure provides regular natural boosters
- Booster may not be needed where reactivation of immune memory by offending pathogen is sufficiently rapid and effective to interrupt microbial invasion (Hep B)

source of the antigen. The 2nd dose of the vaccine is therefore mostly for primary vaccine failures (no uptake of vaccine) and not for secondary vaccine failures (decline in antibodies over time).

Determinants of Intensity and Duration of Immune Responses

The nature of antigen is the primary determinant; broadly speaking live vaccines are superior (exception: BCG and OPV) to protein antigens which in turn are superior to PS vaccines. Adjuvants improve immune responses to inactivated vaccines. Immune response is usually better with higher antigen dose (e.g. hepatitis B). The immune response improves with increasing number of doses and increased spacing between doses.

The long-lasting plasma cells in bone marrow and reactivation of memory B-cells provide longer duration of protection against invading microorganism in an immunized individual.

Technically, 0, 1 and 6 months is the best immunization schedule. The first 2 doses are for induction and the long gap between the 2nd and 3rd dose allows for affinity maturation of B-cells and clonal selection of the fittest B-cells for booster and memory response. Extremes of age and disease conditions lower immune response.

Primary and Secondary Immune Responses

When an antigen is introduced for the first time, the immune system responds primarily after a lag phase of up to 10 days. This is called the "primary response". Subsequently, upon reintroduction of the same antigen, there is no lag phase and the immune system responds by producing antibodies immediately and this is called the "secondary response". However, there are some differences in both these responses: primary response is short-lived, has a lag phase, predominantly IgM type, and antibodies titers are low, whereas secondary response is almost immediate without a lag phase, titers persist for a long time, predominantly of IgG type, and antibodies titers are very high. Figure 9.1.3 describes the background developments at the cellular level and interactions of B-cells, memory B-cells and T-cells at the follicular level in a lymph node. The secondary response is mainly due to booster response and is seen with vaccines that work on a "prime-boost" mechanism inducing T-cells such as conjugate vaccines. On the other hand, non-conjugate, PS vaccines mainly induces primary response and the repeat dose produces another wave of primary response and not acts as a booster since they do not induce T-cells.

Limitations of Young Age Immunization

Young age limits antibody responses to most vaccine antigens since maternal antibodies inhibit antibodies responses but not T-cell response, and due to limitation of B-cell responses.

Immunoglobulin G antibodies are actively transferred through the placenta, via the FcRn receptor, from the maternal to the fetal circulation. Upon immunization, maternal antibodies bind to their specific epitopes at the

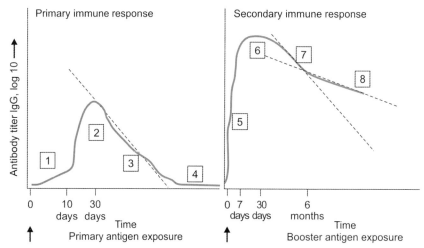

FIG. 9.1.3: correlation of antibody titers to various phases of the vaccine response. The initial antigen exposure elicits an extrafollicular response (1) that results in the rapid appearance of low IgG antibody titers. As B-cells proliferate in germinal centers and differentiate into plasma cells, IgG antibody titers increase up to a peak value (2) usually reached 4 weeks after immunization. The short life span of these plasma cells results in a rapid decline of antibody titers (3), which eventually return to baseline levels (4). In secondary immune responses, booster exposure to antigen reactivates immune memory and results in a rapid (< 7 days) increase (5) of IgG antibody titer. Short-lived plasma cells maintain peak Ab levels (6) during a few weeks after which serum antibody titers decline initially with the same rapid kinetics as following primary immunization. Long-lived plasma cells that have reached survival niches in the bone marrow continue to produce antigen-specific antibodies, which (7) then decline with slower kinetics (8).

Note: This generic pattern may not apply to live vaccines triggering long-term IgG antibodies for extended periods of time.

Source: With permission from Siegrist CA. Vaccine immunology. In: Plotkin SA, Orenstein W, Offit P (Eds). Vaccines, 5th edition. Saunders Elsevier. 2008. pp.17-36.

antigen surface, competing with infant B-cells and thus limiting B-cell activation, proliferation and differentiation. The inhibitory influence of maternal antibodies on infant B-cell responses affects all vaccine types, although its influence is more marked for live attenuated viral vaccines that may be neutralized by even minute amounts of passive antibodies. Hence, antibody responses elicited in early life are short lasting. However, even during early life, induction of B memory cells is not limited.

Early life immune responses are characterized by age-dependent limitations of the magnitude of responses to all vaccines. Antibody responses to most PS antigens are not elicited during the first 2 years of life, which is likely to reflect numerous factors including: the slow maturation of the spleen marginal zone; limited expression of CD21 on B-cells and limited availability of the complement factors. Although this may be circumvented in part by the use of glycolconjugate vaccines, even the most potent glycoconjugate vaccines elicit markedly lower primary IgG responses in young infants.

Although maternal antibodies interfere with the induction of infant antibody responses, they may allow a certain degree of priming, i.e. of induction of memory B-cells. This likely reflects the fact that limited amounts of unmasked vaccine antigens may be sufficient for priming of memory B-cells but not for full-blown GC activation, although direct evidence is lacking.

Importantly, however, antibodies of maternal origin do not exert their inhibitory influence on infant T-cell responses, which remain largely unaffected or even enhanced.

The extent and duration of the inhibitory influence of maternal antibodies increase with gestational age, e.g. with the amount of transferred Igs and declines with postnatal age, as maternal antibodies wane.

9.1.2. ELEMENTARY EPIDEMIOLOGY

DEFINITION, SCOPE AND USES OF EPIDEMIOLOGY

Definition

The word "epidemiology" is derived from the Greek words: epi "upon", demos "people" and logos "study". The study (observation, measurement, analysis, correlation and interpretation) of distribution [how many? in whom? (age group) where? when? season and determinants (why there, why then?)] of diseases (etiology and risk factors) is termed as epidemiology. Epidemiology is the study of the distribution and determinants of disease frequency in man. It is foundation science of public health. It provides insights for applying intervention. It informs if intervention is succeeding. It is the systematic study of the pathogen amplification and transmission systems. Epidemiologies can often pin-point the weak links in the chains of the

source and transmission pathways of the pathogen so that interventions can be directed at those points. Vaccination is one such intervention.

Scope

A focus of an epidemiological study is the population defined in geographical or other terms; for example, a specific group of hospital patients or factory workers could be the unit of study. A common population used in epidemiology is one selected from a specific area or country at a specific time. This forms the base for defining subgroups with respect to sex, age group or ethnicity. The structures of populations vary between geographical areas and time periods. Epidemiological analyses must take such variation into account.

From vaccinology perspective, there are three reasons to learn epidemiology: (1) for the rational choice of vaccines for vaccination programs, (2) to design appropriate intervention program including vaccinations, and (3) to monitor and measure the progress and impact of any vaccination program. Knowledge of epidemiology helps in choosing the appropriate vaccines for inclusion in public health programs after carefully assessing disease burden and economic factors. It also helps in designing disease specific control, elimination or eradication strategies after acquiring exact epidemiological data on prevalence, incidence and transmission characteristics of target pathogens, and their transmission pathways. In the last, it also helps in monitoring intervention success or failure in order to improve performance or efficiency of the vaccination programs.

Population at Risk

An important factor in calculating measures of disease frequency is the correct estimate of the numbers of people under study. Ideally these numbers should only include people who are potentially susceptible to the diseases being studied. For instance, men should not be included when calculating the frequency of cervical cancer (Fig. 9.1.4).

The people who are susceptible to a given disease are called the population at risk, and can be defined by demographic, geographic or environmental factors.

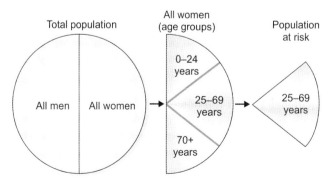

FIG. 9.1.4: Population at risk in a study of carcinoma of the cervix.

For instance, occupational injuries occur only among working people, so the population at risk is the workforce; in some countries brucellosis occurs only among people handling infected animals, so the population at risk consists of those working on farms and in slaughterhouses.

Basic Measures of Disease Frequency—the "Incidence" and "Prevalence"

Basic measures of disease frequency are done by incidence and prevalence. "Incidence" relates to the number of new cases of the disease which occur during a particular period of time (e.g. new TB cases). "Prevalence" relates to total number of cases of a disease in a specified period of time usually during a survey. Often it is expressed as rate which is misnomer and it is actually proportion. In the long run, incidence should be more than the deaths and recoveries for prevalence to accumulate; prevalence of various diseases is a good indicator of the load on health services. Table 9.1.4 displays differences between incidence and prevalence.

Disease Estimation

Where measuring of exact incidence and/or prevalence of a disease is not practical, estimates are developed to have a rough idea about the burden of that particular disease in the community at a given geographic region. Hence, where incidence or prevalence is not "measured" estimation is better than nothing. Estimates are for comparative purpose: intercountry and interdisease.

Comparison is for choice also for example, intervention versus none or vaccination versus other. An estimate is by definition inaccurate, but may be valid or invalid; reliable or unreliable. It is usually expressed in round figures, e.g. 200,000 rabies; 2 million malaria; 3 million HIV infected; 40 million hepatitis B carriers, etc. No estimate is accurate for the actual burden, therefore, arguments against hepatitis B vaccination program for the reason the estimate is inaccurate is an obvious misjudgment. For global leadership in specific diseases gross estimates are used. This is such an example for TB (Fig. 9.1.5).

Population Attributable Risk

The population attributable risk (PAR) is the incidence of a disease in a population that is associated with (or attributed to) an exposure to a risk factor. This measure is useful for determining the relative importance of exposures for the entire population. It is the proportion by which the incidence rate of the outcome in the entire population would be reduced if exposure were eliminated.

Population attributable risk can be estimated by the following formula:

$$PAR = \frac{Ip - Iu}{Ip}$$

Table 9.1.4: Differences between incidence and prevalence.

	Incidence	Prevalence
Numerator	Number of new cases of disease during a specified period of time	Number of existing cases of disease at a given point of time
Denominator	Population at risk	Population at risk
Focus	Whether the event is a new case, time of onset of the disease	Presence or absence of a disease, time period is arbitrary; rather a "snapshot" in time
Uses	Expresses the risk of becoming ill	Estimates the probability of the population being ill at the period of time being studied
	The main measure of acute diseases or conditions, but also used for chronic diseases, more useful for studies of causation	Useful in the study of the burden of chronic diseases and implication for health services

Note: If incident cases are not resolved but continue over time, then they become existing (prevalent) cases. In this sense, prevalence = incidence × duration.

Where,

'Ip' is the incidence of the disease in the total population. Iueu is the incidence of the disease among the unexposed group.

Endemic, Epidemic and Pandemic Patterns of Diseases

"Endemic" refers to normal occurrence of disease in defined population, e.g. cholera, malaria, TB, etc. "Epidemics or outbreaks" is the occurrence of more cases of disease than expected in a given area or among a specific group of people over a particular period of time, e.g. measles, influenza, meningococcal disease. Epidemic or outbreaks: spreading rapidly and extensively by infection and affecting many individuals in an area or a population at the same time. "Pandemic" is global epidemic. Disease originates in one country and then spreads to a number of countries, e.g. AIDS, H1N1, etc.

The difference between epidemic and outbreak is arbitrary. The terms "epidemics" and "outbreaks" are often used similarly; however, latter usually indicates less intensity, e.g. outbreak of salmonella in a neonatal unit. A community-based outbreak meningococcal disease is defined as the occurrence of more than three cases in less than 3 months in the same area who are not close contacts of each other with a primary disease attack rate of more than 10 primary cases/100,000 persons. In terms of the flu, the difference between epidemic and outbreak, and is the percentage of overall deaths caused by the disease. Every week, if the number of flu caused deaths exceeds 7.7% of the total, then the USA officially has an epidemic on its hands (CDC).

Estimated TB incidence rates, 2016

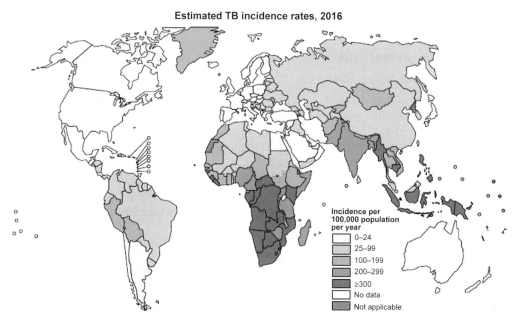

Incidence per
100,000 population
per year
- 0–24
- 25–99
- 100–199
- 200–299
- ≥300
- No data
- Not applicable

FIG. 9.1.5: Estimated TB incidence, 2016.
Source: WHO Global TB Report, 2017.

Vaccine Immunogenicity, Vaccine Efficacy and Vaccine Effectiveness

"Vaccine immunogenicity" is the ability of a vaccine to induce antibodies which may or may not be protective. These antibodies may be of no use in offering protection against the desired disease. The protective threshold for most vaccines is defined. However, there is often controversy about the cut-offs (pneumococcus/Hib). Levels below the limits may be protective due to other reasons such as immune memory/T-cell immunity. "Vaccine efficacy" is the ability of the vaccine to protect an individual. It can be assessed through clinical trials, cohort studies or case control studies. It is calculated as:

$$\text{Vaccine efficacy (VE)} = \frac{\substack{\text{Disease in unvaccinated} - \\ \text{Disease in vaccinated}}}{\text{Disease in unvaccinated}}$$

Vaccine effectiveness is the ability of the vaccine to protect the community and is a sum of the vaccine efficacy and herd effect. It is revealed after a vaccine is introduced in a program. Vaccine effectiveness is a combination of vaccine efficacy, coverage and herd effect. Hence, vaccine efficacy is the protection at the individual level while effectiveness is at the community level. Higher the force of transmission, younger the age at risk greater the need for vaccine effectiveness to reduce R = 1 to R < 1.

Cost Effectiveness of a Vaccine or Vaccination Program

Cost effectiveness is a method of economic evaluation which is carried out by mathematical modelling usually prior to introduction of a vaccine in a national program. It is expressed as cost per infections or deaths or hospitalizations prevented per life years gained.

Force of Transmission, Reproductive Rate and Basic Reproductive Number

The key determinant of incidence and prevalence of infection is depending on force of transmission which is determined by reproductive rate. Reproductive rate is a simple concept in disease epidemiology. Incidence and prevalence of infection depends on reproductive rate. Ro measures the average number of secondary cases generated by one primary case in a susceptible population. Suppose all others were susceptible then how many will be infected? That is basic reproductive number, Ro. Since population is a mix of susceptible and immune persons, one case must attempt to infect more than one person. In the long term, pathogen can survive only if one case reproduces another case (effective reproductive rate, R = 1). If R is less than 1 the disease is declining (e.g. herd effect). If R is more than 1 an outbreak is occurring. For endemic diseases with periodic fluctuations, R may swing from less than 1 to more than 1 but in the long-term the average may remain one. Pathogen can survive if it reproduces. For all endemic infectious diseases (IDs), R = 1 for steady state or for long-term endemicity. The community benefit of a vaccination program is to reduce R to less than 1 and sustain it for long periods. Such beneficial effect, measured as the degree of disease reduction due to a vaccination program is sometimes called vaccine effectiveness to distinguish it from vaccine efficacy which refers to only the direct benefit of immunity in vaccinated individuals. Ro is not a static entity and changes according at different time period even at a same geographic region.

Impact of Vaccination on Natural Epidemiology of an Infectious Disease

Vaccination perturbs epidemiology by removing the vaccinated individual from susceptible pool; so, one less disease case, and by removing individuals from chain of transmission. So, lower incidence or prevalence of the disease. In other words, vaccination program interferes with natural epidemiology of the target disease.

Epidemiologic shift refers to an upward shift in age of infection or disease in communities with partial immunization coverage. Owing to vaccination the natural circulation of the pathogen decreases and the age of acquisition of infection advances. This is especially important for diseases like rubella, varicella and hepatitis A wherein severity of disease worsens with advancing age.

Herd Immunity, Herd Effect and Herd Protection

The term herd immunity has been in use since 1920s, i.e. for about 90 years. In fact, it denotes resistance of a population to the spread of vaccine preventable diseases where causative organisms spread from human-to-human. Because immune individuals act as barrier in spread of infection and lessen the chances of an individual with the disease to come in contact of vulnerable person. Instead of the terms "herd immunity" or "herd effect" contact immunity and herd protection are being used now. Herd immunity is the proportion immune in a herd. This can be deduced from the vaccination coverage. Herd effect is the protection offered to unvaccinated members when good proportion (usually >85%) of the herd is vaccinated. Herd effect is due to reduced carriage of the causative microorganism by the vaccinated cohort and thus is seen only with vaccines against those diseases where humans are the only source (there is no herd effect for tetanus). An effective vaccine is a prerequisite for good herd effect; OPV in India, BCG and unconjugated PS vaccines have no herd effect.

Immunized people provide protection to the unimmunized individuals without inducing immunity, virtually by breaking the transmission of the infection or lessening the chances of susceptible individuals coming in contact with infective individual. In clinical practice, contact immunity does not play significant role, while herd protection plays a major role, although to a limited extent, because unimmunized individuals do not develop immunity, but enjoy the protection because of break in spread of infection. Thus, the herd protection is the major beneficial component of immunization for unimmunized population for the infections which spread from person-to-person. It should be remembered that these unimmunized individuals enjoy protection till they are among immunized and resistant people. As they have not developed immunity, may develop disease if come in direct contact with infected person, in case they shift to the milieu where there is outbreak of the disease.

Phases in Vaccine Development

Phase 1 trials are conducted on small number of healthy human volunteers for assessing vaccine immunogenicity and safety. Phase 2 trials are conducted with a similar objective in larger number of subjects. Phase 3 trials are randomized controlled trials in large number of subjects for assessing vaccine efficacy and safety.

9.1.3. ADVERSE EVENTS FOLLOWING IMMUNIZATION

An adverse event following immunization (AEFI) or vaccine-associated adverse event (VAE) is one that is believed to be caused by immunization. It is defined as an untoward, temporally associated event following immunization that might or might not be caused by the vaccine or the immunization process. Reported adverse event can be true adverse event or an event coincidental to the immunization. These events may be recognized during clinical trials or during postmarketing surveillance. Whenever AEFI are detected, they must be reported on a timely basis so that the cause can be identified.

ADVERSE EVENT FOLLOWING IMMUNIZATION SURVEILLANCE

Adverse events following immunization surveillance is a process that includes detecting, monitoring and responding to AEFI, and implementing appropriate and immediate action to correct any unsafe practices detected through the AEFI surveillance system, in order to reduce the negative impact on the health of individuals and the reputation of the immunization program.

Vaccine reactions are classified as:
- Common minor reactions
- Rare, more serious reactions.

Most vaccine reactions are minor, and include mild side effects, such as local reactions (pain, swelling and/or redness), fever and systemic symptoms (e.g. vomiting, diarrhea, malaise), which can result as part of the normal immune response to the vaccine. Some of the non-antigenic vaccine components (e.g. adjuvants, stabilizers or preservatives) can cause reactions.

SERIOUS VACCINE REACTIONS

A serious adverse event (SAE) is defined as an event which is either (1) fatal or life threatening, or (2) results in

Table 9.1.5: Different types of adverse event following immunization.

Vaccine reaction	Event caused or precipitated by the inherent properties of the vaccine (active component or one of the other components, e.g. adjuvant, preservative, stabilizer) when given correctly
Program errors	Event caused by an error in vaccine preparation, handling or administration
Coincidental	Event that happens after immunization but is not caused by the vaccine. This is due to a chance temporal association
Injection reaction	Event arising from anxiety about, or pain from, the injection itself rather than the vaccine
Unknown	The cause of the event cannot be determined

Box 9.1.2

Emergency management of anaphylaxis.
- The patient must be made to lie down flat and legs must be elevated if possible
- Epinephrine (1:1,000 solution) 0.01 ml/kg/dose (maximum 0.5 ml) by intramuscular (IM) injection must be administered on anterolateral aspect of thigh. It can be repeated after 3–5 minutes if required
- Airway must be cleared, breathing and circulation must be established
- Intravenous (IV) access must be set up
- Wide bore access and IV normal saline 20 ml/kg as a bolus must be given in hypotension
- Oral antihistamines may be given. IV antihistamines are not recommended
- Oral or IV corticosteroids equivalent to prednisolone 1–2 mg/kg may be given, but benefit is not proven

Table 9.1.6: Common minor vaccine reactions.

Vaccine	Local reaction (pain, swelling, redness)	Fever (>38°C)	Irritability, malaise and non specific symptoms
BCG	Common	-	-
Hib	5–15%	2–10%	-
Hepatitis B	Adults up to 15% Children up to 5%	1–6%	-
Measles/MMR	Up to 10%	5–15%	Up to 5% (rash)
Oral polio vaccine (OPV)	-	Less than 1%	Less than 1%[a]
Tetanus/DT/Td	Up to 10%[b]	Up to 10%	Up to 25%
Pertussis (DTP-whole cell)[c]	Up to 50%	Up to 50%	Up to 60%

[a] Diarrhea, headache and/or muscle pains
[b] Rate of local reaction likely by increase with booster closes, up to 50–85%
[c] With whole cell pertussis vaccine. Acellular pertussis vaccine rates are lower
Abbreviations: BCG, bacillus Calmette–Guérin; MMR, mumps, measles, and rubella; OPV, oral polio vaccine; DTP, diphtheria, tetanus and pertussis.

persistent or significant disability, incapacity, or (3) results in or prolongs hospitalization, or (4) leads to congenital anomalies or birth defects.

Important adverse reactions that are not immediately life-threatening or do not result in death or hospitalization but may jeopardize the patient should also be considered as SAEs (Tables 9.1.5 and 9.1.6).

Severe Allergic Reactions

Severe allergy or anaphylaxis or anaphylaxis-like reactions are known to occur following vaccination, these include generalized urticaria, hives, wheezing, swelling of the mouth and throat, difficulty in breathing, hypotension and shock, but these reactions occur very rarely, with a frequency of 1 per 1 million vaccines. These reactions are rarely due to vaccine antigen, they are usually

due to other vaccine constituents like egg, gelatin like stabilizers, antimicrobials like neomycin, streptomycin or preservatives like thiomersal.

A complete detailed history of any past allergies must be obtained. Patients with history of severe allergic reaction to any constituent of the vaccine should not be given the vaccine, except for the children with egg allergy; they can be given measles and MMR vaccines. As occurrence of anaphylaxis cannot be predicted, the vaccine should be observed for 15 minutes after vaccination. The resuscitative equipments like oxygen delivery system, Ambu bag and mask, laryngoscope, endotracheal tubes, IV access devices, epinephrine, hydrocortisone, antihistaminics and inotropes should be kept ready (Box 9.1.2 and Table 9.1.7).

Coincidental Adverse Event Following Immunization

Vaccines are normally scheduled early in life, when infections and other illnesses are common and underlying congenital or neurological conditions may be present. Consequently, many events including deaths are falsely attributed to vaccines (rather than a chance association).

Coincidental events are unrelated to the immunization but medical officers should be encouraged to ensure the proper diagnostic workup and management of the AEFI cases even when not related to the vaccination.

Parents or the community may blame the vaccine, especially if the child was previously healthy. These cases still require investigation to allay public fears and to maintain credibility. Responding to a community's concerns about immunization safety is important in maintaining confidence in the immunization program.

An event is more likely to be coincidental if a similar event affected others in the same age group around the same time, although they did not receive the suspect vaccine(s). There may also be evidence showing that the event is not related to immunization (Table 9.1.8).

Table 9.1.7: Rare serious vaccine reactions, onset interval and rates.

Vaccine	Reaction[a]	Onset interval	Rate per million doses
BCG	Suppurative adenitis BCG osteitis Disseminated BCG itis	2–6 months up to several years 1–12 months	100–1,000 -
Hib	None known	-	-
Hepatitis B	Anaphylaxis	0–1 hour	1–2
Measles/MMR	Febrile seizures Thrombocytopenia (low platelets) Anaphylaxis	5–12 days 30 days 0–1 hour	330 30 1
Oral polio vaccine (OPV)	Vaccine associated paralytic poliomyelitis (VAPP)	4–30 days	Up to 0.4[b]
Tetanus	Brachial neuritis Anaphylaxis Sterile abscess	2–28 days 0–1 hour 1–6 weeks	5–10 1–6 6–10
DTP	Persistent (>3 hours) inconsolable screaming Seizures Hypotonic hyporesponsive episode (HHE) Anaphylaxis/shock	0–48 hours 0–1 days 0–24 hours 0–1 hour	1,000–60,000 600[c] 30–990 1–6
Japanese encephalitis	Serious allergic reaction Neurological event	0–2 weeks 0–2 weeks	10–1,000 1–2.3
Yellow fever	Allergic reaction/anaphylaxis	0–1 hour	5–20

[a]Reactions (except anaphylaxis) do not occur if already immune (90% of those receiving a second dose): children over 6 years are unlikely to have febrile seizures
[b]VAPP risk is higher for 1st dose (12 per 4–3.4 million doses) compared to 1 per 5.9 million for subsequent doses, and 1 per 6.7 million doses for subsequent contacts
[c]Seizures are mostly febrile in origin and rate depends on past history, family history and age, with a much lower risk in infants under the age of four months
Abbreviations: BCG, bacillus Calmette–Guérin; MMR, mumps, measles, and rubella; OPV, oral polio vaccine; VAPP, vaccine associated paralytic poliomyelitis; HHE, hypotonic hyporesponsive episode; DTP, diphtheria, tetanus and pertussis.

Table 9.1.8: Examples of incorrect immunization practices and associated AEFI.

Incorrect practices	Possible severe reaction following immunization
Non-sterile injection: • Reuse of disposable syringe and needle • Improperly sterilized syringe or needle • Contaminated vaccine or diluent	• Infection such as local abscess at injection site • Blood-borne infection transmitted, such as hepatitis, HIV
Reconstitution error: • Inadequate shaking of vaccine • Reconstitution with incorrect diluent • Drug substituted for vaccine or diluents • Reuse of reconstituted vaccine at subsequent session	• Local abscess • Vaccine ineffective • Negative effect of drug, e.g. insulin, oxytocin, muscle relaxants • Death
Injection at incorrect site: • BCG given subcutaneously • DTP/DT/TT too superficial • Injection into buttocks	• Local reaction or abscess • Local reaction abscess • Sciatic nerve damage
Vaccine transportation/storage incorrect: • WM changed color • Clumping of adsorbed vaccine	• Local reaction from frozen vaccine • Vaccine ineffective
Contraindications ignored	Avoidable severe reaction
Vaccine being ineffective is an "effect" it is not strictly an adverse event	

Abbreviations: HIV, human immunodeficiency virus; BCG, Bacillus Calmette–Guérin; DTP, diphtheria, tetanus and pertussis; DT, diphtheria and tetanus; TT, tetanus toxoid.

9.1.4. GENERAL GUIDELINES FOR IMMUNIZATION

While immunizing the children there are many issues, which should be kept in mind. It is important to follow certain guidelines so as to take maximum benefits of available vaccines and to minimize cost and risks associated with vaccination.

Simultaneous Administration of Vaccines

Most of the vaccines available for childhood immunization can be safely and effectively administered simultaneously. There are no contraindications known for simultaneous administration of multiple vaccines routinely recommended for infants and children. It has been observed that immune responses to one vaccine generally do not interfere with immune response to other vaccines administered simultaneously; exceptions include interference among the three oral poliovirus serotypes in trivalent OPV vaccine and concurrent administration of cholera and yellow fever vaccines. Simultaneous administration of multiple vaccines can improve compliance and result in improvement of immunization rates significantly.

The simultaneous administration of the most widely used live and inactivated vaccines does not result in decreased antibody responses or increased rates of adverse reaction. The rate of adverse reactions seen with the combination is usually similar to those seen after the most reactogenic component if given separately. Unless they are licensed for mixing by the authorities individual vaccines should not be mixed in the same syringe.

Recommendations on Spacing of Administration of Different Vaccines

Inactivated vaccines do not interfere with the immune response to other inactivated vaccines or to live vaccines. An inactivated vaccine can be administered either simultaneously or at any time before or after a different inactivated vaccine or live vaccine.

There should be at least 4 weeks interval between live injected vaccines (MMR, varicella) that are not administered on the same day. This is important to reduce or eliminate interference from the vaccine given first on the vaccine given later. If two live injected vaccines are separated by less than 4 weeks interval, it is advisable to repeat the vaccine given second, or confirm that the dose was effective by serologic testing of the recipient.

Live oral vaccines do not interfere with each other if not given simultaneously. These vaccines may be given at any time before or after each other. Injected live vaccines (MMR, varicella) are not believed to have an effect on live vaccines given orally. Live oral vaccines may be given at any time before or after live injected vaccines.

Recommendation on Spacing of Multiple Doses of the Same Vaccine

All vaccines should be administered as close to the recommended schedule as possible to maximize the protection from the vaccine. Recommended spacing between doses should be maintained. If a child is not up-to-date on his or her vaccinations, it may be necessary to "accelerate" the normal schedule in order to catch up. In this situation it is important to know how closely the doses can be spaced and still be effective. Doses of a vaccine given too close together or earlier than the minimum recommended age could reduce the effectiveness of the vaccine and effort should be made to maintain at least the minimum interval between doses and start vaccination at recommended minimum age.

Too frequent administration of some inactivated vaccines, such as tetanus toxoids, can result in increased rates of reactions in some vaccines. Such reactions probably result from formation of circulating antigen-antibody complexes.

Recommendations for Spacing of Administration of Vaccines and Antibody Containing Products

If a circulating antibody is present against a vaccine antigen it may reduce or completely eliminate an immune response to the vaccine. How much will be interference by circulating antibody depends on the type of vaccine administered and the amount of antibody circulating. Killed vaccines are not substantially affected by circulating antibody, so they can be administered before, after or at the same time as the antibody.

It is necessary for live vaccines to replicate to induce an immune response. Antibody against live injected vaccine antigen may interfere with replication. If it is necessary that a live injected vaccine (MMR, its component vaccines or varicella) must be given around the time that antibody is given, the live vaccine and antibody product must be separated by enough interval so that the antibody does not interfere with viral replication. If the live vaccine is given first, it is necessary to wait at least 2 weeks before giving the antibody. If that is not possible and the interval between the vaccine and antibody is less than 2 weeks, the recipient must be tested for immunity or the vaccine dose should be repeated after the appropriate interval. For example, if whole blood is administered less than 14 days after the dose of varicella vaccine, the vaccine should be readministered at least 6 months after the whole blood unless serologic testing indicates an adequate immune response to the initial dose of varicella vaccine.

If the antibody product is given before a dose of live vaccine, it is necessary to wait until the antibody has waned before giving the live vaccine. It was recommended in past that the interval between receipt of antibody (immune globulin or other blood products) and live injected vaccines should be minimum of 6 weeks and preferably 3 months. But recently it has been recommended that the necessary interval between an antibody-containing product and live vaccine vary depending on the concentration of antibody in the product.

Lapsed Immunizations

Because of immunological memory, longer than routinely recommended intervals between doses do not impair the immunologic response to live, and inactivated vaccines that require more than 1 dose to achieve primary immunity. Similarly, delayed administration of recommended booster doses does not adversely affect the antibody response to such doses. Thus the interruption of a recommended primary series or an extended lapse between booster doses does not necessitate reinitiation of the entire vaccination series.

Number of Doses

Administration of 1 dose of live injected vaccines usually provides protection. Immunity following live vaccines is long lasting, and booster doses are not necessary. Multiple doses of some live vaccines are recommended to stimulate an immune response to different types of the same virus, such as poliovirus types 1, 2 and 3 or to induce immunity in persons who failed to mount an immune response to an earlier dose of vaccine, such as measles. These multiple doses constitute a primary vaccination series and are not "booster doses".

First dose of an inactivated vaccine usually does not provide protection. A protective immune response only develops after the 2nd or 3rd dose. Antibody titers may decrease below protective levels after a few years in case of inactivated vaccines. This decrease in antibody titer is most marked for tetanus and diphtheria vaccines. Periodic "boosting" is required for these vaccines. An additional dose is given to raise antibody back to protective levels. All inactivated vaccines do not require boosting throughout life. For example, Hib vaccine does not require boosting because Hib disease is very rare in children older than 5 years of age. Hepatitis B vaccine does not require boosting because of immunologic memory and long incubation period to the vaccine and the long incubation period of hepatitis B.

Recommendations for Children with Unknown or Uncertain Immunization Status

A clinician may come across some children with history of an uncertain immunization status. These children should be taken as susceptible to disease and age appropriate immunizations should be administered. There is nothing to suggest that administration of MMR, varicella, Hib, hepatitis B, or poliovirus vaccine to already immune recipients is harmful.

Recommendations on Site and Route of Immunization

Oral Polio Vaccine

Contrary to popular belief breastfeeding does not interfere with successful immunization with OPV vaccine. A child can be breastfed immediately after receiving a dose of OPV. OPV dose should be repeated if the child immediately spits out, fails to swallow or regurgitates OPV vaccine or vomits within 10 minutes of receiving an OPV dose. Vaccine should be re-administered if the 2nd dose is also not retained.

Injectable Vaccines

The choice of site for giving IM injections depends on the volume of the material to be injected and the size of the muscle. The preferred site in infants is anterolateral aspect of the thigh as it provides the largest muscle mass. The deltoid muscle is preferred site for IM injection in older children. Some clinicians use the anterolateral thigh muscles even for toddlers.

As gluteal region is covered by a significant layer of subcutaneous fat and there are chances of damaging the sciatic nerve, the upper, outer aspect of the buttocks should not be used for active immunization in children. Hepatitis B and rabies vaccines should not be given in the buttock at any age, as there are chances that immunity developed may not be optimal. Those who are given hepatitis B vaccine in the buttock should be tested for immunity and reimmunized if antibody level not found to be adequate (Figs. 9.1.6 to 9.1.10).

Adjuvants containing vaccines like aluminum-adsorbed DTaP, DT, dT, hepatitis B and hepatitis A should not be administered subcutaneously or intradermally because they can cause local irritation, inflammation, granuloma formation and necrosis. These vaccines should be injected deep in the muscle mass. Products for passive immunoprophylaxis like immune globulin, RIG, and other similar products also are injected intramuscularly except when RIG is infiltrated around the site of a bite wound. Subcutaneous injections can be given in the anterolateral aspect of the thigh or the upper arm.

If two or more vaccines are necessary to be given at a single visit it is preferable to use different sites but if necessary, two vaccines can be given in the same limb at a single visit. As thigh has greater muscle mass, it is the preferred site for giving two simultaneous IM injections. There should be distance of at least 1–2 inches between two injection sites. Multiple vaccines should not be mixed in a single syringe unless specifically licensed and labeled

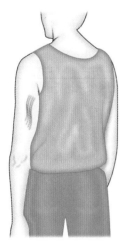

FIG. 9.1.6: Subcutaneous site of administration—triceps
Source: Minnesota Department of Health.

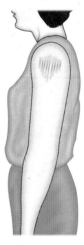

FIG. 9.1.7: Intramuscular site of administration—deltoid
Source: Minnesota Department of Health.

for administering in one syringe. A different needle and syringe should be used for each injection. Bleeding at the injection site for a brief period is common and usually can be prevented or controlled by applying pressure for some time. When used at the recommended sites where no large blood vessels exist, pulling back of the syringe to check for blood is not recommended. The needle should be withdrawn a few seconds after finishing administration of the vaccine (to prevent backflow of vaccine into the needle track) following which the injection site should be pressed firmly for a few seconds with dry cotton. The injection site should not be rubbed following injection (Table 9.1.9).

Contraindications and Precautions to Vaccination

A contraindication is a condition in a recipient that greatly increases the chance of a serious adverse reaction. It is a condition in the recipient of the vaccine, not with the vaccine itself. If the vaccines were given in the presence of that condition, the resulting adverse reaction could seriously harm the recipient. In general, vaccines are never administered when a contraindication is present.

A precaution is similar to a contraindication. A precaution is a condition in a recipient that may increase the chance of a serious adverse reaction, or that may compromise the ability of the vaccine to produce immunity.

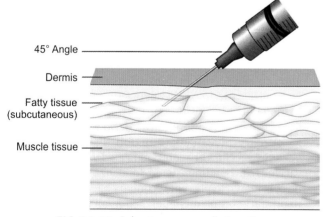

FIG. 9.1.8: Intramuscular or subcutaneous site of administration: anterolateral thigh.
Source: Minnesota Department of Health

90° Angle
Dermis
Fatty tissue (subcutaneous)
Muscle tissue

FIG. 9.1.9: Intramuscular needle insertion.
Source: California Immunization Branch

45° Angle
Dermis
Fatty tissue (subcutaneous)
Muscle tissue

FIG. 9.1.10: Subcutaneous needle insertion.
Source: California Immunization Branch

Table 9.1.9: Injection site, type of needle and technique.

	Site	Type of needle	Comments
Intramuscular injections (needle should enter at 90° angle)			
Preterms and neonates	Anterolateral thigh (junction of middle and lower third)	22–25 gauge, 5/8 inch	Skin should be stretched between thumb and forefinger
Infants (1 to <12 months)	Anterolateral thigh	22–25 gauge, 1 inch	Bunch the skin, subcutaneous tissue and muscle to prevent striking the bone
Toddlers and older children (12 months–10 years)	Deltoid or Anterolateral thigh	22–25 G, 5/8 inch 22–25 gauge, 1 inch	Skin should be stretched between thumb and forefinger Bunch the skin, subcutaneous tissue and muscle
Adolescent and adults (11 years onward)	Deltoid or anterolateral thigh	<60 kg 1 inch >60 kg 1.5 inch	
Subcutaneous injections (needle should enter at 45° to the skin)			
Infants	Thigh	22–25 G, 5/8 inch	
>12 months	Outer triceps	22–25 G, 5/8 inch	
Intradermal injections			
All age	Left deltoid	26/27 G, 0.5 inch	A 5 mm wheal should be raised

Injury could result but the chance of this happening is less than with a contraindication. Under normal circumstances, vaccines are deferred when a precaution condition is present. However, situations may arise when the benefit of protection from the vaccine outweighs the risk of an adverse reaction, and a provider may decide to give the vaccine. For example, prolonged crying or a high fever after a dose of whole cell or acellular pertussis vaccine is considered a precaution to giving subsequent doses of pertussis vaccine to a child. But if the child was at high-risk of pertussis infection (e.g. a pertussis outbreak in the community), a provider may choose to vaccinate the child and treat the adverse reaction if it occurs. In this example, the benefit of protection from the vaccine outweighs the harm potentially caused by the vaccine.

Two conditions are temporary contraindications to vaccination with live vaccines: (1) pregnancy and (2) immunosuppression. Two conditions are temporary precautions to vaccination: (1) moderate or severe acute illness (all vaccines) and (2) recent receipt of an antibody containing blood product (live injected vaccines only).

Children under Antimicrobial/ Antiviral Therapy

Antibiotics do not have an effect on the immune response to a vaccine. With a few exceptions, no commonly used antibiotic or antiviral will inactivate a live virus vaccine. Oral typhoid vaccine (Ty21a) should not be administered to persons receiving antimicrobial agents until 24 hours after the last dose of antimicrobial. If feasible, to avoid a possible reduction in vaccine effectiveness, antibacterial drugs should not be started or resumed until 1 week after the last dose of Ty21a.

Live attenuated influenza vaccine should not be administered until 48 hours after cessation of therapy with antiviral influenza drugs. If feasible, to avoid possible reduction in vaccine effectiveness, antiviral medication should not be administered for 14 days after LAIV administration.

Antiviral drugs active against herpesviruses (e.g. acyclovir or valacyclovir) might reduce the efficacy of live, attenuated varicella and zoster vaccines. These drugs should be discontinued at least 24 hours before administration of vaccines containing varicella zoster virus, including zoster vaccine, if possible. Delay use or resumption of antiviral therapy for 14 days after vaccination. No data exist to suggest that commonly used antiviral drugs have an effect on rotavirus vaccine or MMR.

Breastfed Children and Children with History of Pregnancy in the Household

Breastfeeding does not decrease the response to routine childhood vaccines, including OPV. Breastfeeding also does not extend or improve passive immunity to vaccine preventable disease provided by maternal antibody. All vaccines, including live vaccines (MMR, varicella and yellow fever) can be given to infants or children with

pregnant household contacts. Measles and mumps vaccine viruses produce a noncommunicable infection, and are not transmitted to household contacts. Rubella vaccine virus has been shown to be shed in breast milk, but transmission to an infant has rarely been documented (rubella is not transmitted by oral route). Transmission of varicella vaccine virus is uncommon, and most women are immune from prior chicken pox. OPV virus is shed and can spread, but pregnant contacts are at no greater risk than other household contacts in this situation, and OPV has not been shown to cause fetal defects.

General Principles for Vaccination of the Immunocompromised Individuals

- In severe immunodeficiency, all live vaccines are contraindicated. In mild or moderate immunodeficiency, live vaccines may be given if benefits outweigh the risks. Patients administered live vaccines inadvertently prior to diagnosis of immunodeficiency should be watched for vaccine related adverse effects
- Household contacts of immunocompromised should not receive transmissible vaccines such as OPV but can safely receive other nontransmissible live vaccines such as MMR and varicella. All household contacts should be fully immunized including varicella and influenza to reduce risk of transmission to the immuncompromised
- All inactivated vaccines can be given but immunogenicity and efficacy may be lower
- Higher doses, greater number of doses should be given if indicated (hepatitis B), antibody titers should be checked post immunization/regular basis and regular boosters administered if needed. For major or contaminated wounds tetanus Ig is required in addition to TT even if three or more doses of TT have been received in the past
- Some vaccines including pneumococcal, varicella (depending on degree of immunocompromise and in two doses 4–12 weeks apart), hepatitis A, inactivated influenza vaccines should be given, if resources permit. There is at present insufficient data on the safety and efficacy of the rotavirus vaccine in the immunocompromised
- In B lymphocyte defects there is abnormal humoral response to infections. All live bacterial (BCG and oral typhoid) and live viral (MMR, OPV, measles and varicella) vaccines are contraindicated
- In agammaglobulinemia, pertussis and influenza vaccination are considered. In cases of selective IgG and IgA defects, all live vaccines other than OPV can be considered
- In individuals having primary T lymphocyte defects, all live vaccines are contraindicated. No vaccine is useful
- In primary phagocytic function disorders, all live bacterial vaccines are contraindicated whereas live viral vaccines can be administered. Influenza vaccine can also be considered to prevent secondary bacterial infections
- In primary complement deficiency, all vaccines can be safely administered. These individuals are more prone to pneumococcal and meningococcal infections. In

C1, C4, C2 and C3 deficiency, all vaccines are effective; pneumococcal and meningococcal vaccines should be prioritized. In C5–9, properdin and factor B deficiency, all vaccines are effective. Meningococcal vaccination is recommended in this group of individuals.

9.1.5. VACCINATION SCHEDULES

THE IDEAL IMMUNIZATION SCHEDULE

Ideal immunization schedule should be epidemiologically relevant, immunologically competent, technologically feasible, socially acceptable, affordable and sustainable. It will vary from country to country and from time to time. In order to choose vaccines for vaccination program at government funding, not only incidence, prevalence or disease burden but their implication should be known. For government programs usually it is cost first, efficacy next, safety last. For an individual it is safety first, efficacy next, cost last. Although what is not in the best interests of the individual cannot be in the best interests of the community and what is in the best interests of the community is also in the best interests of the individual. Tables 9.1.10 to 9.1.13 depict the National and IAP immunization schedules.

Table 9.1.10: National immunization schedule (NIS) for infants, children and pregnant women.

Vaccine	When to give	Dose	Route	Site
For Pregnant Women				
TT-1	Early in pregnancy	0.5 mL	Intramuscular	Upper arm
TT-2	4 weeks after TT-1*	0.5 mL	Intramuscular	Upper arm
TT Booster	If received 2 TT doses in a pregnancy within the last 3 years*	0.5 mL	Intramuscular	Upper arm
For Infants				
BCG	At birth or as early as possible till one year of age	0.1 mL (0.05 mL until 1 month of age)	Intradermal	Left upper arm
Hepatitis B—birth dose	At birth or as early as possible within 24 hours	0.5 mL	Intramuscular	Anterolateral side of mid-thigh
OPV-0	At birth or as early as possible within the first 15 days	2 drops	Oral	Oral
OPV 1, 2 and 3	At 6 weeks, 10 weeks and 14 weeks (OPV can be given till 5 years of age)	2 drops	Oral	Oral
Pentavalent 1, 2 and 3	At 6 weeks, 10 weeks and 14 weeks (can be given till one year of age)	0.5 mL	Intramuscular	Anterolateral side of mid-thigh
Rotavirus#	At 6 weeks, 10 weeks and 14 weeks (can be given till one year of age)	5 drops	Oral	Oral
IPV	Two fractional dose at 6 and 14 weeks of age	0.1 mL	Intradermal two fractional dose	Intradermal: Right upper arm
Measles /MR 1st Dose§	9 completed months to 12 months (can be given till 5 years of age)	0.5 mL	Subcutaneous	Right upper arm
JE - 1**	9 completed months to 12 months	0.5 mL	Subcutaneous	Left upper arm
Vitamin A (1st dose)	At 9 completed months with measles—rubella	1 mL (1 lakh IU)	Oral	Oral
For Children				
DPT booster-1	16–24 months	0.5 mL	Intramuscular	Anterolateral side of mid-thigh
Measles/ MR 2nd dose§	16–24 months	0.5 mL	Subcutaneous	Right upper arm
OPV Booster	16–24 months	2 drops	Oral	Oral
JE-2	16–24 months	0.5 mL	Subcutaneous	Left upper arm
Vitamin A* (2nd to 9th dose)**	16–18 months. Then one dose every 6 months up to the age of 5 years	2 mL (2 lakh IU)	Oral	Oral
DPT Booster-2	5–6 years	0.5 mL	Intramuscular	Upper arm
TT	10 years and 16 years	0.5 mL	Intramuscular	Upper arm

*Give TT-2 or Booster doses before 36 weeks of pregnancy. However, give these even if more than 36 weeks have passed. Give TT to a woman in labor, if she has not previously received TT.
**JE vaccine is introduced in select endemic districts after the campaign.
***The 2nd to 9th doses of vitamin A can be administered to children 1–5 years old during biannual rounds, in collaboration with ICDS.
#Phased introduction, at present in Andhra Pradesh, Haryana, Himachal Pradesh and Odisha from 2016 and expanded in Madhya Pradesh, Assam, Rajasthan, and Tripura in February 2017 and planned in Tamil Nadu and Uttar Pradesh in 2017.
§Phased introduction, at present in five states namely Karnataka, Tamil Nadu, Goa, Lakshadweep and Puducherry (As of February 2017).
Source: National immunization Schedule, India (2017). Available from: https://mohfw.gov.in/sites/default/files/245453521061489663873.pdf

Table 9.1.11: IAP recommended immunization schedule for children aged 0-18 years (with range), 2016.

Age ▶ / Vaccine ▼	Birth to 2 weeks	6 weeks	10 weeks	14 weeks	18 weeks	6 months	9 months	12 months	15 months	18 months	19–23 months	2–3 years	4–6 years	7–10 years	11–12 years	13–18 years
BCG	BCG															
Hep B	Hep B1	Hep B2				Hep B3										
Polio	OPV 0	IPV1	IPV2	IPV3		OPV1	OPV2	IPV B1					OPV3			
DTP		DTP 1	DTP 2	DTP 3					DTP B1				DTP B2			
Tdap															Tdap	
Hib		Hib 1	Hib 2	Hib 3				Hib-booster								
Pneumococcal		PCV 1	PCV 2	PCV 3				PCV-booster						PCV		
PPSV23													PPSV			
Rotavirus		RV 1	RV 2	RV 3												
MMR							MMR 1		MMR 2				MMR 3			
Varicella									VAR 1				VAR 2			
Hep A								Hep A1 & Hep A2								
Typhoid							Typhoid CV (TCV)				Booster					
Influenza						Influenza (yearly)										
HPV															HPV	
Meningococcal												Meningococcal				
Cholera								Cholera 1 & 2								
JE								Japanese Encephalitis								
Rabies	Rabies (Pre-EP & PEP)															

	Range of recommended ages for all children		Range of recommended ages for certain high-risk groups
	Range of recommended ages for catch-up immunization		Not routinely recommended

- This schedule includes recommendations in effect as of September 2014.
- These recommendations must be read with the footnotes that follow. For those who fall behind or start late, provide catch-up vaccination at the earliest opportunity as indicated by the green bars in Table 9.1.11.

Footnotes: Recommended immunization schedule for persons aged 0 through 18 Years—IAP, 2016

I. General Instructions:
- Vaccination at birth means as early as possible within 24–72 hours after birth or at least not later than one week after birth
- Whenever multiple vaccinations are to be given simultaneously, they should be given within 24 hours if simultaneous administration is not feasible due to some reasons
- The recommended age in weeks/months/years mean completed weeks/months/years
- Any dose not administered at the recommended age should be administered at a subsequent visit, when indicated and feasible
- The use of a combination vaccine generally is preferred over separate injections of its equivalent component vaccines
- When two or more live parenteral/intranasal vaccines are not administered on the same day, they should be given at least 28 days (4 weeks) apart; this rule does not apply to live oral vaccines
- Any interval can be kept between live and inactivated vaccines
- If given <4 weeks apart, the vaccine given 2nd should be repeated
- The minimum interval between 2 doses of same inactivated vaccines is usually 4 weeks (exception rabies). However, any interval can be kept between doses of different inactivated vaccines

- Vaccine doses administered up to 4 days before the minimum interval or age can be counted as valid (exception rabies). If the vaccine is administered >5 days before minimum period it is counted as invalid dose
- Any number of antigens can be given on the same day
- Changing needles between drawing vaccine into the syringe and injecting it into the child is not necessary
- Once the protective cap on a single-dose vial has been removed, the vaccine should be discarded at the end of the immunization session because it may not be possible to determine if the rubber seal has been punctured
- Different vaccines should not be mixed in the same syringe unless specifically licensed and labeled for such use
- Patients should be observed for an allergic reaction for 15–20 minutes after receiving immunization(s)
- When necessary, 2 vaccines can be given in the same limb at a single visit.
- The anterolateral aspect of the thigh is the preferred site for 2 simultaneous IM injections because of its greater muscle mass
- The distance separating the 2 injections is arbitrary but should be at least 1 inch so that local reactions are unlikely to overlap
- Although most experts recommend "aspiration" by gently pulling back on the syringe before the injection is given, there are no data

Contd...

Contd...

to document the necessity for this procedure. If blood appears after negative pressure, the needle should be withdrawn and another site should be selected using a new needle.

- A previous immunization with a dose that was less than the standard dose or one administered by a nonstandard route should not be counted, and the person should be re-immunized as appropriate for age.

II. Specific instructions:

1. BCG vaccine

Routine vaccination:

- Should be given at birth or at first contact

Catch up vaccination: May be given up to 5 years.

2. Hepatitis B (Hep B) vaccine

Routine vaccination:

- Minimum age: Birth
- Administer monovalent Hep B vaccine to all newborns within 48 hours of birth
- Monovalent Hep B vaccine should be used for doses administered before age 6 weeks
- Administration of a total of 4 doses of Hep B vaccine is permissible when a combination vaccine containing Hep B is administered after the birth dose
- Infants who did not receive a birth dose should receive 3 doses of a Hep B containing vaccine starting as soon as feasible
- The ideal minimum interval between dose 1 and dose 2 is 4 weeks, and between dose 2 and 3 is 8 weeks. Ideally, the final (3rd or 4th) dose in the Hep B vaccine series should be administered no earlier than age 24 weeks and at least 16 weeks after the first dose, whichever is later
- Hep B vaccine may also be given in any of the following schedules: Birth—1 and 6 months, Birth—6 and 14 weeks; Birth—6, 10 and 14 weeks; Birth—6, 10 and 14 weeks, etc. All schedules are protective.

Catch-up vaccination:

- Administer the 3-dose series to those not previously vaccinated.
- In catch up vaccination use 0, 1, and 6 months schedule.

3. Poliovirus vaccines

Routine vaccination:

- Birth dose of OPV usually does not lead to VAPP
- OPV in place of IPV, if IPV is unfeasible, minimum 3 doses
- Additional doses of OPV on all SIAs
- IPV: Minimum age—6 weeks.
- IPV: 2 instead of 3 doses can be also used if primary series started at 8 weeks and the interval between the doses is kept 8 weeks
- No child should leave your facility without polio immunization (IPV or OPV), if indicated by the schedule.

Intradermal vaccination: ACVIP does not approve the use of 'intradermal fractional-dose IPV' (ID-f IPV) for office-practice. However, considering the extreme shortage of IPV and the urgent need of providing immunity against type-2 poliovirus, the committee has now provisionally accepted the immune-protection accorded by two ID-fIPV doses given at 6 and 14-week as moderately effective against type-2 polioviruses. However, another full dose of IM-IPV should be offered at least at 8 weeks interval of the second dose of ID-fIPV.

- If a child has received one dose of ID-fIPV at 6 weeks, two more full doses of IM-IPV should be offered at least 8 weeks after the first dose
- The minimum interval between the 2nd and 3rd dose should also be at least 8 weeks.

Catch-up vaccination:

- IPV catch-up schedule: 2 doses at 2 months apart followed by a booster after 6 months of previous dose.

4. Diphtheria and tetanus toxoids and pertussis (DTP) vaccine

Routine vaccination:

- Minimum age: 6 weeks
- The first booster (4th dose) may be administered as early as age 12 months, provided at least 6 months have elapsed since the third dose
- DTaP vaccine/combinations should preferably be avoided for the primary series

- DTaP may be preferred to DTwP in children with history of severe adverse effects after previous dose/s of DTwP or children with neurologic disorders
- First and second boosters may also be of DTwP. However, considering a higher reactogenicity, DTaP can be considered for the boosters
- ACVIP does not approve the use of Tdap as second booster of DTP schedule!
- If any 'acellular pertussis' containing vaccine is used, it must at least have 3 or more components in the product
- No need of repeating/giving additional doses of whole-cell pertussis (wP) vaccine to a child who has earlier completed their primary schedule with acellular pertussis (aP) vaccine-containing products.

Catch-up vaccination:

- Catch-up schedule: The 2nd childhood booster is not required if the last dose has been given beyond the age of 4 years
- Catch up below 7 years: DTwP/DTaP at 0, 1 and 6 months
- Catch up above 7 years: Tdap, Td, and Td at 0, 1 and 6 months.

5. Tetanus and diphtheria toxoids and acellular pertussis (Tdap) vaccine

Routine vaccination:

- Minimum age: 7 years (Adacel® is approved for 11–64 years by ACIP and 4–64 year olds by FDA, while Boostrix® **for 10 years and older by ACIP and 4 years of age and older by FDA in US)**
- Administer 1 dose of Tdap vaccine to all adolescents aged 11 through 12 years
- *Tdap during pregnancy:* One dose of Tdap vaccine to pregnant mothers/adolescents during each pregnancy (preferred during 27 through 36 weeks gestation) regardless of number of years from prior Td or Tdap vaccination.

Catch-up vaccination:

- Catch up above 7 years: Tdap, Td, Td at 0, 1 and 6 months
- Persons aged 7 through 10 years who are not fully immunized with the childhood DTwP/DTaP vaccine series, should receive Tdap vaccine as the first dose in the catch-up series; if additional doses are needed, use Td vaccine. For these children, an adolescent Tdap vaccine should not be given
- Persons aged 11 through 18 years who have not received Tdap vaccine should receive a dose followed by tetanus and diphtheria toxoids (Td) booster doses every 10 years thereafter
- Tdap vaccine can be administered regardless of the interval since the last tetanus and diphtheria toxoid–containing vaccine
- Tdap vaccine should not be used as second booster for DTP series.

6. *Haemophilus influenzae* type b (Hib) conjugate vaccine

Routine vaccination:

- Minimum age: 6 weeks
- Primary series includes Hib conjugate vaccine at ages 6, 10, 14 weeks with a booster at age 12 through 18 months.

Catch-up vaccination:

- Catch-up is recommended till 5 years of age
- 6–12 months: 2 primary doses 4 weeks apart and 1 booster
- 12–15 months: 1 primary dose and 1 booster
- Above 15 months: Single dose
- If the first dose was administered at age 7 through 11 months, administer the second dose at least 4 weeks later and a final dose at age 12–18 months at least 8 weeks after the second dose.

7. Pneumococcal conjugate vaccines (PCVs)

Routine vaccination:

- Minimum age: 6 weeks
- Both PCV10 and PCV13 are licensed for children from 6 weeks to 5 years of age (although the exact labeling details may differ by country). Additionally, PCV13 is licensed for the prevention of pneumococcal diseases in adults >50 years of age
- Primary schedule (for both PCV10 and PCV13): 3 primary doses at 6, 10, and 14 weeks with a booster at age 12 through 15 months.

Catch-up vaccination:

- Administer 1 dose of PCV13 or PCV10 to all healthy children aged 24 through 59 months who are not completely vaccinated for their age

Contd...

Contd...

- **For PCV 13:** Catch up in 6–12 months: 2 doses 4 weeks apart and 1 booster; 12–23 months: 2 doses 8 weeks apart; 24 months and above: single dose
- **For PCV 10:** Catch up in 6–12 months: 2 doses 4 weeks apart and 1 booster; 12 months to 5 years: 2 doses 8 weeks apart
- **Vaccination of persons with high-risk conditions:**
  - PCV and pneumococcal polysaccharide vaccine [PPSV] both are used in certain high-risk group of children
  - For children aged 24 through 71 months with certain underlying medical conditions, administer 1 dose of PCV13 if 3 doses of PCV were received previously, or administer 2 doses of PCV13 at least 8 weeks apart if fewer than 3 doses of PCV were received previously
  - A single dose of PCV13 may be administered to previously unvaccinated children aged 6 through 18 years who have anatomic or functional asplenia (including sickle cell disease), HIV infection or an immunocompromising condition, cochlear implant or cerebrospinal fluid leak
  - Administer PPSV23 at least 8 weeks after the last dose of PCV to children aged 2 years or older with certain underlying medical conditions.

8. Pneumococcal polysaccharide vaccine (PPSV23)
- Minimum age: 2 years
- Not recommended for routine use in healthy individuals. Recommended only for the vaccination of persons with certain high-risk conditions
- Administer PPSV at least 8 weeks after the last dose of PCV to children aged 2 years or older with certain underlying medical conditions like anatomic or functional asplenia (including sickle cell disease), HIV infection, cochlear implant or cerebrospinal fluid leak
- An additional dose of PPSV should be administered after 5 years to children with anatomic/functional asplenia or an immunocompromising condition.
- PPSV should never be used alone for prevention of pneumococcal diseases amongst high-risk individuals.
- **Children with following medical conditions for which PPSV23 and PCV13 are indicated in the age group 24 through 71 months:**
  - Immunocompetent children with chronic heart disease (particularly cyanotic congenital heart disease and cardiac failure); chronic lung disease (including asthma if treated with high-dose oral corticosteroid therapy), diabetes mellitus; cerebrospinal fluid leaks; or cochlear implant
  - Children with anatomic or functional asplenia (including sickle cell disease and other hemoglobinopathies, congenital or acquired asplenia, or splenic dysfunction)
  - Children with immunocompromising conditions: HIV infection, chronic renal failure and nephrotic syndrome, diseases associated with treatment with immunosuppressive drugs or radiation therapy, including malignant neoplasms, leukemias, lymphomas and Hodgkin disease; or solid organ transplantation, congenital immunodeficiency.

9. Rotavirus (RV) vaccines
Routine vaccination:
- Minimum age: 6 weeks for all available brands [RV-1 (Rotarix), RV-5 (RotaTeq) and RV-116E (Rotavac)]
- Only two doses of RV-1 are recommended
- RV1 should preferably be employed in 10 and 14 week schedule, instead of 6 and 10 week; the former schedule is found to be far more immunogenic than the later
- If any dose in series was RV-5 or RV-116E or vaccine product is unknown for any dose in the series, a total of 3 doses of RV vaccine should be administered.
Catch-up vaccination:
- The maximum age for the first dose in the series is 14 weeks, 6 days
- Vaccination should not be initiated for infants aged 15 weeks, 0 days or older
- The maximum age for the final dose in the series is 8 months, 0 days.

10. Measles, mumps, and rubella (MMR) vaccine
Routine vaccination:
- Minimum age: 9 months or 270 completed days

- Administer the first dose of MMR vaccine at age 9 through 12 months, the second dose at age 15 through 18 months, and final (the 3rd) dose at age 4 through 6 years
- The 2nd dose must follow in 2nd year of life. However, it can be given at anytime 4–8 weeks after the 1st dose
- No need to give stand-alone measles vaccine.
Catch-up vaccination:
- Ensure that all school-aged children and adolescents have had at least 2 doses of MMR vaccine (3 doses if the 1st dose is received before 12 months)
- The minimum interval between the 2 doses is 4 weeks
- One dose if previously vaccinated with one dose (2 doses if the 1st dose is received before 12 months)
- 'Stand-alone' measles/any measles-containing vaccine or MMR can be administered to infants aged 6 through 8 months during outbreaks. However, this dose should not be counted.

11. Varicella vaccine
Routine vaccination:
- Minimum age: 12 months
- Administer the first dose at age 15 through 18 months and the second dose at age 4 through 6 years
- The second dose may be administered before age 4 years, provided at least 3 months have elapsed since the first dose. If the second dose was administered at least 4 weeks after the first dose, it can be accepted as valid
- The risk of breakthrough varicella is lower if given 15 months onwards.
Catch-up vaccination:
- Ensure that all persons aged 7 through 18 years without 'evidence of immunity' have 2 doses of the vaccine
- For children aged 12 months through 12 years, the recommended minimum interval between doses is 3 months. However, if the second dose was administered at least 4 weeks after the first dose, it can be accepted as valid
- For persons aged 13 years and older, the minimum interval between doses is 4 weeks
- For persons without evidence of immunity, administer 2 doses if not previously vaccinated or the second dose if only 1 dose has been administered
- 'Evidence of immunity' to varicella includes any of the following:
  - Documentation of age-appropriate vaccination with a varicella vaccine
  - Laboratory evidence of immunity or laboratory confirmation of disease
  - Diagnosis or verification of a history of varicella disease by a health-care provider
  - Diagnosis or verification of a history of herpes zoster by a health-care provider.

12. Hepatitis A (Hep A) vaccines
Routine vaccination:
- Minimum age: 12 months
- Inactivated Hep A vaccine: Start the 2-dose Hep A vaccine series for children aged 12 through 23 months; separate the 2 doses by 6–18 months
- Live attenuated H2-strain hepatitis A vaccine: Single dose starting at 12 months and through 23 months of age.
Catch-up vaccination:
- Either of the two vaccines can be used in 'catch-up' schedule beyond 2 years of age
- Administer 2 doses of inactivated vaccine at least 6 months apart to unvaccinated persons
- Only single dose of live attenuated H2-strain vaccine
- For catch up vaccination, pre vaccination screening for hepatitis A antibody is recommended in children older than 10 years as at this age the estimated seropositive rates exceed 50%.

13. Typhoid vaccines
Routine vaccination:
- Both Vi-PS conjugate and Vi-PS (polysaccharide) vaccines are available
- Minimum ages:

Contd...

Contd...

- Vi-PS conjugate (Typbar-TCV®): 6 months
- Vi-PS conjugate (Pedatyph®): 6 months
- Vi-PS (polysaccharide) vaccines: 2 years
- Vaccination schedule:

  Typhoid conjugate vaccines (Vi-PS):
  - Typbar-TCV®: Single dose at 9–12 through 23 months followed by a booster at 2 years of age
  - Pedatyph®: Single dose at 9–12 through 23 months followed by a booster at 2 years of age
  - *Vi-PS (polysaccharide) vaccines:* Single dose at 2 years; revaccination every 3 years
- Currently, two typhoid conjugate vaccines, Typbar-TCV® and PedaTyph® **are available in Indian market**
- An interval of at least 4 weeks with the MMR vaccine should be maintained while administering Typbar-TCV® and PedaTyph® **vaccines**
- Typhoid revaccination every 3 years, if Vi-polysaccharide vaccine is used
- No evidence of hyporesponsiveness on repeated revaccination of Vi-polysaccharide vaccine so far. However, typhoid conjugate vaccine should be preferred over unconjugated Vi-PS vaccine.

  Catch-up vaccination:
- Recommended throughout the adolescent period, i.e. up to 18 years of age
- Vi conjugate typhoid vaccine should be preferred over Vi-PS vaccine wherever feasible
- The need and exact timing of the booster doses are not yet determined.

14. Influenza vaccine

Routine vaccination:
- *Minimum age:*
  - 6 months for trivalent inactivated influenza vaccine (IIV)
  - 2 years for live, attenuated influenza vaccine (LAIV)
- IIV: Recommended only for the vaccination of persons with certain high-risk conditions
- LAIV: Recommended for only healthy children aged 2–18 years
- For most healthy children aged 2 through 18 years, either LAIV or IIV may be used
- LAIV should NOT be administered to following category of children:
  - Who have experienced severe allergic reactions to LAIV, any of its components, or to a previous dose of any other influenza vaccine
  - Children 2 through 17 years receiving aspirin or aspirin-containing products
  - Children with immunodeficiency
  - Children 2 through 4 years of age with asthma or who had wheezing in the past 12 months
  - Children who have taken influenza antiviral medications in the previous 48 hours
  - Children who have experienced severe allergic reactions to LAIV, any of its components
- IIV: First time vaccination: 6 months to below 9 years: two doses 1 month apart; 9 years and above: single dose
- Annual revaccination with single dose.
- LAIV: 2–9 years: One or two doses as per the ACVIP annual recommendations; 9 years and above: single dose
- *Dosage*:
  - IIV: Aged 6–35 months 0.25 mL; 3 years and above: 0.5 mL
  - LAIV: See product insert of the available formulation
- For the 2016–2017 season, since the A (H3N2) and B flu viruses have drifted, a child who has received two doses of influenza vaccine (IIV or LAIV) should receive one dose, and those who have received one dose in previous season should receive two doses of new formulation at least 4 week apart. The two doses need not have been received during the same season or consecutive seasons
- For children aged 6 months through 8 years: Administer 2 doses (separated by at least 4 weeks) to children who are receiving influenza vaccine for the first time
- All the currently available IIVs in the country contain the 'Swine flu' or 'A (H1N1)' antigen; no need to vaccinate separately
- LAIV: Not recommended for children with chronic medical conditions

- ACVIP does not endorse the superiority of LAIV over the IIV. There is not adequate data available from the country to recommend discontinuation of LAIV use in healthy individuals contrary to recent CDC ACIP recommendations
- Best time to vaccinate:
  - As soon as the new vaccine is released and available in the market
  - Just before the onset of rainy season
  - Some regions may consider vaccination just prior to onset of winters based on local epidemiology data.

15. Human papillomavirus (HPV) vaccines

Routine vaccination:
- Minimum age: 9 years
- HPV4 [Gardasil®] and HPV2 [Cervarix®] are licensed and available.
- Only 2 doses of either of the two HPV vaccines (HPV4 and HPV2) for adolescent/preadolescent girls aged 9–14 years
- For girls 15 years and older, and immunocompromised individuals 3 doses are recommended
- For two-dose schedule, the minimum interval between doses should be 6 months
- Either HPV4 (0, 2, 6 months) or HPV2 (0, 1, 6 months) is recommended in a 3-dose series for females aged 15 years and older
- HPV4 can also be given in a 3-dose series for males aged 11 or 12 years, but not yet licensed for use in males in India
- The vaccine series can be started beginning at age 9 years
- For three-dose schedule, administer the 2nd dose 1–2 months after the 1st dose and the 3rd dose 6 months after the 1st dose (at least 24 weeks after the first dose).

Catch-up vaccination:
- Administer the vaccine series to females (either HPV2 or HPV4) at age 13 through 45 years if not previously vaccinated.
- Use recommended routine dosing intervals (see above) for vaccine series catch-up.

16. Meningococcal vaccine
- Recommended only for certain high-risk group of children, during outbreaks, and international travelers, including students going for study abroad and travelers to Hajj and sub-Sahara Africa
- Both meningococcal conjugate vaccines (Quadrivalent MenACWY-D, Menactra® *by Sanofi Pasteur* and monovalent group A, PsA–TT, MenAfriVac® *by Serum Institute of India*) and polysaccharide vaccines (bi- and quadrivalent) are licensed in India. PsA–TT is not freely available in market
- Conjugate vaccines are preferred over polysaccharide vaccines due to their potential for herd protection and their increased immunogenicity, particularly in children <2 years of age
- As of today, quadrivalent conjugate and polysaccharide vaccines are recommended only for children 2 years and above. Monovalent group A conjugate vaccine, PsA–TT can be used in children above 1 year of age.

17. Cholera vaccine
- Minimum age: 1 year (inactivated whole cell *Vibrio cholerae* (Shanchol®)
- Not recommended for routine use in healthy individuals; recommended only for the vaccination of persons residing in highly endemic areas and traveling to areas where risk of transmission is very high like Kumbh mela, etc.
- Two doses 2 weeks apart for >1 year old.

18. Japanese encephalitis (JE) vaccine

Routine vaccination:
- Recommended only for individuals living in endemic areas till 18 years of age
- The vaccine should be offered to the children residing in rural areas only and those planning to visit endemic areas (depending upon the duration of stay)
- Three types of new generation JE vaccines are licensed in India: one, live attenuated, cell culture derived SA-14-14-2, and two inactivated JE vaccines, namely '**vero cell culture-derived SA 14-14-2 JE vaccine' (JEEV® by BE India) and 'vero cell culture-derived, 821564XY, JE vaccine' (JENVAC® by Bharat Biotech)**

Contd...

Contd...

- **Live attenuated, cell culture derived SA-14-14-2:**
  - Minimum age: 8 months
  - Two dose schedule, first dose at 9 months along with measles vaccine and second at 16–18 months along with DTP booster
  - Not available in private market for office use
- **Inactivated cell culture derived SA-14-14-2 (JEEV® by BE India) :**
  - Minimum age: 1 year (US-FDA: 2 months)
  - Primary immunization schedule: 2 doses of 0.25 mL each administered intramuscularly on days 0 and 28 for children aged ≥1 to ≤3 years
  - 2 doses of 0.5 mL for children >3 years and adults aged ≥18 years
  - Need of boosters still undetermined
- **Inactivated Vero cell culture-derived Kolar strain, 821564XY, JE vaccine (JENVAC® by Bharat Biotech)**
  - Minimum age: 1 year
  - Primary immunization schedule: 2 doses of 0.5 mL each administered intramuscularly at 4 weeks interval
  - Need of boosters still undetermined.

Catch up vaccination:
- All susceptible children up to 18 years should be administered during disease outbreak/ahead of anticipated outbreak in campaigns

19. Rabies vaccine
- Practically all children need vaccination against rabies
- Following two situations included in 'high-risk category of children' for rabies vaccination and should be offered 'pre-exposure prophylaxis' (Pre-EP):
  - Children having pets in home
  - Children perceived with higher threat of being bitten by dogs such as hostellers, risk of stray dog menace while going outdoor
- Only modern tissue culture vaccines (MTCVs) and IM routes are recommended for both 'postexposure' and 'pre-exposure' prophylaxis in office practice

- Post-exposure prophylaxis (PEP) is recommended following a significant contact with dogs, cats, cows, buffaloes, sheep, goats, pigs, donkeys, horses, camels, foxes, jackals, monkeys, mongoose, squirrel, bears and others. Domestic rodent (rat) bites do not require post-exposure prophylaxis in India.
- *Post-exposure prophylaxis:*
  - MTCVs are recommended for all category II and III bites
  - *Dose:* 1.0 mL intramuscular (IM) in anterolateral thigh or deltoid (never in gluteal region) for Human Diploid Cell Vaccine (HDCV), Purified Chick Embryo Cell (PCEC) vaccine, Purified Duck Embryo Vaccine (PDEV); 0.5 mL for Purified Vero Cell Vaccine (PVRV). Intradermal (ID) administration is not recommended in individual practice
  - *Schedule:* 0, 3, 7, 14, and 30 with day '0' being the day of commencement of vaccination. A sixth dose on day 90 is optional and may be offered to patients with severe debility or those who are immunosuppressed
  - Rabies immunoglobin (RIG) along with rabies vaccines are recommended in all category III bites
  - Equine rabies immunoglobin (ERIG) (dose 40 U/kg) can be used if human rabies immunoglobin is not available
- *Pre-exposure prophylaxis:*
  - Three doses are given intramuscularly in deltoid/anterolateral thigh on days 0, 7 and 28 (day 21 may be used if time is limited but day 28 preferred)
  - For re-exposure at any point of time after completed (and documented) pre or post-exposure prophylaxis, two doses are given on days 0 and 3
  - RIG is not required during re-exposure therapy.

Source: IAP Immunization Schedule 2016. Available from: http://iapindia. org/iap-immunization.php

---

Table 9.1.12: IAPCOI recommended immunization schedule for persons aged 7 through 18 years, 2016 (with range).

Age ▶ Vaccine ▼	7–10 years	11–12 years	13–18 years
Tdap[1]	1 dose (if indicated)	1 dose	1 dose (if indicated)
HPV[2]	See footnote 2	3 doses	Complete 3-dose series
MMR[3]		Complete 2-dose series	
Varicella[4]		Complete 2-dose series	
Hepatitis B[5]		Complete 3-dose series	
Hepatitis A[6]		Complete 2-dose series	
Typhoid[7]		1 dose every 3 years	
Influenza Vaccine[8]		One dose every year	
Japanese Encephalitis Vaccine[9]	Catch-up up to 15 years		
Pneumococcal Vaccine[10]		See footnote 10	
Meningococcal Vaccine[11]		See footnote 11	

▢ **Range of recommended ages for all children**   ▢ **Range of recommended ages for catch-up immunization**

▢ **Range of recommended ages for certain high-risk groups**

Any dose not administered at the recommended age should be administered at a subsequent visit, when indicated and feasible. The use of a combination vaccine generally is preferred over separate injections of its equivalent component vaccines.

---

[1] Tetanus and Diphtheria Toxoids and Acellular Pertussis (Tdap) Vaccine
- Minimum age: 10 years for Boostrix and 11 years for Adacel
- Persons aged 11 through 18 years who have not received Tdap vaccine should receive a dose followed by tetanus and diphtheria toxoids (Td) booster doses every 10 years thereafter
- Tetanus and diphtheria toxoids and acellular pertussis vaccine should be substituted for a single dose of Td in the catch-up series for children aged 7 through 10 years

- Tetanus and diphtheria toxoids and acellular pertussis vaccine can be administered regardless of the interval since the last tetanus and diphtheria toxoid–containing vaccine
- Catch up above 7 years: Tdap, Td, Td at 0, 1 and 6 months
- Tetanus and diphtheria toxoids and acellular pertussis can also be administered safely to pregnant women.

[2] Human papillomavirus (HPV) Vaccines
- HPV4 (Gardasil) and HPV2 (Cervarix)

Contd...

Contd...

- Minimum age: 9 years
- Either HPV4 (0, 2, 6 months) or HPV2 (0, 1, 6 months) is recommended in a 3-dose series for females aged 11 or 12 years
- Human papillomavirus 4 can also be given in a three-dose series for males aged 11 or 12 years
- The vaccine series can be started beginning at age 9 years
- Administer the second dose 1–2 months after the first dose and the third dose 6 months after the first dose (at least 24 weeks after the first dose).

[3] Measles, Mumps, and Rubella (MMR) Vaccine
- The minimum interval between the two doses of MMR vaccine is 4 weeks
- One dose if previously vaccinated with one dose.

[4] Varicella (VAR) Vaccine
- For persons without evidence of immunity, administer two doses if not previously vaccinated or the second dose if only 1 dose has been administered
- For persons aged 7 through 12 years, the recommended minimum interval between doses is 3 months. However, if the second dose was administered at least 4 weeks after the first dose, it can be accepted as valid
- For persons aged 13 years and older, the minimum interval between doses is 4 weeks.

[5] Hepatitis B (Hep B) Vaccine
- Administer the three-dose series to those not previously vaccinated
- For those with incomplete vaccination, the recommended minimum interval between dose 1 and dose 2 is 4 weeks, and between dose 2 and dose 3 is 8 weeks. The final (third or fourth) dose in the Hep B vaccine series should be administered at least 16 weeks after the first dose.

[6] Hepatitis A (Hep A) Vaccine
- Administer two doses at least 6 months apart to unvaccinated persons
- For catch up vaccination, pre vaccination screening for Hepatitis A antibody is recommended in children older than 10 years as at this age the estimated seropositive rates exceed 50%
- Combination of Hep B and Hep A may be used in 0, 1, 6 schedule.

[7] Typhoid Vaccine
- Only Vi-PS (polysaccharide) vaccine is recommended
- Vi-PS conjugate vaccine: data not sufficient to recommend for routine use of currently available vaccine
- A minimum interval of 3 years should be observed between two doses of typhoid vaccine.

[8] Influenza Vaccine
- Administer one dose to persons aged 9 years and older
- For children aged 6 months through 8 years
- For the 2012 season, administer two doses (separated by at least 4 weeks) to those who did not receive at least 1 dose of the 2010–11 vaccine. Those who received at least 1 dose of the 2010–11 vaccine require 1 dose for the 2011–12 season
- Annual revaccination with single dose
- Best time to vaccinate: as soon as the new vaccine is released and available in the market and just before the onset of rainy season.

[9] Japanese Encephalitis Vaccine
- Only in endemic area as catch up
- Currently no type of JE vaccine available in private Indian market
- Live attenuated, cell culture derived SA-14-14-2 JE vaccine should be preferred,
- Dose: 0.5 mL, SC, single dose up to 15 years

[10] Pneumococcal Vaccines
- Pneumococcal conjugate vaccine (PCV) and pneumococcal polysaccharide vaccine (PPSV) both are used in certain high risk group of children
- A single dose of PCV may be administered to children aged 6 through 18 years who have anatomic/functional asplenia, HIV infection or other immunocompromising condition, cochlear implant, or cerebral spinal fluid leak
- Administer PPSV at least 8 weeks after the last dose of PCV to children aged 2 years or older with certain underlying medical conditions, including a cochlear implant
- A single re-vaccination (with PPSV) should be administered after 5 years to children with anatomic/functional asplenia or an immunocompromising condition.

[11] Meningococcal Vaccine
- Recommended only for certain high risk group of children, during outbreaks, travelers to endemic areas, and students going for study abroad.
- Only meningococcal polysaccharide vaccine (MPSV) is available
- Minimum age is 2 years
- Dose schedule: a single dose 0.5 mL SC/IM is recommended
- Revaccination only once after 3 years in those at continued high risk.

Source: IAP Immunization Schedule 2016. Available from: http://iapindia.org/iap-immunization.php

Determinants of Optimal Immunization Schedules

They can be summarized in three heads:

1. Immunological

- Minimum age at which vaccine elicit immune response
- Number of doses required
- Interval between doses, if multiple doses are required.

2. Epidemiological

- Susceptibility for infection and disease
- Disease severity and mortality.

3. Programmatic

- Opportunity to deliver with other scheduled intervention
- Increase coverage by limiting the required contacts.

Balance between immunological and epidemiological determinants is mandatory. One should aim for achieving protective immune response prior to the age when children are most vulnerable. There should be balance between inducing reasonable protection prior to vulnerable age versus inducing optimal immune response. For example, starting late, might induce a higher response, but miss the vulnerable age. Wider intervals between doses give a better response, but delays induction of immunity, leaving children vulnerable in a crucial period of life. Further, the disease epidemiology varies in different populations. A schedule that is used in one population is not the best for another; need to individualize and tailor to suit local needs.

Determinants for Requirement of Doses of Different Vaccines

Number of doses required varies by vaccine: live vaccines induce immunity with a single dose; inactivated vaccines require multiple doses (initial doses to prime and later doses to boost). Some live vaccines induce immunity in small proportion of vaccines, requiring multiple doses to induce good immunity, e.g. OPV.

Number of doses required may also vary by age; more doses of conjugate vaccines required in young infants. In general, a larger interval between doses induces a higher level of antibody (although not provide better

Table 9.1.13: IAP Immunization Timetable 2016.

I. IAP recommended vaccines for routine use

Age (completed weeks/months/years)	Vaccines	Comments
Birth	BCG OPV 0 Hep-B 1	Administer these vaccines to all newborns before hospital discharge
6 weeks	DTwP 1 IPV 1 Hep-B 2 Hib 1 Rotavirus 1 PCV 1	**DTP:** • DTaP vaccine/combinations should preferably be avoided for the primary series • DTaP vaccine/combinations should be preferred in certain specific circumstances/conditions only • No need of repeating/giving additional doses of whole-cell pertussis (wP) vaccine to a child who has earlier completed their primary schedule with acellular pertussis (aP) vaccine-containing products **Polio:** • All doses of IPV may be replaced with OPV if administration of the former is unfeasible • Additional doses of OPV on all supplementary immunization activities (SIAs) • Two doses of IPV instead of 3 for primary series if started at 8 weeks, and 8 weeks interval between the doses • No child should leave the facility without polio immunization (IPV or OPV), if indicated by the schedule • See footnotes under Table titled IAP recommended immunization schedule (with range) for recommendations on intradermal IPV **Rotavirus:** • 2 doses of RV1 and 3 doses of RV5 and RV 116E • RV1 should be employed in 10 and 14 week schedule, 10 and 14 week schedule of RV1 is found to be more immunogenic than 6 and 10 week schedule
10 weeks	DTwP 2 IPV 2 Hib 2 Rotavirus 2 PCV 2	**Rotavirus:** If RV1 is chosen, the first dose should be given at 10 weeks
14 weeks	DTwP 3 IPV 3 Hib 3 Rotavirus 3 PCV 3	**Rotavirus:** • Only 2 doses of RV1 are recommended • If RV1 is chosen, the 2nd dose should be given at 14 weeks
6 months	OPV 1 Hep-B 3	**Hepatitis B:** The final (3rd or 4th) dose in the Hep B vaccine series should be administered no earlier than age 24 weeks and at least 16 weeks after the first dose
9 months	OPV 2 MMR-1	**MMR:** • Measles-containing vaccine ideally should not be administered before completing 270 days or 9 months of life • The 2nd dose must follow in 2nd year of life • No need to give stand-alone measles vaccine
9–12 months	Typhoid conjugate vaccine	• Currently, two typhoid conjugate vaccines, Typbar-TCV® and PedaTyph® **available in Indian market;** either can be used • An interval of at least 4 weeks with the MMR vaccine should be maintained while administering this vaccine
12 months	Hep-A 1	**Hepatitis A:** • Single dose for live attenuated H2-strain Hep-A vaccine • Two doses for all inactivated Hep-A vaccines are recommended
15 months	MMR 2 Varicella 1 PCV booster	**MMR:** • The 2nd dose must follow in 2nd year of life • However, it can be given at anytime 4–8 weeks after the 1st dose **Varicella:** The risk of breakthrough varicella is lower if given 15 months onwards
16–18 months	DTwP B1/DTaP B1 IPV B1 Hib B1	The first booster (4th dose) may be administered as early as age 12 months, provided at least 6 months have elapsed since the third dose. **DTP:** • 1st and 2nd boosters should preferably be of DTwP • Considering a higher reactogenicity of DTwP, DTaP can be considered for the boosters

Contd...

Contd...

18 months	Hep-A 2	**Hepatitis A:** 2nd dose for inactivated vaccines only
2 years	Booster of typhoid conjugate vaccine	• A booster dose of typhoid conjugate vaccine (TCV), if primary dose is given at 9–12 months • A dose of typhoid Vi-polysaccharide (Vi-PS) vaccine can be given if conjugate vaccine is not available or feasible • Revaccination every 3 years with Vi-polysaccharide vaccine • Typhoid conjugate vaccine should be preferred over Vi- PS vaccine
4–6 years	DTwP B2/DTaP B2 OPV 3 Varicella 2 MMR 3	**Varicella:** The 2nd dose can be given at anytime 3 months after the 1st dose **MMR:** The 3rd dose is recommended at 4–6 years of age
10–12 years	Tdap/Td HPV	**Tdap:** It is preferred to Td followed by Td every 10 years **HPV:** • Only 2 doses of either of the two HPV vaccines for adolescent/preadolescent girls aged 9–14 years • For girls 15 years and older, and immunocompromised individuals 3 doses are recommended • For two-dose schedule, the minimum interval between doses should be 6 months. • For 3 dose schedule, the doses can be administered at 0, 1–2 (depending on brand) and 6 months

II. IAP recommended vaccines for high-risk* children (Vaccines under special circumstances)#

1. Influenza vaccine
2. Meningococcal vaccine
3. Japanese encephalitis vaccine
4. Cholera vaccine
5. Rabies vaccine
6. Yellow fever vaccine
7. Pneumococcal polysaccharide vaccine (PPSV 23)

* High-risk category of children
• Congenital or acquired immunodeficiency (including HIV infection)
• Chronic cardiac, pulmonary (including asthma if treated with prolonged high-dose oral corticosteroids), hematologic, renal (including nephrotic syndrome), liver disease and diabetes mellitus
• Children on long-term steroids, salicylates, immunosuppressive or radiation therapy
• Diabetes mellitus, cerebrospinal fluid leak, cochlear implant, malignancies
• Children with functional/anatomic asplenia/hyposplenia
• During disease outbreaks
• Laboratory personnel and healthcare workers
• Travelers
• Children having pets in home
• Children perceived with higher threat of being bitten by dogs such as hostellers, risk of stray dog menace while going outdoor.
#For details see footnotes under Table titled 'IAP recommended immunization schedule (with range)'

Source: IAP Immunization Schedule 2016. Available from: http://iapindia.org/iap-immunization.php

immunity). Duration of immunity and requirement for additional doses is needed either to boost or to reinduce immunity (for T-cell independent antigens). But one needs to differentiate between decay in antibody level and immunity.

Designing vaccination schedules is indeed a trade-off which can be on efficacy, safety or cost. First aim of vaccination program is to prevent serious disease (in absolute numbers, severity or both). Second aim is to reduce the spread of infection.

Considerations in Deciding the Age of Administration of Vaccines

This may vary from place to place and country to country. Optimal response to a vaccine depends on a number of factors:

• Nature of the vaccine-killed, live, PS
• Age and immune status of the recipient, i.e. ability of persons of a certain age to respond to the vaccine and potential interference with the immune response by passively transferred maternal antibody or previously administered antibody containing blood products
• Age-specific risks for disease; age-specific risks for complications.
• Vaccines usually are recommended for members of the youngest age group at risk for experiencing the disease for which efficacy and safety have been demonstrated.

Vaccination schedules for different countries may be different primarily due to prevalence of different communicable diseases in different countries. In India, yellow fever disease is not prevalent, so there is no need to administer vaccine against yellow fever disease. This vaccine is recommended to those persons who have to travel to those countries where this disease occurs, e.g. sub-Saharan countries in Africa and Saudi Arabia during Haj pilgrimage. Similarly, typhoid disease does not occur in many developed countries because of good sanitation and clean drinking water, so typhoid vaccine is not administered in routine, but people are advised to take typhoid vaccine prior to traveling to a place where typhoid disease occurs. Even BCG vaccine is not administered in routine at birth in most of the developed countries. Thus, vaccines are recommended to prevent the vaccine preventable diseases according to the disease burden in a population, so some vaccines may be discontinued while new vaccines may be introduced from time to time as epidemiology of diseases changes. Some vaccines are administered universally, e.g. vaccines against polio, diphtheria, tetanus, pertussis, measles and hepatitis B diseases.

BIBLIOGRAPHY

Principles of Vaccination

1. Epidemiology and Prevention of Vaccine-Preventable Diseases. The Pink Book: Course Textbook, 12th edition (April 2011). [online] Available from http://www.cdc.gov/vaccines/pubs/pinkbook/index.html#chapters [Accessed October 2012].
2. Plotkin SA. Vaccines, vaccination, and vaccinology. J Infect Dis. 2003;187:1349-59.
3. Plotkin SA. Vaccines: correlates of vaccine-induced immunity. Clin Infect Dis. 2008;47:401-9.
4. Siegrist CA. Vaccine immunology. In: Plotkin SA, Orenstein WA, Offit PA (Eds). Vaccines, 5th edition. China: Saunders. 2008.pp.17-36.
5. Vashishtha VM, Kalra A, Thacker N (Eds). FAQs on Vaccines and Immunization Practices, 1st edition. New Delhi: Jaypee Brothers, 2011.
6. Yewale VN, Choudhury P, Thacker N (Eds). IAP Guide Book on Immunization, 5th edition. IAP Committee on Immunization. Mumbai: Indian Academy of Pediatrics, 2011.

Elementary Epidemiology

7. Bonita R, Beaglehole R, Kjellstrom T (Eds). Basic Epidemiology, 2nd edition.World Health Organization; Geneva, 2006.
8. Chen RT, Hausinger S, Dajani AS, et al. Seroprevalence of antibody against poliovirus in inner city preschool children. JAMA. 1996;275:1639-45.
9. Halsey NA, Moulton LH, O'Donovan C, et al. Hepatitis B vaccine administered to children and adolescents at yearly intervals. Pediatrics. 1999;103:1243-7.
10. Paul Y. Herd immunity and herd protection. Vaccine. 2004;22:301-2.
11. Paul Y. Vaccines for whose benefit? Indian J Med Ethics. 2010;7:30-1.
12. Singhal T, Amdekar YK, Agarval RK (Eds). IAP Guide Book on Immunization, 4th edition. IAP Committee on Immunization. New Delhi: Jaypee Brothers, 2009.
13. Thacker N, Shendurkar N. Childhood Immunization-Issues and Options, 1st edition. New Delhi: Incal Communications, 2005.

Adverse Events Following Immunization

14. Rao IM. Adverse events following immunization.Indian J Pediatr. 2006;8(3):208-19.
15. World Health Organization. Immunization, Vaccines and Biologicals-Module 3: Immunization safety. Training manual for mid-level managers (MLM); 2008. [online] Available from: www.who.int/vaccines-documents/(WHO/IVB/08.03).
16. Yewale VN, Choudhury P, Thacker N (Eds). IAP Guide Book on Immunization, 5th edition. IAP Committee on Immunization. Mumbai: Indian Academy of Pediatrics, 2011.

General Guidelines for Immunization

17. American Academy of Pediatrics.Active and passive immunization. In: Pickering LK, Baker CJ, Kimberlin DW, Long SS, (Eds). Red Book: 2009 Report of the Committee on Infectious Diseases, 28th edition. Elk Grove Village, IL: American Academy of Pediatrics, 2009.
18. Atkinson WL, Kroger AT, Pickering LK. General immunization practices. In: Plotkin SA, OrentseinWA, Offit PA (Eds). Vaccines, 5th edition. China: Saunders, 2008.
19. Centers for Disease Control and Prevention (CDC). General Recommendations on Immunization, Recommendations of the Advisory Committee on Immunization Practices (ACIP). MMWR. 2011;60(no. RR-2):1-61. [online] Available from http://www.cdc.gov/mmwr/pdf/rr/rr6002.pdf [Accessed April, 2012].
20. General Recommendations on Immunization. Epidemiology and Prevention of Vaccine-Preventable Diseases, The Pink Book: Course Textbook, 12th edition (April 2011). [online] Available from http://www.cdc.gov/vaccines/pubs/pinkbook/genrec.html [Accessed October, 2012].
21. King GE, Hadler SC. Simultaneous administration of childhood vaccines: an important public health policy that is safe and efficacious. Pediatr Infect Dis J. 1994;13:394-407.

Vaccination in Special Situations

22. American Academy of Pediatrics. Red Book: 2006 Report of the Committee on Infectious Diseases, 27th edition. Elk Grove Village, Ill: AAP, 2006.
23. Mitra M. Vaccination in special situations. In: Vashishtha VM, Kalra A, Thacker N (Eds). FAQs on Vaccines and Immunization Practices, 1st edition. New Delhi: Jaypee Brothers; 2011. pp.54-63.

Vaccination Schedules

24. Agarwal A, Paul Y, Pandya P. Vaccination schedules. In: Vashishtha VM, Kalra A, Thacker N (Eds). FAQs on Vaccines and Immunization Practices, 1st edition. New Delhi: Jaypee Brothers, 2011.pp.32-40.
25. Centers for Disease Control and Prevention. Vaccine schedule.MMWR. 2000;49(No. RR-10):1-147.
26. National Immunization Schedule (NIS) for Infants, Children and Pregnant Women. [online] Available from http://whoindia.org/LinkFiles/Routine_Immunization_National_Immunization_Schedule.pdf.

9.2 IMMUNIZATION IN A NORMAL CHILD

Baldev S Prajapati, Rajal B Prajapati

INTRODUCTION

Immunization is one of the most cost-effective health interventions known to mankind. It is also true that immunization is the most successful, single, child survival strategy to date. As a result of effective and safe vaccines, smallpox has been eradicated; polio is close to worldwide eradication. A successful immunization program is of particular relevance to India, as the country contributes to one-fourth of global under-five mortalities with a significant number of deaths attributable to vaccine preventable diseases. There is no doubt that substantial progress has been achieved in India with wider use of vaccines, resulting in prevention of several diseases. However, lot remains to be done and in some situations, progress has not been sustained. Upgrading immunization is the need of the hour to help bringing down under-five mortalities. It is learnt that in the United States the incidence of most vaccine preventable diseases of childhood has been reduced by >99% from the annual morbidity prior to development of corresponding vaccine. Our country needs implementation of best efforts in the right direction to achieve this goal.

Immunization is the process of inducing immunity against a specific disease. Immunity can be induced either passively through administration of preformed antibodies containing preparations or actively by administering a vaccine or toxoid to stimulate the immune system to produce a prolonged humoral and/or cellular immune response. Passive immunity is achieved by administration of preformed antibodies to offer transient protection against infectious agent. Products used include immunoglobulins (administered by IV or IM route) and specific or hyperimmuneimmunoglobulins. Active immunization is performed by administering vaccines. This chapter includes active immunization in a normal and healthy child.

VACCINES

Vaccines are defined as whole or parts of microorganisms administered to prevent an infectious disease. Vaccines can consist of whole inactivated microorganisms [e.g. injectible polio vaccination (IPV), hepatitis A], parts of the organism [e.g. acellular pertussis, human papillomaviruses (HPV) and Hep B], polysaccharide capsules (e.g. pneumococcal and meningococcal polysaccharide vaccines), polysaccharide capsules conjugated to protein carriers (e.g. Hib, pneumococcal, meningococcal conjugate vaccines), live attenuated microorganisms [measles, mumps, rubella, varicella, oral polio vaccine, rotavirus and live attenuated influenza vaccines and toxoids (tetanus and diphtheria)]. Attenuated vaccines are prepared by nullifying or minimizing pathogenicity (capacity of producing disease) of the organism and maintaining or enhancing its immunogenicity (capacity of producing antibodies).

The vaccines contain a variety of other constituents besides the immunizing agents. Suspending fluids may be sterile water or saline but could be a complex fluid containing small amounts of proteins or other compositions derived from the biologic system used to grow the immunobiologic. Preservatives, stabilizers and antimicrobial agents are used to prevent degradation of the antigen and to inhibit bacterial growth; such components can be gelatin, 2-phenoxyethanol and various antimicrobial agents. Adjuvants are used in some vaccines to enhance the immune response. Mainly aluminum salts are used as adjuvants. Vaccines with adjuvants should be injected deep into muscle mass to avoid local irritation, granuloma formation and necrosis associated with subcutaneous (SC) administration.

Vaccines induce immunity by stimulating antibody formation, cellular immunity or both. Protection induced by most vaccines is thought to be mediated primarily by B lymphocytes which produce antibodies. Most B lymphocyte responses require the assistance of CD_4 helper T lymphocytes. These T lymphocytes-dependent responses tend to induce high levels of functional antibody with high avidity, mature over the time from primarily an IgM response to long-term persistent IgG and induce immunologic memory that leads to enhanced responses upon boosting. T lymphocyte dependent vaccines, which include protein antigens, induce good immune responses even in young infants. In contrast, polysaccharide antigens induce B lymphocyte responses in the absence of T lymphocyte help. These T-cell independent vaccines are associated with poor immune responses in children less than 2 years of age, short-term immunity and absence of an enhanced or booster response on repeat exposure to the antigen. To overcome problems of plain polysaccharide vaccines, conjugate vaccines induce higher avidity antibody, immunologic memory leading to booster responses on repeat exposure to the antigen, long-term immunity and herd immunity by decreasing carriage of the organism.

Serum antibodies may be detected by 7–10 days after injecting the antigen. Early antibodies are usually of the IgM class. IgM antibodies tend to decline as IgG antibodies increase. The IgG antibodies tend to peak approximately 1 month after the vaccination and with most vaccines persist for some time after a primary vaccine course. Secondary or booster responses occur more rapidly and result from rapid proliferation of memory B and T lymphocytes.

Live attenuated vaccines tend to induce long-term immune responses. They replicate often similar to natural infections. Most live vaccines are administered in one or two dose schedules. The purpose of repeat doses is to induce an initial immune response in persons who failed to respond to the first dose. The inactivated vaccines tend to require multiple doses to induce an adequate immune response and are more likely to need booster doses to maintain the immunity. However, some inactivated vaccines appear to induce long-term immunity, perhaps lifelong immunity after a primary series, including hepatitis B and inactivated polio vaccine.

PRACTICAL ASPECTS OF IMMUNIZATION

Communicating with Parents or Care Givers

With several newer vaccines available in the market, it is a difficult task for the pediatricians to offer an ideal advice to parents regarding pros and cons of each vaccine. The pediatricians are required to communicate properly with clarity and appropriate information that should help parents make their own decision appropriately. Risk of developing disease, efficacy of vaccine, safety of vaccine and cost of vaccine should be discussed with the parents.

TECHNICAL ASPECTS OF INJECTION

Sterile Technique and Injection Safety

- Handwashing with soap and water for 2 minutes using standard six steps technique is standard technique. Alcohol based antiseptic hand rub is another alternative. Gloves may not be worn while administering vaccines, unless the person administering the vaccine has open lesions on hands or likely to come in contact with potentially infectious body fluids
- Needles used for injections must be sterile and preferably disposable. Autodisable syringes are single use, self-locking syringes designed in such a way that they are rendered unusable after single use
- A separate needle and syringe should be used for each injection
- Changing needles between drawing vaccine from a vial and injecting it into a recipient is not necessary
- If multidose vials are used, the septum should be swabbed with alcohol prior to each withdrawal. The needle should not be let in stopper in between uses
- Different vaccines should never be mixed in the same syringe unless specifically licensed for such use
- To prevent inadvertent needle-stick injury or reuse, needles and syringes should be discarded immediately after use in labeled, puncture-proof containers located in the same room where vaccine is administered. Needles should not be recapped before being discarded
- It should be checked before using the vaccine that its cold chain is maintained throughout.

Injection Route, Site, Method and Needle Length (Table 9.2.1)

Bacillus Calmette–Guérin (BCG) is given by intradermal (ID) route. Recently antirabies vaccine is also started by intradermal route besides intramuscular (IM) route. The dosages of antirabies vaccine for both the routes are different. Measles, MMR, varicella, meningococcal polysaccharide, Japanese encephalitis and yellow fever vaccines are given by SC route. Rest of the vaccines is given by IM route. Generally, there is no harm done if SC vaccines are given by IM route. However, vaccines recommended to be given by IM route, should not be given by SC route due to risk of side effects (as seen with aluminum adjuvanted vaccines) or reduced efficacy (due to less blood supply in SC tissue and hence reduced immunogenicity).

In children less than 3 years, the vaccines by IM should be given on anterolateral aspect of mid-thigh (middle one-third part from greater trochanter to lateral condyle of femur bone) in vastus lateralis muscle. In older children (> 3 years of age) vaccines by IM route can be given in deltoid muscle (mid-point from acromion process to insertion of deltoid). The gluteal region should never be used for administration of IM vaccines due to ineffective efficacy of vaccines like hepatitis B and rabies vaccines. If a vaccine and immune globulin preparation are administered simultaneously [e.g. Hep B and hepatitis B immune globulin (HBIG)], they should be given on different thighs. If more than one vaccine is given on the same thigh, minimum distance between two vaccines should be kept of more than 2.5 cm so that any local reaction can be differentiated. The location of each injection should be documented in the patient's medical record.

	Site	Type of needle	Comments
Table 9.2.1: Injection site, type of needle and technique.			
Intramuscular injections (needle should enter at 90° angle)			
Infants	Anterolateral thigh (middle-third of greater trochanter to lateral condyle of femur)	23–24 G, 1 inch	Skin should be stretched between thumb and finger
Older children (>3 years)	Deltoid or anterolateral thigh	23 G, 1 inch	Skin should be stretched between thumb and finger
Adolescents and adults	Deltoid or anterolateral thigh	22 or 23 G, 1.5 inch	Skin should be stretched between thumb and finger
Subcutaneous injections (needle should be at 45° to the skin)			
All ages	Thigh	25 G, 0.5 inch	
Intradermal injections (needle should be at 30° to the skin)			
All ages	Left deltoid	26 G, 0.5 inch	5 mm wheal should be raised

When injection site is used as per recommendation, where no large blood vessels exist, confirmation of puncture to blood vessel by pulling the piston is no more recommended. After administering the vaccine, the needle should be withdrawn after 10 seconds to prevent backflow of vaccine into the needle track. The injection site should be pressed firmly for few minutes with cotton swab, and it should not be rubbed.

For IM injections, the 23 gauge, 1 inch long needle is used. The length of needle should be 1.5 inches in adolescents and adults. ID injection should be given by 26 gauge needle and SC by 25 gauge needle.

After giving any vaccine, the recipient should be observed for at least 15 minutes for any adverse effect. All resuscitative equipments should be kept ready for possible anaphylaxis. The parents should be counseled about possible side effects, their management and danger signs before the vaccinee is sent home. For pain and fever, paracetamol in the dose of 15 mg/kg/dose should be prescribed.

The vaccine administrator must record the type of vaccine, brand name, batch number, date of administration of the vaccine, etc. in the patient's medical record file or immunization card. The date for the next vaccine should be written in the record.

IMMUNIZATION SCHEDULE

Expanded Program of Immunization (EPI) and Universal Immunization Program (UIP)

Following the WHO recommendation, India introduced six vaccines [BCG, diphtheria, pertussis, tetanus (DPT), oral polio vaccine (OPV), diphtheria and tetanus (DT), tetanus toxoid (TT) and typhoid] under EPI in 1978 to reduce child mortality. Subsequently in 1985, the Indian government included measles vaccination and launched UIP and a mission to achieve immunization coverage to all infants and pregnant women by the 1990s. The NIP comprises of those vaccines that are given free of cost to all children of the country under UIP.

Bacillus Calmette–Guérin Vaccine

Vaccine

Bacillus Calmette-Guérin vaccine is supplied as a lyophilized (freeze-dried) preparation in vacuum sealed, multidose, dark colored ampoules or 2 mL vials with normal saline as diluent. the BCG vaccine is light sensitive and deteriorates on exposure to ultraviolet rays. In lyophilized form, it can be stored at 2–8°C for up to 12 months without losing its potency. The long necked, BCG ampule, should be cut carefully by gradual filling at the junction of its neck and body as sudden gush of air in the vacuum sealed ampoule may lead to spillage of the contents. Normal saline supplied as diluent should be used to reconstitute it. As the vaccine does not contain preservative, bacterial contamination and subsequent toxic shock syndrome may occur if kept for long after reconstitution. The reconstituted vaccine should be stored at 2–8°C, protected from light and discarded within 4–6 hours of reconstitution, if not used.

Site, Route of Administration and Dosage

It is administered at left shoulder by intradermal route by 26 G needle. The dose is 0.1 mL. Dose does not depend on the age and weight of the baby. The injection site may be cleaned by saline swab. Local antiseptic solutions should not be used. A wheal of 5 mm at injection site indicates successful intradermal administration of the vaccine. Subsequently, the wheal subsides within 30 minutes and it does not show visible changes for several days. Subcutaneous administration of BCG is associated with an increased incidence of BCG adenitis.

Classical BCG Reaction

After 2–3 weeks of BCG vaccination, a papule develops which increases to a size of 4–8 mm by the end of 5–6 weeks. It gets converted into the pustule within few days. The pustule bursts open and again gets sealed off. The bursting open and sealing off may continue for multiple times and at the end it dries up and crust is formed. The crust falls off and a tinny, thin scar of few millimeters is formed. It takes about 6–12 weeks' time. Axillary or cervical lymphadenopathy may develop a few weeks or months after BCG vaccination. The nodes may regress spontaneously and there is no need of antituberculous drug therapy. In some children, there may be an abscess formation which may require surgical removal or repeated needle aspiration, again antituberculous drugs are not recommended. Disseminated BCG infection is unusual but may develop in children with cellular immunodeficiency. BCG should be avoided in immunocompromised children. It may however be given at birth in children born to HIV positive mothers. BCG may be given with all vaccines on same day or at any interval with the exception of measles and MMR vaccines where a gap of 4 weeks between the two vaccines is recommended.

Recommendations for Use

- At birth (for institutional deliveries) or at 6 weeks with other vaccines
- Catch-up vaccination with BCG is recommended till the age of 5 years. Routine tuberculin testing prior to catch-up vaccination is not necessary
- BCG may be repeated once in children less than 5 years of age in the absence of scar presuming that BCG has not been taken up (although most children with absent scars have shown in vitro evidence of cell mediated immunity against tuberculosis). Again, tuberculin testing prior to administration of the second dose of BCG is not necessary.
- Even if BCG scar does not develop following second dose of BCG vaccination, third dose of BCG should not be given.

Polio Vaccines

Two types of polio vaccines are available: (1) Oral polio vaccine (OPV) and (2) inactivated polio vaccine (IPV). The Global Polio Eradication Initiative was launched in 1988 using OPV as the eradication tool and employing a four pronged strategy comprising high routine immunization coverage, supplementary immunization activities (SIAs), pulse immunization, acute flaccid paralysis (AFP) surveillance and Mop-up immunization. The initiative is highly successful with reduction of polio cases. Wild virus type 2 has not been isolated since 1999. In 2005, new monovalent polio vaccines (MOPV) (type 1 and type 3) were licensed and used to enhance the impact of SIAs. Bivalent polio vaccines (bOPV) comprising type 1 and type 3 polioviruses have also been developed since 2010 for pulse immunization. With intelligent use of MOPV and bOPV, the total number of wild polio cases has reduced dramatically.

Vaccines

Oral polio vaccine: OPV is a trivalent vaccine consisting of attenuated poliovirus types 1, 2 and 3 grown in monkey kidney cell cultures and stabilized with magnesium chloride. It is presented in a buffered salt solution, with light pink color indicating the right pH. It is a heat sensitive vaccine and strictly the cold chain should be maintained. It is given orally and the dose is two drops. OPV is contraindicated in immunodeficient children and their household contacts.

Inactivated polio vaccine: IPV is formaldehyde killed poliovirus, grown in monkey kidney cell or human diploid cells. Old IPV contained 20, 8 and 32 D antigen units of types 1, 2 and 3 polioviruses respectively. All currently available IPV vaccines are enhanced potency IPV (eIPV) which contains 40, 8 and 32 D antigen units of types 1, 2 and 3 respectively. The vaccine should be stored at 2–8°C. The dose is 0.5 ml IM. It is highly immunogenic. Seroconversion rates are 90–100% after two doses given after the age of 2 months and at 2 months interval or in the EPI schedule at 6, 10 and 14 weeks. IPV can be administered along with all other childhood vaccines and can be used in combination with DTwP/DTaP, Hib and Hep B vaccines without compromising seroconversion or increasing side effects. It is very safe vaccine. Mucosal immunity and herd effect with OPV and IPV are excellent.

Recommendations for Use

In the light of remarkable achievement in the field of polio eradication in India, the IAP Committee on Immunization (IAPCOI) has decided to adopt a sequential IPV-OPV schedule. This will pave the way to ultimate adoption of all-IPV schedule in future considering the inevitable cessation of OPV from immunization schedules owing to its safety issues (VAPP and cVDPVs). This policy is in accordance with the recent decision taken by global polio eradication initiative (GPEI) where phased removal of Sabin viruses, beginning with highest risk (type 2) would be undertaken. This will result in elimination of VDPV type 2 in 'parallel' with eradication of last wild polioviruses by switching from tOPV to bOPV for routine EPI and campaigns. The sequential schedules that provide IPV first, followed by OPV, can prevent VAPP while maintaining the critical benefits conferred by OPV (i.e. high levels of gut immunity). The committee has retained the birth dose of OPV as recommended earlier. A birth dose of OPV is considered necessary in countries where the risk of poliovirus transmission is high.

The primary schedule: The committee recommends birth dose of OPV, three primary doses of IPV at 6, 10 and 14 weeks, followed by two doses of OPV at 6 and 9 months, another dose (booster) of IPV at 15–18 months and OPV at 5 years.

Alternatively, two doses of IPV can be used for primary series at 8 and 16 weeks, although this schedule is immunologically superior to EPI schedule and the number of IPV doses is reduced, but will be more cumbersome due to extra visits and incompatibility with combination formulations. Further, the child would be susceptible to wild poliovirus (WPV) infection for the first 2 months of life.

Since IPV administered to infants in EPI schedule (i.e. 6 weeks, 10 weeks and 14 weeks) results in suboptimal seroconversion, hence, a supplementary dose of IPV is recommended at 15–18 months. IPV should be given intramuscularly (preferably) or subcutaneously and may be offered as a component of fixed combinations of vaccines. If IPV is unaffordable or unavailable, the primary series must be completed with three doses of OPV given at 6, 10 and 14 weeks. No child should be left without adequate protection against wild poliovirus (i.e. three doses of either vaccine). All OPV doses (monovalent, bivalent or trivalent) offered through supplemental immunization activities (SIAs) should also be provided.

Catch-up schedule: IPV may be offered as 'catch-up vaccination' for children less than 5 years of age who have completed primary immunization with OPV. IPV can be given as three doses; two doses at 2 months interval followed by a third dose after 6 months. This schedule will ensure a long lasting protection against poliovirus disease.

Dose and Schedule

Child who has not received any polio vaccination so far: OPV at birth, OPV and IPV at 6, 10 and 14 weeks. OPV and IPV at 15–18 months and OPV at 5 years. OPV on all NIDs and SNIDs. An alternative to this schedule is birth dose of OPV, OPV at 6 weeks, OPV and IPV at 10 weeks, OPV at 14 weeks and IPV at 18 weeks, OPV and IPV at 15–18 months, OPV at 5 years and OPV on all NIDs and SNIDs. In this schedule through the number of IPV doses have reduced from four to three but it (a) is logistically more demanding as number of visits increase, (b) is not feasible if combination vaccines are chosen.

Child who has completed primary series of OPV: IPV may be offered as catch-up vaccination for children less than 5 years of age who have completed primary immunization with OPV. IPV can be given two doses at 2 months interval. OPV need not be given with these IPV doses. OPV should be given with the first and second boosters of DTP and on all NIDs and SNIDs.

Immunodeficient children and their close contacts: IPV should be the preferred vaccine especially in patients with B-cell immunodeficiency if resources permit. OPV should be avoided. The schedules are as discussed earlier with the exception that a second booster dose of IPV at 5 years is also recommended.

Diphtheria, Tetanus and Pertussis Vaccines

DTwP Vaccine

DTwP vaccine, known as triple antigen, is composed of diphtheria and tetanus toxoids as well as killed whole cell pertussis bacilli adsorbed on insoluble aluminum salts which act as adjuvants. The content of diphtheria toxoid varies from 20 to 30 Lf and that of tetanus toxoid varies from 5 to 25 Lf/dose. It should be stored at 2–8°C. It should never be frozen, if frozen accidentally, should be discarded. The dose is 0.5 mL by deep IM on anterolateral aspect of thigh. Immunity against all three components wanes over the next 6–12 years and therefore regular boosting is needed.

Most adverse effects are due to the pertussis component. Minor adverse effects like pain, swelling and redness at local site, fever, fussiness, anorexia and vomiting are reported in almost half the vaccinees after any of the three primary doses. Serious adverse effects have been reported with DTwP vaccine but are rare. These are fever more than 40.5°C, hypotonic hyporesponsive episodes (HHE), seizures and encephalopathy. The frequency of systemic reactions reduces and that of local reactions increases with increasing number of doses. Children with history of reaction following vaccination are more likely to experience a reaction following future doses. Catastrophic side effects such as sudden infant death syndrome (SIDS), autism, chronic neurologic damage, infantile spasms, learning disorders and Reye's syndrome were attributed to the whole cell vaccine in the past. It has now been proved beyond doubt that whole cell pertussis vaccine is not associated with any of these adverse events.

Absolute contraindications to any pertussis vaccine are history of anaphylaxis or development of encephalopathy within 7 days following previous DTwP vaccination. Events such as persistent inconsolable crying for more than 3 hours duration, hyperpyrexia (fever > 40.5°C), HHE within 48 hours of DTwP administration and seizures with or without fever within 72 hours of administration of DTwP are considered as precautions but not contraindications to future doses of DTwP because these events generally do not recur with the next dose and they have not been proven

to cause permanent sequelae. Progressive neurological illness is relative contraindication to the first dose of DTwP immunization. However, DTwP can be safely given to children with stable neurologic disorders.

Recommendations for use: The standard schedule is three primary doses at 6, 10 and 14 weeks and two boosters at 15–18 months and 5 years. The schedule for catch-up vaccination is three doses 0, 1 and 6 months. The second childhood booster is not required if the last dose has been given beyond the age of 4 years. DTwP is not recommended in children more than 7 years of age due to increased risk of side effects. It is essential to immunize the children recovering from diphtheria, tetanus and pertussis as natural disease does not offer complete protection.

DTaP Vaccine

The components of pertussis bacilli used for preparation of the acellular vaccines include pertussis toxin (PT) as the essential component with or without filamentous hemagglutinin (FHA), pertactin (PRN) and fimbrial hemagglutinins 1, 2 and 3 (FIM). Commercially available vaccines vary in numbers of components, quantity of components and method of inactivation of the components. All currently licensed acellular pertussis vaccines have similar efficacy irrespective of number of components, their concentration and method of inactivation of the components. All DTaP vaccines show better efficacy against severe disease than mild disease. The DTaP vaccines score over whole cell vaccines in term of adverse effects. The incidence of both minor and major adverse effects is reduced by two-thirds with the acellular vaccines. The absolute contraindications to DTaP vaccines are same as those for whole cell vaccines.

Recommendations for use: DTaP vaccines are not more efficacious than DTwP vaccines, but have fewer adverse effects. The schedule is same as with DTwP vaccines. Like DTwP vaccines, DTaP vaccines must not be given in children more than 7 years of age.

Tetanus Toxoid (TT), DT, Td and Tdap Vaccines

Tetanus Toxoid

It contains 5 Lf of toxoid. The dose is 0.5 mL by IM route. Gradually, TT is replaced by Td and Tdap in the practice. TT should be given to all pregnant women for prevention of neonatal tetanus with reference to previous doses of TT received by each woman as follows:

- Those who have not been previously immunized → two doses of TT at least 1 month apart. First dose at the time of first contact or as early as possible → second dose 1 month later (at least 2 weeks before delivery) → 1 dose of TT for subsequent pregnancies that occur in next 5 years

- Those who have received five doses of TT over a period of at least 2.5 years → protection is lasting for rest of reproductive years
- Women who received three primary doses in infancy → two doses of TT during first pregnancy → one more dose during second pregnancy → protection is lasting for rest of reproductive years
- Women who received three primary + one booster in childhood → one dose in first and second pregnancy → protection lasting for rest reproductive years
- Women who received three primary + two boosters in childhood → only 1 dose in first pregnancy
- Women who received three primary + two boosters + one adolescent dose → no further doses are necessary during pregnancy.

Tetanus Toxoids in Wound Management

All patients presenting with skin wounds or infections should be evaluated for tetanus prophylaxis. Cleaning the wound, removal of devitalized tissue, irrigation and drainage is important to prevent anaerobic environment. The indications for TT and tetanus immunoglobulin (TIG) are discussed in Table 9.2.2. Again replacement of TT with Td/Tdap is recommended.

Evidences suggest that tetanus is unlikely in individuals who have received three or more doses of TT in the past and who get a booster dose during wound prophylaxis. Hence, TIG is not indicated in these patients irrespective of wound severity unless the person is immunocompromised. Catch-up vaccination should be as follows:

- Completely unimmunized → three doses of TT at 0, 1 and 6 months
- Partially immunized → at least 3 doses of TT including previous doses
- Children with unknown or undocumented history → as per unimmunized.

It is recommended that the TT booster doses administered at the time of wound management and for catch-up vaccination be replaced with DTwP, DTaP, Td or Tdap depending on the age of the child and nature of previous doses received for more comprehensive protection.

Table 9.2.2: Indications for TT and TIG.

History of tetanus toxoid doses	Clean, minor wounds		All other wounds	
	TT/Td	TIG*	TT/Td	TIG*
Unknown, ≤3, immunodeficient	Yes	No	Yes	Yes
≥3 doses	No**	No	No***	No

*TIG, tetanus immunoglobulin (250–500)
**Yes, if more than 10 years since last dose
***Yes, if more than 5 years since last dose

Diphtheria and Tetanus Vaccine

It comprises of diphtheria and tetanus toxoid in similar amounts as in DTwP or DTaP. The dose is 0.5 mL by IM route. It is recommended in children below 7 years of age where pertussis vaccination is contraindicated. Its practical utility nowadays is rare in the practice.

Tetanus Diphtheria Vaccine

Td contains the usual dose of tetanus toxoid and only two units of diphtheria toxoid. It is stored at 2–8°C. The dose is 0.5 mL by IM route. It is used as replacement for DTwP, DTaP or DT for catch-up vaccination in those aged more than 7 years (along with Tdap) and as replacement for TT in all situations where TT is given.

Tetanus, Diphtheria and Acellular Pertussis Vaccine

Tdap contains tetanus toxoid 5 Lf, diphtheria toxoid 2 Lf and the three acellular pertussis components, namely PT 8 µg, FHA 8 µg and PRN 2.5 µg. It contains aluminum hydroxide as adjuvant and no preservative. It should be stored at 2–8°C. The dose is 0.5 mL by IM route.

Recommendations for use:

- Those who received three primary + two boosters of DTwP or DTaP → Tdap single dose at the age of 10–12 years. Catch-up vaccination till the age of 18 years. Tdap may also be used as replacement for Td or TT booster in adults of any age if they have not received Tdap in the past
- As a replacement for Td or TT in wound management of children aged 10 and above if they have not received Tdap in the past, and at least 5 years have elapsed since receipt of Td or TT vaccines
- Children who have missed second booster of DTwP or DTaP and who are 7 years of age or more → Tdap single dose
- Those who have not completed primary doses of DTwP or DTaP and are more than 7 years of age → one dose of Tdap and 2 doses of Td at 0, 1 and 6 months, respectively
- Single booster dose of Tdap may be followed by Td booster every 10 years.

Measles Vaccine

Measles vaccine is live attenuated vaccine. Currently used live attenuated measles vaccine strains originate from the original Edmonston strain and include Schwarz, Edmonston Zagreb, Moraten and Edmonstan B strains. Indian measles vaccines are formulated from the Edmonston Zagreb strain. It is supplied as freeze-dried in single dose or multidose vials with distilled water as a diluent. It should be stored frozen at 2–8°C. Reconstituted vaccine is destroyed by light and is heat labile. It is susceptible to contamination as it does not have any preservative. For these reasons, reconstituted vaccine should be protected from light, kept at 2–8°C and used within 4–6 hours of reconstitution. The dose is 0.5 mL by SC route at the age of 9 months in our country.

Vaccine immunogenicity and efficacy are best if the vaccine is administered beyond the age of 12 months. However, in India a significant proportion of measles cases occur below the age of 12 months. Hence, in order to achieve the best balance between these competing demands of early protection and high seroconversion, completed 9 months of age has been recommended as the appropriate age for measles vaccination in India. In case of outbreak, however, the vaccine can be given to infants ats young as completed 6 months. The vaccine should be given irrespective of prior history of measles as any exanthematous illness is often confused as measles. In view of about 15% cases of primary vaccine failures with the first dose of the vaccine, an additional dose of measles vaccine preferably as MMR vaccine at the age of 15 months is required for durable and possibly lifelong protection against measles.

Mumps, Measles, and Rubella Vaccine

Measles, mumps, and rubella vaccine is supplied in lyophilized form should be frozen for long-term storage. Reconstituted vaccine should be stored at 2–8°C, protected from light and used within 4–6 hours. The dose is 0.5 mL by SC route. It can be given along with all other vaccines except BCG vaccine. Currently, two doses are recommended: First at the age of 12–15 months, and second at 4–6 years of age or at any time 8 weeks after the first dose. In a child who has not received measles vaccine, two doses of MMR at 8 weeks interval suffices.

Haemophilus influenzae Type B (Hib) Conjugate Vaccine

All Hib vaccines are conjugated vaccines where the Hib capsular polysaccharide is conjugated with a protein carrier so as to provide protection in early years of life when it is most needed. The vaccines should be stored at 2–8°C. The dose is 0.5 mL by IM route. The Hib vaccine is recommended to all children. The vaccine schedule consists of three primary doses at 6, 10 and 14 weeks with a booster at 18 months. If it is initiated between 6 and 12 months, two primary doses and one booster at 18 months are recommended. If child is brought for vaccination at the age of 12–15 months, 1 dose as primary and booster at 18 months are recommended. For children aged more than 15 months, a single dose may suffice. It is not recommended for healthy children above 5 years of age. However, the Hib vaccine should be given to all individuals with functional or anatomical asplenia irrespective of age. Hib vaccines are now used mostly as combination vaccines with DTwP/DTaP/Hep B/IPV, etc.

Hepatitis B (Hep B) Vaccine

The currently available Hep B vaccine contains surface antigen of hepatitis B, produced by recombinant technology in yeast and adjuvanted with aluminum salts and preserved with thiomersal (thiomersal-free vaccine is also available). It is available as single and multidose vials and should be stored at 2–8°C. It should not be frozen, frozen vaccine should be discarded. The dose in children and adolescents (aged <18 years) is 0.5 mL (10 µg) and in those more than 18 years of age is 1 mL (20 µg). It should be injected by IM route on anterolateral thigh or deltoid and never on gluteal region.

Schedules

- Birth, 1 and 6 months
- Birth, 6 and 14 weeks
- Birth, 6, 10 and 14 weeks
- Birth, 6 weeks and 6 months
- No booster dose is required
- Catch-up vaccination 0, 1 and 6 schedule.

Management of an Infant Born to Hepatitis B Positive Mother

Pregnant women should be counseled and encouraged to opt for HBsAg screening. If the mother is HBsAg negative, Hep B vaccine can be given along with other vaccines at 6, 10 and 14 weeks.

If the mother's HBsAg status is not known, Hep B vaccination should be started within a few hours of birth to prevent perinatal transmission. The schedule may be birth, 6 and 14 weeks or birth, 6 weeks and 6 months.

If the mother is HBsAg positive, the baby should be given HBIG along with Hep B vaccine within 12 hours of birth, using two separate syringes and on separate sites. The dose of HBIG is 0.5 mL IM. HBIG may be given up to 7 days of birth but the efficacy of HBIG after 48 hours is not known. Two more doses of Hep B vaccine at 1 month and 6 months of age are needed. The closely spaced schedule should not be used. If HBIG is not available (or not affordable) Hep B vaccine may be given at 0, 1 and 2 months with an additional dose between 9 and 12 months. All infants born to HBsAg positive mothers should be tested for HBsAg and anti-HBsAg antibodies at the age of 9–15 months to identify carriers or non-responders.

Combination Vaccines

A combination vaccine consists of two or more separate immunogens that have been physically combined in a single preparation. This is different from simultaneous vaccination where the multiple vaccines are administered concurrently but are physically separate. Combination vaccines currently licensed in India. These vaccines are:

- DTwP + Hib, DTwP + Hep B, DTwP + Hib + Hep B

- DTaP + Hib, DTaP + Hib + IPV
- Hep A + Hep B

The advantages of combination vaccines are many and include decreases injection pricks, reduced burden on cold chain, reduced requirement of syringes and needles and easier record keeping.

Typhoid Vaccines

Several vaccines have been available against typhoid or paratyphoid fever. Whole cell inactivated typhoid or paratyphoid vaccines (TA/TAB) and oral live attenuated Ty21a vaccine are no longer available in India.

Vi-capsular Polysaccharide Vaccine

The vaccine contains highly purified antigenic fraction of Vi-capsular polysaccharide antigen of *Salmonella typhi* which is virulence factor of the organism. Each dose contains 25 µg of purified polysaccharide in 0.5 mL of phenolic isotonic buffer for IM use. It should be stored at 2–8°C and should not be frozen. Since, it is a pure polysaccharide vaccine, it is not immunogenic in children below 2 years of age and has no immune memory. The vaccine does not interfere with the interpretation of the Widal test. The Vi polysaccharide vaccine is recommended for use as a single dose in children aged 2 years and above and can safely be given with all other childhood vaccines. Revaccination is recommended every 3 years. It can be safely given in the immunocompromised including HIV infected.

Vi-conjugate Typhoid Vaccines

Vi-PS Conjugate vaccine conjugated with *Pseudomonas aeruginosa* exotoxin A

The limitations of the currently available typhoid vaccines include noneffectiveness below the age of 2 years, limited efficacy (of around 60%), T cell independent response which lacks immune memory and is not boostable, and finally no protection against paratyphoid fever. Conjugation of the Vi antigen with a protein carrier is hence desirable as it would induce a T cell dependent immune response.

Vi-PS Conjugate vaccine conjugated with Tetanus Toxoid

This vaccine has been developed in India. It is a conjugate vaccine using tetanus toxoid as the carrier protein with a dose of 5 µg of Vi-PS antigen.

Vi-polysaccharide conjugate vaccine conjugated with Tetanus Toxoid

Vi-capsular polysaccharide conjugate typhoid vaccine conjugated with tetanus toxoid. The manufacturer has used a dose of 25µg/0.5 mL of Conjugate Vi Content polysaccharide which is the highest having been used in other trials as well on conjugate vaccine the world over.

Recommendations for use

Individual use

Vi-capsular polysaccharide (Vi-PS) vaccine

- IAP ACVIP recommends the administration of the currently available Vi polysaccharide vaccine 0.5 mL IM every three years beginning at the age of 2 years. A child with history of suspected/confirmed enteric fever may be vaccinated 4 weeks after recovery if he/she has not received the vaccine in the past 3 years.
- Considering the typhoid epidemiology in the country and analyzing the available data of the vaccine, IAP recommends the use of new conjugate vaccine below one year of age, preferably between 9–12 months (minimum age 6 months). Since the incompatibility data with measles vaccine is not available, there should be an interval of at least 4 weeks either before or after the former. The initial dose should be followed by a booster dose in the second year. Only one dose is required if started above 2 years.

Varicella Vaccine

Varicella vaccines are derived from the original Oka strain but the virus contents may vary from one manufacturer to another. The recommended dose is 0.5 mL by SC route and the minimum infectious virus content should be 1,000 plaque forming units. It is available as lyophilized vaccine. It should be protected from light and needs to be used within 30 minutes of its reconstitution. It may be given with all other childhood vaccines.

The IAPCOI recommends offering the vaccine to all healthy children with no prior history of varicella with special emphasis in all children belonging to certain high-risk groups. Varicella vaccine is licensed for 12 months and above. However, the risk of breakthrough varicella is lower if given 15 months onward. Hence, the IAPCOI recommends the administration of varicella vaccine in children aged 15 months or older. After a single dose of varicella vaccine, approximately 15% of vaccines remain at risk of developing breakthrough varicella disease. Two doses of varicella vaccinees offer superior individual protection as compared to a single dose. It is now recommended two doses of varicella vaccine for children with all age groups. For primary immunization, the first dose should be given at the age of 15 months and second dose at 4–6 years. For catch-up vaccination, children below the age of 13 years should receive two doses 3 months apart and those aged 13 years or more should receive two doses at interval of 4–8 weeks.

Varicella zoster immunoglobulin provides passive immunity against varicella and is indicated for post-exposure prophylaxis (PEP) in susceptible individuals with significant contact with varicella or herpes zoster who are at high risk for severe disease.

Hepatitis A Vaccines

Inactivated Vaccines

Most of the currently available vaccines are derived from HM 175/GBM strains and grown on MRC_5 human diploid cell lines. The virus is formalin inactivated and adjuvanted with aluminum hydroxide. The vaccine is stored at 2–8°C. The vaccines are given in a two-dose schedule, 6 months apart by IM route. Immunity is lifelong due to anamnestic response and no boosters are recommended at present in the immunocompetent. The protective efficacy is around 90–100% and onset of protection is 2–4 weeks after the first dose of the vaccine. A liposomal adjuvanted hepatitis A vaccine is now available. The efficacy and safety profile is nearly similar to the other inactivated vaccines.

Live Attenuated Vaccine

The vaccine is derived from the H2 strain of the virus attenuated after serial passage in human diploid cell (KMB 17 cell line). It has been in use in China since the 1990s in mass vaccination programs. The vaccine meets requirements of the Chinese Drug Authority and WHO. It is also now licensed and available in India. The recommended dose is 1 mL SC in children aged 1–15 years. Immunogenicity studies with single dose show seroconversion rates of more than 98%, 2 months after vaccination and persistence of protective antibodies in more than 80% of vaccinees at 10 years follow-up. Two immunogenicity studies from India in 143 and 505 children respectively have demonstrated greater than 95% seroconversion with single dose of the live attenuated vaccine with persistence of antibodies on follow-up. Some studies have reported inability of single dose of the live vaccine to protect against subclinical infection. The IAPCOI recommends two doses of even the live attenuated vaccine. The hepatitis A vaccine may be offered to all healthy children with special emphasis in risk groups. The IAPCOI recommends initiating hepatitis A vaccine at the age of 12 months.

Rotavirus Vaccines

Currently two live oral vaccines are licensed and marketed worldwide: human monovalent live vaccine and Human Bovine pentavalent live vaccine. Human monovalent live vaccine is a monovalent attenuated human rotavirus vaccine derived from Human Rotavirus strain 89-12 grown in vero cells and contains the G1P1(8) strain administered orally in a two-dose schedule to infants of 2 and 4 months of age. Human bovine pentavalent live vaccine is a human bovine reassortant vaccine and consists of five reassortants between the bovine WC3 strain and human G1, G2, G3, G4 and P1A(8) rotavirus strains grown in vero cells and administered orally in three dose schedule at 2, 4 and 6 months. Regardless of which vaccine is used, the first dose should be given between 6 weeks and 14 weeks 6 days of age.

Immunization should not be initiated in infants 15 weeks or older because of insufficient safety data for vaccines use in older children. All the doses of either of the vaccines should be completed within 32 weeks of age. Both the vaccines are available in India. They have shown excellent protective efficacy against severe rotavirus gastroenteritis. Both the vaccines have been demonstrated safe with no increased risk of intussusception as compared to placebo.

Rotavirus vaccination should be strictly as per schedule as there is a potentially high risk of intussusception if vaccines are given to older infants. Rotavirus vaccination should be avoided if age of the infant is uncertain. There are no restrictions on the infant's consumption of food or liquid, including breast milk, either before or after the vaccination. It may be administered during minor illnesses. Though there are limited evidences on safety and efficacy of rotavirus vaccines in preterm infants, vaccination should be considered for these infants if they are clinically stable and at least 6 weeks of age as preterms are susceptible to severe rotavirus gastroenteritis. Vaccination should be postponed in infants with acute gastroenteritis as it might compromise efficacy of the vaccine. Risk versus benefits of vaccination should be considered while deciding vaccination for infants with chronic gastrointestinal diseases, gut malformation, previous intussusception and immunocompromised infants.

Human Monovalent Live Vaccine

Human monovalent live rotavirus vaccine contains one strain of live attenuated human strain 89-12 [type G1P1A(8)] rotavirus. It is provided as lyophilized powder that is reconstituted before administration. The vaccine should be administered promptly after reconstitution as 1 mL orally. The first dose can be administered at the age of 6 weeks and should be given not later than the age of 12 weeks. The interval between two doses should be at least 4 weeks.

Human Bovine Pentavalent Vaccine

Human bovine pentavalent live vaccine contains five reassortant rotaviruses developed from human and bovine penta rotaviruses. The vaccine is available as a liquid virus mixed with buffer and no reconstitution is needed. It should be stored at 2–8°C. The recommended schedule is three oral doses at ages 2, 4 and 6 months. The first dose should be administered between ages 6 and 12 weeks and subsequent doses at intervals of 4–8 weeks. The manufacturer does not recommend readministration of vaccine if a dose is spit out or regurgitated. Both the vaccines should not be frozen. Rotavirus vaccine must not be injected. Programatic errors have been reported. Ideally, the rotavirus vaccine series should be completed with the same product. However, vaccination should not be deferred because the product used for previous dose is unavailable. In such cases, the series should be continued with the product that is available. If any dose in the series was human bovine pentavalent vaccine or if the product is unknown for any dose in the series, a total of three doses should be administered. It is not necessary to restart the series or add doses because of a prolonged interval between doses with either of the vaccines.

Indian Neonatal Rotavirus Live Vaccine, 116 E

This vaccine developed in India is a live, naturally attenuated vaccine containing monovalent, bovine-human reassortant strain characterized as G9P [11], with the VP4 of bovine rotavirus origin, and all other segments of human rotavirus origin. The vaccine strain was isolated from asymptomatic infants, with mild diarrhea by Indian researchers in 1985 at AIIMS, New Delhi. Follow-up of these infants indicated that they were protected against severe rotavirus diarrhea for up to 2 years. This strain was sent for vaccine development to the NIH by DBT-India and later transferred to Bharat Biotech International Limited in 2001 for further development. This vaccine is licensed in India. The recommended schedule is 3 oral doses.

Human Bovine Rotavirus Vaccine

Human bovine rotavirus vaccine containing genotypes G1, G2, G3, G4, G9 has also been licensed in India. The recommended schedule is 3 oral doses starting at 6 weeks of age with a gap of 4 weeks. Each dose of 2.5 mL contains live, human bovine reassortant strains of rotavirus serotypes G1, G2, G3, G4 and G9 x10 5.6 FFU of each serotype. Diluent is citrate bicarbonate buffer prepared using 9.6 mg/mL citric acid and 25.6 mg/mL sodium bicarbonate. It can be stored at 25°C.

Pneumococcal Vaccines

Currently, three types of pneumococcal vaccines (PCV) are available in the market for use in the practice. They are 13 valent pneumococcal conjugate vaccine (PCV13), 10 valent pneumococcal conjugate vaccine (PCV10) and unconjugated pneumococcal polysaccharide vaccine (PPSV23).

Pneumococcal Polysaccharide Vaccine

The unconjugated pneumococcal polysaccharide vaccine is a 23 valent vaccine (PPSV23). It is a T-cell independent vaccine that is poorly immunogenic below the age of 2 years, has low immune memory, does not reduce nasopharyngeal carriage and does not provide herd immunity. It is stored at 2–8°C and the dose is 0.5 mL SC or IM. It is a safe vaccine with occasional local side effects. Not more than two lifetime doses are recommended, as repeated doses may cause immunologic hyporesponsiveness.

Pneumococcal Conjugate Vaccines

Conjugate PCV were developed primarily to address the problem of low immunogenicity of the polysaccharide vaccine in children below the age of 2 who are at high risk of pneumococcal disease. Conjugation of the pneumococcal polysaccharide of varying number of serotypes has been done with diphtheria toxoid cross reactive material 197 (CRM 197) proteins, protein D of non-capsulated Hib, DT and TT, and finally Men OMP.

Pneumococcal Vaccines 13

Pneumococcal vaccines 13 was developed as a successor to the currently registered PCV7. It contains polysaccharides of the capsular antigens of *Streptococcus pneumoniae* serotypes 1, 5, 7F, 3, 6A and 19A in addition to serotypes in PCV7. PCV13 is administered by IM route as a 0.5 mL dose and is available in latex free, single dose prefilled syringes. PCV13 can be administered at the same time as other routine childhood vaccines. The safety and efficacy of concurrent administration of PCV13 and PPV23 has not been studied and concurrent administration is not recommended.

Pneumococcal Vaccines 10

Pneumococcal vaccines 10 contains three additional serotypes besides PCV7 and they are 1, 5, 7F. Three different carrier proteins are used in this formulation. PCV10 is a preservative free vaccine and adsorbed on aluminum phosphate. It is available in the form of prefilled syringe containing one dose (0.5 mL) given by IM route.

Recommended Schedule for Use of PCV13 and PCV10 (Table 9.2.3)

- Minimum interval between two doses is 4 weeks for children vaccinated at the age less than 12 months whereas for those vaccinated at the age more than 12 months, the minimum interval between doses is 8 weeks
- Minimum age for administration of first dose is 6 weeks
- Routine use of PCV13 and PCV10 is not recommended for healthy children aged more than 5 years
- For children who have begun a series of PCV7, replace all remaining doses with PCV13 or PCV10
- For children who have completed a 4 dose or other age appropriate series of PCV7, given one additional dose of PCV13 or PCV10 to all the healthy children who have not yet reached their fifth birthday.

Table 9.2.3: Schedule for use of PCV13 and PCV10.

Age	Primary doses	Booster
6 weeks to 6 months	3 doses	1 dose at 12–15 months
7–11 months	2 doses	1 dose at 12–15 months
12–23 months	2 doses	-
24–59 months	1 dose	-

Human Papillomavirus Vaccines

Two HPV vaccines have been licensed globally, a quadrivalent and a bivalent vaccine. Both are manufactured by recombinant DNA technology that produces non-infectious virus like particles comprising of the HPV L1 protein, the major capsid protein of HPV. Quadrivalent vaccine available in India is a mixture of L1 proteins of HPV serotypes 16, 18, 6 and 11 with aluminum containing adjuvant. The bivalent vaccine is a mixture of L1 proteins of HPV serotypes 16 and 18 with ASO4 as an adjuvant.

The IAPCOI recommends offering HPV vaccine to all females in the schedules. Since protection is seen only when the vaccine is given before infection with HPV, the vaccine should be given prior to sexual debut. Both the vaccines are equally efficacious and safe for protection against cervical cancer and percutaneous lesions as of currently available data. The quadrivalent vaccine additionally protects against anogenital warts.

The vaccines should be stored at 2–8°C and must not be frozen. The dose is 0.5 mL by IM route in deltoid. The recommended age for initiation of vaccine is 10–12 years. As of current licensing regulations in India, catch-up vaccination is permitted up to age of 45 years. Three doses at 0, 2 and 6 months are recommended with quadrivalent vaccine (minimum interval between first and second dose is 4 weeks and second and third dose is 12 weeks) and 0, 1 and 6 months with the bivalent vaccinee. HPV vaccine can be given by SC route with other vaccines, such as hepatitis B and Tdap. As a precaution against syncope following any vaccinee in adolescents, the vaccinee should be counseled prior to vaccination, vaccine be administered in a sitting or lying down position and the patient observed for 15 minutes post vaccination. Both the vaccines are contraindicated in those with history of previous hypersensitivity to any vaccine component and should be avoided in pregnancy.

Influenza Vaccines

Two types of influenza vaccines are available: (1) inactivated and (2) live attenuated.

Inactivated Influenza Vaccines

The inactivated influenza vaccines are produced from virus growth in embryonated hen's eggs and are of three types: (1) whole virus; (2) split product and (3) subunit surface antigen formulations. Whole virus vaccines have more adverse reactions, especially in children and are currently not used. Most influenza vaccines are split-product vaccines, produced from detergent treated, highly purified influenza virus or surface antigen vaccines containing purified hemagglutinin and neuraminidase.

Inactivated influenza vaccines are trivalent or monovalent. Trivalent vaccines contain 15 µg of each of WHO recommended two influenza A strains (H1N1 and H3N2) and one influenza B strain. Monovalent vaccines contain 15 µg of novel H1N1 2009 strain. They should be stored at 2–8°C and never be frozen. The trivalent vaccines are licensed for use in children aged 6 months and above. The current seasonal trivalent vaccines contain A/California/7/2009 (H1N1)-like, A/Perth/16/2009 (H3N2)-like and B/Brisbane/60/2008-like antigens. The dosage schedule has been discussed in Table 9.2.4.

Side effects are mild and include fever, rash and pain at injection sites. It should be avoided in patients with history of Guillain-Barré syndrome and who are not at high risk of severe influenza related complications.

Live Attenuated Influenza Vaccine (LAIV)

The vaccine is composed of the live attenuated reassortant of the three WHO recommended strains and is administered as a nasal spray. It is currently not available in India.

In the current scenario of post-pandemic phase, the IAPCOI recommends using the influenza vaccine in all children with high-risk factors like immunodeficiency, chronic cardiac, pulmonary, renal, liver diseases and diabetes mellitus, children on long-term aspirin therapy, asthma requiring oral steroids and also in healthy children wherein the vaccine is desired by parents after discussing with them the benefits and limitations of the vaccine.

Cholera Vaccines

The parenteral killed vaccine which had a 3 month efficacy of 45% is no longer recommended. The WC-rBS vaccine available internationally as Dukoral and widely used in travelers is a vaccine comprising of killed *Vibrio cholerae* 01 with recombinant to subunit of cholera toxoid. It is an oral vaccine with buffer, has to be stored at 2–8°C and is administered as two doses one week apart. It is licensed for those aged 2 years and above. The inclusion of new killed whole cell oral cholera vaccine in the national immunization schedule is being considered by the policy makers, in those areas where cholera is highly endemic, particularly the states of West Bengal and Orissa. For office practice purposes, the cholera vaccine should be used in special situations. These include travel to or residence in a highly endemic area and circumstances where there is risk of an outbreak such as during pilgrimages like Kumbh Mela, etc. The protection is available after 2 weeks of the second dose.

Table 9.2.4: Dosage and schedule of inactivated trivalent influenza vaccine.

Age	6–35 months	3–8 years	From 9 years of age
Dose	0.25 mL	0.5 mL	0.5 mL
No. of doses	1 or 2*	1 or 2*	1

*For children who have not previously been vaccinated a second dose should be given after an interval of at least 4 weeks.

Meningococcal Vaccines

Unconjugated Meningococcal Polysaccharide Vaccine (MPSV)

They are either bivalent (A + C) or quadrivalent (A, C, Y and W-135) and contain 50 µg of each of the polysaccharide antigen, available in lyophilized form, reconstituted with sterile water and stored at 2–8°C. They are indicated for adults and children above the age of 2 years. The protective antibody levels are usually achieved within 10–14 days of vaccination.

Conjugated Meningococcal Polysaccharide Vaccine

A conjugate meningococcal serogroup C vaccine (conjugated to CRM 197 or TT) has been a part of routine immunization in UK. The dosing schedule is three doses at interval of 4–8 weeks in children below 6 months, two doses in 6–12 months age group and single dose in older children along with the routine childhood vaccines.

A quadrivalent A, C, Y and W-135 conjugate vaccine has been licensed for use of individuals aged 11–55 years in the USA (2–55 years in Canada). A single dose of 0.5 mL IM is recommended.

The IAPCOI recommends the use of meningococcal vaccines only in certain high-risk situations in children above the age of 2 years:

- During outbreaks, if caused by serogroups included in the vaccine
- Children with complement deficiency
- Children with asplenia
- Travelers to Saudi Arabia for Haj (Mandatory)
- Travelers to African meningitis belt
- Students going to abroad (Mandatory in USA).

The quadrivalent vaccine is a preferred for Haj pilgrims, international travelers and students. A single dose 0.5 mL SC/IM is recommended.

Yellow Fever Vaccine

It is a live attenuated vaccine derived from 17D strain of the virus grown in chick embryo cells. It is available as a freeze dried preparation in single or multidose vials that should be stored at 2–8°C (must not be frozen) along with sterile saline as diluent. The reconstituted vaccine is heat labile, must be stored at 2–8°C and discarded within an hour of reconstitution, if not used. The dose is 0.5 mL SC. It can safely be given along with all other childhood vaccines. Immunogenicity and efficacy are more than 90%. Protective immunity is attained by 10 days of vaccination and lasts for at least 10 years. Adverse reactions are minor and are seen in only 25% of vaccinees. It is contraindicated in infants below the age of 6 months. The vaccine is mandatory for all travelers to yellow fever endemic zones as per International

Health Regulations. The list of endemic countries should be confirmed. All vaccinees receive an international certificate for vaccination duly dated, stamped and signed by center administering the vaccine. The certificate is valid from the 10th day of the vaccination for a period of 10 years. Individuals with medical contraindications for vaccination are advised to avoid or postponed travel. In case travel is unavoidable, an exemption certificate or waiver letter should be taken from the treating physician and vector control measures should be practiced. The waiver letter does not guarantee entry and the person may face refusal of entry, quarantine or on site vaccination. In Indian context, a valid certificate is required for all individuals aged more than 6 months entering India after travel to yellow fever endemic zones even if it was mere transit. This vaccine is currently available only at selected government centers and not at private clinics.

Japanese Encephalitis Vaccines

Mouse Brain Derived Inactivated Vaccine

This vaccine is prepared from either the Nakayama/Beijing strain of JE virus grown in mice brain, purified, inactivated by formalin and preserved with thiomersal. The vaccine is given by SC route 0.5 mL in children 1–3 years and 1 mL in older children. Primary immunization consists of three doses given on 0, 7 and 30 days. Short schedule 0, 7 and 14 days may be used. Two does 7 days apart may be used in travelers for logistic reasons. For long-term protection regular boosters every 2–3 years are recommended. Owing to high cost, complicated dosing schedule and availability of better vaccines, its use has markedly declined

Inactivated Mouse Brain Derived Vaccine SA-14-14-2 Vaccine

It is the second generation vaccine based on attenuated JEV strain SA 14-14-2. The vaccine is produced on Vero cells, purified, inactivated and alum adjuvanted. It is given in two dose schedule, 0.25 mL for pediatric use and 0.5 mL for adult use.

Kolar 821564XY Strain Vaccine

Isolated and characterized by the National Institute of Virology, adapted to Vero cells. It has been found to be safe, well tolerated and immunogenic against homologous and heterologous JE virus strains. The immune response is adequate (100% seroconversion) with two dose vaccination.

JE vaccine should not be used as an outbreak response vaccine. Government has implemented universal immunization with this vaccine in all children in JE endemic states. It is also recommended for travellers to JE endemic areas provided they are expected to stay for a minimum of 4 weeks in rural areas in the JE season.

Rabies Vaccines

The nerve tissue vaccines are no longer available and stopped to use due to its poor efficacy and life-threatening adverse effects like neuroparalytic reactions. The currently available vaccines are modern tissue culture vaccines (MTCV) and they are purified chick embryo cell (PCEC) vaccine, human diploid cell vaccine (HDCV), purified vero cell rabies vaccine (PVRV) and purified duck embryo vaccine (PDEV). These vaccines are available in lyophilized form with sterile water as diluent. They are stored at 2–8°C and should be used within 6 hours of reconstitution. All modern tissue culture vaccines have almost equal efficacy and any one of them can be used. These vaccinees induce protective antibodies in more than 99% of vaccines following preexposure or postexposure prophylaxis. The main adverse effects are local swelling, pain and tenderness and less commonly fever, headache and dizziness. Along with proper wound care and rabies immunoglobulin (RIG), PEP is effective 100% in preventing rabies cases. Failure occurs due to delay in initiation or nonuse of RIG in spite of indication.

Rabies Immunoglobulin and Rabies Monoclonal Antibody

Rabies immunoglobulin (RIG) contains specific antirabies antibodies that neutralize the rabies virus and provide passive protection till active immunity is generated. Two types of RIGs are available: (1) human rabies immunoglobulin (HRIG) and (2) equine rabies immunoglobulin (ERIG). HRIG is preferable and close is 20 IU/g body weight, maximum 1,500 IU. The dose of ERIG is 40 IU/kg body weight. Skin testing prior to ERIG is not recommended. RIG is indicated in all cases of category 3 wounds. RIG should be infiltrated thoroughly into and around the wound. The remaining part of RIG may be administered by IM route into the deltoid or anterolateral aspect of thigh away from the vaccine site. If the quantity of RIG is small, it can be diluted with normal saline for wide infiltration. If RIG could not be given initially, it can be administered up to 7th day of starting the vaccine. RIG is not indicated in individuals who have received pre-exposure or postexposure prophylaxis in the past. Rabies monoclonal antibody (RMAb) is the latest development in passive immunization against rabies. The dose required is lesser than RIG.

Postexposure Prophylaxis

Post-exposure prophylaxis is a dire medical emergency and is indicated following a defined contact with any warm blooded animal. Pregnancy, lactation and infancy are never contraindications for PEP. Persons presenting several days or months or years after the bite should be managed in a similar manner as a person who has been bitten recently (with RIG, if indicated), as rabies have a long incubation

Table 9.2.5: Categories of rabies exposure.

Category	Description	Recommended treatment
I	Touching of feeding of animals, licks on intact skin	None if information is reliable
II	Nibbling of uncovered skin, minor scratches or abrasions without bleeding licks on broken skin	Vaccination
III	Single or multiple transdermal bites or scratches, contamination of mucous membrane with saliva or exposure to bats	RIG + Vaccination

period and the window opportunity for prevention remains. Rabies exposure may be classified as per WHO into three categories which are discussed in Table 9.2.5.

- First step is thorough cleansing the wound with soap and flushing under running water for 10 minutes
- Irrigation with a virucidal agent, such as 70% alcohol or povidone iodine
- Antimicrobials and tetanus toxoid, if indicated
- RIG if indicated
- Suturing of the wound should be avoided. If suturing is unavoidable, minimum suturing after infiltration of the wound with RIG
- Modern tissue culture rabies vaccine. The dose is same at all ages and is 1 mL for HDCV, PCEV, PDEV and 0.5 mL for PVRV.

The standard (Essen protocol) is five doses on days 0, 3, 7, 14 and 30. Day '0' being the day of commencement of vaccination. A sixth dose on day 90 is optional and may be offered to patients with severe debility or those who are immunosuppressed. Interchange of vaccines is permitted only in special circumstances but should not be done routinely. If RIG is not available, two doses of the vaccine may be given on day 0. If the animal remains healthy over a 10-day observation period, further vaccination may be discontinued.

Several other schedules of rabies vaccination have been proposed. Intradermal vaccination is cost-effective alternative to IM route as the dose required is only 0.1 mL. Based on recommendations of the expert group as well as WHO, Drug Controller General of India (DCGI) has recently decided to allow ID route administration of tissue culture based antirabies vaccine for PEP in a phased manner in certain government centers. Vaccines currently recommended for ID route administration in India are PVRV and PCEV. The ID route should not be used for immunocompromised patients and those on chloroquine therapy.

Preexposure Prophylaxis

Preexposure prophylaxis is important where the exposure may be unrecognized (laboratory) or unreported (children). Preexposure prophylaxis eliminates need for RIG. It also reduces PEP to two doses only. Preexposure prophylaxis is scheduled as three doses by IM route on deltoid or anterolateral thigh on days 0, 7 and 28. For pre-exposure at any point of time after completed preexposure or postexposure prophylaxis, two doses are given on days 0 and 3.

IMMUNIZATION OF ADOLESCENTS

IAP Recommendations for Adolescent Immunization (10–18 years)

Vaccine	Schedule
Tdap/Td	10 years
HPV	10–12 years

- Tdap is preferred to Td, followed by repeat Td every 10 years (Tdap to be given once only)
- HPV is for females, three doses at 0, 1, 2 or 0, 1, 6 months schedule depending upon the vaccine used.

IAP Recommendations for Catch-up Immunization in Adolescents

IAP recommendations for catch-up immunization in adolescents have been discussed in Table 9.2.6.

Table 9.2.6: IAP recommendations for catch-up immunization in adolescents.

Vaccine	Schedule
MMR	2 doses at 4–8 weeks interval
Hepatitis B	3 doses at 0, 1 and 6 months
Hepatitis A	2 doses at 0 and 6 months
Typhoid	1 dose every 3 years
Varicella	2 doses at 4–8 weeks interval

Table 9.2.7: IAP recommendations for adolescent travelers.

Vaccine	Place of travel	Dose recommended
Meningococcal vaccine	USA/UK/Endemic areas of Saudi Arabia and Africa	2 doses 4–8 weeks apart
Yellow fever	Endemic countries	10 days before travel
Oral cholera vaccine	Endemic areas or area with an outbreak	2 doses, one week apart
Japanese encephalitis	Endemic areas	Single dose
Rabies vaccine pre-exposure prophylaxis	Going on trekking	0, 7, 28

IAP Recommendations for Adolescent Travelers

IAP recommendations for adolescent travellers have been discussed in Table 9.2.7.

BIBLIOGRAPHY

1. Indian Academy of Pediatrics Committee on Immunization (IAPCOI).Consensus recommendations on immunization, 2012. Indian Pediatr. 2012;49:550-64.
2. Kliegman RM, Stanton BF, Geme III, JW, et al. Nelson Textbook of Pediatrics, 19th edition. Gurgaon, India: Elsevier Saunders; 2011.
3. Manual of Advancing Science of Vaccinology. Indian Academy of Pediatrics; 2009.
4. Plotkin SA, Orenstein WA, Offit PA. Vaccines, 5th edition. Printed in China: Saunders Elsevier; 2008.
5. Thacker N, Shah NK (Eds). Immunization in Clinical Practice. New Delhi: Jaypee Brothers; 2005.
6. Vashistha VM, Kalra A, Thacker N. FAQs on Vaccines & Immunization Practices. New Delhi: Jaypee Brothers Medical Publishers (P) Ltd; 2011.
7. Yewale V, Choudhury P, Thacker N. IAP Guide Book on Immunization Edition 2011, Mumbai: India Academy of Pediatrics; 2009.

A Parthasarathy, Hitt Sharma

9.3 IMMUNIZATION OF THE IMMUNE COMPROMISED CHILDREN AND ADOLESCENTS

INTRODUCTION

Immunization of immune compromised children and adolescents is an important aspect of pediatric and adolescent immunization. Because of immune deficient they should not be denied vaccination. Instead it should be realized that they are at greater risk for certain diseases than normal children, e.g. children with congenital asplenia/splenectomy, sickle cell anemia, etc. are at high risk for pneumococcal disease. However, the immunogenicity and safety of vaccinating these children depends on the nature and degree of immunosuppression.

PRIMARY VERSUS SECONDARY IMMUNE DEFICIENCY

The immune deficiency disorders can be primary or secondary. Primary immune deficiency is inherited, e.g. B lymphocyte (humeral), T lymphocyte (cell mediated), compliment and phagocytic function and other abnormalities of innate immunity. Secondary immune deficiency disorder is acquired, e.g. HIV/AIDS, malignant neoplasm, organ transplants, splenectomy, children and adolescents receiving immunosuppressants, antimetabolic and radiation therapy, etc.

LIVE VERSUS INACTIVATED VACCINES FOR IMMUNE COMPROMISED

Whereas, live vaccines like tOPV, LAIV, yellow fever vaccines, etc. are contraindicated the inactivated vaccine formulations to protect these diseases can safely be used in immune compromised. The nature and degree of immune suppression should be taken into consideration before administering these vaccines. For example, HIV infected child/adolescent can still receive tOPV, whereas child suffering from AIDS can receive only inactivated polio vaccine. Live virus vaccines should be administered at least 3 months after immune suppressive cancer therapy.

Immunocompromised Host and Specific Vaccines

Live Vaccines

Rotavirus
Rotavirus vaccine should be avoided in infants with Severe Combined Immunodeficiency (SCID), but is recommended for infants with HIV infection. Majority of the children with other immunocompromising conditions are likely to benefit, by potentially avoiding the severe outcome associated with a natural rotavirus infection.

Varicella
Two monovalent vaccine containing live attenuated 'OKA' strains are available. The vaccine is recommended for varicella seronegative HIV positive patients with CD4 counts of more than 15%. If immunosuppressive therapy is planned in seronegative patients, vaccine should be administered 3–4 weeks before treatment.

Influenza
UK guidelines recommend live attenuated influenza vaccine (LAIV) in 2–18 year oldchildren with stable HIV infection receiving antiretroviral therapy and high risk children who are receiving inhaled corticosteroids or low-dose systemic corticosteroids.

MMR
MMR vaccine is recommended in HIV infected children with CD4 count > 15%. The vaccine should be avoided for all T cell and combined immunodeficiencies. If immunosuppressive therapy is planned, primary immunization should be done before start of the treatment.

Conjugated Vaccines

Immunocompromised children should receive all the routine nonlive (include toxoids and other purified proteins, purified polysaccharide, protein–polysaccharide conjugate vaccines).

Meningococci
MenB and MenACWY vaccines are recommended in all children with congenital or acquired complement deficiency or asplenia.

Pneumococcal
Advisory Committee on Immunization Practice (ACIP) Pneumococcal Work Group has concluded that benefits of broader serotype protection achieved through use of both PCV13 and PPSV23 among immunocompomised children 6 through 18 years old outweighs the undesirable consequences.

Household Contacts
Routine OPV doses should not be administered to normal children in the same household where immune deficient

children are living, since OPV virus can get transmitted to the immune deficient contacts and cause poliomyelitis in them. However, if indicated, MMR, varicella, rotavirus vaccines can be administered routinely since these vaccine viruses do not get transmitted to the household contacts. Similarly LAIV can be administered to infants more than 6 months old.

VACCINE RECOMMENDATIONS FOR SPECIFIC CONDITIONS

Each immunocompromised person is different and presents unique considerations regarding immunization. The relative degree of immunodeficiency is variable depending on the underlying condition. Tables 9.3.1 and 9.3.2 summarize the vaccine administration strategies adapted from CDC Atlanta, USA and AAP recommendations for specific immunodeficiency conditions.

HEMATOPOIETIC CELL AND OTHER TRANSPLANT RECIPIENTS

Many factors like the donors' immunity status, type of transplantation (autologus or allogenic, blood or hematopoietic stem cell) and interval since the transplantation receipt of immunosuppressive medications, and presence of graft versus host disease (GVHD), etc. Inactivated or subunit vaccines, like pertussis, Hib, influenza, hepatitis B, hepatitis A, IPV and pneumococcal and meningococcal conjugate and polysaccharide vaccines, can be administered until 5 weeks after transplant.

SOLID ORGAN TRANSPLANT

Routine immunization of children and adolescents with the required vaccines should be done before transplantation. Live vaccines should be given at least 1 month before

Table 9.3.1: Vaccination of persons with primary immune deficiencies.				
Category	**Specific immunodeficiency**	**Contraindicated vaccines[1]**	**Risk-specific recommended vaccines[1]**	**Effectiveness and comments**
B-lymphocyte (humeral)	Severe antibody deficiencies (e.g. X-linked agammaglobulinemia and common variable immunodeficiency)	OPV[2] Smallpox LAIV BCG Ty21a (live oral typhoid) Yellow fever	Pneumococcal Influenza (TIV) Consider measles and varicella vaccination	The effectiveness of any vaccine will be uncertain if it depends only on the humeral response; IGIV interferes with the immune response to measles vaccine and possibly varicella vaccine
	Less severe antibody deficiencies (e.g. selective IgA deficiency and IgG subclass deficiency)	OPV[2] BCG Ty21a (live oral typhoid) Other live vaccines appear to be safe	Pneumococcal influenza (TIV)	All vaccines probably effective. Immune response may be attenuated
T-lymphocyte (cell-mediated and humeral)	Complete defects [e.g. severe combined immunodeficiency (SCID) disease, complete DiGeorge syndrome]	All live vaccines[3,4]	Pneumococcal influenza (TIV)	Vaccines may be ineffective
	Partial defects (e.g. most patients with DiGeorge syndrome, Wiskott-Aldrich syndrome, ataxia telangiectasia)	All live vaccines[3,4]	Pneumococcal Meningococcal Hib (if not administered in infancy) Influenza (TIV)	Effectiveness of any vaccine depends on degree of immune suppression
Complement	Deficiency of early components (C1-C4), late components (C5-C9), properdin, factor B	None	Pneumococcal Meningococcal Influenza (TIV)	All routine vaccines probably effective
Phagocytic function	Chronic granulomatous disease, leukocyte adhesion defects and myeloperoxidase deficiency	Live bacterial vaccines[3]	Pneumococcal[5] Influenza (TIV) (to decrease secondary bacterial infection)	All inactivated vaccines safe and probably effective. Live viral vaccines probably safe and effective

[1]Other vaccines that are not specifically contraindicated may be used if otherwise indicated

[2]OPV is no longer licensed in the United States, and therefore is not recommended for routine use

[3]Live bacterial vaccines: BCG, and Ty21a *Salmonella typhi* vaccine

[4]Live viral vaccines: MMR, OPV, LAIV, yellow fever, varicella (including MMRV and zoster vaccine) and vaccinia (smallpox). Smallpox vaccine is not recommended for children or the general public

[5]Pneumococcal vaccine is not indicated for children with chronic granulomatous disease

Table 9.3.2: Vaccination of persons with secondary immune deficiencies.

Specific immunodeficiency	Contraindicated vaccines[1]	Recommended vaccines[1]	Effectiveness and comments
HIV/AIDs	OPV[2] Smallpox BCG LAIV Withhold MMR and varicella in severely immunocompromised persons	Influenza (TIV) Pneumococcal Consider Hib (if not administered in infancy) and meningococcal vaccination	MMR, varicella and all inactivated vaccines, including inactivated influenza, might be effective[3]
Malignant neoplasm, transplantation, immuno-suppressive or radiation therapy	Live viral and bacterial, depending on immune status[4,5]	Influenza (TIV) Pneumococcal	Effectiveness of any vaccine depends on degree of immune suppression
Asplenia	None	Pneumococcal Meningococcal Hib (if not administered in infancy)	All routine vaccines probably effective
Chronic renal disease	LAIV	Pneumococcal Influenza (TIV) Hepatitis B	All routine vaccines probably effective

[1]Other vaccines that are not specifically contraindicated may be used if otherwise indicate.

[2]OPV is no longer licensed in the United States, and therefore is not recommended for routine use.

[3]HIV-infected children should receive IG after exposure to measles, and may receive varicella and measles vaccine if CD4+ lymphocyte count is ≥ 15%. If HAART is indicated, delay vaccination until both viral load <50 cp/ml and CD4>15%for 6 months.

[4]Live viral vaccines: MMR, OPV, LAIV, yellow fever, varicella (including MMRV and zoster vaccine) and vaccinia (smallpox). Smallpox vaccine is not recommended for children or the general public

[5]Live bacterial vaccines: BCG, and Ty21a Salmonella typhi vaccine.

Abbreviations: AIDS, acquired immunodeficiency syndrome; BCG, bacilli Calmette–Guérin vaccine; Hib, *Haemophilus influenza* type b vaccine; HIV, human immunodeficiency virus; IGIV, immune globulin intravenous; IG, immunoglobulin; LAIV, live attenuated influenza vaccine; MMR, measles, mumps, and rubella vaccine; OPV, oral poliovirus vaccine (live); TIV, trivalent (inactivated) influenza vaccine.

Source: Modified from American Academy of Pediatrics. Passive immunization. In: Pickering LK, Baker C, Long S, McMillen J, (Eds). Red Book 2009 Report of the Committee on Infectious Diseases. 27th edition. Elk Grove Village. It American Academy of Pediatrics 2006: (71-72) and CDC General Recommendations on Immunization Recommendations of the Advisory Committee on Immunization Practices (ACIP) MMWR 2006:55(No RR-15).

transplantation since immunosuppressive drugs can alter their immunogenicity if given after transplantation. Passive immunization with immune globulin preparations should be administered on the basis of serological evidence of susceptibility and exposure to the disease. However, household contacts and healthcare contacts of transplant recipients should have been protected with MMR, varicella, polio, influenza and hepatitis A vaccines well before the transplant is planned for siblings in the household.

SUMMARY

The safety and effectiveness of vaccines in immuno-compromised children are determined by the type of immunodeficiency and degree of immunosuppression. In summary, immunization of the immune-compromised should be judged on the basis of safety profile from severe adverse reactions, effectiveness of the vaccines administered. Vaccines should be administered judiciously and with caution adopting the right strategy with the right vaccine at the right time.

BIBLIOGRAPHY

1. Alkinson, Wolfe S, Hamborsky J, McIntyre I (Eds). Centre for Disease Control and Prevention, Epidemiology and Prevention of Vaccine Preventable Diseases, 11th edition. Washington DC: Public Health Foundation; 2009 (Tables A18 and A19).

2. CDC. Grading of Recommendations, Assessment, Development, and Evaluation (GRADE) for Pneumococcal Vaccines for Immunocompromised Children Aged 6 through 18 Years. Available at https://www.cdc.gov/vaccines/acip/recs/grade/pneumo-immuno-child.pdf Accessed on 9 October 2017.

3. Pickering LK, Baker CJ, Long SS, McMillan JA (Eds). Immunization in Special Clinical Circumstances. Red Book; 2009 Report of Committee on Infectious Diseases, 28th edition. Elk Grove Village, IL: American Academy of Pediatrics; 2009. pp.72-82.

4. Pinto MV, Bihari S, Snape MD. Immunisation of the immunocompromised child. J Infect. 2016;72 Suppl:S13-22.

9.4 | ADOLESCENT IMMUNIZATION

A Parthasarathy, Hitt Sharma

For many reasons, disease management, prevention and elimination goals are likely to be achieved by additional immunization activities and extra doses of vaccine which involve adolescents. Targeting adolescents for immunization would result in direct benefit of protection and to help in wider diseases controlling activities. Mainly it will help in continuing the protection which the adolescent achieved in his early years of life and infancy.

Before planning the adolescents' vaccination, careful weighing of the advantages and disadvantages is essential. Because only very few vaccines have been recommended for wide spread use in adolescent. Parents need to be fully informed about the risk, safety and relevance of vaccination. Many times children would also ask questions; interact meaningfully and rationally with the physician. Best efforts needs to be taken to relive their anxiety and obtain consent. In this chapter we have addressed goals and objectives, recommended schedule, catch up vaccines and a number of barriers for adolescent immunization.

INTRODUCTION AND BACKGROUND

WHO defines adolescents as young people between the 10 and 19 years of age. Today, 1.2 billion adolescents stand at the crossroads between childhood and the adult world. Around 243 million of them live in India.[1] Vaccines recommended for adolescents are underused, leaving our nation's teens vulnerable to serious illness. Healthcare providers should make every effort to vaccinate adolescents according to the National Immunization Schedule to benefit adolescents, their close contacts, and society at large. In the last two decades, the expanded program on immunization (EPI) has achieved a high vaccine coverage especially against the target diseases like tuberculosis, tetanus, diphtheria, pertussis, polio, measles, yellow fever, hepatitis B and, *Haemophilus influenzae* type b. In the recent years, a strong need has been felt to expand immunization activities beyond infancy, thereby representing the adolescent population as the target group. This need can be fulfilled either as a part of routine National Immunization Program or as disease eradication measures.

Disease control objectives, financial capacity, medical facilities and administrative commitment are different for each country. Number of factors such as the age-specific incidence of disease, response to vaccination, compatibility with other recommended vaccines, cost and risk benefit ratio, determine the age at which vaccine should be administered. All these factors need to be evaluated before considering any new or existent vaccine for delivery to adolescents.[2]

THE GOALS AND OBJECTIVES OF ADOLESCENT IMMUNIZATION

The reason for approaching adolescents for immunization is to boost immunity that is waning, especially in the absence of "natural" boosting from exposure to the infectious agent. Another objective is to accelerate control of specific disease during the outbreaks or to counter-specific risk. Immunization initiatives in adolescents frequently cover a wide age range, with the aim to increase herd immunity, interrupt spread of infectious diseases and providing opportunity to those children who have missed the immunization in the past. This may result to a direct benefit to the adolescents themselves, or may be part of wider disease control strategy. Thus, long-term control of infectious diseases and their elimination need supplementary immunization in adolescent.

The twin objectives of adolescent immunization in India are administration of age-specific boosters (e.g. Td vaccine every 10 years for 10–12 years age group), newly recommended vaccines (e.g. like Tdap/HPV), epidemic response vaccines like Japanese encephalitis in endemic regions as well as combined seasonal and swine flu vaccine following pandemic recommendations (Table 9.4.1).[3] Secondly, catch-up vaccination for those adolescents who were not immunized/partially immunized during their childhood, e.g. MMR, Hepatitis B, varicella vaccines.

Chickenpox during childhood is considered as a harmless self-limiting infection; it can result in severe complications and may even add to mortality figures in adolescents between 10 years and 18 years of age. Thus, the goal of adolescent immunization is also to protect them from the dreaded complications of childhood vaccine preventable diseases (e.g. measles, mumps, pertussis, diphtheria) when they occur during adolescence.

Table 9.4.1: IAP recommended immunization schedule for persons aged 7 through 18 years, 2016[3] (with range).

Age ▸ Vaccine ▾	7–10 years	11–12 years	13–18 years
Tdap[1]	1 dose (if indicated)	1 dose	1 dose (if indicated)
HPV[2]	See footnote 2	2 doses	Complete 3-dose series for girls 15 years and older
MMR[3]	Complete 2-dose series		
Varicella[4]	Complete 2-dose series		
Hepatitis B[5]	Complete 3-dose series		
Hepatitis A[6]	Complete 2-dose series		
Typhoid[7]	1 dose every 3 years		
Influenza Vaccine[8]	One dose every year		
Japanese Encephalitis Vaccine[9]	Catch-up up to 18 years		
Pneumococcal Vaccine[10]	See footnote 10		
Meningococcal Vaccine[11]	See footnote 11		
Cholera[12]	Cholera 1 and 2		
Rabies[13]	Rabies (Pre-EP and PEP)		

Range of recommended ages for all children	Range of recommended ages for certain high-risk groups
Range of recommended ages for catch-up immunization	Not routinely recommended

Any dose not administered at the recommended age should be administered at a subsequent visit, when indicated and feasible. The use of a combination vaccine generally is preferred over separate injections of its equivalent component vaccines.

1. **Tetanus and diphtheria toxoids and acellular pertussis (Tdap) vaccine**
   - Minimum age: 10 years for Boostrix and 11 years for Adacel
   - Persons aged 11 through 18 years who have not received Tdap vaccine should receive a dose followed by tetanus and diphtheria toxoids (Td) booster doses every 10 years thereafter
   - Tdap vaccine should be substituted for a single dose of Td in the catch-up series for children aged 7 through 10 years
   - Tdap vaccine can be administered regardless of the interval since the last tetanus and diphtheria toxoid-containing vaccine
   - Catch up above 7 years: Tdap, Td, Td at 0, 1 and 6 months
   - Tdap can also be administered safely to pregnant women.
2. **Human papillomavirus (HPV) vaccines**
   - HPV4 (Gardasil) and HPV2 (Cervarix)
   - Minimum age: 9 years
   - Either HPV4 (0, 2, 6 months) or HPV2 (0, 1, 6 months) is recommended in a 3-dose series for females aged more than 15 years
   - Administer the second dose 1 to 2 months after the first dose and the third dose 6 months after the first dose (at least 24 weeks after the first dose)
   - In the age group 9–15 years 2 doses are recommended (0, 6 months).
3. **Measles, mumps, and rubella (MMR) vaccine**
   - The minimum interval between the 2 doses of MMR vaccine is 4 weeks
   - One dose if previously vaccinated with one dose.
4. **Varicella (VAR) vaccine**
   - For persons without evidence of immunity, administer 2 doses if not previously vaccinated or the second dose if only 1 dose has been administered
   - For persons aged 7 through 12 years, the recommended minimum interval between doses is 3 months. However, if the second dose was administered at least 4 weeks after the first dose, it can be accepted as valid
   - For persons aged 13 years and older, the minimum interval between doses is 4 weeks.
5. **Hepatitis B (HepB) vaccine**
   - Administer the 3-dose series to those not previously vaccinated
   - For those with incomplete vaccination, the recommended minimum interval between dose 1 and dose 2 is 4 weeks, and

between dose 2 and 3 is 8 weeks. The final (third or fourth) dose in the HepB vaccine series should be administered at least 16 weeks after the first dose.
6. **Hepatitis A (Hep A) vaccine**
   - Administer 2 doses at least 6 months apart to unvaccinated persons
   - For catch up vaccination, prevaccination screening for Hepatitis A antibody is recommended in children older than 10 years as at this age the estimated sero-positive rates exceed 50%
   - Combination of Hep B and Hep A may be used in 0, 1, 6 schedule
7. **Typhoid vaccine**
   - Both typhoid conjugate and typhoid polysaccharide vaccine are available
   - Typhoid conjugate vaccine to be preferred over Vi polysaccharide vaccine both for booster and catchup vaccination
   - Polysaccharide vaccine needs revaccination every 3 years
   - Up to 18 years of age single dose of Vi conjugate typhoid vaccine. The need of booster dose not yet determined.
8. **Influenza vaccine**
   - Administer 1 dose to persons aged 9 years and older
   - For most healthy children aged 2 through 18 years, either LAIV or IIV may be used
   - IIV: 9 years and above single dose
   - Annual revaccination with single dose
   - LAIV: 9 years and above: Single dose
   - Best time to vaccinate: As soon as the new vaccine is released and available in the market and just before the onset of rainy season.
9. **Japanese encephalitis (JE) Vaccine**
   - Recommended only for individuals living in endemic areas till 18 years of age
   - Currently 3 type of JE vaccine available in India
   - Live attenuated, cell culture derived SA-14-14-2 JE vaccine should be preferred
   - Dose: 0.5 mL SC
   - 2 doses 9 months and 16 to 18 months
   - Inactivated Vero cell culture SA 14-14-2 IXIARO
   - Schedule: 2 doses 0 and 28 days. 0.25 mL age >1–3 years. 0.5 mL age >3 years

Contd...

Contd...

- Inactivated, vero cell culture. Strain isolated from NIV Pune.
- Schedule: Primary dose schedule 0.5 mL, 2 dose, 4 week apart.

10. **Pneumococcal vaccines**
    - Pneumococcal conjugate vaccine (PCV) and pneumococcal polysaccharide vaccine (PPSV) both are used in certain high-risk group of children
    - A single dose of PCV may be administered to children aged 6 through 18 years who have anatomic/functional asplenia, HIV infection or other immunocompromising condition, cochlear implant, or cerebral spinal fluid leak
    - Administer PPSV at least 8 weeks after the last dose of PCV to children aged 2 years or older with certain underlying medical conditions, including a cochlear implant
    - A single revaccination (with PPSV) should be administered after 5 years to children with anatomic/functional asplenia or an immunocompromising condition.

11. **Meningococcal vaccine**
    - Recommended only for certain high-risk group of children, during outbreaks, travelers to endemic areas, and students going for study abroad

- Only meningococcal polysaccharide vaccine (MPSV) is available
- Minimum age: 2 years
- Dose schedule: A single dose 0.5 mL SC/IM is recommended
- Revaccination only once after 3 years in those at continued high risk.

12. **Cholera vaccine**
    - Minimum age: One year (inactivated whole cell *Vibrio cholerae*)
    - Recommended only for the vaccination of persons residing in highly endemic areas and traveling to areas where risk of transmission is very high
    - Two doses 2 weeks apart for >1 year old.

13. **Rabies vaccine**
    - Following two situations included in 'high-risk category of children' for rabies vaccination and should be offered 'pre-exposure prophylaxis' (Pre-EP):
      ◆ Children having pets in home
      ◆ Children perceived with higher threat of being bitten by dogs such as hostellers, risk of stray dog menace while going outdoor.

THE TRUE ADOLESCENT VACCINES

Achieving and maintaining high immunization rates is critical for disease prevention.

In adolescent vaccine category, Tdap and HPV are the two true adolescent's vaccines—Tdap as a single booster for children above 7 years and from 10 to 18 years and HPV the female specific vaccine from 10 to 45 years.

The single adolescent vaccine for inclusion in the National Immunization Program is Td in place of TT as a first step, and if resources permit, Tdap on a later date.

Td is now the WHO recommended immunogen for antenatal boosters and for wound prophylaxis at all ages including for adolescents, in view of (a) increase in incidents of diphtheria cases[3] and (b) waning immunity to the diphtheria component resulting in more severe disease during adolescence and even adulthood with fatal complications like myocarditis.

PERTUSSIS VACCINATION

The epidemiology of pertussis is changing, with a clear increase in the number of cases diagnosed in adolescents as it is known that the humoral and cellular immunity evoked by vaccines tends to wane after some years. Infected adolescents may serve as an important reservoir of infection for neonates and others at higher risk of serious illness or pertussis-related death. Pertussis vaccination in adolescents has many advantages including significant lowering of new cases among vaccinated subjects. Tdap is a highly effective vaccine that replaces the Td vaccine as the booster at 11–12 years of age or in older adolescents who need a Td booster.[4,5]

HUMAN PAPILLOMAVIRUS VACCINATION IN ADOLESCENT

Human papillomavirus (HPV) vaccination in adolescents also deserves special attention as HPV is closely associated with the development various anogenital and oropharyngeal cancers, of which cervical cancer is the most frequent; and most infections are acquired very early during adolescence, at the time of initial sexual activities. Cervical cancer ranks as the 2nd most frequent cancer among women and the 2nd most frequent cancer among women between 15 and 44 years of age. About 5.0% of women in the general population are estimated to harbor cervical HPV-16/18 infection at a given time, and 83.2% of invasive cervical cancers are attributed to HPVs 16 or 18.[6]

Disease progression; from HPV infection to cervical cancer is a process, which may take 10–20 years. One of the first histological signs of HPV infection is the presence of koilocytosis; epithelial cell with distinctive large, clear vacuoles around the nucleus. Thus, when the immune system fails to clear an oncogenic HPV infection, a persistence infection develops. This persistent oncogenic HPV infection are more likely to progress towards invasive cervical cancer if they are left untreated. 36.1% of Indian women per one lakh population suffer from cervical cancer. While sero type 16 and 18 account for 76.4% incidence, type 45 and 31 responsible for a small percentage. Over 40 sero types identified as oncogenic. Every sexually active women is at risk of oncogenic HPV infection. Of the estimated 50–80% of women who will accrue an HPV infection in their life lime, 50% are infected with oncogenic HPV type. Young woman aged 16–25 years are at greatest risk of oncogenic HPV infection.

Prophylactic HPV vaccination has provided a powerful tool for primary prevention of cervical cancer and other HPV-related diseases. Currently, two vaccine formulations are licensed in India: bivalent (against HPVs 16/18), quadrivalent (against HPVs 6/11/16/18). Two doses of HPV vaccine are advised for adolescent/pre-adolescent girls aged 9–14 years; for girls 15 years and older, current three dose schedule will continue. For two-dose schedule, the minimum interval between doses should be 6 months. For both vaccines, no boosters are recommended.

National Technical Advisory Group on Immunization (NTAGI) has formed a subcommittee to explore the feasibility of including HPV vaccine in the National Immunization program. With assistance from GAVI, HPV vaccine is being introduced in selected pilot project areas in National Immunization Program. Punjab state and New Delhi Capital Territory have introduced HPV vaccination in 2016.[7,8] Coverage for the first dose in two districts in Punjab (initial introduction districts) exceeded 95% with excellent safety and acceptability profile. Haryana government is planning to introduce in immunization program.

Adolescent Vaccines for Catch-up Vaccination

More than half of parents are not aware of a catch-up vaccination program, which could prevent many infectious diseases to which children are highly vulnerable. Therefore, to ensure that children who have missed out on the previously scheduled immunization, the catch-up schedule is an opportunity to get protected as early as possible. Every hospital visit of adolescent should be taken as opportunity to check history of immunization and catch up missing schedule. However, the appropriateness of a booster or additional dose in adolescence will depend on how the infant vaccination program is followed.

Even though children against diseases like pertussis may have already been vaccinated, they should get another dose as immunity weans. Thus, vaccines are not just for infants and young children but they are important for adolescent too. Also, as kids get older they are more at risk catching diseases like meningitis and HPV, so they need the protection (Tables 9.4.2 and 9.4.3).

Issues to be Considered when Planning Catch-up Vaccination[9]

- Consideration of history of previous immunization
- Vaccine doses should not be administered at appropriate age and interval
- Be very vigilant on interchangeability of vaccines brands
- If vaccinated prior to recommended age, those should not be counted as valid doses
- For incomplete vaccination, schedule from previous documented record should be taken forward
- As the age increase, the required number of doses may be reduced, e.g. from 12 months of age, only single dose of Hib vaccine is essential
- Plan to keep minimal hospital visits, if more than one vaccine is overdue.

Travel-related Adolescent Vaccines

Children and adolescents are at increased risk for travel-related illness. For adolescent traveler, the immunization schedule must be personalized. There can not be a single schedule of vaccination for travelers. This personalized

Table 9.4.2: Recommendation for catch up vaccination.

Vaccine	Schedule
MMR	2 doses at 4–8 weeks interval[@]
Hepatitis B	3 doses at 0, 1 and 6 months*
Hepatitis A	2 doses at 0 and 6 months** (prior check of anti HAV IgG may be cost effective)
Typhoid	1 dose every 3 years[#]
Varicella	2 doses at 4–8 weeks interval
Influenza	1 dose every year
Japanese encephalitis	Catch up to 18 years[##]
PPSV23 (pneumococcal)	2 doses 5 years apart[$]
Rabies	As soon as possible after exposure

[@] One dose if previously vaccinated with 1 dose
*, ** combination of Hep A and Hep B can be used at 0, 1 and 6 schedule
[#] Minimum interval of 3 years should be observed between two doses
[##] Only in endemic area as a catch up
[$] Maximum number of doses two

Table 9.4.3: Mandatory adolescent vaccines.

- MMR and varicella vaccines in 2 doses at 4–8 weeks interval if not immunized during childhood
- HEP A and HEP B Vaccine at 0, 1 and 6 months schedule if not immunized previously
- Typhoid boosters every 3 years maximum of 6 boosters
- Tdap single booster followed by Td boosters every 10 years
- Epidemic related varicella, hepatitis A and typhoid vaccines for hostellers
- High-risk group vaccines like pneumococcal vaccine
- Annual combined FLU vaccine
- Travel-related adolescent vaccines like yellow fever, meningococcal vaccines, etc.
- Japanese B encephalitis vaccine in endemic areas ahead of anticipated epidemic in campaign approach

schedule is followed according to the immunization history of traveler, duration and time of travel and country to be visited. The immunization should start early enough, to allow sufficient time for adequate immunity to develop and minimize any adverse events around the time of departure. All age appropriate vaccines should be completed before travel, in addition to those listed below (Table 9.4.4).

Barriers for Adolescent Vaccination in India

Vaccines recommended for adolescents are underused and the main reason is concept of adolescent vaccine is not yet established in India. There is a lack of clarity on disease burden of vaccine preventable diseases and very limited adolescent surveillance data is available. Also, epidemiological studies are very few which hinders the true assessment of economic impact and vaccine importance. Also criteria and process to include new vaccines and schedule in unclear in India and bounded by constrains.

Table 9.4.4: Travel vaccine for adolescent.

Vaccine	Place of travel	Dose recommended
Meningococcal	USA/UK/Endemic areas Saudi Arabia and Africa#	2 doses 4 B weeks apart
Yellow fever ^	Yellow fever endemic zones**	10 days before travel
Oral cholera	Endemic area or area with an outbreak	2 doses 1 week apart
Japanese B encephalitis	Endemic areas for JE	Single dose up to 15 years
Rabies (pre-exposure prophylaxis)	For adolescents going on trekking	Day 0, 7, 28

#Quadravalent vaccine for those traveling to the US and bivalent (A+C) or quadravalent for those traveling to the UK

^ Mandatory for all travelers to yellow fever endemic zones as per International Health Regulations

**The list of endemic countries can be obtained at http://wwwn.cdc.gov/ travel yelowBookch4,YellowFever.aspx currently available only at select government controlled centers in India

e.g. introduction of non-life-threatening diseases is uncertain.

Use of antibiotics, antiviral medicines and others is preferred, in comparison to using a vaccine. Diseases like typhoid, influenza are often treated and very low importance is given to prevention. Many of the general physicians and doctors from other specialties have a very limited knowledge about vaccine introduction; efficacy and dosage as pharmaceutical sales team do not approach them. This results in a low awareness and trust amongst patients. Due to lack of literature, sero-epidemiological studies and epidemiological patterns, doctors also are not convinced about vaccine efficacy and hesitant to promote the product.

In comparison to infants, adolescents often play an important role in decision making and thus, awareness about the vaccine preventable diseases is very important at the school level. Therefore, education and outreach is required to change the behavior among adolescents and their parents or guardians. Also, in India, most of the medical insurance policies do not cover vaccines, unlike developed countries and china. This cost burden also leads to prevent the vaccine uptake as these newer vaccines and several vaccines are expensive considered only in high-risk situations.

SUMMARY AND RECOMMENDATIONS

Successful implementation of immunization program has resulted in significant decline of targeted vaccine preventable diseases.[10] However, the shift has occurred only for vaccines like measles, diphtheria, pertussis, etc. Newly registered vaccines like Td, Tdap and HPV merit consideration for inclusion in the national immunization program. The catch-up immunization should be increased for providing much greater benefits. Misinformation on safety of newly registered vaccines by some experts should be countered by professional bodies with evidence-based approach. Also, other barriers for adolescent immunization should be eliminated by effective adolescent immunization awareness campaigns. State and central government should be addressed to boost awareness and introduce adolescent friendly, need-based vaccines in the National Immunization Programme.

ACKNOWLEDGMENTS

The authors are indebted to Dr Sameer Parekh, and Dr Pramod Pujari, Serum Institute of India Pvt. Ltd., Pune, Maharashtra, India, for help rendered in the preparation of this section.

REFERENCES

1. The State of the World's Children 2011. Adolescence: An Age of Opportunity. https://www.unicef.org/adolescence/files/SOWC_2011_Main_Report_EN_02092011.pdf. Accessed on 20 July 2017.
2. Global strategies, policies and practices for immunization of adolescents. World Health Organization. WHO/V&B/99.24.
3. IAP Immunization Schedule 2016: Detailed recommendations. Advisory Committee on Vaccines and Immunization Practices. http://acvip.org/professional/columns/detailed-recommendations-iap-immunization-schedule-2016.
4. Lee, Hyo-Jin, Jung-Hyun Choi. Tetanus–diphtheria–acellular Pertussis Vaccination for Adults: An Update. Clinical and Experimental Vaccine Research. 2017;6(1):22-30.
5. Murhekar MV, Bitragunta S, Hutin Y, et al. Immunization coverage and immunity to diphtheria and tetanus among children in Hyderabad, India. Journal of Infection. 2009;58: 191-6.
6. Bruni L, Barrionuevo-Rosas L, Albero G, et al. ICO Information Centre on HPV and Cancer (HPV Information Centre). Human Papillomavirus and Related Diseases in India. Summary Report 19 April 2017. [Accessed on 19th July 2017]
7. http://www.searo.who.int/india/mediacentre/events/2016/Punjab_HPV_vaccine/en/) [Accessed on 8th Aug 2017]
8. Sankaranarayanan R, Bhatla N, Basu P. Current global status and impact of human papillomavirus vaccination: Implications for India. Year 2016;144(2):169-80.
9. Catch-up vaccination. http://www.nevdgp.org.au/info/immunisation/catch_up_vac.htm.
10. Andre FE, Booy R, Bock HL, et al. Vaccination greatly reduces disease, disability, death and inequity worldwide. Bulletin of the World Health Organization. 2008;86:2.

9.5   FUTURE VACCINES

Srinivas G Kasi

INTRODUCTION

Vaccines have been hailed as one of the greatest public health achievements of the 20th century. Smallpox has been eradicated, polio is on the verge of eradication, diphtheria, tetanus, pertussis, measles, *Haemophilus influenzae* type B (Hib) and pneumococcal diseases have been largely controlled in most of the developed world. Over 10 million deaths annually worldwide are attributable to infectious diseases and these can be prevented by wider use of existing vaccines, while most of these deaths would be preventable by the development of effective new vaccines.

The next few decades will witness a revolution in the way vaccines are made, used and the diseases targeted for control or elimination.

Conventionally, vaccines have targeted only infectious diseases. Efforts are on to develop vaccines against non-infectious diseases like cancer, autoimmunity, allergies and other conditions. Both preventive and therapeutic vaccines will improve outcome in a variety of chronic conditions.

NEWER TECHNOLOGIES IN VACCINE DEVELOPMENT

Technologies in vaccine development have passes through different phases (Fig. 9.5.1):

Vaccinology in the Genomics Era

This era began with the characterization of the entire genome of the *H. influenzae* in 1995 (Fig. 9.5.2). Subsequently the genomes of over 2,000 bacteria and 3,000 viruses have been characterized. This has enabled the identification of a growing number of potential vaccine targets. Once the complete genome sequence of the organism is available,

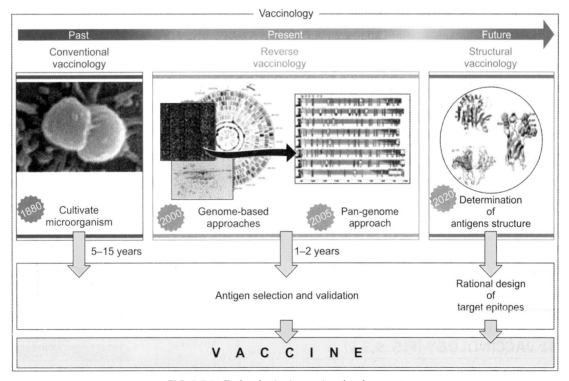

FIG. 9.5.1: Technologies in vaccine development.

The past involved conventional approaches of cultivation of the microorganism in laboratory conditions, inactivation or attenuation of the microorganism, purification testing for immunogenicity and safety and injecting it. This method was empirical, laborious and took 5–15 years for development of a vaccine. The present, in the genomic era, involves choosing the most appropriate antigen from the virtual catalogue of all the potential vaccine candidates available in the genomic and pangenomic data of microorganisms and use of reverse vaccinology to produce a vaccine in 1–2 years. The future involves the use of structural vaccinology, to construct the most appropriate antigen and personalizing vaccines based on "vaccinomics".

Source: Reproduced with permission from Serruto D, Rappuoli R. FEBS Letters. Elsevier Ltd. 2006;580:2985-92.

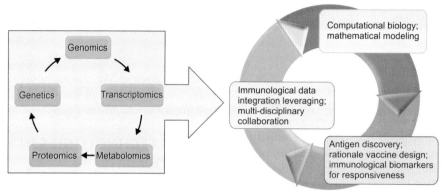

FIG. 9.5.2: Systems biology approaches for vaccine studies interactions and implications on translational research. Systems biology is a term used to describe the study of the interactions between the components of biological systems, and how these interactions give rise to the function and behavior of that system. This diagram illustrates the use of systems biology for vaccine development.
Source: Reproduced from Buonaguro et al. BMC Systems Biology. 2011;5:146.

high-throughput approaches can be used to screen for target molecules. Transcriptomics, functional genomics, proteomics, immunomics, structural genomics and immunogenetics are other spinoffs of the genomic era, which are revolutionizing the way vaccines are made. Vaccinomics refers to the investigation of heterogeneity in host genetic markers at the individual or population level that may result in variations in the immune responses to vaccines, with the hope of predicting and optimizing vaccine outcomes and "personalizing vaccines". This will help in making vaccines more effective and safe.

Advances in the fields of physics, chemistry, electronics, biotechnology and engineering were amalgamated with omics to invent a new entity called structural biology. The application of structural biology to vaccines is called structural vaccinology. Structural vaccinology enables the study of the complex pathways of cell interactions in the immune response. It also enabled the atomic resolution of antigen structure, enabling rational design of specific target epitopes for use as vaccine candidates, made to order vaccine antigens.

In the coming years, vaccines are set to have even greater impact on world health than they currently do.

Reverse vaccinology, DNA vaccines, vectored vaccines, edible vaccines and needle free devices are some of the recent advances that will be discussed.

REVERSE VACCINOLOGY (FIG. 9.5.3)

Reverse vaccinology is a novel and new method in vaccinology, pioneered by Rino Rappuoli and first used successfully in developing a vaccine against group B *Meningococcus.*

In reverse vaccinology, an entire pathogen genome sequence is screened using bioinformatics, to identify several candidate protective antigens and these are tested for their suitability as vaccine candidates. These proteins

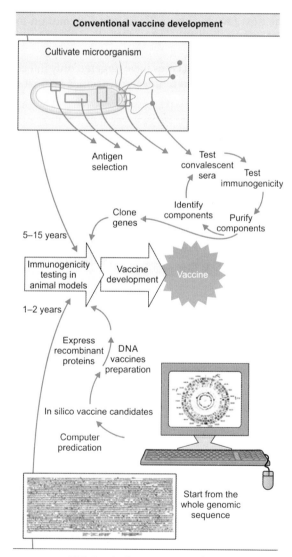

FIG. 9.5.3: Reverse vaccinology.
Source: Reproduced with permissions from Rappuoli R. Current Opinion in Microbiology. 2000;3:445-50. © 2000 Elsevier Science Ltd. All rights reserved.

then undergo conventional testing in the laboratory for immune responses. Since the process of vaccine discovery starts in silico using the genetic information rather than the pathogen itself, this process has been named reverse vaccinology. Reverse Vaccinology (RV), has provided a paradigm change in the perspective of vaccine design.

The major advantages of this technology include: the identification of antigens not seen by the conventional methods and the identification of novel antigens that work on totally different mechanisms. In addition it is a quick and efficient method for identifying antigen candidates for vaccines.

A vaccine against the group B *Meningococcus* is the first successful application of this technology. Reverse vaccinology identified 350 genes from the *Neisseria meningitidis* genome as potential vaccine candidates, which were then evaluated for their ability to elicit bactericidal antibodies. Five of these 350 genes with the most favorable attributes were combined to develop a vaccine which has proved to be safe and immunogenic in human trials. Vaccines against malaria, human immunodeficiency virus (HIV), tuberculosis (TB), hepatitis C, syphilis, *Pneumococcus, Streptococcus, Staphylococcus, Escherichia coli,* etc. are being investigated using this technology.

DNA VACCINES

DNA vaccination was discovered in the 1990s. A DNA vaccine contains a nucleotide sequence encoding a key antigenic determinant from a given pathogen or a tumor antigen that is injected into a host via a plasmid (Figs. 9.5.4 and 9.5.5).

The plasmid vector is taken up into cells and transcribed in the nucleus. The host cell translates the encoded DNA into protein in the cytoplasm. The DNA vaccine-derived protein antigen is then degraded by proteasomes into intracellular peptides. The vaccine derived-peptide, being foreign, is recognized as non-self. They bind to major histocompatibility complex (MHC) class I molecules which are presented on the cell surface and induce a cell-mediated immune response. As DNA vaccines generate cell-mediated immunity, the hope is that they will be effective against some difficult viruses even as standard vaccines have failed to work.

Although there are no US Food and Drug Administration (FDA)-approved DNA vaccines for use in humans, they are the newest vaccine platform currently in development and have already had success in veterinary medicine. While DNA based vaccines showed promising results in animals, in humans the immune response was lower than that observed with conventional vaccines. To enhance the immune response, novel approaches such as DNA delivery by electroporation and stimulation of the immune system via the use of genetic adjuvants have been used in human clinical trials with encouraging preliminary results.

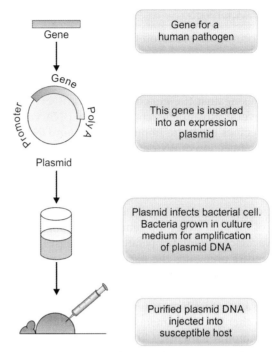

FIG. 9.5.4: How DNA vaccines are prepared.

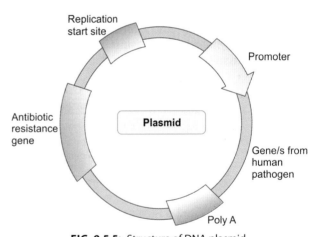

FIG. 9.5.5: Structure of DNA plasmid.

Status Report

Four DNA vaccines for larger animals were licensed for veterinary use. Two of them target infectious diseases, like West Nile virus in horses, and aquatic Rhabdovirus called infectious hematopoietic necrosis in salmon; one is a cancer vaccine for melanoma in dogs; and the last one has a therapeutic purpose in swine.

DNA vaccines currently under investigation are targeting viruses such as HIV-1, hepatitis B virus (HBV) and malaria, or cancer cells like melanoma. Amongst bacterial infections TB, typhoid fever and anthrax DNA vaccines are the most popular candidates for entering clinical trials.

RNA VACCINES

RNA vaccines are based on mRNA and self-amplifying RNA replicons of the vaccine antigen which when injected intramuscularly in mice resulted in local production of an encoded reporter protein and induction of immune responses against the encoded antigen. RNA vaccines have several advantages compared to DNA vaccines. RNA vaccines are more immunogenic than DNA-based vaccines. Injection of RNA presents no risk of disrupting the cell's natural DNA sequence.

The efficiency and thermostability of RNA-based vaccines have been increased through the use of viral-particle engineered to express a heterologous antigen in place of the viral structural gene enabling the storage of RNA vaccines at room temperature for at least 18 months. This feature precludes the necessity of maintaining the cold chain, making RNA vaccines particularly practical for developing countries.

mRNA vaccines have entered human clinical trials as immunotherapeutic in metastatic melanoma and renal cell carcinoma patients. Clinical trials have also been performed with RNA replicon vaccines packaged in viral particles encoding for cytomegalovirus (CMV) gB and pp65/IE1 proteins.

RNA vaccines are also being developed to prevent infectious diseases. A vaccine against rabies is currently in clinical trials, while vaccines against influenza, HIV and tuberculosis are still at the research stage.

VIRAL VECTORS FOR VACCINES

Viral vector vaccines use live viruses to carry DNA/RNA into human cells. The inserted DNA/RNA encodes antigens that, once expressed in the infected human cells, elicit an immune response. Viral vectored vaccines have the distinct advantage of inducing a broad based immune response, including a strong cell mediated immune response. Moreover, they also have the potential to replicate like live attenuated vaccines.

Viral vector vaccines are being used in a strategy called heterologous prime-boost strategy in which vector vaccines are being pursued as both prime and boost vaccines.

There are 12 viral vector vaccines currently in use for veterinary diseases. The approved viral vectors in humans include adenovirus, fowlpox virus, attenuated yellow fever (YFV-17D) and vaccinia virus.

CHIMERIC VACCINES (FIG. 9.5.6)

Chimeric vaccines are created by cloning pieces of one virus into another virus and deriving a "chimer." Usually, yellow fever virus is used as a replicative backbone but carries the structural proteins of another virus, forming a **chimeric** structure. Chimeric vaccines against Japanese encephalitis and dengue are in clinical usage.

Chimeric vaccines against tick borne encephalitis, Chikungunya, malaria, *Clostridium* difficile are in various stages of clinical development.

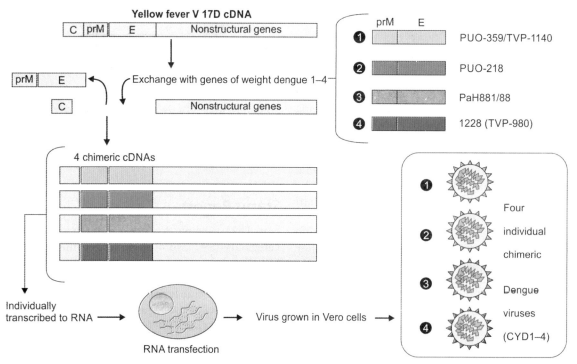

FIG. 9.5.6: Construction of the tetravalent yellow fever/dengue chimeric vaccine.

Source: Guy B,* Saville M Lang J. Human vaccines. 2010;6:696-705. © 2010 Landes Bioscience. (*Permission obtained from Guy B through Email)

NEWER ADJUVANTS

New adjuvants are important, as the currently approved vaccine adjuvants are not always potent enough to induce an efficient protective immune response against different target pathogens.

Some future adjuvants are:
MF59: This is a water-in-oil emulsion which induces a Th2-type immune response. MF59 and ASO3 are licensed in Europe and are included in the influenza vaccines.

Liposomes: It can encapsulate antigens and act as a vehicle adjuvant. Several liposomal vaccines based on viral membrane proteins (virosomes) have been extensively evaluated and are approved in Europe for hepatitis A influenza.

Immunopotentiating reconstituted influenza virosomes (IRIV) have been registered for use in hepatitis A vaccine in Europe, South America and Asia.

Saponins: These are derived from the bark of a Chilean tree, Quillaja saponaria. Saponins act by induction of cytokines. Saponins are part of the proprietary ASO2, which is the adjuvant being used for the *Plasmodium falciparum* vaccine, RTS.S.

Toll-like receptor (TLR) agonists: Monophosphoryl lipid A (MPL A) is a derivative of lipopolysaccharide (LPS) primarily from Salmonella minnesota, which retains much of the immune-stimulatory properties of LPS without its inherent toxicity. MPL interacts with TLR4 and stimulates IL-12 production by DCs and macrophages. It also activates nuclear factor-kB (NF-kB) and production of proinflammatory cytokines. ASO2 is a combination of MPL, alum and QS-21, while ASO4 is a combination of MPL and alum. MPL-based adjuvants, including AS01B and AS02A, have been evaluated in clinical trials in malaria vaccines, TB and Leishmania vaccines. Other adjuvants being investigated include chitosan, recombinant cytokines, Thymosin alpha-1 and the TLR9 agonist CpG oligonucleotide.

EDIBLE VACCINES

Edible vaccines involve the introduction of selected genes into the genome of plants and inducing them to produce the desired proteins (Fig. 9.5.7). This process is called "transformation" and such plants are called "transgenic" plants.

Edible vaccines stimulate both mucosal and systemic immune responses. This would be particularly beneficial for protection against pathogens which gain entry through mucosal surfaces, e.g. tuberculosis, organisms causing diarrhea, pneumonia, sexually transmitted diseases (STD) and HIV.

Multiple antigens can be inserted and antigens corresponding to biological adjuvants can be inserted to produce second-generation edible vaccines (Table 9.5.1).

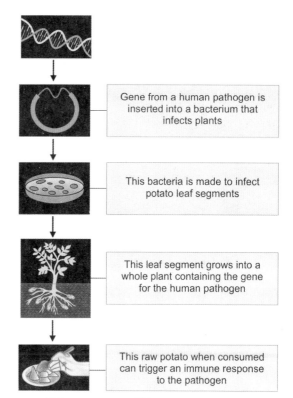

FIG. 9.5.7: How edible vaccines are made?

Table 9.5.1: Edible vaccines under development.

Pathogen	Vector
Hepatitis B virus	Potato, tobacco
Rabies virus	Tobacco
Corona virus	Maize
HIV	Tomato
Vibrio cholerae	Potato
Measles virus	Tobacco
Anthrax	Tobacco

Needle-free Vaccine Delivery

Advantages of needle-free vaccine delivery include ease and speed of delivery, improved safety and compliance, decreasing costs, and reducing pain associated with vaccinations. Needle-free vaccine delivery systems include needle-free injection devices, transcutaneous immunization (TCI) and mucosal immunization (Figs. 9.5.8 and 9.5.9).

Jet injectors are needle-free devices that deliver a liquid vaccine through a narrow orifice and penetrate the skin with a high-speed narrow stream. Jet injectors using powders may render the need for a cold chain unnecessary.

In TCI the vaccine antigen with or without adjuvant is applied to the skin, using a patch or "microneedles". This can induce both systemic and mucosal immunity. Mucosal

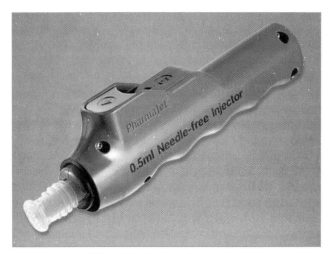

FIG. 9.5.8: A needle-free injector.

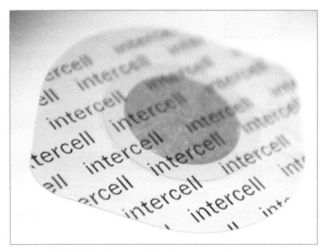

FIG. 9.5.9: Intercell intradermal vaccine patch.

immunization has thus far been focused on oral, nasal and aerosol vaccines. Transgenic plant "edible" vaccines are an exciting new area as discussed above.

MALARIA, TUBERCULOSIS AND AIDS VACCINE

Malaria, tuberculosis and AIDS collectively cause more than five million deaths per year, but have so far eluded conventional vaccine development. They represent one of the major global public health challenges of the 21st century.

Vaccines against Malaria

The majority of malarial deaths are due to *P. falciparum*. The importance of *P. vivax* infection, particularly in Southeast Asia, and the severity of some infections caused by this malaria parasite have been underestimated but are now receiving more attention. Over 1.5 million cases of malaria were reported in India in 2009.

Multiple antigens at different stages of the mosquito life cycle, antigenic variations, absence of correlates of protection and complexity of conducting clinical and field trials are some reasons for this failure to develop a successful vaccine against malaria.

Classification of vaccines against malaria:

- *Pre-erythrocytic vaccines:* Antigens under investigation include irradiated sporozoites, circumsporozoite protein (CSP) or peptides, liver stage antigens-1 (LSA-1).
- *Asexual blood-stage (erythrocytic) vaccine:* It will inhibit the development of the parasite in RBCs.
- *Sexual stage vaccines:* Antigens being investigated include Pfs 25, 48/45k, Pfs 230.
- *Combined vaccine (cocktail):* Based on incorporation of antigens from different stages. Antigens being investigated include SPf 66 (based on pre-erythrocytic and asexual blood stage proteins of Pf). The CDC/NII Malvac-1 vaccine has included nine different malaria antigen combined into one synthetic gene.

The RTS,S/AS01 Vaccine

This vaccine is a hybrid molecule expressed in yeast, that consists of the tandem repeat tetrapeptide (R) and C-terminal T-cell epitope containing (T) regions of CSP fused to the hepatitis B surface antigen (S), plus unfused S antigen with the adjuvant AS01. RTS,S is several years ahead of any other vaccine in terms of assessment of its efficacy in clinical trials.

The most advanced malaria vaccine candidate in development globally, RTS,S/AS01, completed Phase III clinical testing in 2014. The final study results were published in 2015 . These final results demonstrated that vaccination with the three-dose primary series reduced clinical malaria cases over the length of the study by 28% in young children (over a median follow-up of 48 months after first dose across trial sites) and 18% in infants (over a median follow-up of 38 months after first dose across trial sites). A booster dose of RTS,S, administered 18 months after completion of the primary series, reduced the number of cases of clinical malaria in young children (aged 5–17 months at first vaccination) by 36% over the entire study period and in infants (aged 6–12 weeks at first vaccination) by 26% over the study period. These results were achieved on top of existing malaria interventions, such as ITNs, which were used by approximately 80% of the trial participants.

On January 29, 2016 the World Health Organization (WHO) recommended large-scale pilot implementations of RTS,S in children 5–9 months of age in African settings of moderate-to-high parasite transmission. Similar endorsement has been made by the European Medicinal Agency (EMA).

Of the over 20 candidate vaccines none have reached phase III trials.

HUMAN IMMUNODEFICIENCY VIRUS VACCINES

The first phase I trial of an HIV vaccine was conducted in the year 1987. Some two hundred HIV vaccine candidates/regimens have been clinically tested since 1986, yet efficacy trials were completed for only four vaccines, only one of which demonstrated modest efficacy in preventing HIV acquisition.

The HIV-1 Env gp120 proteins vaccine (sponsored by VaxGen) and the STEP and Phambili trials-MRKAd5 HIV-1 Gag/Pol/Nef were suspended as no protective responses were seen. Moreover, the vaccinated cohorts had a higher incidence of HIV acquisition.

Novel Vaccinal Approaches

Peptides, fusion proteins and long lipopeptides in multiepitopic combinations also are at an early stage of clinical development, either alone or in prime-boost combinations with live vector-based recombinant vaccines. Lipopeptides whose sequence corresponds to that of CTL epitopes-rich regions in the Gag and Nef viral proteins are in phase II trials in the USA and in France (NIAID/ANRS).

Finally, nonstructural viral proteins, such as Tat, Rev, Vif and Nef, are being developed as candidate vaccines using viral vectors such as MVA or Ad5 (bioMérieux/Transgene), fowlpox virus (AVC), DNA recombinant proteins or fusion proteins or polyepitopic peptides.

The development of a safe, effective and affordable HIV vaccine remains a formidable scientific and public health challenge.

NEWER TUBERCULOSIS VACCINES

Over the past decade, 12 vaccine candidates have left the laboratory stage and entered clinical trials. These vaccines are either aimed at replacing the present vaccine, bacillus Calmette-Guérin (BCG) or at enhancing immunity induced by BCG.

The future TB vaccines include:

- *Pre-exposure TB vaccines:* Intended for use in newborns or young infants to replace or amplify BCG early in life and before exposure to TB, these vaccines are intended to prevent TB in people who have not been infected with tuberculosis
- *Postexposure TB vaccines:* Given post-infancy, typically to school children, adolescents or adults, who have either been vaccinated or latently infected with the TB bacteria or both, these vaccines reduce progression to active disease
- *Therapeutic vaccines:* These vaccines are given to individuals with active TB in conjunction with TB drug therapy with the aim of shortening the duration of the drug therapy.

The new generation of TB vaccines may work best using a heterologous prime-boost strategy. Three vaccine candidates: (1) M72, (2) AERAS-402/CrucellAd35, and (3) MVA85A/AERAS-485 are in phase II/IIb clinical trials (Table 9.5.2).

Table 9.5.2: TB vaccines in development.

Agent	Strategy	Type	Sponsor(s)	Status
M. vaccae	Immunotherapeutic	Whole-cell *M. vaccae*	AnHui Longcom	Phase III
M72/AS01	Prime-boost	Protein/adjuvant	GlaxoSmithKline, Aeras	Phase IIb
H4 + IC31	Prime-boost	Protein/adjuvant	Statens Serum Institut (SSI), Sanofi Pasteur, Valneva, Aeras	Phase IIa
H 56 + IC31	Prime-boost	Protein/adjuvant	SSI, Valneva, Aeras	Phase IIa
MTBVAC	Prime	Live genetically attenuated *M. tuberculosis* (MTB)	University of Zaragoza, Biofabri, Tuberculosis Vaccine Initiative (TBVI)	Phase IIa
VPM1002	Prime	Live recombinant rBCG	Serum Institute of India, Vakzine Projekt Management, TBVI, Max Planck Institute for Infection Biology	Phase IIa
Dar-901	Prime-boost	Whole-cell *M. vaccae*	Dartmouth University, Aeras	Phase IIa
ID93 + GLA-SE	Prime-boost	Protein/adjuvant	Infectious Disease Research Institute, Aeras	Phase IIa
RUTI	Immunotherapeutic	Fragmented MTB	Archivel Farma	Phase IIa
Ad5Ag85A	Prime-boost	Viral vector	McMaster University, CanSino	Phase I
ChAdOx1.85A + MVA85A	Prime-boost	Viral vector	Oxford University	Phase I
MVA85A (aerosol)	Prime-boost	Viral vector	Oxford University	Phase I
MVA85A-IMX313	Prime-boost	Viral vector	Oxford University, Imaxio	Phase I
TB/FLU-04L	Prime-boost	Viral vector	Research Institute for Biological Safety Problems	Phase I

Source: Adapted from Stop TB partnership working group on new TB vaccines

Tuberculosis (TB) vaccine research and development (R&D) is entering a period of basic science. After years of focusing on phase II clinical trials, the focus is shifting to the beginning of the pipeline—basic discovery and preclinical development. This change is motivated by a growing consensus that the guiding assumptions of the last 10 years of TB vaccine research require updating in the face of emerging evidence from the clinic and the lab.

FUTURE VACCINES AGAINST RESPIRATORY PATHOGENS

While effective vaccines exist against many of the respiratory pathogens, their usage is limited by high cost, lack of universal serotype coverage and the need to change the formulation yearly.

Major viral pathogens, like respiratory syncytial virus (RSV) and parainfluenza, are not preventable with any available vaccine.

RESPIRATORY SYNCYTIAL VIRUS VACCINES

The Respiratory syncytial virus (RSV) is a major etiological agent of viral lower respiratory tract illness in infants and children globally. Presently, no vaccine is available to protect these infants and children.

A number of RSV vaccine candidates using a variety of technologies has emerged in recent years. These include:

- *Live-attenuated RSV vaccines:* Engineered viruses that are attenuated but still immunogenic, such as the M2-2 deletion mutant.
- Protein-based vaccine including whole-inactivated virus, subunit antigens that associate to form aggregate particles, and nonparticle based subunit antigens
- Viral vectors encoding RSV surface antigens (including replication-competent and -deficient variations)
- Nucleic acid vaccines

There are now 60 RSV vaccine candidates in development. Sixteen of these have reached the stage of clinical development.

Live Vaccines

Recombinant RSV A2 cp248/404/1030/DSH is a recombinant temperature-sensitive RSV with a deletion of SH gene. This is the first LAV to enter human clinical trials. Other LAV candidates under development include recombinant RSV A2 cpts248/404/DNS2 and recombinant RSV A2 cpts530/1009DNS2, which include a deletion in the NS genes.

Vector Vaccines

This vector vaccine candidate is a recombinant bovine or human parainfluenza virus type 3 (PIV3)/RSV F2 (MEDI-534) which delivers RSV F using a bovine or human chimeric parainfluenza type 3 genome. Safety was demonstrated in a phase I study of RSV-seropositive adults. This candidate vaccine is being investigated as a combined vaccine against PIV and RSV.

Subunit Vaccines

The following subunit vaccines have advanced to clinical trials:

- Respiratory syncytial virus F subunit vaccines (purified F protein 1–3)
- Combined subunit vaccine containing F, G and M proteins (Sanofi Pasteur)
- BBG2Na, a G peptide conjugated to streptococcal protein G.

PARAINFLUENZA VIRUS VACCINES

Using reverse genetics systems, several live-attenuated human parainfluenza virus (HPIV) have been generated and evaluated as intranasal vaccines in adults and in children. Two vaccines against HPIV3 were found to be well tolerated, infectious and immunogenic in phase I trials in HPIV3-seronegative infants and children and should progress to proof-of-concept trials. Vaccines against HPIV1 and HPIV2 are less advanced and have just entered pediatric trials.

NEWER INFLUENZA VACCINES

Several innovative influenza vaccine candidates are currently in preclinical or early clinical development. These vaccines aim to induce more broad based protection across serotypes. Well-conserved influenza proteins, such as nucleoprotein and the matrix protein M2e are being targeted as vaccine candidates.

Adjuvanted Vaccines

MF59 adjuvanted influenza vaccines are now approved for use in Europe and several other countries but not in the USA. Purified bacterial outer membrane protein (OMP), TLRs and a variety of TLR agonists (bacterial carbohydrates, lipids, proteins and nucleic acids) have also shown promise as adjuvants for influenza vaccines.

Next Generation of Influenza Vaccines

Recombinant DNA techniques will shorten the time for vaccine production.

Recombinant Proteins

A recombinant trivalent hemaglutinin (HA) protein-based influenza vaccine is in the late stages of clinical development in the United States.

Virus-like Particles

Multiple virus-like particles candidates have shown promise in studies in animals, and at least one has advanced to phase II clinical trials.

Viral Vectors

Influenza HA genes from seasonal or H5N1 viruses, or both, have been cloned into carrier viruses, including vaccinia virus, alphaviruses, adenoviruses, Newcastle disease virus, baculoviruses and vesicular stomatitis virus.

Universal Vaccines

Highly conserved external domain of the influenza matrix 2 (M2) protein and conserved epitopes from the influenza NP, matrix 1 (M1) and HA proteins are potential candidates. Priming with a DNA-based HA vaccine followed by a boost with an inactivated, attenuated or adenovirus-vector based vaccine is expected to result in the generation of broadly cross-neutralizing antibodies.

NEWER PNEUMOCOCCAL VACCINES

A number of strategies are being pursued to develop safe, affordable and effective vaccines across serotypes. These include targeting conserved surface epitopes common to most or all pneumococcal strains. The targeted common proteins include pneumolysin, pneumococcal surface protein A (PspA), pneumococcal surface protein C (PspC), pneumococcal surface antigen A (PsaA), neuraminidase enzymes, and histidine-triad proteins, with the aim of inducing broader cross-serotype protection than current PCVs. Pneumococcal proteins in expressed in attenuated Salmonella strains as vectors have demonstrated encouraging results in preclinical studies.

Amongst the Pneumococcal conjugate vaccines (PCVs), the15 valent PCV (Merck & Co.), 12 valent PCV (GlaxoSmithKline [GSK]), 10 valent PCV (Panacea Biotech, Ltd.) and the 10 valent PCV (Serum Institute of India, Ltd.) are in phase II trials. The Multivalent PCV (SK Chemicals and Sanofi Pasteur) and Multivalent PCV (Pnuvax) are in preclinical studies.

Amongst the Common protein vaccines, the Pneumococcal whole cell vaccine (PATH/Boston Children's Hospital) and the PhtD/pneumolysoid/PcpA common protein vaccine (Sanofi Pasteur) are in phase II studies. The Trivalent protein (Genocea Biosciences) and the Live Recombinant Attenuated Salmonella Vaccine (Arizona State University) are in phase I studies while the two or more pneumococcal proteins loaded on bacterium-like-particles (Mucosis B.V.) is in preclinical studies.

Amongst the PCVs incorporating common proteins, the PhtD/pneumolysoid common protein vaccine (GSK) is in phase II studies while the Particle based PCV (Liquidia Technologies) and the novel conjugation technology using common protein carriers (Affinivax, Inc.) are in preclinical studies.

NEWER PERTUSSIS VACCINES

It is hoped that the newer pertussis vaccines will provide longer-term protection, at least as long as that estimated theoretically for recovery from natural infection estimated at 20 years.

DNA Vaccines

These include a genetically inactivated pertussis toxin pcDNA3.1-based DNA vaccine and a recombinant pertussis DNA vaccine expressing the pertussis toxin subunit 1 (PTS1), filamentous hemagglutinin (FHA) gene and pertactin (PRN). Boosting DNA vaccine-primed mice with pertussis toxoid yielded excellent antibody as well as cell-mediated immune responses.

Biodegradable Micro- and Nano-particle Vaccines

Oral and parenteral delivery of purified pertussis toxoid and filamentous HA encapsulated in poly-lactide-co-glycolide (PLG) polymers were demonstrated to protect mice from an aerosol-induced *Bordetella pertussis* infection.

Live Attenuated Vaccines

A live attenuated *B. pertussis* mutant strain (BPZE1 was reported to induce protection in young mice after a single nasal administration and reported to be safe. A metabolite deficient (aroQ), nonreverting deletion mutant of *B. pertussis* as a LAV candidate was immunogenic in adult interferon-γ receptor deficient adult mice.

FUTURE VACCINES AGAINST ENTERIC PATHOGENS

Enterotoxigenic *Escherichia coli* Vaccines

Two cellular vaccine candidates, ETVAX (a mixture of four inactivated strains) and ACE527 (a mixture of three live attenuated strains), have been found to be safe and immunogenic in Phase 1/2 trials. ETVAX is undergoing descending-age studies in Bangladesh. Other ETEC vaccine candidates based on protein subunits, toxoids (both LT and ST), or novel, more broadly conserved ETEC antigens are also under development.

Shigella Vaccines

Cellular candidates guaBA-based live attenuated (CVD 1208, CVD 1208S)] and virG-based live attenuated (WRSS1, WRSs3, WRSf3) are in phase I and II trials respectively.

A Heat Killed Multi Serotype Shigella (HKMS) vaccine and a 34 kDa OmpA vaccine based on a conserved and cross reactive major outer membrane protein (MOMP) of Shigella flexneri 2a being developed by NICED, Kolkata are in preclinical studies.

Cholera Vaccines

The focus of cholera vaccines development is on live attenuated, oral vaccines, several of which are in various stages of development.

Peru15 is a live attenuated oral *V. cholerae* O1 El Tor Inaba strain with deletions of the ctx A and the rtx A genes, inactivation of the recA gene and deletion of the attRS1 sequences. This vaccine was shown to be safe, immunogenic and protective in the United States, and among adults and children in a cholera-endemic area in Bangladesh. This vaccine was recently reformulated to make it stable at higher temperatures.

Vibrio cholerae 638, another live attenuated oral vaccine, derived from a *V. cholerae* O1 El Tor Ogawa strain by deletion of the entire CTXF genetic element and by insertion of the Clostridium thermocellum endoglucanase A gene into the HA/protease hapA gene. Studies have shown the vaccine to be safe, immunogenic and protective in Cuban volunteers.

A combined Bsubunit bivalent O1/O139 vaccine is also currently being developed in Sweden.

Two other *V. cholerae* O1 derived vaccines under development are the VA1.3 and the IEM 108. CVD 112 and Bengal15 are other candidate vaccines derived from *V. cholerae* O139.

Typhoid and Paratyphoid Vaccines

S. Paratyphi A vaccines in clinical development are based on either whole cell live-attenuated strains or repeating units of the lipopolysaccharide O-antigen (O:2) conjugated to different protein carriers. An O-specific polysaccharide (O:2) of S. Paratyphi A conjugated to tetanus toxoid (O:2-TT), was initially developed by NIH and subsequently undergoing further development , in combination with Vi-TT, by Chengdu and Lanzhou Institutes of Biological Products in China. This vaccine is undergoing phase II trials.

A combination vaccine of O:2,12-CRM197 + Vi-CRM197, being jointly developed by Biological E and SVGH] and a O:2,12-DT + Vi DT vaccine by the International Vaccine Institute are in preclinical stage.

A combination oral vaccine CVD 1902 + CVD 909 being jointly developed by UMB and Bharat Biotech is in phase I development

Subunit vaccines being developed include outer membrane proteins of Salmonella, flagellin and fimbria as a potential vaccine antigen using mouse models.

Other live attenuated typhoid vaccines in development include CVD908, CVD htrA, CVD 909, Ty 800 and ZH9.

FUTURE VACCINES AGAINST VECTOR BORNE DISEASES

Japanese Encephalitis Vaccines

Live Recombinant Vaccines

The ALVAC and the NYVAC strains of viral vectors were used to express the membrane proteins of JEV. The vaccine as found to be safe is poorly immunogenic.

DNA Multivalent Vaccines

A single intramuscular (IM) dose of a combined DNA vaccine against West Nile virus and the JEV was found to be protective against virus challenge in mice and horses.

Multivalent DNA vaccine against multiple flaviviruses is a promising area of development.

Dengue Vaccines

In addition to CYD-YFV (DengVaxia™), which was licensed for clinical usage recently, six other candidates are in clinical development using a variety of technological approaches (Fig. 9.5.10).

Live Attenuated Vaccines

The Walter Reed US Army Institute of Research (WRAIR) tetravalent LAV, produced by serial passage in dog kidney cells, was tested in Thai children. The vaccine was then licensed to GlaxoSmithKline (GSK), which continued clinical trials and is presently going through phase II trials.

The US National Institutes of Health (NIH) also have developed attenuated DV strains, using reverse genetics to create an attenuating 30-nucleotide deletion in the 3' untranslated region of the genome of the four DV strains. The four attenuated virus strains should eventually be combined together and tested as a tetravalent LAV candidate.

Chimeric Live Attenuated Vaccines

A homotypic chimeric virus has been developed by the US Center for Disease Control and Prevention (CDC) by inserting the structural protein genes from DV1, DV3 and DV4 into an attenuated PDK53 DV2 genome that had been attenuated by replacing a portion of the DV terminal 3' stem and loop structure with that of West Nile virus. The clinical development of these DV2-based chimeras is being carried yR Inviragen, in collaboration with the US CDC and Shantha Biotechnic.

Another DEN-YF chimeras were developed by Acambis by replacing the M and E structural protein-coding

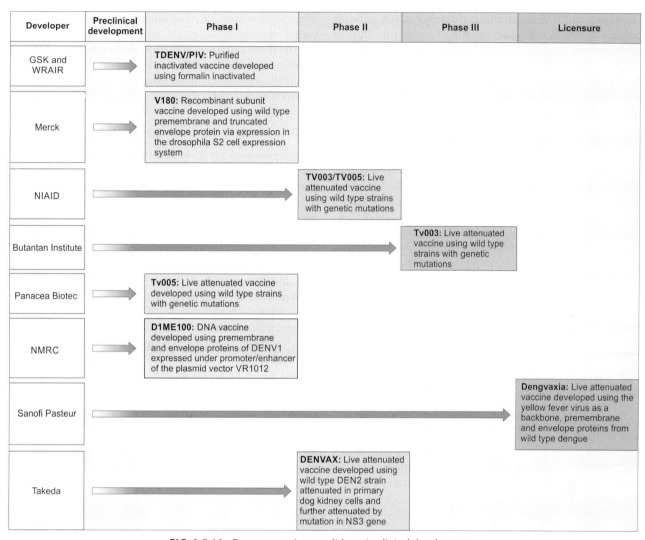

Developer	Preclinical development	Phase I	Phase II	Phase III	Licensure
GSK and WRAIR	→	**TDENV/PIV:** Purified inactivated vaccine developed using formalin inactivated			
Merck	→	**V180:** Recombinant subunit vaccine developed using wild type premembrane and truncated envelope protein via expression in the drosophila S2 cell expression system			
NIAID	→→→→		**TV003/TV005:** Live attenuated vaccine using wild type strains with genetic mutations		
Butantan Institute	→→→→→			**Tv003:** Live attenuated vaccine using wild type strains with genetic mutations	
Panacea Biotec	→	**Tv005:** Live attenuated vaccine developed using wild type strains with genetic mutations			
NMRC	→	**D1ME100:** DNA vaccine developed using premembrane and envelope proteins of DENV1 expressed under promoter/enhancer of the plasmid vector VR1012			
Sanofi Pasteur	→→→→→→				**Dengvaxia:** Live attenuated vaccine developed using the yellow fever virus as a backbone, premembrane and envelope proteins from wild type dengue
Takeda	→→→→		**DENVAX:** Live attenuated vaccine developed using wild type DEN2 strain attenuated in primary dog kidney cells and further attenuated by mutation in NS3 gene		

FIG. 9.5.10: Dengue vaccine candidates in clinical development.

sequences in the YFV genome with those from either the four DV serotypes and licensed to Sanofi Pasteur.

The chimeric viruses were tested and found to be safe and immunogenic in humans. This vaccine, ChimeriVax-Den, was shown to induce a transient and low-grade viremia in non-human primate and in human volunteers, followed by a robust immune response against the four serotypes with some strains showing dominant immunogenicity. A dose adjustment for the DV2 chimera resulted in a more balanced response. A phase II trial is taking place in the USA and Latin America and a phase IIb pediatric trial has been launched by Sanofi Pasteur in early 2009 in Thailand.

Live Recombinant, DNA and Subunit Vaccines

Dengue virus genes were inserted into a non-replicative adenovirus vector (Ad5) to engineer double recombinants expressing the prM and E sequences from both DV1 and DV2 and DV3 and DV4 respectively. Evaluation in a phase I study is ongoing.

Subunit dengue vaccine has been developed with the truncated amino-terminal 80% of the E glycoprotein from each serotype plus the entire NS1 protein from DV2 formulated in a proprietary adjuvant. Another dengue subunit vaccine candidate consists of a consensus dengue virus envelope protein domain III (cEDIII). Several groups are developing subunit vaccines based on domain III of the DV E protein, a strategy that is aimed at reducing the induction of cross-reactive antibodies.

Chikungunya Vaccines

Several heterogeneous strategies including live attenuated, inactivated, subunit, DNA, VLPs, chimeric and recombinant vectors are being pursued. Only two candidates have recently qualified to enter clinical phase II trials, a chikungunya virus-like particle-based vaccine and a recombinant live attenuated measles virus-vectored vaccine.

A formalin inactivated, whole virus vaccine based on multiple Indian strains is in the stage of pre-clinical development by Bharat Biotech International. A subunit vaccine by NIV, Pune is also in the phase of pre-clinical development.

FUTURE HEPATITIS VACCINES

Hepatitis E Vaccine

Recombinant protein hepatitis E vaccines (HEV) under study are based on recombinant proteins derived from immunogenic parts of the HEV capsid gene expressed in *E. coli*, insect expression systems or other systems. Other approaches, such as DNA-based vaccines or transgenic tomatoes, have also been developed.

Two vaccine candidates, the rHEV vaccine expressed in baculovirus and the HEV 239 vaccine, expressed in *E. coli*, were successfully evaluated in phase II/III trials.

The 56-kDa baculovirus-expressed ORF2 protein was evaluated in humans by the WRAIR. This vaccine has been field-tested in Nepal in 1,794 volunteers from the Nepalese Army who received three doses of the vaccine or placebo at 0, 1 and 6 months in a phase II trial. VE against clinically apparent disease was 95% and the only adverse event was injection-site pain. The efficacy of this vaccine against asymptomatic infection is unknown and there is no information on the duration of immunity.

The recombinant hepatitis E vaccine, HEV 239 was studied in a randomized, double-blind, placebo-controlled, phase III trial. Vaccine efficacy after three doses was 100% (95% CI 72.1–100.0). Adverse effects attributable to the vaccine were few and mild. No vaccination-related serious adverse event was noted.

Hepatitis C Vaccines

Vaccine Approaches: Current Status

Only a small fraction of animal hepatitis C vaccine (HCV) studies have progressed to human trials. The majority of these trials have evaluated potential therapeutic vaccines in HCV-infected patients. A smaller number have assessed vaccines in healthy volunteers.

Four main vaccine strategies have been investigated in human clinical studies: (1) recombinant protein vaccines, (2) peptide vaccines, (3) DNA vaccines, and (4) vector vaccines.

The prophylactic vaccine, MVA-NSmut/AdCh3-NSmut, developed by NAIDH/NIH, is in phase II trials, while the Ad6-Nsmut/AdCh3-Nsmut is in phase I trial.

Three therapeutic vaccines, Peptide vaccine IC41, MVA vaccine TG4040 and GI-5005 combined with Peg-IFNa/RBV are in phase II trials.

Cytomegalovirus Vaccines

A phase II study of a purified, recombinant vaccine based on adjuvanted glycoprotein B demonstrated an efficacy of approximately 50% against acquisition of human cytomegalovirus (HCMV) infection in a clinical trial in young women.

The results of a phase II clinical trial of bivalent HCMV DNA vaccine will be available and will provide information about the safety and immunogenicity of this vaccine in transplant recipients.

Sabin-inactivated Poliovirus

Development of Sabin-inactivated poliovirus (Sabin-IPV) will be critical in the post-oral polio vaccine (OPV) cessation period. The use of attenuated Sabin strains instead of wild-type Salk polio strains will provide additional safety during vaccine production and obviate the need for high levels of biosafety enabling it's manufacture in low and middle income countries. This will result in reduced cost of production.

The type 2 poliovirus strain in Sabin-IPV is less immunogenic than the type 2 strain in wIPV (3–4 times less), the type 1 Sabin-IPV strain appears to be more immunogenic than the type 1 strain in wIPV (1.5 times more), and a comparable immunogenicity is observed for type 3 in both vaccines. Comparative studies have shown that the acceptable composition of S-IPV would be 10DU–16DU–s32DU of types 1, 2 and 3 respectively. Since $Al(OH)_3$ adjuvantation would increase the potency twofold, the composition of the adjuvanted vaccine would be 5DU–8DU and 16DU respectively. Studies done in Japan, China and the Netherlands have shown that the middle antigen content as indicated above elicit VNTs comparable to that by wtIPV.

In collaboration with the RIVM, Netherlands, clinical lots of S-IPV seed-strains have been prepared. This new technology will be transferred to China National Biotec Group (CNBG) and Serum Institute of India. Earlier two other companies, Panacea Biotec, Ltd., in India and the LG Life Sciences Republic of Korea, were selected for this technology transfer.

In a phase III study conducted in China 3 doses of sIPV resulted in seroconversion rates of 100%, 94.9% and 99.0% (types I, II, and III, respectively), and 94.7%, 91.3% and 97.9% in those receiving Salk-IPV, at one month after the completion of primary immunization. An anamnestic response for poliovirus types I, II, and III was elicited by a booster in both groups. Except in the case of fever, other adverse events were similar between the two groups.

Japan is the first country in the world to develop and introduce Sabin-derived IPVs (sIPVs) for routine immunization in November 2012. While standalone sIPV is not marketed, it is available as a DTaP-sIPV combination.

VACCINES AGAINST THE NEGLECTED TROPICAL DISEASES

Leishmaniasis

Only one second-generation vaccine is in clinical development. This is the LEISH-F1 + MPL-SE vaccine, consisting of three recombinant Leishmania polyprotein LEISH-F1 antigens (TSA-LmSTI1-LeIF), together with the adjuvant monophosphoryl lipid and squalene in a stable emulsion (MPL-SE). An initial phase I safety and immunogenicity trial was conducted in the USA followed by several phase II studies initiated in Latin America and recently in India. While LEISH-F2, an improved version of LEISH-1, is in phase II studies, LEISH-3 is in phase I studies.

Three other vaccines are in preclinical development in Europe. These are the synthetic vaccine RAPSODI and two DNA vaccines. One of these is based on a viral vector.

Schistosomiasis

A phase I safety trials of one vaccine candidate, the 14-kDa fatty acid-binding protein (Sm14) against *Schistosoma mansoni* is ongoing. The other vaccine candidate to have entered clinical trials, a 28-kDa glutathione-S-transferase (Sh28GST, also known as BILHVAX), is derived from *Schistosoma haematobium*, has completed phase II and III trials in West Africa. The results are pending.

Human Hookworm Vaccine

The Sabin Vaccine Institute announced the start of a phase I clinical trial of its *Na*-GST-1 antigen, a candidate for the first human hookworm vaccine. The trial began in January 2012 in Brazil. Vaccine based on the antigen, *Na*-APR-1 is also in phase I trials.

Leptospirosis

Leptospira external membrane protein LipL32 cloned and expressed in mycobacterial vectors, LigA and LigB have been found to be immunogenic and protective to hamsters. At least two DNA vaccines, one encoding hemolysis-associated protein (Hap1) and the other endoflagella gene (fl aB2) have been tested. The advent of leptospiral genome sequences has allowed a reverse vaccinology approach for vaccine development.

OTHER FUTURE VACCINES

Staphylococcal Vaccines

Currently there are no licensed prophylactic vaccines for human use for the prevention of *Staphylococcus aureus* disease.

The reformulated StaphVAX (CP5, CP8, type 336, a-hemolysin and PVL, conjugated to mutant nontoxic recombinant *Pseudomonas aeruginosa* exotoxin) has been taken over by GSK for further development.

Pfizer's SA4Ag candidate, comprising 4 antigens, is currently the most advanced and is undergoing phase II trials.

There are at least seven active vaccine efforts in various stages of clinical development (GlaxoSmithKline/ Nabi, Pfizer/Inhibitex, Sanofi Pasteur/Syntiron, Novartis, Novadigm, Integrated Biotherapeutics and Vaccine Research International).

Group A Streptococcal Vaccine

Only two GAS vaccines have entered clinical trials. These are the N-terminal M protein-based multivalent vaccines (26-valent and 30-valent vaccines) and conserved M protein vaccines (the J8 vaccine and the StreptInCor vaccine).

Several vaccine candidates against GAS infection are in varying stages of preclinical and clinical development.

Group B Streptococcal Vaccine

A tetanus toxoid-CPS conjugates: monovalent, and bivalent vaccines are in phase II trials. CRM197-CPS conjugate monovalent and trivalent vaccines are also in phase II trials.

In addition, preventive vaccines against H.simplex, Nipah virus, Ebola virus, Zika virus, Norovirus, EV-71, MERS and Chagas disease are in the phase of preclinical development and phase I – II trials.

Vaccines against Novel and Emerging Pathogens

One of the main public health concerns of emerging viruses is their introduction into and sustained circulation among populations of immunologically naïve, susceptible hosts resulting in significant morbidity and mortality. Conventional approaches to develop vaccines against these emerging pathogens have significant limitations, the most significant being the long time frame for production. In these situations there is a demand for the rapid production of safe and effective vaccines.

This is particularly true for the very real threat of "novel pathogens" such as the avian-origin influenzas H7N9 and H5N1, thenew coronaviruses such as hCoV-EMC, Zikavirus, Ebolavirus,etc.

The application of computational vaccine design tools and rapid production technologies can make it possible to engineer vaccines for novel emerging pathogen in record time. These new tools are being applied to produce vaccines against some of the recent novel pathogens. The initial design process, genome to gene sequence and ready to insert in a DNA plasmid can now be accomplished in less than 24 hours. This FastVax vaccine design may yield a utilizable vaccine within 4–6 weeks.

Therapeutic Vaccines

Vaccines are being investigated against cancers, autoimmune diseases and chronic infections e.g. HBV, human papillomavirus (HPV), HCV.

Cancer Vaccines

Various types of therapeutic cancer vaccines are under investigation:

- Based on specific tumor associated antigens (TAA) for induction of anti-TAA antibodies, e.g. pancreatic and breast cancers, melanomas, nonround cell lung cancers
- Peptide, DNA and recombinant virus vaccines against defined TAAs
- Vaccines based on anti-idiotype antibodies against defined TAAs
- Allogenic vaccines
- Autologous vaccines.
  A few of these vaccines are in phase III trials.

Tumor associated antigens based vaccines raise the possibility of preventing these cancers in genetically susceptible individuals. However, the thrust of research is in therapeutic cancer vaccines.

Provenge, a vaccine designed to treat prostate cancer, was the first vaccine to receive USFDA approval for use in the treatment of advanced prostate cancer patients on April 29, 2010.

Oncophage, a vaccine to treat a subset of patients with renal carcinomas, received approval by the drug authorities in Russia.

Autoimmune Disorders

The goal of vaccination is the antigen and tissue-specific suppression of pathological inflammation that underlies immune-mediated inflammatory disorders like autoimmune diseases and allograft rejection. These include immunoregulatory DNA vaccines coding for autoantigens such as insulin and glutamic acid decarboxylase for type 1 diabetes, myelin-associated proteins for multiple sclerosis, and heat shock protein 60 for rheumatoid arthritis. The objective is to induce a homeostatic-like regulatory immune response to suppress pathological inflammation.

Copolymer 1 (glatiramer acetate), used today as a therapeutic vaccine against multiple sclerosis, is the first vaccine for an autoimmune disease.

Chronic Infections

Great effort is being devoted to develop therapeutic vaccines against AIDS, hepatitis B, hepatitis C, HPV, tuberculosis, malaria and *Helicobacter pylori.*

Vaccine for Prevention of Asthma

Oral administration of transgenic rice seeds containing an immunodominant fragment of the Der p 1 (45–145) was studied in a murine model of asthma.

It was observed that production of Th2-type cytokines by peripheral CD4 + T-cells in vitro was significantly reduced but not Th1-type cytokines. In addition, allergen-induced infiltration by eosinophils and neutrophils into the airways, and bronchial hyper-responsiveness were also inhibited.

Vaccines against Bioterrorism

Variola major virus, the *Bacillus anthracis,* is at the apex of potential pathogens that could be used in a bioterror attack to inflict mass casualties.

The cytokine IL-15 was integrated into the Wyeth strain of vaccina virus derived from the licensed smallpox vaccine resulting in the development of a smallpox vaccine candidate (Wyeth/IL-15) with superior efficacy and immunogenicity. The PA gene of *Bacillus anthracis* was inserted into this platform to create a dual vaccine against smallpox and anthrax. This dual vaccine conferred superior protection against inhalation of anthrax in both mice and rabbits.

A Vaccine for Obesity

Neutralization of ghrelin through an anti-ghrelin vaccine might prove to be a useful tool for obesity treatment to be used in association with diet and exercise.

CONCLUSION

The rapid pace of development of new technologies has enabled the development of effective vaccines against many new pathogens, improved the safety and efficacy of the existing vaccines, and targeted diseases such as chronic infectious diseases and cancer. Vaccines are expected to cater to the need of all age groups, not just infants and children. With the pioneering efforts of organization like the Bill and Melinda Gates Foundation, the development, introduction and supply of vaccines focused on the needs of developing countries are becoming a reality. Vaccines have saved more lives and will continue to save more lives in the years to come.

BIBLIOGRAPHY

1. 2016 Pipeline Report. Tuberculosis (TB) Edition .www. pipelinereport.org
2. Anderson RP, Jabr R. Vaccine against autoimmune disease: antigen-specific immunotherapy. Curr OpinImmunol. 2013; 25(3):410-7. doi:10.1016/j.coi.2013.02.004.
3. Birkett AJ. Status of vaccine research and development of vaccines for malaria. Vaccine. 2016;34:1915-20.
4. Blanco JC, Boukhvalova MS, Shirey KA, et al. New insights for development of a safe and protective RSV vaccine. Hum Vaccin. 2010;6(6):482-92.
5. Chackerian B, Frietze KM. Moving towards a new class of vaccines for non-infectious chronic diseases. Expert Review of Vaccines. 2016;15:5:561-3; DOI: 10.1586/14760584.2016.1159136

6. De Groot AS, Einck L, Moise L, et al. Making vaccines "on demand" A potential solution for emerging pathogens and biodefense? Human Vaccines and immunotherapeutics. 2013;9(9):1877-84; © 2013 Landes Bioscience.

7. Finco O, Rappuoli R. Designing vaccines for the twenty-first century society. Frontiers in Immunology. 2014;5:12.

8. Hagana T, Nakayab HI, Subramaniama S, et al. Systems vaccinology: Enabling rational vaccine design with systems biological approaches. Vaccine. 2015;33:5294-301.

9. Higgins D, Trujillo C, Keech C. Advances in RSV vaccine research and development—A global agenda. Vaccine. 2016;34:2870-5

10. Ingolotti M, Kawalekar O, Shedlock DJ, et al. DNA vaccines for targeting bacterial infections. Expert Rev Vaccines. 2010;9 (7):747-63.

11. Lambert LC, Fauci AS. Influenza vaccines for the future. N Engl J Med. 2010;363:2036-4.

12. Larrañeta E, McCrudden MTC, Courtenay AJ, et al. A New Frontier in Nanomedicine Delivery. Pharm Res. 2016; 33:1055-73.

13. Malabadi RB, Meti NT, Mulgund GS, et al. Recent advances in plant derived vaccine antigens against human infectious diseases. Research in Pharmacy. 2012;2(2):08-19.

14. Melief CMJ, van Hall T, Arens R, et al. Therapeutic cancer vaccines. J Clin Invest. 2015;125(9):3401-12. doi:10.1172/JCI80009

15. Montomoli E, Piccirella S, Khadang B, et al. Current adjuvants and new perspectives in vaccine formulation. Expert Rev Vaccines. 2011;10(7):1053-61.

16. Safrit JT, Fast PE, Gieber L, et al. Status of vaccine research and development of vaccines for HIV-1. Vaccine. 2016;34:2921-5.

17. Schwameis M, Buchtele N, Wadowski PA, et al. Chikungunya vaccines in development. Human Vaccines and Immunotherapeutics. 2016;12(3):716-31, DOI: 10.1080/21645515.2015.1101197

18. Schwartz, Lauren M, et al. The dengue vaccine pipeline: Implications for the future of dengue control. Vaccine. 2015;33(29):3293-8.

19. Scorza FB, Tsvetnitsky V, Donnelly JJ. Universal influenza vaccines: Shifting to better vaccines. Vaccine. 2016;34:2926-33.

20. Seib KL, Zhao X, Rappuoli R. Developing vaccines in the era of genomics: a decade of reverse vaccinology. Clin. Microbiol Infect. 2012;18 (Suppl. 5):109-16.

21. Shimizu H. Development and introduction of inactivated poliovirus vaccines derived from Sabin strains in Japan. Vaccine. 2016;34:1975-85.

22. Ura T, Okuda K, Shimada M. Developments in Viral Vector-Based Vaccines. Vaccines. 2014;2:624-41.

23. Verdijk P, Rots NY, Bakker WA. Clinical development of a novel inactivated poliomyelitis vaccine based on attenuated Sabin poliovirus strains. Expert Rev Vaccines. 2011;10(5):635-44.

24. WHO Product Development for Vaccines Advisory Committee (PDVAC) Pipeline Analyses for 25 Pathogens. Vaccine. 2016;34(26):2863-3006.

9.6 VACCINE STORAGE AND HANDLING

Digant D Shastri

INTRODUCTION

Immunization programs have had a major impact on the health status of the world population, by preventing many cases of infectious disease through immunization. Efficient vaccine storage and handling is a key component of immunization programs. Proper vaccine storage and handling is a shared responsibility from the time the vaccine is manufactured until it is administered. The majority of vaccine storage and handling mistakes are easily avoidable.

Cold chain breaches can occur even in well-designed and well-managed systems as a result of technical malfunctions but if there are good procedures in place, problems will be detected and effectively managed so that effective protection can be extended to its recipients and vaccine losses can be prevented. Efficient vaccine storage management is an essential quality assurance measure for vaccine service providers.

WHAT IS THE COLD CHAIN?

The "cold chain" is the system of transporting and storing vaccines within recommended temperature from the place of manufacture to the point of administration. It has three main components: (1) personnel, (2) equipment, and (3) procedures.

- Trained personnel
- Transport and storage equipment
- Efficient management procedures.

Above three discussed components combine to ensure proper vaccine transport, storage and handling. The optimum temperature for refrigerated vaccines is between +2°C and +8°C. For frozen vaccines the optimum temperature is –15°C or lower. In addition, protection from light is a necessary condition for some vaccines.

WHY SHOULD WE BE CONCERNED ABOUT PROPER COLD CHAIN?

Vaccines and toxoids are made up of proteins, nucleic acids, lipids and carbohydrates which may become less effective or even destroyed, when exposed to temperatures, outside the recommended range. As healthcare personal it becomes our professional and moral duty to ensure that the people receive effective healthcare product. Vaccines are costly and limited available biological products and replacing them now and then because of cold chain breach leads to wastage of national/individual resources. Giving the damaged vaccines inadvertently is even worse a condition for the society. Thus, efficient vaccine storage management is good quality assurance. Proper vaccine storage and management is responsibility of all those dealing with them right from manufacturer, transporter, stockiest, retailers to doctors and paramedic staff. Along with them the government and regulatory authorities have their own responsibilities to share.

Cold-sensitive vaccines experience an immediate loss of potency following freezing. Vaccines exposed to temperatures above the recommended temperature range experience some loss of potency with each episode of exposure. Repetitive exposure to heat episodes results in a cumulative loss of potency that is not reversible.

Proper vaccine storage and management is the responsibility of all those dealing with them right from manufacturer, transporter, stockist, retailers to doctors and end users.

Different surveys, studies and site visits have found that about 17–37% of healthcare providers expose vaccines to improper storage temperatures. Refrigerator temperatures are more commonly kept too cold rather than too warm (Table 9.6.1).

VACCINE STORAGE EQUIPMENT SUPPLIED UNDER THE IMMUNIZATION PROGRAM

Walk-in-freezers

Walk-in-freezers (WIF) are used for bulk storage of OPV vaccines and also to prepare and store frozen ice packs at state stores. They maintain a temperature of –18°C to –20°C.

Vaccine	**Exposure to heat/light**	**Exposure to cold**	
Table 9.6.1: Summary of vaccine sensitivities.			
Heat and light sensitive vaccines			
BCG	Relatively heat stable, but sensitive to light	Not damaged by freezing	+2°C to +8°C
OPV	Heat sensitive	Not damaged by freezing	+2°C to +8°C
Measles	Sensitive to heat and light	Not damaged by freezing	+2°C to +8°C
Freeze sensitive vaccines			
DPT	Relatively heat stable	Freezes at –3°C	+2°C to +8°C
Hep B	Relatively heat stable	Freezes at –0.5°C	+2°C to +8°C
DT	Relatively heat stable	Freezes at –3°C	+2°C to +8°C
TT	Relatively heat stable	Freezes at –0.5°C	+2°C to +8°C

Abbreviations: BCG, bacillus Calmette–Guérin; OPV, oral poliomyelitis vaccine; DPT, diphtheria, pertussis and tetanus; Hep B, hepatitis B; DT, diphtheria and tetanus; TT, tetanus toxoid.

Walk-in-coolers

Walk-in-coolers (WIC) made up of modular, prefabricated physical unclonable function (PUF) insulated panels with floor of either stainless steel panels or modular floor panels with an aluminum chequered plates. These cold rooms are typically controlled between 2°C and 8°C. It has digital light emitting device/light crystal device (LED/LCD) temperature display and temperature recorder. It is fitted with an audio-video alarm system to warn of high or low temperature. These are used for bulk storage of vaccines at state and regional stores.

Walk-in-coolers/WIF stores three months of requirement of vaccines +25% buffer stock for the districts they cater.

Deep Freezers

Deep freezers have either top opening lid or front door. Deep freezers supplied under immunization program have a top opening lid. The cabinet temperature is maintained between –18°C and –20°C. This is used for storing of OPV at district and also for freezing ice packs.

Ice Lined Refrigerator

These types of refrigerators are top opening. Inside the ice lined refrigerator (ILR) there is a lining of water containers (ice packs or tubes) fitted all around the walls and held in place by frame. While refrigerator is operating, the water in the containers freezes and if the electricity supply fails then the ice lining keeps the inside temperature of the refrigerator at a safe level for vaccines. It can keep vaccine safe with as little as 8 hours continuous electricity supply in a 24-hour period.

Hence, it is suitable for use in the area with poor power supply. ILR has two sections—the top and the bottom. The bottom of the refrigerator is the coldest place. OPV and measles vaccine can be placed at the bottom of the ILR. The DPT, DT, TT, and hep B vaccines should not be kept directly on the floor of the refrigerator as they can freeze and get damaged, and they should be stored in basket along with diluents (Figs. 9.6.1 to 9.6.3).

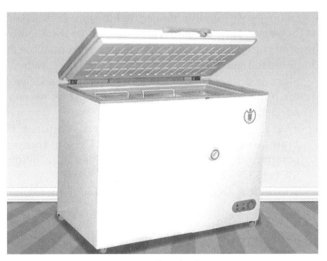

FIG. 9.6.1: Ice-lined refrigerator.

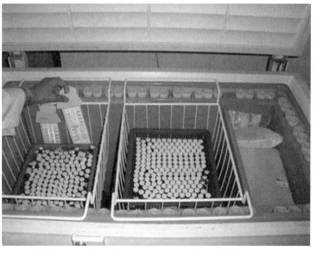

FIG. 9.6.2: Vaccine storage in ice-lined refrigerator.

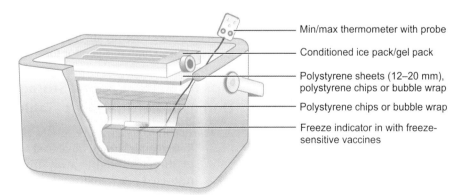

Min/max thermometer with probe

Conditioned ice pack/gel pack

Polystyrene sheets (12–20 mm), polystyrene chips or bubble wrap

Polystyrene chips or bubble wrap

Freeze indicator in with freeze-sensitive vaccines

FIG. 9.6.3: Vaccine storage in cooler ice-lined refrigerator.

Automatic Voltage Stabilizer

The function of the voltage stabilizer is to control the range of fluctuations in the main voltage of 220 volts (+10 volts). *No electrical cold chain equipment should be used/operated without a voltage stabilizer.*

Cold Boxes (Coolers)

Cold boxes are big insulated boxes with ice packs. They are mainly used for transportation of vaccines from district store to the primary health Centre (PHC). In emergency, they can also be used to store vaccines and frozen ice packs. Before placing vaccines in the cold boxes first put fully frozen ice packs at the bottom and sides of the cold box. The vials of DPT, DT, hep B and TT vaccines should not be placed in direct contact with frozen ice packs place it in cartoon or plastic bag.

Vaccine Carriers

It is used by health workers for carrying vaccines (16–20 vials) to sub-centers or to villages. They maintain the cold chain during transport from the PHC for one day's use in the field. The inside temperature is maintained between +2°C and –8°C with four frozen ice packs for one day (if not opened frequently) (Table 9.6.2).

Domestic Refrigerator

Majority of the vaccination service providers in private sector use domestic refrigerator to store the vaccines. The domestic refrigerator is designed and built to store fresh or frozen food and drinks and not for the special storage temperature need of vaccines. They do not have accurate temperature controlling system and hence, it can place the safety of vaccines at risk. For vaccine storage the domestic refrigerator has following drawbacks:

- Temperature varies significantly every time the door is opened
- Temperature rises during defrosting in cycle in cyclic defrost and frost-free refrigerator
- Cabinet temperature is easily affected by ambient temperature
- Temperature setting using dial is crude and inaccurate.

However, if domestic refrigerator is the only alternative to store the vaccines in that it is acceptable to store vaccines provided that the refrigerator and freezer compartments have separate external doors. There are two types of domestic refrigerators: (1) frost-free refrigerator and (2) manual and cyclic defrost refrigerator. The frost-free refrigerators have no heating cycles but have low level warming cycles and hence, it provides more uniform temperatures than manual and cyclic defrost models and may be more suitable for vaccine storage. The manual and cyclic defrost model refrigerator and bar refrigerator (dormitory style) should not be used to store the vaccine as they have wide fluctuations in the temperature in the internal compartment. Safe vaccine storage is possible in domestic refrigerators if following points are observed:

- Store vaccine in a dedicated refrigerator especially for biologics. *Do not store food or drink in vaccine refrigerators.*
- The refrigerator compartment temperatures is maintained between 2°C and 8°C and freezer compartment temperatures maintained at or below 5°F (–15°C)
- The door seals are in good condition and are sealing tightly
- The door closes properly automatically on leaving it free
- The refrigerator has separate freezer compartment
- The refrigerator compressor is quiet
- The refrigerator is free from any coolant or water leak
- Vaccination clinic staff is well aware about vaccine storage plans.

If the above criteria cannot be met with that one should go for purpose built refrigerator for storing the vaccine.

Tips for Better Vaccine Storage in Domestic Refrigerators (Table 9.6.3)

A. *Placement of refrigerator*
   - Refrigerator should be placed away from exposure to direct sunlight, away from heat and with restricted accessibility only to the vaccination staff so as to minimize unnecessary door opening and preventing accidental switch off of power supply

Table 9.6.2: Summary of cold chain equipment used under expanded program on immunization.

Equipment	Temperature	Storage capacity	Holdover time
Electrical			
Deep freezer	–15°C to –25°C	200 ice packs or OPV stock for 3 months	43°C for 18 hours 32°C for 22 hours
ILR	+2°C to +8°C	BCG, DPT, DT, TT, measles, hep B vaccine stock for 3 months	43°C for 18 hours 32°C for 22 hours
Nonelectrical			
Cold box (large)	+2°C to +8°C	All vaccines stored for transport or in case of power failure	43°C for 6.5 days 32°C for 10 hours
Vaccine carrier	+2°C to +8°C	All vaccines carried for 12 hours	43°C for 34 hours 32°C for 51 hours

Abbreviations: BCG, bacillus Calmette–Guérin; OPV, oral poliomyelitis vaccine; DPT, diphtheria, pertussis and tetanus; DT, diphtheria and tetanus; TT, tetanus toxoid; ILR, ice-lined refrigerator

Table 9.6.3: Checklist for preventive maintenance of vaccine refrigerator.

External	Internal	Technical
• The exterior is clean • Its sides are at least 10 cm away from walls • It is away from direct sunlight • It is opened only when necessary	• Doors seals properly without gap • The door seal is clean • Ice packs are in proper position • Vaccines are neatly placed with space for air circulation • DPT, TT, hep B and DT are not touching the cooling surface • Thermometer has been kept amongst the vaccine • Temperature is recorded twice a day	• Temperature is within prescribed limit (if not, set the thermostat) • Voltage stabilizer is working properly and equipment are connected through it • Plug of the voltage stabilizer is fitted properly to the power line • There is no abnormal noise • Compressor mounting bolts are tight

Abbreviations: DPT, diphtheria, pertussis and tetanus; TT, tetanus toxoids; hep B, hepatitis B; DT, diphtheria and tetanus.

B. *Recognize individual vaccine refrigerator*
   – Before starting storing the vaccines identify which are the cold and warm areas in refrigerator?
C. *Stabilize the temperature of the refrigerator before stocking*
   – The refrigerator temperature needs to be stabilized before start using for vaccine storage
D. *Monitoring temperatures inside the refrigerators*
   – Monitor internal temperature regularly with thermometer—preferably Celsius digital minimum/maximum thermometer. Place the thermometer in a central location within the storage compartment (Fig. 9.6.4)
E. *Safeguard the power source*
   – Ensure the power source is marked clearly in a way to prevent the refrigerator from being accidentally unplugged or turned off (Fig. 9.6.5).
F. *Increase cool mass*
   – Place water bottles or ice packs/gel packs in the refrigerator to increase the cool mass; these will assist in stabilizing the temperature in refrigerator compartment and reduces warming periods when the refrigerator is opened. This is also useful if there is a short time power cut or refrigerator failure (Fig. 9.6.6).
G. *Ideal storage method*
   – Store vaccines in enclosed plastic labeled containers or basket. This will allow easy identification of vaccines and minimizes the time spent with the door opened searching for vaccines
   – Store vaccines in original packing as it can provide some protection from very short-term fluctuations
   – Do not crowd the vaccines by overfilling the shelves. Allow space between containers and gap of at least 4 cm from all refrigerator walls to allow free air circulation
   – Never store any vaccine in the door of the refrigerator
   – Place freeze-tolerant vaccines (measles, mumps, rubella, OPV and BCG) in the top shelf and freeze-sensitive vaccines (DTP containing vaccines; *Haemophilus influenzae* type B (Hib),

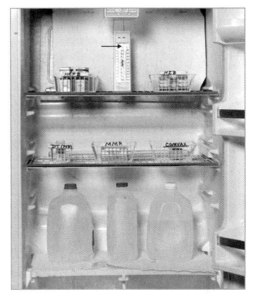

FIG. 9.6.4: Temperature monitoring.

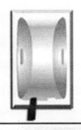
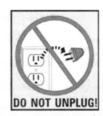
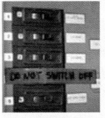
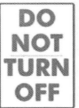

FIG. 9.6.5: Safeguard the power source.

pneumococcal, influenza, hepatitis, inactivated polio vaccine (IPV) and some varicella vaccines) on middle shelf (Figs. 9.6.7 and 9.6.8).

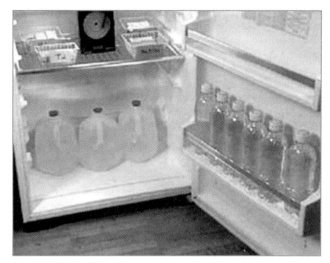

FIG. 9.6.6: Water bottles to increase cool mass.

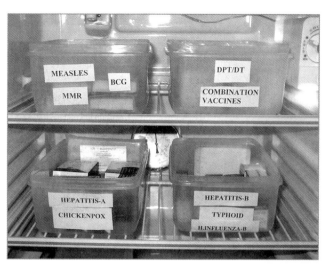

FIG. 9.6.7: Vaccine storage pattern.

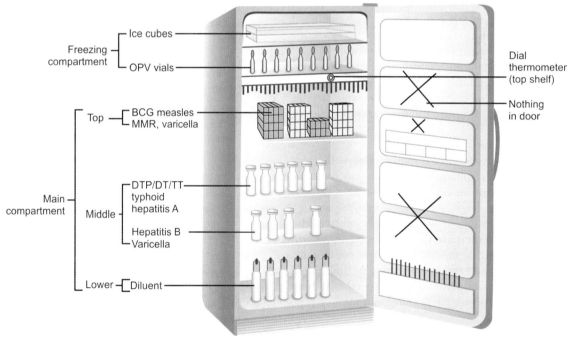

FIG. 9.6.8: Storage protocol in domestic fridge.

H. *Keep the door closed as much as possible*
   - Reducing door opening helps to keep internal temperatures stable
   - Vaccine refrigerators should have a sticker to remind staff of avoiding unnecessary door opening
   - Stick a basic map of vaccine locations outside of the refrigerator door so staff can go 'straight' to the vaccine when the door is opened
   - Do not open the door fully while using, keep it to minimum sufficient for the need.

I. *Training and assigning staff*
   - Good vaccine storage and handling depends on knowledge and habits of the staff
   - Training ensures that everyone handling vaccines knows how to protect them
   - Ensure that one person is responsible for adjusting refrigerator controls and who is responsible for cold chain management to enable consistency.

J. *Maintenance of the vaccine refrigerator*
   - Report breakdowns immediately and arrange for alternative storage for vaccines while the refrigerator is repaired (Table 9.6.3)
   - Defrost refrigerator regularly. This also aids in the efficient functioning of refrigerator.

K. *Power failure*
   - During a power failure of 4 hours or less the refrigerator door should be kept closed

– If the backup generator facility is lacking, identify an available unit at another nearby site

– If a refrigerator with a backup generator has not been located or is not working, and for power failures more than 4 hours store vaccines in a cooler with conditioned ice packs/gel packs.

Purpose-built Vaccine Refrigerator

Purpose-built vaccine refrigerator is preferred refrigerator for vaccine storage. It is used by hospitals, pharmacies and larger general practices. It has following advantages over the domestic refrigerator (Fig. 9.6.9):

• Do not require to modify for vaccine storage

• Programmed to maintain an internal temperature between 2°C and 8°C

• Cabinet temperature is not affected by ambient temperature and is stable and uniform

• Evaporator operates at 2°C–8°C, preventing vaccine from freezing

• Defrost cycle allowing defrosting without rise in cabinet temperature

• Even distribution of temperature because of on going air circulation

• Have external temperature reading display, maximum/minimum temperature continuous display, and an out of range temperature alarm

• Good temperature recovery–when the fridge is open to access the vaccines.

Types of Temperature Monitoring Devices

To measure the temperature during storage of vaccines, different types of thermometers are used. The only thermometers and temperature recording devices recommended for monitoring the temperatures within vaccine storage units are thermometers that provide continuous recording or minimum or maximum thermometers that are properly monitored. These types of thermometers are preferred because they provide an indication of the length of time a storage compartment has been operating outside recommended temperature ranges when a cold chain break occurs.

Data Loggers

Digital data loggers are miniature, battery-powered, stand-alone temperature monitors that record hundreds or thousands of temperature readings. These are the ideal temperature monitors because they can indicate when the exposure occurred and how long the vaccines were exposed to the minimum or maximum temperatures. Data loggers may be single use and used only in transport, or they may be multiple use (Fig. 9.6.10).

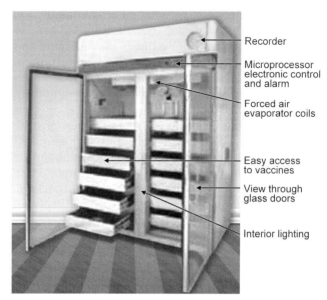

Recorder

Microprocessor electronic control and alarm

Forced air evaporator coils

Easy access to vaccines

View through glass doors

Interior lighting

FIG. 9.6.9: Purpose built refrigerator.

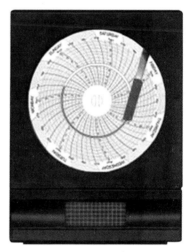

FIG. 9.6.10: Data logger.

Chart Recorders

Chart recorders consist of a graph wheel with replaceable graph paper and ink pens. The pens mark the temperature on the graph paper as the wheel turns. Temperatures are recorded continuously, 24 hours a day. The graph paper has a Fahrenheit or Celsius scale on it and the temperature is read where the ink line falls on the scale. The graph paper must be changed when it completes a full circle, usually weekly. As with other thermometers, temperature readings should be checked and recorded at least twice daily.

Minimum or Maximum Thermometer

Minimum or maximum thermometers are available in fluid-filled and digital forms. They show the current temperature and the minimum and maximum temperatures that have been reached since the last time the thermometer was reset. Temperature fluctuations outside the recommended range can be detected by referring to the minimum and maximum temperature readings. It is important to manually reset the minimum and maximum temperatures to the current temperature each time the temperatures are recorded.

The minimum or maximum thermometer must be reset regularly (after properly recording temperatures) for meaningful readings. The most effective minimum or maximum thermometer is a digital type with a probe. Place the probe directly in contact with a vaccine vial or package. The thermometer battery must be checked and replaced time-to-time.

A limitation of minimum or maximum thermometers is that readings do not indicate when the exposure occurred and the exact length of time the vaccines were exposed to the out of range temperatures (Fig. 9.6.11).

Digital Thermometers

Digital thermometers have a screen in which the temperature is displayed. Two types of digital thermometers are available; one with digital display of only current temperature, and second one those with digital display of current temperature as well as display of the minimum and maximum temperatures. The other one is a preferred type for temperature monitoring. Some digital thermometers have two components—a display that mounts to the outside of the unit and a probe on a cord (usually 1–3 m long) that is placed inside a vaccine or a diluent box inside the unit. This arrangement allows the temperature to be read without opening the door of the storage unit.

Digital thermometers with a minimum or maximum feature are easy to read because they display a number indicating the temperature and do not require interpretation. Temperature fluctuations outside the recommended range can be detected by referring to the minimum and maximum temperature readings. The digital thermometer must be reset regularly (after properly recording temperatures) for meaningful readings (Fig. 9.6.12).

Thermometers that are not Recommended for Monitoring Temperatures Inside Vaccine Storage Units

Fluid-filled bio-safe liquid (bottle) thermometers, bimetal stem thermometers, and household thermometers are not recommended for temperature monitoring in vaccine storage units. They can be difficult to read and only indicate the temperature at the precise time they are read; therefore, temperature fluctuations outside the recommended range may not be detected. Similarly the "Dial Thermometer"

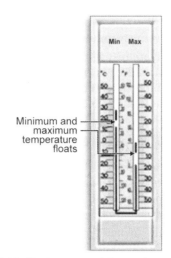

FIG. 9.6.11: Maximum or minimum thermometer.

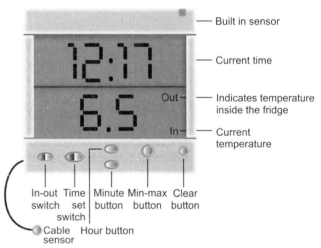

FIG. 9.6.12: Digital thermometers.

although used commonly is not much accurate and hence not recommended for use.

Thermometer Placement

The thermometer should be placed in the center of the compartment away from the coils, walls, door, floor and fan, and the temperature probe should be placed in the vaccine box. In the refrigerator compartment, the thermometer should be placed on the middle shelf adjacent to the vaccine. In the freezer, the thermometer should be placed on a box (or other item) adjacent to the vaccine so that it is in the middle of the compartment, not on the floor of the freezer.

Vaccine Vial Monitor

A Vaccine vial monitor (VVM) is a label containing a heat sensitive material, which is placed on a vaccine vial to register cumulative heat exposure over time. A VVM enables the health worker to know whether vaccine has been damaged by exposure to heat. The VVM is a circle with a small square inside it. The inner square of the VVM is made of heat sensitive material that is light at the starting point (Fig. 9.6.13).

The combined effect of time and temperature causes the inner square of the VVM to darken gradually. The color change is irreversible. A direct relationship exists between rate of color change and temperature. Thus, lower the temperature, slower the color change and higher the temperature, faster the color change. VVMs are not substitutes for expiry dates. Different types of VVM depending upon the heat stability of four different types are designed (Figs. 9.6.13 and 9.6.14).

EFFICIENT VACCINE MANAGEMENT PROTOCOLS

Routine Vaccine Storage and Handling Protocols

Routine protocols should include all aspects of day to day vaccine management, from ordering vaccines, controlling inventory, handling vaccines and monitoring storage conditions. It should include following four elements:
1. *Ordering and accepting vaccine deliveries:*
   - Order vaccines to maintain an adequate stock to meet the needs of the vaccination unit
   - Ensure that the "ordered vaccine stock" is delivered when the vaccination unit is open. Vaccine shipments should be delivered when staff is available to unpack and store
   - Store vaccines at the recommended temperatures, immediately on arrival, refrigerated vaccines between 2°C and 8°C and frozen vaccines between –50°C and 15°C
   - Maintain a vaccine inventory log including:
     * Vaccine name and number of doses received
     * Date vaccine received
     * Condition of vaccine on arrival
     * Vaccine manufacturer and lot number
     * Vaccine expiration date.
2. *Storing and handling vaccines (as discussed above).*
3. *Managing inventory:*
   - Rotate vaccine stock so vaccine and diluent with the shortest expiration date is used first
   - Place vaccine with the longest expiration date behind the vaccine that has short expiry
   - Remove expired vaccine and diluent from usable stock
   - Keep vaccine stock well-organized
   - Stick a basic map of vaccine locations outside of the refrigerator door so staff can go "straight" to the vaccine when the door is opened

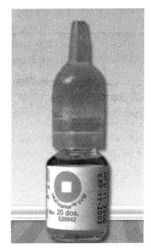

FIG. 9.6.13: Vaccine vial monitor (VVM).

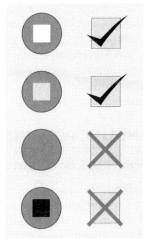

FIG. 9.6.14: Decision to use vaccine based on vaccine vial monitor.

   - Inspect the storage unit daily. A physical inspection helps to ensure vaccines and thermometers are placed appropriately within the unit
   - Dispose of all vaccine materials using medical waste disposal procedures.
4. *Managing potentially compromised vaccines:*
   - Identify and isolate all potentially compromised vaccines and diluents
   - Label these vaccines "DO NOT USE" and store separately from uncompromised vaccines and diluents in the recommended temperature range
   - Contact vaccine manufacturers and/or state immunization program for appropriate actions that should be followed for all potentially compromised vaccines and diluents.

Emergency Vaccine Retrieval and Storage

Various situations like equipment failures, power outages or natural disasters may compromise vaccine storage conditions and its important that all the staff involved in the immunization activity is aware of the probable adverse affect of such situations on vaccine storage conditions. Ensure that all staff has appropriate training so that they understand the urgent vaccine storage and handling protocols and their responsibility in maintaining the cold chain. Emergency vaccine retrieval and storage plan should include the following components:

- Designate an alternate site where vaccines and diluents can be safely stored. While choosing an alternate site consider availability of types of storage unit(s), temperature monitoring capabilities and backup generator.
- Obtain and store an adequate packing containers and materials (e.g. frozen or refrigerated gel packs, bubble wrap) in the facility that will be needed to pack vaccines for safe transport.
- Include written directions for packing vaccines and diluents for transport. A calibrated thermometer should be placed in each packing container near the vaccine
- Incorporate written procedures for managing potentially compromised vaccines
- Include contact information for vaccine manufacturers and/or the immunization program.

VACCINE HANDLING PERSONNEL

Designated Vaccine Coordinators Staff

Each vaccination clinic should designate one staff member to be the primary vaccine coordinator and another staff member as a backup in case the primary coordinator is unavailable. The designated person will be responsible for ensuring that all vaccines are handled correctly, that procedures are documented, and that all personnel receive appropriate cold chain training. Designated vaccine coordinators should be fully trained in routine and urgent vaccine storage and handling protocols.

Other Staff

All staff members should be familiar with the policies and procedures for vaccine storage and handling. This especially includes staff members, such as receptionists who accept vaccine shipments. Written policies and procedure documents should be available near the vaccine storage units for easy reference.

Training Personnel

All staff that handle or administer vaccines should be trained in proper vaccine storage and handling practices. All staff should be trained to have an understanding of the importance of cold chain maintenance and basic practices so they are aware of their responsibilities to the cold chain. Staff who monitor and record vaccine storage unit temperatures should immediately report inappropriate storage conditions (including exposure to inappropriate temperature or light exposures) to the designated vaccine coordinator.

BIBLIOGRAPHY

1. Getting started with VVMs. VVM for all, Technical Session on Vaccine Vial Monitors. WHO Publication 27/3/2002. Geneva.
2. Gupta SK, Shastri DD, Cold Chain & Vaccine Storage, IAP Textbook of Vaccines, 1st edition. Jaypee Brothers 2014. pp. 89-99.
3. Safety of vaccines affected by a power outage. Quick Clinical Notes, Disaster management and response. 2004;2:62-3 CDC.
4. Shastri DD, Vaccine Storage & Handling, IAP Textbook of Pediatrics, 5th edition, Jaypee Brothers Medical Publishers, New Delhi.
5. Shastri DD, Vaccine Storage & Handling, IAP Textbook of Pediatrics Infectious Diseases, 1st edition. Jaypee Brothers 2013 .pp. 493-501.
6. Strive for 5, National Vaccine Storage Guidelines. Australian Government Department of Health and Aging.
7. Target-5, Guide to Vaccine Storage & Handling, 1st edition, 2006.
8. "Thermostability of Vaccines" 1998 by A Galazka, J Milstien, M Zaffran. WHO (Global Programme for Vaccines and Immunization).
9. Vaccine Management, recommendations for handling and storage of selected biologicals. Department of Health and Human Services, CDC. Atlanta.
10. WHO, Immunization in Practice, WHO/EPI/PHW/84.01 to 84.07.

10

Miscellaneous Topics

Sailesh Gupta

10.1   PERIODIC FEVER

Kheya Ghosh Uttam

INTRODUCTION

Febrile illnesses are very common in children. A child may have up to 10 episodes of limited febrile illnesses per year in his first 2–3 years of life. Children attending day care usually have more frequent febrile illness. Recurrent fever with each episode lasting from few days to few weeks and the episodes being separated by symptom free intervals of variable duration is called periodic fever. These febrile illnesses are mostly due to some infective etiology. Recurrent episodes of self-limited viral infection, urinary tract infections and sinopulmonary infections are quite common in children. Systematic diseases also give rise to periodic fever, e.g. hematological disorder (cyclic neutropenia), various immunodeficiency disorders and autoimmune diseases (juvenile idiopathic arthritis, inflammatory bowel disease, Behçet disease) manifest as recurrent fever.

Thus, it is important to take a careful medical history and do a detailed physical examination in a child with recurrent fever to differentiate the above mentioned causes. If periodic fever comes with similar set of symptoms and signs with a predictable course along with history of similar illnesses in the family hereditary cause of periodic fever or periodic fever syndrome should be suspected. In most of these diseases, the episodes have consistent periodicity whereas in some they do not.

As most of the causes of periodic fever are described elsewhere we have restricted our discussion to periodic fever syndrome in this chapter. Table 10.1.1 differentiates between infective, autoimmune and hereditary causes of periodic fever (periodic fever syndrome).

PERIODIC FEVER SYNDROME

Periodic fever syndromes are rare disorders of immune system characterized by episodes of systemic inflammation. Several periodic fever syndromes are well described. The four common periodic fever syndromes with their main features are summarized in Table 10.1.2.

Table 10.1.1: Differentiating features to detect the etiology of periodic fever.

Sl. No	History	Recurrent infections	Autoimmune disorder	Periodic fever syndrome
1.	Periodicity of episodes	Irregular	Irregular	Usually clockwise periodicity
2.	Characteristic of episodes	Waning and waxing of single illness (EBV) or multiple self-limited illness (recurrent viral respiratory tract, AOM, UTI). Course as expected for the infective agent	Waning and waxing of single disease (JIA inflammatory bowel disease). Course prolonged	Episodes with similar symptoms and signs and predictable course
3.	Clustering of episodes	Concurrent illness in school home	Nil	Nil
4.	Family history	Negative	May be positive	Positive
5.	Interval between episodes	Completely well	Lingering symptoms, unless treated	Completely well
6.	Weight gain and energy	Normal	Usually poor	Variable

Abbreviations: EBV, Epstein-Barr virus; AOM, acute otitis media; UTI, Urinary tract infection; JIA, juvenile idiopathic arthritis.

Table 10.1.2: Cardinal features of periodic fever syndrome.

Periodic fever	Genetics	Febrile episodes	Characteristic signs	Treatment
Familial Mediterranean fever	AR MEFV gene on chromosome 16	Short (2–3 days), irregular, unpredictable	Serositis, abdominal pain, oral ulcers, arthritis, erysipelas rash	Colchicine
TRAPS	AD TNFRSF1A gene on chromosome 12	Usually >7 days, interval being 1week to months	Localized migratory myalgia, arthralgia Cellulitis like skin rash, conjunctivitis	Corticosteroids Etanercept
HIDS	AR MVK gene on chromosome 12	Lasting 3–7 days Interval 1–2 months	Lymphadenopathy, abdominal pain, hepatosplenomegaly, arthralgia	Etanercept Anakinra
PFAPA	Not known	Lasting 3–5 days with striking periodicity (3–8 weekly)	Mouth ulcers, pharyngitis, tonsillitis, lymphadenopathy	Corticosteroid tonsillectomy

Abbreviations: AR, autosomal recessive; MEFV, Mediterranean fever; AD, autosomal dominant; TRAPS, tumor necrosis factor receptor associated periodic syndrome; HIDS, hyperimmunoglobulinemia D and periodic fever syndrome ; PFAPA, periodic fever, aphthous stomatitis, pharyngitis and adenitis.

FAMILIAL MEDITERRANEAN FEVER

Epidemiology

Familial Mediterranean Fever (FMF) is the most prevalent periodic fever syndrome. FMF predominantly affects eastern Mediterranean people, prevalence varies from 1/250 in Jewish to 1/1,073 in Turkish population. FMF also occurs in other European populations (e.g. Italians, Greeks).

Genetics

Familial Mediterranean fever is an autosomal recessive disease. Mutation of MEFV gene is responsible for the disease; till now 152 mutations have been identified. The five most common mutations are: (1) M694V, (2) M680I, (3) V726A, (4) M694I and (5) E148Q. A severe disease pattern is seen in patients with homozygosity for the M694V mutation. Some patients have definite clinical picture of FMF but no identifiable MEFV gene mutation. On the other hand, some homozygous patients may be asymptotic. Eighty-five percent of FMF patients have two mutations.

Clinical Features

The condition is characterized by short attacks of fever and serositis (peritonitis, pleuritis or arthritis). Febrile episodes are irregular above 39°C, lasting for 2–3 days. Two-thirds of affected individuals have manifestation before 10 years and in 90% of cases, the first attack occurs before 20 years. Eighty-five percent of patients presents with severe abdominal pain (peritonitis). Thirty-five to sixty-five percent of patients presents with joint involvement (oligoarthritis involving knee, hip or ankle joint). Chronic peritoneal inflammation or joint involvement is rare. More than 50% of patients present with oral ulcers and 10–40% have erysipelas like rashes mainly on the ankles, shinbone or feet. Less common features are headache, chest pain (unilateral pleuritis or rarely pericarditis), orchitis,

splenomegaly, diarrhea, nausea and myalgia. Stress, exercise, menstruation and dietetic factors have been identified as triggers. The ongoing inflammation may lead to amyloidosis of kidneys, intestine, liver and spleen. Renal involvement results in proteinuria, nephrotic syndrome and eventually renal failure. The diagnostic criteria for FMF are suggested in Table 10.1.3.

Investigation

Acute phase reactants, C-reactive protein (CRP), erythrocyte sedimentation rate (ESR), neutrophils, fibrinogen, interleukin (IL)-6, tumor necrosis factor-alpha (TNF-α) and serum amyloid A protein are known to be elevated during febrile episodes. Proteinuria suggests amyloidosis. Genetic testing is the confirmatory test for FMF.

Treatment

Since 1972, colchicines have been the first line treatment for patients with FMF. It reduces symptoms in 95% of cases. The drug is concentrated in neutrophils where it arrests microtubule polymerization, inhibits neutrophil chemotaxis and phagocytosis, thus decreasing inflammation. Lifelong adherence to therapy is important

Table 10.1.3: Diagnostic criteria for familial Mediterranean fever.

Sl. No.	Major criteria	Minor criteria
1.	Recurrent febrile (>38°C) episodes (≥3 attacks of 12 hours to 3 days duration) accompanied by peritonitis, synovitis or pleuritis (unilateral)	Recurrent febrile episodes
2.	Amyloidosis of the AA type without predisposing disease	Erysipelas like erythema
3.	Favorable response to continuous colchicine treatment	Familial Mediterranean fever in a first degree relative

The clinical diagnosis of FMF requires two major or one major and two minor criteria.

as discontinuation can result in recurrence of episodes. Till now, there is no consensus regarding the second line drug in cases not responding to colchicines. Steroids have shown to relieve abdominal pain. Anakinra, the IL-1 receptor antagonist, has been successfully used in colchicines resistant patients.

Prognosis

The prognosis for patients with FMF is determined mainly by the presence or absence of AA amyloidosis. Before the introduction of colchicine amyloidosis was the main cause of death in above 40 years, when more than 60% of the patients developed renal failure due to amyloidosis. Even if colchicines therapy does not prevent febrile attacks, it arrests amyloidosis and reverse proteinuria. Asymptomatic children with known FMF mutation should undergo regular urine analysis for proteinuria as in this group the risk of developing amyloidosis is not unknown.

TUMOR NECROSIS FACTOR RECEPTOR ASSOCIATED PERIODIC SYNDROME

Tumor necrosis factor receptor associated periodic syndrome (TRAPS) previously known as familial Hibernian fever was first described in 1982 in a large Irish family. It is the second most common hereditary periodic fever with an incidence of approximately 1/million in the UK.

Genetics

Tumor necrosis factor receptor associated periodic syndrome is an autosomal dominant disorder caused by the mutations in the TNFRSF1A (TNF-α receptor super family 1A) or chromosome 12p13.

About 50 mutations have been identified. Mutations at cysteine residues are linked with severe disease. Fifty percent of cases may have no family history especially P46L or R92Q variant where the disease is milder. Like FMF, there are cases with symptoms suggesting TRAPS but no TNFRSF1A mutation identified.

Clinical Features

Tumor necrosis factor receptor associated periodic syndrome usually presents before 4 years of age. Although age of onset may vary from few weeks to older than 40 years. Boys and girls are equally affected. Febrile attack usually lasts for more than 7 days and is usually high (about 40°C). Fever is associated with severe localized pain and tightness of muscle group, which becomes migratory in nature. Arthralgia, painful conjunctivitis, periorbital edema and skin rashes are often present. The arthralgia is mono or oligo articular affecting usually knee, shoulder or elbow joints. More than 60% of patients have erythematous macules or plaques simulating cellulitis, due

to perivascular and interstitial mononuclear cell infiltrate. Other symptoms like mouth ulcers, lymphadenitis, pleuritic pain, abdominal and testicular pain and central nervous system (CNS) manifestation are less specific but reported. Acute myocarditis has been described in a patient with TRAPS. The prolonged attacks, conjunctivitis and localized migratory myalgias help to differentiate TRAP from other causes of periodic fever syndrome.

Investigation

During attack blood test show neutrophilia, thrombocytosis with raised CRP, ESR and mild complement activation. Elevated serum immunoglobulins (Ig), including IgA and IgD, can present but the value is never very high. The most discriminatory laboratory finding is low serum level of the soluble type 1 TNF receptor along with increased TNF-α levels.

Treatment

High dose oral steroids given at the start of an episode dramatically reduce the severity of attack. Colchicine has no effect in TRAPS. Etanercept, an anti-TNF-α dimeric recombinant TNF receptor fusion protein, is highly effective. Treatment with Etanercept given subcutaneously twice a week is effective in about 50% of cases. Conversely, infliximab—another TNF antagonist—can worsen the on going inflammation and is contraindicated.

Prognosis

Like FMF the prognosis is determined mainly by the presence or absence of amyloidosis. AA amyloidosis occurs in about 10–25% of cases depending on the type of mutation and duration of illness. Amyloid deposits generally lead to renal impairment but hepatic failure has also been noted.

HYPER-IgD PERIODIC FEVER SYNDROME OR MEVALONATE KINASE DEFICIENCY

Hyper-IgD periodic fever syndrome (HIDS) was first described as a separate disease entity in 1984. Most patients with the hyper-IgD syndrome are white and are from Western European countries (especially the Netherlands and France). In the Dutch population, the carrier rate is about 1/350.

Genetics

This autosomal recessive defect was identified in 1999. Mutation in the mevalonate kinase (MVK) gene on long arm of chromosome 12 results in significant reduction of MVK activity. Partial deficiency of this enzyme causes HIDS due to increased secretions of interleukins leading to inflammation. Less than 1% of patients suffer from complete deficiency of the enzyme resulting in the lethal disease mevalonic aciduria. About 60 mutations have been identified, V3771 being the most common.

Clinical Features

The age of onset is usually within the first year of life. A typical febrile episode is heralded by chills, followed by a sharp rise in body temperature ($\geq 39°C$) and lasts for 4–6 days, with gradual defervescence. It is often triggered by immunization, injury or stress. The attacks are associated with tender firm lymphadenopathy (in 90% of cases) mainly cervical, and abdominal pain with nausea, diarrhea, hepatomegaly and splenomegaly. Arthritis, arthralgia, recurrent aphthous oral or genital ulcers and skin rash are less common features. Skin rash is typically seen on extremities (in 70% of cases) and are in the form of erythematous macules, papules or urticaria. Patients are well between attacks and growth is unimpaired. As the age increases frequency severity of febrile episodes tend to decrease.

Investigation

Hyper-IgD periodic fever syndrome should be suspected if there is characteristic clinical findings and continuously high level of serum IgD (defined as >200 mg/mL). However, elevated IgD is not specific for HIDS as it is also seen in 10–13% of patients with TRAPS and FMF. Moreover, all children with characteristic fever and MVK mutation do not have raised IgD level. In approximately, 80% of cases of HIDS raised IgA levels are seen during attacks. During an attack, there is a brisk rise of acute phase reactants like CRP, neutrophils and ESR.

Treatment

No uniformly successful treatment of the HIDS is available. Anti-TNF-α therapy with Etanercept improved attacks. Similar results is found using Anakinra, a soluble IL-1 receptor antagonist.

Prognosis

Frequency of attacks is highest in childhood and adolescence. As age increases patients become free of attack for months or even years. Very few cases have been reported to develop amyloidosis.

PERIODIC FEVER, APHTHOUS STOMATITIS, PHARYNGITIS AND ADENITIS OR MARSHALL'S SYNDROME

Periodic fever, aphthous stomatitis, pharyngitis and adenitis (PFAPA) is a non-hereditary condition occurring sporadically and was first described by Marshall et al. in 1987. The pathogenesis of PFAPA is not fully understood. Rise of inflammatory markers during febrile episodes and remarkable response to corticosteroid therapy points toward abnormality of cytokine regulation as a probable mechanism.

Clinical Features

Age of onset is usually before 3 years and almost always before 5 years. Boys are affected more than girls. The fever is usually high (>39°C) lasting for 3–5 days, poorly responsive to antipyretics and has a striking periodicity. Aphthous ulcers occur in 39–60% of these children during the febrile episode. The lesions are typically round, small and shallow, surrounded by erythema and heals without scarring. Sixty-one to eighty-five percent cases have cervical lymphadenopathy and most cases have pharyngitis and tonsillitis. Abdominal pain is also reported in 50–65% of patients. Other less common features are headache, malaise, chills, arthralgia, vomiting and hepatosplenomegaly. The diagnostic criteria were proposed by Marshall et al. in the year 1989 which were modified in the year 1999 by Thomas et al. The modified diagnostic criteria are shown in Box 10.1.1.

Investigation

Investigations are essential to rule out other periodic febrile illness. Cultures from the throat swab, chest radiography, serial blood counts (to rule out cyclic neutropenia) and Epstein-Barr virus serology are essential. Sometimes immunoglobulin C3, lymphocyte T4/T8 ratio, IgG subset and IgD are done to rule out immunodeficiency disorder.

Raised white blood cell (WBC) count, ESR and CRP are seen during febrile episodes. High serum IgD (>100 U/mL) is seen in some children, even between the episodes.

Treatment

Use of oral steroids causes a dramatic resolution of febrile episodes, although it does not prevent recurrence. Antibiotics, non-steroidal anti-inflammatory and antiviral

---

Box 10.1.1

Diagnostic criteria for PFAPA syndrome (Thomas et al. 1999).
Regularly recurring fevers with an early age of onset (<5 years of age)
Symptoms in the absence of upper respiratory tract infection with at least one of the following:
- Aphthous stomatitis
- Cervical lymphadenitis
- Pharyngitis
Exclusion of cyclic neutropenia
Completely asymptomatic between episode
Normal growth and development

therapy are ineffective. Tonsillectomy with/without adenoidectomy remains controversial as the studies shown effectiveness of it had very small number of cases and short follow-up.

Prognosis

Spontaneous remission has been seen in most cases followed up to 5 years. Episodes eventually become less frequent and finally resolves. No long-term sequelae have been reported.

Apart from these four common disorders, there are other rare causes of periodic fever syndrome. Familial cold urticaria, cryopyrin associated periodic fever syndrome, pyogenic sterile arthritis pyoderma gangrenosum and acne syndrome are three rare autosomal dominant diseases which are also included in the list of hereditary periodic fever. Cryopyrin associated periodic fever syndrome includes three diseases with overlying features and the mutation is in the same gene, NLRP3/CIAS1 located on chromosome 1q44 which encodes the protein cryopyrin.

They are familial cold auto-inflammatory syndrome (FCAS), Muckle-Wells syndrome (MWS), chronic infantile neurological cutaneous and articular (CINCA) syndrome.

Thus, to summarize a high degree of suspicion together with thorough investigation is required to diagnose a child with periodic fever. Periodic fever syndromes are rare immunological disorders with characteristic features and typical prevalence in certain population. Identification of the involved genes has lead to effective therapy in some of these cases.

BIBLIOGRAPHY

1. Drenth JPH, van der Meer JWM. Hereditary periodic fever. N Engl J Med. 2001;345:1748-56.

2. Long SS. Distinguishing among prolonged, recurrent and periodic fever syndromes: approach of pediatric infectious disease subspecialist. PediatrClin North Am. 2005;52:811-35.

3. Mushtaq F, Hildebrandt T, Jolles S. Periodic fever syndromes. Pediatrics and child health. 2010;20:503-8.

10.2 SEXUALLY TRANSMITTED DISEASES IN ADOLESCENTS

S Yamuna

INTRODUCTION

All boys and girls between 10 and 19 years are referred to as adolescents by the World Health Organization (WHO). Adolescents are in a phase of transition from childhood to adulthood. They are in the process of emancipating from their parents and are in the course of forming an identity for themselves. This phase has numerous physical, emotional, sexual and social changes taking place in the growing children. These changes expose the adolescents to plenty of challenges which have to be overcome by the adolescents by making use of their life skills which may/may not be developed adequately.

Developmentally, after a phase of sexual latency between 6 years and puberty, all adolescents are tuned to realize their sexuality and are endowed with motivation to experiment and practice adult sexual behavior as a result of the hormonal inputs from the gonads. Sexual activity during adolescence is usually not planned, and hence protection against sexually transmitted infections (STIs) takes a back seat. Use of mind altering substances like alcohol makes the adolescents forget the importance of usage of barrier protection in spite of adequate knowledge of using the same.

GLOBAL SCENARIO

Globally, it is understood that consensual sexual activities by adolescents above 15 years have been exposing them to STIs and diseases. More than 50% of new STIs happen in adolescents. Adolescents may be exposed to sexual interactions either in the context of marriage, outside the context of marriage in a consensual relationship or may be exploited by authority figures without consent in an abusive situation.

NATIONAL SCENARIO

Sexual Activity within Marriage

In India, the legal age of marriage has been recommended as 18 years for females and 21 years for males. National Family Health Survey (NFHS) 3 that concluded in 2006 gives us a disturbing figure that 47% of women aged between 20 and 24 years were married before they turned 18 years, thus exposing the girls to early sexual activity, early pregnancy and STIs from their older married partners who may have been sexually experienced earlier than the marriage. Thirteen percent of the young women have had their sexual début before 15 years.

Premarital Sexual Activity

Premarital sexual activity has been increasing in urban and rural India. According to NFHS 3, the median age at first marriage in men is 23 years and the median age at first sexual intercourse is 22.6 years. The discrepancy in the age denotes premarital sexual activity. Another study on male sexual début from Orissa states that 36.1% of urban men and 26.3% of rural men have had sex before marriage. Youth in India, situation and needs study (2006–2008) states that 9–17% of young men and 2–7% of young women had engaged in premarital sex, among whom, fewer than 10% had used condom during the previous sexual act. 14.5% of men from Uttar Pradesh, 13.9% in Bihar, 16.6% in Jharkhand, 15.5% in Rajasthan, 16.4% in Andhra Pradesh had self-reported premarital sexual activity.

Heterosexual partners of young men at sexual debut in Orissa comprised of married women, single women and sex workers; 75% with girl friends or acquaintances; 16% with relatives; 4% with sister-in-law; less than 2% with sex workers (sexual debut by men above 20 years); less than 10% were under the influence of alcohol with nonsex workers; 40% under the influence of alcohol, if with sex workers.

High-risk sexual activity is the highest among adolescents in detention like in observation homes; high-risk behaviors usually occur as a cluster. Homosexual experiences among themselves and with care takers, have been self-reported by boys from juvenile homes in Chennai.

PREVALENCE OF SEXUALLY TRANSMITTED INFECTIONS IN ADOLESCENTS

According to NFHS 3, 11% women aged 15–19 years reported some kind of STI symptoms. More women than men report having a STI (1.4% compared to 0.8% in men) or its symptoms (10.9%). A higher percentage of younger men (15–19 years) reported STI symptoms compared to older men. Women generally reported of abnormal genital discharge while a higher percentage of men report genital sore or ulcer. Seventy-five percent of clients at an STD clinic in Mumbai were 18–19 years of age (1999).

Risk and Protective Factors

(Adapted from risk and protective factors affecting adolescent reproductive health in developing countries WHO, 2004)

Box 10.2.1

Risk factors that expose adolescents to sexually transmitted infections.

Biological risk factors
- Early puberty
- Early age of sexual debut
- Microabrasions
- Immature cervix/cervical ectopy
- Sex during menstruation
- Unprotected anal sex
- Untreated genitourinary disease
- History of sexually transmitted infections
- Female genital mutilation
- Not circumcised

Sociocultural risk factors
- Early marriage
- School drop out
- Taboo about sex education
- Lack of family life education
- Lack of life skills education
- Coercive sex/sexual abuse
- Unstable family environment

Individual risk factors
- Older adolescent
- Male
- Urban residence
- Employed
- Substance abuse/alcohol use
- Multiple sexual partners
- Watching/reading X-rated material
- Talks about sexual and reproductive health (SRH) issues with friends
- Perceived sexual behavior of friends
- Lack of knowledge about condom availability and accessibility
- Barriers to use condom
- Partner's negative attitude about condom use

Economic risk factors
- Abuse in the work setting
- Survival sex
- Sugar daddies
- Early age at becoming a commercial sex worker
- Being a commercial sex worker in a brothel
- To sustain drug behavior
- No money to buy condom

Box 10.2.2

Protective factors against exposure of adolescents to sexually transmitted infections.

Sociocultural protective factors
- Higher education
- Universality of marriage
- Education on sexual and reproductive health (SRH) issues
- Life skills education in schools
- Knowledge about availability and accessibility of condoms
- Living with both parents
- Stable family environment

Individual protective factors
- Older adolescent
- Higher educational aspirations
- Feeling valued
- High self-esteem
- Spiritual beliefs
- Sense of future
- Abstinence from using substances like alcohol, etc.
- Refusal skills for unsafe sex
- Knowledge on condom usage
- Knowledge on where to access/buy condoms
- Positive attitude about using condoms
- Regular use of condoms
- Self efficacy in using condoms
- Perceived effectiveness of using condoms
- Perceived risk of exposure to STIs
- Single faithful partner
- Talks about protection with partners
- Partner approval of condoms
- Talks about SRH issues with teachers and parents

Economic protective factors
- Employed
- Financially sound to buy condoms

predispose to increased susceptibility to acquisition and transmission of human immunodeficiency virus (HIV). In female adolescents pelvic inflammatory disease (PID) is a complication that could be accompanied by fertility issues in future due to block in the fallopian tubes and adnexal tissue inflammation. Thus knowledge about an approach to STIs in adolescents would help pediatricians in limiting the spread of STIs in adolescents.

Approach to Sexually Transmitted Diseases in Adolescents

As STIs in adolescents is a topic of high public health relevance, especially in view of its increased association with the spread of HIV, let us approach the same with a public health perspective.

Adolescents are in need of Specialized Services

As depicted above adolescents are susceptible to STIs at higher rates than adults in view of their vulnerability. Adolescents are transitioning from concrete thought processes that are oriented to the current moment to abstract

By definition factors are called "protective" if they increase the likelihood of positive health behaviors or outcomes (e.g. using condoms) or curb, control and discourage behaviors that might lead to negative health outcomes (e.g. having sex with many partners). Similarly, factors are labeled "risk" if they increase the likelihood of negative health behaviors and outcomes or inhibit positive behaviors that might prevent them.

Factors that make adolescents vulnerable to exposure to STIs are given in Box 10.2.1. Factors that protect adolescents against exposure to STIs are given in Box 10.2.2.

Thus, Indian adolescents are vulnerable to acquire STIs due to social, biological and economic reasons. To include a chapter on sexually transmitted diseases (STDs) in adolescents in this textbook is relevant because adolescents come under the care of pediatricians. Untreated STIs

thought processes which acknowledge the continuity of past, present and future. Psychosocially they are in a phase where experimentation is ecstatic. In emotionally loaded situations impulsivity decides their actions. In the event of consequences to their high-risk activities, hesitations, shame, guilt, remorse, anger are the predominant emotions. Seeking help from professionals is resorted to only when it is absolutely necessary and only when they are assured of audio-visual privacy, confidentiality and non-judgmental attitude from the providers.

The adolescent friendly health services will have to be accessible, approachable, affordable, and available when adolescents are in need of them. Nonmoralistic, non-threatening approach by the healthcare providers would attract more adolescents to the services. Reproductive and child health clinics cater to young women and children. Adolescent boys are in need of healthcare centers where they can interact with healthcare providers of same gender in a manner where all their health needs including concerns about their sexual health and development can be addressed with maintenance of confidentiality.

In primary healthcare, regular healthcare consultations do not focus on the sexual health of the clients. Sexual behaviors, risk proneness of the sexual practices are usually not discussed. Thus lack of knowledge about the sexual practices in the clients reduces the need to offer risk reduction counseling to the subjects. For the same reason, routine screening for STIs is also not carried out. Early detection, treatment of the person followed by partner tracing, identification and treatment are not taking place in spite of the high prevalence of STIs in adolescents.

A shift in the planning and provision of sexual health services in an adolescent friendly manner is expected to curtail the spread of STIs among the boys and girls. Early diagnosis and treatment would reduce complications of STIs in adolescents. An approach toward establishment of responsible sexual behavior including secondary abstinence and usage of protection in a correct and consistent manner would help in reducing the prevalence of STIs among adolescents.

Adolescent Friendly Health Services in India

Adolescent friendly healthcare is slowly expanding in India with the creation of adolescent friendly sexual and reproductive health (SRH) clinics in government medical college hospitals and primary health centers where integrated counseling and treatment centers for early detection of HIV are being conducted. A few clinics run by private practitioners are catering to almost 75–80% of the health needs of adolescents where the general practitioners are the first line healthcare providers. Only in the last decade specialist pediatricians are being trained to expand their services to cater to the adolescents.

Box 10.2.3

Role of Pediatricians in the Reduction of Sexually Transmitted Infections in Adolescents.

The agenda before us are to:
- Reduce the vulnerability of our adolescents to sexual exposure
- Equip them with awareness about various consequences of unprotected sexual exposure
- Empower them with skills to protect themselves with adequate training on life skills
- Train them to use barrier protection continuously and consistently against infections
- Prepare them to identify and report to health services in the event of symptoms
- Provide them with adolescent friendly health services with maintenance of privacy and confidentiality
- Make treatment available to adolescents in all these centers so that early treatment would limit the spread of infection and protect against complications
- Help in treating their partners and thus reduce the chance of a reinfection
- Endow them with life skills to choose abstinence until marriage with a stable partner
- Educate them to channelize their sexual energy in other activities

---

Awareness among public about the availability of adolescent friendly SRH services within the premises of the pediatricians office is gradually expanding. An adolescent reporting to clinicians with symptoms suggestive of STI is fortunately or unfortunately not the norm yet. We can consider ourselves as fortunate that we have not been seeing adolescents with symptoms of STIs because we can blissfully assume that indiscriminate transmission and acquisition of STIs is not happening among our adolescents. On the other side, we should also not forget that adolescents with symptoms may not be reaching us in view of lack of awareness about our openness to treat them, fear of maintenance of confidentiality from their parents, perceived lack of experience and knowledge among all of us to treat STIs.

Sexually transmitted infections are usually concentrated among out of school adolescents with the stated risk factors (Box 10.2.3). Recently, there is an increased sexual activity among school or college students in committed relationships prior to the context of marriage. Many adolescents are involved either in serial monogamy or have multiple sexual partners among their regular associates. Some of them have sex with casual contacts who have been introduced through the wide social networks, especially under the influence of mind altering substances. Most of these sexual activities are not protected because of the belief that the partners are "Not Strangers" and they are "Healthy to look at".

ETIOLOGY OF SEXUALLY TRANSMITTED INFECTIONS

Sexually transmitted infections are caused by bacteria, viruses and parasites.

Common Bacterial Infections

- *Neisseria gonorrhoeae*: Urethritis, cervicitis, PID
- *Chlamydia trachomatis*: Urethritis, cervicitis, PID
- *Treponema pallidum* (syphilis): Ulcerative disease, chancre, secondary syphilis, tertiary syphilis, neurosyphilis, etc.
- *Haemophilus ducreyi* (chancroid): Ulcerative disease
- *Klebsiella granulomatis* (previously known as *Calymmatobacterium granulomatis* causes donovanosis).

Common Viral Infections

- Human immunodeficiency virus (AIDS, refer Chapter 5.16)
- Herpes simplex virus (HSV) type 2 (genital herpes): ulcerative disease
- Human papillomavirus (HPV) (genital warts and certain subtypes lead to cervical cancer in women)
- Hepatitis A, B and C virus (hepatitis and chronic cases may lead to cancer of the liver)
- Cytomegalovirus (causes inflammation in a number of organs including the brain, the eye and the bowel).

Parasites

- *Trichomonas vaginalis* (vaginal trichomoniasis): vaginal discharge
- *Candida albicans* [vulvovaginitis in women; inflammation of the glans penis and foreskin (balanoposthitis) in men].

Ectoparasites

- Scabies
- Pediculosis pubis.

PATHOGENESIS

Pubertal estrogens cornify the vaginal epithelium with a rise in the glycogen content that makes the vaginal pH to fall. This offers resistance to infection by gonococci but increases susceptibility to candida and trichomonas. Cervical ectopy at the squamocolumnar junction is another reason for increased vulnerability to infection. With maturation this involutes. Thus, an adolescent girl has a ten times higher chance of having an ascending infection with subsequent PID with *N. gonorrhoeae* compared to an adult female. Early sexual debut, multiple partners and inadequate treatment of infections increase the propensity for complications due to STIs in adolescents.

Clinical Approach to Sexually Transmitted Infections in Adolescents

Adolescents who require the attention of healthcare providers for STIs can be married adolescents, unmarried adolescents who are sexually active, adolescents who have been sexually abused, adolescents who are marginalized including boys who have sex with men/boys, commercial sex workers, injectable drug users, street children, adolescents in detention facilities, etc. Usually adolescents report by self or are accompanied by their parents (urban private providers' clinics), partners, friends, well wishers, servants, etc.

History Taking

Adolescents who reach the clinicians for symptoms suggestive of STIs are usually shy and guilty. After establishment of rapport, the adolescent should be assured of audio-visual privacy and confidentiality. Clinical history taking is to be conducted with a high degree of empathy and non-judgmental attitude with unconditional positive regard for the adolescent all through their stay within the chambers. Depending on the comfort level of the adolescent, it is essential to have a chaperone during the clinical care. The chaperone can be either the same sex parent or the nursing staff in the center as approved by the adolescent.

Whether to inform the parents or not is a question that has to be handled with care keeping the legal implications of the same. In India, any sexual activity in boys and girls less than 16 years is considered abuse. Sexual activity between 16 and 18 years is not a crime as of now, it can be considered consensual; but there is a move to consider it as a crime and a Bill is being under process to protect adolescents from consequences of early sexual activity.

Exceptions to maintenance of confidentiality are when there is suspected physical, sexual or emotional abuse, and/or the presence of risk for harm to self or others.

After the listing of complaints, it is essential to conduct a home education, activities drugs, suicide, sexuality, safety spirituality (HEADSSSS) screening to assess the psychosocial environment of the adolescent (Box 10.2.4). Similarly, it is useful to assess the strengths using the strength, school home, activities drugs, emotions, sexuality, safety (SSHADESS) tool (Box 10.2.5). Simultaneously Partners, prevention of pregnancy, protection from STDs, practices and past history of STDs as the "FIVE Ps" (Box 10.2.6).

Box 10.2.4

HEADSSSS Screening.
- *Home (H):* Conflicts with or between parents predispose to early sexual activity
- *Education/Employment/Eating (E):* School drop outs have higher rates of early sexual debut
- *Activities (A):* Exposure to pornography through print and electronic media promotes sexual activity
- *Drugs (D):* Mind altering substances alter the sense of judgment
- *Suicidality/Depression (S):* Low mood promotes ecstasy seeking
- *Sexuality/Sexual behavior (S):* Orientation, practices to be explored with gentleness
- *Safety (S):* Poor knowledge about protection against STIs
- Spirituality (optional) (S)

Box 10.2.5

SSHADDESS tool.
- *Strength or interests (S):* Interest in academics, sports, music, etc.
- *School (S):* School connectedness, school-based sexual health clinics
- *Home (H):* Parents being the providers of sex education
- *Activities (A):* Team activities, nature walks, etc. preclude
- *Drugs/Substance use (D):* Abstinence from mind altering substances
- *Emotions/Depression (E):* Sense of well-being, high self-esteem, focused approach to achievement
- *Sexuality (S):* Cross gender friendships versus romantic relationships
- *Safety (S):* Knowledge of protection against the consequences of impulsive behaviors. Center for Disease Control and Prevention, Atlanta, USA, in the Sexually Transmitted Diseases Treatment Guidelines, 2010 recommends clinicians to ask specific questions on the following headings to understand the sexual behavior and practices of the clients reaching the sexual health clinics

Box 10.2.6

FIVE Ps in history.
1. *Partners*:
   - Whether the partners have been boys/men, girls/women or both
   - The number of sexual partners in the last two months
   - The number of sexual partners in the previous 12 months
   - Chance for any of the client's current sexual partners to have had sex with another person outside the current sexual relationship with the client
2. *Prevention of pregnancy*: Precautions that are taken to prevent pregnancy
3. *Protection from sexually transmitted diseases:* Precautions that are taken to protect self against STI and HIV
4. *Practices*:
   - Knowledge about the kind of sex the adolescent usually experiences helps in risk assessment
   - Whether it is penile-vaginal, anal or oral sex has to be understood
   - If anal sex, whether it is penetrative or receptive, has to be explored
   - Knowledge about use of barriers to protect against STIs like the usage of condoms
   - If condoms are used, the consistency and the correctness of use
   - If condoms are not used, the reasons for not using the same
5. *Past history of sexually transmitted diseases*:
   - Past history of STD in self
   - Past history of STD in any of the partners so far
   - Knowledge about the use of injectable drugs by self or partners
   - Whether self or partners have exchanged money or drugs for sex
   - Any other relevant information about the sexual practices followed by the client

Clinical Presentation

Urethral discharge, vaginal discharge, dysuria, dyspareunia, genital ulcer, scrotal swelling, inguinal swelling, lower abdominal pain are some of the common complaints with which adolescents may reach the healthcare services.

Urethral or vaginal discharge and ulcers are more common during adolescence than the rest.

As adolescents seek help only when absolutely essential it is necessary that we treat them completely at the first visit as the rates of adherence to follow-up visits is very poor. Clinicians usually do not get time to find an etiological diagnosis of the condition they are treating. Tests that are necessary to establish an etiological diagnosis of the sexually acquired infections are also expensive.

Clinical Examination

Adolescents are usually shy and hesitant to submit themselves to physical examination. In the presence of symptoms that are of concern and distress they do not hesitate to seek help from an adolescent friendly healthcare provider. With the establishment of audio-visual privacy, in the presence of a chaperone and with the provision for bed linen to protect one's modesty, adolescents are requested to undress for examination of their genitourinary system. The approach is described in accord with the presenting symptoms.

Urethral Discharge

Urethral discharge in boys or young men can be accompanied by burning and increased frequency of micturition. Penis has to be examined for discharge. If not present massage along the ventral aspect of the shaft of the penis brings the discharge to the meatus. Common causative organisms are *N. gonorrhoeae* and *C. trachomatis*.

Vaginal Discharge

Vaginal discharge may be accompanied by burning and increased frequency of micturition, vaginal itching and dyspareunia (pain during sexual intercourse). Vulvar pruritic, swelling and edema may also accompany the discharge.

Unusual vaginal discharge can be due to vaginitis or cervicitis. Clinical differentiation of one from the other is difficult. Speculum examination may/may not be necessary. Speculum examination may be useful in differentiating vaginitis from cervicitis, but difficult even for a trained eye. Etiological diagnosis depending on the type of vaginal discharge, its color, odor, etc. is done away with as the descriptions are subjective and thus can mislead the clinicians.

Organisms that are commonly implicated are *N. gonorrhoeae*, *C. trachomatis* for cervicitis, and *T. vaginalis*, *Candida albicans* and Bacterial vaginosis for vaginitis.

Genital Ulcer

Single or multiple sores or ulcers on or near the genitals are some of the common symptoms in adolescents that indicate a genital ulcerative disease. Genital ulcers are well seen in boys, but the presence of ulcers in girls may go unnoticed and may remain asymptomatic. Ulcerative disease increases the chances of acquisition and transmission of HIV manifold.

Herpes simplex is more common in adolescents. Ulcers are usually well seen after a first infection but subsequent shedding can be asymptomatic. The organisms remain in the body forever with frequent eruptions even after a course of antivirals.

Chancroid and syphilis are less common during adolescence.

Scrotal Swelling

Boys may present with acute painful swelling of the scrotum. The scrotum becomes swollen, warm and tender to examination. This usually happens as a complication of the infections with *N. gonorrhoeae* and *C. trachomatis*.

Lower Abdominal Pain in Girls

Pain in the hypogastrium and iliac regions of the lower abdomen is attributed to PID. This is usually accompanied by fever and pain during or after sexual intercourse. This is associated with adnexal tenderness and cervical motion tenderness. This indicates the inflammation of parts above the cervix and present as endometritis, salpingitis, tubo-ovarian abscess and peritonitis.

Neisseria gonorrhoeae, *C. trachomatis* and anaerobic bacteria have been implicated in the causation of PID.

Future complication of PID is ectopic pregnancy in the presence of tubal blockage and/or infertility.

Inguinal Bubo

Painful enlargement of inguinal lymph nodes with or without abscess formation can be a presenting feature. Sometimes fistulae from the swollen inguinal lymph nodes are also seen. Lymphogranuloma venereum and chancroid have been the working diagnoses.

Screening Recommendations for Sexually Active Young People

Routine annual screening for *N. gonorrhoeae* and *C. trachomatis* is recommended for all sexually active men and women less than 25 years.

Screening for HIV for all sexually active young people is also recommended. Injection drug users are also suggested screening for HIV.

Pap smear screening for HPV is recommended to begin by 21 years for all sexually active young women.

DIAGNOSIS AND TESTING FOR SEXUALLY TRANSMITTED INFECTIONS

Depending on the time of sexual exposure and the respective incubation period of the likely organisms, tests have to be requested to screen as well diagnose the infection.

Urethral discharge is:

- Mucoid or purulent
- More than and equal to 5 WBC per high-power field on microscopic examination
- More than and equal to 10 WBC per high-power field on microscopic examination of first-void urine (FVU) specimen or
- Positive FVU leukocyte esterase test.
- The presence of gram-negative intracellular diplococci on microscopy confirms the diagnosis of gonococcal urethritis.
- Vaginal discharge due to *T. vaginalis* is usually diffuse, malodorous, yellow-green in color. Discharge in vulvo-vaginal candidiasis is thick, white and curdy.
- Vaginal discharge is usually tested for pH and microscopy
- pH of more than 4.5 is common with bacterial vaginosis and trichomoniasis
- Saline preparation reveals motile or dead *T. vaginalis* or clue cells of bacterial vaginosis
- Potassium hydroxide (KOH) preparation identifies the yeast or Pseudohyphae of *Candida species*.

Sexually Transmitted Infection Testing in Postpubertal Girls

Vulval or vaginal swabs taken by the girls themselves or by clinicians are used if speculum is not used.

If speculum is used, endocervical swab is the preferred one.

Sexually Transmitted Infections Testing in Boys

Meatal swab from prepubertal boys and urethral swab from postpubertal boys is tested for:
- Microscopy for pus cells
- Gonococcal culture
- *Chlamydia trachomatis* culture, if available.

Urine Sample

Nucleic acid amplification test (NAAT) for gonococci (GC) and *C. trachomatis* (CT).

Rectal Swab

If there is anal sex:
- Nucleic acid amplification test for GC and CT
- Gonococci culture
- *Chlamydia trachomatis* culture, if available.

Pharyngeal Swab

If there is oral sex:
- Nucleic acid amplification test for GC and CT
- Gonococci culture
- *Chlamydia trachomatis* culture, if available.

Genital Blisters or Ulcers

- Swab for HSV culture or polymerase chain reaction (PCR) (more sensitive than culture)
- Herpex simplex virus serology for IgM and IgG
- Swab for bacterial culture
- Dark ground microscopy
- Polymerase chain reaction swab for syphilis, if available
- Serological tests for syphilis like venereal disease research laboratory (VDRL), rapid plasma regain (RPR), etc.

Genital Warts

- Pap smear
- Colposcopy
- Polymerase chain reaction.

MANAGEMENT OF INDIVIDUAL SEXUALLY TRANSMITTED DISEASES

Treatment of adolescents with STIs poses following challenges to the clinicians like they ignore or trivialize the symptoms, postpone attention to symptoms with hope to self healing, do self treatment, hesitate to disclose partners (identification), poor compliance, poor adherence to treatment duration, poor follow-up.

Poor adherence to abstinence from sexual activity until the completion of treatment schedule.

Therefore, adolescents are treated with regimens on the same day as clinical evaluation and are given single dose schedules as far as possible. Abstinence from sexual activity is recommended at least for 7 days.

Although partner evaluation and treatment should be done with appropriate clinical examination, in most instances, the index client is motivated to procure and provide the treatment for the partner also to prevent re-infection. This is referred to as expedited partner therapy and has helped in the reduction of STIs and its complications in the community.

Centers for disease control and prevention: 2010 Sexually Transmitted Diseases Treatment Guidelines, 2010 MMWR is the document that gives the treatment schedule for all STIs. The suggestions are grouped as recommended regimens and alternate regimens in the event of treatment failure. Readers are asked to consult this document for expanding the knowledge about the recent recommendations.

Here, an attempt is made to give only the recommended regimens (and also alternate regimens in conditions that are common during adolescence) so that in the event of identification of an STI the first line management can be offered to our clients from our health services.

Recommended Regimens
Nongonococcal Urethritis

Azithromycin 1 g orally in single dose or doxycycline 100 mg orally twice a day for 7 days.

Alternative Regimens

Erythromycin base 500 mg orally four times a day for 7 days or erythromycin ethylsuccinate 800 mg orally four times a day for 7 days or levofloxacin 500 mg orally once daily for 7 days or ofloxacin 300 mg orally twice a day for 7 days.

Chlamydia trachomatis

Azithromycin 1 g orally in a single dose or doxycycline 100 mg orally twice a day for 7 days.

Uncomplicated Gonococcal Infections of the Cervix, Urethra and Rectum

Ceftriaxone 250 mg intramuscular (IM) in a single dose or if not an option, cefixime 400 mg orally in a single dose or single-dose injectable cephalosporin regimens and azithromycin 1 g orally in a single dose or doxycycline 100 mg orally twice a day for 7 days.

Chancroid

Azithromycin 1 g orally in a single dose or ceftriaxone 250 mg IM in a single dose or ciprofloxacin 500 mg orally twice a day for 3 days or erythromycin base 500 mg orally three times a day for 7 days. Ciprofloxacin is contraindicated for pregnant and lactating women.

First Clinical Episode of Genital Herpes

Acyclovir 400 mg orally three times a day for 7–10 days, or acyclovir 200 mg orally five times a day for 7–10 days or famciclovir 250 mg orally three times a day for 7–10 days or valacyclovir 1 g orally twice a day for 7–10 days. Treatment can be extended if healing is incomplete after 10 days of therapy. Young people with HSV infection should be informed about the lifelong natural course of the disease and the chances of recurrence with/without symptoms. The chances of having asymptomatic infection that is likely to increase the acquisition and transmission of HIV should also be informed. The advantages of the usage of barrier protection should be insisted upon.

Primary Syphilis

Benzathine penicillin G 2.4 million units IM in a single dose.

Vaginal Discharge/Bacterial vaginosis

Metronidazole 500 mg orally twice a day for 7 days or metronidazole gel 0.75%, one full applicator (5 g) intravaginally, once a day for 5 days or clindamycin cream 2%, one full applicator (5 g) intravaginally at bedtime for 7 days.

Alternative Regimens

Tinidazole 2 g orally once daily for 2 days or tinidazole 1 g orally once daily for 5 days or clindamycin 300 mg orally twice daily for 7 days or clindamycin ovules 100 mg intravaginally once at bedtime for 3 days.

Trichomoniasis

Metronidazole/Tinidazole 2 g orally in a single dose.

Vulvovaginal Candidiasis

Butoconazole 2% cream, 5 g intravaginally for 1 day or nystatin 100,000 unit vaginal tablet, one tablet for 14 days or terconazole 0.4% cream 5 g intravaginally for 7 days or terconazole 0.8% cream 5 g intravaginally for 3 days or terconazole 80 mg vaginal suppository, one suppository for 3 days.

Oral agent: Fluconazole 150 mg oral tablet, one tablet in single dose.

PELVIC INFLAMMATORY DISEASE

Recommended Parenteral Regime A

Cefotetan 2 g intravenous (IV) every 12 hours or cefoxitin 2 g IV every 6 hours plus doxycycline 100 mg orally or IV every 12 hours.

Recommended Parenteral Regimen B

Clindamycin 900 mg IV every 8 hours and gentamicin loading dose IV or IM (2 mg/kg of body weight), followed by a maintenance dose of gentamicin (1.5 mg/kg) every 8 hours. Single daily dosing (3–5 mg/kg) can be given for maintenance.

Oral Treatment

Ceftriaxone 250 mg IM in a single dose and doxycycline 100 mg orally twice a day for 14 days with/without metronidazole 500 mg orally twice a day for 14 days or cefoxitin 2 g IM in a single dose and probenecid, 1 g orally administered concurrently in a single dose plus oxycycline 100 mg orally twice a day for 14 days with or without metronidazole 500 mg orally twice a day for 14 days or other parenteral third-generation cephalosporin (e.g. ceftizoxime or cefotaxime) plus doxycycline 100 mg orally twice a day for 14 days with/without metronidazole 500 mg orally twice a day for 14 days.

HUMAN PAPILLOMAVIRUS

External Genital Warts

Patient-Applied

Podofilox 0.5% solution or gel or imiquimod 5% cream or sinecatechins 15% ointment.

Provider-Administered

Cryotherapy with liquid nitrogen or cryoprobe. Repeat applications every 1–2 weeks or podophyllin resin 10–25% in a compound tincture of benzoin or trichloroacetic acid (TCA) or bichloroacetic acid (BCA) 80–90% or surgical removal either by tangential scissor excision, tangential shave excision, curettage or electrosurgery.

Proctitis

Ceftriaxone 250 mg IM plus doxycycline 100 mg orally twice a day for 7 days (Boys who have sex with boys/men).

Pediculosis Pubis

Permethrin 1% cream rinse applied to affected areas and washed off after 10 minutes or pyrethrins with piperonyl butoxide applied to the affected area and washed off after 10 minutes.

Scabies

Permethrin cream (5%) applied to all areas of the body from the neck down and washed off after 8–14 hours or ivermectin 200 µg/kg orally, repeated in 2 weeks.

Adolescents Who Have Undergone Sexual Assault

Although this category of adolescents who have been subjected to exploitation is not addressed in detail in this chapter, a brief note on treatment is being provided for completion.

In addition to emergency contraception, ceftriaxone 250 mg IM in a single dose or cefixime 400 mg orally in a single dose plus metronidazole 2 g orally in a single dose and azithromycin 1 g orally in a single dose. The other option is doxycycline 100 mg orally twice a day for 7 days.

COMPLICATIONS OF SEXUALLY TRANSMITTED INFECTIONS

- Chronic PID
- Infertility
- Strictures of urethra
- Pregnancy with STI complicating the pregnancy
- Cancer cervix.

PREVENTION OF SEXUALLY TRANSMITTED INFECTIONS IN YOUNG PEOPLE

Prevention of STIs in adolescents can be approached by the following ways:

Primordial Prevention

- Overall well-being of an adolescent with respect to growth, development, nutrition, prevention of anemia, immunization, maintenance of mental health, etc.
- Establishment of adolescent friendly health services all over the country.
- Training of more pediatricians to include services for STI prevention and management among adolescents.

Primary Prevention

Health promotion and specific protection (for vulnerable adolescents):
- Information and education on reproductive and sexual health issues like health risks of early sexual debut, early marriage, unprotected sexual intercourse and multiple sex partners
- Life skills training
- Information and education on substance use and the associated hazards
- Anticipatory guidance on maintenance of responsible sexual behavior which includes abstinence
- Imparting skills to access and negotiate condom usage for all adolescents
- Information and education on correct and consistent use of condoms
- Access to condom for sexually active adolescents like sex workers, street youth, men who have sex with men (MSMs), attendees of STI clinics
- *Harm reduction:* Needle exchange program for injectable drug users
- Vaccines against vaccine preventable STIs, like HPV, hepatitis B, hepatitis A, for all adolescents to prevent genital warts, serum hepatitis B and hepatitis A (among those who practice oral or anal intercourse) infection respectively.

Secondary Prevention

Early Diagnosis and Treatment

- Early diagnosis and treatment of STIs using the syndromic approach recommended by the WHO
- Partner identification and treatment to prevent re-infection and to stall spread in the community
- Counseling on HIV testing.

Tertiary Prevention

Disability Limitation

- Monitoring the progress of the disease during the asymptomatic carrier state
- Advice on use of barrier contraception especially in viral genito-ulcerative diseases.

Rehabilitation

- Promotion of secondary abstinence
- Rehabilitation services for drug use behavior
- Psychosocial support.

CONCLUSION

Sexually transmitted infections spread from person-to-person due to voluntary involvement in high-risk sexual activity. Exposure to organisms that are responsible for the various syndromes need not happen in an adolescent's life if the person practices a responsible sexual behavior and prevent infection to self and to all his or her sexual partners. Avoidance of STIs is a matter of individual choice. The best course of action is to stay away from exposure by abstaining from sexual activity until a faithful partner is available. If this is not feasible at least knowledge and commitment to protect self by using barrier protection like condoms at every sexual encounter is very helpful in preventing the acquisition as well as transmission. Curtailing the spread of STIs is thus an individual's responsibility. To help adolescents achieve this pediatrician will have to provide appropriate information, create awareness and guide in the maintenance of responsible sexual behavior.

BIBLIOGRAPHY

1. Bustein GR. Sexually transmitted infections. In: Kliegman RM, Stanton BMD, Geme JS, Schor N, Behrman RE (Eds). Nelson Textbook of Pediatrics, 19th edition. New Delhi: Reed Elsevier India Private Limited; 2011. pp. 705-14.
2. Dehne KL, Reidner G. Sexually Transmitted Infections Among Adolescents. In: Berer M (Ed) The Need for Adequate Health Services. 2005.
3. Greydanus DE, Bhave SY, Patel DR. Reproductive tract infections and sexually transmitted diseases. In: Bhave S (Ed). Bhave's Textbook of Adolescent Medicine, 1st edition. New Delhi: Jaypee Brothers Medical Publishers (P) Ltd, 2006. pp. 199-210.
4. Reproductive and sexual health of young people in India. Secondary analysis of data from national family health surveys 1, 2 and 3 (1996–2006) for the age group of 15–24 years. Ministry of Health and Family Welfare.GOI. 2009.
5. Rogstad K, Thomas A, Williams O, et al. UK National guideline on the management of sexually transmitted infections and related conditions in children and young people (2009). Int J STD AIDS. 2010;21:229-41.
6. Rompalo A. Preventing sexually transmitted infections: back to basics. J Clin Invest. 2011;121(12):4580-3.
7. Workowski KA, Berman S. Centers for disease control and prevention: sexually transmitted diseases treatment guidelines. MMWR Recomm Rep. 2010;59(RR-12):1-110.
8. World Health Organization: Guidelines for the Management of Sexually Transmitted Infections, 2003.

10.3 **INFECTION ASSOCIATED HEMOPHAGOCYTIC LYMPHOHISTIOCYTOSIS**

Priyankar Pal

INTRODUCTION

Hemophagocytic lymphohistiocytosis (HLH) is a potentially fatal condition that occurs due to an uncontrolled and ineffective hyperinflammatory response to different precipitants. They are a heterogenous group of clinical syndromes characterized by activation and uncontrolled non-malignant proliferation of T-lymphocytes and macrophages, leading to a cytokine storm that accounts for the main clinical features of acute febrile illness, hepatosplenomegaly, multiorgan dysfunction and fulminant pancytopenia resembling severe sepsis.

TYPES OF HEMOPHAGOCYTIC LYMPHOHISTIOCYTOSIS

Hemophagocytic lymphohistiocytosis comprises two different conditions that may be difficult to distinguish from one another—a primary (familial) form and a secondary (reactive) form. The familial form of HLH was first described by Farquhar and Claireaux in 1952 when they reported it as familial hemophagocytic reticulosis. Initially thought by the original authors to be a red cell membrane defect, HLH is now known to be a rare disorder of the immune system. The incidence is about 1.2 in every 1 million children under the age of 15 years.

The primary or familial form is an autosomal recessive disorder, typically having its onset during infancy or early childhood, and is a fatal disease with a median survival of less than 2 months after diagnosis, if untreated. Despite its name, family history is often negative, and the onset and recurrence of the disease may be triggered by infections.

Secondary HLH develops as a result of strong immunological activation of the immune system which may be caused by a severe infection, a viral infection in an immunocompromised host or malignancy.

Since the most common triggers of reactive HLH are viruses, particularly the Epstein-Barr virus (EBV), the disease was previously known as virus associated hemophagocytic syndrome (VAHS). It is now known that severe infections with bacteria or parasites may also cause HLH. Thus, infection associated hemophagocytic syndrome (IAHS) is a more accepted term now. Other infections ranging from typhoid, tuberculosis, malaria, kala-azar to histoplasmosis, human immunodeficiency virus (HIV) have all been reported to trigger off secondary HLH. Although secondary HLH are known to occur more commonly in immunocompromised hosts, however, one must remember that most patients with the secondary form are not obviously immunosuppressed.

The underlying causes of reactive HLH are:

Malignancy: Acute lymphocytic leukemia (ALL) (T-cell), Hodgkin's and Non-Hodgkin's lymphoma, histiocytosis and more rarely solid tumors like rhabdomyosarcoma and neuroblastoma.

Rheumatological illness: Systemic lupus erythematosus (SLE), systemic onset juvenile idiopathic arthritis (Still's disease) and Kawasaki disease.

Infections: (i) EBV associated: Mimics T-cell lymphomas and requires cytotoxic chemotherapy and (ii) Others: A number of bacterial, viral, fungal and protozoal diseases have been reported (hepatitis A, *Brucella*, typhoid, tuberculosis, leishmaniasis, HIV, etc.).

Drugs: Immunosuppressants and chemotherapeutics.

Henceforth, we shall restrict our discussions to infection associated HLH (IAHLH).

CLINICAL MANIFESTATIONS

Infection associated HLH can occur at any age, and is variable in severity and outcome. The most typical presentation is with fever which fails to respond to broad spectrum antibiotics, along with hepatosplenomegaly and cytopenias. There may be associated varying degrees of multiorgan dysfunction, ranging from myocarditis and congestive cardiac failure, hepatic and renal dysfunction, to coagulopathy with a disseminated intravascular coagulation (DIC) like picture. Neurological features include encephalopathy, meningism, cranial nerve palsies and seizures, with some patients having a primary neurological presentation. Other less common findings include lymphadenopathy, skin rash and mucositis.

Epstein-Barr virus associated HLH usually occur in previously healthy children (and rarely in X-linked lymphoproliferative disease). Some children have a prolonged infectious mononucleosis like illness, while others have a very aggressive rapidly fatal course. In other infection-related HLH syndromes, the findings of hepatosplenomegaly and fever may be due to the underlying infection and/or due to HLH, and a high index of suspicion is required for accurate diagnosis, as treatment of both the infection and of HLH is vital.

INVESTIGATIONS

The diagnostic guidelines are provided in Box 10.3.1. Any child presenting with a prolonged fever, showing inadequate response to broad spectrum antibiotics with

Revised diagnostic guidelines for hemophagocytic lymphohistiocytosis.

The diagnosis hemophagocytic lymphohistiocytosis (HLH) can be established if one of either 1 or 2 below is fulfilled:

1. A molecular diagnosis consistent with HLH
2. Diagnostic criteria for HLH fulfilled (5 out of the 8 criteria below)
   A. Initial diagnostic criteria (to be evaluated in all patients with HLH):
      ◆ Fever
      ◆ Splenomegaly
      ◆ Cytopenias (affecting 2 of 3 lineages in the peripheral blood):
         ▶ Hemoglobin <90 g/L (in infants <4 weeks of age,
         ▶ Hemoglobin <100 g/L), Platelets <100 × 10⁹/L
         ▶ Neutrophils <1.0 × 10⁹/L
      ◆ Hypertriglyceridemia and/or hypofibrinogenemia:
         ▶ Fasting triglycerides 3.0 mmol/L (i.e. ≥265 mg/dL)
         ▶ Fibrinogen ≤1.5 g/L
         ▶ Hemophago cytosis in bone marrow or spleen or lymph nodes
         ▶ No evidence of malignancy
   B. New diagnostic criteria:
      ◆ Low or absent NK-cell activity (according to local laboratory reference)
      ◆ Ferritin ≥500 µg/L
      ◆ Soluble CD25 (i.e. soluble IL-2 receptor) ≥2,400 U/mL

organomegaly, and multisystem involvement, developing cytopenias with a falling erythrocyte sedimentation rate (ESR), should arouse suspicion. Associated elevated levels of ferritin, triglycerides, D-dimer; hypofibrinogenemia, with prolonged activated partial prothrombin time (APTT) and prothrombin time (PT), raised hepatic transaminases; point toward the diagnosis. Spinal fluid pleocytosis (mononuclear cells) and/or elevated spinal fluid protein, a histological picture in the liver resembling chronic persistent hepatitis, may provide strong supportive evidence. Demonstration of hemophagocytosis in bone marrow, or spleen or lymph nodes, confirms the diagnosis. However, only 60–80% of initial bone marrow aspirate shows hemophagocytosis. Dyserythropoiesis is frequently the only initial manifestation. Serial marrow aspirates over time may be helpful in demonstrating hemophagocytosis. Absence of histological proof in the presence of clinical and biochemical markers should not delay treatment initiation.

Thus, the investigations to be ordered in a child with suspicion of HLH are a complete blood count with ESR and C-reactive protein (CRP), serum ferritin, fibrinogen, D-dimer, triglycerides, PT and APTT, liver function tests (LFT) and renal function tests with electrolytes, and a bone marrow aspiration study. Microbiological studies should be based on clinical suspicion regarding the nature of the primary infection.

PATHOPHYSIOLOGY

Although the exact pathogenic mechanisms involved are not fully known it appears that there is an underlying abnormality in immunoregulation that contributes to the lack of control of an exaggerated immune response.[4] Indeed, the clinical findings during the acute phase can largely be explained as a consequence of the prolonged production of cytokines and chemokines originating from activated macrophages and T-cells. Indeed, excess of circulating interleukin (IL)-1β, tumor necrosis factor (TNF), IL-6, IL-18 and interferon (IFN)-g is likely to contribute to the findings of fever, hyperlipidemia, endothelial activation responsible for the coagulopathy, as well as the pathognomic feature of hemophagocytosis.

To understand the pathophysiology, one has to recollect the normal immune response induced by a viral infection. Natural killer (NK) cells provide the first line of defense by inducing lysis of virally infected cells, thus limiting the extent of viral replication. Antigen specific CD-8 cells become subsequently important as they eliminate infected cells and secrete proinflammatory cytokines such as IFN-that activate other immune cells, including macrophages. Subsequently the CD-8 cells are eliminated through mechanisms that presumably involve NK-cells and/or perforin.

Increasing evidence suggests that depressed NK-cell activity, often associated with abnormal perforin expression, may be important for the pathogenesis of HLH. In at least some familial HLH patients, the development of the symptoms has been linked to the mutation in the gene encoding perforin. Perforin is a protein that NK-cells and cytotoxic CD-8 cells utilize to kill tumors or cells infected by intracellular microbes such as viruses.

In HLH, NK-cells fail to limit the extent of viral replication at early stages leading to increased viral load, and massive expansion of cytotoxic CD-8 cells. At later stages, due to perforin deficiency and/or poor NK-cell function cytotoxic CD-8 cells are not eliminated even if the infection is cleared. They continue to survive and secrete proinflammatory cytokines. Prolonged stimulation of macrophages with cytokines leads to their excessive activation and proliferation associated with hemophagocytic activity. Hemophagocytosis of blood elements in the bone marrow lead to peripheral cytopenias probably be attributed primarily to high concentrations of TNF-α and INF-γ. Production of procoagulant tissue factor combined with TNF-α effects on vascular endothelial cells contribute to the development of coagulopathy.

MANAGEMENT

In 1991, the histiocyte society presented the first set of diagnostic guidelines for HLH, and in 1994 the first prospective international treatment protocol (HLH 94) was introduced. The cumulative experiences from HLH 94 have led to the development of a new treatment protocol HLH 2004.

The HLH 2004 protocol in designed for the patients of HLH, with/without evidence of familial or genetic disease, regardless of suspected or documented viral infections. The complete protocol is available at www.histio.org/society/protocols.

The immediate aim in the treatment of any patient with reactive HLH is to suppress the severe hyperinflammation that is responsible for the life-threatening symptoms. A second aim is to kill pathogen-infected antigen-presenting cells to remove the stimulus for the ongoing, but ineffective activation of cytotoxic cells. The third and ultimate aim in genetic cases of HLH is stem cell transplantation to exchange the defective immune system by normally functioning cells.

All experts have advocated maximal supportive therapy prior to initiation of specific treatment. These measures include the elimination of known or suspected triggers, and infection control with administration of antibiotics, antifungals and antivirals, as indicated. Some authors have suggested that aggressive supportive management be combined with a course of high dose steroids as initial step, followed in refractory disease by second line therapies such as cyclosporine A, etoposide, and the administration of intravenous immunoglobulin. It is important to note that though infection acts as a trigger, administration of specific infective measures are just not sufficient to control the hyperinflammation in the majority; with the exception of leishmaniasis and certain bacterial infections like salmonella and rickettsia where specific antileishmanial/antibiotic therapy only is usually sufficient to control the disease process.

Epstein-Barr virus associated HLH requires cytotoxic therapy. Mild cases of acquired, non-EBV infection related HLH may be self limiting in nature with resolution on treatment of the primary disease; however, immunomodulatory therapy is indicated in most cases and may be lifesaving in severe cases where late recognition and lack of specific therapy may be fatal. Reported best responses in such cases have been with high dose steroids, which should be continued until biochemical and hematological abnormalities subside.

Hyperinflammation, caused by hypercytokinemia, can be suppressed successfully by corticosteroids, which are cytotoxic for lymphocytes, inhibit the expression of cytokines and chemokines, and also interfere with the production of CD95 ligand and differentiation of dendritic cells. Since dexamethasone crosses the blood brain barrier better than prednisolone, it is preferred for treatment. Cyclosporin A inhibits activation of T-lymphocytes by interfering with the cyclophilin pathway. Immunoglobulins probably act by generating cytokine and pathogen-specific antibodies. Etoposide, a pro-apoptotic agent, which was introduced for the treatment of HLH in 1980, is highly active in monocytic and histiocytic diseases.

The following is an overview of the HLH 2004 protocol.

Initial Therapy

The initial therapy covers the first 8 weeks of treatment and is based on etoposide, dexamethasone and cyclosporine A; only selected patients will receive intrathecal therapy with methotrexate and prednisolone. Chemotherapy is initiated with dexamethasone 10 mg/m^2 daily for 2 weeks, 5 mg/m^2 for 2 weeks, 2.5 mg/m^2 for 2 weeks, 1.25 mg/m^2 for 1 week, and then tapered and discontinued in the 8th week. In patients without a known family history who achieve complete resolution of the disease after 8 weeks of therapy, treatment is stopped.

Continuation Therapy

Patients with a family history of HLH and nongenetic patients with persistent activity are recommended to start continuation therapy with dexamethasone, etoposide and cyclosporin till 24 weeks.

Hematopoietic Stem Cell Transplantation

Patients with genetically verified or familial disease or those having persistent nonfamilial disease with reactivation on stopping treatment should undergo stem cell transplantation as curative treatment. Results are equal with matched related or unrelated transplants.

Although this three tier therapy has been advocated by the HLH 2004 protocol, but majority of the IAHLH patients show an excellent response to dexamethasone only without the inclusion of other cytotoxics. The complete regimen is best used in suspected genetic HLH and some cases with Epstein-Barr associated HLH who show inadequate response to the steroid only protocol.

Resolution of the disease is indicated by:

- No fever
- No splenomegaly
- No cytopenia (Hb >9 g/dL, platelet >100,000/mL, absolute neutrophil count >1000/mL)
- No hypertriglyceridemia
- No hyperferritinemia
- Normal cerebrospinal fluid (CSF).

It cannot be overemphasized that to treat a febrile and pancytopenic child with corticosteroids, immunosuppressive drugs and cytostatics is a highly unusual experience for a pediatrician and may take a lot of conviction and willpower. However, immediate unfaltering institution of therapy can be a choice between life and death.

KEY MESSAGES

- Any infection behaving with unusual toxicity with multisystem involvement, falling counts and decreasing ESR—think of IAHLH.

- Though a potentially life-threatening condition but prompt diagnosis and immediate steroid administration can reverse the disease process.
- Do not be overwhelmed by the elaborate treatment protocol advocated by the histiocytic society. Majority of IAHLH do strikingly well with just corticosteroids and supportive therapy.

BIBLIOGRAPHY

1. Ambruso DR, Hays T, Zwartjes WJ, et al. Successful treatment of lymphohistiocytic reticulosis with phagocytosis with epipodophyllotoxin VP 16-213. Cancer. 1980;45:2516-20.
2. Filipovich HA. Hemophagocytic lymphohistocystosis. Immunol Allergy Clin N AM. 2002;22:281-300.
3. Fruman DA, Burakoff SJ, Bierer BE. Immunophilins in protein folding and immunosuppression. Faseb J. 1994;8:391-400.
4. Galon J, Franchimont D, Hiroi N, et al. Gene profiling reveals unknown enhancing and suppressive actions of glucocorticoids on immune cells. Faseb J. 2002;16:61-71.
5. Giri PP, Pal P, Ghosh A, et al. Infection associated hemophagocytic lymphohistiocytosis: a case series using steroids only protocol for management. Rheumatology Int. 2011.
6. Henter JI, Aricò M, Egeler M, et al. HLH-94: a treatment protocol for hemophagocytic lymphohistiocytosis. Med Pediatr Oncol. 1997;28:342-7.
7. Henter JI, Ehrust A, Anderson J, et al. Familial hemophagocytic lymphohistiocytosis and viral infections. Acta Paediatr. 1993;82:369-72.
8. Henter JI, Horne A, Aricó M, et al. HLH-2004: diagnostic and therapeutic guidelines for hemophagocytic lymphohistiocytosis. Pediatr Blood Cancer. 2007;48: 124-31.
9. Imagawa T, Katakura S, Mori M, et al. A case of macrophage activation syndrome developed with systemic onset juvenile rheumatoid arthritis. Ryumachi. 1997;37:487-92.
10. Ross C, Svenson M, Nielsen H, et al. Increased in vivo antibody activity against interferon alpha, interleukin-1 alpha, and interleukin-6 after high dose Ig therapy. Blood. 1997;90:2376-80.
11. Stéphan JL, Koné-Paut I, Galambrun C, et al. Reactive haemphagocytic syndrome in children with inflammatory disorders. A retrospective study of 24 patients. Rheumatology. 2001;40(11):1285-92.
12. Woltman AM, Massacrier C, de Fijter JW, et al. Corticosteroids prevent generation of CD34+-derived dermal dendritic cells but do not inhibit Langerhans cell development. J Immunol. 2002;168:6181-8.

10.4 SAFE INJECTION PRACTICES

SS Kamath

INTRODUCTION

Injection is defined as a skin piercing event performed by a syringe and a needle to introduce a vaccine or a curative substance into a patient by various routes such as intravenous (IV), intramuscular (IM), subcutaneous (SC), intradermal (ID), etc.

A safe injection, phlebotomy (drawing blood), lancet procedure or IV device insertion is one which does not harm the recipient, does not expose the provider to any avoidable risk and does not result in any waste that is dangerous for other people.

Unsafe injection practices are a powerful engine to transmit blood-borne pathogens, including hepatitis B virus (HBV), hepatitis C virus (HCV) and human immunodeficiency virus (HIV). Because infection with these viruses initially presents no symptoms, it is a silent epidemic. However, the consequences of this are increasingly recognized. HBV is highly infectious and causes the highest number of infections: in developing and transitional countries 21.7 million people become infected each year, representing 33% of new HBV infections worldwide. Unsafe injections are the most common cause of HCV infection in developing and transitional countries, causing two million new infections each year and accounting for 42% of cases. Globally, nearly 2% of all new HIV infections are caused by unsafe injections. In South Asia, up to 9% of new cases may be caused in this way. Such proportions can no longer be ignored.

Hepatitis B virus, HCV and HIV cause chronic infections that lead to disease, disability and death a number of years after the unsafe injection. Those infected with HBV in childhood will typically present with chronic liver disease by the age of 30 years, at the prime of their life. This has a dramatic effect on national economies.

SAFE AND APPROPRIATE USE OF INJECTIONS

Safe and appropriate use of injection is not difficult. It can be achieved very easily. Table 10.4.1 shows the risk associated with injection giving.

Unsafe injection practices are often viewed as a chronic problem with no easy solution. However, safe and appropriate use of injections can be achieved by adopting a three-part strategy.

Changing Behavior of Healthcare Workers and Patients

Knowledge of HIV among patients and healthcare workers in some countries has driven consumer demand for safe injection equipment and irreversibly improved injection practices. With growing knowledge of HCV and HBV, similar patterns of consumer demand for safe injections should emerge. HIV prevention programs can be expanded to include injection safety components.

Ensuring Availability of Equipment and Supplies

Simply increasing the availability of safe injection equipment can stimulate demand and improve practices. Because the cost of safe disposable syringes is low (<5 US cents per unit) when compared to the fee paid for receiving an injection (50 US cents on average), patients are usually willing to pay a little extra for safety once they personalize the risks.

Managing Waste Safely and Appropriately

As waste disposal is frequently not an integral part of health planning, unsafe waste management is common. However,

Table 10.4.1: Examples of conditions causing risk: steps related to injection giving.

Patients or clients	*Health workers who give injections or collect blood*	*Community or other health workers*
Unnecessary injections Reuse of injection equipment Nonsterile or reprocessed syringes and needles Poor hand hygiene Cross-contamination through: • Poor hand hygiene • Medication vials Improper injection technique or site Sharps in hospital linen or other unexpected places	Unnecessary injections Two-handed recapping of needles Manipulation of used sharps Lack of sharps box within arm's reach Poor positioning of patient Poor phlebotomy technique Two-handed transfer of blood Unsafe transport of blood Poor hand hygiene Nonsegregated sharps waste	Increased waste from unnecessary injections Unsafe disposal of sharps waste: • Outside safety boxes • Mixed with hospital linen • In nonsecure disposal sites Lack of protective clothing (boots, gloves, etc.) for waste handlers Reuse of needles or syringes

when it is appropriately planned, significant results ensure. National healthcare waste management strategies require a national policy to manage healthcare waste, a comprehensive system for implementation, improved awareness and training of health workers at all levels, as well as the selection of appropriate options for the local solutions.

SPECIFICS OF SAFE INJECTION PRACTICES

Medical treatment is intended to save life and improve health, and all health workers have a responsibility to prevent transmission of healthcare associated infections. Adherence to safe injection practices and related infection control is part of that responsibility and it protects patients and health workers.

Do's and Don'ts of Injection Safety

Do's

- Carry out hand hygiene (use soap and water or alcohol rub) and wash carefully, including wrists and spaces between the fingers for at least 30 seconds
- Use one pair of nonsterile gloves per procedure or patient
- Use a single-use device for blood sampling and drawing
- Disinfect the skin at the venipuncture site
- Discard the used device (a needle and syringe is a single unit) immediately into a robust sharps container where recapping of a needle is unavoidable, and use the one-hand scoop technique
- Seal the sharps container with a tamper-proof lid
- Place laboratory sample tubes in a sturdy rack before injecting into the rubber stopper
- Immediately report any incident or accident linked to a needle or sharp injury and seek assistance; start postexposure prophylaxis (PEP) as soon as possible, following protocols.

Don'ts

- Forget to clean your hands
- Use the same pair of gloves for more than one patient
- Wash gloves for reuse
- Use a syringe, needle or lancet for more than one patient
- Recap a needle using both hands
- Touch the puncture site after disinfecting it
- Leave an unprotected needle lying outside the sharps container
- Overfill or decant a sharps container
- Inject into a laboratory tube while holding it with the other hand
- Delay PEP after exposure to potentially contaminated material; beyond 72 hours, PEP is not effective.

The essential steps for safe injection practices are clean work space for injection preparations (free from any blood contamination) and appropriately done hand hygiene as described below.

Hand hygiene is a general term that applies to either hand washing, antiseptic hand wash, antiseptic hand rub or surgical hand antisepsis.

It is the best and easiest way to prevent the spread of microorganisms. Hand hygiene should be carried out as indicated below; either with soap and running water (if hands are visibly soiled) or with alcohol rub (if hands appear clean).

PRACTICAL GUIDANCE ON HAND HYGIENE

Perform hand hygiene before
- Starting an injection session (i.e. preparing injection material and giving injections)
- Coming into direct contact with patients for healthcare related procedures
- Putting on gloves (first make sure hands are dry).

Perform hand hygiene after
- An injection session
- Any direct contact with patients
  - Removing gloves. You may need to perform hand hygiene between injections, depending on the setting and whether there was contact with soil, blood or body fluids. Avoid giving injections if your skin integrity is compromised by local infection or other skin conditions (e.g. weeping dermatitis, skin lesions or cuts), and cover any small cuts.

KEY STEPS OF HAND WASHING

The six steps of proper hand washing are shown in Figure 10.4.1.

Injection Site Preparation

Injection site should be cleaned in a scientific manner as shown in Figure 10.4.2.

To disinfect skin, use the following steps:
- Apply a 60–70% alcohol-based solution (isopropyl alcohol or ethanol) on a single-use swab or cotton-wool ball. Do not use methanol or methyl-alcohol as these are not safe for human use
- Wipe the area from the center of the injection site working outward, without going over the same area
- Apply the solution for 30 seconds then allow it to dry completely.

Do not use presoak cotton wool in a container—these become highly contaminated with hand and environmental bacteria.

Do not use alcohol skin disinfection for administration of vaccinations.

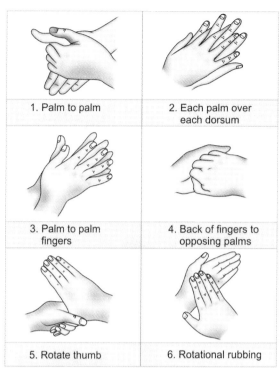

FIG. 10.4.1: Steps of hand washing.

1. Palm to palm
2. Each palm over each dorsum
3. Palm to palm fingers
4. Back of fingers to opposing palms
5. Rotate thumb
6. Rotational rubbing

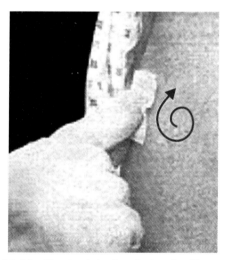

FIG. 10.4.2: Cleaning injection site in scientific manner.

Preventing Injection Equipment from Contamination

Contamination of injection equipment should be prevented by not touching certain parts as shown in Figure 10.4.3. The used needles and syringes should be disposed as per biomedical waste management (BWM) rules.

Rational Injection Therapy

People may have different perceptions and meanings regarding the term "rational drug use". However, the

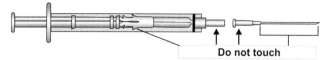

Do not touch

FIG. 10.4.3: Prevention of contamination of injecting equipment.

conference of experts on the rational use of drugs, convened by the WHO in Nairobi in 1985 defined that "Rational use of drugs requires that patients receive medications appropriate to their clinical needs, in doses that meet their own individual requirements for an adequate period of time, at the lowest cost to them and their community".

A review of essential drug lists and management guidelines of common illnesses shows that injections are recommended only for acute care (emergency setting) and immunization. The reasons given for injection over use are that patients and health workers believe injections are more effective, act fast and course of management is short.

These are wrong notions. There is need to promote rational injection therapy among all prescribers. It can be achieved through following steps:

- Defining effective and safe protocols
- Promoting minimal essential injection practices
- Promoting rational drug or injection therapy
- Reduction in procurement of injectable drugs at health facilities
- Encouraging prescription auditing at all health facilities, public as well as private sectors
- Continuing medical education (CME) for health workers
- Community awareness regarding harmful effects of injections.

BEST INJECTION TECHNIQUES

General Principles

- Give injections only when indicated
- Emergency equipment should be kept ready to use in emergency situations like anaphylactic reactions
- Oxygen bag and mask, laryngoscope and endotracheal tubes as well as emergency drugs, such as adrenaline, volume expanders, hydrocortisone, dopamine, should be available. IV cannulae, syringes and needles are also essential
- Check the appropriate drug or vaccine and its date
- Make sure that vial or ampoule contains right medication, its appropriate concentration and doses
- The drug or vaccine should be kept sterile during the procedure
- Clean the injection site properly
- Use disposable or sterile needle and syringe, preferable with reuse prevention feature
- Do not touch the parts of needle and syringe in which come in contact with injectable drug and body
- If you accidentally touch these parts, discard the syringe-needle

- Take care to avoid air bubble in the syringe or bulb
- While injecting take care to prevent needle stick injury (report immediately if you get injured as this is for your own safety)
- Used needles and syringes should be disposed as per standard guidelines
- Observe the child for 15 minutes, after giving injection
- Talk to the parents regarding drug or vaccine given by injection, necessary precautions, possible adverse reactions, necessary remedial measures in case of adverse reactions
- Guide them to give information to medical person in case of major problems.

Important Points

Don'ts

- Allow the needle to touch any contaminated surface
- Reuse a syringe, even if the needle is changed
- Touch the diaphragm after disinfection with the 60–70% alcohol (isopropyl alcohol or ethanol)
- Enter several multidose vials with the same needle and syringe
- Re-enter a vial with a needle or syringe used on a patient if that vial will be used to withdraw medication again (whether it is for the same patient or for another patient)
- Use bags or bottles of IV solution as a common source of supply for multiple patients (except in pharmacies using laminar flow cabinets).

Intramuscular Injection

Common Sites

Muscles commonly used for intramuscular (IM) injections are: vastus lateralis, deltoid and gluteus medius.

Children do not have well-developed gluteus medius and therefore, it is not the site of preference for IM injections in children. It has been documented that some vaccines like hepatitis B and antirabies vaccines administered at gluteal region produce very poor antibody response.

The vastus lateralis (anterolateral aspect of thigh) is preferred site in infants. The specific site in vastus lateralis is the middle third of the area between the greater trochanter and lateral femoral condyle.

In case of deltoid, the site for injection is midway between acromion process and deltoid insertion; it comes to 3–5 cm below the acromion process. This site may be used in children above 5 years and adults. The quantity of drug should be less than 5 mL. Only watery injections with less viscosity should be injected at deltoid region.

WHO Technique

- The site of injection should be exposed well
- For anterolateral aspect of thigh, the child may be laid supine or be held in mother's lap

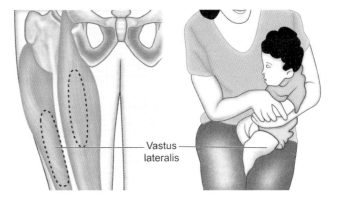

FIG. 10.4.4: A child held in mother's lap for IM injection.

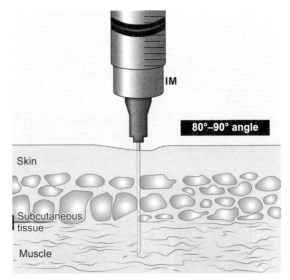

FIG. 10.4.5: Intramuscular (IM) injection.

- For deltoid, child may be held in mother's lap or may sit as shown in Figure 10.4.4
- The muscle selected for injection should be relaxed
- The skin over injection site should be cleaned with spirit. A circular motion of swab is used proceeding from puncture site and extending outward for 5 cm
- Let the spirit evaporate and skin become dry, otherwise spirit entering into tissues is painful
- The syringe is filled with the medicine
- In children usually 23 Gneedle with 25 mm length is used for IM injections
- Stretch the skin flat and push the needle down at 90° (Fig. 10.4.5)
- Aspiration before injecting the vaccine is not required
- Inject the vaccine at the rate of 1 mL/10 seconds
- The needle is withdrawn and injection site is pressed for few seconds
- Do not rub the injection site
- Needle should be withdrawn smoothly with steady movement

- Discard the needle and syringe as per standard guidelines.
- Alternative to WHO technique, advisory committee on immunization practices (ACIP) technique may be used. It is also called bunching technique. In this technique, bunch the muscle and direct needle inferiorly along long axis of leg at an angle of 45°. It stabilizes leg and increases the muscle mass.

Subcutaneous Injection

Drugs or vaccines are injected subcutaneously when slow absorption and long duration of action are desired. Another indication of SC route is a coagulopathy which makes IM injection hazardous, for fear of development of IM hematoma. Insulin and heparin like drugs as well as measles, varicella, mumps, measles and rubella (MMR), etc. vaccines are given by SC route.

Technique

- Common sites are arm, anterior abdominal wall and thighs. Atrophic and injected areas are avoided
- The skin is cleaned and disinfected with spirit
- 26G needle with 13 mm length is commonly used for SC injection
- The skin is raised into a fold with thumb and index finger of the left hand
- The midpoint of the fold is pierced with the needle held at 45° with its surface (Fig. 10.4.6)
- The tip of the needle is advanced into the subcutaneous tissue
- Aspiration is not required
- Drugs or vaccine is injected, needle is withdrawn and site is pressed for few minutes.

Intradermal Injection

Indications for ID injections are:
- Bacillus Calmette-Guérin (BCG) vaccination
- Mantoux test
- Skin tests for allergy
- Test for sensitization of certain drugs like penicillin, etc.

Technique

- Ventral (volar) aspect of forearm is commonly used for ID injection except during BCG vaccination
- Skin is cleaned with spirit or clean water
- A measured amount of antigen (usually 0.1 mL) is drawn into the syringe
- 26G or 27G needle with 1/4 to 1/2 inch (6.35–12.7 mm) length needle is used for ID injection
- The skin is held taut between thumb and index finger of the left hand. The syringe is held at an angle of 10–15° with the skin (Fig. 10.4.7)
- Needle is inserted for about 2 mm, so that entire needle bevel penetrates the skin and the injected solution raises a small bleb of about 5 mm in diameter. The development of perifollicular puckering (Peau d' orange) indicates successful ID injection
- The needle is withdrawn
- The site is circled and it is recorded in patient's chart
- The reaction is observed in defined time.

NEEDLESTICK INJURY AND POST-EXPOSURE PROPHYLAXIS

Needlestick Injuries

Needlestick injuries (NSI) can be defined as an accidental exposure through needles which may occur before, during

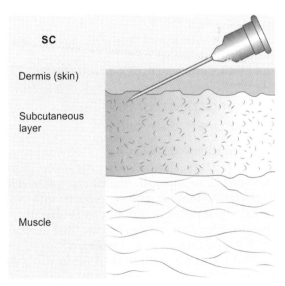

FIG. 10.4.6: Subcutaneous injection.

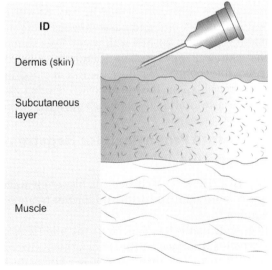

FIG. 10.4.7: Intradermal injection.

or after the process of injection giving. It might place healthcare professional or worker (HCP/HCW) at risk of bloodborne infections like hepatitis B, hepatitis C or HIV and many others.

Globally, NSIs are the most common source of occupational exposures to blood and the primary cause of bloodborne infections of HCWs.

The two most common causes of NSIs are two handed recapping and the unsafe collection and disposal of sharps waste.

Determinants of Needlestick Injuries

Determinants of NSIs include:
- Overuse of injections and unnecessary sharps
- *Lack of supplies:* disposable syringes, safer needle devices and sharps-disposal containers
- Lack of access to and failure to use sharps containers immediately after injection
- Inadequate or short staffing
- Recapping of needles after use
- Lack of engineering controls such as safer needle devices
- Passing instruments from hand to hand in the operating suite
- Lack of awareness of hazard and lack of training.

Determinants of Transmission of Infection

The risks of transmission of infection from an infected patient to the HCW following an NSI are: hepatitis B 3–10%, hepatitis C 3% and HIV 0.3%.

Immediate Management of Needlestick Injuries

The exposure site should be cleaned immediately. This is the most important part of PEP. Puncture wounds and other cutaneous injury sites should be washed with soap and water. Exposed oral and nasal mucous membranes should be vigorously flushed with water. Eyes should be irrigated with clean water or saline. There is no evidence that antiseptics for wound care reduce the risk of blood-borne pathogen transmission. The use of bleach or other caustic agents that cause local tissue trauma are not recommended.

Postexposure Prophylaxis for Hepatitis B (Flowchart 10.4.1)

- If the HCP/HCW is vaccinated and his serum antibody titer is more than 10 IU/mL, no further treatment is required
- If antibody titer is less than 10 IU/mL and HCP/HCW is hepatitis B surface antigen (HbsAg) negative or the source is unknown, then one course of three doses of vaccine is repeated and then antibody titer is re-checked

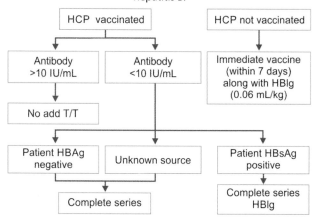

FLOWCHART 10.4.1: Postexposure prophylaxis (PEP) for hepatitis B.

- If HCP/HCW is HbsAg positive then both hepatitis B vaccine is repeated and hepatitis B immune globulin is given within hours of exposure
- If HCP/HCW is not vaccinated then vaccination series is started within 7 days.

MANAGEMENT OF EXPOSURE TO HEPATITIS C VIRUS

The following are recommendations for follow-up of occupational HCV exposures:
- For the source, perform anti-HCV
- For the person exposed to HCV positive source:
  - Perform baseline testing for anti-HCV and ALT activity and
  - Perform follow-up testing at 4–6 months for anti-HCV and ALT activity.
  - If earlier diagnosis of HCV infection is desired, testing for HCV RNA may be performed at 4–6 weeks.
- Confirm all anti-HCV results reported positive by enzyme immunoassay, using supplement anti-HCV testing
- Immunoglobulins and antiviral agents are not recommended
- For PEP after exposure to HCV positive blood.

Recommendations for HIV Postexposure Prophylaxis

- Indian Academy of Pediatrics (IAP) endorses the National AIDS Control Organization (NACO) guidelines. These should be implemented all over India
- If any HCP/HCW or citizen reports with NSI to emergency services in a public health facility, it is recommended that immediate care, free testing and free PEP medicines should be provided
- A nodal contact person should be in place in all facilities with 24 hours access to deal with immediate management of NSIs/other exposures

- Healthcare workers should ensure that a start up pack of PEP medication is available in their place of work.
- For HIV PEP, as per NACO guidelines, first define exposure code (EC) indicating degree of exposure to infectious materials, then decide HIV status of exposure source (ES) and follow PEP regimen as per recommendations.

DISPOSAL OF INJECTION WASTE (SYRINGES AND NEEDLES)

Biomedical waste management is a process starting from the point of use of a device till its final disposal. It is not only an issue of technology but also requires lot of changes in the way we think. Healthcare waste is hazardous both to the HCP, patients and public at large.

Government of India under the provision of Environmental Act, 1988, notified the BMW Rules in 1988, which regulates the disposal of all biomedical waste with an objective to ensure safety of health and environment. All healthcare facilities are required to segregate, disinfect, transport and dispose off the biomedical waste in an environmental friendly manner. Biomedical waste shall not be mixed with other wastes.

As per the schedule-I, rule 5 of BMW Rules, sharp-wastes are classified in category 4, which says, sharp-wastes mean needles, syringes, scalpel blades, glass, etc. that may cause puncture and cuts. This includes both used and unused sharps, which should be treated. As per schedule-II, color coding of the container for disposal sharps is a must. Blue or white translucent colored puncture proof container has to be used and disposed as per the schedule.

Section 4 of the Act has given policy statement. The following steps should be followed:
- Minimization
- Segregation
- Handling
- Storage of hospital waste
- Disposal.

Sharp Waste Minimization

As far as possible minimize the use of sharps. Emphasize the rational use of injections in the treatment of illness. The use of disposable syringes and needles has increased considerably, generating potentially infectious waste with limited options for treatment and disposal. The use of plastic disposables should be limited as far as possible because plastics are not degradable and more likely to cause reuse.

Segregation of Sharps

Sharps should be segregated at source. The clinical staff is responsible for segregating the waste at source. Blue or white translucent puncture proof containers should be placed at strategic and easily accessible locations. Needles should not be recapped, removed and transported by hand. Sharps should be disinfected. Hub-cutters or needle and syringe destroyer should be used at the site of generation to reduce the bulk, to disinfect and to prevent reusing.

Handling

Sharp containers should be picked-up and carried by the handle provided. They should not be supported at the bottom. Sharp containers should not be carried on back and should not be dropped or thrown. Containers should be labeled. Vehicles used to transport sharp containers should be authorized.

Containers

Sharps decontaminating units (SDU) for syringes and needles are made of plastic and are puncture proof, they can be foot operated with an inner perforated container with secured handles. They should be filled 1/3 with 1% hypochlorite solution (refer to the recent central pollution board guidelines). Sharps in inner containers after treatment with hypochlorite solution should be transferred to puncture proof containers for shredding. They should be labelled as sharps only.

Mutilation/Destruction/Shredding

Types of waste required to be mutilated are needles, syringes, plastic disposables, etc. Shredders are equipment to cut the waste into small pieces to reduce the volume. They must have safety provisions to prevent contamination. They must be placed in a separate room. Waste must be properly disinfected before feeding into shredder.

Treatment and Disposal

It is necessary to treat certain waste before disposal to prevent hazards to human health and environment. Immediately after use, syringes with needles should be dropped into sharp decontaminating unit so that both parts are completely immersed in disinfectant. When SDU is one-third full, after contact time of 30 minutes the inner perforated container contents are drained into puncture proof containers for shredding. Heat disinfection, encapsulation, smelting, burial, incineration are modes for disposal of sharp wastes in mass.

The education and awareness of HCW and public is important. The general public coming to hospital and in the community should know the medical risks of hospital waste so that they keep away from risks and also to demand the proper care, services from the hospital.

NEWER TECHNOLOGIES

Technology plays a supportive role in enhancing the quality of patient care in our day-to-day working. This has over a period of time helped healthcare professionals to deliver services effectively and efficiently. Most of the technological advances have happened as a response to the demands of the healthcare provider. These technologies for ease of understanding can be divided into three different kinds: auto-disable syringes, prefilled AD devices and healthcare worker safety devices.

Auto-disable Syringes

These are disposable syringes that lock once the medication has been injected and hence physically cannot be reused, since these syringes prevent reuse and they present the lowest risk of patient-to-patient transmission of blood-borne pathogens. These are available as prefixed 0.5 mL syringes and are presently available for immunization only (Fig. 10.4.8).

Syringe with different mechanisms are commercially available. These can be broadly divided into two types of auto-disable mechanisms:

Active Mechanism

- Requires the user to "actively" disable the syringe or device after use
- Disadvantage—chances of reuse if mechanism is not activated.

Passive Mechanism

The device is disabled as soon as the drug is fully injected out. The user has no control over the mechanism.

No chance of reuse as user has no control over mechanism.

WHO-UNICEF-UNFPA joint statement issued in 1999 on the use of auto-disable syringes in immunization services has urged countries to use only AD syringes for immunization after 2003. It is also recommended that in the curative sector also, injection devices with re-use prevention mechanisms should be used.

PREFILLED VACCINE DEVICES OR POUCH AND NEEDLE DEVICES

Prefilled vaccine devices or pouch and needle devices were also developed by PATH and are used by the pharmaceutical companies and vaccine manufacturers to fill vaccines

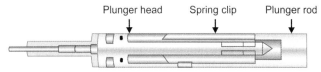

Plunger head   Spring clip   Plunger rod

FIG. 10.4.8: Auto-disable syringes.

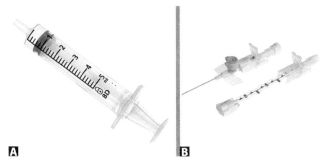

FIGS. 10.4.9A AND B: Safety engineered products.

into them and supply. They combine the benefit of prefilled device with that of auto-disable technologies. Minimally trained volunteers can use them. Several vaccines are now available with this technology.

HEALTHCARE WORKER SAFETY DEVICES

With the identification of the spread of blood-borne pathogens due to needlestick injuries and a needle stick safety and prevention act passed in the US in 2000, the trend, globally, is shifting toward use of safety engineered products. Now a range of products which help to prevent accidental NSIs are available (Figs. 10.4.9A and B). These products are now widely available in India.

BIBLIOGRAPHY

1. Abdel-Aziz F, Habib M, Mohamed MK, et al. Hepatitis C virus (HCV) infection in a community in the Nile Delta: population description and HCV prevalence. Hepatology. 2000;32:111-5.
2. Adegboye AA, Moss GB, Soyinka F, et al. The epidemiology of needlestick and sharp instruments accidents in a Nigerian hospital. Infect Control Hosp Epidemiol. 1994;15:27-31.
3. Battersby A, Feilden R, Nelson C. Sterilizable syringes: excessive risk or cost-effective option. Bull World Health Organ. 1999;77:812-9.
4. Battersby A, Fellden R, Stoeckel P, et al. Strategies for safe injections. Bull World Health Organ. 1999;77:996-1000.
5. Bhattarai MD, Wittet S. Perceptions about injections and private sector injection practices in Central Nepal. General Welfare Pratisthan and Gates Children's Vaccine Program. 2000.
6. Birungi H. Injections and self-help: risk and trust in Ugandan health care. Social Science and Medicine. 1998;47:1455-62.
7. Centers for disease control and prevention. National institute for occupational safety and health (NIOSH) NIOSH alert: preventing needlestick injuries in health care settings [online]. Available from http://www.cdc.gov/niosh/docs/2000-108/ [Accessed November 2012].
8. Chowdhury A, Santra A, Chaudhuri S, et al. Prevalence of hepatitis B infection in the general population: a rural community-based study. Trop Gastroenterol. 1999;20:75-7.
9. Consten E, van Lanschot JJ, Henny PC, et al. A prospective study on the risks of exposure to HIV during surgery in Zambia. AIDS. 1995;9:585-8.

10. Darwish MA, Faris R, Darwish N, et al. Hepatitis C and cirrhotic liver disease in the Nile delta of Egypt: a community-based study. Am J Trop Med Hyg. 2001;64:147-53.

11. Dicko M, Oni A, Ganivet S, et al. Safety of immunization injections in Africa: not simply a problem of logistics. Bull World Health Organ. 2000;78:163-9.

12. Drucker E, Alcabes PG, Marx PA. The injection century: massive unsterile injections and the emergence of human pathogens. The Lancet. 2001;358:1989-92.

13. El-Sayed NM, Gomatos PJ, Rodier GR, et al. Hepatitis C virus, human immunodeficiency virus, and *Treponema pallidum* infections: association of hepatitis C virus infections with specific regions of Egypt. Am J Trop Med Hyg. 1996;55: 179-84.

14. El-Sayed NM, Gomatos PJ, Rodier GR, et al. Seroprevalence of Egyptian tourism workers for hepatitis B virus, injection safety promotion in low-income countries 101. Downloaded from http://heapro.oxfordjournals.org/ by guest on April 15, 2012.

15. Frank C, Mohamed MK, Strickland GT, et al. The role of parenteral antischistosomal therapy in the spread of hepatitis C virus in Egypt. Lancet. 2000;355:887-91.

16. Gumodoka B, Favot I, Berege ZA, et al. Occupational exposure to the risk of HIV infection among health care workers in Mwanza Region, United Republic of Tanzania. Bull World Health Organ. 1997;75:133-40.

17. Hutin YJ, Chen RT. Injection safety: a global challenge. BullWorld Health Organ. 1999;77(10):787-8.

18. Hutin YJ, Hauri AM, Armstrong GL. Use of injections in health care settings worldwide, 2000: literature review and regional estimates. BMJ. 2003;327:1075.

19. IAP Guide Book on Safe Injection Practices. In: Kamath SS, Bhave S, Shah RC (Eds). IAP National Task Force on Safe Injection Practices; 2005.

20. Kamath SS. IAP workshop on safe injection practices: recommendations and IAP plan of action. Indian Pediatr. 2005;42:155-61.

21. Kane A, Lloyd J, Zaffran M, et al. Transmission of hepatitis B, hepatitis C and human immunodeficiency viruses through unsafe injections in the developing world: model-based regional estimates. Bull World Health Organ. 1999;77(10):801-7.

22. Lakshman M, Nichter M. Contamination of medicine injection paraphernalia used by registered medical practitioners in South India: an ethnographic study. SocSci Med. 2000;51: 11-28.

23. Lala KR, Lala MK. Intramuscular injection: review and guidelines. Indian Pediatr. 2003;40:835-45.

24. Management of wastes from immunization campaign activities. Practical guidelines for planners and managers. [Online].Available from www.healthcarewaste.org [Accessed November 2012].

25. Marcus R and the CDC Cooperative Needle Stick Surveillance Group. Surveillance of health care workers exposed to blood from patients infected with the human immunodeficiency virus. N Eng J Med. 1988;319:1118-23.

26. Prajapati BS. Essential Procedures in Pediatrics, 1st edition. New Delhi: Jaypee Brothers Medical Publishers (P) Ltd, 2003. pp. 64-71.

27. Prüss-Ustün A, Rapiti E, Hutin Y. Estimation of the global burden of disease from sharps injuries to health-care workers. Geneva, Switzerland: World Health Organization, 2003 (WHO Environmental Burden of Disease Series, No. 3). Am J Ind Med. 2005;48:482-90.

28. Royal college of pediatrics and child health, position statement in injection technique. March, 2002.

29. Safety of injections in immunization programmes. WHO recommended policy.Global Programme for vaccines and immunization, 1998. WHO; JiWI/LHIS/96.05Rev.I.

30. Simonsen L, Kane A, Llyod J, et al. Unsafe injections in the developing world and transmission of blood borne pathogens: a review. Bull World Health Organ. 1999;77(10):789-800.

31. UNAIDS/WHO Position paper on modes of transmission of HIV with particular reference to Sub-Saharan Africa and unsafe injections.

32. WHO best practices for injections and related procedures toolkit: March 2010. Printed by the WHO document production services, Geneva, Switzerland.

33. World Health Organization. Aide-Memoire for a Strategy to Protect Health Workers from Infection with Bloodborne Viruses. Geneva, Switzerland: WHO, November 2003.

34. Zaffran M, Lloyd J, Clements J, et al. A drive to safer injections. EPI: Report: GPV/SAGE. WHO/GPV and I 97/WP05.

Annexures

ANNEXURE 1: DRUG DOSAGE FOR PEDIATRIC INFECTIONS

Jesson Unni

Drug	Brand name	Dosage	Contraindications	Drug interaction	Side effects
Antibiotic					
Amikacin	Amicin, Amitax, Mikacin	Many dose regimens exist depending on target concentration aimed for and patient groups treated. The doses mentioned are accepted initial doses and dose adjustments done depending on serum levels. *Newborn:* Loading dose of 10 mg/kg then 7.5 mg/kg every 12 hrs intravenous (IV)—less than 35 weeks up to 14 days 10 mg/kg once daily and more than 14 days 10 mg/kg loading dose followed by 7.5 mg/kg per dose 2 times daily; more than 35 weeks less than 14 days 15 mg/kg as single dose daily and more than 14 days 10 mg/kg loading dose followed by 7.5 mg/kg per dose two times daily. Extended interval dose regimen by slow IV injection or IV infusion—15 mg/kg every 24 hrs. *Children (1 month to 18 years):* IV/intramuscular (IM) 7.5 mg/kg per dose two times daily up to maximum of 500 mg/dose. Child more than 12 years with life-threatening infection: 1.5 g/day in three divided doses for up to 10 days may be given. Aim for 1 hr post-dose (peak) of 15–30 mg/L. Once daily dose regimen (nct for endocarditis or meningitis) child 1 month to 18 years: initially 15 mg/kg, then adjusted according to serum-ar-ikacin concentration.	Myasthenia gravis. Child should be well hydrated and renal function monitored. Hearing test done, if child has received repeated courses.	Increased risk of ototoxicity and nephrotoxicity with cephalosporins, vancomycin, cyclosporin, cisplatin, diuretics, such as furosemide (frusemide), amphotericin. Enhances effects of non-depolarizing muscle relaxants (calcium IV may reverse this effect). Antagonizes effect of neostigmine and pyridostigmine.	As with all aminoglycosides, nephrotoxicity and ototoxicity can occur, if optimum blood levels are exceeded.
Amoxicillin	Biomoxil, idimox, pexomox	*Oral:* 20–50 mg/kg per day in two or three divided doses. Higher dose of 80–90 mg/kg in acute suppurative otitis media (maximum of 500 mg 2–3 times daily). *In uncomplicated gonorrhea:* 3 g with 1 g probenecid.	See ampicillin monograph.		See ampicillin monograph.
Ampicillin	Aristocillin, Roscillin	*Neonate:* 50 mg/kg per dose less than 7 days, 12th hourly, 7–21 days 8th hourly, more than 21 days, 6th hourly. 100 mg/kg per dose for suspected meningitis and Gr B streptococcal infection. *Children:* Oral: 1 month to 2 years, 12.5 mg/kg per dose, 2–12 years 250 mg/dose and 12–18 years, 500 mg/dose; IV/IM 25 mg/kg per dose (maximum 1 g/dose); IV infusion 100 mg/kg per dose (maximum 3 g/dose)—all given four times daily.	Hypersensitivity to penicillins or cephalosporins. A high percentage of patients with infectious mononucleosis develop a rash with aminopenicillins and ampicillin should preferably not be used in these patients. Monitor renal and hepatic function especially if prolonged therapy, high doses or preexisting renal or hepatic insufficiency.	With allopurinol increased frequency of skin rashes. Chloroquine reduces ampicillin absorption. Probenecid increases ampicillin levels. With warfarin prolongation of prothrombin time. Ampicillin decreases efficacy of estrogen containing oral contraceptives.	Gastrointestinal upsets (nausea, diarrhea), urticarial penicillin hypersensitivity rash; erythematous, maculopapular rash in 10% of children. Incidence of rash may be higher in HIV patients.

Contd...

Contd...

Drug	Brand name	Dosage	Contraindications	Drug interaction	Side effects
Azithromycin	Azee, Azithral, Zithrox	6 months to 12 years 10 mg/kg per day once daily for 3 days up to maximum of 200 mg (3–7 years), 300 mg (8–11 years), 400 mg (12–14 years) and 500 mg less than 14 years. Alternatively, 10 mg/kg per day once on first day followed by 5 mg/kg per day once daily from 2nd to 5th day. Group A beta-hemolytic streptococcal (GAS) pharyngitis and tonsillitis (primary prophylaxis of rheumatic fever)—12.5 mg/kg per day—single dose for 5 days. (Not recommended for secondary prophylaxis of rheumatic fever) chlamydial infection, such as non-gonococcal urethritis (NGU) or cervicitis due to susceptible strains of Chlamydia trachomatis. Adolescents: Single dose of 1 g orally. Bacterial endocarditis prophylaxis: 15 mg/kg (single dose max 500 mg) 30–60 minutes before procedure in children and adolescents allergic to penicillin. Treatment and post-exposure pertussis prophylaxis—(For post-exposure prophylaxis, administer to close contacts within 3 weeks of exposure, especially in high-risk patients (e.g. women in 3rd trimester, infants <12 months). Oral dosage: Infants more than 6 months and children 10 mg/kg per day (maximum 500 mg) on day 1, then 5 mg/kg per day (maximum 250 mg) on 2nd to 5th day. Infants less than 6 months—10 mg/kg per day for 5 days. Monitor for infantile hypertrophic pyloric stenosis in infants less than 1 month old. Uncomplicated typhoid fever. Orally: Adolescent 8–10 mg/kg per day once daily for 7 days; 1,000 mg on first day, followed by 500 mg once daily for 6 days. Children: 10 mg/kg per day once daily for 7 days or 5 days regimen of 20 mg/kg per day. Continued treatment may be needed to prevent relapse in cryptosporidiosis. Sexually transmitted disease (STD) caused by Chlamydia trachomatis: 12–18 years 1 g as single dose.	Avoid patients with hepatic disease. Use with caution in severe renal failure. Observe for signs of bacterial/fungal superinfection.	Antacids: Administer azithromycin at least 1 hr before and 2 hrs after antacids. May enhance effects and toxicity of carbamazepine, cyclosporin, digoxin and theophylline—monitor levels. Terfenadine: Possible risk of hazardous arrhythmias. Effect of warfarin may be enhanced—monitor INR.	Nausea, abdominal discomfort (pain/cramps), vomiting, flatulence, diarrhea, rash and photosensitivity, reversible elevation in liver transaminases, transient reduction in neutrophil count, reversible hearing impairment and cholestatic jaundice (rare). Serious allergic reactions, e.g. angioneurotic edema and anaphylaxis reported rarely.
Aztreonam	Azenam	Intravenous over 3–5 min or IV infusion less than 7 days old, 30 mg/kg 12th hourly; rest of neonatal period and up to 12 years, 30 mg/kg 6–8th hourly. In severe infection and cystic fibrosis in 2–12 year olds, may increase up to 50 mg/kg 6–8th hourly (maximum 2 g 6th hourly); 12–18 years, 1 g 8th hourly or 2 g 12th hourly (severe infection with Pseudomonas aeruginosa or pulmonary infection in cystic fibrosis). Renal impairment—Cr Cl 10–30 mL/min/1.73 m², no change in first dose but subsequent doses to be halved; Cr Cl less than 10 mL/min/1.73 m², no change in first dose but subsequent doses to be reduced to 1/4th usual dose.		Might enhance anticoagulant effect of coumarins; small risk of reducing contraceptive effect of estrogens.	Nausea, vomiting, diarrhea, abdominal pain, oral ulceration, jaundice, flushing, allergic rash, thrombocytopenia, neutropenia, and rarely hypotension, headache, bad breath and breast tenderness.

Contd...

Contd...

Drug	Brand name	Dosage	Contraindications	Drug interaction	Side effects
Benzathine penicillin	Penidure	Infants and children, Gr A streptococcal upper respiratory infection (URI): 25,000–50,000 units/kg as single dose, maximum 12 lakh units/dose or child less than 27 kg, 3–6 lakh units as single dose and more than 27 kg, 9 lakh units as single dose. *Adolescents*: 12 lakh units as single dose. *Prophylaxis of rheumatic fever*: Indian academy of pediatrics (IAP) recommends. Children less than 27 kg, 6 lakh units every 15 days; more than and equal to 27 kg, 1.2 lakh units every 21 days. *Congenital syphilis*: 50,000 units/kg per dose (max 24 lakh units) once a week for 3 weeks. *Early syphilis in adolescents*: 24 lakh units as single dose in two injection sites. If present for more than 1 year, 24 lakh units as single dose in two injection sites once weekly for three doses.	Hypersensitivity to penicillin or other components. Caution in child with impaired renal function, impaired cardiac function, preexisting seizure disorder or hypersensitivity to cephalosporins.	Probenecid increases serum conc. of penicillin. Synergistic antibacterial effect when given with aminoglycosides. Tetracyclines, chloramphenicol and erythromycin may antagonize the activity of penicillin.	Central nervous system (CNS) —Convulsions, giddiness, confusion, lethargy and fever. Skin rash. *Blood*: Hemolytic anemia. 242 *Local*: Severe pain at site. Musculoskeletal myoclonus. *Renal*: Interstitial nephritis. *Others*: Hypersensitivity reactions, anaphylaxis and Jarisch-Herxheimer reaction.
Benzylpenicillin (penicillin G)		*Newborn*: 25 mg/kg per dose two times daily up to 7 days age and three times daily thereafter. Dose doubled if meningitis diagnosed. *Child*: 25 mg/kg per dose four times daily. In severe infection and meningitis 50 mg/kg per dose six times daily to maximum single dose of 2.4 g and daily dose of 14.4 g/day. In moderate renal failure (creatinine clearance 10–50 mL/minute/1.73 m²), dosage interval may be increased to 8–12 hrs and in severe renal failure (<10 mL/minute/1.73 m²) to every 12 hrs.	Allergy to penicillins. Very large dose may cause hypokalemia and hypernatremia.	Increased levels of benzylpenicillin if given with probenecid.	Anaphylactic reactions, immediate and delayed hypersensitivity reactions. Rare reports of paresthesia and hematological disorders in prolonged use.
Carbapenems		*Meropenem newborn*: 40 mg/kg per day in two divided doses less than 7 days and in three divided doses more than 7 days. Double dose in meningitis and severe infection. *Children*: UTI, gynecological infections, skin and soft tissue infection, 30 mg/kg in three divided doses (max 500 mg/ dose). Pneumonia, periton tis, neutropenia, septicemia 60 mg/kg per day in three divided doses (max 1 g/dose). Meningitis and life-threatening infections 120 mg/kg per day in three divided doses (max 2 g/dose). *In renal impairment*: Cr Cl (mL/min/1.73 m²); 25–50 give full dose but at 12 hrs intervals, 10–25, 50% dose at 12 hrs intervals less than 10–50% dose at 24 hrs interval. Imipenem with cilastin, newborn IV 20 mg/kg per dose in the frequency less than 7 days, 7–21 days and more than 21 days at two times, three times and four times daily, respectively. *Children*: IV less than 3 months 80 mg/kg per day, 3 months to 2 years 60 mg/kg per day, 12–18 years 2 g/day in four divided doses (max/dose <12 years 500 >12 years 1 g).			

Contd...

Contd...

Drug	Brand name	Dosage	Contraindications	Drug interaction	Side effects
Cefaclor	Distaclor, Keflor	Orally, less than 1 year, 62.5 mg; 1–5 years, 125 mg; 6–18 years, 250 mg/dose three times daily. Dose doubled in severe infection with susceptible organisms.	Hypersensitivity to cephalosporins. Caution in patient hypersensitive to penicillin, particularly type 1 reactions and in renal impairment as the half-life is extended in moderate/severe impairment.	*Warfarin:* Increased prothrombin time; monitor INR and adjust dose as necessary. Renal excretion of cofactor is inhibited by probenecid. False-positive Coombs' test. False-positive reaction for glucose in urine with Benedicts' or Fehlings' solution. Absorption of modified release tablets reduced by aluminum or magnesium containing antacids.	*Gastrointestinal:* Diarrhea, nausea, vomiting. Skin: rash, urticaria, pruritus. *Hematological:* Eosinophilia. May cause serum sickness like reactions in susceptible individuals.
Cefadroxil	Bicef, Cefadrox	*Children:* Orally, 30 mg/kg per 24 hrs in two divided doses (maximum 2 g/day); adolescent 250–500 mg, 8th–12th hourly.	Hypersensitivity to cephalosporins. Caution in patients with a history of penicillin allergy.	Probenecid raises serum levels which may increase nephrotoxicity. Urine form patients receiving cefadroxil may give false-positive glycosuria reaction when tested with Benedicts' or Fehlings' solution-does not occur with enzyme-based tests. False-positive Coombs' reaction may occur.	Rash, pruritus, urticaria, angioneurotic edema (rare). Nausea, vomiting, diarrhea, dyspepsia, abdominal discomfort, dizziness, headache. Reversible neutropenia, minor elevation in transaminases and Stevens–Johnson syndrome.
Cefdinir	Adcef, Aldinir, Oceph, Zefdinir	14 mg/kg per day in two divided doses.	Patients with known hypersensitivity to cephalosporins.	*Antacids:* Cefdinir rate and extent of absorption is reduced in presence of antacid. *Probenecid:* It inhibits renal excretion of cefdinir and may prolong plasma levels by competitively inhibiting renal tubular secretion. *Iron:* Concomitant administration of cefdinir with therapeutic iron supplement reduces absorption. *Loop diuretics:* Risk of nephrotoxicity may be increased.	Abdominal pain, diarrhea, nausea, vomiting, flatulence, dyspepsia, anorexia, constipation. Headache, dizziness, insomnia, somnolence, confusion. Vaginal moniliasis, vaginitis, rash, pruritus. Hypotension, anxiety, palpitation, anaphylaxis, angioedema.

Contd...

Contd...

Drug	Brand name	Dosage	Contraindications	Drug interaction	Side effects
Cefepime	Biopime, maxicef	Neonates less than 14 days 30 mg/kg per dose twice daily IV/ IM. Neonates more than 14 days 50 mg/kg per dose twice daily IV/IM. Children IV 50 mg/kg every 8 hrs (maximum 2 g/dose). Intraperitonial 15 mg/kg per dose. In peritoneal dialysis associated with peritonitis 1,000 mg/24 hours. However, not yet licensed for use in children under 12 years in UK and US.	Patients who have shown immediate hypersensitivity reactions to cefepime, other cephalosporins, penicillins or other beta-lactam antibiotics.	No clinically significant drug interactions reported. However, renal functions has to be monitored carefully if high doses of aminoglycosides are to be administered with cefepime because of increased potential of nephrotoxicity and ototoxicity of aminoglycosides antibiotics. Nephrotoxicity has been reported following concomitant administration with potent diuretics, such as furosemide.	Cefepime is a relatively safe drug with good safety profile. The most common adverse events are, however, headache, diarrhea, nausea, vomiting, pruritus and rash. Rarely, reversible cefepime induced encephalopathy has been seen in adult patients, with a peculiar electroencephalogram pattern characterized by semiperiodic diffuse triphasic waves and other neurological symptoms, including confusion, hallucinations, agitation, convulsions, tremor, delirium and coma with regression of symptoms within 2–7 days after stopping antibiotic treatment. Almost all these patients had renal failure and the dose of cefepime was high for the level of renal failure. There is a mild risk of superinfections with organisms like *Candida*, *Enterococcus*, methicillin resistant *Staphylococcus aureus* (MRSA), *Pseudomonas aeruginosa*, *Clostridium difficile*, etc. while on cefepime.
Cefixime	Taxim-O, C-Tax O, Extacef, Gramocef-O	8 mg/kg per 24 hrs in one to two divided doses; adolescent: 400 mg/24 hrs in one to two divided doses.	Hypersensitivity to cephalosporins and known hypersensitivity to penicillins and those with marked renal impairment.	Urine from patients receiving cefixime may give fasle-positive glycosuria reaction when tested with Benedicts' or Fehlings' solution–does not occur with enzyme based tests. False-postitive Coombs' reaction may occur.	*Pruritus and vaginitis:* Mild transient changes in liver and renal function tests. Diarrhea, abdominal pain, nausea, vomiting, rash and headache. Thrombocytopenia, leukopenia, eosinophilia, pseudomembranous colitis (rare) and hypersensitivity reactions.

Contd...

Contd...

Drug	Brand name	Dosage	Contraindications	Drug interaction	Side effects
Cefoperazone	Cefomycin, Magnamycin	50–200 mg/kg per day in two or more divided doses (max in adolescent 1–2 g/IM/IV 12th hourly)	Hypersensitivity to cephalosporins, hepatic disease and severe biliary obstruction.		Skin rash, urticaria, transient rise in hepatic enzymes, reversible neutropenia. Pseudomembranous colitis can occur during use or following discontinuance of cefoperazone, but this reaction is rare.
Cefotaxime	C-Tax, Taxim	Newborn (severe infections like meningitis): 50 mg/kg per dose less than 7 days two times; 7–21 days 3 times; 21–30 days 3–4 times. one month to 12 years 50 mg/kg per dose and 12–18 years 1–3 g two times daily. Dosage adjustment in renal impairment due to extrarenal elimination; it is only necessary to reduce dose in severe renal impairment (creatinine clearance <10 mL/minute/1.73 m²). A normal single dose should be given as a loading dose then the daily dose should be halved without a change in frequency.	Allergy to cephalosporins/ penicillins (particularly type 1 penicillin hypersensitivity).	High doses should be given with caution to patients receiving aminoglycosides or potent diuretics due to the combination having an adverse effect on renal function. A positive Coombs' test may be seen.	Generally infrequent, mild and transient. Effects reported include candidiasis, rashes, fever, transient rises in liver transaminase and/or alkaline phosphatase and diarrhea. Pseudomembranous colitis may occur rarely—stop drug. Changes in renal function have been observed rarely with high doses. Hypersensitivity reactions include skin rashes, drug fever and vary rarely anaphylaxis. Granulocytopenia and more rarely agranulocytosis may occur. Eosinophilia, neutropenia, thrombocytopenia and hemolytic anemia have been reported, if treatment is for longer than 10 days monitor full blood count. Transient pain may be experienced at the site of injection.
Cefpodoxime	Cefoprox, Spectratil	9 mg/kg per day in two divided doses (maximum single dose, 200 mg). The dose frequency should be reduced in renal impairment. Creatinine clearance 10–40 mL and less than 10 mL/min per 1.73 m², frequency of dosing once in 24 hrs and once in 48 hrs, respectively.	Hypersensitivity to cephalosporin antibiotics or type 1 hypersensitivity to penicillins. Suspension contains aspartame thus contraindicated in patients with phenylketonuria.	Absorption decreased by antacids or histamine H₂ antagonists.	Diarrhea, nausea, vomiting and abdominal pain can occur. Occasional reports of headache, allergic reactions.

Contd...

Drug	Brand name	Dosage	Contraindications	Drug interaction	Side effects
Ceftazidime	Fortum, Spectrazid	*Neonates*: Less than 7 days and more than 7 days less than 1,200 g 100 mg/kg per 24 hrs in two divided doses IV/IM; more than 7 days more than 1,200 g 150 mg/kg per day divided 8th hourly IM/IV. Children 150 mg/kg per 24 hrs divided 8th hourly. Maximum 6 g/day. Single dose more than 1 g to be given through IV only. Dose adjustment in renal failure: In mild impairment give a dose in every 12 hrs, in moderate impairment (creatinine clearance 10–50 mL/minute/1.73 m²) give a dose once daily and in severe impairment (creatinine clearance <10 mL/minute/1.73 m²) give 50% of dose once daily. Levels may be monitored, if clinically indicated. *In hemodialysis*: The appropriate maintenance dose should be repeated after dialysis. In peritoneal dialysis: 125–250 mg may be added to 21 of dialysis fluid, and given in addition to the IV dose.	Contraindicated in patients with a known sensitivity to cephalosporins. Special caution in patients with type 1 or immediate hypersensitivity to penicillin.	Possible antagonism of effect of ceftazidime if given with chloramphenicol. Caution when given with nephrotoxic drugs.	Infusion related phlebitis, thrombophlebitis and pain on injection. Via nebulization-sensitivity reactions and local effects.
Ceftriaxone	C Tri, Monocef, Xone, injection	*Neonates*: 50–75 mg/kg once daily IM/IV. Infuse over 10–30 minutes. Avoid in premature, acidotic or hyperbilirubinemic neonates. Children 50–75 mg/kg once daily IV/IM. Meningitis loading dose 75 mg/kg followed by 80–100 mg/kg per 24 hrs once or divided 12th hourly. Maximum 4 g/day. In severe renal failure reduce dose to a maximum of 2 g or 50 mg/kg. No dose adjustment required in hepatic impairment. If both hepatic and severe renal impairment monitor serum concentrations. In patients undergoing dialysis no supplemental dose required but serum concentration monitoring advisable.	As for cefotaxime. Use with caution in preexisting disease of biliary tract, gallbladder, liver or pancreas. Ceftriaxone may displace bilirubin from albumin binding site and should not be used in jaundiced, hypoalbuminemic or acidotic newborn infants. Should probably not be used in premature infants for this reason.	*As for cefotaxime*: Interferes with cupric sulfate method for urinary glucose determination. Glucose oxidase method unaffected. May displace phenytoin from albumin binding site.	As for cefotaxime. Urinary precipitates of calcium ceftriaxone have occurred rarely; immobile, dehydrated and young patients are most at risk. A similar precipitate has been reported in the gallbladder and may be seen on ultrasound as shadows. If biliary symptoms develop, ceftriaxone should be discontinued and ultrasound performed. Biliary precipitates generally disappear on discontinuation and non-surgical management is recommended. Those most at risk are patients with preexisting renal hepatic disease, dehydration or receiving concurrent parenteral nutrition.
Cefuroxime	Spectraxime	*Neonates*: 40–100 mg/kg per 24 hrs divided 12th hourly IM/IV. *Children*: 200–400 mg/kg per 24 hrs divided 8th hourly IM/IV; 20–30 mg/kg per day divided 8th hourly orally. Maximum of 1.5 g/dose IV or 6 g/24 hours.	Known hypersensitivity to cephalosporins. Cross sensitivity to penicillin has been reported, particularly in type 1 or intermediate hypersensitivity to penicillin.	High doses should be given with caution with other nephrotoxic drugs, e.g. diuretics/aminoglycosides.	Hypersensitivity reactions, including rashes and fever. Gastrointestinal disturbances and rarely transient rises in liver function tests.

Contd...

Contd...

Drug	Brand name	Dosage	Contraindications	Drug interaction	Side effects
Cephalexin	Phexin, Sporidex, Sporidex AF	*Children*: 25–100 mg/kg per 24 hrs in 3–4 divided doses; adolescent 250–500 mg four times daily (maximum 4 g/ 24 hrs. Reduce dose in severe renal impairment (creatinine clearance <10 mL/minute per 1.73 m²) by reducing dose frequency. Removed by dialysis thus an additional dose may be required after dialysis.	Hypersensitivity to cephalosporins. Caution in those with hypersensitivity to penicillins.	Urine form patients receiving cephalexin may give false-positive glycosuria reaction when tested with Benedicts' or Fehlings' solution—does not occur with enzyme based tests. False-positive Coombs' reaction may occur.	*Gastrointestinal*: Diarrhea, dyspepsia, abdominal pain, rarely nausea and vomiting. Hypersensitivity: allergic reactions in the form of rash, urticaria and angioedema have been reported. Other effects reported include headache, dizziness and fatigue.
Cephalosporins		*First-generation cephalosporins* *Dose*: Cephalexin for children, 25–100 mg/kg per 24 hrs in 3–4 div ded doses and 12–18 years, 250–500 mg four times daily (maximum 4 g/day). *Cefadroxil*: For children, 30 mg/kg per 24 hrs in two divided doses maximum 2 g/day) and in 12–18 years, 250–500 mg 8–12th hourly. Second generation cephalosporins. *Dose*: Cefuroxime for neonates 40–100 mg/kg per day IM/ IV given 12th hourly; children 200–400 mg/kg per day, 8th hourly IM/IV and 20–30 mg/kg per day, three times a day orally. Maximum dose not to exceed 1.5 g/dose IV or 6 g/24 hours. *Cefaclor*: Orally; less than 1 year, 62.5 mg, 1–5 years, 125 mg; 6–18 years, 250 mg/dose three times daily. Dose doubled in severe infection with susceptible organisms. Third-generation cephalosporins. *Dose*: Cefixime for children, 8 mg/kg per 24 hrs in one to two divided doses. In adolescent: 400 mg/24 hrs in one to two divided doses. *Cefpodoxime*: For children, 9 mg/kg per 24 hrs in two divided doses (maximum single dose, 200 mg). In adolescent: 200 mg two times daily. *Cefdinir*: In children, 7 mg/kg per dose two times daily. 12–18 years 300 mg/dose two times daily. Fourth-generation cephalosporins. *Cefpirom*: Children 12–18 years IV injection or infusion 1 g 12th hourly and increased to 2 g 12th hourly in severe infections and infections in immunocompromised children. *Cefepime*. Children IV 50 mg/kg every 8 hrs (maximum 2 g/ dose).			
Chloramphenicol	Chloromycetin	Neonates less than 14 days 12.5 mg/kg per dose twice daily; more than 14 days 12.5 mg/kg per dose, two to four times daily—monitor levels. *Children*: 50 mg/kg per day (maximum 1 g/day) four divided doses, double dose for meningitis, septicemia).		Increases plasma levels of warfarin, phenytoin and sulfonylureas. Phenobarbital (phenobarbitone) and	Blood disorders, peripheral or optic neuritis, headache, depression, dry mouth, nausea and vomiting, diarrhea, urticaria.

Contd...

Contd...

Drug	Brand name	Dosage	Contraindications	Drug interaction	Side effects
		Eardrops: Two to three drops and two to three times daily. Eye ointment may be used in the ear. *Eyedrop:* One drop 4–6 times daily (1–2 hourly in severe infections). In addition, a small amount of ointment may be applied at bedtime. *Eye ointment:* Apply four times daily (1–2 hourly in severe infections). Continue treatment till 48 hrs after the eye is clinically normal.		rifampicin decrease chloramphenicol levels. Chymotrypsin eye drops would be inactivated if given at the same time as chloramphenicol eyedrops.	Superinfection with *Candida*. Sensitivity reactions to the eardrop vehicle may occur.
Ciprofloxacin	Alcipro, Ciplox	*Neonates:* 10 mg/kg 12 hourly orally or IV; children 15–30 mg/kg per 24 hrs in two divided doses oral or IV (maximum single dose IV 400 mg and oral 750 mg). Dose adjustment in renal or liver failure: In severe impairment (creatinine clearance < 20 mL/minute/1.73 m²) total daily dosage may be reduced by half, although monitoring serum levels provides the most reliable basis for dose adjustment. No adjustment in impaired hepatic function. *Corneal ulcers:* Apply throughout the day and night. First day, two drops in every 15 minutes for 6 hrs followed by two drops every 30 minutes for the rest of the day. Second day, two drops every hour and from 3rd to 14th day, two drops 4th hourly. One to two drops four times daily till 48 hrs after the eye is clinically norma (use for max of 21 days).	In children and growing adolescents use only where the benefits outweigh the risk of arthropathy. Contraindicated in hypersensitivity to ciprofloxacin or other quinolones. Use with caution in epilepsy or CNS disorders seizure threshold may be reduced by ciprofloxacin. Patients receiving ciprofloxacin should be well hydrated and excessive alkalinity of the urine avoided prevent crystalluria. Patients with a familial history of G6PD activity may be prone to hemolysis.	Ciprofloxacin tablets should not be administered within 4 hrs of medication containing magnesium, aluminum, calcium or iron salts. Theophylline dose should be reduced when concomitant therapy given. Prolonged bleeding times reported on concomitant administration of oral anticoagulants. Metoclopramide may accelerate the absorption of ciprofloxacin. Increased risk of nephrotoxicity with cyclosporine.	*Gastrointestinal (GI) disturbances:* Rarely pseudomembranous colitis, central nervous system (CNS) disturbances. Hypersensitivity skin reactions-rarely erythema nodosum, Steven-Johnson syndrome. Transient hepatic disturbances. Reversible arthralgia, joint swelling and myalgia. Reversible hematological disorders. Eyedrops may cause local itching and burning, lid margin crusting and taste disturbance.
Clarithromycin	Crixan, Synclar	Oral 15 mg/kg per 24 hrs in two divided doses up to maximum of 500 mg twice daily for 5–10 days. *Helicobacter pylori:* 1–2 years 125 mg; 2–6 years 250 mg; 6–9 years 375 mg; 9–12 years 500 mg; and 12–18 years 1 g/day in two divided doses along with amoxicillin and omeprazole or amoxicillin and lansoprazole or metronidazole and omeprazole. Community, acquired pneumonia (CAP) and pharyngitis in children due to *Chlamydophila pneumoniae*, *Mycoplasma pneumoniae* or *Streptococcus pneumoniae* give for 10 days. *Bacterial endocarditis prophylaxis:* 15 mg/kg (single dose max 500 mg) 30–60 minutes before procedure in children and adolescents allergic to penicillin. Treatment and post-exposure pertussis prophylaxis: For post-exposure prophylaxis, administer to close contacts within 3 weeks of exposure, especially in high-risk patients (e.g. women in 3rd trimester, infants <12 months).	Known hypersensitivity to macrolides or excipients. Monitor for signs of bacterial/fungal superinfection.	*Theophylline:* Increased serum levels and potential theophylline toxicity. Digoxin, warfarin, carbamazepine, reduced rate of excretion of these drugs, potentiation of effect; monitor levels; monitor prothrombin time for warfarin. Terfenadine, astemizole and cisapride—risk of cardiac arrhythmias, avoid concurrent use. Ergot derivatives and clarithromycin should not be coadministered; ergotism reported.	Nausea, vomiting, diarrhea, abdominal pain, taste perversion, stomatitis and glossitis. Headache, allergic reactions-mild urticaria to Stevens–Johnson syndrome (rare). CNS effects including dizziness, anxiety, insomnia, bad dreams, pseudomembranous colitis (rare), altered liver function tests (LFTs).

Contd...

Contd...

Drug	Brand name	Dosage	Contraindications	Drug interaction	Side effects
		Oral dosage: Infants more than 6 months and children— 15 mg/kg per day up to maximum of 500 mg twice daily for 7 days. Not used in neonates. Patients with renal impairment: Cr Cl more than 60 mL/min: no dosage adjustment needed. Cr Cl 30—60 mL/min: no dosage adjustment needed except in patients receiving concurrent ritonavir. In these patients, reduce the recommended clarithromycin dose by 50%. Cr Cl less than 30 mL/min: reduce recommended dose by 50%. In patents receiving ritonavir, decrease the recommended clarithromycin dose by 75%.			
Clindamycin	Clincin	*Neonates:* Less than 7 days less than 2,000 g 10 mg/kg per day divided 12th hourly IV/IM; less than 7 days more than 2,000 g 15 mg/kg per day divided 8th hourly IV/IM; more than 7 days less than 1,200 g 10 mg/kg per day divided 12th hourly IV/IM; 1,200—2,000 g 15 mg/kg per day divided 8th hourly; more than 2,000 g 20 mg/kg per day divided 8th hourly IV/IM. *Children:* 10—40 mg/kg per day divided 8th hourly IV/IM or orally: 12—18 years 150—300 mg up to maximum of 450 mg/dose four times daily. Falciparum malaria (alternate therapy) with 20 mg/kg per day for 5 days. Acne topical application as thin film two times daily with lotion and once with gel. Dose adjusted in hepatic failure: Dose reduced and liver function monitored. Not readily removed by dialysis or peritoneal dialysis.	Should only be used in the treatment of severe infections and contra indicated in diarrheal states. Discontinue immediately if diarrhea or colitis develops. Cases of diarrhea have been reported during or even two or three weeks following treatment. When used topically avoid concurrent application of benzyl peroxide.	Drug interactions include antagonism of neostigmine and pyridostigmine and enhancement of nondepolarizing muscle relaxants.	*Diarrhea:* Discontinue treatment. Nausea and vomiting, antibiotic associated colitis, jaundice and altered LFTs, blood dyscrasias and erythema multiforme have been reported. With topical use—skin dryness and irritation can occur.
Cloxacillin	Bioclox, Klox	*Newborn:* IV/oral less than 7 days 50—100 mg/kg per day in two divided doses; 7—21 days 75—150 mg/kg per day in three divided doses, more than 21 days 100—200 mg/kg per day in four divided doses. May be increased to 100 mg/kg per dose in severe infection (meningitis, cerebral abscess, staph osteitis). Oral used only for minor infections. Children: IV/IM 50—100 mg/kg per day in four divided doses (max single dose 1 gm—may be doubled in severe infection). Oral less than 1 year 250 mg/day; 1—5 years 500 mg/day; 5—18 years 1 g in four divided doses. Doses may be doubled in severe infection. In renal failure, if creatinine clearance less than 10 mL/min per 1.73 m², increase dosage interval to 8th hourly.	Penicillin hypersensitivity.	With warfarin prothrombin time may be increased.	Gastrointestinal effects, particularly at high oral doses. Skin rash; treatment should be discontinued. Hepatitis and cholestatic jaundice; may occur up to several weeks after stopping treatment. Pseudomembranous colitis has been reported rarely in combination with other antibiotics.
Co-amoxiclav (amoxicillin and clavulanic acid)	Moxclav, Moxclav BD, Moxclav DS	Dosed on amoxicillin content. *Neonates:* 30 mg/kg per day in two divided doses. Children 20—45 mg/kg in two to three divided doses. Higher doses of 80 mg/kg per day may be required in otitis media. Administration	See amoxicillin monograph. Caution in hepatic impairment (monitor hepatic function). Also see side-effects section of this monograph.	See ampicillin monograph.	See ampicillin monograph. Also hepatitis, cholestatic jaundice; CSM has advised that cholestatic jaundice has been identified as an adverse reaction occurring during or shortly after, the use of co-amoxiclav.

Contd...

Contd...

Drug	Brand name	Dosage	Contraindications	Drug interaction	Side effects
		Oral: Give at the start of a meal. Dispersible tablets should be stirred into a little water before taking. IV: reconstitute a 600 mg vial with 10 mL water for injections (final volume 10.5 mL) and a 1.2 g vial with 20 mL (final volume 20.9 mL). Give by slow IV injection (over 3–4 minutes, within 20 minutes of reconstitution) or infuse over 30–40 minutes and complete infusion within 4 hrs of reconstitution. For infusion the reconstitutec injection can be diluted to five times its volume in NaCl 0.9%. Do not infuse in glucose solutions, as co-amoxiclav is less stable in infusions containing glucose.			An epidemiological study has shown that the risk of acute liver toxicity was about six times greater with co-amoxiclav than with amoxicillin; these reactions have only rarely been reported in children. Jaundice is usually self-limiting and very rarely fatal. The duration of treatment should be appropriate to the indication and not normally exceed 14 days. Erythema multiforme (including Stevens–Johnson syndrome), toxic epidermal necrolysis, exfoliative dermatitis, and vasculitis have been reported. Rarely, prolongation of bleeding time, headache, dizziness, convulsions, superficial staining of the teeth with the suspension and phlebitis at injection site.
Colistin	Colygyl, Walamycin	Nebulized along with oral ciprofloxacin for *Pseudomonas* lung infection in cystic fibrosis less than 1 year 500,000 units, 1–10 years 1 million units, more than 10 years 2 million units two times daily. IV for early *Pseudomonas* infections not cleared by ciprofloxacin and nebulized colistin or mod; severe infection or multiresistant strains along with aminoglycosice where other regimens fail (IV preparation not available in India).	Contraindicated in patients with known hypersensitivity to colistin or collistimethate sodium. Bronchospasm may occur when nebulized–treat with beta-agonist. Caution in acute porphyria.	Enhanced muscle relaxant effect with muscle relaxants. Increased risk of ototoxicity and nephrotoxicity with loop diuretics, aminoglycosides, ciclosporin (cyclosporin), amphotericin and cisplatin.	Bronchospasm if inhaled. Other side-effects are minimal with nebulization but the following have been noted with IV administration: impaired renal function, muscle weakness, facial paresthesia, slurred speech, visual disturbance and apnea.
Co-trimoxazole	Bactrim, Septran	*Children:* Orally: 6–20 mg TMP/kg per 24 hrs divided 12th hourly (maximum 160 mg TMP 12th hourly). *Pneumocystis carinii* pneumonia oral/IV15–20 mg TMP/kg per 24 hours divided 12th hourly. *P. carinii* prophylaxis orally 5 mg TMP/kg per 24 hrs or three times/week. The use of co-trimoxazole is not generally recommended under 6 weeks of age but some neonatologists feel that there is no specific reason for this caution other than the risk of hemolytic anemia in babies with G6PD deficiency and the risk of kernicterus because	Hypersensitivity to sulfonamides, trimethoprim or co-trimoxazole; marked liver parenchyma damage; severe renal insufficiency where repeated measurements of the plasma concentration cannot be performed. Avoid in patients	Potentiates the anticoagulant activity of warfarin. Prolongs the half-life phenytoin. If considered appropriate therapy in patients receiving other antifolate drugs, e.g. methotrexate, a folate supplement should be considered.	Most are mild and comprise nausea with or without vomiting and skin rashes. Fatalities, although rare, have occurred due to severe reactions, including Stevens–Johnson syndrome, Lyell syndrome (toxic epidermal necrolysis), fulminant hepatic necrosis,

Contd...

Contd...

Drug	Brand name	Dosage	Contraindications	Drug interaction	Side effects
		sulfamethoxazole competes for the protein binding sites usually available to bilirubin in babies with jaundice. If co-trimoxazole is used in newborn infants it is given in the same dosage as for six weeks to five months but trimethoprim on its owr is now usually preferred to co-trimoxazole.	with serious hematological disorders except under specialist supervision; regular monthly blood counts are advisable when given for long periods; discontinue immediately if blood disorders or rash develops. A folate supplement should also be considered with prolonged high dosage. Infusion contains sulfite which may cause allergic type reactions, including anaphylaxis.		agranulocytosis, aplastic anemias. The majority of hematological changes are mild and reversible when treatment is stopped. The changes are mainly leukopenia, neutropenia, thrombocytopenia and less commonly, agranulocytosis, megaloblastic anemia and purpura, co-trimoxazole may induce hemolysis in certain most are mild and comprise nausea, with or without vomiting, and skin rashes. Fatalities, although rare, have occurred due to severe reactions, including Stevens–Johnson syndrome, Lyell syndrome (toxic epidermal necrolysis), fulminant hepatic necrosis, agranulocytosis, aplastic anemias. The majority of hematological changes are mild and reversible when treatment is stopped. The changes are mainly leukopenia, neutropenia, thrombocytopenia and less commonly, agranulocytosis, megaloblastic anemia and purpura, co-trimoxazole may induce hemolysis in certain susceptible G6PD deficient patients. At the high dosages used for the therapy of PCP, rash, fever neutropenia, thrombocytopenia and raised liver enzymes have been reported, necessitating cessation of therapy. Concomitant administration of IV chlorpheniramine may permit continued infusion.

Contd...

Contd...

Contd...

Drug	Brand name	Dosage	Contraindications	Drug interaction	Side effects
Erythromycin	Althrocin, Erytop	*General indications neonates:* Orally/IV less than 7 days age 20 mg/kg per day two times daily; more than 7 days less than 1,200 g 20 mg/kg per day two times daily; more than 7 days more than 1,200 g 30 mg/kg per day three to four times daily. *Children:* Orally; 30–50 mg/kg per day in three to four divided doses maximum 250 mg four times daily may be given; 12–18 years, 250–500 mg four times daily. IV: 1 month to 18 years 12.5 mg/kg per dose four times daily or as a continuous infusion. *Maximum dose:* 4 g/day. Replace by oral dosage as soon as possible. *Special Indications* *Topical (acne vulgaris):* Wash and apply twice daily directly to the affected area. Secondary prevention of rheumatic fever: when child is sensitive to penicillin, oral 20 mg/kg per day max 500 mg twice daily (contraindicated in liver disorder). *Chlamydia trachomatis* pneumonia in infants and neonates: Oral 50 mg/kg per day (erythromycin base) in four divided doses for 14 days. Ophthalmia neonatorum caused by *Chlamydia trachomatis.* *Neonates:* Oral 50 mg/kg per day in four divided doses for 14 days. If chlamydial conjunctivitis recurs after discontinuing therapy, the erythromycin dosage regimen should be repeated. GAS pharyngitis (primary rheumatic fever prophylaxis as an alternative to penicillin in children allergic to penicillin)—40 mg/kg/day in 4 divided doses × 10 days. Cardiology Subchapter of IAP does not recommend using erythromycin for this indication. Uncomplicated urethral, endocervical, or rectal gonorrhea, penicillinase-producing *Neisseria gonorrhoeae,* or for gonorrhea during pregnancy. *Adolescent:* 500 mg PO four times per day for 7 days. Treatment and post-exposure pertussis prophylaxis— (For post-exposure prophylaxis, administer to close contacts within 3 weeks of exposure, especially in high-risk patients (e.g. women in 3rd trimester, infants <12 months). *Oral dosage:* Infants, children, and adolescents—40–50 mg/kg/per day PO (maximum 2 g/day) in four divided doses for 14 days. *For neonates:* Azithromycin is the preferred. If azithromycin is unavailable, erythromycin 40–50 mg/kg/per day PO in four divided doses may be used. Monitor for infantile hypertrophic pyloric stenosis. Pneumococcal prophylaxis: 1 month and 2 years; 250 mg/day; 2–8 years; 500 mg/day, more than 9 years 1 g/day in two divided doses. *Gastric stasis:* Oral/IV 1 month and 18 years 3 mg/kg 4 times daily.	Known hypersensitivity to erythromycin. Contraindicated with terfenadine, cisapride, astemizole, ergotamine and dihydroergotamine. Concurrent topical acne therapy should be used with caution because a cumulative irritant effect may occur.	Increased risk of cardiotoxicity with terfenadine, cisapride or astemizole. Increased serum concentrations of carbamazepine, digoxin, warfarin, phenytoin, theophylline, cyclosporin, disopyramide, midazolam and alfentanil.	Nausea, abdominal pain, vomiting, diarrhea. Reversible hearing loss with high doses. Allergic reactions anaphylaxis is rare. Cardiac arrhythmias have been very rarely reported and isolated reports of chest pain, dizziness and palpitations. Venous irritation can occur with IV administration, but if the injection is diluted and given slowly as outlined above, pain and venous trauma are minimized.

Contd...

Contd...

Drug	Brand name	Dosage	Contraindications	Drug interaction	Side effects
Furazolidone	Furoxone	*Oral:* 1 month to 12 years 6 mg/kg per day in four divided doses and 12–18 years 400 mg/day in four divided doses. 7–10 days for giardiasis and for 4–6 days after defervescence in typhoid fever.	Prior sensitivity to furazolidone. Furazolidone may cause mild, reversible intravascular hemolysis in G6PD deficient patients. Such patients should be closely observed and furazolidone treatment stopped if any evidence of hemolysis occurs. Furazolidone should not be given to infants less than 1 month of age (who have immature enzyme systems and glutathione instability) because of the possibility of producing hemolytic anemia. Furazolidone is a monoamine oxidase inhibitor (MAOI) and the cautions advised for MAOIs regarding the concomitant administration of other drugs, especially indirect acting sympathomimetic amines, and the consumption of food and drink containing tyramine should be observed; however, there appear to be no reports of hypertensive crisis in patients receiving furazolidone. Darkening of the urine due to the presence of metabolites.	*Alcohol:* A disulfiram like reaction has been reported in patients consuming alcohol whilst on furazolidone; alcohol should be avoided for the duration of treatment and for 4 days thereafter to prevent this reaction.	Nausea and vomiting are the most common side-effects and abdominal pain, diarrhea, headache and malaise occur occasionally. Hypersensitivity reactions including a fall in blood pressure, urticaria, fever, arthralgia, and a vesicular morbilliform rash have occurred in a small number of patients.
Gentamicin	Garamycin, Genticyn Eye/Ear, G-Mycin	Many dose regimens exist for aminoglycosides depending on target concentration aimed for and patient groups treated. The dose regimens shown here are generally accepted initial doses and dose adjustments should be made in the light of serum concentration measurement. *Neonates:* IV/IM less than 7 days 1,200–2,000 g 2.5 mg/kg once in 12–18 hrs and more than 2,000 g 2.5 mg/kg once in 12 hrs; more than 7 days 1,200–2,000 g 2.5 mg/kg once in 8–12 hrs and more than 2,000 g 2.5 mg/kg once in 8 hrs. Extended interval dose regimen by slow intravenous injection or intravenous infusion: less than 32 weeks gestation 4–5 mg/kg every 35 hrs; more than 32 weeks gestation 4–5 mg/kg every 24 hrs.	Known hypersensitivity to gentamicin, myasthenia gravis. Patients should be well hydrated during therapy and renal function monitored. In patients with impaired renal function dosage and/or frequency of administration must be adjusted in response to serum drug concentrations and the extent of renal impairment. The 'child single daily dose regimen' is not recommended in children with renal impairment.	Increased risk of ototoxicity and nephrotoxicity with cephalosporins, vancomycin, cyclosporin, cisplatin, diuretics, such as frusemide, amphotericin, indomethacin. Enhances effects of non-depolarizing muscle relaxants. Calcium IV may reverse this effect. May antagonize effects of neostigmine and pyridostigmine. Contra-indicated in myasthenia gravis. Aminoglycosides have a magnesium-like effect	Nephrotoxicity and ototoxicity can occur if optimum blood levels are exceeded; unlikely if nebulized. Bronchospasm can occur with nebulized gentamicin. Epithelial toxicity may occur with high doses or prolonged use of eyedrops.

Contd...

Drug	Brand name	Dosage	Contraindications	Drug interaction	Side effects
		Children: Less than 12 year 7.5 mg/kg/day and 12–18 year 3–6 mg/kg/per day in 3 divided doses. Plasma levels done after 3–4 doses to achieve predose level of less than 2 mg/L and 1 hr post dose peak of 5 mg/L. Alternatively 5–7.5 mg/kg/24 hr IV once daily. Plasma levels done 18–24 hr after 1st dose to achieve predose level of less than 1 mg/l and 1 hr post dose peak of 16–20 mg/L. Once daily dose regimen (not for endocarditis or meningitis) by intravenous infusion—child 1 month–18 years—initially 7 mg/kg, then adjusted according to serum-gentamicin concentration. Intrathecal/ventricular-preservative free preparation. *Newborn:* 1 mg/24 hr; children 1–2 mg/24 hr; 16–18 year. Pseudomonal lung infection in cystic fibrosis. By inhalation of nebulized solution. Child: 1 month–2 years 40 mg twice daily; Child: 2–8 years; 80 mg twice daily; Child: 8–18 years, 160 mg twice daily. 0.3% eye drops—1–2 drops up to 6 times/day. In severe infections 1 drop every 15–20 min and gradually decreasing frequency as infection gets controlled till 48 hrs after healing. 1.5% eye drops for severe eye infection. Ear drops: 2–3 drops 3–4 times daily and at night; children and adults.	Ear drops should not be used if there is perforation of the ear drum. Hearing tests are recommended for cystic fibrosis patients having repeated courses of aminoglycosides. Care must be taken in children with hepatic and renal impairment as systemic absorption occurs when eye drops are given in high doses.	acting at the neuromuscular junction prejunctionally to reduce transmitter release and postjunctionally to reduce receptor sensitivity.	
Imipenem with cilastatin	Zienam	*Newborn:* IV 20 mg/kg/per dose in the frequency—less than 7 days, 7–21 days and more than 21 days at 2 times, 3 times and 4 times daily, respectively. *Children:* IV less than 3 months 80 mg/kg/per day, 3 month; 12 years 60 mg/kg/day, 12–18 years 2 g/day in 4 divided doses. (max/dose < 12 years 500 > 12 year 1 g).	Caution in beta-lactam allergy as partial cross-sensitivity has been demonstrated. Monitor LFTs carefully in patients with preexisting liver disease	Use with caution with nephrotoxic drugs. May cause positive Coombs' test without hemolysis. Probenecid inhibits renal excretion of cilastatin. General seizures with ganciclovir. Little evidence of other interactions though no formal studies have been done.	Local irritation at injection site, skin rashes, gastrointestinal upset, pseudomembranous colitis reported rarely, reversible neutropenia, thrombocytopenia, eosinophilia, and thrombocytosis reported, raised LFTs may occur. Adverse CNS effects, such as seizures have been reported, particularly in patients with underlying CNS disorders, bacterial meningitis or poor renal function.
Linezolid	Linox, Linospan	Intravenous (IV) infusion over 30–120 min: Pre-term neonates less than 7 days old (gestational age <34 weeks): 10 mg/kg 12th hourly for 14–28 days; 10 mg/kg 8th hourly in those with a suboptimal Clinical response; neonates, infants, and children less than 12 years: 10 mg/kg 8th hourly for 14–28 days. Linezolid is not recommended for empiric treatment of acute CNS infections. Children exhibit variability in drug clearance and systemic exposure. Those with VP shunts achieve variable cerebrospinal fluid (CSF) therapeutic concentrations; more than and equal to 12 years: 600 mg 12th hourly for 14–28 days. May give aztreonam or aminoglycosides concurrently if indicated.	Hypersensitivity	Linezolid is a reversible, nonselective inhibitor of monoamine oxidase. When vasopressor or dopaminergic agents are co-administered, the initial doses should be reduced and titrated to achieve the desired response and reduce the incidence of serotonin syndrome. Adrenergic drugs, such as dopamine, epinephrine,	Diarrhea, headache, nausea, abnormal liver function test, fever, moniliasis, vaginal and oral moniliasis, skin rash, thrombocytopenia, vomiting, constipation, dizziness, dysgeusia, insomnia, anemia, bone marrow depression, leukopenia and pancytopenia, pseudomembranous colitis.

Contd...

Contd...

Drug	Brand name	Dosage	Contraindications	Drug interaction	Side effects
		Oral: Acolescents, and children more than and equal to 12 years: 600 mg 12th hourly for 10–14 days. *Term:* Neonates, infants, and children less than 12 years: 10 mg/kg 8th hourly for 10–14 days. Pre-term neonates less than 7 days old (gestational age <34 weeks): 10 mg/kg 12th hourly for 10–14 days; 10 mg/kg 8th hourly in those with a suboptimal clinical response.		phenylpropanolamine, psuedoephedrine may cause hypertension. Monitor blood pressure and heart rate. Increased blood pressure may occur when linezolid is used with diet high in tyramine.	
Meropenem	Meronem	*Newborn:* 40 mg/kg/day in two divided doses less than 7 days and in three divided doses more than 7 days. Double dose in meningitis and severe infection. Children UTI, gynecological, skin and soft tissue infection: 30 mg/kg in three divided doses (max 500 mg/dose) Pneumonia, peritonitis, neutropenia, septicemia: 60 mg/kg/ per day in three divided doses (max 1 g/dose) Meningitis and life-threatening infections: 120 mg/kg/day in 3 divided doses (max 2 ɡ/dose). In renal impairment: Cr Cl (mL/min/1.73 m²) 25–50 give full dose but at 12 hrs intervals, 10–25, 50% dose at 12 hrs intervals less than 10–50% dose at 24 hour interval.	Caution in beta-lactam allergy as partial cross-sensitivity between penicillins and cephalosporins has been demonstrated. Monitor LFTs carefully in patients with preexisting liver disease.	Use with caution with nephrotoxic drugs. May cause positive Coombs' test without hemolysis. Probenecid inhibits renal excretion of meropenem. Little evidence of other interactions though no formal studies have been done.	Local irritation at injection site, skin rashes, gastrointestinal upset, pseudomembranous colitis reported rarely, reversible neutropenia, thrombocytopenia, eosinophilia, and thrombocythemia reported, raised LFTs may occur, adverse CNS effects such as seizures have been reported particularly in patients with underlying CNS disorders, bacterial meningitis or poor renal function.
Minocycline	Cynomycin	*Oral:* 50 mg/dose two times daily for minimum of 6 weeks.	Contraindicated in children less than 12 years. Avoid in complete renal failure. Use with caution in patients with hepatic dysfunction.	With oral contraceptives possibility of contraceptive failure. Do not use with penicillins. Reduced doses of concomitant anticoagulants may be necessary. Absorption impaired by antacids. Iron, calcium, magnesium, aluminum and size salts.	*Gastrointestinal:* Nausea, vomiting, diarrhea. *Skin:* Severe exfoliative rashes; photosensitivity-hyperpigmentation. Hypersensitivity reactions including urticaria, anaphylaxis, SLE.
Netilmicin	Netromycin	Newborn IV 3 mg/dose 12th hourly. Increase to 8th hourly after 1 week age postnatal. Monitor after 3rd dose for 1 hr post dose peak of 8–12 mg/L and a trough of < 3 mg/L. Prolong dose interval in PDA, prolonged hypoxia and indomethacin therapy. *Children:* IV/IM less than 12 years 7.5 mg/kg/day and more than 12 years 6 mg/kg/ per day in three divided doses or 1 month–18 years 7.5 mg/kg as single dose daily. Intraperitoneal 7.5–10 mg/L in peritoneal dialysis fluid.	Hypersensitivity to other aminoglycosides. Contraindicated in myasthenia gravis. Aminoglycosides have a magnesium-like effect acting at the neuromuscular junction prejunctionally to reduce transmitter release and postjunctionally to reduce receptor sensitivity.	Increased risk of ototoxicity and nephrotoxicity with cephalosporins, vancomycin, cyclosporin, cisplatin, diuretics such as frusemide, amphotericin. Enhances effects of nondepolarizing muscle relaxants. Calcium IV may reverse this effect. Antagonizes effects of neostigmine and pyridostigmine.	As with all aminoglycosides nephrotoxicity and ototoxicity can occur if optimum blood levels are exceeded. May be a more potent neuromuscular blocking agent.

Contd...

Contd...

Drug	Brand name	Dosage	Contraindications	Drug interaction	Side effects
Nitrofurantoin	Furadantin, Niftran	Contraindicated in infants less than 3 month age. UTI treatment 3 month–12 years 5–7 mg/kg/per day and in 12–18 year 200–400 mg/day in four divided doses. *UTI prophylaxis:* 1–2.5 mg/kg/day in at bedtime or in two divided doses (max 100 mg/24 hrs).	Nitrofurantoin should not be given to infant less than 3 months of age or to pregnant patients at term (during labor and delivery) because of the theoretical possibility of hemolytic anemia in the fetus or the newborn infant due to immature erythrocyte enzyme systems. It is also contraindicated in patients with a creatinine clearance less than 60 mL/minute per 1.73 m² and in anyone with hypersensitivity to nitrofurantoin or other nitrofurans. Contraindicated in patients with G6PD deficiency.	Concurrent administration with magnesium trisilicate reduces absorption. Uricosuric drugs, such as probenecid and sulfinpyrazone may inhibit renal tubular secretion of nitrofurantoin; the resulting increase in serum levels may increase toxicity and decreased urinary levels could lessen the efficacy of nitrofurantoin as a urinary tract antibacterial. There may be decreased antibacterial activity in the presence of carbonic anhydrase inhibitors and urine alkalinizing agents.	*Gastrointestinal:* Nausea, anorexia and less commonly vomiting, abdominal pain and diarrhea. *Respiratory:* Acute and chronic pulmonary reactions (may be associated with lupus erythematosus-like syndrome). *Hepatic:* Rarely cholestatic jaundice and hepatitis. *Neurological:* Peripheral neuropathy reported infrequently. *Hematological:* Agranulocytosis, leukopenia, granulocytopenia, hemolytic anemia, thrombocytopenia, G6PD deficiency, megaloblastic anemia and eosinophilia have occurred. *Hypersensitivity:* Allergic skin reactions including pruritus; exfoliative dermatitis and erythema have been reported rarely. *Other:* Benign intracranial hypertension, transient alopecia. Superinfections by fungi or resistant organisms, such as *Pseudomonas* may occur, limited to the genitor-urinary tract.
Ofloxacin	Of, Oflox Eye, Zenflox E/E drops	*Eyedrops:* More than 1 year one drop 2–4 hourly for 1st 48 hrs and then 4 times daily till 2 days after healing is achieved (max 10 days). *Eardrops:* Otitis externa; 1–12 year 5 drops and 12–18 year 10 drops to affected ear(s) 2 times daily for 10 days. CSOM: More than 12 years 10 drops to affected ear(s) 2 times daily for 14 days. AOM with perforation or with tympanostomy tubes; 1–12 year, 5 drops to affected ear(s) 2 times daily for 10 days. IV and oral: 10–15 mg/kg/per day in a single dose or divided twice daily. *Systemic use:* it is replaced by levofloxacin which is an S-isomer of ofloxacin and has less side effects.	Avoid in kidney disease, children with epilepsy; or those with a history of head injury or brain tumor. Hypersensitivity to quinolones. Should not take antacids that contain magnesium or aluminum, sucralfate, didanosine, and vitamin or mineral supplements that contain iron or zinc within the 2 hrs before or after administering ofloxacin orally. Taking these		Ofloxacin may cause upset stomach, diarrhea, vomiting, stomach pain, headache, dizziness, numbness, restlessness, difficulty falling asleep or staying asleep, skin rash, itching, difficulty breathing or swallowing, swelling of the face or throat, yellowing of the skin or eyes, dark urine, pale or dark stools, blood in urine, unusual tiredness, sunburn, seizures, vaginal infection,

Contd...

Contd...

Drug	Brand name	Dosage	Contraindications	Drug interaction	Side effects
			other medicines too close to oral ofloxacin can make the antibiotic much less effective.		vision changes, pain, inflammation, or rupture of a tendon. Eye drops may cause transient ocular irritation, including photophobia and burning. Otic use may be associated with pruritus, local irritation, burning, taste perversion, dizziness and earache.
Oxytetracycline	Oxytetracycline, Terramycin, Terramycin SF	*Acne:* Oral: 12–18 years 250–500 mg/dose 12th hourly. *Infections:* 250–500 mg/dose 6th hourly.	Avoid in liver or renal impairment. Contraindicated in children less than 12 years as it adversely affects tooth development (discoloration and enamel hypoplasia).	Absorption may be impaired by aluminum, calcium, magnesium, zinc or iron salts. Long-term therapy depresses plasma prothrombin activity so anticoagulant dose may need to be reduced. Concurrent use of oral contraception-possibility of reduced contraceptive effect.	*Gastrointestinal:* Nausea, vomiting, diarrhea. *Skin:* Maculopapular and erythematous rashes. Photosensitivity: discontinue if erythema occurs. *Hypersensitivity reactions:* Urticaria, anaphylaxis. *Blood:* Hemolytic anemia, thrombocytopenia, neutropenia and eosinophilia.
Penicillins (Benzylpenicillin/ Penicillin G)	Benzylpenicillin	Given IV. n newborn—25 mg (approx 40,000 units)/ kg/ per dose 2 times daily up to 7 days of age and 3 times daily thereafter. Dose is doubled in meningitis. In children 25 mg/ kg/per dose 4 times daily. Double dose is given in meningitis 6 times daily to a maximum single dose of 2.4 g (approx 40 lakh units) and a maximum daily dose of 14.4 g (approx 2.3 crore units).	Hypersensitivity to beta-lactam. Cautious use in renal and hepatic impairment.	Oral contraceptives—interferes with enterohepatic circulation of these pills and thus reduce efficacy. Probenecid retards renal excretion of penicillin.	Hypersensitivity— rash, urticaria, fever, bronchospam, vasculitis, serum sickness, exfoliative dermatitis, Stevens–Johnson syndrome and anaphylaxis.
Phenoxymethyl-penicillin (Penicillin V)	Kaypen	Oral: 250 mg/day, 1–5 year; 500 mg/day, 6–12 year and 1 g/ day and 12–18 years 2 g/day (severe infection 3 g/day) in four divided doses. Pneumococcal infection prophylaxis— half the above daily dose in two divided doses. *Rheumatic fever prophylaxis:* 500 mg/day in two divided doses.	Penicillin hypersensitivity.	*Guar gum:* Reduced absorption of phenoxymethylpenicillin; probenecid, reduced excretion of penicillins; oral contraceptives possibility of reduced contraceptive effect.	Hypersensitivity reactions, including urticaria, fever, joint pains, rashes, angioedema, anaphylaxis, serum sickness-like reactions, hemolytic anemia, and interstitial nephritis, neutropenia, thrombocytopenia, coagulation disorders and central nervous system toxicity reported (especially with high doses or in severe renal impairment); paresthesia with prolonged use; diarrhea and antibiotic-associated colitis have also been reported.

Contd...

Drug	Brand name	Dosage	Contraindications	Drug interaction	Side effects
Piperacillin with tazobactam	Pipracil, Pipzo, Piptaz, Piprapen Injection	Newborn IV 90 mg/kg per dose three times daily. Children IV 90 mg/kg per dose four times daily (max single dose 4.5 g).	Allergy to penicillins or hypersensitivity to any ingredients of the preparation.	Possible prolonged prothrombin time with warfarin. May prolong the action of neuromuscular blocking agents, e.g. vecuronium. May reduce excretion of methotrexate.	Serious and occasionally fatal anaphylactic reactions have occurred. Rarely liver disorders, blood dyscrasias and dermatological manifestations have been reported. Rarely renal failure may occur.
Rifampicin	Ticin, Zucox	*Tuberculosis in combination with other drugs:* Oral 10 mg/kg (max 600 mg/day) as single morning dose. Meningococcal infection prophylaxis and staphylococcal infections: Oral less than 5 year 5 mg/kg/per dose and more than 1 year 10 mg/kg/per dose (max 600 mg/dose) 2 times daily for 2 days for meningococcal infection prophylaxis and for 10–14 days for staphylococcal infections. *H. influenzae prophylaxis:* Oral less than 3 months 10 mg/kg and more than 3 months 20 mg/kg/per dose (max 600 mg/dose) once daily. *Cholestasis:* Pruritus—5–10 mg/kg (max 600 mg) once daily. Dose adjustment in liver failure. Avoid altogether, or reduce doses for tuberculosis and prophylaxis to 8 mg/kg daily.	Patients who are hypersensitive to rifamycins. Although not recommended for use in patients with jaundice, the therapeutic benefit should be weighed against the possible risks.	Induces liver enzymes reducing plasma levels of many drugs, e.g. anticoagulants, cyclosporin, phenytoin, phenobarbital (phenobarbitone), theophylline, digoxin, most benzodiazepines, fluconazole and dose adjustment of these may be necessary if they are given concurrently with rifampicin.	*Gastrointestinal:* These include anorexia, nausea, vomiting, abdominal discomfort, diarrhea; pseudomembranous colitis has been reported. *Skin:* Flushing, urticaria, rash. *Hematological:* Thrombocytopenia with or without purpura, leukopenia, eosinophilia. Reactions occurring mainly on intermittent therapy and probably of immunological origin include 'flu-like symptoms (with chills, fever, dizziness, bone pain), shortness of breath and wheezing, acute hemolytic anemia, acute renal failure and thrombocytopenic purpura, alterations of liver function. Other side effects have included edema, muscular weakness, and menstrual disturbances.
Roxithromycin	Biorox, Roxid, Roxyrol	*Dosage:* Adolescents 150 mg twice daily at least 15 minutes before meals. *Children:* 5–8 mg/kg per day in two divided doses for not more than 10 days.	Concomitant use of ergotamine type compounds.	*Digoxin:* Increases absorption. *Midazolam:* Increases its half-life. *Terfenadine:* Serum levels elevated leading to ventricular arrhythmias *Disopyramide:* Displaced from its protein bound sites.	Nausea, vomiting, diarrhea, skin rash and transient rise in liver transaminase.

Contd...

Contd...

Drug	Brand name	Dosage	Contraindications	Drug interaction	Side effects
Spiramycin	Rovamycin	Pregnant women with suspected or confirmed toxoplasma infection: 1.5 g (4.5 million international units) orally twice daily until term if the fetus is not infected.	Previous sensitivity to spiramycin. Use with caution in patients with a hypersensitivity to other macrolide antibiotics as cross-sensitivity between erythromycin and spiramycin has been reported (cutaneous reactions); liver disease as spiramycin is potentially hepatotoxic; those with gastrointestinal disorders as these may be exacerbated; cardiac disease as spiramycin may be capable of inducing adverse cardiovascular effects, including adverse cardiovascular effects, including QT interval prolongation.	None of significance.	Relatively infrequent and include nausea, vomiting, diarrhea, epigastric pain, dizziness, headache, and cutaneous hypersensitivity reactions. Hepatotoxicity, thrombocytopenia, vasculitis, colitis, and QT prolongation have been reported, rarely.
Streptomycin	Ambistryn-S	*Adolescents:* 0.75–1 g daily by IM route. *Children:* 20–40 mg/kg per day IM.	Diseases of ear, hypersensitivity.	Aminoglycosides, amphotericin B, bacitracin, cisplatin, cephalothin, vancomycin, methoxyflurane ethacrynic acid, frusemide, bumetanide and mannitol: increased ototoxic, neurotoxic or nephrotoxic affects. Anesthetics, neuromuscular blocking agents (tubocurarine, gallamine): Risk of neuromuscular blockade and respiratory paralysis. Penicillin, cephalosporins, carbenicillin, ticarcillin—exert antibiotic synergism, especially useful in *Pseudomonas* infections. *Lab tests:* Aminoglycoside serum levels, guard against *in vitro* inactivation of aminoglycosides by beta-lactum antibiotics in patients on combination therapy.	Pain at injection site, ototoxicity, nephrotoxicity, skin rash, fever, exfoliative dermatitis and eosinophilia. Anaphylaxis rarely seen. Optic nerve dysfunction.

Contd...

Contd...

Drug	Brand name	Dosage	Contraindications	Drug interaction	Side effects
Sulfadiazine	Sulfadiazine	Less than 12 years, 100–200 mg/kg per day and 12–18 years 4–6 g/day in four divided doses.	Patients with a history of sulfonamide sensitivity; those with G6PD deficiency as it may precipitate hemolysis; acute porphyria; renal or hepatic failure. Caution in hepatic and renal impairment. Avoid sun exposure. Give calcium folinate (folinic acid) during long-term therapy.	Warfarin effects enhanced. Phenytoin antifolate effect and plasma concentration increased. Methotrexate displaced from albumin binding sites; increases the risk of methotrexate toxicity. Avoid ascorbic acid as the likelihood of crystalluria and renal damage is increased when the urine is acid. Pyrimethamine antibacterial action potentiated by sulfadiazine. Cyclosporin plasma concentration possibly reduced.	Nausea, vomiting, rash (including rarely Stevens–Johnson syndrome; discontinue if rash occurs), liver damage, blood disorders, discontinue therapy, nephrotoxicity including crystalluria; maintain high fluid intake, serum-sickness type of reaction (3–17 days after start of therapy), headache, dizziness.
Teicoplanin	Ticocin	*Newborn:* Loading 16 mg/kg and 24 hrs later start maintenance 8 mg/kg per day as single dose; children 10 mg/kg per dose two times daily × 3 doses and then once daily in same dose for severe infection and 6 mg/kg per day once for mod infection. Orally for pseudomembranous colitis 10 mg/kg per dose two times daily. May be given intraventricular and intraperitoneal.	Previous hypersensitivity reaction to teicoplanin. Cross hypersensitivity to vancomycin may occur but vancomycin-induced 'red man syndrome' is not a contraindication to teicoplanin.	No specific interactions known. No evidence of synergistic toxicity with other neurotoxic or nephrotoxic agents. However, monitoring of renal and auditory function is advised when such combinations are used.	Local irritation on injection is the most frequent side effect. Allergic and anaphylactic reactions, such as rash and fever. Transient increase in serum creatinine and liver enzymes. Thrombocytopenia (especially at higher than recommended doses) and other blood dyscrasias rarely reported.
Tetracycline	Hostacycline, Resteclin	*Acne:* Topical application 2 times daily for max 10–12 weeks/ may be repeated after 12 weeks interval. *Aphthous ulceration:* Local mouth wash with contents of 250 mg cap of tetracycline in water 3–4 times daily for 2–3 min each time (do not swallow) for 3 days.	Hypersensitivity. Avoid in renal impairment. Tetracycline is contraindicated in children less than 12 years of age.		*Topical preparation:* Some patients may experience stinging or tingling sensations, skin rashes and skin discoloration. *Mouthwash:* Fungal superinfection.
Tobramycin	Tobacin, Tobraneg	*Newborn:* IV less than 32 weeks 4–5 mg/kg 36 hourly and more than 32 weeks 4–5 mg/kg once in 24 hrs. Patent ductus arteriosus (PDA), prolonged hypoxia, indomethacin treatment necess tate increased dose intervals. Extended interval dose regi nen by intravenous injection over 3–5 minutes or by intravenous infusion. Neonate less than 32 weeks postmenstrual age 4–5 mg/kg every 36 hrs; neonate 32 weeks and over postmenstrual age 4–5 mg/kg every 24 hrs. Child:IV/IM 2.5 mg/kg per dose three times daily or 7 mg/kg as single daily dose. Once daily dose regimen by intravenous infusion.	Patients with known hypersensitivity to tobramycin. Bronchospasm may occur when nebulized treatment with a beta-agonist. Hearing tests are recommended for cystic fibrosis patients receiving repeated courses of aminoglycosides. Monitor baseline renal function when on regular nebulization and then every 6 months.	Negligible when nebulized or given orally as systemic absorption very low. For details of interactions when given parenterally, see gentamicin monograph.	Bronchospasm can occur, if nebulized. Impaired renal function and ototoxicity can occur if optimum blood levels are exceeded. Minimal risk of these effects if nebulized or given orally. Eye-drops may cause epithelial toxicity.

Contd...

Drug	Brand name	Dosage	Contraindications	Drug interaction	Side effects
		Child: 1 month to 18 years, initially 7 mg/kg, then adjusted according to serum-tobramycin concentration. Pseudomonal lung infect on in cystic fibrosis. *Child*: 1 month to 18 years 8–10 mg/kg per daily in three divided doses. Once daily dose regimen by intravenous infusion over 30 minutes: Child: 1 month to 18 years, initially 10 mg/kg (max. 660 mg), then adjusted according to serum-tobramycin concentration. Chronic pulmonary *Pseudomonas aeruginosc* infection in patients with cystic fibrosis: by inhalation of nebulized solution. *Child*: 6–18 years 300 mg every 12 hours for 28 days, subsequent courses repeated after 28 days interval without tobramycin nebulizer solution. *Intraventricular*: Newborn 1 mg/day, child 1–2 mg/day, adolescent 2–4 mg/day. *Eye drops*: One drop 2 hourly and then reduce frequency as infection is controlled. To continue till 2 days after healing.			
Vancomycin	Vancocin CP, Vancoled, Vansafe, Vanlid, Vancogen	*Newborn*: V 15 mg/kg per dose less than 28 weeks once daily, 29–35 weeks twice daily and more than 35 weeks three times daily. Intrathecal all newborn 2.5–5 mg once daily child IV 15 mg/kg loading dose followed by 10 mg/kg per dose four times daily (max 2 g/day). Intrathecal 1 month to 4 years 5 mg; 4–15 years 10 mg and more than 15 years 20 mg; once daily. Children with enlarged ventricles need higher doses. Adjust dose according to Cerebrospinal fluid (CSF) levels aiming fo a trough level of less than 10 mg/L.	Hypersensitivity to vancomycin. Too rapid infusion may be associated with 'redman' syndrome. Not for IM use. Interactions 1. Concurrent administration with other nephrotoxic drugs (e.g. aminoglycosides, amphotericin B) requires careful monitoring of renal function as the nephrotoxicity may be additive. 2. Diuretics such as frusemide may enhance ototoxicity. 3. Vancomycin may enhance neuromuscular blockade produced by drugs such as suxamethonium and vecuronium.	Concurrent use of other potentially nephrotoxic drugs, such as aminoglycosides and amphotericin B requires careful monitoring. Concurrent administration of vancomycin and anesthetic agents has been associated with erythema, histamine-like flushing and anaphylactoid reactions.	Nephrotoxicity; ototoxicity (enhanced by aminoglycoside therapy) rarely if serum levels are kept below 30 mg/L. *Rash and hypotension*: Usually related to duration of infusion and resolves with increasing infusion time. *Neutropenia*: Reported after prolonged administration (> 3 weeks). *Phlebitis*: May be minimized with slow infusion related events ('redman' syndrome); miscellaneous; see manufacturers statistical process control (SPC) for details.
Antileprotic					
Dapsone	Dapsone	*Leprosy*: Oral 1–2 mg/kg per day as single dose in combination with rifampicin. Blistering skin conditions: Start at 500 μg/kg per day and increase or decrease as necessary in 12.5 mg increments.	Use with caution in cardiac or pulmonary disease, anemia (treat severe anemia first), G6PD deficiency.	Plasma concentration reduced by rifamycins. Probenecid reduces dapsone excretion-increased risk of side effects.	Dose related. CNS: Peripheral neuropathy, insomnia, headache. *Dermatologic*: Exfoliative dermatitis. *Gastrointestinal*: Nausea, vomiting, cholestatic jaundice.

Contd...

Contd...

Drug	Brand name	Dosage	Contraindications	Drug interaction	Side effects
					Hematological: Hemolytic anemia, methemoglobinemia, leukopenia, agranulocytosis. Hepatic: Hepatitis. *Ocular:* Blurred vision. *Otic:* Tinnitus. May develop dapsone hypersensitivity syndrome (fever, rash, lymphadenopathy, liver dysfunction)—a rare idiosyncratic reaction, within the first 6 weeks of therapy and lasting for up to 4 weeks.
Antituberculous drug					
Ethambutol	Albutol, Combutol	Following oral administration, absorption is approximately 80%. The drug is well distributed throughout the body with high concentrations in kidneys, lungs, saliva and red blood cells. Half-life is approximately 2.5–3.6 hours but this can be up to 7 hours or longer with renal impairment. 20% metabolism in the liver to inactive metabolite. Approximately, 50% excreted in the urine and 20% in the feces as unchanged drug.	Patients known to be hypersensitive to the drug; patients with known optic neuritis unless clinical judgment determines that it may be used. Patients who cannot understand warnings about visual side-effects should, if possible, be given an alternative drug. In particular, ethambutol should be used with caution in children until they are at least 5 years old capable of reporting symptomatic visual changes accurately. Patients should undergo a full ophthalmic examination before starting treatment. This should include visual acuity, color vision, perimetry and ophthalmoscopy. Thereafter, routine ophthalmological examinations may be considered desirable when treating young children (for the reasons outlined above) and older children/adults should be informed of the importance of reporting any change in vision.	Aluminum salts can decrease ethambutol levels.	Optic neuritis, red/green color blindness, peripheral neuritis, rarely rash, pruritus, urticaria, thrombocytopenia. Gastrointestinal symptoms such as nausea, vomiting and diarrhea have been reported in patients on multiple-drug antituberculous therapy but not in patients receiving ethambutol as sole therapy.

Contd...

Contd...

Drug	Brand name	Dosage	Contraindications	Drug interaction	Side effects
Isoniazid	Isokin, Sonex	5 mg/kg per day.	Should not be given patients with a history of isoniazid sensitivity. Baseline LFTs and then monitor hepatic function in all patients, use with caution in hepatic impairment. Use with caution in renal impairment; dosage adjustments are generally not necessary until creatinine clearance falls to 10 mL/minute per 1.73 m²; such patients, and patients with slow acetylator status may require a dose reduction to maintain trough plasma levels of 1mg/L.	The metabolism of phenytoin, carbamazepine and diazepam may be reduced by isoniazid. The absorption of isoniazid may be reduced by concurrent administration of antacids. Corticosteroid effects of prednisolone may be enhanced.	Isoniazid is generally well tolerated; the only common side-effect is peripheral neuropathy which is more likely to occur if there are preexisting risk factors such as malnutrition, chronic renal failure, diabetes and HIV infection. In children, supplemental pyridoxine is not necessary, except for breast-fed infants and malnourished children. When given, the daily pyridoxine prophylaxis dosage in neonates is 5 mg, children 5–10 mg, adults 10 mg. The following have been reported less frequently; nausea, vomiting, optic neuritis, convulsions, psychotic episodes, hypersensitivity reactions, allergic skin reactions, hyperglycemis, hepatitis. Although hepatitis occurs only rarely, patients and their carers should be told how to recognize signs of liver disorder and to seek medical attention, if symptoms such as persistent nausea, vomiting, malaise or jaundice develop.
Para-amino-salicyclic-acid (PAS)	Monopas, Q-PAS	*Adolescents:* 14–16 g/day in 2–3 divided doses. *Children:* 275–420 mg/kg per day in 3–4 divided doses.	Severe hypersensitivity to aminosalicylate sodium and its congeners.	*Digoxin:* Oral absorption of digoxin reduced with subsequent reduction in serum levels of PAS. Vitamin B_{12}: PAS interferes with GI absorption of vitamin B_{12} leading to deficiency. Parenteral vitamin B_{12} may be required.	Nausea, vomiting, diarrhea, abdominal pain.

Contd...

Contd...

598 Textbook of Pediatric Infectious Diseases

Drug	Brand name	Dosage	Contraindications	Drug interaction	Side effects
Pyrazinamide	Pyzina, PZA Ciba	Oral children 15–40 mg/kg per 24 hours as single dose or in two divided doses (max 2 g/day) for the first 2 months of the standard 6 months regimen. 12–18 years less than 50 kg 1.5 g/day and more than 50 kg 2 g/day as single dose or in two divided doses (max 2 g/day) for the first 2 months of the standard 6 month regimen.	Caution with use in children due to hepatotoxicity. Monitor liver function before and during treatment. Baseline and regular monitoring of liver function is required in patients with known chronic liver disease and in those known to be hepatitis B or C antigen positive. In such patients surveillance should be particularly frequent in the first 2 months of treatment (weekly liver function tests for the first 2 weeks, and then at 2 weekly intervals). Use with caution in patients with renal failure or gout.	Antagonises the effect of probenecid and sulfinpyrazone.	A hepatic reaction is the most common side-effect of pyrazinamide. This varies from a symptomless abnormality of hepatic cell function, through a mild syndrome of fever, anorexia, malaise, liver tenderness, hepatomegaly and splenomegaly, to more serious reactions such as clinical jaundice and rare cases of progressive fulminating acute yellow atrophy and death. Patients and their carers should be told how to recognize signs of liver disorder and to seek medical attention if symptoms such as persistent nausea, vomiting, malaise or jaundice develop. Other side-effects include active gout, sideroblastic anemia, arthralgias, anorexia, nausea and vomiting, dysuria, malaise, fever, urticaria, aggravation of peptic ulcer.
Rifampicin	Ticin, Zucox	*Tuberculosis in combination with other drugs:* Oral 10 mg/kg (max 600 mg/day) as single morning dose. Meningococcal infection prophylaxis and staphylococcal infections: Oral less than 5 years 5 mg/kg per dose and more than 1 year 10 mg/kg per dose (max 600 mg/dose) two times daily for 2 days for meningococcal infection prophylaxis and for 10–14 days for staphylococcal infections. *Haemophilus influenzae* prophylaxis: Oral less than 3 months 10 mg/kg and more than 3 months 20 mg/kg per dose (max 600 mg/dose) once daily for 4 days. Cholestasis: Pruritis 5–10 mg/kg (max 600 mg) once daily. Dose adjustment in liver failure. Avoid altogether, or reduce doses for tuberculosis and prophylaxis to 8 mg/kg daily.	Patients who are hypersensitive to rifamycins. Although not recommended for use in patients with jaundice, the therapeutic benefit should be weighed against the possible risks.	Induces liver enzymes reducing plasma levels of many drugs, e.g. anticoagulants, cyclosporin, phenytoin, phenobarbital (phenobarbitone), theophylline, digoxin, most benzodiazepines, fluconazole and dose adjustment of these may be necessary, if they are given concurrently with rifampicin.	*Gastrointestinal:* These include anorexia, nausea, vomiting, abdominal discomfort, diarrhea; pseudomembranous colitis has been reported. *Skin:* Flushing, urticaria, rash. *Hematological:* Thrombocytopenia with or without purpura, leukopenia, eosinophilia. Reactions occurring mainly on intermittent therapy and probably of immunological origin include 'flu-like symptoms (with chills, fever, dizziness, bone pain), shortness of breath and

Contd...

Contd...

Drug	Brand name	Dosage	Contraindications	Drug interaction	Side effects
					wheezing, acute hemolytic anemia, acute renal failure and thrombocytopenic purpura, alterations of liver function. Other side-effects have included edema, muscular weakness, and menstrual disturbances.
Antimalarial					
Artemisinin and its derivatives	Aartee, Aba, Duther, Falcigo, Larither	Expert advice should be sought for optimum treatment including choice of preparation and dosage.	First trimester of pregnancy.	Caution with drugs that prolong the QT interval, such as quinine and halofantrine.	Generally, well tolerated at therapeutic doses; usually signs and symptoms cannot be differentiated from malaria-related effects. Neurotoxicity and cardiotoxicity have been demonstrated in high dose animal studies.
Artesunate + Lumefantrine	Arte Plus, Falcinil LF, Falcinil LFX, Lumerax	Treatment of uncomplicated *P. falciparum* and other plasmodium malaria. *Oral:* Infant or child 5–14 kg initially one tablet followed by five further doses of one tablet each at 8, 24, 36, 48 and 60 hours (total six tablets over 60 hours); 15–24 kg initially two tablets followed by five further doses of two tablets each at 8, 24, 36, 48 and 60 hours (total 12 tablets over 60 hours); 25–34 kg initially three tablets followed by five further doses of three tablets each at 8, 24, 36, 48 and 60 hours (total 18 tablets over 60 hours); over 34 kg initially four tablets followed 2y five further doses of four tablets each at 8, 24, 36, 48 and 6C hours (total 24 tablets over 60 hours). *Renal impairment:* severe; caution; monitor electrocardiogram (ECG) anc plasma potassium. *Hepatic irr pairment:* Severe—caution; monitor ECG and plasma p3tassium. Nondispersible tablets may be crushed. If the dose is vomited within 1 hour of taking, the dose should be repeated.	First trimester of pregnancy; history of arrhythmias; history of clinically relevant bradycardia; history of congestive heart failure accompanied by reduced left ventricular ejection fraction; family history of sudden death or of congenital prolongation of QTc interval. Use cautiously in presence of electrolyte disturbances; concomitant administration of drugs that prolong QT interval; patients unable to take food (monitor for greater risk of recrudescence); severe renal impairment or hepatic impairment.	Avoid/cautious use with amitriptyline, azithromycin, chloroquine, chlorpromazine and ciprofloxacin. Metabolism of artemether and lumefantrine may be inhibited by simultaneous ingestion of grapefruit juice. Quinine increases risk of ventricular arrhythmias. May also avoid concomitant administration of erythromycin, fluconazole, fluoxetine, haloperidol, levofloxacin, lopinavir, mefloquine, ofloxacin, primaquine, proguanil, pyrimethamine, ritonavir, saquinavir and sulfadoxine + pyrimethamine.	*Common:* Abdominal pain, anorexia, diarrhea, nausea and vomiting, headache, dizziness, sleep disorders, palpitation, arthralgia, myalgia, cough, asthenia, fatigue, pruritus, rash. *Infrequent:* Paresthesia, ataxia. *Rare:* hepatitis, hypersensitivity.
Chloroquine	Lariago, Nivaquine-P	*Doses expressed as chloroquin base:* Malaria prophylaxis 1 month to 12 years 5 mg/kg; 12–18 years 300 mg once weekly. Start 1 week before entering and 4 weeks after leaving endemic area. Malaria treatment (*P. vivax, P. ovale* and sensitive *P. falciparum*). *Oral/IV:* 1 month to 12 years, initially 10 mg/kg followed by 5 mg/kg 6–8 hours later and then daily once for 2 days. 12–18 years initially 600 mg followed by 300 mg 6–8 hours later and then daily once for 2 days.	There are no absolute contraindications. Caution in renal or hepatic impairment— reduced dose in renal failure. Full blood counts at regular intervals, as bone marrow suppression may rarely occur. Caution is advised in G6PD	Absorption may be reduced by antacids administer at least 4 hours apart. Absorption of ampicillin may be reduced. Chlorpromazine, cyclosporin, digoxin and penicillamine levels may be increased. Cimetidine may increase	Retinal damage may occur, particularly if treatment duration is greater than 1 year, but is unlikely with doses less than 4 mg/kg per day. Short-term blurring of vision or difficulty in accommodation may occur at the start of therapy.

Contd...

Contd...

Drug	Brand name	Dosage	Contraindications	Drug interaction	Side effects
			deficiency, and epilepsy (chloroquine may provoke seizures). Exacerbates psoriasis and myasthenia gravis. Chloroquine long-term (>12 months continuously or at weekly intervals for >3 years) should undergo ophthalmic examination before treatment and at 3 monthly intervals.	chloroquine levels—monitor for toxicity. Increased risk of ventricular arrhythmias with amiodarone and halofantrine. Antagonism of anticonvulsant effect with antiepileptics. Increased metabolism of levothyroxine (thyroxine). Increased risk of convulsions with mefloquine.	Headache, gastrointestinal disturbances, pruritus and skin eruptions, depigmentation or loss of hair, ECG changes, dyskinesias, hematological effects; thrombocytopenia, agranulocytosis, aplastic anemia.
Mefloquine	Mefliam, Mefloc	*Treatment:* Oral 15 mg; 15 mg/kg followed by 10 mg/kg 8–12 hours later (max 1.25 g). Prophylaxis: Oral 1st dose 1 week before entering malarious area (may be started earlier to make sure drug is tolerated) and given weekly on same day for 6 weeks a nd continued for 4 weeks after return from malarious area. 3 month to 3 years 6–16 kg 62.5 mg (1/4th tab); 4–7 years 16–25 kg 125 mg (1/2 tab); 8–12 years 25–45 kg 187.5 mg (3/4th tab) and more than 13 years more than 45 kg 250 mg (1 tab).	*Contraindications:* Prophylactic use in patients with renal insufficiency or severe impairment of liver function; a history of psychiatric disturbances or convulsions. Known hypersensitivities to mefloquine or related products, e.g. quinine. Because of lack of experience, prophylactic use in young children (body weight of < 5 kg) is not recommended. In patients with epilepsy, mefloquine should be used only for curative treatment and only if compelling reasons exist. Avoid pregnancy during and for 3 months after taking mefloquine. *Cautions:* Mefloquine should be taken with caution in patients suffering from cardiac conduction disorders.	Mefloquine must not be administered concurrently with quinine or related compounds, e.g. choloroquine, since this could increase the risk of convulsions and ECG changes. In severe cases, however, patients may be treated initially for one or more days with quinine given IV, and subsequently with mefloquine after a period of 12 hours. Because of the danger of a potentially fatal prolongation of the QTc interval, halofantrine must not be given simultaneously with or subsequent to mefloquine. Concomitant use of mefloquine with anticonvulsants may reduce seizure control by lowering the plasma levels of the anticonvulsant. For oral live typhoid vaccines, attenuation of the immunization induced by such vaccines cannot be excluded. Therefore, vaccination should be completed at least 3 days before the first intake to mefloquine, keeping in mind that mefloquine prophylaxis should be started	At the doses given for acute malaria, adverse reactions to mefloquine may not be distinguishable from symptoms of the disease itself. Because of the long half-life of mefloquine, adverse reactions may occur or persist up to several weeks after the last dose. Obtain medical advice before the next weekly dose if any concerning or neuropsychiatric symptoms develop. Discontinuation should be considered, particularly is neuropsychiatric reactions occur. Common side-effects include nausea, vomiting, dizziness or vertigo, loss of balance, headache, somnolence, sleep disorders (insomnia, abnormal dreams), loose stools or diarrhea and abdominal pain.

Contd...

Contd...

Contd...

Drug	Brand name	Dosage	Contraindications	Drug interaction	Side effects
				1 week before arrival in a malarious area. Increased risk of cardiotoxicity with digoxin, beta-blockers, calcium-channel antagonists, amiodarone and primozide.	
Primaquine	Pmq-Inga, Primacap	Oral: 1–12 years 0.25 mg/kg per day and 12–18 years 15 mg once daily for 14 days. For G6PD patients: 1–12 years 0.5–0.75 mg/kg and 12–18 years 30 mg once in a week for 8 weeks.	Acutely ill patients who have systemic diseases associated with granulocytopenia, e.g. rheumatoid arthritis, lupus erythematosus; patients with an underlying condition compromising bone marrow function or taking medication capable of depressing the myeloid elements of bone marrow; children aged less than 1 year. Use with caution and follow the weekly dosing regimen in patients with G6PD deficiency, as acute hemolytic anemia can occur.		Generally well tolerated at the doses used for treatment of recurrent malaria although nausea, vomiting, abdominal cramps and gastric distress can occur. Methemoglobinemia may occur occasionally and hemolytic anemia can occur in persons with G6PD deficiency. Headache, pruritus, and interference with visual accommodation have been reported and rarely hypertension, cardiac arrhythmias and leukopenia.
Proguanil	Laveran	Oral: 0–12 weeks less than 6 kg 25 mg 1/4th tab; 12 weeks 11 months 6–10 kg 50 mg ½ tab; 1–3 years 10–16 kg 75 mg 3/4th tab; 4–7 years 16–24 kg 100 mg 1 tab; 8–12 years 25–44 kg 150 mg 1 ½ tab; more than 13 years more than 45 kg 200 mg 2 tab. To be given once daily starting 1 week before entering endemic area and continue till 4 weeks after return.	Renal impairment: No data in children suggest half dose, if creatinine clearance is below 60 mL/min per 1.73 m²; quarter recommended dose on alternate days if creatinine clearance is below 20 mL/min per 1.73 m².	Antacids may reduce absorption separate dosing by 2–3 hours. May enhance anticoagulant effects of warfarin-monitor INR.	Mild gastric upset; occasional stomatitis and mouth ulcers; rarely skin rash and reversible hair loss. Hematological changes have been reported in patients with severe renal impairment.
Pyrimethamine		Toxoplasmosis in pregnancy: If toxoplasma infection is diagnosed in early pregnancy and the fetus is not infected, spiramycin is given (see spiramycin monograph). If the fetus is found to be infected then pyrimethamine 50 mg once daily, sulfadiazine 1 g 3 times daily and calcium folinate (folinic acid) 15 mg 3 times per week are given until delivery. Toxoplasmosis in infants: Pyrimethamine along with sulfadiazine (50 mg/kg two times daily) and calcium folinate (folinic acid) (15 mg/kg three times in a week) are given for 12 months. Pyrimethamine is started with loading dose of 1 mg/kg per dose two times daily for 2 days, then 1 mg/kg per dose once daily for 6 months followed by 1 mg/kg per dose thrice in a week for 6 months. Prednisolone at 0.5/kg/dose	History of pyrimethamine sensitivity. Avoid large loading doses in patients with a history of seizures.	The antifolate properties of pyrimethamine may exacerbate those of other antifolates such as co-trimoxazole, trimethoprim, methotrexate and phenytoin. Sequential blockade of folate pathways by sulphone or sulphonamide plus pyrimethamine results in considerable potentiation in the treatment of malaria and toxoplasmosis.	These can include gastrointestinal symptoms, such as atrophic glossitis, abdominal pain and vomiting; hematological effects such as megaloblastic anemia, leukopenia, thrombocytopenia and pancytopenia and CNS effects, including headache, dizziness, and insomnia. Calcium folinate (folinic acid) should be given concurrently to prevent the hematological effects.

Contd...

Drug	Brand name	Dosage	Contraindications	Drug interaction	Side effects
		2 times daily is also given until signs of CNS inflammation (CSF protein >10 g/L) or active chorioretinitis have settled and then tapered. Ocular toxoplasmosis, reactivation of toxoplasmosis during HIV infection and toxoplasmosis in immunocompromised child with protracted or incapacitating illness. 2 mg/kg loading dose for 2 days followed by 1 mg/kg in less than 12 years and 25–100 mg in 12–18 years o ds for 6 weeks to prevent relapse in HIV patients followed by maintenance of a quarter to half of starting dose indefinitely.			
Pyrimethamine with sulfadoxine	Laricox	*Oral:* 2 month to 4 years half tab; 5–6 years one tab, 7–9 years one and half tab. 10–14 years 2 tab and more than 14 years three tabs as a single dose after quinine therapy.	*Contraindications:* Sulphonamide hypersensitivity, severe renal or hepatic failure, blood dyscrasias. Treatment must be discontinued immediately upon the appearance of any mucocutaneous signs or symptoms. Premature babies and during the first 2 months of life. Precautions: excessive exposure to the sun should be avoided. Regular blood counts if used for over 3 months (but it is not recommended for prophylaxis).	Avoid other preparations containing folate antagonists (e.g. co-trimoxazole, trimethoprim, methotrexate, anticonvulsants).	Skin reactions, gastrointestinal reactions, hematological changes.
Quinine	Quininga, Rez-Q	*Oral: birth:* 12 years 30 mg/kg per day (sulfate) and 12–18 years 1.8 g/day (sulfate) in three divided doses for 7 days. IV infusion over 4 hours initial loading dose of 20 mg/kg (max 1.4 g), then 10 mg/kg (max 0.7 g) every 12 hours for 48 hours and then maintenance of 5–7 mg/kg once in 8 hours if IV is needed after 48 hours. As soon as possible change to oral.	Caution in reduced liver function (more significant adverse effects) and in patients with cardiac conduction defects and optic neuritis.	Increased risk of arrhythmias with amiodarone, flecainide, halofantrine, cisapride and certain antipsychotics. Increased risk of convulsions with mefloquine–separate administration by 12 hours. Increased plasma-quinine concentration with cimetidine. Plasma concentration of digoxin increased.	Expect symptomatic adverse effects-called 'cinchonism' (tinnitus, headache, nausea, visual disturbances). Sometimes effects are more marked-vertigo, reduced hearing, blurred vision, diplopia, night blindness, visual field defects; but most are reversible. Cardiac side-effects include prolonged QT interval, AV block, sinus arrest, ventricular tachycardia. Hypoglycemia as quinine stimulates insulin secretion-monitor blood glucose levels.

Contd...

Contd...

Contd...

Drug	Brand name	Dosage	Contraindications	Drug interaction	Side effects
Antiviral					
Acyclovir	Acivir DT, Ocuvir	The cream and ophthalmic ointment may be used five times daily for herpes simplex infection and herpes simplex keratitis respectively of the skin. Continue the eye ointment for 3 days after healing. *Newborn:* IV infusion at 10 mg/kg three times daily for 10 days. *Children:* Orally 100 mg less than 2 years and 200 mg 2–18 years five times daily; IV infusion 10 mg/kg less than 3 months, 250 mg/sq meter 3 months to 12 years and 5 mg/kg 12–18 three times daily. Double dose for immunocompromised. *Herpes simplex prophylaxis:* 100 mg 1 month to 2 years; 200 mg 2–18 years four times daily. Double dose for immunocompromised.	Hypersensitivity to acyclovir. Polyuric renal failure reported with high doses. Hence, ensure adequate hydration; avoid dehydration.	May produce extreme lethargy with zidovudine. Increased levels and risk of toxicity with probenecid and cimetidine. Risk of renal damage is increased with concurrent use of other nephrotoxic drugs.	Severe local inflammatory reactions and phlebitis have occurred at the site of injection. Reversible neurological reactions reported.
Amantadine	Amantrel	*Influenza a virus infection:* Oral, children more than and equal to 10 years. 5 mg/kg per day per os (PO) in two divided doses, not to exceed 200 mg/day (100 mg PO twice daily in children who weigh ≥40 kg). *Children less than 10 years:* 5 mg/kg per day PO (up to 150 mg/day) in two divided doses. Primary influenza prophylaxis (influenza virus type A only) *Oral:* Adults less than 65 years and adolescents: 200 mg/day PO as a single dose or two divided doses; begin as soon as possible after initial exposure and continue for at least 10 days after exposure. *Elderly:* No more than 100 mg PO once daily; begin as soon as possible after initial exposure and continue for at least 10 days after exposure. HIV-infected adults, adolescents, and children more than and equal to 10 years: as an alternative to influenza vaccination amantadine 100 mg PO twice daily be considered for primary prophylaxis during outbreaks of influenza A. Monitor these patients closely. Children more than and equal to 10 years 5 mg/kg per day PO in two divided doses; begin as soon as possible after initial exposure and continue for at least 10 days after exposure. Do not exceed 200 mg/day. *Children less than 10 years:* 5 mg/kg per day PO (up to 150 mg/day) given in two divided doses; begin as soon as possible after initial exposure and continue for at least 10 days after exposure. In all above mentioned scenarios, prophylaxis may be continued for up to 90 days for repeated or suspected exposures if influenza virus vaccine is unavailable. If used with the influenza virus vaccine, continue amantadine for 2–3 weeks until vaccine protection develops.	Amantadine is contraindicated in patients with a known amantadine hypersensitivity, rimantadine hypersensitivity or hypersensitivity to any agent in the adamantine class. Renal impairment or renal failure, including dialysis, requires dosage adjustment. Renal function should be monitored closely and the dose adjusted accordingly. Children with congestive heart failure, orthostatic hypotension or peripheral edema should be cautiously treated with amantadine as the drug induces a redistribution of fluid within the body (rather than an actual increase in total body water) and thereby worsens these conditions. Recurrent eczema or rash can be aggravated during treatment. Patients with a history of seizures should be monitored closely when amantadine is initiated as it may increase seizure activity. Patients with preexisting	Although the mechanism of amantadine is not clear, it appears, it potentiates the actions of dopamine. Since butyrophenones (e.g. haloperidol), and metoclopramide, phenothiazines and thiothixene are dopamine antagonists, these drugs should be avoided. Amantadine may exhibit anticholinergic activity. Other medications with significant anticholinergic activity may include: clozapine, disopyramide sedating H 1-blockers, olanzapine, orphenadrine, and tricyclic antidepressants. Observe patients for additive effects. Patients receiving bupropion concurrently with amantadine developed neurologic side effects such as restlessness, agitation, gait disturbance and dizziness. Amantadine can increase the efficiency of levodopa and psychostimulants by its action on central nerve	Primarily associated with the CNS includes dizziness, anxiety, impaired coordination, insomnia, and nervousness. Effects can appear after a few hours or several days of therapy or after an increase in dosage. Generally mild. Some experience headache, irritability, nightmares, depression, ataxia, confusion, drowsiness, agitation, fatigue, and hallucinations and rarely psychosis, abnormal thinking, weakness, amnesia, dysarthria (slurred speech), and hyperkinesia. Occasional reports of increased frequency of seizures, suicidal ideation, and neuroleptic malignant syndrome (NMS). Nausea/vomiting may occur. Rarely diarrhea, constipation, anorexia, and xerostomia. Some respond to dose reduction. Diffuse, white, subendothelial corneal opacification that resolve

Contd...

Contd...

Drug	Brand name	Dosage	Contraindications	Drug interaction	Side effects
			psychoses should be treated with caution. Patients should avoid driving or operating machinery until they know how amantadine affects their vision and muscle control.	terminals. Mental status changes have been reported after sulfamethoxazole; trimethoprim, SMX-TMP was administered to a patient taking amantadine. Amantadine toxicity when used with quinidine or quinine as they inhibit renal tubular secretion of amantadine. Trivalent inactivated influenza vaccine may be administered with amantadine but it inhibits replication of the live attenuated intranasal influenza vaccine.	within a few weeks of stopping drug. Antimicrobial resistance can occur during therapy with amantadine due to the development of viral mutations. Drug effectiveness may be diminished by resistance mutations or other factors such as viral virulence. Drug susceptibility patterns should be assessed when determining appropriateness of treatment with amantadine.
Didanosine (ddi, DDI)	Dinex, Dinex EC, Virosin DR		Hypersensitivity to the components. Use with caution if there is a previous history of pancreatic disease or elevation of pancreatic amylase or triglycerides. Suspend treatment if pancreatitis is suspected or pancreatic enzymes are raised significantly during treatment even if asymptomatic. The tablets contain phenylalanine (from aspartame) and caution is advised in patients with phenylketonuria; use in such patients only if clearly indicated. Retinal or optic nerve changes have been reported in children and regular eye examinations are recommended at least 6 monthly or if vision disturbance occurs. Suspend treatment if any of the following become clinically significant; peripheral neuropathy, hyperuricemia, raised liver enzymes, rapidly elevating aminotransferase levels, progressive	Buffers and antacids present in didanosine formulations may reduce absorption of some drugs such as ciprofloxacin, itraconazole, ketoconazole and dapsone. This occurs either by direct interaction with aluminum/ magnesium in the antacids or due to the raising of gastric pH. Avoid taking such drugs within 2 hours of didanosine. Use with caution with other drugs that may be associated with pancreatic toxicity or peripheral neuropathy.	Pancreatitis and elevation of serum amylase and lipase have been reported. Pancreatitis, which may be fatal, is more frequent with high doses, in advanced HIV disease and if there is a previous history of pancreatitis. It usually appears at 1–6 months after the start of treatment and resolves within 3 weeks of discontinuation of didanosine. Peripheral neuropathy has been associated with didanosine and may require dose modification. Abnormal liver function tests have been reported. Rare reports of liver failure. Also rare reports of lactic acidosis and hepatomegaly with steatosis have been reported with other dideoxynucleoside antivirals. Asymptomatic hyperuricemia has been reported which may require discontinuation, if there is no response to measures

Contd...

Contd...

Drug	Brand name	Dosage	Contraindications	Drug interaction	Side effects
			hepatomegaly, hepatitis or lactic acidosis of unknown origin.		aimed at reducing uric acid levels. Gastrointestinal symptoms such as nausea, vomiting, abdominal pain, diarrhea, constipation and taste disturbance have been reported. Dry mouth may also occur. Sensitivity reactions such as rash, pruritus, allergic reactions and anaphylaxis have occurred. Hematological effects such as leukopenia, thrombocytopenia and anemia may be more common in children. Retinal or optic nerve changes have been reported in children and regular eye examinations are recommended at least 6 monthly or if vision disturbance occurs. Rare reports of diabetes mellitus and hypokalemia.
Foscarnet sodium	Foscavir	*Dosage description:* Usually, in combination with ganciclovir IV more than 1 month, 18 years induce therapy for CMV rhinitis with 180 mg/kg per day in three divided doses and for mucocutaneous HSV with 120 mg/kg per day in three divided doses and follow it up with maintenance therapy of 90 mg/kg as single dose.	Hypersensitivity to foscarnet. Monitor renal function regularly during treatment as renal impairment may occur. Ensure adequate hydration. Monitor serum calcium and magnesium as foscarnet may chelate divalent metal ions and lead to an acute decrease in ionized calcium/ magnesium.	Concurrent nephrotoxic drugs may cause additive renal toxicity. Drugs known to reduce serum calcium (pentamidine, frusemide, may potentiate hypocalcemia).	Renal function impairment. Genital irritation or ulceration. Serum electrolyte changes including hypocalcemia, hypomagnesemia, hypophosphatemia, hypokalemia, hyperphosphatemia, and reductions in serum iron and zinc. Hypocalcemia may be acute, symptomatic and related to rate of infusion. Convulsions have occurred during foscarnet therapy and in some cases may be related to acute hypocalcemia. Skin rashes may occur during treatment. Decrease in hemoglobin concentration has been observed. CNS effects such as paresthesia, headache,

Contd...

Contd...

Drug	Brand name	Dosage	Contraindications	Drug interaction	Side effects
					dizziness, involuntary muscle contractions, tremor, ataxia and neuropathy may occur. Anorexia, anxiety, nervousness, confusion, psychosis and aggression have also been reported. Other less common adverse effects reported include gastrointestinal effects (nausea, vomiting, diarrhea and constipation) pancreatitis, increases in serum amylase, alkaline phosphatase, hyponatremia. Foscarnet is not generally myelosuppressive but monitoring of white cell count is advisable. Thrombocytopenia, increases in serum alanine aminotransferase (ALT), aspartate aminotransferase (AST) and gamma GT, ventricular arrhythmia and diabetes insipidus also reported rarely.
Ganciclovir	Ganguard	Cytomegalovirus (CMV) retinitis: Induction therapy 10 mg/kg per 24 hours IV (over 1–2 hours) divided into two doses given 12th hourly for 14–21 days followed by maintenance of 5–6 mg/kg per 24 hours IV once daily. CMV disease and prophylaxis (solid organ transplant): Induction 10 mg/kg per 4 hours IV divided into two doses given 12th hourly for 7–14 days followed by maintenance of 5–6 mg/kg per 24 hours IV once daily.	Contraindicated in those patients with a known hypersensitivity to ganciclovir or acyclovir. Contraindicated in pregnancy and lactation. Ensure adequaet hydration when using IV. Avoid if neutrophil count less than 500 cell per microliter. Increased risk of thrombocytopenia if platelet count less than 25,000 per microlitre. Regular monitoring of white blood cell count is advised. Ganciclovir should be considered potentially mutagenic, carcinogenic and teratogenic.	Drugs that inhibit replication of rapidly dividing cells: potential additive toxicity. Patients receiving immunosuppressive agents may require decreased doses or temporary withdrawal of these drugs to prevent excessive suppression of the bone marrow or immune system. Dapsone, pentamidine, flucytosine, amphotericin, cotrimoxazole; potential for additive toxicity. Zidovudine; severe neutropenia likely if used concurrently. Regular monitoring advised. Probenecid and other drugs that inhibit renal tubular	Leukopenia and thrombocytopenia occur in 10–40% of patients given IV ganciclovir. Anemia, fever, rash and abnormal LFTs occur in up to 2% of patients. Chills, edema, confusion ataxia, nervousness, paresthsia, psychosis, tremor, hypotension, hypertension, cardiac arrhythmias, gastrointestinal effects including hemorrhage, eosinophilia, decreased blood glucose, alopecia, pruritus, urticaria, hematuria, increases in serum creatinine and urea also reported.

Contd...

Drug	Brand name	Dosage	Contraindications	Drug interaction	Side effects
				secretion or reabsorption may reduce renal clearance of ganciclovir. Imipenem cilastatin; seizures have been reported when used in combination with ganciclovir.	
Interferon alfa	Alferon	Subcutaneous (SC) less than 12 years 3 million units/m²; more than 12 years 3–10 million units/m² usually three times/week (daily for hemangioma) for 4–6 months.	Interferon A should not be used in the neonatal period, due to possibility of fatal reactions to the benzylalcohol excipient. Hypersensitivity to interferon alfa or any component of the individual formulation. Severe preexisting cardiac disease, severe renal, hepatic or myeloid dysfunction. Epilepsy and/or compromised CNS function. Patients with preexisting psychiatric condition or history of severe psychiatric disorder. Chronic hepatitis with advanced cirrhosis or decompensated hepatic disease. Chronic hepatitis in patients currently or recently treated with immunosuppressive agents (excluding corticosteroids). Autoimmune hepatitis or history of autoimmune disease. Immunosuppressed transplant recipients and patients for whom allogenic bone marrow transplantation is planned or possible in the immediate future. Thyroid disease unless well controlled.	Narcotic drugs, hypnotics and sedatives should be used with caution due to the risk of interferon affecting CNS function. May interfere with oxidative metabolism; concurrent use of drugs metabolized by this route, such as theophylline, should be undertaken with caution. Monitor serum theophylline levels. May reduce the activity of the cytochrome P 450 enzyme system. Drugs metabolized by this enzyme system, including cimetidine, phenytoin, diazepam, propranolol, warfarin, cyclophosphamide and doxorubicin should be used with caution due to a risk of enhanced effects and/or toxicity. Concurrent administration with vinblastine or busulfan may produce severe myelosuppression. Concurrent administration with acyclovir may enhance the risk of progressive renal failure, although the combination is reported as beneficial in hepatitis B infection.	The most commonly reported adverse effects are flu-like symptoms such as fever, fatigue, headache and myalgia. These acute side-effects tend to diminish with continued therapy or dose reduction and can be reduced by administration of paracetamol. Other common adverse effects include rigors, anorexia and nausea. Less common effects include vomiting, diarrhea, arthralgia, asthenia, somnolence, dizziness, dry mouth, alopecia, back pain, malaise, increased sweating, altered taste, insomnia, impaired concentration and hypotension. Abnormalities of liver function, hypo and hyperthyroidism and ocular adverse effects have occurred rarely. Baseline assessment of liver and thyroid function and visual acuity is recommended. Pulmonary infiltrates, pneumonitis and pneumonia have been observed rarely and may lead to fatality. Any patient developing fever, cough, dyspnea or other respiratory symptoms should be investigated. If chest X-ray shows evidence of pulmonary infiltrates or impairment of function, the patient should be closely monitored and

Contd...

Drug	Brand name	Dosage	Contraindications	Drug interaction	Side effects
			Caution should be exercised in patients with debilitating conditions, including pulmonary disease, diabetes mellitus prone to ketoacidosis, coagulation disorders, and mild-to-moderate renal, hepatic or myeloid disease. Patients with chronic hepatitis B, with evidence of deteriorating synthetic function.		discontinuation considered. A wide variety of other adverse effects has been reported rarely: see manufacturers SPC for further details.
			Clinical decompensation may follow a flare of aminotransferases and the risks of treatment should be weighed against the possible benefits. Patients with a history of congestive heart failure and/or previous or current arrhythmic disorders should be closely monitored. A baseline ECG is advised, with monitoring as appropriate throughout treatment. Cardiac arrhythmias, usually supraventricular, respond to conventional therapy but may necessitate discontinuation of interferon alfa. Adequate hydration must be maintained to prevent fluid depletion and hypotension.		
Interferon gamma-1b (immune interferon)		Subcutaneous surface area less than 0.5 m² 21.5 µg/kg per dose and surface area more than 0.5 m² 50 µg/kg per dose three times in a week. Avoid in children less than 6 months.	Contraindicated in patients who have hypersensitivity to interferon gamma or known hypersensitivity closely related interferons. Cautioned in seizure disorders and/or compromised CNS function; preexisting cardiac disease (including ischemia, congestive heart failure and arrhythmias); severe hepatic or renal impairment. Monitor before and during treatment;	Simultaneous administration of interferon gamma-1b with other heterologous serum protein preparations or immunological preparations (e.g. vaccines) should be avoided because of the risk for unexpected amplified immune response.	Fever, headache, chills, myalgia or fatigue; nausea and vomiting, arthralgia, rashes and injection-site reactions.

Contd...

Contd...

Drug	Brand name	Dosage	Contraindications	Drug interaction	Side effects
			hematological tests [including full blood count (FBC), differential white cell count and platelet count, blood chemistry tests (including renal and LFTs) and urinalysis.		
Lamivudine	Ladiwin, Lamidac 100	*Adolescents (weight >= 40 kg):* 300 mg/day. Safe and effective use has not been established in adolescent less than 40 kg and in children. Patients with renal impairment: CrCl less than and equal to 50 mL/min. Lamivudine requires dose adjustment in the presence of renal insufficiency.	Not for use in adolescent less than 40 kg and in children. Use cautiously in patients with peripheral neuropathy. Patients with peripheral neuropathy can experience exacerbations during lamivudine therapy. Avoid in renal impairment or adjust dose.	Co-administration of lamivudine with nelfinavir results in increased lamivudine concentrations of 1–20%. No changes in nelfinavir levels are noted. Dosage adjustments for lamivudine or zidovudine are not required. Concomitant administration of zalcitabine and lamivudine is not recommended. Co-administration of lamivudine is contraindicated in patients receiving emtricitabine; tenofovir due to similarities between emtricitabine and lamivudine. Co-administration results into component duplication.	Headache, fatigue, nausea, anorexia, abdominal pain. Rarely, pancreatitis, hyperglycemia, lactic acidosis, hepatitis are reported. Hypersensitivity reactions with fever, rash, nausea, hypotension and bronchospasm limits its use.
Nevirapine	Neve, Nevimune	Treatment of HIV infection in combination with other antiretroviral agents. For adolescents, the initiation of antiretroviral therapy ART is recommended in any patient: with a history of an AIDS-defining infection; with a CD4 less than 350/mm³; who is pregnant; who is being treated for hepatitis B virus (HBV) infection. For children, the initiation of ART is recommended in any symptomatic patient. For asymptomatic or mildly symptomatic children more than and equal to 5 years, the initiation of ART is recommended for patients with HIV RNA more than and equal to 100,000 copies/mL and CD4 less than 350/mm³. For asymptomatic or mildly symptomatic children 1–5 years, the initiation of ART is recommended for patients with HIV RNA more than and equal to 100,000 copies/mL and CD4 less than 25%. For infants, the initiation of ART is recommended in any infant regardless of clinical status, CD4 percentage or viral load. *Adolescents:* 200 mg PO once daily for the first 14 days, then 200 mg PO twice daily. If mild-to-moderate rash with constitutional symptoms is observed during the first	Hypersensitivity, hepatic or renal failure. Liver functions to be monitored periodically.	Phenobarbitone, phenytoin, carbamazepine, methadone, estrogen, containing drugs—metabolism of these drugs are increased.	Rash, hepatitis, nausea, vomiting, abdominal pain, diarrhea, headache, drowsiness, fatigue, fever, elevated liver enzymes, myalgia, arthralgia. Somnolence, paresthesia, Stevens–Johnson syndrome and granulocytopenia.

Contd...

Contd...

Drug	Brand name	Dosage	Contraindications	Drug interaction	Side effects
		14 days of therapy, do not increase the dose until the rash has resolved; if the rash does not resolve by treatment day 28, discontinue nevirapine and use an alternative treatment regimen. Permanantly discontinue treatment if severe hepatotoxicity, severe cutaneous reactions or hypersensitivity reactions occur. Adolescents in early puberty (Tanner I–II) should be dosed using pediatric schedules. *Neonates:* More tnan and equal to 15 days old, infants, and children: 150 mg/m² (not to exceed 400 mg) PO once daily for the first 14 days then 150 mg/m² (not to exceed 400 mg) twice daily. Alternatively, the following volume recommendations per dose of nevirapine 50 mg/5 mL oral suspension, based on body surface area, can be used: more than 1.25 m² 20 mL; 1.08–1.25 m² 17.5 mL; 0.92–1.08 m² 15 mL; 0.75–0.92 m² 12.5 mL; 0.58–0.75 m² 10 mL; 0.42–0.58 m² 7.5 mL; 0.25–0.42 m² 5 mL; 0.12–0.25 m² 2.5 mL; and 0.06–0.12 m² 1.25 mL. Same rules as for adolescent in case of rash or appearance of indication for discontinuation of therapy. Neonates less than 15 days old: dosing information is unavailable. (HIV) prophylaxis to prevent perinatal transmission of HIV to neonates born to HIV-infected women in labor who have had no prior antiretroviral therapy.			
		Oral dosage (nevirapine single agent): Pregnant females, intrapartum; The addition of single-dose maternal/infant nevirapine to an ongoing highly active combination antiretroviral therapy regimen does not provide additional efficacy in reducing perinatal transmission and may result in nevirapine resistance in the mother, and is therefore not recommendec. In patients who are not receiving any antiretroviral treatment prior to labor, administer 200 mg PO as a single dose at the onset of labor. Neonates more than and equal to 34 weeks gestation—the CDC recommends 2 mg/kg PO as a single dose 48–72 hours after birth. If the mother received nevirapine <1 hr prior to delivery, the infant should be given 2 mg/kg PO as soon as possible after birth and again at 48–72 hours. *Oral dosage (nevirapine and zidovudine combination):* Pregnant females, intrapartum: Due to synergistic inhibition of HIV with the combination in vitro, the following regimen has been suggested: nevirapine 200 mg PO as a single dose at the onset of labor plus zidovudine (2 mg/kg IV bolus followed by 1 mg/kg/hour IV continuous infusion until delivery). During or immediately after intrapartum treatment with nevirap ne and zidovudine, consider initiation of maternal zidovudine and lamivudine, continuing for 3 to 7 days, to potentially reduce development of nevirapine resistance.			

Contd...

Drug	Brand name	Dosage	Contraindications	Drug interaction	Side effects
		Neonates: More than equal to 34 weeks gestation: Due to synergistic inhibition of HIV with the combination in vitro, the following regimen has been suggested: nevirapine 2 mg/kg PO as a single oral dose at 48–72 hours plus zidovudine (2 mg/kg PO every 6 hours for 6 weeks). Maximum *dosage limits: Adolescents:* 400 mg/day PO. *Children:* 300 mg/m², up to 400 mg, per day PO. *Infants:* 300 mg/m², up to 400 mg, per day PO. Neonates more than and equal to 15 days old: 300 mg/m², up to 400 mg, per day PO. Neonates <15 days old: Safe and effective use not established.			
Oseltamivir	Tamiflu	*Prevention of influenza:* Oral: 13–18 years, 75 mg once daily for at least 7 days after exposure or for up to 6 weeks during an epidemic. Treatment of influenza: oral, for children above 1 year age up to 16 kg 30 mg, 16–23 kg 45 mg; 23–40 kg 60 mg and more than 40 kg 75 mg and every 12 hours for 5 days.	*Renal impairment:* Reduce dose, if creatinine clearance is 10–30 mL/min per 1.73 m² and avoid if creatinine clearance is less than 10 mL/min per 1.73 m².		Nausea, vomiting, abdominal pain, dyspepsia, diarrhea, skin rash, conjunctivitis, insomnia, dizziness, headache, fatigue, epistaxis and occasionally hypersensitivity reactions, hepatitis and Stevens–Johnson syndrome.
Zidovudine (azidothymidine or AZT)	Retrovir, Zidovir	*Newborn:* Prevention of feto-maternal transmission oral 2 mg/kg ɔer dose four times daily started within 12 hours of birth and continued for 6 weeks. IV 1.5 mg/kg per dose four times daily. *Child:* oral 180 mg/m² two times daily (max 250 mg/dose). IV 120 mg/m² four times daily.	Hypersensitivity to zidovudine or components. Contraindicated in neonates with hyperbilirubinemia requiring treatment other than phototherapy or if serum transaminases are more than five times normal levels. Avoid if hemoglobin less than 7.5 g/dL or neutrophil counts less than 0.75 × 109/L.	Alterations in phenytoin plasma levels may occur, normally a decrease in levels although increase has been reported; monitor carefully. Increased incidence of neutropenia reported with paracetamol, but the mechanism is unclear. It has been suggested that short-term paracetamol use is acceptable, but with close monitoring. Other drugs that inhibit or competes for glucuronidation or inhibit hepatic microsomal enzymes should be used with caution as they may alter the metabolism of zidovudine; use with caution and monitor closely. Concurrent therapy with other potentially nephrotoxic or myelosuppressive drugs may have additive effects	Reversible anemia, neutropenia and leukopenia occur, usually after 4–6 weeks of therapy but potentially earlier. Regular monitoring is advised. Patients with preexisting bone marrow depression are particularly at risk. Dose reduction or suspension of treatment may be required. Lactic acidosis and severe hepatomegaly with steatosis have been reported. Although a causal relationship is unclear monitoring of liver enzymes is advised and treatment should be suspended if necessary. Headache, nausea, vomiting and other gastrointestinal effects reported. Myalgia, myopathy or polymyositis have been reported generally after 6–12 months therapy in adults.

Contd...

Contd...

Drug	Brand name	Dosage	Contraindications	Drug interaction	Side effects
				(pentamidine, ganciclovir, dapsone, amphotericin, pyrimethamine and flucytosine). Ribavirin (tribavirin) antagonizes zidovudine anti-viral activity in vitro. Similar data has been reported for ganciclovir. Rifampicin may decrease plasma levels of zidovudine. Probenecid increases half-life and area under plasma concentration time curve by decreasing glucuronidation and reducing renal excretion. Sodium valproate, fluconazole or methadone may increase plasma concentrations of zidovudine; monitor carefully for zidovudine-related adverse effects.	Hypersensitivity reactions, including anaphylaxis, have occurred rarely. Skin rashes also reported. Capsules swallowed at night while lying down have reportedly caused esophageal ulceration in some adults.
Antiretroviral drug					
Abacavir	Abamune	Human immunodeficiency virus (HIV) infection in combination with at least two other antiretroviral medicines, by mouth, adolescent 300 mg twice daily; 3 months to 16 years, 8 mg/kg twice daily (maximum, 600 mg daily). For adolescents, the initiation of antiretroviral therapy (ART) is recommended in any patient with a history of an AIDS-defining infection; with a CD4 less than 350/mm³; who is pregnant; who has HIV associated nephropathy; or who is being treated for HBV infection. For children, the initiation of ART is recommended in any symptomatic patient. For asymptomatic or mildly symptomatic children more than and equal to 5 years, the initiation of antiretroviral therapy is recommended for patients with HIV RNA more than and equal to 100,000 copies/mL and CD4 less than 350/mm³. For asymptomatic or mildly symptomatic children 1–5 years, the initiation of antiretroviral therapy is recommended for patients with HIV RNA more than and equal to 100,000 copies/mL and CD4 less than 25%. For infants, the initiation of antiretroviral therapy is recommended in any infant regardless of clinical status, CD4 percentage, or viral load.	Chronic hepatitis B or C, hepatic impairment; renal impairment; exercise caution in patients (particularly obese women) with hepatomegaly, hepatitis, liver enzyme abnormalities or risk factors for liver disease and hepatic steatosis (including alcohol abuse) and discontinue if rapid deterioration in liver function tests, symptomatic hyperlactatemia, progressive hepatomegaly or lactic acidosis occurs. To reduce the risk of hypersensitivity reactions, perform HLA-B*5701 testing before initiating an abacavir-containing treatment regimen. Do not prescribe/administer abacavir to an HLA-B*5701-positive patient, and clearly record the positive	Life-threatening hypersensitivity reactions characterized most commonly by fever or rash and possibly nausea, vomiting, diarrhea, abdominal pain, dyspnea, cough, lethargy, malaise, headache, and myalgia, less frequently by mouth ulceration, edema, hypotension, sore throat, adult respiratory distress syndrome, paresthesia, arthralgia, conjunctivitis, lymphadenopathy, lymphocytopenia, renal failure, and anaphylaxis and rarely by myolysis have been reported. Laboratory abnormalities may include raised liver enzymes and creatine kinase. Symptoms

Contd...

Contd...

Drug	Brand name	Dosage	Contraindications	Drug interaction	Side effects
			status as an abacavir allergy in the patient's medical record. If HLA-B*5701 screening is not readily available, initiation of abacavir is reasonable with appropriate clinical counseling and monitoring for any signs of hypersensitivity reaction.		usually appear in the first 6 weeks, but may occur at any time; monitor patients for symptoms every 2 weeks for 2 months; discontinue immediately if any symptom of hypersensitivity develops and do not rechallenge (risk of more severe hypersensitivity reaction); also discontinue if hypersensitivity cannot be ruled out, even when other diagnoses possible (if rechallenge is necessary, it must be carried out in a hospital setting). If abacavir is stopped for any reason other than hypersensitivity, exclude hypersensitivity reaction as the cause and rechallenge only if medical assistance is readily available; care is needed with concomitant use of drugs which are known to cause skin toxicity. Potentially life-threatening lactic acidosis and severe hepatomegaly with steatosis have been reported. Blood disorders; lipodystrophy; pancreatitis; very rarely Stevens–Johnson syndrome and toxic epidermal necrolysis; rash and gastrointestinal disturbances more common in children.

Contd...

Contd...

Drug	Brand name	Dosage	Contraindications	Drug interaction	Side effects
Efavirenz	Efavir, Efferven, Estiva	*Children less than 3 years:* There are no pharmacokinetic data available on the appropriate dose of efavirenz in children less than 3 years. *Treatment of HIV infection:* Children PO more than and equal to 3 years, 32.5–39.9 kg: 400 mg; 25–32.4 kg, 350 mg; 20–24.9 kg 300 mg; 15–19.9 kg, 250 mg; 10–14.9 kg, 200 mg; more than and equal to 40 kg, 600 mg PO once daily at bedtime. For children who can swallow capsules combine efavirenz with either 1) zidcvudine plus lamivudine, emtricitabine or didanosine or 2) didanosine plus lamivudine or emtricitabine. Adolescents more than 40 kg 600 mg PO once daily at bedtime. Combine efavirenz with either lamivudine or emtricitabine plus either zidovudine or tenofovir. HIV postexposure prophylaxis: The CDC recommends that efavirenz once daily at bedtime (or nelfinavir, indinavir or abacavir) be added to the basic two-drug regimen in situations where exposure is associated with an increased risk of HIV transmission (e.g. severe percutaneous exposure (e.g. large-bore hollow needle, deep puncture, visible blood on device or need e used in patient's artery or vein) from a Class 1 or 2 HIV+ source; or a large volume exposure to mucous membranes or nonintact skin exposures from a Class 2 HIV+ source); or if the source person's virus is known or suspected to be resistant to one or more antiretrovirals. In all cases, therapy should be initiated as soon as possible and continued for 4 weeks. Although animal studies suggest postexposure prophylaxis started more than 24–36 hours following exposure is substantially less effective, the interval after which no ber eft is derived for humans is undefined. Therefore, if appropriate for the exposure, prophylaxis should be started even when the interval following exposure is more than 36 hours. The dose is the same as for treatment of HIV given above. *Patients with hepatic impairment:* Dosing in patients with hepatic impairment has not been studied. *Patients with renal impairment:* No dosage adjustment is required.	In patients with a known or suspected history of hepatitis B or hepatitis C, and in patients treated concurrently with other hepatotoxic drugs, monitoring of liver enzymes is recommended during efavirenz therapy. In patients with persistent elevations of serum transaminases to more than five times the upper limit of normal, the benefit of continued therapy with efavirenz must be weighed against the unknown risks of significant liver toxicity.		
Lamivudine	Ladiwin, Lamidec 100	*Adolescents (weight ≥40 kg):* 300 mg/day. Safe and effective use has not been established in adolescent less than 40 kg and in children. Patients with renal impairment: CrCl less than and equal to 50 mL/min. Lamivudine requires dose adjustment in the presence of renal insufficiency.	Not for use in adolescent less than 40 kg and in children. Use cautiously in patients with peripheral neuropathy. Patients with peripheral neuropathy can experience exacerbations during lamivudine therapy. Avoid in renal impairment or adjust dose.	Co-administration of lamivudine with nelfinavir results in increased lamivudine concentrations of 1–20%. No changes in nelfinavir levels are noted. Dosage adjustments for lamivudine or zidovudine are not required. Concomitant	Headache, fatigue, nausea, anorexia, abdominal pain. Rarely, pancreatitis, hyperglycemia, lactic acidosis, hepatitis are reported. Hypersensitivity reactions with fever, rash, nausea, hypotension and bronchospasm limits its use.

Contd...

Contd...

Drug	Brand name	Dosage	Contraindications	Drug interaction	Side effects
				administration of zalcitabine and lamivudine is not recommended. Co-administration of lamivudine is contraindicated in patients receiving emtricitabine; tenofovir due to similarities between emtricitabine and lamivudine. Co-administration results into component duplication.	
Nevirapine	Neve, Nevimune	Treatment of HIV infection in combination with other antiretroviral agents. For adolescents, the initiation of ART is recommended in any patient: with a history of an AIDS-defining infection; with a CD4 less than 350/mm³; who is pregnant; who has HIV-associated nephropathy or who is being treated for HBV infection. For children, the initiation of ART is recommended in any symptomatic patient. For asymptomatic or mildly symptomatic children more than and equal to 5 years, the initiation of ART is recommended for patients with HIV RNA more than and equal to 100,000 copies/mL and CD4 less than 350/mm³. For asymptomatic or mildly symptomatic children 1–5 years, the initiation of ART is recommended for patients with HIV RNA more than and equal to 100,000 copies/mL and CD4 less than 25%. For infants, the initiation of ART is recommended in any infant regardless of clinical status, CD4 percentage or viral load. *Adolescents:* 200 mg PO once daily for the first 14 days, then 200 mg PO twice daily. If mild-to-moderate rash with constitutional symptoms is observed during the first 14 days of therapy, do not increase the dose until the rash has resolved; if the rash does not resolve by treatment on 28th day, discontinue nevirapine and use an alternative treatment regimen. Permanently discontinue treatment if severe hepatotoxicity, severe cutaneous reactions or hypersensitivity reactions occur. Adolescents in early puberty (Tanner I–II) should be dosed using pediatric schedules. *Neonates:* More than and equal to 15 days old, infants and children: 150 mg/m² (not to exceed 400 mg) PO once daily for the first 14 days, then 150 mg/m² (not to exceed 400 mg) twice daily.	Hypersensitivity, hepatic or renal failure. Liver functions to be monitored periodically.	Phenobarbitone, phenytoin, carbamazepine, methadone, estrogen, containing drugs—metabolism of these drugs are increased.	Rash, hepatitis, nausea, vomiting, abdominal pain, diarrhea, headache, drowsiness, fatigue, fever, elevated liver enzymes, myalgia, arthralgia. Somnolence, paresthesia, Stevens–Johnson syndrome and granulocytopenia.

Contd...

Contd...

Contd...

Drug	Brand name	Dosage	Contraindications	Drug interaction	Side effects
		Alternatively, the following volume recommendations per dose of nevirapine 50 mg/5 mL oral suspension, based on body surface area, can be used: more than 1.25 m², 20 mL; 1.08–1.25 m², 17.5 mL; 0.92–1.08 m², 15 mL; 0.75–0.92 m², 12.5 mL; 0.58–0.75 m², 10 mL; 0.42–0.58 m², 7.5 mL; 0.25–0.42 m², 5 mL; 0.12–0.25 m², 2.5 mL; and 0.06–0.12 m², 1.25 mL. Same rules as for adolescent in case of rash or appearance of indication for discontinuation of therapy. *Neonates:* Less than 15 days old. Dosing information is unavailable. (HIV) prophylaxis: to prevent perinatal transmission of HIV to neonates born to HIV-infected women in labor who have had no prior antiretroviral therapy. Oral dosage (nevirapine single agent). *Pregnant females Intrapartum:* The addition of single-dose maternal/infant nevirapine to an ongoing highly active combination ART regimen does not provide additional efficacy in reducing perinatal transmission and may result in nevirapine resistance in the mother, and is therefore not recommended. In patients who are not receiving any antiretroviral treatment prior to labor, administer 200 mg PO as a single dose at the onset of labor. Neonates more than and equal to 34 weeks gestation: The CDC recommends 2 mg/kg PO as a single dose 48–72 hours after birth. If the mother received nevirapine less than 1 hour prior to delivery, the infant should be given 2 mg/kg PO as soon as possible after birth and again at 48–72 hours. *Oral dosage (nevirapine and zidovudine combination):* Pregnant females, intrapartum. Due to synergistic inhibition of HIV with the combination in vitro, the following regimen has been suggested: nevirapine 200 mg PO as a single dose at the onset of labor plus zidovudine (2 mg/kg IV bolus followed by 1 mg/kg/per hour IV continuous infusion until delivery). During or immediately after intrapartum treatment with nevirapine and zidovudine, consider initiation of maternal zidovudine and lamivudine, continuing for 3–7 days, to potentially reduce development of nevirapine resistance. Neonates more than and equal to 34 weeks gestation: Due to synergistic inhibition of HIV with the combination in vitro, the following regimen has been suggested: nevirapine 2 mg/kg PO as a single oral dose at age 48–72 hours plus zidovudine (2 mg/kg PO every 6 hours for 6 weeks). Maximum *Dosage limits: adolescents:* 400 mg/day PO. *Children:* 300 mg/m², up to 400 mg, per day PO. *Infants:* 300 mg/m², up to 400 mg, per day PO. *Neonates more than and equal to 15 days old:* 300 mg/m², up to 400 mg, per day PO. Neonates less than 15 days old: Safe and effective use not established.			

Drug	Brand name	Dosage	Contraindications	Drug interaction	Side effects
Zidovudine (azidothymidine or AZT)	Retrovir, Zidovir	*Newborn:* Prevention of fetomaternal transmission. *Oral:* 2 mg/kg/per dose 4 times daily started within 12 hours of birth and continued for 6 weeks. IV 1.5 mg/kg/per dose 4 times daily. *Child:* Oral 180 mg/m² 2 times daily (max 250 mg/dose). IV 120 mg/m² 4 times daily.	Hypersensitivity to zidovudine or components. Contra-indicated in neonates with hyperbilirubinemia requiring treatment other than phototherapy or if serum transaminases are more than 5 times normal levels. Avoid if hemoglobin less than 7.5 g/dL or neutrophil counts < 0.75 × 10⁹/L.	Alterations in phenytoin plasma levels may occur, normally a decrease in levels although increase has been reported; monitor carefully. Increased incidence of neutropenia reported with paracetamol, but the mechanism is unclear. It has been suggested that short-term paracetamol use is acceptable, but with close monitoring. Other drugs that inhibit or competes for glucuronidation or inhibit hepatic microsomal enzymes should be used with caution as they may alter the metabolism of zidovudine; use with caution and monitor closely. Concurrent therapy with other potentially nephrotoxic or myelosuppressive drugs may have additive effects (pentamidine, ganciclovir, dapsone, amphotericin, pyrimethamine and flucytosine). Ribavirin (tribavarin) antagonizes zidovudine anti-viral activity in vitro. Similar data has been reported for ganciclovir. Rifampicin may decrease plasma levels of zidovudine. Probenecid increases half-life and area under plasma concentration time curve by decreasing glucuronidation and reducing renal excretion. Sodium valproate, fluconazole or methadone may increase plasma concentrations of zidovudine; monitor carefully for zidovudine-related adverse effects.	Reversible anemia, neutropenia and leukopenia occur, usually after 4–6 weeks of therapy but potentially earlier. Regular monitoring is advised. Patients with preexisting bone marrow depression are particularly at risk. Dose reduction or suspension of treatment may be required. Lactic acidosis and severe hepatomegaly with steatosis have been reported. Although a causal relationship is unclear monitoring of liver enzymes is advised and treatment should be suspended if necessary. Headache, nausea, vomiting and other gastrointestinal effects reported. Myalgia, myopathy or polymyositis have been reported generally after 6–12 months therapy in adults. Hypersensitivity reactions, including anaphylaxis, have occurred rarely. Skin rashes also reported. Capsules swallowed at night while lying down have reportedly caused esophageal ulceration in some adults.

Contd...

Drug	Brand name	Dosage	Contraindications	Drug interaction	Side effects
Antifungal					
Amphotericin	Abelcet, AmBisome, Amfotex, Amphocil, Mycol	No dose reduction is generally required in preexisting renal failure. Dose reduction may be advisable if amphotericin is suspected of causing nephrotoxicity. Lipid complex formulations should also be considered in such situations. In renal dialysis patients, administration of amphotericin should commence only when dialysis is completed. *Children*: 2.5–5 mg/kg IV infused over 1–2 hours once a day. May use higher doses of 7.5–10 mg/kg per 24 hours if indicated and tolerated.	Lipid formulations, particularly liposomal amphotericin, less likely to cause severe side-effects, still advisable to monitor for hypersensitivity to amphotericin or any constituents of the formulations. Renal impairment may occur and discontinuation or reduction should be considered if urea or serum creatinine exceed twice the upper limit of normal. Monitor serum potassium, magnesium and phosphate as low serum levels may occur. Monitor LFTs and consider discontinuation if seriously deranged. Avoid concurrent nephrotoxic drugs, antineoplastic agents if possible and also corticosteroids unless necessary to control drug reactions. Hyperkalemia and arrhythmias can result if administered too rapidly.	Increased nephrotoxicity with concurrent use of other nephrotoxic drugs. Amphotericin-induced hypokalemia may potentiate toxicity of digitalis glycosides and enhance effects of skeletal muscle relaxants. Corticosteroids may enhance potassium depletion. Flucytosine toxicity may be enhanced by increased cellular uptake and/or impaired renal function. *Zidovudine*: Effects on bone marrow and renal function may be enhanced. Concomitant administration with cyclosporin has reportedly resulted in increased cyclosporin levels. Acute pulmonary reactions have occurred when amphotericin is given during or shortly after leukocyte transfusions.	*Conventional formulation:* Acute infusion reactions are the most frequent adverse reactions such as fever, shaking, chills, nausea, vomiting, headache, dyspnea, tachypnea, gastrointestinal effects, muscle and joint pains, pain at site of injection. These reactions are most severe and occur most frequently with initial doses and often lessen with subsequent doses. Febrile reactions may be managed by IV administration of hydrocortisone but keep dose and duration to a minimum. Other reactions may be decreased by use of antihistamines or paracetamol. Nephrotoxicity occurs to some degree in more than 85% of patients. Hypokalemia, hypomagnesemia, azotemia, renal tubular acidosis, nephrocalcinosis and hyposthenuria can occur. Increased urea and serum creatinine, decreased creatinine clearance, glomerulose of filtration rate (GFR) and decreased renal blood flow occur in many patients receiving conventional amphotericin. Renal function generally improves within a few months though some degree of permanent impairment may occur. Patients with higher serum low density lipoprotein (LDL)

Contd...

Contd...

Contd...

Drug	Brand name	Dosage	Contraindications	Drug interaction	Side effects
					concentrations may be more susceptible to renal toxicity. Less common renal toxicity reactions are: anuria, oliguria, hematuria, urinary incontinence and acute renal failure.
Fluconazole	Forcan, Zocon	*Newborn: Systemic candidiasis and cryptococcosis.* Oral/IV 6–12 mg/kg every 72 hours in less than 14 days, every 48 hours in 14–28 days and every 24 hours in more than 28 day olds. Mucosal candidiasis 3 mg/kg in same intervals. *Children mucosal candidiasis:* Oral/IV loading dose 6 mg/kg followed by 3 mg/kg once daily for 7–14 days. *Systemic candidiasis and cryptococcosis:* 6–12 mg/kg daily once (max 400 mg), dose dependent on severity of infection. Prophylaxis of fungal infection in immunocompromised 3–12 mg/kg once daily (max 400 mg) dose dependent on extent and duration of neutropenia.	Contraindicated in known hypersensitivity to azole compounds. In some patients, particularly those with underlying serious diseases, such as HIV or malignancies, hepatic, renal, hematological and biochemical abnormalities may be exaggerated. Patients with AIDS are considered at higher risk of developing severe cutaneous reactions. Co-administration of cisapride or terfenadine contraindicated.	Fluconazole enhances effects or plasma levels of warfarin, sulphonylureas, phenytoin, theophylline, zidovudine and rifabutin. Potential increase in levels of midazolam and cyclosporin is less clear. Plasma levels measured where appropriate. Plasma concentration of fluconazole reduced by rifampicin; 25% decrease in area under coverage (AUC) and 20% shorter half-life. Consider dose increase. Hydrochlorothiazide may increase plasma fluconazole concentration by up to 40%. Due to potentially serious interactions with terfenadine and cisapride leading to significantly increased levels of these drugs and an increased risk of various cardiac adverse events, fluconazole combination with either of these drugs is contraindicated.	*Gastrointestinal:* nausea, diarrhea and flatulence, headache, skin rashes, seizures, leucopenia rarely reported. Toxic epidermal necrolysis and Stevens–Johnson syndrome reported rarely. Occasional abnormalities in liver enzymes, usually mild and transient, reported in 5–7% of patients. Higher increases reported in 1% of patients. Eosinophilia, anemia, thrombocytopenia rarely reported. Hypokalemia has been reported (see warnings section).
Flucytosine		*Newborn:* IV/oral 100 mg/kg per day less than 7 days and 100–200 mg/kg per day more than 7 days in four divided doses. *Children:* IV/oral 200 mg/kg per day (100–140 mg/kg per day if organism sensitive) in four divided doses. *In renal impairment:* CrCl in mL/min per 1.73 m², 20–40, 50% daily dose in two divided doses; 10–20, 25% of daily dose once daily; less than 10, 50 mg/kg as single dose and adjust dose according to serum levels.	Hypersensitivity to flucytosine or any excipients. Monitoring of blood count and liver enzymes advisable before and during therapy. Use with particular care in patients with preexisting bone marrow depression.	Cytarabine may reduce plasma flucytosine concentrations; plasma concentration monitoring advisable.	Nausea, vomiting, diarrhea and skin rash. Rarely, confusion, hallucinations, convulsions, sedation and headache. Generally, reversible elevations of liver enzymes have been reported although hepatitis and hepatic necrosis have occurred. Bone marrow depression with leukopenia, thrombocytopenia,

Contd...

Contd...

Textbook of Pediatric Infectious Diseases

620

Drug	Brand name	Dosage	Contraindications	Drug interaction	Side effects
					agranulocytosis or aplastic anemia has occurred, generally when plasma levels are high in renal impaired patients treated concurrently with amphotericin. Other adverse effects: pyrexia, hypoglycemia, hypokalemia, muscle weakness, cardiac arrest and respiratory arrest. Side-effects more likely if serum level is more than 100 µg/mL.
Flumazenil		*Dosage description:* IV bolus over 15 seconds less than 12 years 10 µg/kg (max 200 µg) and more than 12 years 200 µg as single dose, repeated every minimum to maximum total dose of 40 µg/kg. IV infusion less than 12 years 2–10 µg/kg per hours (max 400 µg dose/hr) and more than 12 years 100–400 µg/kg per hours.	See warning above. Contraindicated in patients who have been given a benzodiazepine for control of a life-threatening condition. Use is not recommended in epileptic patients who have been receiving benzodiazepine treatment for a prolonged period. Use with caution in patients with head injury.	The effects of non benzodiazepines acting via the benzodiazepine receptor (e.g. zopiclone) are blocked by flumazenil.	Generally well tolerated. Nausea and vomiting are the most common adverse effects and dizziness is a common CNS effect. Rare reports of seizures, especially in epileptics. Benzodiazepine withdrawal symptoms may be experienced in patients who have received benzodiazepines for long periods. In mixed overdose, administration of flumazenil may unmask adverse effects of other psychotropic drugs. Cardiac arrhythmias are reported rarely.
Griseofulvin	Fluvin, Grisovin-FP	1 month to 12 years 10 mg/kg and 12–18 years 500 mg once daily.	Liver failure, lupus erythematosus, porphyria. Males should not father children within 6 months of treatment.	Accelerates metabolism of warfarin and oral contraceptives. Phenobarbital (Phenobarbitone) accelerates griseofulvin metabolism. Plasma cyclosporin levels may be reduced.	Headache, nausea, vomiting, rashes, photosensitivity, dizziness, fatigue, agranulocytosis and leukopenia.
Itraconazole	Canditral, Sporanox	*Oral:* Less than 12 years 3–5 mg/kg and 12–18 years 100 mg once daily for 15 days in tinea corporis, tinea cruris and oropharyngeal candidiasis and 30 days for tinea pedis and tines manuum. *Aspergillosis:* Allergic bronchopulmonary 3–5 mg/kg in two divided doses.	Avoid in liver disease. For treatment longer than 1 month, liver function tests required. Caution with renal disease-decreased bioavailability. Absorption reduced in AIDS and neutropenia. Discontinue, if peripheral neuropathy occurs.	Increased plasma levels of terfenadine, astemizole and cisapride-risk of serious arrhythmias, avoid concurrent use. Increased plasma levels of midazolam prolonged sedation, concurrent oral use contraindicated. Increased	Nausea, abdominal pain, dyspepsia, constipation (diarrhea with oral liquids). Headache, dizziness, raised hepatic enzymes, menstrual disorders. Allergic reactions including pruritus, rash, urticaria and angioedema.

Contd...

Contd...

Drug	Brand name	Dosage	Contraindications	Drug interaction	Side effects
				levels of digoxin, warfarin and ciclosporin (cyclosporin) have been reported monitor levels. Phenytoin, rifampicin and carbamazepine greatly reduce the oral bioavailability of itraconazole.	
Ketoconazole	Ketovate Shampoo, Nizral	*Pityriasis versicolor:* Use daily for a maximum of 5 days. Seborrhe c dermatitis and dandruff: use twice weekly for 2–4 weeks, Candidiasis, candiduria or chromomycosis. Oral: Adolescent 200 mg PO once daily. Serious infection may require 400 mg PO once daily. Children more than and equal to 2 years of age: 3.3–6.6 mg/kg PO once daily. Children ess than 2 years of age: Safety and efficacy have not been established. Oropharyngeal candidiasis (thrush) in HIV-infected children. *Oral in children:* 3–7 mg/kg per day for 5–49 days till cured. Vulvovaginal candidiasis. *Nonpregnant adolescent females:* 200–600 mg PO once daily for 3–6 days. For recurrent vulvovaginal candidiasis, topical or oral therapy daily for 2 weeks, then 6 months of therapy that could include ketoconazole 100 mg PO every day. Not recommended in pregnancy are tinea capitis, tinea corporis, tinea cruris, tinea pedis, tinea manuum, tinea unguium (onychomycosis) caused by *Trichophyton species, Microsporum spp.* or epidermophyton species, and tinea versicolor. *Adolescent:* 200 mg PO once daily. Serious infection may require 400 mg PO once daily. Children more than and equal to 2 years of age: 3.3–6.6 mg/kg PO once daily.	Hypersensitivity to any of ingredients. Avoid oral drug in hepatic disease. Due to its potent inhibition of the CYP3A4 enzyme system, oral ketoconazole co-administration with other drugs should be done with extreme caution, if at all (check drug interactions). When stopping long-term topical corticosteroids, use the topical corticosteroid with the shampoo and then gradually withdraw the steroid therapy over 2–3 weeks. Keep out of eyes. If adolescent develops drowsiness, care to be taken when driving or operating machinery.		Nausea/vomiting, hepatotoxicity, urticaria, anaphylactoid reactions, drowsiness, dizziness, headache and photophobia reported. Inhibits testosterone secretion at doses of 200–400 mg/day and can inhibit cortisol synthesis in doses of 400–600 mg/day. Inhibition of testosterone synthesis has led to cases of gynecomastia, libido decrease, and impotence (erectile dysfunction). Serum testosterone concentrations return to baseline and gynecomastia and impotence usually abate after ketoconazole therapy is stopped. Local burning sensation, itching, irritation and oily/dry hair reported on topical application. Discoloration of chemically damaged hair observed.
Nystatin	Mycostatin	*Newborn:* Treatment and prophylaxis against oral *Candidia*, 1 mL three to four times daily. *Children:* Intestinal and oral candida 1 mL three to four times daily; oral candida in immunocompromised 1 mL 46 times; esophageal/ intestinal candida 5 ml or one tablet four to six times daily.	Hypersensitivity to nystatin has been reported. Some nystatin oral suspension preparations contain sugar and are unsuitable for children with disaccharide intolerance. Use sugar-free bands.	None known.	*Infrequent and generally mild and transient:* Nausea, vomiting, gastrointestinal distress, diarrhea, very rarely rashes and Stevens–Johnson syndrome.
Terbinafine	Tebina		*Cream:* avoid contact with eyes. *Tablets:* caution in renal and hepatic impairment.	Terbinafine plasma concentration reduced by rifampicin, increased by cimetidine.	*Oral use:* Gastrointestinal-loss of appetite, nausea, diarrhea, mild abdominal pain; others are: rash, urticaria, arthralgia and myalgia. *Topical use:* redness, itching or stinging; rarely allergic reactions.

Contd...

Contd...

Drug	Brand name	Dosage	Contraindications	Drug interaction	Side effects
Antihelminthic					
Ivermectin	Ivermectol	Five to eighteen years 0.15 mg/kg as single dose to repeat every 6–8 months. Strongyloidosis: Five to eighteen years 0.2 mg/kg for 2 days as single dose and repeat every 6–12 months, if necessary. Filariasis: Ivermectin has no lethal effects against adult worms and therefore it is to be given in dose of 150 μg/kg once a year for 10 years. If symptoms recur, then dose is given every 3 months instead of once a year. Ivermectin is also effective against lymphatic filaria caused by W. bancrofti. In endemic areas, for mass treatments single dose of albendazole 400 mg + ivermectin 200 mg/kg every 12 months is highly effective in controlling filariasis. Its effect is more sustained than diethylcarbamazine for elimination of microfilaria from skin and ocular tissues. Ivermectin is not used against filariasis caused by Loa loa due to risk of encephalopathy (in Loa loa diethylcarbamazine and albendazole are first and second line drug of choice). Scabies and pediculosis: Recently single dose of ivermectin (200 μg/kg) has been found to be highly effective in treatment of scabies and head lice. Ivermectin is typically helpful in treatment of crusted scabies found in patient with immunosuppression (e.g. HIV and leukemia, etc.). It is used to prevent and cure the outbreak of scabies in institution.	Contraindications: History of hypersensitivity to ivermectin; children <5 years of age; severe concurrent illness (delay treatment); pregnancy. Cautions: Individuals with CNS disorders, e.g. epilepsy, meningitis or trypanosomiasis; nursing mothers. Monitor for ophthalmic and other hypersensitivity reactions when onchocerciasis is being treated.		Fever, pruritus, arthralgia, myalgia, postural hypotension, edema, lymphadenopathy, gastrointestinal symptoms, sore throat, cough and headache. Less severe than those occurring with diethylcarbamazine.
Levamisole	Vermisol	Roundworm (ascariasis): Less than 12 years 2.5–3 mg/kg and 12–18 years 150 mg as single dose. Hookworm (ankylostomiasis): Less than 12 years 2.5 mg/kg and 12–18 years 150 mg as single dose. Repeat after 7 days if severe infection. Adults: 300 mg for 1–2 days. Nephrotic syndrome: 2.5 mg/kg on alternate days for 12–18 months.	Contraindicated in patients demonstrating previous hypersensitivity to levamisole. Also patients with preexisting blood disorders. Caution in rheumatoid arthritis, Sjögren syndrome, epilepsy and liver disease where dose adjustment may be necessary.	Warfarin and phenytoin-some evidence that levamisole can increase effects of these drugs but clinical importance uncertain. There have been reports that levamisole can produce a disulfiram-like reaction with alcohol.	When given in single doses for the treatment of worm infestations it is generally well tolerated and side-effects are limited to nausea, vomiting, diarrhea, abdominal pain, dizziness and headache (affects approximately 1% of patients). When given for longer periods for other indications (immunostimulant effect) may get more serious side-effects including hypersensitivity reactions, hematological reactions (consult an expert nephrologist for advice on monitoring blood counts during treatment).

Contd...

Contd...

Contd...

Drug	Brand name	Dosage	Contraindications	Drug interaction	Side effects
Mebendazole	Mebex, Wormin	*Oral:* More than 6 months 100 mg as single dose for all members of the family, may be repeated after 2 weeks. All other susceptible worm infestation: 100 mg two times daily for three consecutive days. Better than albendazole for trichuris infestation. *Hydatid disease:* 200–400 mg bid or tid for 3–4 weeks, less effective than albendazole. Reduction in dose for hepatic impairment	*Contraindications:* pregnancy, breastfeeding of children less than 2 years of age and in patients with known hypersensitivity to the product or its components.	Increased plasma mebendazole concentration with cimetidine. Plasma concentrations may be lowered with concurrent administration of phenytoin or carbamazepine.	Rarely, transient abdominal pain and diarrhea—only reported in cases of massive infestation and expulsion of worms. Hypersensitivity reactions, e.g. exanthema, rash, urticaria and angioedema. Rare reports of convulsions in children less than 1 year.
Antiprotozoal					
Diloxanide furoate		Oral: Two to twelve years 20 mg/kg per day and 12–18 years 1.5 g in three divided doses.	Hypersensitivity to diloxanide furoate.		No serious side-effects have been reported. Flatulence, vomiting, urticaria and pruritus may occur.
Furazolidone	Furoxone	*Oral:* One month to 12 years 6 mg/kg per day in four divided doses and 12–18 years 400 mg/day in four divided doses. 7–10 days for giardiasis and for 4–6 days after defervescence in typhoid fever.	Prior sensitivity to furazolidone. Furazolidone may cause mild, reversible intravascular hemolysis in G6PD deficient patients. Such patients should be closely observed and furazolidone treatment stopped if any evidence of hemolysis occurs. Furazolidone should not be given to infants less than 1 month of age (who have immature enzyme systems and glutathione instability) because of the possibility of producing hemolytic anemia. Furazolidone is a monoamine oxidase inhibitor (MAOI) and the cautions advised for MAOIs regarding the concomitant administration of other drugs, especially indirect acting sympathomimetic amines, and the consumption of food and drink containing tyramine should be observed;	*Alcohol:* a disulfiram like reaction has been reported in patients consuming alcohol whilst on furazolidone; alcohol should be avoided for the duration of treatment and for 4 days thereafter to prevent this reaction.	Nausea and vomiting are the most common side-effects and abdominal pain, diarrhea, headache and malaise occur occasionally. Hypersensitivity reactions including a fall in blood pressure, urticaria, fever, arthralgia, and a vesicular morbilliform rash have occurred in a small number of patients.

Contd...

Drug	Brand name	Dosage	Contraindications	Drug interaction	Side effects
			however, there appear to be no reports of hypertensive crisis in patients receiving furazolidone. Darkening of the urine due to the presence of metabolites.		
Metronidazole	Flagyl, Metrogyl	*Newborn:* IV 15 mg/kg as loading dose followed 24 hours later by 7.5 mg/kg per dose two times daily. Anaerobic infections and propionic and methylmalonic acidemia. Oral/IV 7.5 mg/kg per dose (max 400–500 mg) three times daily. *Giardiasis:* Oral 40 mg/kg (max 2 g) once daily for 3 days. *Trichomoniasis:* 5 mg/kg per dose (max 300–499 mg/day) three times daily for 7 days. Amebiasis (5–10 days), balantidiasis (5 days): Oral 10 mg/kg (max 400–800 g). *H. pylori* oral 1–6 years 100 mg, 6–12 years 200 mg and 12–18 years 400 mg/dose three times daily for 14 days with either amoxicillin/omeprazole or clarithromycin/omeprazole. Increase dose interval to 12 hours in renal impairment (Cr Cl < 20 mL/min per 1.73 m². Reduce dose in hepatic impairment and avoid in hepatic encephalopathy.	Use with caution and reduce dose in severe hepatic impairment. In patients with preexisting blood dyscrasia leukocyte counts are advised.	Potentiates anticoagulant effect of warfarin. No effect on heparin. Increased levels of lithium may lead to lithium toxicity. Increased levels of phenytoin may occur and levels should be monitored. Cimetidine reduces hepatic metabolism of metronidazole leading to increased serum levels and potentially increased incidence of side-effects. Phenobarbital (phenobarbitone) may significantly decrease serum levels. Possible potentiation of vecuronium action has been reported. Disulfiram reaction may occur with alcohol and the alcohol content of concurrently administered medication should be considered.	Nausea, vomiting, unpleasant taste and gastrointestinal disturbances are most common, and darkening of urine may occur. CNS effects such as drowsiness, dizziness, headache and ataxia occur rarely. Skin rashes, urticaria, myalgia and arthralgia have been reported. During intensive or prolonged therapy, seizures or peripheral neuropathy have occurred. Mild leukopenia and thrombocytopenia have also been reported rarely.
Nitazoxanide	Nitacure	*Amebiasis, giardiasis, cryptosporidiosis and helminthiasis:* 12–47 months, 100 mg 12 hourly for 3 days; 4–11 years 200 mg 12 hourly for 3 days; adolescents: 500 mg 12 hourly for 3 days.	Prior hypersensitivity to nitazoxanide. It should be used with caution in patients with hepatic and renal disease. Diabetic patients should be aware that oral suspension contains 1.48 g of sucrose per 5 mL.	Nitazoxanide inhibits the cytochrome P450C9 enzyme and therefore it affects metabolism of drugs like warfarin, phenytoin, etc. Tizoxanide is highly bound to plasma proteins (more than 99%) and hence should be used carefully with other plasma protein bound drugs.	Usually well tolerated with minimal side effects like headache, nausea and mild abdominal discomfort. Abdominal pain (7.8%), diarrhea (2.1%), vomiting (1.1%), headache (1.1%)—all symptoms transient in nature. Pruritus, pale yellow discoloration of eye, rhinitis, dizziness are observed in less than 1% of cases.

Contd...

Contd...

Drug	Brand name	Dosage	Contraindications	Drug interaction	Side effects
Pyrimethamine		*Toxoplasmosis in pregnancy*: If toxoplasma infection is diagnosed in early pregnancy and the fetus is not infected, spiramycin is given (see spiramycin monograph). If the fetus is found to be infected then pyrimethamine 50 mg once daily, sulfadiazine 1 g 3 times daily and calcium folinate (folinic ac d) 15 mg 3 times per week are given until delivery. *Toxoplasmosis in infants*: pyrimethamine along with sulfadiazine (50 mg/kg 2 times daily) and calcium folinate (folinic ac d) (15 mg/kg 3 times in a week) are given for 12 months. Pyrimethamine is started with loading dose of 1 mg/ kg per dose two times daily for 2 days, then 1 mg/kg per dose once daily for 6 months followed by 1 mg/kg per dose thrice in a week for 6 months. Prednisolone at 0.5/ kg per dose two times daily is also given until signs of CNS inflammation (CSF protein >10 g/L) or active chorioretinitis have settled and then tapered. Ocular toxoplasmosis, reactivation of toxoplasmosis during HIV infection and toxoplasmosis in immunocompromised child with protracted or incapacitating illness: 2 mg/kg loading dose for 2 days followed by 1 mg/kg in less than 12 years and 25–100 mg in 12–18 years olds for 6 weeks to prevent relapse in HIV patie ts followed by maintenance of a quarter to half of starting c ose indefinitely.	History of pyrimethamine sensitivity. Avoid large loading doses in patients with a history of seizures.	The antifolate properties of pyrimethamine may exacerbate those of other antifolates such as co-trimoxazole, trimethoprim, methotrexate and phenytoin. Sequential blockade of folate pathways by sulfone or sulfonamide plus pyrimethamine results in considerable potentiation in the treatment of malaria and toxoplasmosis.	These can include gastrointestinal symptoms, such as atrophic glossitis, abdominal pain and vomiting; hematological effects such as megaloblastic anemia, leukopenia, thrombocytopenia and pancytopenia and CNS effects, including headache, dizziness, and insomnia. Calcium folinate (folinic acid) should be given concurrently to prevent the hematological effects.
Sodium stibogluconate	Sodium stibogluconate	IV/IM 1 month to 18 years, 20 mg/kg (max 850 mg) daily once for 20–30 days. Total daily dose may be given in two divided doses 12 hours apart.	Severe hepatic and renal impairment (cautious use in mild-moderate impairment) and previous serious reaction to stibogluconate are absolute contraindications. Some hepatic derangement is seen in leishmaniasis and in these cases the benefit of treatment outweighs the risk of medicating. Heart disease, cautious use and monitor ECG biweekly. IM injections are very painful.	None reported	Arthralgias and myalgias that ranged from mild discomfort to activity-limiting effects. Abdominal pain and nausea/vomiting were usually reported in the first week and were associated with elevated serum amylase and lipase concentrations. Hepatic abnormalities involved elevated SGPT and SGOT. Hepatic impairment may be rapidly reversed upon discontinuation of sodium stibogluconate. Other side effects included fatigue, anorexia, headache and rash. Hematologic suppression may be characterized by decreased white blood cell, hematocrit, and/or platelet counts. ECG changes have been documented in treated

Contd...

Contd...

Drug	Brand name	Dosage	Contraindications	Drug interaction	Side effects
					patients, predominately flattening and/or T-wave inversion when compared with baseline. ECG abnormalities resolve within 6 weeks after completion of treatment. QT prolongation and sudden death have been documented with dose of more than 20 mg/kg per day or when treatment given for greater than 30 days. Thrombophlebitis may be expected. If cough, vomiting or chest pain (retrosternal) occur, administration should be stopped immediately.
Tinidazole	Tini, Tiniba	*Oral:* One month to 12 years 50–60 mg/kg and 12; 12 years 2 g, single dose for *Trichomonas vaginitis* and amebiasis, 3 days for amebiasis and colitis and 5 days for liver abscess.	Contraindicated during the first trimester of pregnancy, in patients with organic neurologic disorders and in those with known hypersensitivity to tinidazole	*Alcohol:* Disulfiram-like reaction is possible.	Generally infrequent, mild and self-limiting and can include nausea, vomiting, anorexia, diarrhea, metallic taste, abdominal pain, and rarely headache, tiredness and hypersensitivity reactions (occasionally severe with rash, urticaria, pruritus and angioneurotic edema).
Antiparasitic					
Diethylcarbam-azine	Banocide, Hetrazan	*Filariasis and loiasis:* Oral 300 µg/kg per dose on day 1 and increased over 3 days to 2 mg/kg per dose three times daily for 3 weeks. Tropical pulmonary eosinophilia: oral 6 mg/kg per day in three divided doses for 21 days. Toxocariasis (visceral larva migrans): Oral 160 µg/kg per dose on day 1 and 2 and increased over 3 days to 2 mg/kg per dose three times and given for further 7–10 days.	Hypersensitivity to diethylcarbamazine. Severe allergic reactions can occur especially in patients with onchocerciasis or Loa loa infection. In the event of severe hypersensitivity reaction, administration of a corticosteroid is recommended. Encephalitis may occur in patients with loiasis. Monitor for eye changes in patients with onchocerciasis. Impaired renal function: dose reduction may be required.	Concurrent use of diethylcarbamazine with corticosteroids may reduce the antifiliarial activity of diethylcarbamazine. Urinary alkalinizers can reduce the loss of diethylcarbamazine in the urine, whereas urinary acidifiers can increase the loss.	Headache, lassitude, weakness, general malaise are seen most commonly. Nausea, vomiting, skin rash, occasionally observed. Severe allergic phenomenon can occur in conjunction with the skin rash, in patients with onchocerciasis severe allergic reactions may occur. Facial edema and pruritus, especially of the eyes, are often encountered.

Contd...

Contd...

Contd...

Drug	Brand name	Dosage	Contraindications	Drug interaction	Side effects
Gamma Benzene Hexachloride	Gab, Scaboma	*Scabies:* Apply to whole body surface below neck. Scrub baths after 12–24 hours. If required, one more application may be repeated after a week. *Pediculosis:* Massage scalp with emulsion at night and cover with a piece of cloth. Following morning, head bath should be taken ensuring that medication does not enter eyes.		*Oil:* Enhances absorption of gamma benzene hexachloride. Therefore avoid simultaneous applications of creams, ointment and oils.	As it is highly lipophilic drug, systemic absorption and toxicity may occur. The manifestations are convulsions, vertigo, ataxia, tremor. Local skin irritation.
Ivermectin	Ivermectol	5–18 years 0.15 mg/kg as single dose to repeat every 6–8 months. *Strongylo dosis:* 5–18 years, 0.2 mg/kg for 2 days as single dose and repeat every 6–12 months, if necessary. *Filariasis:* Ivermectin has no lethal effects against adult worms and therefore it is to be given in dose of 150 µg/kg once a year for 10 years. If symptoms recur, then dose is given every 3 months instead of once a year. Ivermectin is also effective against lymphatic filaria caused by *W. bancrofti*. In endemic areas, for mass treatments single dose of albendazole 400 mg + ivermectin 200 mg/kg every 12 months is highly effective in controlling filaria. Its effect is more sustained than diethylcarbamazine for elimination of microfilaria from skin and ocular tissues. Ivermectin is not used against filaria caused by Loa loa due to risk of encephalopathy (in Loa loa diethylcarbamazine and albendazole are first and second line drug of choice). *Scabies and pediculosis:* Recently single dose of ivermectin (200 µg/kg) has been found to be highly effective in treatment of scabies and head lice. Ivermectin is typically helpful in treatment of crusted scabies found in patient with immunosuppression (e.g. HIV and leukemia, etc.). It is used to prevent and cure the outbreak of scabies in institution.	*Contraindications:* History of hypersensitivity to ivermectin; children less than 5 years of age; severe concurrent illness (delay treatment); pregnancy. *Cautions:* individuals with CNS disorders, e.g. epilepsy, meningitis or trypanosomiasis; nursing mothers. Monitor for ophthalmic and other hypersensitivity reactions when onchocerciasis is being treated.		Fever, pruritus, arthralgia, myalgia, postural hypotension, edema, lymphadenopathy, gastrointestinal symptoms, sore throat, cough and headache. Less severe than those occurring with diethylcarbamazine.
Niclosamide	Niclosan	Tenia solium (pork) tenia saginata (beef), diphyllobothrium latum (fish); Oral less than 2 years 500 mg, 2–6 year 1 gm, more than 7 years 2 g once daily; give the dose in two divided doses one before breakfast and the rest 1 hour later. Hymenolepis nana (dwarf tapeworm): Oral single dose on first day followed by ½ that dose daily once for the next 6 days. Initial day dose for less than 2, 2–6 and 7–18 year are 500 mg, 1 g and 2 g, respectively. No purgative is needed.	*Contraindications:* Hypersensitivity to niclosamide. *Warnings:* In infection with Tenia solium there is always a danger of cysticercosis. A drastic purge is therefore recommended to eject the lower segment of the tapeworm containing mature eggs. For other warnings refer to the manufacturers SPC.	Alcohol may possibly increase the side effects of niclosamide.	Mild transient gastrointestinal effects, e.g. nausea, retching and abdominal pain, light-headedness, pruritis.

Contd...

Drug	Brand name	Dosage	Contraindications	Drug interaction	Side effects
Nitazoxanide	Nitacure	Amebiasis, giardiasis, cryptosporiodiosis and helminthiasis: 12–47 months, 100 mg 12 hourly for 3 days; 4–11 years, 200 mg 12 hourly for 3 days; adolescents: 500 mg 12 hourly for 3 days.	Prior hypersensitivity to nitazoxanide. It should be used with caution in patients with hepatic and renal disease. Diabetic patients should be aware that oral suspension contains 1.48 g of sucrose per 5 mL	Nitazoxanide inhibits the cytochrome P4502C9 enzyme and therefore it affects metabolism of drugs like warfarin, phenytoin, etc. Tizoxanide is highly bound to plasma proteins (more than 99%) and hence should be used carefully with other plasma protein bound drugs	Usually well tolerated with minimal side effects like headache, nausea and mild abdominal discomfort. Abdominal pain (7.8%), diarrhea (2.1%), vomiting (1.1%), Headahce (1.1%)—all symptoms transient in nature. Pruritus, pale yellow discoloration of eye, rhinitis, dizziness are observed in less than 1% of cases.
Permethrin	Perlice, Permite, Scabper cream, Scabper lotion	Scabies (dermal cream). Single topical application of up to: 1 tube for children more than 12 years. Half a tube for children aged 6–12 years. A quarter of a tube for children aged 1–5 years. An 8th of a tube for children aged 2 months to 1 year. Medical supervision required for children less than 2 years of age. If necessary a second application may be given not less than 7 days after the initial application. Apply to whole body excluding head. Wash off after 8–12 hours. Children less than 2 years old should also have the cream applied to the face, neck, scalp and ears. If hands or any part are washed, the treatment must be reapplied. *Pediculosis:* Head lice (cream rinse). Apply to clean damp hair, leave on for 10 minutes, rinse and dry. Not affected by chlorine in swimming pools.	Avoid contact with eyes. Do not use on broken or secondarily infected skin.	None known.	Pruritus, erythema and stinging.
Antimicrobial eye					
Framycetin sulfate	Soframycin	*Eye drops:* One to two drops 2 hourly and reducing gradually as infection gets controlled to 48 hours after the eye is clinically normal. *Eye ointment:* Three times daily when given alone or at bedtime along with eye drops given during the day. *Cream:* Apply one to three times daily.	Caution is advised in using framycetin in children allergic to streptomyces derived antibiotics (e.g. aminoglycosides). Care must be taken in children with hepatic and renal impairment as systemic absorption occurs when eye drops are given in high doses. Avoid if eardrum is perforated and fungal and viral infections of the eye. Avoid skin cream in viral and tuberculous lesions and in varicella and vaccinia. If large areas of skin are being treated, ototoxicity may be a hazard in children, especially in those with renal impairment.	Coadministration with gentamicin eye drops reduces the risk of selecting resistant organisms.	If large areas of skin are being treated, ototoxicity may be a hazard in children, especially those with renal impairment. Sensitization, contact dermatitis, local irritation and itching.

Contd...

Contd...

Drug	Brand name	Dosage	Contraindications	Drug interaction	Side effects
Topical antibacterial / ANTIBIOTIC					
Neomycin sulfate	Methacin, Neomycin sulfate	*Adolescents:* 0.25–1 g four times. *Children:* 12.5 mg/kg per dose oral in diarrhea and 3 g/m² per day q 6 hours oral in hepatic coma. *Eye drops:* Superficial eye infection, 1 drop two to four times daily, severe infection one drop every 15–20 minutes initially then reducing frequency as infection gets controlled. *Eye ointment:* Three to four times daily. Treatment to continue till 2 days after condition is cured.	Renal failure, hypersensitivity.	Aminoglycosides, vancomycin, methoxyflurane enflurane cephaloridine: increased nephrotoxic affects. *Loop diuretics:* The auditory toxicity appears to be increased. Anesthetics, neuromuscular blocking agents (tubocurarine, gallamine): Risk of neuromuscular blockade and respiratory paralysis. Penicillin V, methotrexate, 5-fluorouracil, oral Vitamin B₁₂ *Digoxin:* Oral neomycin inhibits the GI absorption of these drugs. *Coumarin:* Oral, neomycin enhances effect of coumarin.	Ototoxicity and nephrotoxicitly. Urticaria, rash, erythema, dermatitis contact syndrome conjunctivitis.
Potassium permanganate		Cleansing and deodorizing suppurating eczematous reactions and wounds for wet dressings or baths, use approximately 0.01% (1 in 10,000) solution OR 1 granule dissolved in 300 mL (2 1/2 glasses) of water.	Not for oral use. Use with particular care in patients with extensive erosive or ulcerated skin lesions, especially if they have renal failure, due to theoretical risk of absorption. Irritant to mucous membranes. Stains skin and clothing. Do not use in ceramic basin or bath as staining will occur.		
Povidone-iodine	Betadine	*Antiseptic paint:* Apply twice daily. *Dry powder:* Use for minor wounds and infections. *Ointment:* Apply once or twice daily for up to 14 days. *Shampoo.* Use as shampoo twice weekly until improvement noted then once weekly. *Skin cleanser:* Retain on infected skin for 3–5 minutes before rinsing. Repeat twice daily. Solutions, tinctures and scrub: use undiluted for skin disinfection.	Most products not licensed to be used less than 2 years. Hypersensitivity. Avoid in patients with thyroid disorders or on lithium therapy. Exercise special care when applying to broken skin and in patients with renal insufficiency.	May interfere with thyroid function tests.	*Skin irritation:* Application to large wounds may produce metabolic acidosis, hypernatremia and impairment of renal function.

Contd...

Contd...

Drug	Brand name	Dosage	Contraindications	Drug interaction	Side effects
Framycetin sulfate	Soframycin	*Eye drops:* One to two drops 2 hourly and reducing gradually as infection gets controlled to 48 hours after the eye is clinically normal. *Eye ointment:* Three times daily when given alone or at bedtime along with eye drops given during the day. *Cream:* Apply 1–3 times daily.	Caution is advised in using framycetin in children allergic to streptomyces derived antibiotics (e.g. aminoglycosides). Care must be taken in children with hepatic and renal impairment as systemic absorption occurs when eye drops are given in high doses. Avoid if eardrum is perforated and fungal and viral infections of the eye. Avoid skin cream in viral and tuberculous lesions and in varicella and vaccinia. If large areas of skin are being treated, ototoxicity may be a hazard in children, especially in those with renal impairment.	Coadministration with gentamyicin eye drops reduces the risk of selecting resistant organisms.	If large areas of skin are being treated, ototoxicity may be a hazard in children, especially those with renal impairment. Sensitization, contact dermatitis, local irritation and itching.
Mupirocin	Bactroban, T-Bact	*Dosage description:* *Topical cream:* Apply to affected area three times daily for up to 10 days; nasal ointment apply to the inner surface of each nostril 2–3 times a day for 5–7 days; ointment-apply to affected area 2–3 times daily for up to 10 days.	Hypersensitivity to mupirocin or constituents. Avoid application to the eyes. Ointment (not nasal ointment) contains polyethylene glycol (PEG) which may be absorbed from open wounds and damaged skin. PEG is excreted renally and caution is needed in moderate or severe renal impairment, in neonates and burns patients. Prolonged use may result in overgrowth of non-susceptible organisms.		Rarely minor local irritation reactions, hypersensitivity.
Silver sulfadiazine (sulfadiazine)	Silver sulfadiazine, silvindon	*Burns:* After cleaning the wound apply over the affected areas to a depth of 3–5 mm, using a sterile gloved hand or sterile spatula. Where necessary, re-apply to any area from which it has been removed by patient activity. Re-apply at least every 24 hours or more frequently if the volume of exudates is large. *Hand burns:* Apply to the burn and enclose the whole hand in a clear plastic bag or glove which is then closed at the wrist. The patient should be encouraged to move the hand and fingers and the dressing should be changed when an excessive amount of exudates has accumulated in the bag.	Should not be used at or near term pregnancy, on premature infants or newborn infants during the first month of life, due to the risk of causing kernicterus. Patients who are hypersensitive to silver sulfadiazine (sulphadiazine) or to components of the preparation. Concurrent use of enzymatic debriding agents. Leg or pressure ulcers that is very exudative.	Should not be used with enzymatic debriding agents as they can be inactivated by silver. In large-area burns where serum sulfadiazine levels may approach therapeutic levels, it should be noted that the effects of systemically administered drugs might be altered. This can especially apply to oral hypoglycemic agents and to phenytoin. It is recommended that phenytoin blood levels are monitored as its effects can be potentiated.	Local reactions such as burning, itching and skin rash may occur in about 2% of patients. Leucopenia has been reported in 3–5% of burns patients treated with silver sulfadiazine. Systemic absorption of silver sulfadiazine may vary rarely result in any of the adverse reactions attributable to systemic sulfonamide therapy.

Contd...

Contd...

Annexures 631

Drug	Brand name	Dosage	Contraindications	Drug interaction	Side effects
		Leg ulcers/pressure sores: The cavity of the ulcer should be filled with cream to a depth of at least 3–5 mm, followed by application of an absorbent pad or dressing, with further application of pressure bandaging as appropriate. Dressings should be changed daily, but if less exudates every 48 hours may be sufficient. *Finger-tip injuries:* Hemostasis of the injury should be achieved prior to the application of a 3–5 mm layer of cream, and then the finger covered with a finger dressing or the finger of a plastic glove. Dressings should be changed every 2–3 days. In all cases, use the contents of the tube or pot on one person only. Discard 50 g tubes 7 days after opening. Discard 250 g and 500 g pots 24 hours after opening.			
Topical antifungal					
Amorolfine		*Cream:* Apply once daily after cleansing in the evening for at least 2–3 weeks (up to 6 weeks for foot mycosis) continuing for 3–5 days after lesion has healed. *Nail lacquer:* Apply to infected nails one to two times weekly after filing and cleaning; allow to dry (approximately 3 minutes). Treat finger nails for 6 months; toe nails for 9–12 months. Review 3 monthly.	Avoid contact with eyes, ears and mucous membranes.		Occasional transient burning sensation, erythema and pruritus.
Clotrimazole	Candid, Candid mouth paint, Candid-B, Candid-TV, Candid-V, Candid-V6, Candid-V6/V3/V1	Apply 2–3 times daily continuing for 14 days after lesions have healed. *Oral thrush:* 10–20 drops gently apply to buccal mucosa (covering all lesions) four times daily for 5–7 days. *Vaginal candidiasis:* Apply 2% vaginal gel 5 g deep into vagina at bedtime for six consecutive nights (not to be used during menstruation). Or alternatively 100 mg vaginal pessaries for 6 days, 200 mg for 3 days or 500 mg single dose at bedtime. *Scalp seborrhea:* Apply to liquid with selenium to scalp, massage gently, leave for 5 minutes and then rinse well with water for two to three times/week. *Otomycosis:* Instill four to five drops in ear 3–4 times daily till 2 weeks after infection subsides.	Hypersensitivity to clotrimazole.		Occasional skin irritation or sensitivity.
Econazole	Ecanol	Apply 2–3 times daily continuing for 14 days after lesions have healed.	Avoid contact with eyes.		Occasional skin irritation or sensitivity.
Miconazole	Daktarin, Fungitop, Micogel	Topical or skin apply on affected area two times daily for 10 days after lesions have healed. Oral thrush less than 1 month 1.25 mL, up to 2 years 2.5 mL, 2–12 years 5 mL and 12–18 years 5–10 mL, two to four times daily. Use in the mouth after food and retain as long as possible.			Occasional skin irritation or sensitivity.

Contd...

Contd...

Drug	Brand name	Dosage	Contraindications	Drug interaction	Side effects
Tolnaftate	Tinaderm	Apply evenly to affected area and rub gently two to three times daily.	Hypersensitivity, deep infections.	None reported	Stinging sensation, irritation, sensitization, contact dermatitis.
Topical antiparasitic					
Crotamiton	Crotorax	*Topical:* After patient has a warm bath and dried well, the preparation should be rubbed into the entire body surface excluding face and scalp. The application should be repeated once daily preferably in the evening for a total of 3–5 days. Children less than 3 years of age should not apply crotamition more than once a day.	Avoid use near eyes and broken skin. Acute exudative dermatoses.		
Malathion		*Topical:* Medical supervision is required for children less than 6 months of age. Scabies: apply to whole body excluding head and neck, allow to dry, wash off after 24 hours. Children less than 2 years should have a thin film applied to scalp, face and ears, avoiding eyes and mouth. If hands or any other part are washed, the treatment must be reapplied. Head lice-rub liquid gently into dry hair until all hair is thoroughly moistened. Comb and allow to dry naturally, away from heat or sunshine. A contact time of 12 hours or overnight is recommended. Repeat after 7 days only if live lice are found again.	Avoid contact with eyes. Do not use on broken or secondarily infected skin. Do not use more than once a week for 3 weeks at a time. Alcoholic lotion not recommended for head lice in severe eczema, asthma or in small children.		Skin irritation.

ANNEXURE 2: FLUID THERAPY IN INFECTIOUS DISEASES

Shivananda, Prabhas Prasun Giri

INTRODUCTION

Water is the most plentiful and essential constituent of the human body electrolytes complement to maintain life. The other components of the body include protein, minerals, fat and a small amount of carbohydrate. Total body water (TBW) as a percentage of bodyweight varies with age. TBW in healthy term neonates at birth is 75–80% of the bodyweight; this gradually declines to 60–65% by 1 year of age. In adolescent boys, TBW is 60% of bodyweight, while in adolescent girls, it is about 55% of the bodyweight.

The TBW is divided into two main compartments: (1) the fluid inside cells [intracellular fluid (ICF)] and (2) the fluid outside cells [extracellular fluid (ECF)]. The ICF remains relatively constant at 40% of the bodyweight, while ECF as a proportion of bodyweight reduces with age. The ECF is further divided into the intravascular (or plasma) volume and the interstitial fluid by the capillary membrane. In addition, ECF also includes the transcellular fluid, i.e. cerebrospinal fluid (CSF), intraocular fluid, synovial fluid, and the pleural and peritoneal fluids. The plasma water is normally about 5% of bodyweight. The blood volume, given a hematocrit of 40%, is usually close to 8% of bodyweight, although it is higher in newborns and young infants.

The composition of the solutes in the ICF and ECF are very different. Sodium and chloride are the dominant cations and anions in the ECF. The sodium and chloride concentrations in the ICF are much lower. Potassium is the most abundant caution in the ICF, almost 30 times higher within the cells. Proteins, phosphorus are the dominant anions in the ICF.

Children normally have large variations in their daily intake of water and electrolytes. Patients lose water, sodium and potassium in their urine and stool; water is also lost from the skin and lungs. Fluids are given to replace these losses and therefore avoid the development of dehydration and deficiencies of sodium or potassium. Maintenance solutions consist of water, glucose, sodium, potassium and chloride. They are simple, cheap, easy to store and compatible.

Healthy children can tolerate significant variations in intake because of the many homeostatic mechanisms that can adjust absorption and excretion of water and electrolyte.

The glucose in maintenance fluids provides approximately 20% of the normal caloric needs of the patient. This is enough to prevent the development of starvation ketoacidosis and diminishes the protein degradation that would occur, if the patient received no calories.

Maintenance fluids do not provide adequate calories, protein, fat, minerals or vitamins. This is typically not problematic for a patient receiving intravenous fluids for a few days. But it is important to remember that a patient on maintenance intravenous fluids is receiving inadequate calories and will actually lose 0.5–1% of weight each day. Thus, it is imperative that patients not remain on maintenance therapy indefinitely; total parental nutrition should be used for children who cannot be fed enterally for more than a few days. This is especially important in a patient with underlying malnutrition. They do not supply other electrolytes like calcium, phosphorus magnesium and bicarbonates.

Water is a crucial component of fluid therapy. This is because of the obligatory water losses that occur during the day. These losses are both measurable (urine and stool) and not measurable (insensible losses from the skin and lungs). Failure to replace these losses leads to dehydration indicated by irritable and thirsty child. The goal of fluid therapy is to provide enough water to replace these obligatory losses. Urinary losses are approximately 60% of the total water. However, the normal kidney has the ability to markedly modify water losses.

NORMAL REQUIREMENT OF FLUID AND ELECTROLYTES

The normal requirements of water and electrolytes consist of the amounts necessary to replace the urinary and insensible water losses and provide water for metabolism. These can be calculated on the basis of bodyweight, body surface area or metabolic rate. The "Caloric method" suggested by Holliday and Segar is the most accurate to determine the fluid and electrolyte requirements. They observed that the insensible loss of water and urinary water loss roughly parallel energy metabolism. The net requirement of water is usually 100–110 mL for 100 Cal metabolized. The approximate requirements for Na^+ are 3 mEq/100 Cal, K^+ about 2 mEq/100 Cal and Cl^{-}2 mEq/100 Cal that are utilized.

The maintenance requirements are usually met using N/5 saline in 5% dextrose with 1 mL of 15% KCl per 100 mL of intravenous fluid. But this fluid is basically hypotonic and does not suit in older children and most of the sick children and sometimes leads to fatal hyponatremia. That is why current consensus is to use more isotonic fluid (N/2 or normal saline with 5% dextrose, i.e. either ½ DNS or DNS) as a maintenance fluid.

But there are no strict and fixed protocol for using the maintenance fluid and electrolytes. It should be changed depending upon the clinical situation. Many of the infectious diseases can derange the homeostasis of the fluid dynamics lead to dyselectrolytemia. This may be due to loss of body fluids as in acute diarrhea, increase in insensible loss as in pneumonia. Deficiency of fluid and electrolytes also occur due to deficient intake during acute illness and fever.

The knowledge of fluid dynamics is critical in managing infectious diseases in children as they are more vulnerable to disorders in fluid homeostasis. It is helpful to consider the sources of normal water loss and determine whether any of these sources is being modified in a specific patient. It is then necessary to adjust maintenance water and electrolyte calculations.

It is difficult to review the fluid therapy in whole gambit of infectious diseases. An attempt is made here to put epitomized presentation of management of common infections in day to day practice. Readers are requested to refer appropriate references.

Fluid in Febrile Children

Fever increases evaporative losses from the skin. These losses are somewhat predictable, leading to a 10–15% increase in maintenance water needs for each 1°C increase in temperature above 38°C. These guidelines are for a patient with a persistent fever; a 1 hour fever spike does not cause an appreciable increase in water needs. All children with fever are required to be given adequate quantity of fluids which should be sufficient to compensate the insensible water loss. Extra water and electrolytes are given in the form of fruits to avoid asthenia and weakness. Sufficient allowances are to be made depending on the environment. Children from tropics require more fluids and electrolytes and climate also determine the need for fluids.

Fluid Therapy in Diarrhea

Diarrheal disease are common in children below 2 years of life, second common leading cause of death in children accounting for 1 billion episodes in the world per year and is the leading cause of malnutrition.

With available newer laboratory methods still 15–20% cases etiology is not discernible, while majority are viral diarrheas, accounts for nearly 65%. Among them Rotadiarrheas are common, *Escherichia coli* diarrhea is next.

Oral rehydration therapy (ORT) is the cornerstone for the management of dehydration associated with diarrhea.

Dehydration

The most severe threat posed by diarrhea is dehydration. During a diarrheal episode, water and electrolytes (sodium, chloride, potassium and bicarbonate) are lost through liquid stools, vomit, sweat, urine and breathing. Frequently they are complicated with severe acidosis. In nearly 70–80% of cases, isonatremic dehydration occurs where the losses of water and sodium are proportionate. About 10–15% of patients will have hyponatremic dehydration

where the loss of sodium is out of proportion of water in the stools. Hypernatremia may results in 15–20% when disproportionately large quantity of water lost compared with loss of electrolytes.

The dehydration status in diarrheal children is simplified by using three terms:
1. Diarrhea with no dehydration
2. Diarrhea with some dehydration
3. Diarrhea with severe dehydration

Dehydration is not evident up to 80–85% of cases of diarrhea. In 10–15% of cases, there is some dehydration. Severe dehydration occurs only less than 5% of cases. Death can follow severe dehydration if body fluids and electrolytes are not replenished, either through the use of oral rehydration salts (ORS) solution or through an intravenous drip.

The treatment of dehydration in case of diarrhea is universally managed by the World Health Organizations (WHO) guidelines by three plans of management.

Treatment Plan A
(Patients without Physical Signs of Dehydration)

The child should be fed with culturally appropriate home available fluids (sugar and salt solution, rice water with salt, butter-milk with salt, etc.) and ORS. The mother should be asked to take the child to the health worker if the child does not get better in 3 days or develops any of the following danger signs:
- Many watery stools
- Repeated vomiting
- Marked thirst
- Eating or drinking poorly
- Fever and blood in stool.
- Not passed urine in last 6–8 hours.

Treatment Plan B
(Patients with Physical Signs of Dehydration)

All cases with obvious signs of dehydration need to be treated in a health center or hospital. However, oral fluid therapy must be commenced promptly and continued during the transport. The fluid therapy has three components:
1. Correction of existing water and electrolyte deficit (rehydration therapy)
2. Replacement of ongoing losses (maintenance therapy)
3. Provision of normal daily fluid requirements.

Rehydration therapy: requires 75 mL/kg of ORS in the first 4 hours.

Maintenance fluid therapy: This begins when the signs of dehydration disappear. ORS should be continued in volume equal to diarrhea losses; approximately 10–20 mL/kg bodyweight for each liquid stool. Feeding should be uninterrupted during the maintenance fluid therapy. Plain water should be offered in between the feed and ORS. Another 4-hour treatment should be repeated if the child continues to have some dehydration after 4 hours. Younger infants are offered breastfeeds in between ORS feeds.

Treatment Plan C
(Children with Severe Dehydration)

- Start the intravenous (IV) fluid immediately
- Ringer's lactate or normal saline is the fluid of choice. Ideal preparation would be Ringer's lactate with 5% added dextrose
- Give 100 mL/kg of fluid in following manner:

Age	First	Then
Less than 12 months	30 mL/kg in 1 hour	70 mL/kg in 5 hours
12 months to 5 years	30 mL/kg in 30 minutes	70 mL/kg in 2.5 hours

- Oral rehydration ORS solution should be started as soon as possible when the child is able to drink
- Monitoring: Frequent monitoring (every 15–20 minutes) is very essential in all cases of severe dehydration. If the hydration is not improving in usual manner, IV fluid should be given more rapidly. When the full amount of IV fluid has been given, reassess the child's hydration status and follow the action plans like:
  - If the signs of severe dehydration still present, repeat the IV fluid infusion as outlined earlier
  - If the child improves, but still there are features of some dehydration, discontinue IV fluid, start ORT and follow plan B.

WHO Meeting of Experts concluded in 2001 that there are programmatic advantages of using a single rehydrating solution globally for all causes of diarrhea in all ages. Evidence from large, well-conducted, randomized controlled trials, including those in India, showed that low osmolarity ORS with 75 mEq/L of sodium and 75 mmol/L of glucose, osmolarity of 245 osmol/L is effective in children with non-cholera diarrhea and in adults and children with cholera. The need for unscheduled supplemental intravenous therapy in children given the new ORS fell by 33%. An analysis of this and other recent studies of reduced osmolarity ORS solutions (osmolarity 210–268 mOsm/L, sodium 50–75 mEq/L) found that stool output decreased by about 20% and vomiting by about 30%. The reduced osmolarity (245 mOsm/L) solution also appeared to be as safe and effective as standard ORS for use in children with cholera. This new improved ORS was recommended by the WHO/UNICEF as the universal solution for all ages and all types of diarrhea. It was also included in the national policy by the Government of India in 2004.

Revised Guidelines for Management of Diarrhea

The revised guidelines for management of diarrhea issued by the Government of India and the Indian Academy of Pediatrics recommend low osmolarity ORS, zinc (10 mg/day elemental zinc for infants 2–6 months and 20 mg/day for children ≥ 6 months for 14 days) and continued feeding of energy dense feeds in addition to breastfeeding. The guidelines emphasize the importance of home available fluids, hand washing and other hygiene practices. Antimicrobials are recommended only for gross blood in stools or Shigella positive culture, cholera, associated systemic infection or severe malnutrition.

Fluid Therapy in Respiratory Tract Infection

Children with respiratory infections need more fluids. Tachypnea or a tracheostomy increases evaporative losses from the lungs. Severe pneumonia needing hospital admission and IV antibiotics demands more fluid and most of the times, IV fluid is needed, especially in smaller infants.

Acute respiratory distress syndrome (ARDS) is another fatal illness that occurs as a result of infectious or non-infectious lung injury. It is particularly characterized by pulmonary edema caused by an increase in pulmonary capillary permeability. It is considered that limiting pulmonary edema or accelerating its resorption through the modulation of fluid intake or oncotic pressure could be beneficial. Fluid management with the goal to obtain zero fluid balance in ARDS patients without shock or renal failure significantly increases the number of days without mechanical ventilation. On the other hand, patients with hemodynamic failure must receive early and adapted fluid resuscitation. Liberal and conservative fluid strategies are therefore complementary and should ideally follow each other in time in the same patient whose hemodynamic state progressively stabilizes. At present, albumin treatment does not appear to be justified for limitation of pulmonary edema and respiratory morbidity.

A humidified ventilator causes a decrease in insensible losses from the lungs and can even lead to water absorption via the lungs. Thus, a ventilated patient has a decrease in maintenance water requirements. A mist tent decreases evaporative losses from both the skin and the lungs. Unfortunately, in all of these situations, it is difficult to quantify the changes that take place in the individual patient.

Fluid Therapy in Central Nervous System Infection

Meningitis and encephalitis and cerebral malaria these three are the principal fatal central nervous system (CNS) infection in children. Most of these children are severely sick and needed in patient's therapy and IV fluids. All the recent studies do not support the conventional views of fluid restriction. Full maintenance fluid should be given. Hypovolemia can lower the cerebral perfusion pressure

(CPP) and lead to worse intracranial pressure (ICP) due to autoregulatory vasodilation. What must be restricted are hypotonic fluids such as N/5 saline in 5% dextrose (Isolyte-P/Arolyte-P).

The question of fluid restriction comes when dealing with a case of hyponatremia due to syndrome of inappropriate antidiuretic hormone (SIADH) in the settings of meningitis or encephalitis. Hyponatremia is a frequent finding in patients with CNS infection mostly due to SIADH. However, it may be due to volume contraction rather than water retention. So, we have to keep in mind that the hyponatremia may be due to dehydration or water retention as in SIADH. The circulatory compromise caused by hypovolemia is as dangerous as cerebral edema caused by water retention. So the cause of hyponatremia should be assessed along with clinical signs of volume depletion and biochemical settings, i.e. serum and urine osmolarity and if there is clinical or laboratory evidence that the patient is suffering from SIADH, two-thirds of maintenance fluids are started and symptomatic management of hyponatremia instituted. Full maintenance requirement of sodium should be given as hyponatremia impairs cerebrovascular reactivity.

Another problem that may be encountered in the setting of CNS infection is the cerebral salt wasting. Here, there is the combination of hypovolemia, hyponatremia, excessive renal sodium losses and marked elevation of plasma atrial natriuretic hormone. Treatment includes volume—for volume replacement of urinary sodium losses and oral sodium supplementation after discharge from the hospital to correct and maintain the normal fluid balance.

Fluid Therapy in Dengue Fever

World Health Organization (WHO) in the recent communication has issued the guidelines for management of dengue fever which has standardized the management. Following its implementation in all levels, there is marked decrease in mortality and morbidity. Oral rehydration therapy is recommended for patients with moderate dehydration caused by high fever and vomiting during the febrile phase of dengue.

The patients who have diagnosed as Dengue fever (DF) without warning signs are classified as group A they may be sent home unless they have some social reasons.

Usually these patients tolerate oral fluids orally and as urine frequently they should be given clear advice on the care that should be given at home, i.e. bed rest and frequent oral fluids. Patients with ≥3 days of illness should be reviewed daily for disease progression (indicated by decreasing white blood cell and platelet counts and increasing hematocrit, defervescence and warning signs) until they are out of the critical period. Those with stable hematocrit can be sent home but should be advised to return to the nearest hospital

immediately if they develop any of the warning signs and to adhere to the following action plan:

- Adequate oral fluid intake may reduce the number of hospitalizations. Encourage oral intake to replace fluid loss from fever and vomiting. Small amounts of oral fluids should be given frequently for those with nausea and anorexia. The choice of fluids should be based on the local culture: coconut water in some countries, in others rice water or barley water. Oral rehydration solution or soup and fruit juices may be given to prevent electrolyte imbalance. Commercial carbonated drinks that exceed the isotonic level (5% sugar) should be avoided. They may exacerbate hyperglycemia.

Sufficient oral fluid intake should result in a urinary frequency of at least 4 to 6 times per day. A record of oral fluid and urine output could be maintained and reviewed daily in the ambulatory setting.

Group B

These are patients who should be admitted for in-hospital management for close observation as they approach the critical phase. These include patients with warning signs, those with coexisting conditions that may make dengue or its management more complicated (such as pregnancy, infancy, old age, obesity, diabetes mellitus, hypertension, heart failure, renal failure, chronic hemolytic diseases such as sickle-cell disease and autoimmune diseases), and those with certain social circumstances (such as living alone, or living far from a health facility without reliable means of transport). Rapid fluid replacement in patients with warning signs is the key to prevent progression to the shock state. If the patient has dengue with warning signs or signs of dehydration, judicious volume replacement by intravenous fluid therapy from this early stage may modify the course and the severity of disease.

- Obtain a reference hematocrit before intravenous fluid therapy begins. Give only isotonic solutions such as 0.9% saline, Ringer's lactate solution. Start with 5–7 mL/kg/hour for 1–2 hours, then reduce to 3–5 mL/kg/hour for 2–4 hours, and then reduce to 2–3 mL/kg/hour or less according to the clinical response.
- Reassess the clinical status and repeat the hematocrit. If the hematocrit remains the same or rises only minimally, continue at the same rate (2–3 mL/kg/hour) for another 2–4 hours.
- If the vital signs are worsening and the hematocrit is rising rapidly, increase the rate to 5–10 mL/kg/hour for 1–2 hours. Reassess the clinical status, repeat the hematocrit and review fluid infusion rates accordingly.
- Give the minimum intravenous fluid volume required to maintain good perfusion and an urine output of about 0.5 mL/kg/hour. Intravenous fluids are usually needed for only 24–48 hours. Reduce intravenous fluids

gradually when the rate of plasma leakage decreases towards the end of the critical phase. This is indicated by urine output and/or oral fluid intake improving, or the hematocrit decreasing below the baseline value in a stable patient.

- Patients with warning signs should be monitored by health-care providers until the period of risk is over. A detailed fluid balance should be maintained. Parameters that should be monitored include vital signs and peripheral perfusion (1–4 hourly until the patient is out of the critical phase), urine output (4–6 hourly), hematocrit (before and after fluid replacement, then 6–12 hourly), blood glucose and other organ functions (such as renal profile, liver profile, coagulation profile, as indicated). If the patient has dengue with coexisting conditions but without warning signs, the action plan should be as follows:

- Encourage oral fluids. If not tolerated, start intravenous fluid therapy of 0.9% saline or Ringer's lactate with or without glucose at the appropriate maintenance rate (Textbox H). Use the ideal body weight for calculation of fluid infusion for obese and overweight patients (Textboxes J and K). Patients may be able to take oral fluids after 27 a few hours of intravenous fluid therapy. Thus, it is necessary to revise the fluid infusion frequently. Give the minimum volume required to maintain good perfusion and urine output. Intravenous fluids are usually needed only for 24–48 hours. Patients should be monitored by health-care providers for temperature pattern, volume of fluid intake and losses, urine output (volume and frequency), warning signs, hematocrit, white blood cell and platelet counts.

Group C

These are patients with severe dengue who require emergency treatment and urgent referral because they are in the critical phase of the disease and have:

- severe plasma leakage leading to dengue shock and/or fluid accumulation with respiratory distress;
- severe hemorrhages;
- severe organ impairment (hepatic damage, renal impairment, cardiomyopathy, encephalopathy or encephalitis).

All patients with severe dengue should be admitted to a hospital with access to blood transfusion facilities.

Judicious intravenous fluid resuscitation is the essential and usually sole intervention required.

The crystalloid solution should be isotonic and the volume just sufficient to maintain an effective circulation during the period of plasma leakage.

Plasma losses should be replaced immediately and rapidly with isotonic crystalloid solution: in the case of hypotensive shock, colloid solution is preferred If

possible, obtain hematocrit levels before and after fluid resuscitation. Continue replacement of further plasma losses to maintain effective circulation for 24–48 hours. All shock patients should have their blood group taken and a cross-match carried out. Blood transfusion should be given only in cases with established severe bleeding, or suspected severe bleeding in combination with otherwise unexplained hypotension. Fluid resuscitation must be clearly separated from simple fluid administration. This is a strategy in which larger volumes of fluids (e.g. 10–20 mL/kg boluses) are administered for a limited period of time under close supervision, to evaluate the patient's response and to avoid the development of pulmonary edema. These fluids should not contain glucose. The degree of intravascular volume deficit in dengue shock varies. Input is typically much greater than output, and the input/output ratio is of no help in judging fluid resuscitation needs during this period.

The goals of fluid resuscitation include:

- improving central and peripheral circulation, i.e. decreasing tachycardia, improving BP and pulse volume, warm and pink extremities, a capillary refill time < 2 seconds;
- improving end-organ perfusion, i.e. achieving a stable conscious level (more alert or less restless), and urine output ≥0.5 mL/kg/hour or decreasing metabolic acidosis.

Treatment of shock: (4–8) The action plan for treating patients with compensated shock is as follows:

- Obtain a reference hematocrit before starting intravenous fluid therapy. Start intravenous fluid resuscitation with isotonic crystalloid solutions at 10–20 mL/kg/hour over one hour in infants and children. Then reassess the patient's condition (vital signs, capillary refill time, hematocrit, urine output).

- If the condition in the infant or child improves, intravenous fluids should be reduced to 10 mL/kg/hour for 1–2 hours; then to 7 mL/kg/hour for 2 hours; 5 mL/kg/hour for 4 hours and then to 3 mL/kg/hour, which can be maintained for up to 24–48 hours. Consider reducing intravenous fluid earlier if oral fluid intake improves. The total duration of intravenous fluid therapy should not exceed 48 hours.

- If vital signs are still unstable (i.e. shock persists), check the hematocrit after the first bolus.

  Treatment of profound shock (hypotensive; undetectable pulse and BP). All patients (infants, children and adults) with hypotensive shock should be managed more vigorously. The action plan for treating patients with hypotensive shock is outlined below. For all patients (infants, children), initiate intravenous fluid resuscitation with crystalloid or colloid solution at 20 mL/kg as a bolus given over 15–30 minutes to bring the patient out of shock as quickly as possible. Colloids may be the preferred choice if the BP has to be restored urgently, i.e. in those with pulse pressure less than 10 mm Hg. Colloids have been shown to restore the cardiac index and reduce the level of hematocrit faster than crystalloids in patients with intractable shock. The intraosseous route should be attempted if peripheral venous access cannot be obtained.

- If the patient's condition improves:
  - In infants and children, give colloid infusion of 10 mL/kg/hour for 1 hour. Then continue with crystalloid 10 mL/kg/hour for 1 hour, then to 7.5 mL/kg/hour for 2 hours, to 5 mL/kg/hour for 4 hours and to 3 mL/kg/hour, which can be maintained for up to 24–48 hours.

Consider reducing intravenous fluid earlier if oral fluid intake and urine output improve.

The total duration of intravenous fluid therapy should not exceed 48 hours.

- For all patients, if vital signs are still unstable (i.e. shock persists), review the hematocrit obtained before the first bolus.
  - If the hematocrit was normal or low (<30–35% in infants, this may indicate bleeding. Look for severe bleeding. Cross-match fresh whole blood or fresh packed red cells and transfuse if there is severe overt bleeding. If there is no bleeding, give a second bolus of 10–20 mL/kg of colloid over 30 minutes to 1 hour, repeat clinical assessment and hematocrit level plus a review by senior staff to consider blood transfusion (see treatment for hemorrhagic complications).
  - If the hematocrit was high compared to the baseline value (if not available, use population baseline), change intravenous fluids to colloid solutions at 10–20 mL/kg as a second bolus over 30 minutes to 1 hour. After the second bolus, reassess the patient. If the condition improves, reduce the rate to 7–10 mL/kg/hour for 1–2 hours, then change back to crystalloid solution and reduce the rate of infusion as mentioned above.
- If the condition is still unstable, repeat the hematocrit after the second bolus.
  - If the hematocrit decreases compared to the previous value (<35% in infants, this indicates bleeding and the need to cross-match and transfuse blood as soon as possible (see 2.2.3.3 for hemorrhagic complications).
  - If the hematocrit increases compared to the previous value or remains very high (>50%), continue colloid solutions at 10–20 mL/kg as a third bolus over 1 hour. After this dose, reduce the rate to 7–10 mL/kg/hour for 1–2 hours, then change back to 32 crystalloid solution and reduce the rate of infusion

as mentioned above when the patient's condition improves. If the condition is still unstable, repeat the hematocrit after the third bolus.

Further boluses of fluids may need to be given during the next 24 hours. The rate and volume of each bolus infusion should be titrated to the clinical response. Patients with severe dengue should be admitted to the high-dependency or intensive care area and be managed by senior staff.

- Clinicians who take care of dengue shock infants should remember that an infant with a low baseline hematocrit of 30%, presenting with dengue shock and a hematocrit of 40%, is relatively more hemoconcentrated than another child with a baseline value of 42% and hematocrit of 50% at the time of shock.
- Patients with dengue shock should be monitored frequently until the danger period is over. A detailed fluid balance of all inputs and outputs should be maintained.
- Parameters to be monitored include: Alertness and comfort levels, vital signs and peripheral perfusion (every 15–30 minutes until the patient is out of shock then 1–2 hourly).
- Colloids at the rate of 10–20 mL/kg may be started when the child requires higher rate of infusion of crystalloids to maintain the blood pressure and to mitigate the danger of fluid overload.

When to stop intravenous fluid therapy Recognizing when to decrease or stop intravenous fluids as part of the treatment of severe dengue is crucial to prevent fluid overload.

When any of the following signs are present, intravenous fluids should be reduced or discontinued:
- signs of cessation of plasma leakage;
- stable BP, pulse and peripheral perfusion;
- hematocrit decreases in the presence of a good pulse volume;
- apyrexia (without the use of antipyretics) for more than 24–48 hours;
- resolving bowel/abdominal symptoms;
- improving urine output.

Continuing intravenous fluid therapy beyond the 48 hours of the critical phase will put the patient at risk of pulmonary edema and other complications such as thrombophlebitis.

Electrolyte and Acid-base Imbalances

Hyponatremia is a common observation in severe dengue; the underlying mechanism is not fully understood. It could be related to gastrointestinal losses through vomiting and diarrhea or the use of hypotonic solutions for resuscitation and correction of dehydration. The use of isotonic solutions for resuscitation will prevent and correct this condition.

Hyperkalemia is observed in association with severe metabolic acidosis or acute renal injury. Appropriate volume resuscitation will reverse the metabolic acidosis and the associated hyperkalemia. Life-threatening hyperkalemia, in the setting of acute renal failure should be managed with Resonium A and infusions of calcium gluconate and/or insulin-dextrose. Renal support therapy may have to be considered.

Hypokalemia is often associated with gastrointestinal fluid losses and the stress-induced hypercortisol state; it is usually encountered towards the later part of the critical phase. It should be corrected with potassium supplements in the parenteral fluids. Serum calcium levels should be monitored and corrected when large quantities of blood have been transfused or if sodium bicarbonate has been used.

(Readers are requested to see the WHO guidelines for management of dengue for further details and the flow diagrams.)

Patients with dengue hemorrhagic fever or dengue shock syndrome may be discharged from the hospital when they meet the following criteria:
* Afebrile for 24 hours without antipyretics
* Good appetite, clinically improved condition
* Adequate urine output
* Stable hematocrit level
* At least 48 hours since recovery from shock
* No respiratory distress
* Platelet count greater than 50,000 cells/µL
* Development of rashes.

Fluid Therapy in Septic Shock

Infectious organisms release toxins that affect fluid distribution, cardiac output, and so on primary pump failure produces inadequate tissue perfusion; results in metabolic acidosis which further impairs cardiac function. Neurologic disturbances may cause uneven distribution of fluids, leading to acidosis.

Adequate volume resuscitation is the most important step in management of septic shock. Preload needs to be optimized to improve cardiac output and thus oxygen delivery. The circulating volume must be replaced in boluses of 20 mL/kg within minutes since rapid restoration of cardiac output and tissue perfusion reduces the chances of serious end organ damage.

Choice of Fluid

There is an age old debate regarding the ideal fluid for resuscitation in septic shock. The controversy of choice of fluid between crystalloids and colloids perhaps continue for a decade more. But most of the recent pediatric data supports the use of crystalloids over colloids as the initial fluid for resuscitation. Colloids usually does not add any advantage over the crystalloids in pediatric septic shock except in those cases where there is a pre-existing low plasma oncotic pressure such as Protein–energy malnutrition (PEM), nephrotic syndrome, acute severe burns or liver disease, in patients with malaria and dengue shock syndrome. Actually, it is the volume of fluid and how quickly the fluid started is more important than the choice of fluid.

The isotonic crystalline solution (normal saline or Ringer's lactate) are the initial choice of fluid.

Colloids

Several studies have looked at the role of colloids in the early management of septic shock.

Human Albumin

There is no literature to suggest that 5% albumin administration improved outcome in regards to sepsis mortality. Albumin administration may be most useful in patients who are hypoalbuminemic.

Packed Red Blood Cells

The optimal hemoglobin for patients in septic shock has not been established. In the early management of sepsis in adults, maintaining a hemoglobin of 7–9 g/dL in order to improve oxygen-carrying capacity will improve sepsis survival by improve tissue perfusion. But packed red blood cells (PRBC) can never be used as a fluid for resuscitation.

Starch

Complex starches are considered colloids and have been considered as alternatives to blood products. The complex starches, however, have been associated with undesirable effects. Hydroxyethyl starches have been shown to have effects on coagulation, with predominant exerting inhibitory effects on platelet aggregation, but the newer starches have less of an effect on coagulation. Hydroxyethyl starch (6%) has been associated with an increased rate of acute renal failure. These synthetic products can be rather expensive and have not been shown to be consistently superior to current fluid strategies.

Fresh Frozen Plasma

Fresh frozen plasma (FFP) is practically important in the settings where initial resuscitation has already been done with crystalloids and there is a coagulation abnormality [like disseminated intravascular coagulation (DIC)] and the clotting factors is to be replaced.

Amount of Fluid

The amount of fluid to be administered depends upon the volume status and ongoing loses of the patient. Initial fluid resuscitation usually requires 40–60 mL/kg but can be as much as 200 mL/kg in septic shock. Children who receive more than 40 mL/kg of intravenous fluid in the first hour have greater survival and far less likely to be persistently hypovolemic at 6 hours after presentation than those who receive less than 40 mL/kg. Therapeutic endpoints include objective measures such as normal pulses, warm extremities, urine output more than 1 mL/kg/per hour, normal mental status, normal blood pressure (target mean BP >65 mm Hg) and capillary refill less than 2 seconds. Close observation is needed to monitor the features of fluid overload such as pulmonary edema or hepatomegaly.

At present a judicious mixture of crystalloids, colloids and blood products to maintain hemoglobin and clotting factors, and colloids to maintain colloid oncotic pressure seems most appropriate and reasonable.

If shock lasts more than 1 hour despite aggressive fluid resuscitation vasopressor support becomes mandatory.

Fluid management in children with infectious diseases require the knowledge of the basics of fluid therapy, pathogenesis of the infectious diseases which cause fluid disregulations and designated protocols for appropriate management for better survival of children.

BIBLIOGRAPHY

1. Alderson P, Bunn F, Lefebvre C, et al. Human albumin solution for resuscitation and volume expansion in critically ill patients. Cochrane Database Syst Rev. 2002;1:CD001208.
2. Alderson P, Schierhout G, Roberts I, et al. Colloids versus crystalloids for fluid resuscitation in critically ill patients. Cochrane Database Syst Rev. 2000;2:CD000567.
3. Behrman K, Stanton J. Nelson Text Book of Pediatrics, 19th edition. Philadelphia, PA. Saunders; 2011.
4. Boldt J, Haisch G, Suttner S, et al. Effects of a new modified, balanced hydroxyethyl starch preparation (Hextend) on measures of coagulation. Br J Anaesth. 2002;89:722-8.
5. Brown LW, Feigin RD. Bacterial meningitis: fluid balance and therapy. Pediatr Ann. 1994;23(2):93-8.
6. Bunn F, Trivedi D, Ashraf S. Colloid solutions for fluid resuscitation. Cochrane Database Syst Rev. 2008;1:CD001319.
7. Darrow DC, Pratt EL. Fluid therapy, relation to tissue composition and expenditure of water and electrolytes. JAMA. 1950;143:432-9.
8. Dengue. Guidelines for diagnosis, treatment prevention and control. WHO. 2009.
9. Duke T, Mokela D, Frank D, et al. Management of meningitis in children with oral fluid restriction or intravenous fluid at maintenance volumes: a randomised trial. Ann Trop Pediatr. 2002;22(2):145-57.
10. Feigin R, Kaplan S. Inappropriate secretion of antidiuretic hormone in children with bacterial meningitis. Am J ClinNutr. 1977;30(9):1482-4.
11. Finberg L. Water metabolism and regulation. In: Finberg L, Kravath RE, Hellerstein S (Eds). Water and Electrolytes in Pediatrics: Physiology, Pathology, and Treatment, 2nd edition. Philadelphia, PA: WB Saunders; 1993. pp. 17-21.
12. Finfer S, Bellomo R, Boyce N, et al. A comparison of albumin and saline for fluid resuscitation in the intensive care unit. N Engl J Med. 2004;350:2247-56.
13. Friis-Hansen B. Body water compartments in children: changes during growth and related changes in body composition. Pediatrics. 1961;28:169-81.
14. Holliday MA, Segar WE, Friedman A. Reducing errors in fluid therapy management. Pediatrics. 2003;111:424-5.
15. Holliday MA, Segar WE. The maintenance need for water in parenteral fluid therapy. Pediatrics. 1957;19:823-32.
16. Martin GS, Mangialardi RJ, Wheeler AP, et al. Albumin and furosemide therapy in hypoproteinemic patients with acute lung injury. Crit Care Med. 2002;30:2175-82.
17. Mecham N. Early recognition and treatment of shock in the pediatric patient. J Trauma Nurs. 2006;13:17-21.
18. Mehta D, Bhattacharya J, Matthay MA, et al. Integrated control of lung fluid balance. Am J Physiol Lung Cell Mol Physiol. 2004;287:L1081-90.
19. Murphy CV, Schramm GE, Doherty JA, et al. The importance of fluid management in acute lung injury secondary to septic shock. Chest. 2009;136:102-9.
20. Neville K, Verge C, Rosenberg A, et al. Isotonic is better than hypotonic saline for intravenous rehydration of children with gastroenteritis: a prospective randomised study. Arch Dis Child. 2006;91:226-32.
21. Patwari AK, Singh BS, Manorama DEB. Inappropriate secretion of antidiuretic hormone in acute bacterial meningitis. Ann Trop Pediatr. 1995;15:179-83.
22. Ranjit S, Kissoon N, Jayakumar I. Aggressive management of dengue shock syndrome may decrease mortality rate: a suggested protocol. PediatrCrit Care Med. 2005;6:412-9.
23. Schierhout G, Roberts I. Fluid resuscitation with colloid or crystalloid solutions in critically ill patients: a systematic review of randomised trials. Br Med J. 1998;316:961-4.
24. Shafiee MAS, Bohn D, Hoorn EJ, et al. How to select optimal maintenance intravenous fluid therapy. QJM. 2003;96:601-10.
25. Simmons RS, Berdine GG, Seidenfeld JJ, et al. Fluid balance and the adult respiratory distress syndrome. Am Rev Respir Dis. 1987;135:924-9.
26. Sparrow A, Hedderley T, Nadel S. Choice of fluid for resuscitation of septic shock. Emerg Med J. 2002;19:114-6.
27. Vincent JL, Gerlach H. Fluid resuscitation in severe sepsis and septic shock: an evidence-based review. Crit Care Med. 2004;32(11 Suppl):S451-54.
28. Wallace WM. Quantitative requirements of infant and child for water and electrolytes under varying conditions. Am J ClinPathol. 1953;23:1133-41.
29. WHO Diarrheal Disease FACT SHEET n33o Aug 2005.
30. Zimmerman JL. Use of blood products in sepsis: an evidence-based review. Crit Care Med. 2004;32(11 Suppl):S542-7.

Index

Page numbers followed by, b refer to box, f refer to figure, fc refer to flowchart, and t refer to table.